Pathology of bone tumours

Personal experience

Springer

Paris
Berlin
Heidelberg
New York
Barcelona
Budapest
Hong Kong
London
Milan
Santa Clara
Singapore
Tokyo

André Mazabraud

Pathology of bone tumours

Personal experience

Preface by Professor M. Postel

with 1,100 illustrations

Springer

André Mazabraud, MD
Former Head of Department
of Pathological Anatomy, Institut Curie, Paris
Centre de Pathologie
20, avenue de la Gare
91570 Bièvres
France

Translation:
David Le Vay, MD
6, Garstons, High Street
Burwash, East Sussex, TN 197EZ, UK

Revision:
Prof. Sir Colin Berry, Dsc, MD, PhD, FRCPath, FRCP, FFPM
St Bartholomew's & the Royal London
School of Medicine & Dentistry
Royal London Hospital
London E1 1BB, UK

Original French edition
Anatomie pathologique osseuse tumorale

ISBN-13: 978-3-642-95841-0 e-ISBN-13: 978-3-642-95839-7
DOI: 10.1007/978-3-642-95839-7

Library of Congress Cataloging-in-Publication Data
Mazabraud, André
[Anatomie pathologique osseuse tumorale, English]
Pathology of bone tumours: personal experience / André Mazabraud; preface by M. Postel.
p. cm.
Includes bibliographical references and index.
ISBN-13: 978-3-642-95841-0
1. Bones--Tumors. I. Title
[DNLM: 1. Bone Neoplasms--pathology. 2. Neoplasms, Connective Tissue--pathology. WE 258 M475a 1997a]
RC280. B6M3913 1997
616.99'27107--dc21
DNLM/DLC
for Library of Congress 97-29696
CIP

Softcover reprint of the hardcover 1st edition 1998

SPIN: 10555382 90/2918 - 5 4 3 2 1 0 Printed on acid-free paper

Contents

Preface

The production of a textbook of the pathology of bone tumours is a hard task to embark upon, but André Mazabraud has certainly succeeded.

It is the outcome of a very long experience, provided initially by his hospital training, then by his collaboration with Rutishauser at the Institut de Pathologie at Geneva and with Dahlin at the Mayo Clinic. The bonds he forged then have never been loosened.

Subsequently, his duties as head of the department of pathology at the Institut Curie directed him finally towards tumour pathology. At the Institute, he was not satisfied with routine examinations but very soon linked up with the research team and worked especially on Ewing's sarcoma and the problems of ultrastructure, particularly of giant-cell tumours and clear-cell chondroma. His interest in osteogenic sarcoma lead him to work with isotopic markers to refine their classification.

In this book, the author takes up a firm position about the difference between osteoid osteoma and osteoblastoma, about "tumoral associations" and about the so-called malignant forms of disorders described as benign. His personal stamp is evident throughout the various chapters.

Certainly, treatment in the area is rapidly changing and advancing, but this book does not risk obsolescence since treatment is not its focus. The extent and nature of the author's experience explain the essentially anatomo-pathological orientation taken by this seminal book. It also provides valuable clinical information and a good radiological study.

M. Postel

Foreword

This book is intended primarily for physicians, surgeons and pathologists who have to deal with the problems posed by bone pathology. It does not claim to cover the entirety of this pathology. These are "chosen morsels" selected from the everyday personal experience of some forty years. It aims especially to relate the difficulties encountered and to help the practitioner to resolve them by stressing the value of a multidisciplinary approach and of close anatomo-clinical collaboration.

It is true that the new techniques of radiological and microscopic imaging, such as MRI, immunocytology and the data recently provided by genome studies have supplied a rich and exciting harvest of new facts that are usefully employed in diagnosis and decisions as to treatment. However, in the majority of cases these new methodologies have confirmed the value and reality of the classical entities laid down by the anatomo-clinical findings established by our predecessors. The story of Ewing's tumour, which in less than 50 years has seen the identification of this disorder, and the discovery (by the teams of Alain Auras and Gilles Thomas) of its specific genomic analysis, is the best and most gratifying example of this.

Unfortunately, experience shows that, despite the support provided by these new techniques, urgent problems of diagnostic identification or therapeutic approaches emerge almost daily. Their source is complex. Often enough, we are ourselves to blame: a radiological survey that is incomplete or provides only a partial view of the lesions, inadequate biopsy, poor fixation, hasty or poorly performed decalcification or, more simply, ignorance of the elementary clinical data. Further, it is related to the very nature of the tumour, its heterogeneity or its very undifferentiated nature. In our experience, the multiplication of biopsies, the performance of new planes of section, help to clarify difficult situations and allow us to wait more serenely for the confirmation of histochemical and molecular studies.

However, it has to be acknowledged that the increasing use of trocar or needle biopsies has added to the frequency of these situations. It is in the operating-room, at the time of biopsy, that one must plan for the preservation of tumour fragments with an eye to complementary investigations and also with the aim of constructing series of rigorously classified tumours which will lend themselves to subsequent research studies.

The first thirty-eight chapters of this book are devoted to tumours and pseudotumours of bone. One chapter is reserved for tumours of the craniofacial skeleton, where the embryology and the relations with the dental organ confer particular reactive modalities. In the last three chapters, are mentioned the principal lesions which gravitate around bony tumour pathology, to which they are usually related by imaging. The brief clinical reviews that accompany the descriptions of these latter lesions, most of which form part of complex syndromes, have no other aim than to remind the pathologist of the essential concepts allowing him to reinforce his diagnostic opinion.

Besides these typical forms, and not really raising diagnostic problems, are stressed certain anatomo-clinical variants and some of the particular circumstances that sometimes accompany requests for a report and serve rather to distract from than to point to the true diagnosis.

The chapters are followed by lists of references, some recent, others older, on which our current knowledge has been built.

I trust that all my clinical and pathological teachers will find here the expression of my profound gratitude. I would mention Professors de Sèze, Merle d'Aubigné, Padovani and their co-workers, and particularly Professor Postel and Drs Ordonneau and Djian.

It is a pleasure for me to thank my colleagues at the Institut Curie- clinicians, pathologists and researchers- and specially Jean-Paul Thiery and Alain Aurias, whose fundamental studies are reported in this book, as well as my friend Jean Dubousset for his close collaboration. My thanks, too, to Jeanine Dumont for her irreplaceable collaboration in the pathology department and her efficient aid in the editing of some chapters of this book. It was the competence and spirit of research of Bernard Perdereau which led us to assess the functional differentiation of the cell by isotopic studies.

The erudition of the pathologists J Delarue, E Vermès and E Rutishauser as well as the friendship of David C Dahlin and the judicious advice of my friend Christian Nezelof have played a determining part in my career.

The production of this book has been facilitated by the collaboration of Jean-Marc Guinebretière in the department of my colleague and friend Geneviève Contesso, and by the efficient co-operation of Dr E Baviera and his co-workers, who placed at my disposal the technical and bibliographic resources of the diagnostic center at Bièvres. I warmly thank my colleague, Dr Hatcherian, for his helpful advice and Agnès Vignes for her effective help with the illustrations.

My sincere thanks also go to all those anonymous helpers whose daily work ensures the metamorphosis from biopsy to photomicrography and from ideas to publication.

In memory of my friend, Wolfgang Bechtoldt,
orthopaedic surgeon (Frankfort-am-Main),
Founder of the European Academy for Medical Training,
President of the Fédération Européenne des médecins salariés
from 1975 to 1986

Cartilaginous tumours: preamble to an anatomo-pathological study of cartilaginous neoplasms (Chapters 1 and 2)

- Knowledge of the age, precise location, radiographic image and clinical history.

- Tumour not subjected to previous treatment, radiation or chemotherapy, which render the examination practically valueless.

- Thin sections immediately on removal; too often, fixation of the cartilaginous tissue is defective.

- The nature of a bulky tumour is not necessarily revealed at biopsy: polymorphism, mixed bony and cartilaginous neoformations, and localised malignant transformation may not have been included in the sample.

- There may be major difficulties in the interpretation of tumours of a low degree of malignancy.

This underlines the importance of the nuances that must in many circumstances be sprinkled through the pathologist's report, specially if one bears in mind that an incompletely removed benign cartilaginous tumour invariably recurs: a nightmare for the pathologist, a problem for the orthopaedist and an anxiety for the patient.

The ultrastructural photographs have been reduced by 20% when compared with the originals.

1. Chondroma

General considerations

A true chondroma may be regarded as a harmartoma, a cartilaginous proliferation of mature appearance and moderate size, developing within or alongside the bone. Chondromas represent around 10 to 12% of benign tumours of bone and 2.8% of all bone tumours in the statistics of the Mayo Clinic [Dahlin & Unni 1986]. Both sexes are equally affected. Solitary chondromas are detected between the 2nd and 5th decades, multiple lesions during the first three decades. All the long bones of cartilaginous origin may be affected. Besides the long bones of the hands and feet, which account for 50% of cases, we may note the metaphyses of the long bones of the limbs, the short bones of the hands and feet, the vertebrae, the base of the skull, rarely the flat bones of the limb girdles. Samilsons et al (1968) found only 4 chondromas as against 34 chondrosarcomas in a review of the literature relating to 247 tumours of the scapula.

Clinical features and course

This lesion is often discovered radiologically. The diagnosis is suggested by localised osteolysis in a bone which may be "ballooned" with annular calcification situated at the periphery of the lobules [Ragsdale et al 1989]. The tumour may be revealed by a swelling if the involved bone is superficial, rarely by a spontaneous fracture or by mild pain.

Chondromas of the long bones of the hands (Table 1)

Case history

The sole abnormality noted by Marie-José M., aged 27 years, was a slight, barely painful swelling on the back of the right hand, present for some months. On examination, it was obvious that this firm swelling arose from the diaphyseal portion of the 2nd metacarpal. In the radiograph (fig. 2) the bone was slightly ballooned in its middle portion. The cortices were thinned and the spongy bone replaced by a clear image. This central zone of osteolysis was spotted by some calcifications. The boundaries of this lesion, particularly the proximal boundary, did not have the regularity of those of a cyst. There was no other bony lesion in this young patient. At operation, this tumour was not enucleable; it consisted of chondromyxoid tissue (figs. 22, 23) infiltrating the cavities of the spongy bone. The histological report mentioned the presence of young stellate or fusiform chondrocytes in a matrix that was in places more mucoid than hyaline. Careful examination revealed some chondrocytes with double nuclei. Lastly, at the periphery, minute cartilaginous foci were infiltrating the alveoli of the spongy bone.

It was surprising that the conclusion stated that, despite the cytological anomalies observed and the immature appearance of this cartilage but with due regard for the site, this was a chondroma. The report of this cautious pathologist ended by asking for local surveillance to detect any possible recurrence.

Table 1

Chondromas of the long bones of the hands and feet
- 50% of chondromas, especially the phalanges
- 99% benign, despite their immature appearance

Differential diagnosis (radiological)
- Cyst of unknown aetiology
- Osteoblastoma
- Bone invasion by nodule of villonodular synovitis, glomus tumour, metastasis

General features and course

Sites in the long bones of the hands and feet account for some 50% of chondromas. The radiographs (figs. 1-5) strongly suggest the diagnosis of benign chondroma, particularly the images of annular calcifications enclosing small cartilaginous nodules which, if not pathognomonic, are at least highly suggestive of benign chondroma. Localisation in the phalanges is commonest, sometimes revealed by a fracture, in which case the immature chondroid tissue may infiltrate the soft tissues. The histological picture is typical, as we have seen in the case quoted.

In cartilaginous tumours of the metacarpals and phalanges, the probability of benign behaviour associated with the site largely exceeds that of a progressive lesion wrongly attributed to it by the immature histological picture (fig. 23). More rarely, the appearance is that of a chondroma of nodular architecture and partly calcified (fig. 21). Chondrosarcomas at the same site are very rare; less than 1% at this site [Roberts & Price 1977].

Chondromas of the long bones of the limbs (Table 2)

Table 2

Chondroma in the adult (excluding the long bones of the hands and feet)
A rare tumour of small size, mature hyaline cartilage. No cells with large nuclei

Differential diagnosis
- Chondrosarcoma grade 1, clinically and cytologically progressive, especially at the periphery of the nodules. A fractured chondroma further complicates the problem because of the special cytological features of the callus.
- A fracture callus may mask a true underlying tumour and must not be confused with a simple fractured chondroma
- Sessile exostosis; to be distinguished from a juxta-osseous chondroma.

Ensure whether or not the chondroma belongs to one of the following syndromes:
- Enchondromatosis (Ollier's dyschondroplasia)
- Maffucci's syndrome (chondromatosis + angiomas)
- Maffucci-Kaast syndrome (Maffucci + pigmentary anomalies)

Case history

Ms B., a teacher aged 44, consulted a diagnostic center for localised pain in the right knee, noticed at night, when she felt tired. The history revealed nothing remarkable and clinical examination detected no specific bone or skin lesion (angioma, pigmentation, etc.). Frontal and lateral radiographs of the femur showed the joint to be uninvolved, but in the lower femoral metaphysis there were small, clear, well-circumscribed and rounded images, situated a few millimeters from each other and extending over 3-4 cm. Within these clear images calcifications of annular appearance were noted. A skeletal survey revealed no other lesion. Some weeks later, a surgical approach to the lower end of the femur allowed removal of white tissue with bluish glints, of elastic cartilaginous consistency.

Macroscopically, the small chondroid nodules were embedded in bony compartments hollowed out in the spongy bone. On section, the appearance was of glistening hyaline cartilage, except for small dull calcified zones of a whitish-grey hue.

Microscopically, the histological sections showed homogeneous hyaline cartilage in which well-differentiated chondrocytes, with small central nuclei, were embedded in well-marked chondroplastic cavities with defined borders.

Surgical intervention with careful curettage was followed by cure without recurrence after 15 years.

Clinical features and course

Chondromas of the long bones of the limbs represent about 30% of chondromas of bone. Complete removal is followed by cure.

Pathological anatomy and histopathology

Macroscopically and histologically, these chondromas are formed of nodules of hyaline cartilage; Mirra et al (1985) stress their nodular architecture. These nodules are separated from each other by intervals of normal osteomedullary tissue and are often bounded by a osteoid or bony border (figs. 13, 25). The chondrocytes are few, of small size, and embedded in a well-marked chondroplast. Rarely, there may be double nuclei. There is no necrosis, but some small calcified areas may be seen. Apart from the nodular architecture, the diagnosis of (benign) chondroma as a lesion of the long bones of the limbs in adults, can in our view, be made only on the basis of a radiologically and anatomically well-circumscribed tumour of nodular bounded appearance, of moderate dimensions and where hyaline cartilage encloses mature chondrocytes whose nucleo-cytoplasmic ratio is similar to that of chondrocytes of articular cartilage.

Table 3

Varieties according to site

- Root of limbs, limb-girdles, trunk
  - Tumour 1-2 cm in diameter: benign chondroma if the cartilage is well-differentiated
  - Bulky tumour: consider common or clear-cell types of chondrosarcoma
- Base of skull
  - Prognosis guarded
  - Exclude chondrosarcoma grade 1, chordoma, chordoid chondroma (cf Chapter 20)
- Juxta-osseous
  - Exclude sessile exostosis, periosteal chondrosarcoma, myxoma, juxtacortical myxoma

Anatomo-clinical variants (Table 3)

Tumours of the base of the limbs, limb-girdles and trunk

Authentic benign chondromas may be found in the supra-acetabular region; they are small in size and usually discovered by chance. All too frequently, a bulky tumour of slow and painless growth, covered by major muscle masses, is ominous from the outset. Apart from rare exostoses, I do not recall ever having examined a large tumour of the trunk whose course was benign.

Tumours of the base of the skull

Because of their situation, these lesions may be serious, Their diagnosis from chordoma may be difficult with standard staining. However, though labelling with anti-S100 protein is positive in both cartilaginous tumours and chordomas, only the latter give a positive reaction with epithelial membrane anti-cytokeratin and anti-antigen.

Juxtaosseous tumours (figs. 16-18)

Periosteal chondroma may be formed of hyaline cartilage of elastic consistency or sometimes of immature mucoid cartilage. In the latter case, low magnification examination may suggest a myxoma; the cells are then few, round or stellate. There may also be an osteogenic reaction of the periosteum, which tends to envelop the cartilaginous formation [Rockwell et al 1972].

It is easy to exclude a sessile exostosis by the radiological images and a properly performed biopsy. In X-rays, a periosteal chondroma makes its mark by a slight excavation of the cortex of a long bone; an exostosis is grafted on the parent bone like a branch on a trunk.

If we accept the possibility of cytologic anomalies in authentic periosteal chondromas, as is usually the case, the necessary corollary is great difficulty in recognising periosteal chondrosarcomas of low malignancy. Argument on the basis of the post-therapeutic course is invalid; complete ablation will ensure cure, if necessary after local reinterventions.

Childhood tumours

Before the age of 5 years, cellular proliferation and immaturity are commonplace appearances. The tumour-like hypertrophy of the anterior tuberosity of the tibia, supposedly due to trauma, or partial avulsion, is an example (fig. 6). No frank anomalies are to be found in this richly cellular cartilage. This type of cartilaginous hypertrophy, probably secondary to some mechanical cause which often goes unrecognised, is more logically classed among the chondrohamartomas than the exostoses.

The case illustrated in figure 19 is more frankly tumour-like. The "tumour" is bounded by a neocortex, the whole ensheathing the tibia. A biopsy fragment of the lesion of this young girl of 15 months was submitted to leading pathologists on the occasion of an international congress; their conclusions were totally diverse.

At the age of 5, this child was operated for a cyst of the ovary, and during the subsequent months developed multiple cutaneous myxomas, but without cardiac involvement. Resection-reconstruction of the tibia was not followed by recurrence.

Neither of the two reports of this condition by Carney et al (1985, 1986), which relate to 51 and 40 patients respectively, nor the report of Atherton et al (1980), mention of bony localisation, but it is nevertheless very tempting to class this case with this syndrome.

Chondromatosis and Maffucci's syndrome

Chondromatosis is characterised by a multiplicity of the bony sites for the chondromas. Ollier insisted on the asymmetry of the lesions, though it is not possible to specify a frankly unilateral form [Maroteaux 1995].

The Maffucci (or Kaast-Maffucci) syndrome combines multiple chondromas and angiomas; its prognosis is more guarded than that of chondromatosis because of the frequency of a chondrosarcomatous course [Lascombes & Mainard 1996].

References

The references for Chapters 1 and 2 are given together at the end of Chapter 2, p. 22

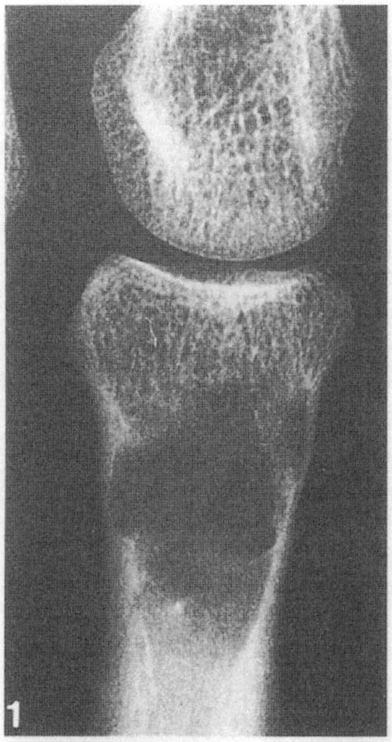

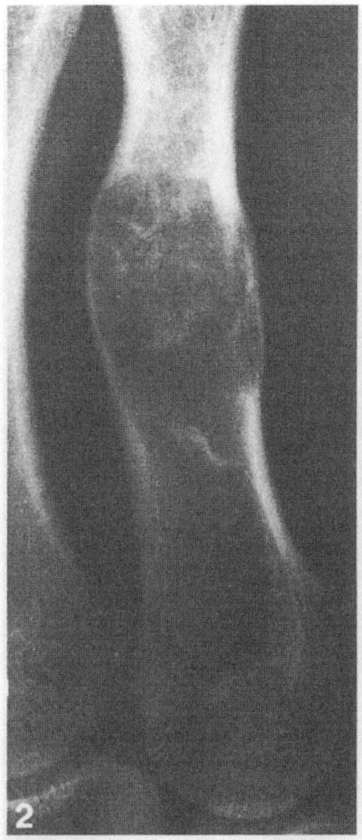

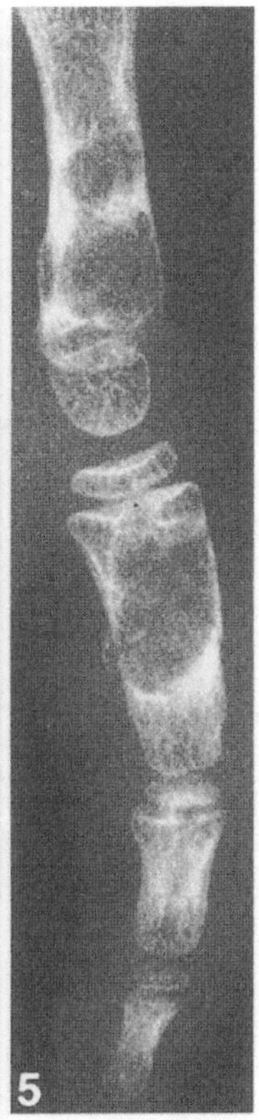

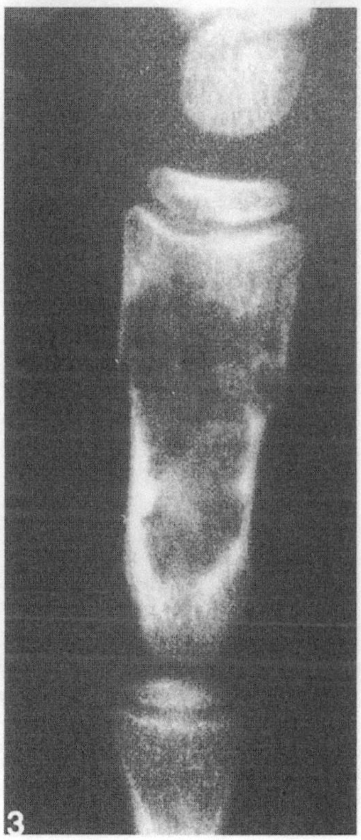

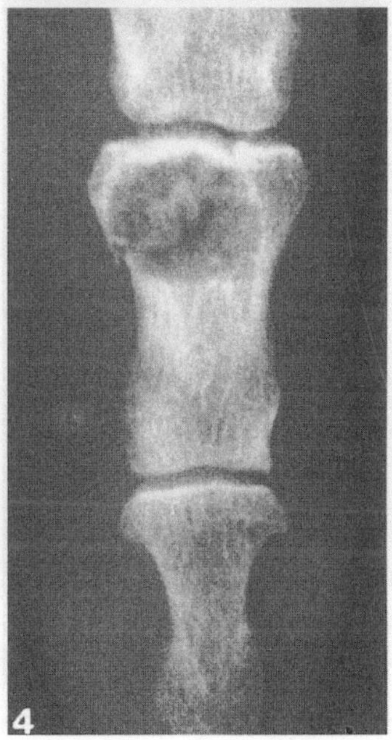

Figs. 1, 2. Base of the first phalanx of the ring finger and diaphysis of the 2nd metacarpal. The osteolysis of these two chondromas spares the cortices. The first phalanx is virtually undeformed, but the metacarpal is ballooned

Figs. 3, 4. Two chondromas revealed by fracture. The first phalanx of the ring finger (3) is almost completely destroyed

Fig. 5. Chondromatosis of 5th ray. Girl aged 6 years

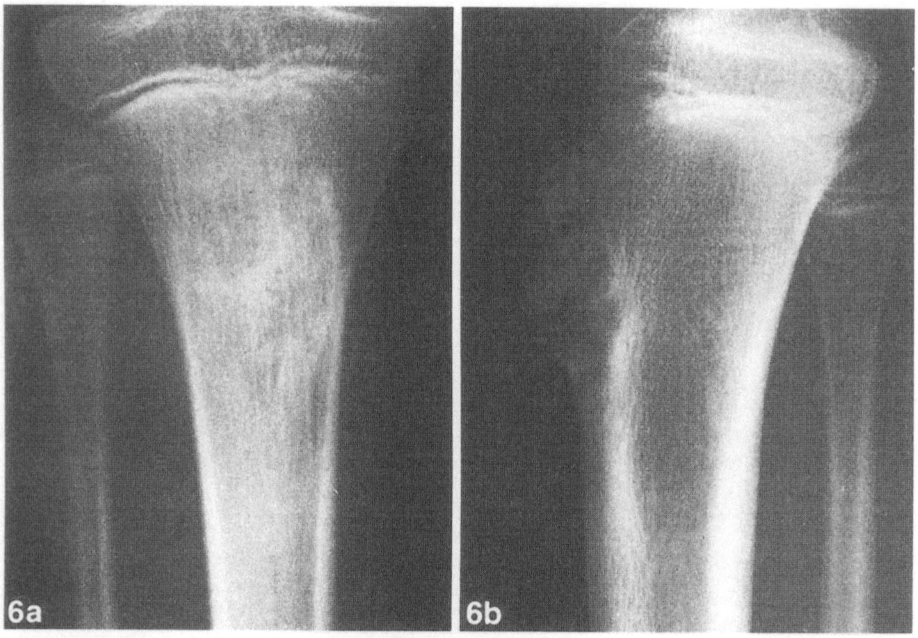

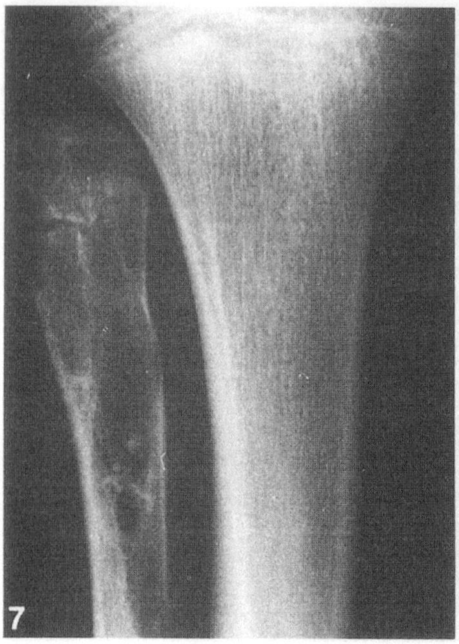

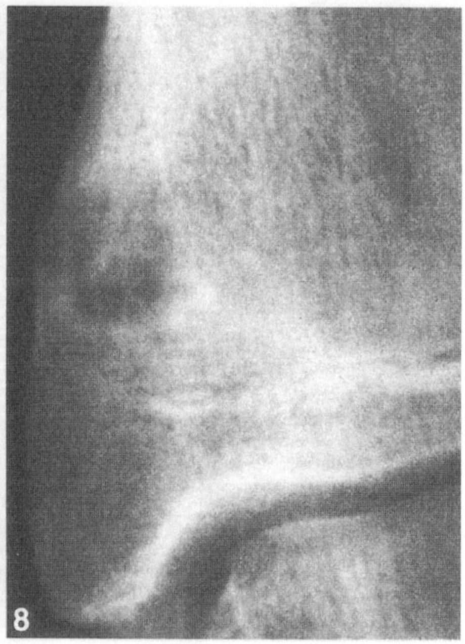

Fig. 6 a, b. Hamartochondroma of anterior tuberosity of tibia: child aged 10 years

Fig. 7. Enchondroma of upper third of fibula, tumour extensive but well circumscribed. Child of 11 years

Fig. 8. Chondroma of lower end of tibia; the radiological appearance is not characteristic. The lesion is very near the growth cartilage. Adolescent aged 17 years

→

Fig. 9 a-c. In these two chondromas of the upper third of the humerus, the images of annular calcifications are visible in the standard films (**a, b**). A CT section shows the extent of the calcifications, related to small zones of infarction (**c**)

Fig. 10 a, b. In this chondroma of the upper third of the tibia, the MRI demonstrates the boundaries of the lesion

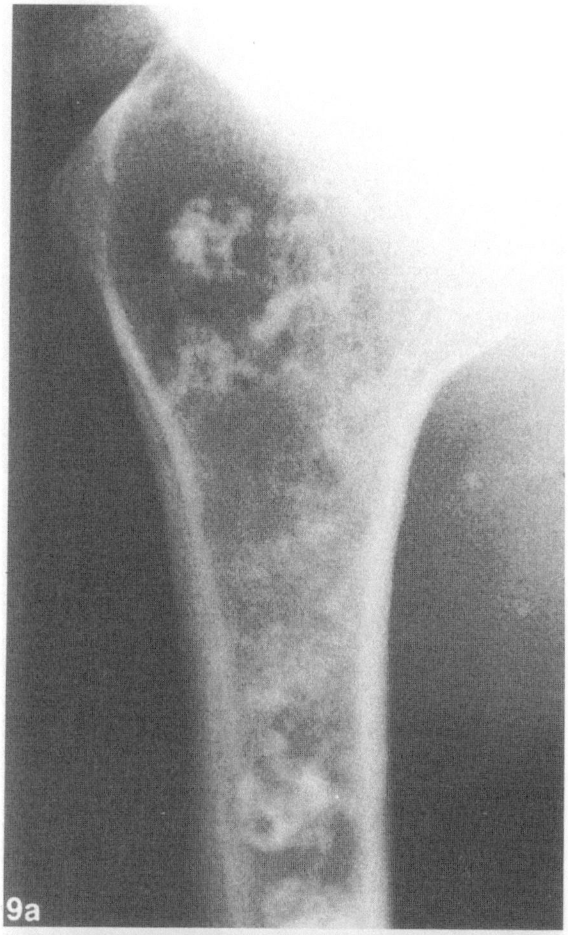
9a

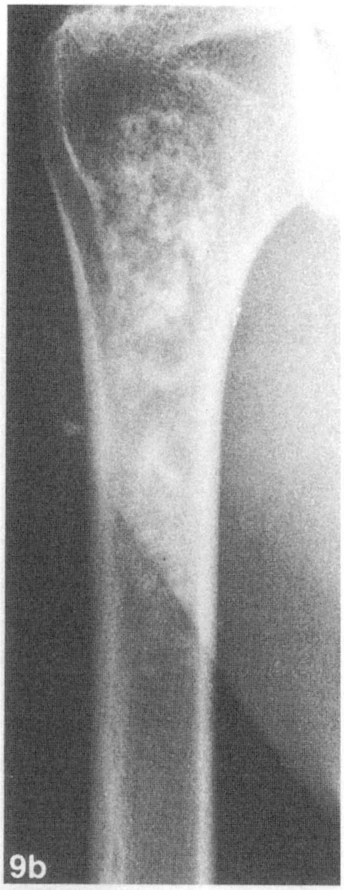
9b

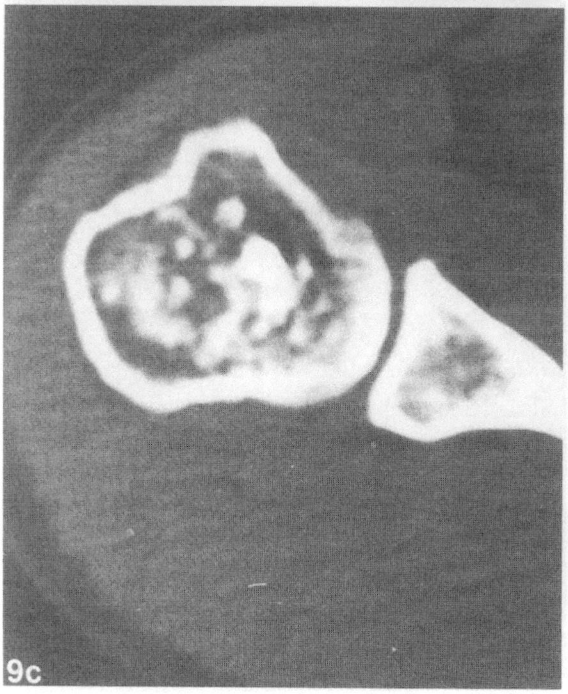
9c

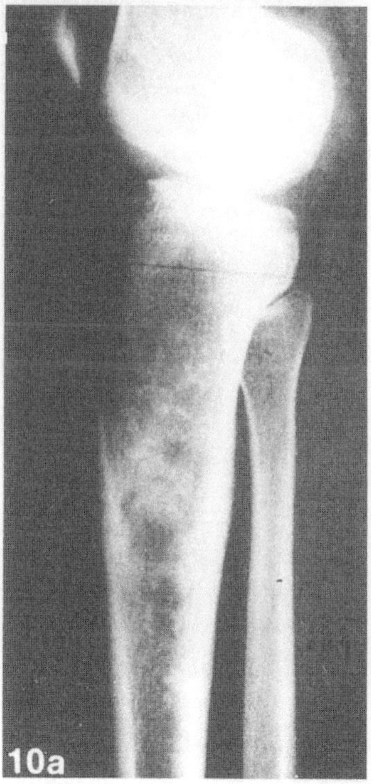
10a

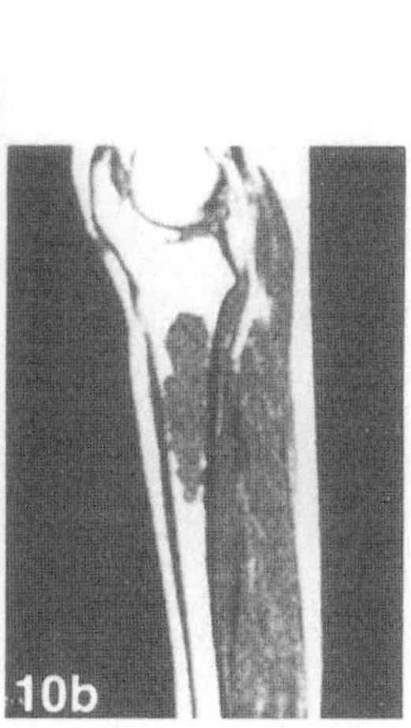
10b

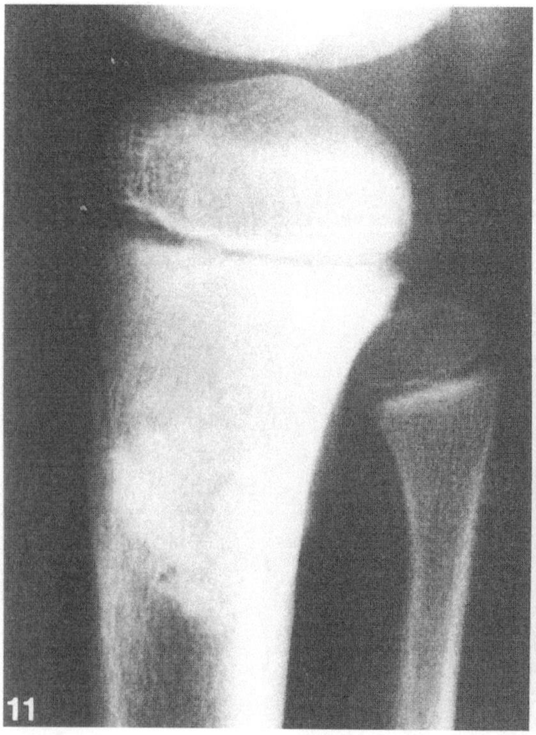

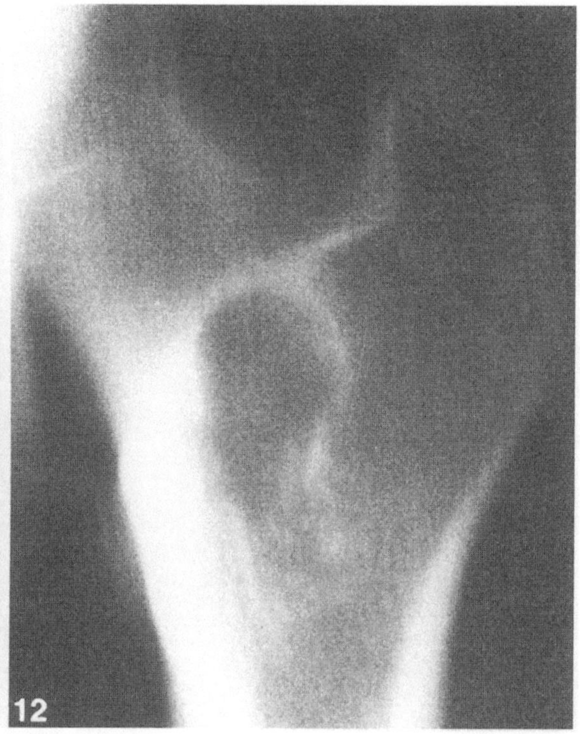

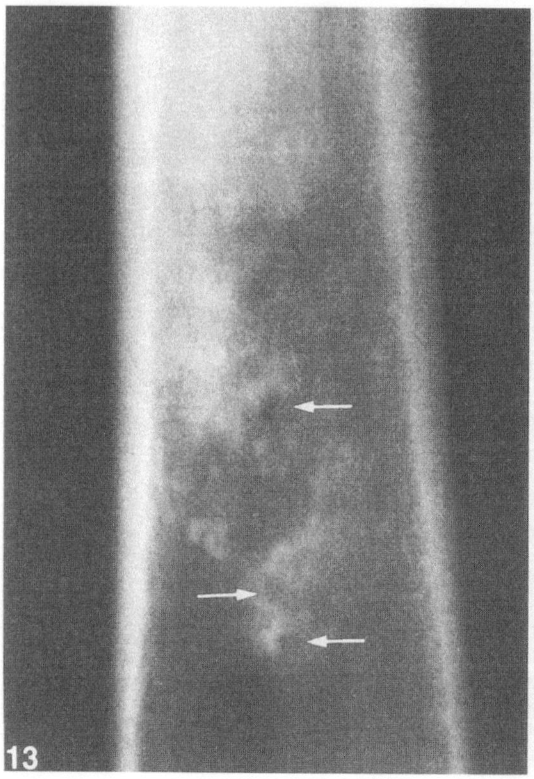

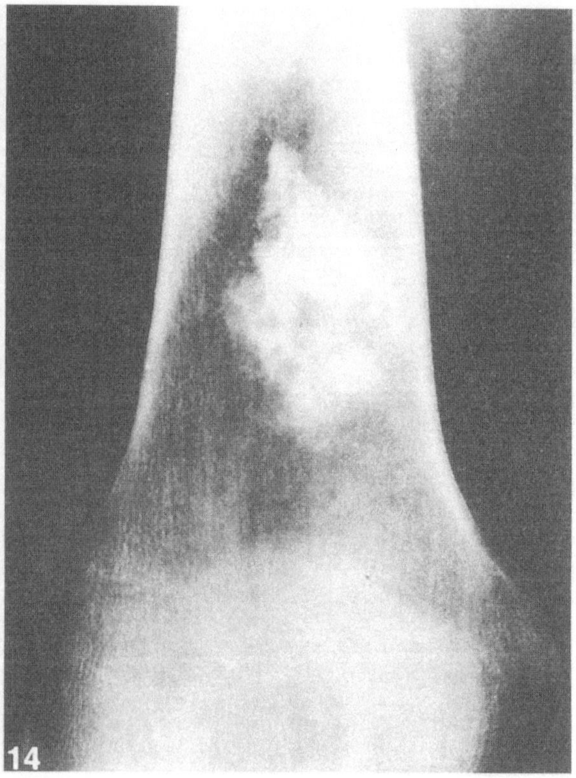

Fig. 11. In contrast to the preceding images, this standard radiograph is suggestive of the diagnosis of chondroma of the upper third of the tibia but does not define its extent. Child of 8 1/2 years

Fig. 12. Chondroma of upper metaphysis of femur with dense boundaries. Some calcified zones in its lower part

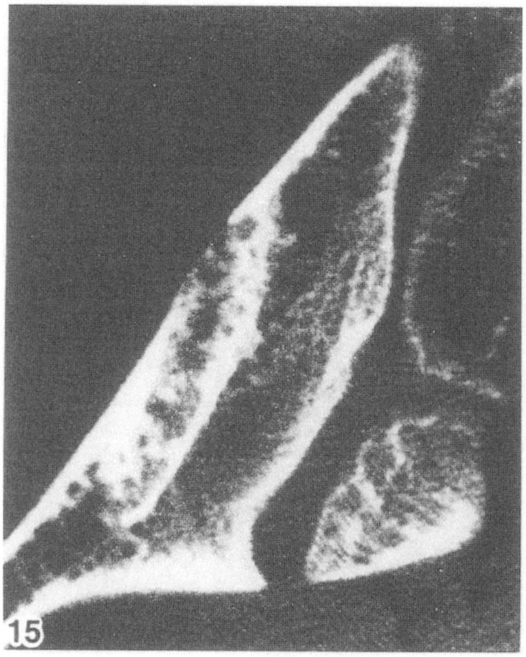

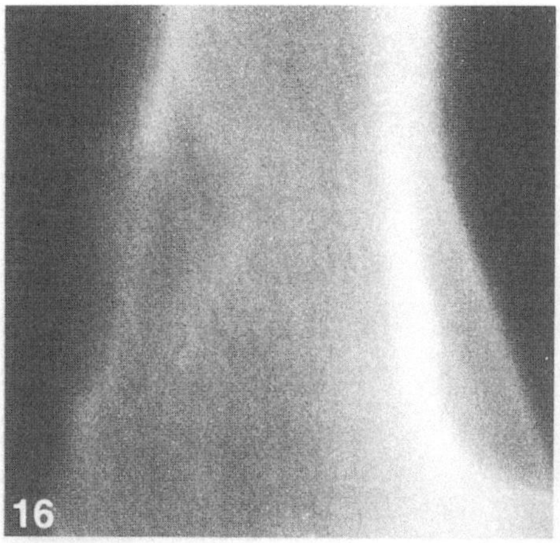

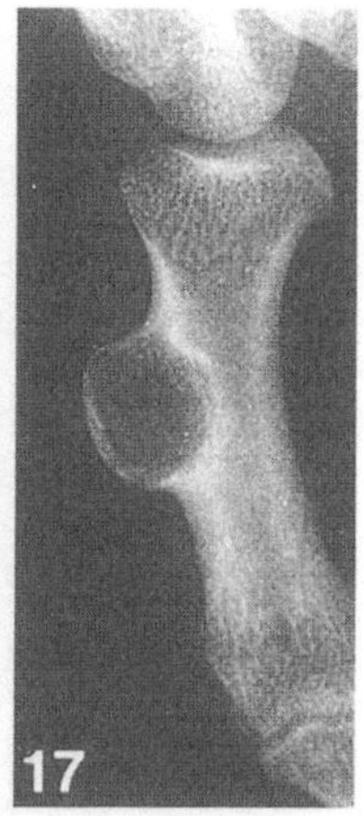

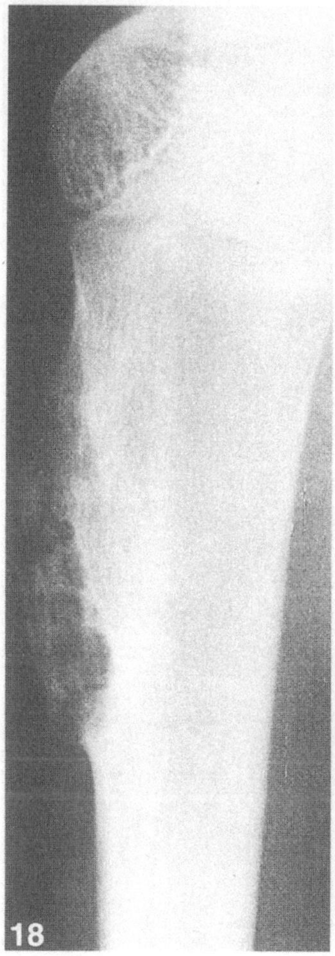

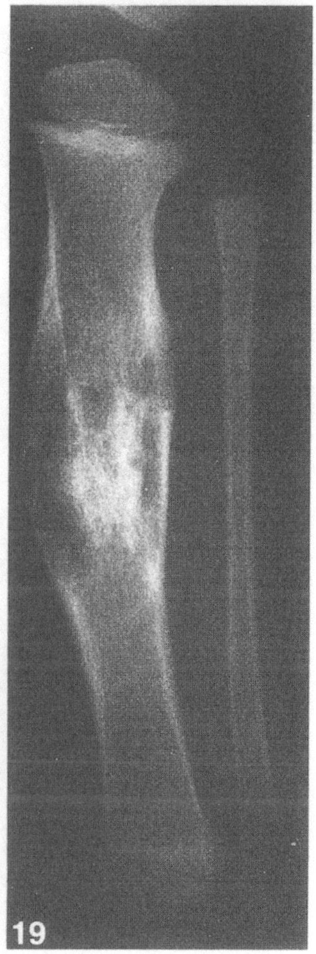

Fig. 15. Hamartochondroma of ilium, CT section. Child aged 7 years

Figs. 16-18. Three appearances of subperiosteal chondroma. **16** lower end of femur in a 42-year-old man; **17** first phalanx of right index finger; **18** juxtacortical humeral lesion in child of 12 years

Fig. 19. Child of 15 months. Cartilaginous tumour of tibia, initial manifestation of Carney's syndrome (cf "Case history"). This case was kindly supplied by Dr Boccon-Gibod

Fig. 13. Chondroma of lower metaphysis of tibia. The areolar appearance of the calcifications (*arrows*) corresponds to peripheral osteogenesis in the cartilaginous lobules. Child aged 8 years

Fig. 14. The areolar appearance given by the cartilaginous lobules is particularly evident in this radiograph of a chondroma of the lower femoral metaphysis

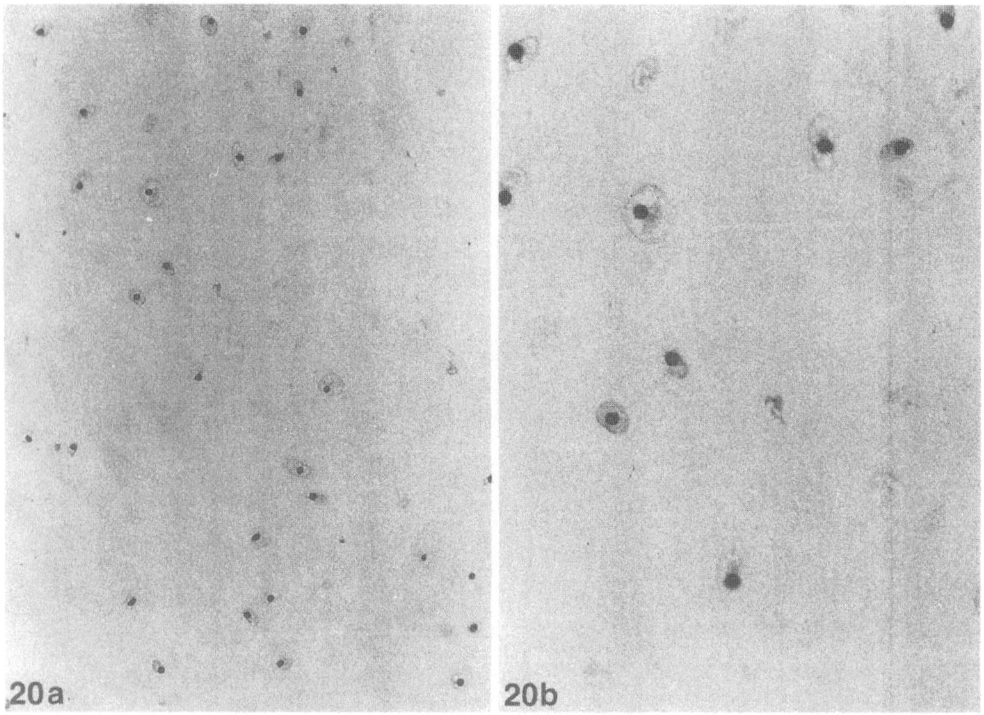

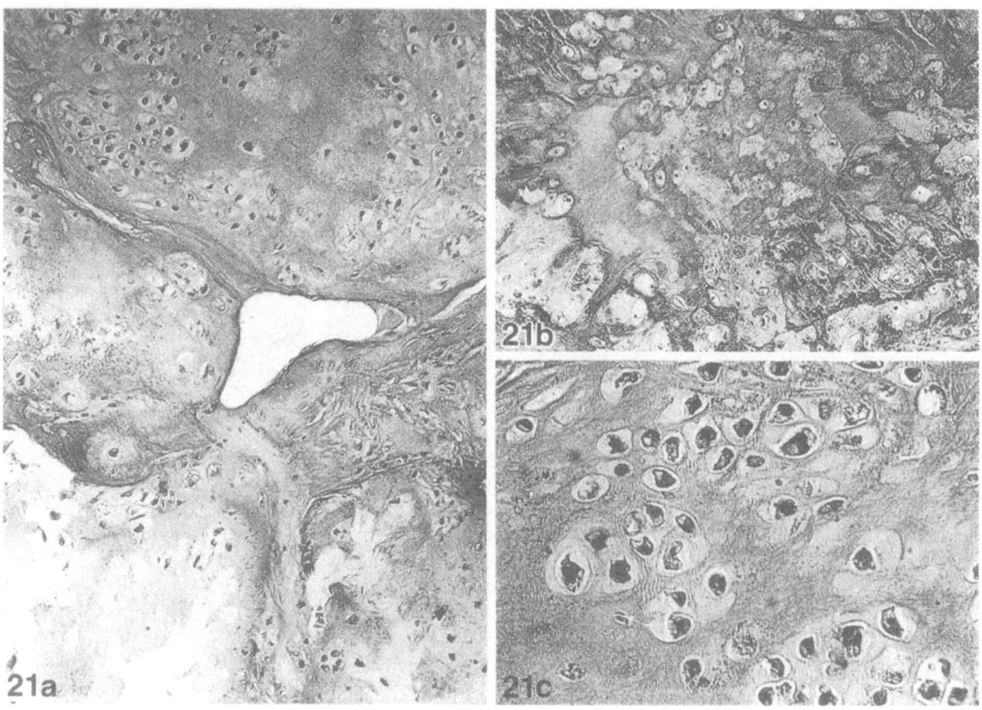

Fig. 20 a, b. Chondrohamartoma of iliac crest (see fig. 15). Chondrocytes sparse, round or slightly ovoid, with round very chromophil nuclei embedded in well-defined chondroplasts in a uniform hyaline matrix. Child aged 7 years

Fig. 21 a-c. Chondroma of metacarpal. **a** The lobular aspect is evident under low magnification. **b** Calcified zone at periphery of lobule. **c** High magnification: the nuclei of the chondrocytes are strongly stained but the nucleo-cytoplasmic ratio is maintained; the chondroplasts are well-marked. Man of 54 years

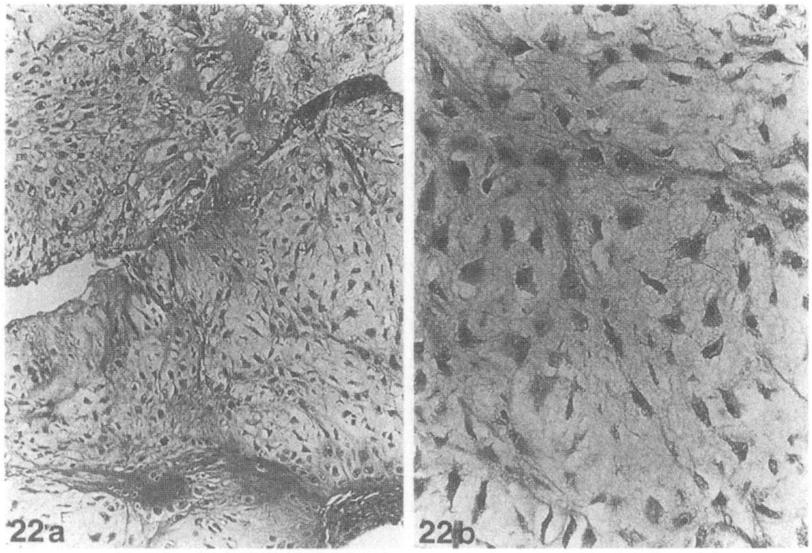

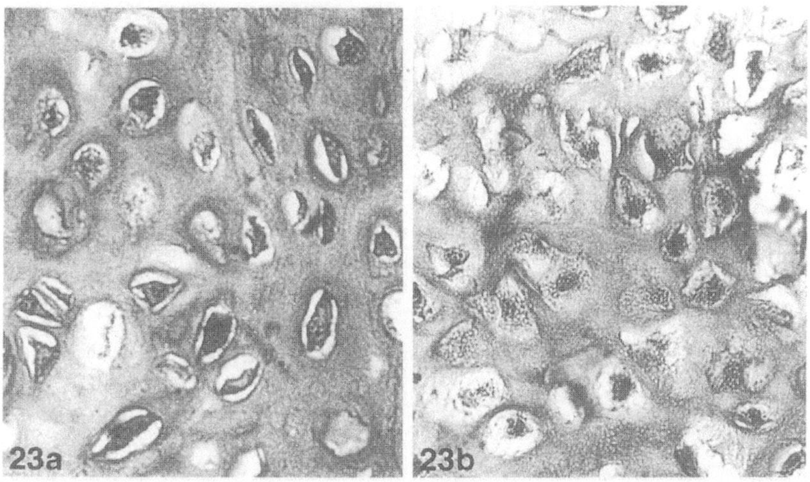

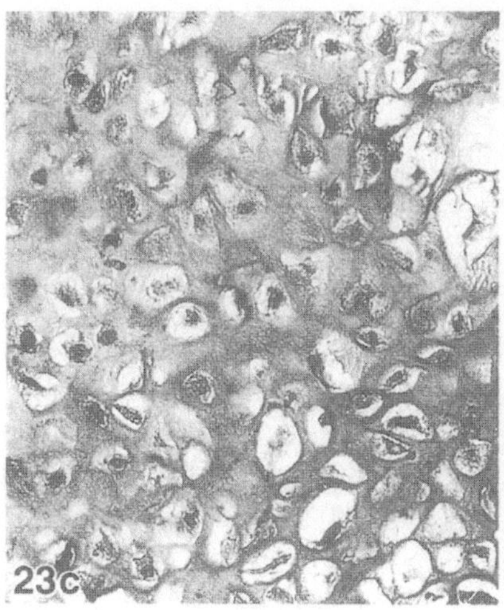

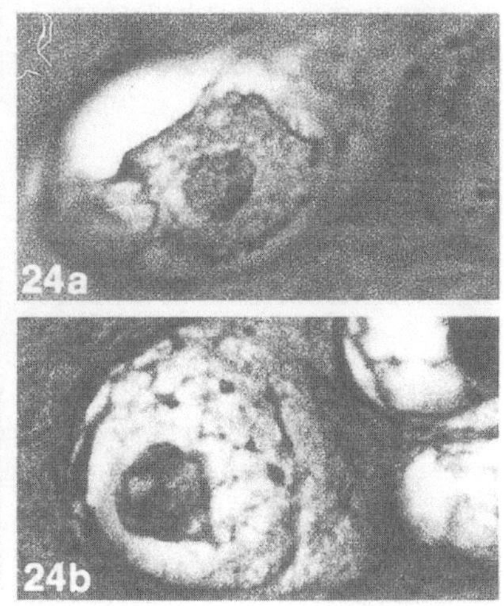

Fig. 22 a, b. Chondroma of first phalanx of 5th finger. In this tumour the chondrocytes have the immature appearance very often seen in chondromas of the digits: irregular shape and differing size, relatively numerous, in a loose poorly-staining matrix. The whole has a myxoid appearance. Man of 29 years

Fig. 23 a-c. Very cellular islets in chondroma of phalanx. Numerous ballooned degenerate chondrocytes. Girl aged 6 years

Fig. 24 a, b. For purposes of comparison: chondrocytes of articular cartilage (immersion)

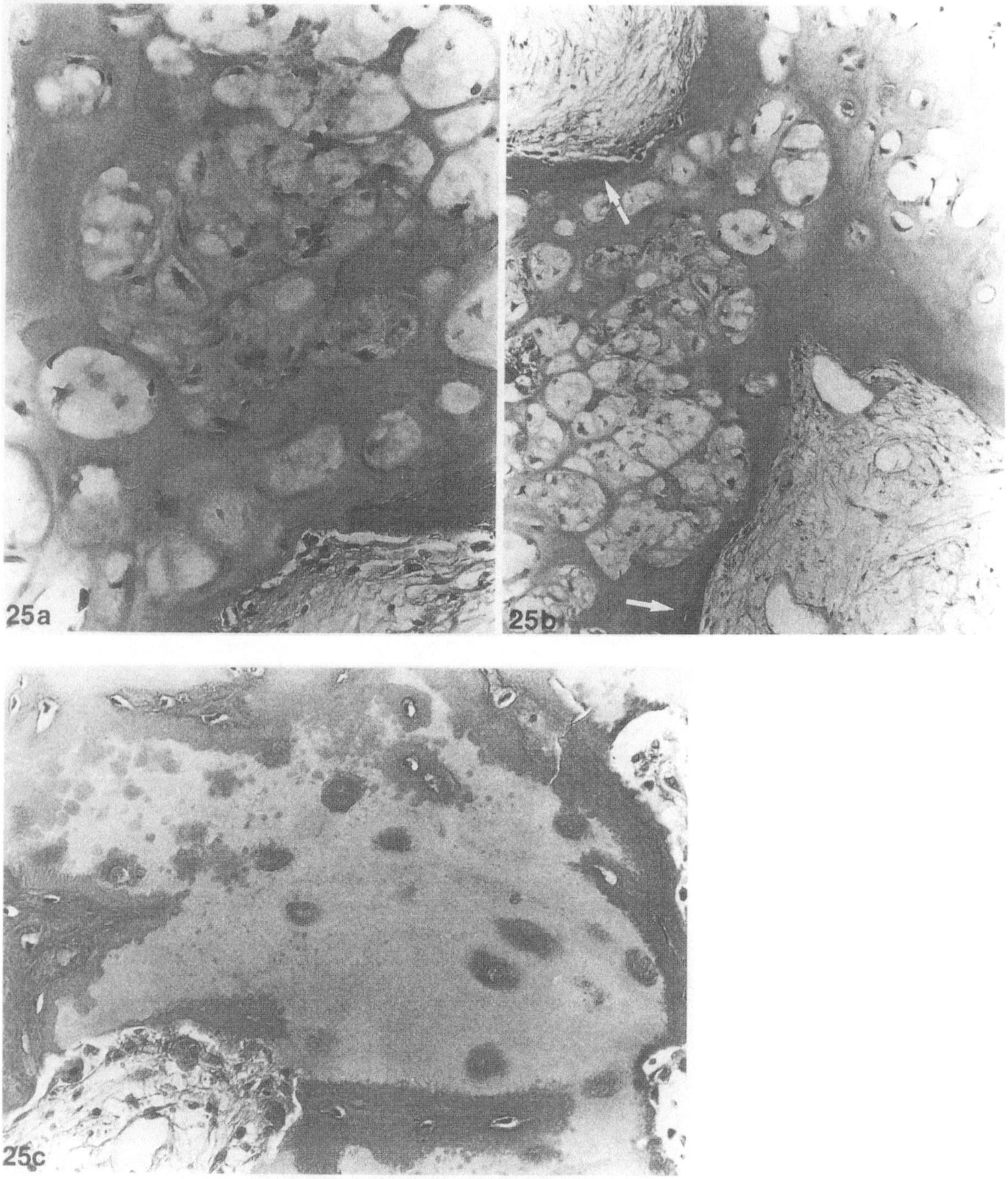

Fig. 25 a-c. Chondroma of humerus. **a** Ballooned chondrocytes undergoing necrosis, with punctiform nuclei; **b** the marrow between the cartilaginous lobules is fibrous, the margins of the lobules have few cells, in places undergoing ossification (*arrows*); **c** cartilaginous nodule, few cells, bounded by calcified cartilage, partly ossified

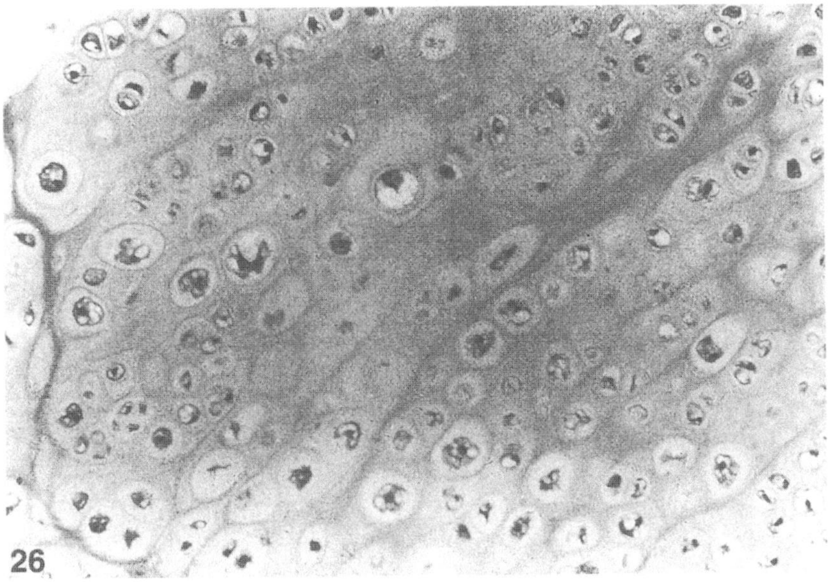

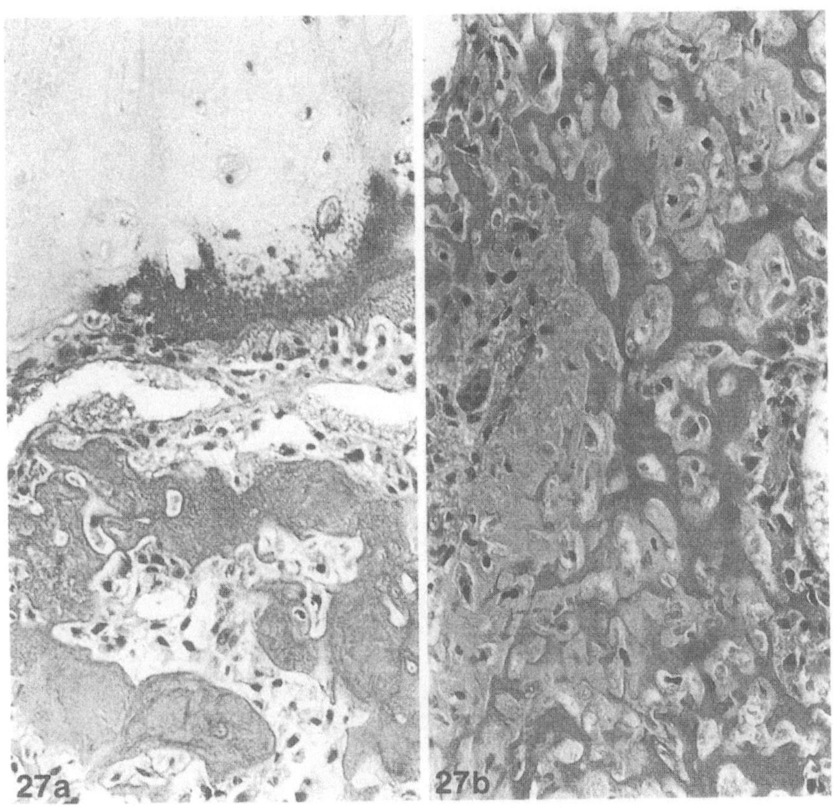

Fig. 26. Irradiated cartilaginous tumour, in all probability a chondroma. After irradiation, sections of this cartilaginous tumour are uninterpretable

Fig. 27 a, b. Osteosarcoma developing in preexisting chondroma. **a** The upper third is occupied by a cartilaginous plaque representing the margin of a partly calcified cartilaginous lobule of the preexisting chondroma. **b** Plexiform tumour-like osteogenesis, cells irregularly distributed and atypical with bulky hyperchromatic nuclei, small foci of necrosis

2. Chondrosarcoma

General considerations

These represent around 10% of malignant tumours of bone. There is a slight masculine predominance. The age distribution extends from the 2nd to 8th decades, with a peak towards the 6th decade. In 75% of cases, the tumour develops in the vertebrae, ribs, iliac bones (at this site in 31% of cases according to Huvos, 1979) and scapulae (more than 20% of malignant tumours of the scapula). The head and limbs account for 25% of cases. Around 50% of chondrosarcomas develop in a preexisting chondroma or exostosis, either spontaneously or, exceptionally, following irradiation.

It is usually impossible to determine on examining a bulky tumour, whether it may have originated from a preexisting exostosis or chondroma. Conversely, malignant transformation of an exostosis as shown by the development of pain and/or rapid increase in size allows the diagnosis of sarcomatous transformation. Rare cases of chondrosarcoma have been diagnosed in healthy bones situated in the field of irradiation of an adjacent tumour [Aprin et al 1986, Fitzwater et al 1976].

Clinical features and course

Pain, the recent appearance of a swelling or the increase in size of a known swelling and more rarely fracture, are possible presenting features. Current imaging techniques provide valuable data for diagnosis: osteolysis with or without cortical destruction, intratumour calcifications are seen with expansion into the soft tissues, a virtually certain sign of malignancy. There is some relationship between the course of chondrosarcomas and their histological appearance (Table 1) and this defines the importance of reference systems expressing the histological grading of malignancy [O'Neal & Ackerman 1952, Evans et al 1977, Larson et al 1979, Ishida et al 1991].

Classification of chondrosarcomas

Grade 1

Chondrosarcoma of grade 1 is a localised lesion and is distinguished by an abnormal abundance of cells, often limited to patchy areas, in which the chondrocytes shows an increase in the nucleo-cytoplasmic ratio and some double nuclei.

It is evident that cytological study allows better cytonuclear assessment, but it is not possible to dispense with a topographical study of the histological sections [Sanerkin 1980, Jelthi et al 1987]. Whereas a chondroma is preceded in its slow course by osteoclastic osteolysis, chondrosarcoma is in direct contact with the bony trabeculae and includes residues of partly destroyed trabeculae at the advancing margin.

Grade 2

Chondrosarcoma of grade 2 is above all a cartilaginous tumour in which examination with a magnification of the order of 40 x 10 reveals the undeniable presence of malignant cells that would not have been suspected at a lower magnification: numerous bulky nuclei, multiple nuclei and increased cellularity are seen (figs. 17, 18).

Grade 3

The grade 3 chondrosarcoma has more or less retained its nodular character. Some nodules are very cellular,

Table 1.

	Peripheral zone	Mitoses	Increased nuclear cyto-plasmic ratio	Binucleate cells
Enchondroma	Osteoid	#0	+ (?)	+
Chondrosarcoma grade 1	Cellular +	+	++	+
Chondrosarcoma grades 2 and 3	Cellular ++	++	+++	+++

others more so peripherally and chondrocytic differentiation is less marked there. The centers of some nodules are necrotic. Cytonuclear anomalies are evident with bulky nuclei and double or triple nuclei. In places the matrix has lost its uniform appearance, which is replaced by a sort of plexus in which the cells are polymorphic, without chondroplasts, the whole assuming the myxoid appearance of an undifferentiated sarcoma. The development of these myxoid zones is very variable from case to case. In some tumours, the diagnosis of sarcoma is obvious, that of its cartilaginous origin more difficult (fig. 25).

Correlations between histological appearance and prognosis

Prognostic evaluation is difficult, particularly with minor degrees of malignancy. Even allowing for variations in surgical treatment we must accept that our histological classifications are not 100% reproducible in clinical terms. Thus, tumours classed as grade 1 are regarded by some as locally and only locally aggressive [Evans et al 1977], whereas others report metastases in 5% of cases and death in 29% [Sanerkin 1975]. For grade 2 chondrosarcomas, metastases vary between 10 and 15% with a mortality of the order of 50%, and for grade 3 metastases are around 70-75% with a mortality exceeding 80%. In 1995, the studies of Coughlan et al and those of Adler et al showed a high rate of aneuploidy and a strongly positive expression of gene p 53 in chondrosarcomas of grade 3 histological malignancy; unfortunately, these studies do not provide a prognostic factor for minor degrees of malignancy.

Metastases, essentially by the venous route, first affect the lungs. The arterial route is rarer; in one of our cases, multiple small nodules developed in the fine arterioles of the finger pulp secondary to surgical intervention for a large chondrosarcoma of the upper end of the humerus. A feature quite specific to chondrosarcomas is their formidable ability to engraft along the path of a surgical approach.

It is evident that the prognosis is a function of the surgical procedure, itself largely determined by the site and size of the tumour [Larson et al 1979]. Global results expose the inefficacy of current methods of treatment [Ucla et al 1991]. Radiotherapy for inoperable tumours has yielded some remissions; more recently, cryosurgery has been attempted [Pidhorz et al 1987], but not without local difficulties.

Chondrosarcoma of low histological malignancy: grade 1 (Table 2)

Case history

This was a young girl of 8 years in whom a radiograph performed for vague pains in the right knee showed small clear images with sinuous outlines at the upper and lower metaphyses of the tibia. Examination of the biopsy led to a diagnosis of chondrosarcoma and the treatment proposed was amputation through the thigh. In a film including the entire leg, there were virtually identical clear images extending along the long axis of

Table 2. Chondrosarcoma grade 1: differential diagnosis

Chondroma, appearance of mature cartilage. Minimal treatment justified
Chondrosarcoma grade 2 or 3, distinction relatively easy; necessary to examine the maximum number of sections. The histological report determines the magnitude of the surgical procedure
Chondromyxoid fibroma; clinical features and imaging are important aids to diagnosis.
Variants in age and site occur

the bone into the lower metaphysis. A review of the sections led us to consider that this was a cartilaginous formation exhibiting some cellular anomalies, particularly very rare large nuclei, but in which the degree of malignancy remained low (grade 1). Complete resection of the tibial shaft and the interposition of the left fibula between the two epiphyses, an ideal graft, very soon allowed the resumption of normal physical activity. There is now a disease-free interval of more than 15 years.

Imaging

While examination of the standard films remains the initial investigation for all cartilaginous tumours, they are often deceptive for minor grades of malignancy: MRI supplies more significant findings [de Beuckeleer et al 1996]. CT defines the boundaries of the osteolysis, the cortical involvement, and the presence of calcification.

Histology

With the exception of cartilaginous tumours of the phalanxes and chondromas in children, the immature aspect of the cartilage must attract attention. The cells are more numerous than in a chondroma and are irregularly distributed. Some double nuclei and rare cells with bulky nuclei may be noted. The marrow spaces are invaded by the tumour, which comes into direct contact with the bony tissue in places, without the interposition of evident osteoclastic activity [Sanerkin 1980]. There is no necrosis and the presence of some ballooned cells does not aid the diagnosis.

For pathologists accustomed to this type of lesion, a cytological study clearly demonstrates increase in the nuclear-cytoplasmic ratio.

Chondrosarcomas of histological malignancy: grades 2 and 3

(Table 3, figs. 18-20, 27)

Case history

Miss B. was at the start of a brilliant career when she experienced mild pain in the right thigh, localised at its mid-portion. The clinical examination and history revealed nothing to aid in diagnosis.

Table 3. Chondrosarcomas grades 2 and 3

These justify an extensive, even mutilating, procedure
Prognosis guarded
Differential diagnosis:
- Chondrosarcoma grade 1, excluded by the number of atypical cells, mitoses, and large-nucleated cells in chondrosarcomas grades 2 and 3
- A clear-cell chondrosarcoma containing zones of grades 2 or 3, which alter the prognosis and treatment
- Biopsy by cytological aspiration of a zone with clear cells may promote metastasis

The radiographs showed a clear central diaphyseal image, eroding the inner wall of the femoral cortex. The lesion was not bounded but poorly confined along the axis of the bone, not exceeding 20 mm in diameter. Macroscopically, the cortex was not destroyed. The tumour, situated in the medullary canal, was of gelatinous mucoid consistency. The pathologist diagnosed a chondrosarcoma, of largely myxoid appearance. The patient's refusal of any aggressive surgical procedure explains why curettage was the sole treatment.

Nine years later, after several recurrences for which mutilating procedures were refused, the patient was admitted to the orthopaedic department with the femur almost totally invaded by the tumour. Appearance of pulmonary metastases soon put an end to further developments.

Comparison of the sections made from the disarticulation specimen with those of the first biopsy showed few changes in this grade 2 chondrosarcoma. In addition to the myxoid appearance of the matrix there was great irregularity of cell distribution, the presence of some double nuclei, and especially an increase in the nuclear-cytoplasmic ratio of numerous cells.

Clinical features and course

In 80% of cases, chondrosarcomas of grades 2 and 3 are revealed by pain, often not severe, which may not lead to consultation until 15-18 months after its onset; the tumour has usually then reached 4-6 cm in diameter and sometimes much more.

Imaging

The radiological signs are virtually pathognomonic: rupture of the cortex, invasion of the soft tissues, multiple nodular opacities due to calcification.

Pathological anatomy and histopathology

Macroscopically, the tumour is adherent to the tendino-aponeurotic structures and the bone, from which it is inseparable.

On section, the bluish-white cartilaginous nodules are riddled here and there with necrotic cavities. Other zones are calcified. As it extends, the tumour engulfs some relics of the bony trabeculae, mature bone oriented with the general architecture of the bone, and easy to distinguish from tumour osteogenesis [Jelthi et al 1987]. The cytological anomalies are obvious. In some tumours there exist tumour plaques whose cells have a nucleus that is depressed peripherally by a clear vacuole. Some authors [Demetrick et al 1991] have suggested listing these chondrosarcomas with cells like signet-rings as a new entity (figs. 25, 26). Nuclear monstrosities and cellular polymorphism are characteristic of grade 3, but mitoses in grades 2 and 3 have to be sought in the peripheral zone of proliferation.

Figure 21 shows the relative frequency of anaplastic areas in grade 3 chondrosarcoma.

Undifferentiated chondrosarcoma

(Table 4, figs. 21, 22)

Case history

A biopsy of a lymph node arrived at the laboratory of the orthopaedic department accompanied by the following note: "right inguinal adenopathy in man aged 61, Case record N°...", a record that I was at leisure to consider and a patient I could also visit and interrogate.

Table 4. Undifferentiated chondrosarcoma

Some pitfalls to avoid:

- Undifferentiated zone in a chondrosarcoma of grade 1 or 2
- Biopsy taken from a primary tumour or metastasis exclusively involving a sarcomatous proliferation of fusiform cells: the diagnosis of a cartilaginous origin is impossible to confirm
- Confusion of an undifferentiated chondrosarcoma with a mesenchymal chondrosarcoma (each has a guarded prognosis, but the course is usually different) (cf Chapter 4)

The result of the histological examination was reported as follows: "Virtually complete destruction of the lymphoid tissue, replaced by a proliferation of fusiform cells with bulky nuclei and frequent mitoses". Perusal of the case notes showed that 12 years previously, in the same department, this patient had undergone the ablation of a chondrosarcoma (grade 2) of the sole of the foot, then 8 years later of a metastatic lesion in the popliteal fossa (grade 2/3). In this completely undifferentiated nodal lesion the cartilaginous origin was impossible to suggest without a knowledge of the history.

Clinical features and course

Dahlin and Unni (1986) state that the percentage of "dedifferentiation" (see Glossary) in chondrosarcomas is of the order of 10%. In 40% of cases, the anaplastic tumour consists of fusiform cells. Development of an osteosarcoma or malignant histiocytofibroma may also be seen. This dedifferentiation appears in diverse circumstances, listed in table 3. The basis of this dedifferentiation may be a chondrosarcoma of grade 2 or 3, but also a chondrosarcoma of low malignancy. The transition between the chondrosarcoma and the anaplastic tissue is usually abrupt; as for the metastatic lesions, these, as in the case quoted above, consist usually of fusiform cells (figs. 21, 26), sometimes of osteosarcomatous type.

Table 5. Chondrosarcoma: anatomo-clinical variants

Localisation at the limb-girdles, particularly the pelvic girdle, diagnosis often delayed, biopsy more or less representative. Course often very grave

Localisation juxtaosseous: distinguish a chondroma with cytological anomalies from a chondrosarcoma of low malignancy

Localisation in the sole of the foot. This tumour often infiltrates deeply

Epiphyseal chondrosarcoma of chondroblastic type: diagnosis very difficult, based on clinical features, imaging and cytology. Often impossible to distinguish from a chondroblastoma (cf Chapter 5)

Exostosis: aggressive and painful course; careful study of cartilaginous cap

Chondroma: recent modifications, study of multiple sections

Exuberant fracture callus: ascertain if there has been an injury causing loss of consciousness, even of short duration

Sternoclavicular and chondrosternal swellings (rheumatic, Tietze's syndrome) are clinically and histologically problematic

Irradiated chondroma: diagnosis impossible

Anatomo-clinical variants (Table 5)

Chondrosarcoma of the limb-girdles

Case history

A man aged 45, robust and active, came to consultation for a tumour he found in the right groin, slow-growing and painless; for months he had put off this consultation. Examination revealed a bulky firm tumour, connected with the iliac bone and palpable in the iliac fossa. It extended into the ilio-pubic region. The radiographs showed a half-tone opacity, dotted with several dense patches of calcification, with sharp limits, effacing the lower third of the iliac wing and the outer part of the ilio-pubic ramus. Biopsy indicated relatively well-differentiated cartilaginous tissue; there were bulky nuclei but peripheral mitotic activity was limited. An interilio-abdominal disarticulation was rapidly followed by progressive regional recurrence and pulmonary metastases.

Remarks

Localisation in the limb-girdles is associated with a high rate of histological malignancy but authentic benign chondromas of the pelvic girdle do exist. They are usually very small.

Juxtaosseous chondrosarcoma (figs. 13, 24)

This problem was discussed in the previous chapter. While well-characterised chondrosarcomas exist, it is sometimes difficult to distinguish between grade 1 chondrosarcoma and a chondroma exhibiting some cytological anomalies.

Cartilaginous tumour of the sole of the foot

A frequently encountered pitfall, this is a tumour which infiltrates between the metatarsals and involves the entire thickness of the foot. The sequence of events is characteristic of chondrosarcoma, requiring a mutilating procedure.

Chondrosarcoma in childhood and adolescence

As we have noted, chondrosarcoma is virtually non-existent before the age of 4 years. In a child of 12-14 years, chondrosarcoma may be found in the long bones of the limbs. The problem posed by the report of a cartilaginous sarcoma from a biopsy is that of the representative nature of the biopsy. The various imaging procedures help in recognising a predominantly cartilaginous osteosarcoma and favour verification, if necessary by a second biopsy, given the importance of the proper planning of treatment.

Histological variants

Chordoid appearance

Some chondrosarcomas resemble peripheral chordomas. An epithelioid appearance and the grouping of small columns of tumour cells may cause confusion between an epitheliomatous metastasis and a primary cartilaginous tumour. In such cases, it is simple to ascertain that the immunohistological reactions for epithelial markers are negative and those for vimentin and the S100 protein positive.

Liposarcomatous appearance

Another cellular appearance in chondrosarcoma, noted by Demetrick et al (1991) may at first sight suggest a liposarcoma. The tumour is characterised by so-called "signet-ring" cells (figs. 25, 26).

Epiphyseal chondroblastic chondrosarcoma

This tumour is better known by the name of "metastasising chondroblastoma" (cf Chapter 5). A slowly growing tumour, tending to local recurrence(s) after curettage, then to malignant transformation. This course, which is continuous, extends over 8-12 years. The histological diagnosis of this type of chondroblastic chondrosarcoma is particularly difficult, and usually impossible with conventional methods. It is probable that the information provided by CT and MR imaging, and perhaps by DNA and cytogenetic studies, will direct greater attention to the histocytological anomalies and so justify resection of the tumour. This type of chondrosarcoma is certainly rare, but too many instances have been reported (aggressive chondroblastoma, metastasising chondroblastoma, malignant transformation of a chondroblastoma) for it not to be singled out as a definite entity.

References (chapters 1 and 2)

Abdelwahab IF, Hermann G, Lewis M, Klein MJ (1990) Intracortical chondroma of the left femur. Skeletal Radiol 19: 59-61

Adler CP, Herget GW, Neuburger M (1995) Cartilaginous tumours prognostic applications of cytophotometrie DNA analysis. Cancer 76: 1176-1180

Aparisi T, Arborgh B, Ericsson JL, Göthlin, G, Nilsonne U (1978) Contribution to the knowledge of the fine structure of chondrosarcoma of bone. With a note on the localization of alkaline phosphatase and (ATPase). Acta Pathol Microbiol Scand Sect A 86: 157-167

Aprin H, Calandra J, Mir R, Youl Lee J (1986) Radiationinduced chondrosarcoma of the clavicle complicating hodg- kints disease. A case report. Clin Orthop 209: 189-193

Atherton DJ, Pitcher DW, Well RS, McDonald DM (1980) A syndrome of various cutaneous pigmented]esions, myxoid neurofibromata and atrial myxoma: the name syndrome. Br J Dermatol 103: 421-429

Barnes R, Catto M (1966) Chondrosarcoma of bone. J Bone Joint Surg 48B: 729-764

Bertoni F, Boriani S, Laus M, Campanacci M (1982) Periosteal chondrosarcoma and periosteal osteosarcoma: two distinct entities. J Bone Joint Surg 64B: 370-376

Beuckefeer (de) LHL, Schepper (de) AMA, Ramon F (1996) Magnetic resonance imaging of cartilaginous tumors: is it useful or necessary? Skeletal Radiol 25: 137-141

Cannon SR, Sweetnan DR (1985) Multiple chondrosarcomas in dyschondroplasia (Ollier's disease). Cancer 55: 836-840

Carney JA (1985) Differences between nonfamilial and familial cardiac myxoma. Ann Surg Pathol 9: 53-55

Carney JA, Gordon H, Carpenter PC, Shenoy BR, Vay Liang Wgo (1985) The complex of myxomas, spotty pigmentation and endocrine overactivity. Medicine 64: 270-283

Colley B, Higinbotham NL (1954) Secondary chondrosarcoma. Ann Surg 139: 547-557

Coughlan B, Feliz A, Ishida T, Czerniak B, Dorfman H (1995) p53 expression and DNA ploidy of cartilage lesions. Hum Pathol 26: 620-624

Cremer H, Gullota F, Wolf L (1981) The Maffucci-Kaast syndrome. Dyschondroplasia with hemangiomas and frontal lobe astrocytoma. Cancer Res Clin Oncol 101: 231-237

Dahlin DC, Beabout JW (1971) Dedifferentiation of low-grade chondrosarcoma. Cancer 28: 461-466

Dahlin DC, Salvador AH (1974) Chondrosarcomas of bones of the hands and feet. A study of 30 cases. Cancer 34: 755-760

Dahlin DC, Unni KK (1986) Bone tumors general aspects and data on 8,542 cases, 4th edn. Charles C Thomas Publisher, Springfield

Demetrick DJ, Kneafsey PD, Hwang WS (1991) Signet ring chondrosarcoma: a new morphologic entity. Hum Pathol 22: 1175-1179

Desantos LA, Spjut HJ (1981) Periosteal chondroma: a radiographic spectrum. Skeletal Radiol 6: 15-20

Eng J, Sabanathan S, Pradhan GN, Mearns AJ (1990) Primary bony chest wall tumors. J R Coll Surg Edinb 35: 44-47

Erlandson RA, Huvos AG (1974) Chondrosarcoma: a light and electron microscopic study. Cancer 31: 1642-1652

Evans HL, Ayala AG, Marvin M, Romsdhal MM (1977) Prognostic factors in chondrosarcoma of bone. A clinicopathologic analysis with emphasis on histologic grading. Cancer 40: 818-831

Fitzwater JE, Cabaud HE, Farr GH (1976) Irradiation-induced chondrosarcoma. A case report. J Bone Joint Surg 58A: 1037-1039

Fuentes JM, Benezech J, Iborra F, Marty M, Monthieu JY (1990) Les tumeurs rachidiennes primitives: résultats d'une enquête nationale. Rachis 2: 301-310

Garrington GE, Collet WK (1988) Chondrosarcoma I. A selected literature review. J Oral Pathol 17: 1-11

Grimer RJ, Davies AM, Starkie CM, Sneath RS (1989) Chondrosarcome chez un patient porteur d'ostéopoïkilie. Rev Chir Orthop 75: 188-189

Henderson ED, Dahlin DC (1963) Chondrosarcoma of bone. A study of two hundred and eighty-eight cases. J Bone Joint Surg 45A: 1450-1458

Huvos AG (1979) Bone tumors. Diagnosis, treatment and prognosis. WB Saunders, Philadelphia

Huvos AG, Marcover RC (1987) Chondrosarcoma in the young. A clinicopathologic analysis of 79 patients younger than 21 years of age. Am J Surg Pathol II: 930-942

Ishida T, Kikuchi F, Machinami R (1991) Histological grading and morphometric analysis of cartilaginous tumors. Virchows Arch Pathol Anat 418: 149-155

Jelthi A, Forest M, Tomeno B, Abelanet R (1987) Résorption et remodelage osseux dans les chondrosarcomes des membres et des ceintures. Valeur diagnostique à propos de 84 cas. Ann Pathol 7: 198-208

Jokl P, Albright JA, Goodman AH (1971) Juxtacortical chondrosarcoma of the hand. J Bone Joint Surg 53 A: 1370-1376

Kindblom LG, Angervall L (1975) Histochemical characterization of mucosubstances in bone and soft tissue tumors. Cancer 36: 965-994

Kreicbergs A, Boquist L, Borssen B, Larsson SE (1982) Prognostic factors in chondrosarcoma. A comparative study of cellular DNA content and clinicopathologic features. Cancer 50: 577-583

Lambes P, Mainard L (1996) Chondromes et chondromatoses multiples in: Les tumeurs bénines de l'enfant. Sauramps medical edn

Larsson SV, Borssen R, Boquist L (1979) Chondrosarcoma. A multifactorial clinical and histopathological study with particular regard to therapy and survival. Int Orthop (Sicot) 2: 333-341

Lichtenstein L, Jaffe HL (1953) Chondrosarcoma of bone. Ann J Pathol 19: 553-589

Lichtenstein L, Bernstein D (1959) Unusual benign and malignant chondroid tumors of bone. Cancer 112: 1142-1157

Marcove RG, Huvos AG (1971) Cartilaginous tumors of the tibia. Cancer 27: 794-801

Maroteaux P, Lamy M (1960) Dyschondroplasie, chondromatose multiple du squelette. Sem Hôp Paris 36: 182-193

Maroteaux P (1995) Maladies osseuses de l'enfant, 3rd edn. Flammarion Médecine-Sciences, Paris

McCarthy EF, Dorfman HD (1982) Chondrosarcoma of bone with dedifferentiation: a study of eighteen cases. Hum Pathol 13: 36-40

Mirra JM, Gold R, Downs J (1985) A new histogic approach to the differentiation of enchondroma and chondrosarcoma of the bones. A clinicopathologic analysis of 51 cases. Clin Orthop 201: 214-237

Mirra JM, Marcove RC (1974) Fibrosarcomatous dedifferentiation of primary and secondary chondrosarcoma. Review of five cases. J Bone Joint Surg 56A: 285-296

Mourao PAS, Michelacci YM, Toledo OMS (1979) Glycosaminoglycans and proteoglycans of normal and tumoral cartilages of humans and rats. Cancer Res 39: 2802-2806

Nakajima H, Ushigome S, Fukuda J (1988) Chondrosarcoma (grade 1) arising from the right second toe in patient wiht multiple enchondromas. Skeletal Radiol 17: 289-292

Nakamura Y, Becker LE, Marks A (1983) S-100 protein in tumors of cartilage and bone. An immunohistochemical study. Cancer 52: 1820-1824

O'Neal LW, Ackerman LV (1952) Chondrosarcoma of bone. Cancer 5: 551-577

Ollier M (1920) Sur une nouvelle affection: la dyschondroplasie. Rev Chir 21: 396-398

Pachter MR, Alpert M (1964) Chondrosarcoma of the foot skeleton. J Bone Joint Surg 46A: 601-607

Peimer CA, Yuan HA, Sagerman RH (1976) Postradiation chondrosarcoma. A case report. J Bone Joint Surg 58A: 1033-1036

Perspectives on cartilaginous tumors (1989) Nomenclature, nosology, and neologism symposium. Hum Pathol 20: 927-963

Pidhorz L, Le Nay P, Boscher Y, François H (1987) Traitement des chondrosarcomes du tibia par cryochirurgie. A propos de 2 observations. Rev Chir Orthop 73: 401-406

Ragsdale BD, Sweet DE, Vinh TN (1989) Radiology as gross pathology in evaluating chondroid lesions. Hum Pathol 20: 930-951

Remagen W, Jani L, Luthi A, Schuman L (1981) Atypical (dedifferentiated) chondrosarcoma or osteosarcoma with preponderant chondroblastic differentiation. Cancer Res Clin Oncol 101: 177-182

Roberts PH, Price CHG (1977) Chondrosarcoma of the bones of the hand. J Bone Joint Surg 59B: 213-221

Rockwell MA, Saiter EA, Enneking WF (1972) Periosteal chondroma. J Bone Joint Surg 54A: 102-108

Samilson RL, Morris JM, Thompson RW (1968) Tumors of the scapula. A review of the literature and an analysis of 32 cases. Clin Orthop 58: 105-115

Sanerkin NG (1980) The diagnosis and grading of chondrosarcoma of bone. A combined cytologic and histologic approach. Cancer 45: 582-594

Schajowicz F, Cabrini RI, Samis RJ (1974) Ultrastructure of chondrosarcoma. Clin Orthop 100: 378-381

Schajowicz F (1977) Juxtacortical chondrosarcoma. J Bone Joint Surg 59B: 473-480

Sinkovics JG, Shirato E, Martin RG, Cabiness Jr, White EC (1971) Chondrosarcoma. Immune reactions of a patient to autologous tumor. Cancer 27: 782-793

Sissons HA (1979) Dedifferentiated chondrosarcoma of the tibia. Skeletal Radiol 3: 257-260

Spjut HJ, Nelson PW (1980) Periosteal (parosteal juxtacortical) chondroma of tibia. Skeletal Radiol 5: 47-50

Steiner GC (1979) Ultrastructure of benign cartilaginous tumors of intraosseous origin. Hum Pathol 10: 71-86

Trias A, Basora J, Sanghez G Madarnas P (1978) Chondrosarcoma of the hand. Clin Orthop 134: 297-301

Ucla E, Tomeno B, Forest M (1991) Facteurs du pronostic tumoral dans les chondrosarcomes de l'appareil locomoteur. A propos de 180 cas. Rev Chir Orthop 77: 301-311

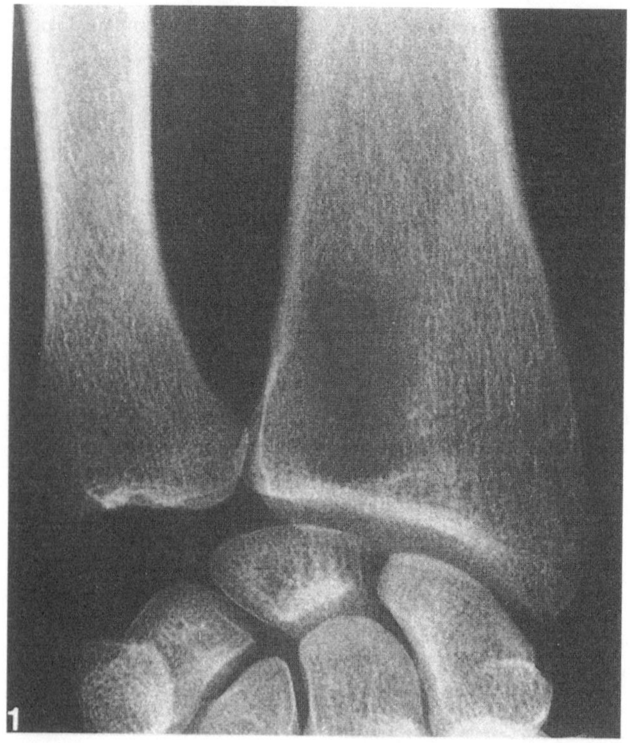

Fig. 1. Image of osteolysis with fuzzy borders at distal end of radius. Woman aged 35

Fig. 2 a, b. This inferior metaphyseal tumour has "ballooned" and then destroyed the anterior cortex of the femur and extended towards the epiphysis. Its boundaries are difficult to detect in a standard radiograph. Male patient aged 52

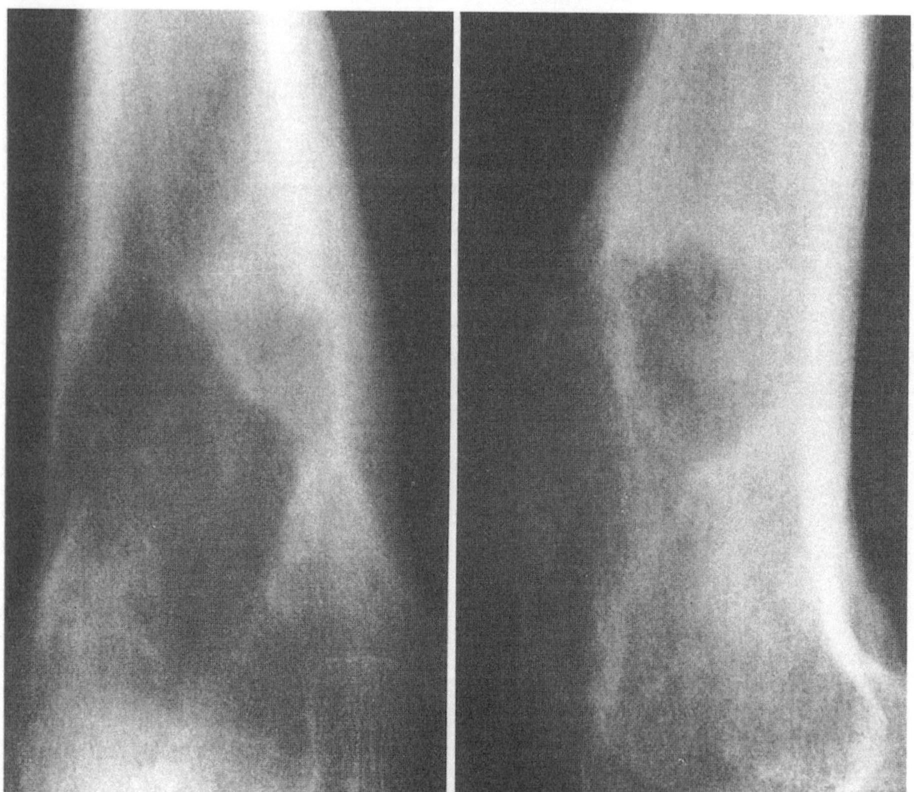

Fig. 3. Chondrosarcoma of upper end of tibia with marked calcification, especially of its medial portion, transgressing the cortex behind and below the head of the fibula. The lower limit is indistinct and the upper part extends into the joint near the tibial spines

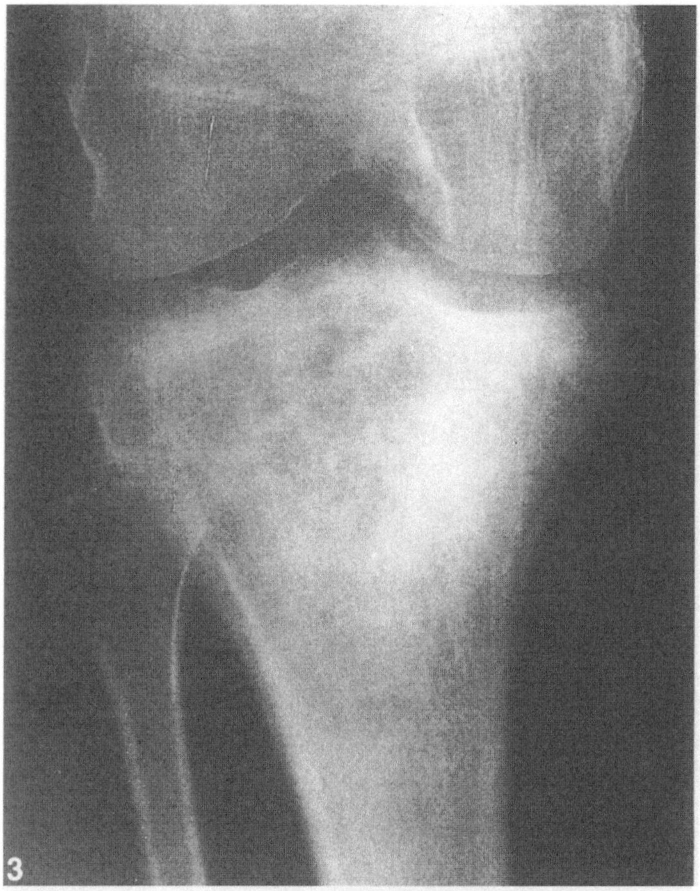

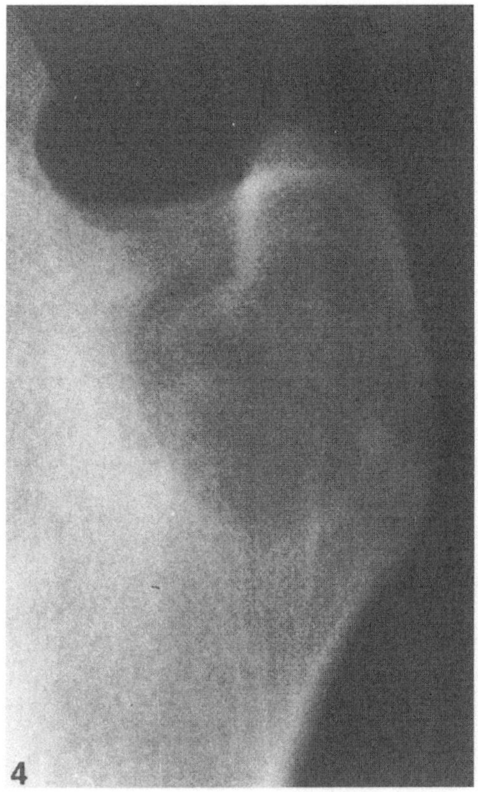

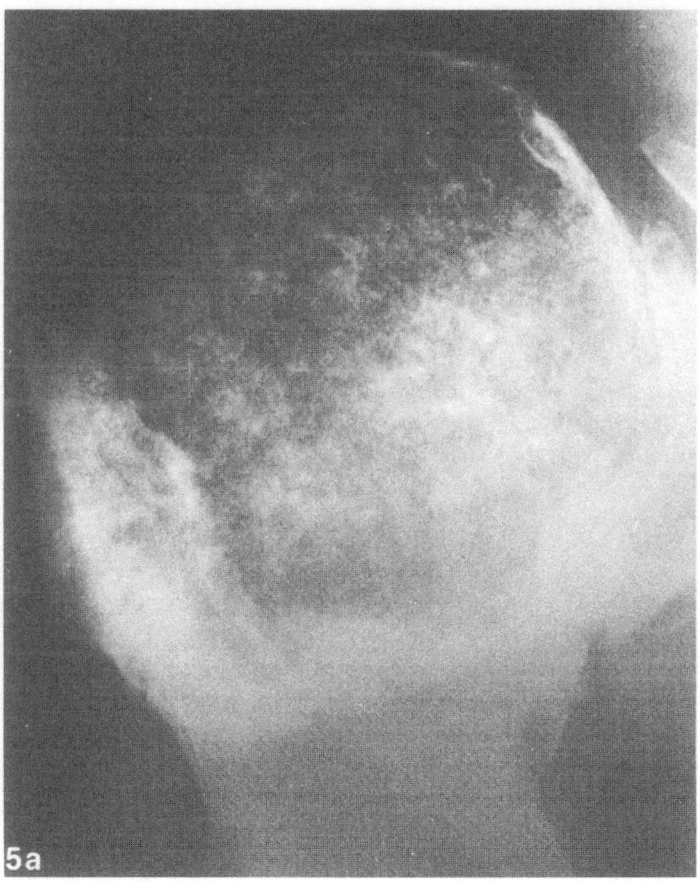

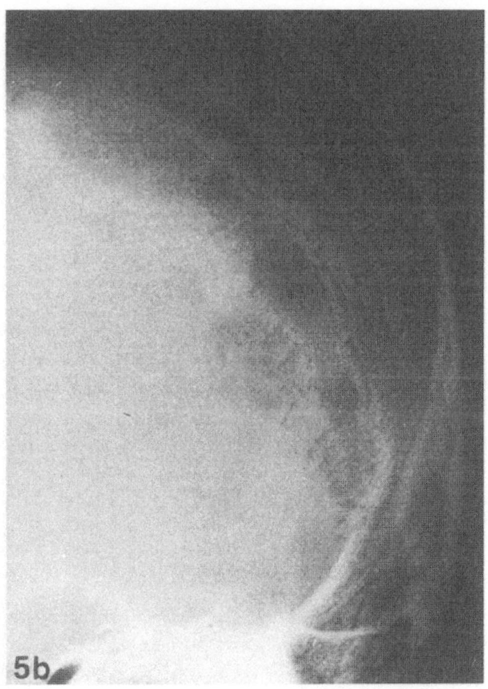

Fig. 4. Chondrosarcoma of low malignancy invading the great trochanter

Fig. 5 a, b. Chondrosarcoma of the iliac wing (**a**) in an adolescent of 16 years giving rise to bony metastases, some cranial (**b**)

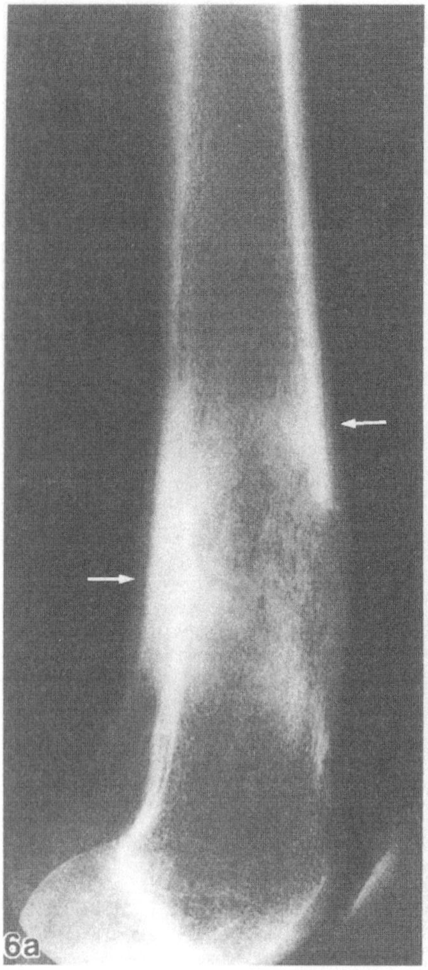

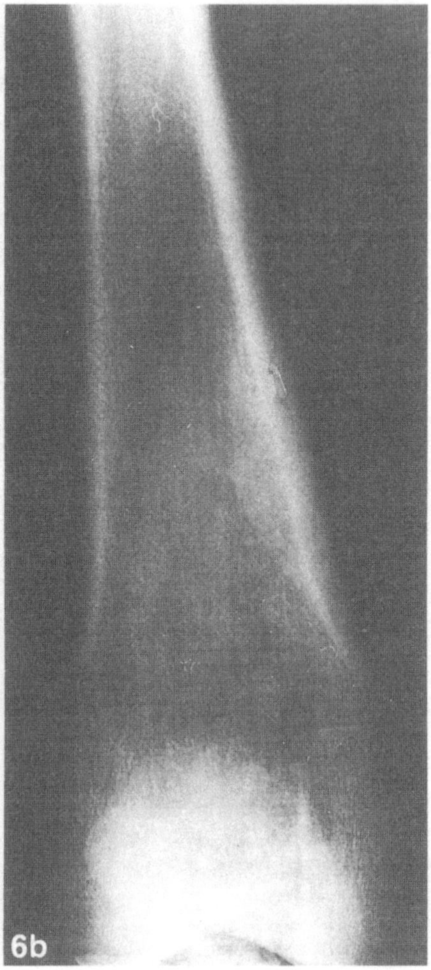

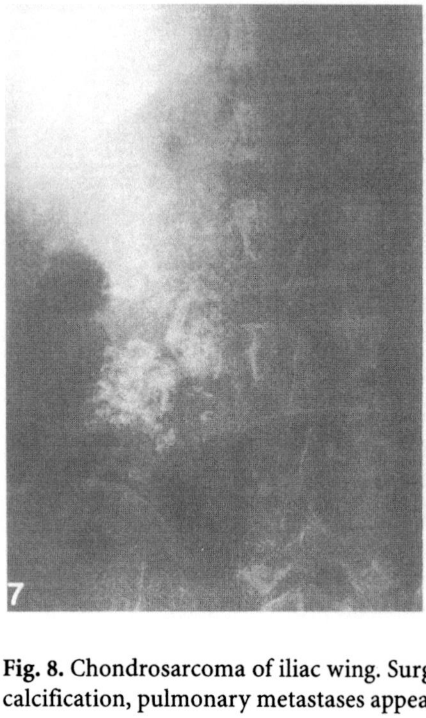

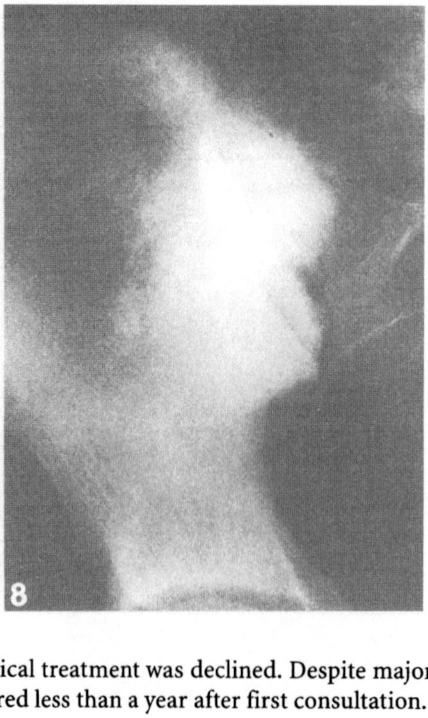

Fig. 6 a, b. Heterogeneous appearance of chondrosarcoma of lower third of femur. Marked periostal reaction (*arrows*). The boundaries in the long axis of the bone are indistinct in these standard radiographs

Fig. 7. Chondrosarcoma of lateral border of L3 invading the lumbar region and ascending as far as L1. Man aged 56

Fig. 8. Chondrosarcoma of iliac wing. Surgical treatment was declined. Despite major irradiation followed by obvious calcification, pulmonary metastases appeared less than a year after first consultation. Adolescent aged 17

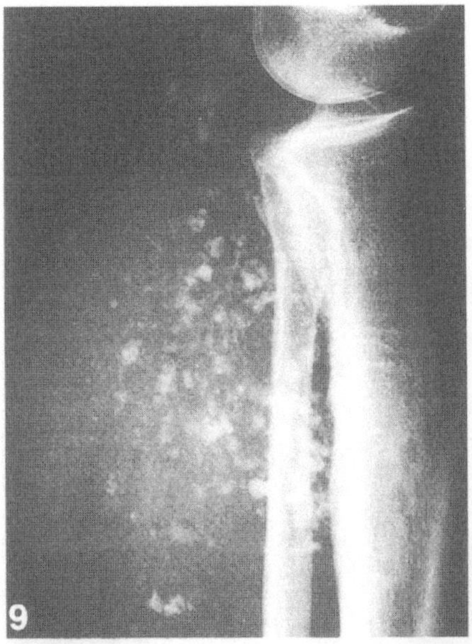

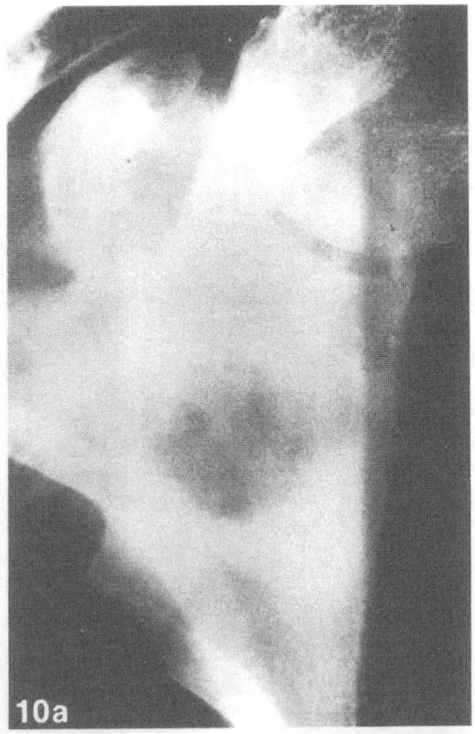

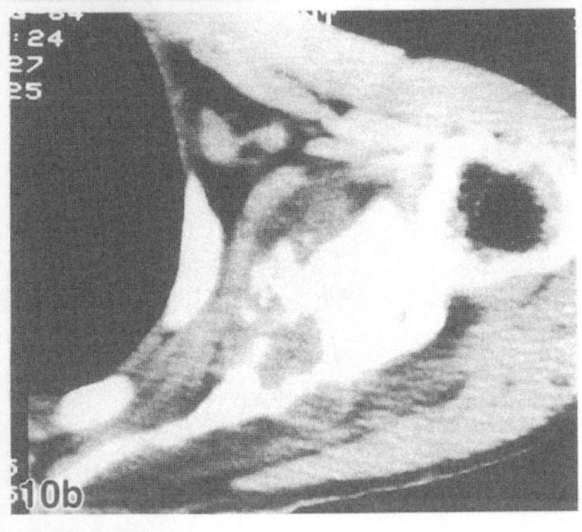

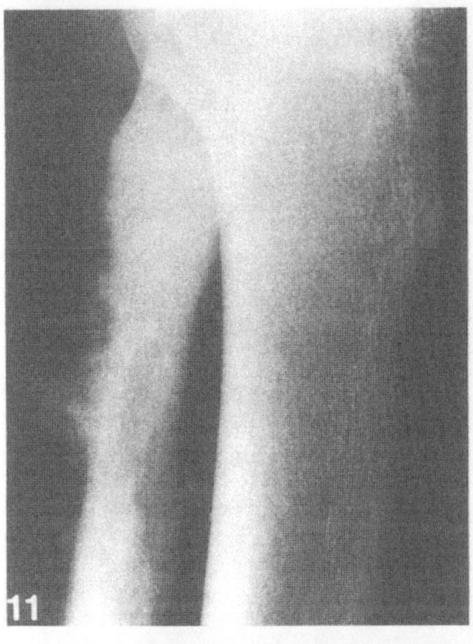

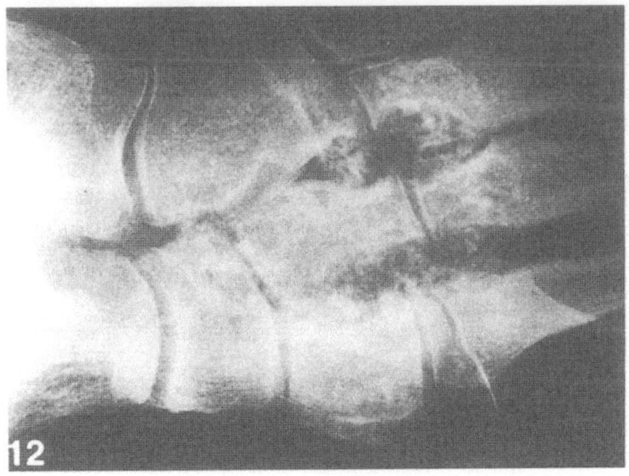

Fig. 9. Large sarcoma of upper end of tibia, man aged 45. The tumour, which has developed mainly outside the bone, contains numerous calcified foci. Histology: low-grade malignancy

Fig. 10. **a** Large lytic tumour of the scapula, man aged 54. **b** The CT section shows destruction of the scapula and invasion of the adjacent soft tissues

Fig. 11. Grade 2 chondrosarcoma developing superficially at the upper end of fibula. Girl aged 14

Fig. 12. Chondrosarcoma invading tarsus and metatarsus. There are often aggressive appearances thought to be recurrences of an inadequately treated chondrosarcoma of the sole of the foot

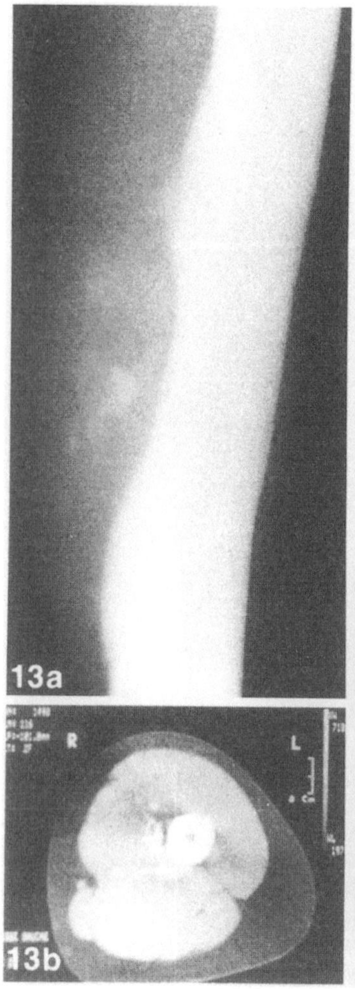

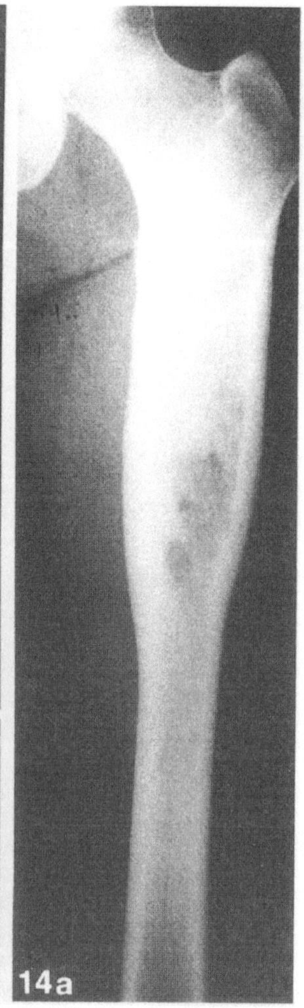

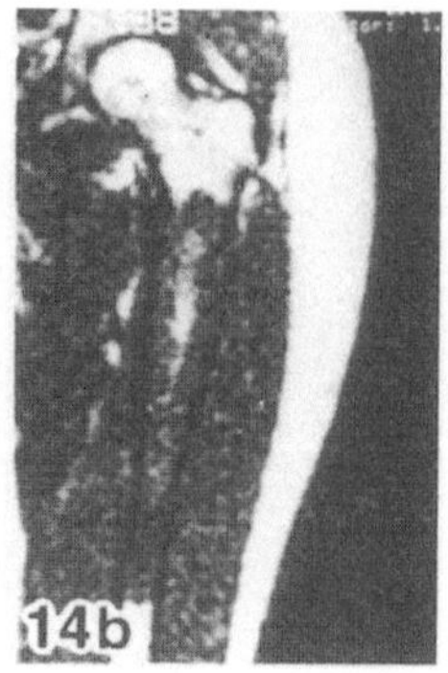

Fig. 13. **a** Periosteal chondrosarcoma of femur. Wide resection was followed by cure. **b** CT section shows invasion of soft tissues around femur. Woman aged 20 years

Fig. 14. **a** Chondrosarcoma ballooning the proximal half of femoral shaft. **b** CT allows assessment of extent and shows destruction of femoral cortex

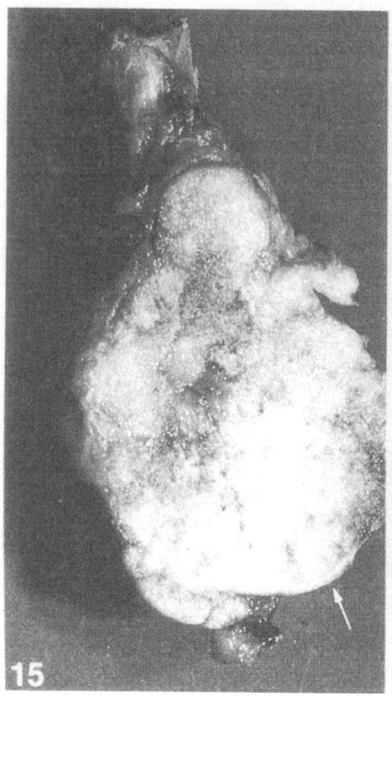

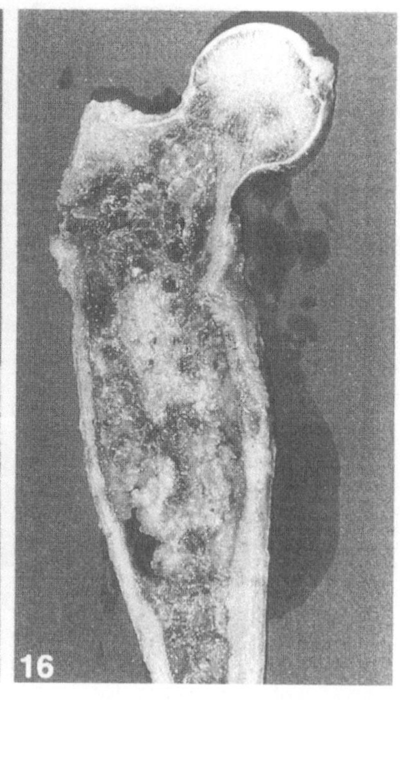

Fig. 15. Chondrosarcoma of lower end of femur, man aged 58. Section shows mingling of translucent gelatinous zones and more definitely chondroid zones, calcified in places; the section surface is both uniform and heterogeneous. Only the middle part of the condylar cartilage remains (*arrow*) while in front of and behind this cartilage the tumour invades the joint cavity

Fig. 16. The slow growth of this chondrosarcoma of the upper end of the femur has allowed the laying down of periosteal bony lamellae leading to swelling of the bone at the level of the tumour, even as destruction of the deep surface of the cortex proceeds. The sectional surface is non-uniform, hollowed out in places by necrotic cavities which are partly filled by haemorrhagic coagulum

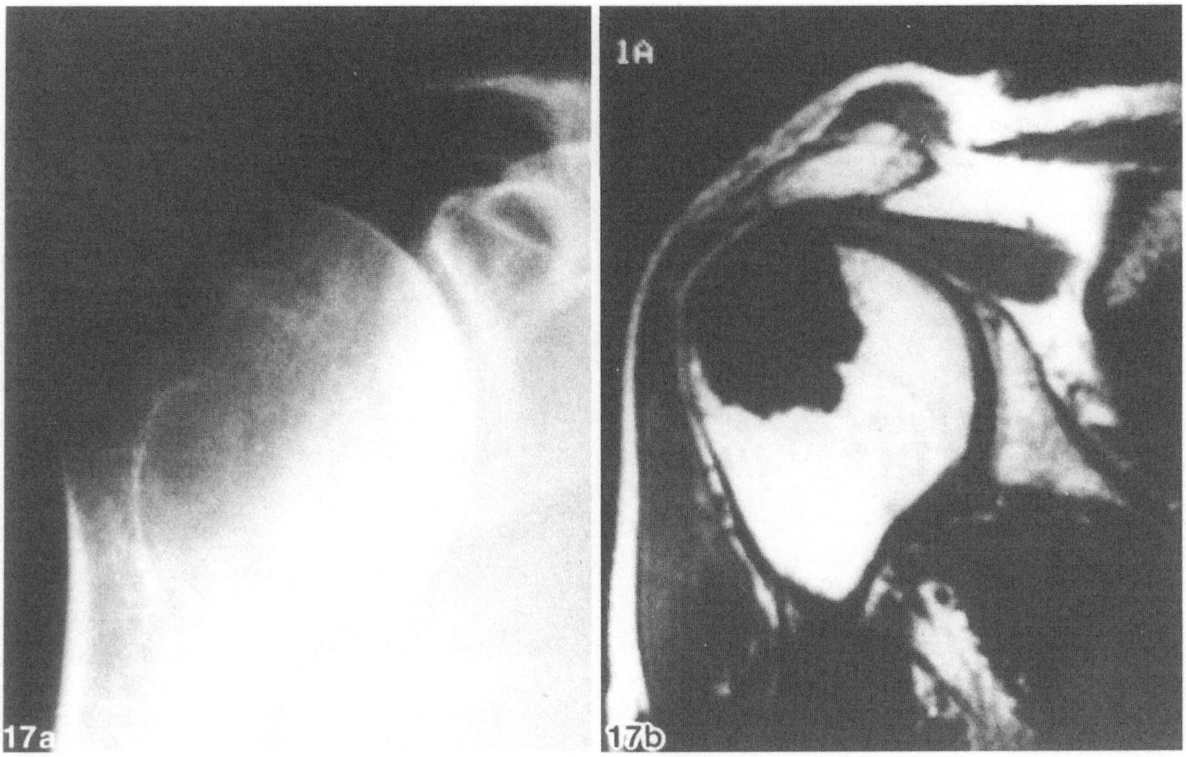

Fig. 17 a, b. MRI shows sharp lower and medial boundaries of this chondrosarcoma (grade 2) compared with the fuzzy imprecise margins seen in the standard radiograph (case kindly supplied by Dr Quillard)

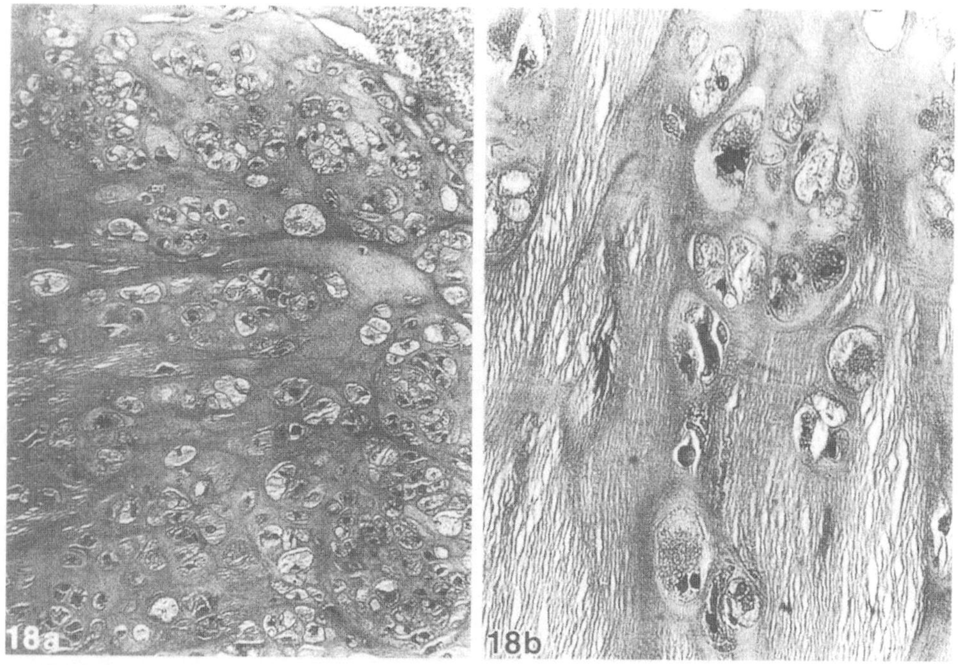

Fig. 18 a, b. Chondrosarcoma of scapula, man aged 17. A degree of cellular abundance, with (**b**) chondrocytes of unequal size with heavily staining large nuclei and of atypical forms allows, despite a relatively uniform matrix (**a**), a diagnosis of grade 2 chondrosarcoma. Shortly after resection of the scapula a tumour nodule developed in the subcutaneous tissue. This nodule had a hyaline chromophile matrix; the tumour cells lacked chondroplastic compartments and were immature, polygonal or stellate, indicating histological deterioration

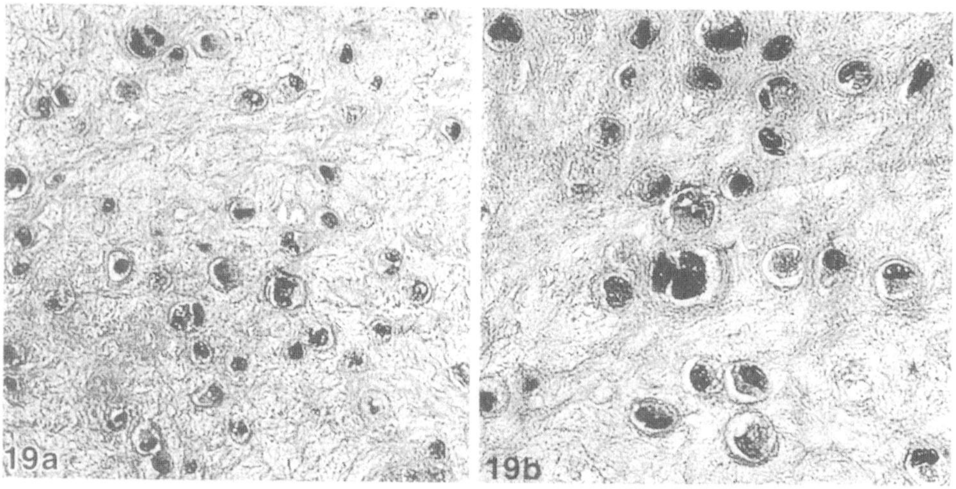

Fig. 19 a, b. Chondrosarcoma of iliac wing, cytonuclear monstrosities, fibrillary matrix. Malignancy is obvious, as is its chondrocytic origin: chondrosarcoma grade 2

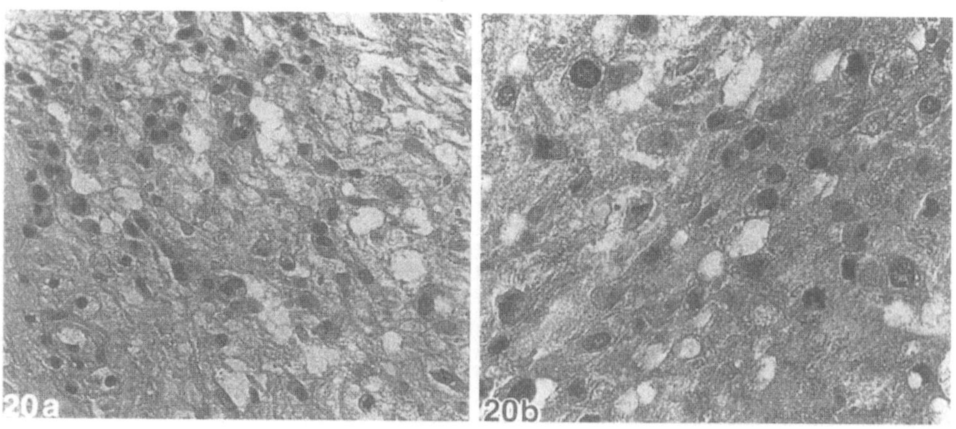

Fig. 20 a, b. Chondrosarcoma of lower end of femur. Immature cells, and marked increase of nuclear-cytoplasmic ratio. The secretion of ground substance by these immature cells is only rudimentary. Chondrosarcoma grade 3. Man aged 18

Fig. 21 a, b. Chondrosarcoma of upper end of humerus. Tumour of undifferentiated appearance in which the intercellular matrix is only remotely akin to that of normal cartilage. Bulky hyperchromatic nuclei, marked anisocytosis. Chondrosarcoma grade 3. Man aged 78

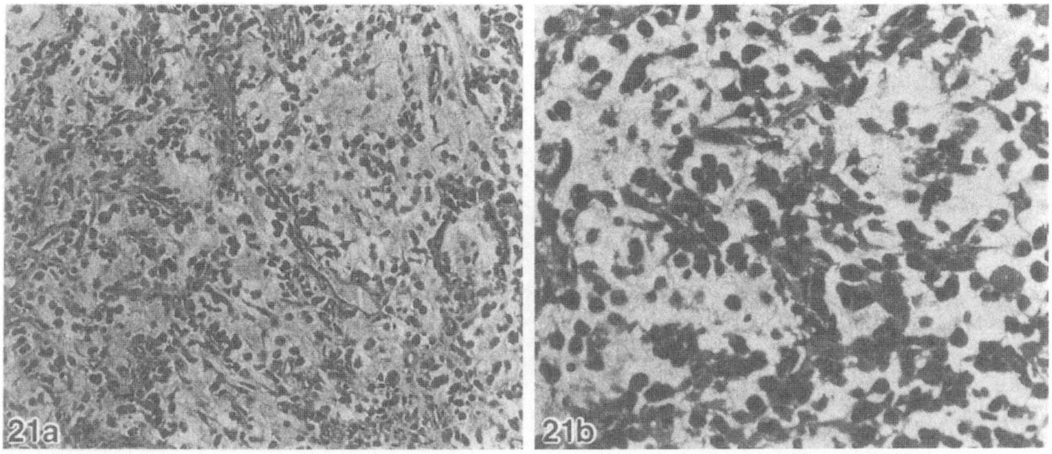

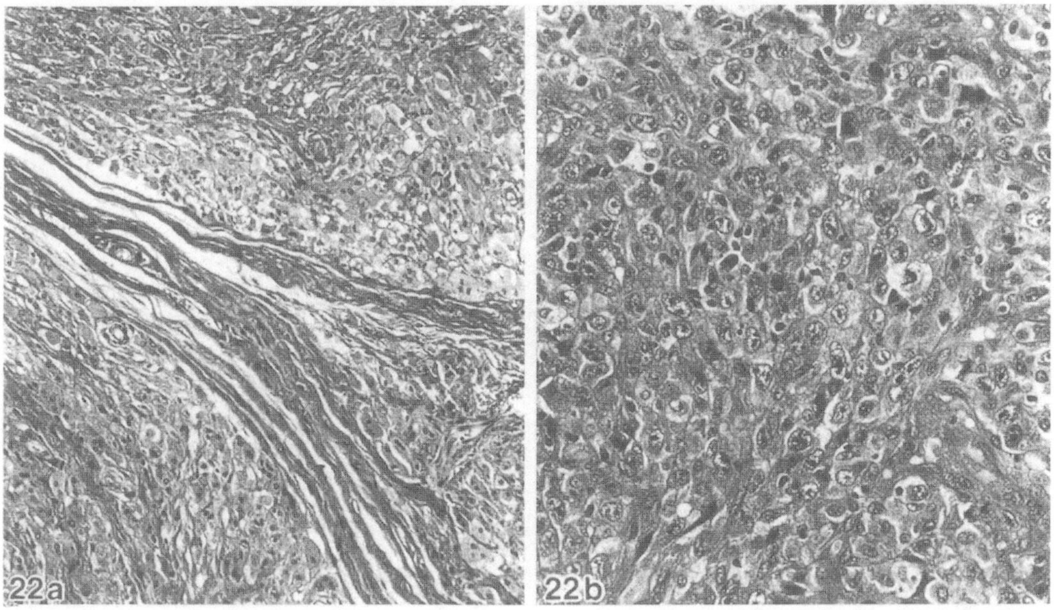

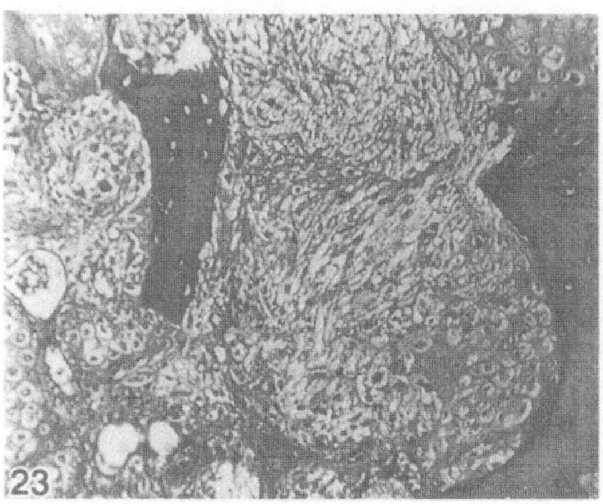

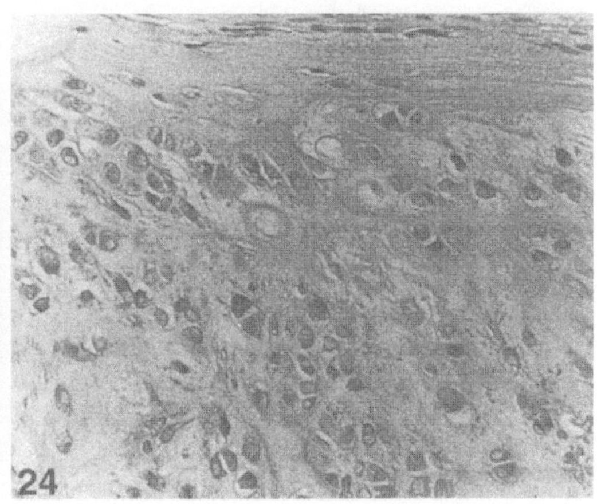

Fig. 22 a, b. Undifferentiated chondrosarcoma. Low magnification (**a**), cellular proliferation without secretion of ground substance, obvious cytonuclear anomalies (**b**). The difficulty is to recognise the chondroblastic origin of these tumours; sometimes a chondroid zone persists but some metastases are purely sarcomatous with fusiform cells

Fig. 23. Chondrosarcoma of tarsus, cellular anomalies and areas of proliferation devoid of matrix: tumour grade 3. Man aged 31

Fig. 24. Subperiosteal sarcoma; apart from the cell density, the diagnosis is based essentially on the increased nuclear-cytoplasmic ratio and the major anisocytosis. The ground substance is completely heterogeneous

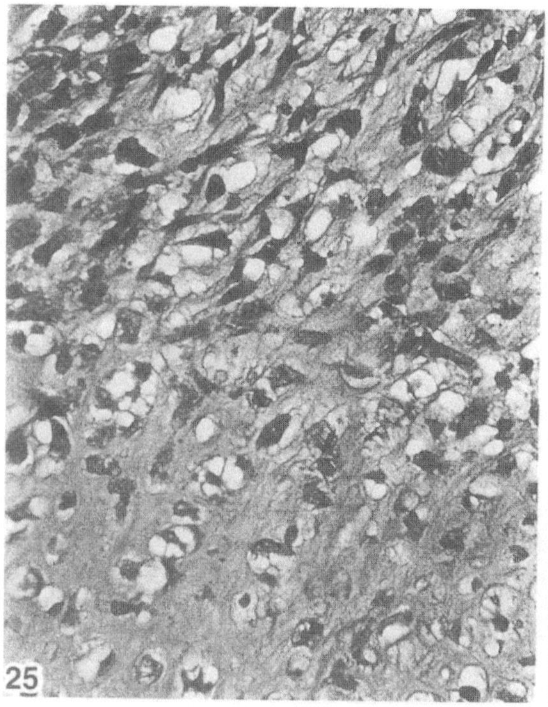

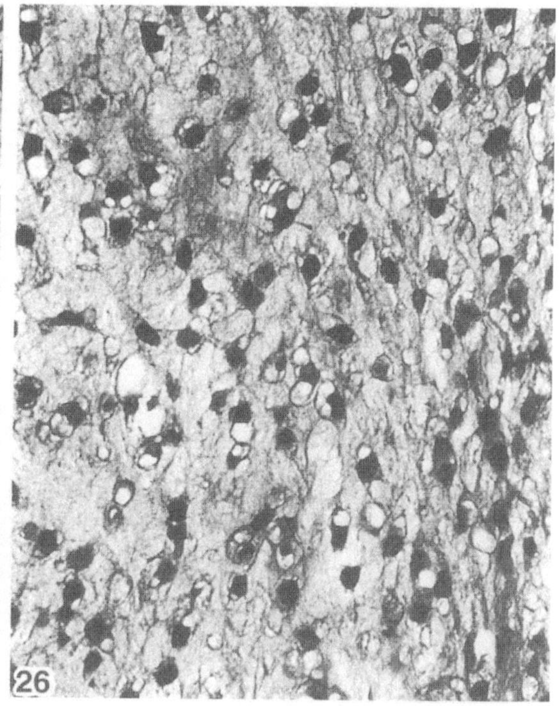

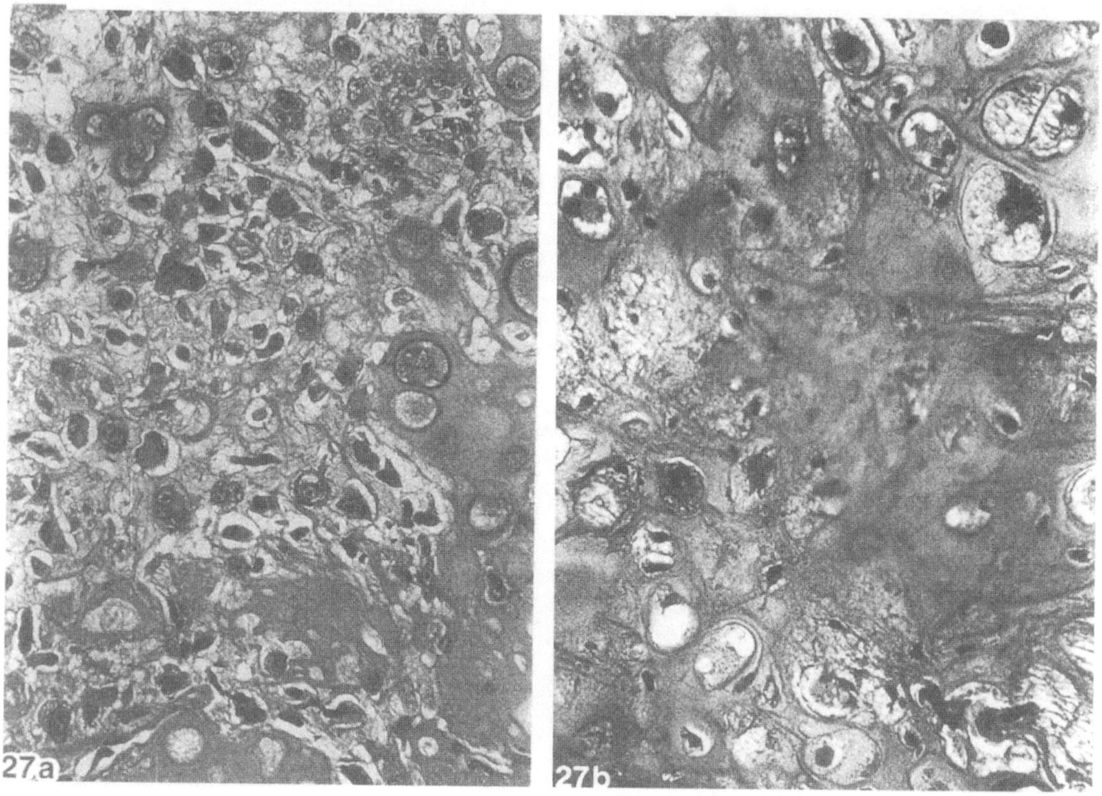

Fig. 25. Chondrosarcoma of lower end of tibia composed mainly of atypical deformed cells with large hyperchromatic nuclei displaced by a clear vacuole; some more chondroid zones allow this sarcoma to be attributed to the group of chondrosarcomas, grade 3

Fig. 26. Chondrosarcoma of upper end of humerus. As in the microphotograph shown in figure 25, there are cells whose nucleus occupies one pole as if displaced by clear cytoplasmic vacuoles: the signet-ring form with lipid vacuole

Fig. 27 a, b. Chondrosarcoma of maxilla. The numerous cytonuclear abnormalities and the non-secretion of ground substance in large zones of undifferentiated cells justify classification of this tumour as a grade 3 malignancy. Woman aged 46

3. Clear-cell chondrosarcoma

This is a definite clinical, radiological and histological entity. While all chondrosarcomas have clear cells at one time or another, the clear cells in this discrete entity have very special features.

Case history

In June a woman of 20 came for a surgical opinion, complaining of pain on lifting the right arm. The history revealed that the patient, a secretary, had felt slight inconstant pain since January of the previous year, a discomfort attributed to fatigue. Active abduction now evoked severe pain, localised to the upper end of the limb.

The clinical examination revealed little, but locally there was slight swelling compared with the left side. The radiological appearances (fig. 1) were more striking. The entire upper end of the humerus was the site of osteolysis of speckled appearance. The entire humeral head, whose articular surface remained perfectly defined, the large and small tubercles as well as the shaft were involved in the process. Some more opaque spots were interpreted as calcification. The bone was not ballooned, but small areas of calcification projected into the soft tissues at the lower limit and medial to the humeral head.

This appearance suggested a cartilaginous tumour. The site in this young patient aroused suspicion of a possible chondroblastoma. However, benign chondroblastoma, whether epiphyseal or apophyseal, is usually discovered before attaining such a degree of development.

In this patient, the spread towards the shaft, the presence of extraosseous calcification and the alveolar appearance of the metaphysis indicative of invasion of the spongy bone, all suggested that despite the age of 20 years, a diagnosis of malignant cartilaginous tumour should be made. The general examination, the chest X-ray and a study of the biochemical parameters added nothing to the diagnosis.

This, then was a tumour of malignant appearance presenting the radiological features of a cartilaginous neoplasm, whose history extended for over 18 months. The diagnosis considered most likely was that of a clear-cell chondrosarcoma, despite the fact that this tumour is commoner in males and is found mainly after the age of 30.

The diagnosis was easily confirmed by examination of a biopsy, which showed a clear-cell chondrosarcoma in its purest form. To complete this case history, we may add that activity was rapidly restored after resection-prosthesis and that the cure was permanent.

General considerations

In 1976, Unni et al reported 16 cases of a variant of chondrosarcoma which they labelled clear-cell chondrosarcoma. Its main features were the clear and relatively abundant cytoplasm of the tumour cells, whose boundaries are usually well-defined, plus the presence of giant cells. By 1983, Volpe et al could find only 29 well-documented cases in the literature and added 2 personal cases. This is a rare cartilaginous tumour, representing less than 0.5% of malignant tumours of bone. The male-female ratio is of the order of 2: 1 and the maximum incidence is after the age of 30, in the 4th and 5th decades.

The tumours are generally found in the epiphyses, apophyses and adjacent metaphyses of the long bones: the upper epiphysis of the femur and humerus, upper ends of the ulna and tibia and more rarely the vertebrae, ribs and pelvis. Cases involving several bones have been reported [Unni et al 1976].

Clinical features and course

Swelling and moderate pain affecting joint function are the clinical features at onset, often more than a year before the first consultation. Complete resection of the tumour is usually followed by cure.

Imaging

The radiological aspect was mentionned in the description of the above case: it could be either an alveolar aspect (figs. 1, 2) or a vast clear lacuna (fig. 3). CT scan can precise the limits of osteolysis, the involvement of cortical substance and the presence of calcification.

Pathological anatomy and histopathology

At *macroscopic examination* of the resection, the cartilaginous nature of the tumour is obvious. The tumour is glistening pearly-white in appearance and elastic in consistency; it destroys the bony tissue, of which only rare irregular strands are left, mainly in the peripheral zone. Within the tumour, some dull whitish zones, some of chalky appearance, represent zones of calcification or rudimentary ossification. There are also some "cystic" cavities of necrobiotic origin. The nodular arrangement of the cartilaginous islets was clearly visible mainly at the periphery. The cortex, though thinned, is almost entirely intact except for the inferomedial part of the humeral head, in the vicinity of small cartilaginous islets situated in the soft tissues and included in the resection.

At *histological examination*, the presence of great areas of bulky cells with clear cytoplasm, together with little or no formation of ground substance is characteristic (fig. 4). This clear appearance and the generally large size of the cells do not exclude a certain degree of polymorphism and inequality of distribution. The nuclei are also bulky, usually in central position, more rarely eccentric. Because of their distended appearance, some cells may simulate those of a chordoma (figs. 5, 6). There are also some rare multinucleate giant cells. In some tumours we have noted a sort of cytoplasmic gelification reminiscent of chondroid substance (figs. 8, 9). In some cells positive staining with PAS and with alcian blue demarcates a localised ring against the cell membrane. At the center of some lobules, degenerative zones may be seen, some of which undergo cystic necrosis. In these degenerative areas, the persistence of the cell membranes reveals the outlines of cells which are in direct contact with each other without the interposition of ground substance. A search in multiple sections for the coexistence of zones of chondrosarcoma of the ordinary type fails to detect such formations. It is not uncommon, in these cases, to detect the presence of small newly-formed bony or neo-osteoid trabeculae, on studying large surfaces unconnected with the peripheral osteogenesis.

Ultrastructurally, the nucleolus is prominent; the paranuclear zone is often surrounded by an area of small vacuoles. The deposits of glycogen are situated between this vacuolated area, which they surround, and the nuclear membrane. Ultrastructural studies [Forest et al 1978, Faraggiana et al 1981] show that intercellular substance is rare or absent. At the periphery, the cells bristle with numerous villosities. On the whole, the cytoplasmic organelles are poorly developed. Glycogen forms an abundant deposit at the periphery of the cell (figs. 12, 13). The Golgi apparatus is often surrounded by numerous small vacuoles. Angervall et al (1980) have demonstrated the presence of chondroitin 4 and 6 sulfate without keratosulfate. According to Thiery [Volpe et al 1983] the cell accumulates the substances it synthesises in the cytoplasm. Thus it is the non-secretion of these components of the intercellular substance which is responsible for the very specific appearance of these tumour cells.

In the clear cells, there is a strongly positive reaction for anti-osteonectin, which substance cannot be demonstrated in other types of chondrosarcoma [Bosse et al 1991]. Liang-Tang and Tze-Chun (1993) hypothesise that the clear cells are the outcome of anaplastic modifications of chondroblastoma cells.

Diagnosis

The diagnosis is not always as obvious, as in the case we have reported (Table 1). There must be a systematic search for the coexistence of zones of chondrosarcoma of the usual type, which worsens the prognosis: this is the critical point. The appearance of zones of chondro-

Table 1. Clear-cell chondrosarcoma

Three main pitfalls: - Failure to recognise the presence of areas of chondrosarcoma grade 2 or 3 - The exclusion of a metastasis with clear cells from an unidentified tumour - With an axially located lesion, a chordoma must be excluded
Beware of zones simulating osteosarcoma, chondroblastoma, aneurysmal cyst, or giant-cell tumour

sarcoma of the common type during a recurrence of clear-cell chondrosarcoma is evidence of an exacerbation of the lesion. Conversely, some clear-cell zones may be observed in the ordinary type of chondrosarcoma; this is without practical implications; it is the histological grade of malignancy found in the common type of chondrosarcoma which must be noted.

From the theoretical viewpoint, the hypothesis of the transformation of a primary clear-cell chondrosarcoma into the common type may be envisaged, but nothing in these skeletogenic sarcomas excludes the possible coexistence of different appearances. One must still be strict about the morphology of these clear cells and reject a simple cellular clarification, which is very common and which, in a malignant form, is sometimes reminiscent of the so-called "cartilage with a capsular stroma" of the histologists.

Virtually any carcinoma may exhibit a clear-cell type; metastasis from a carcinoma of the kidney may present problems in differential diagnosis. In fact, the endocrine tumour-like appearance, the abundant vascularisation and the cellular monomorphism suffice to determine its origin. Immunohistological stains may be necessary to establish the origin of the lesion.

The diagnosis of chordoma should be considered only for a tumour situated along the axis of the body. Here, too, the immunohistological reactions (positive anti-keratin test in chordoma, positive anti-protein S100 in cartilaginous tumours and in chordoma) help to decide in favour of one or other diagnosis. The very rare intraosseous liposarcoma, has histochemical and histoimmunological reactions and cytological features which are very different.

Apart from these differential diagnoses, the observation of 47 cases at the Mayo Clinic has led Bjornsson et al (1984) to describe the presence of structures that may direct the diagnosis towards another benign or malignant bony lesion. Osteoid zones, in plexiform or compact zones, may suggest an osteosarcoma or an osteoblastoma respectively. In certain tumours, cavities filled with blood and bordered by fibro-osteoid tissue may simulate an aneurysmal bone cyst. Sometimes, compact zones of eosinophils cells or an abundance of multinucleate cells simulate chondroblastoma or giant-cell tumour.

Treatment

The treatment of this tumour of grade 1 histological malignancy, calls for a wide resection to secure definitive cure since the lesion is more often intracompartmental (1A) than extracompartmental (1B), according to the classification of Enneking et al (1980). It is certain that the common juxta-articular localisation may lead to serious articular sequelae of surgery. The prognosis is good on the whole, but in the 47 patients of the Mayo Clinic, 7 died from their tumour (a metastatic course in 15%).

References

Angervall L, Kindblom L (1980) Clear cell chondrosarcoma. A light and electron-microscopic and histochemical study of two cases. Virchows Arch Pathol Anat 389: 27-41

Bagley L, Kneeland HB, Dalinka MK, Bullough P, Brooks J (1993) Unusual behavior of clear chondrosarcoma. Skeletal Radiol 22: 279-282

Bjornsson J, Beabout MD, Unni KK, Sim FH, Dahlin DC (1984) Clear cell chondrosarcoma of bone. Observations in 47 cases. Am J Surg Patnol 8: 223-230

Bosse A, Veda Y, Wuisman P, Jones DB, Vollmer E, Rœssner A (1991) Histogenesis of clear cell chondrosarcoma: an immunohistochemical study with osteonectin, a non-collagenous structure protein. J Cancer Res Clin Oncol 117: 43-49

Faraggiana T, Sender B, Glicksman P (1981) Light and electron microscopic study of clear cell chondrosarcoma Am J Clin Pathol 75: 117-121

Forest M, Le Charpentier Y, Postel M, Tomeno B, Roux JP, Mazabraud A, Dahdouh B, Abelanet R (1978) Une nouvelle variété de chondrosarcome: les sarcomes dits "chondroblastiques" ou chondrosarcomes "à cellules claires". Etude anatomoclinique et ultrastructurale de 5 observations. Arch Anat Cytol Pathol 26: 5-11

Le Charpentier Y, Forest M, Postel M, Tomeno B, Abelanet R (1979) Clear-cell chondrosarcoma. A report of five cases including ultrastructural study. Cancer 44: 622-629

Liang-Tang W, Tze-chung L (1993) Clear cell chondrosarcoma of bone. A report of three cases with immunohistochemical and affmity histochemical observations. Pathol Res Pract 189: 411-415

Present D, Bacchini P, Pignatti G, Picci P, Bertoni F, Campanacci M (1991) Clear cell chondrosarcoma of bone. A report of 8 cases. Skeletal Radiol 20: 187-191

Salzer-Kuntschik (1981) Clear-cell chondrosarcoma Cancer. Res Oncol 101: 171-176

Sreekantaiati C, Long SPI, Davis JR, Sandberg AA (1991) Cytogenetic and flow cytometry analysis of a clear cell chondrosarcoma. Cancer Genet Cytogenet 52: 193-199

Unni KK, Dahlin DC, Beabout JW, Sim FH (1976) Chondrosarcoma: clear-cell variant. J Bone Joint Surg 58A: 676-683

Volpe R, Mazabraud A, Thiery JP (1983) Clear cell chondrosarcoma. Report of a new case and review of literature. Pathologica 75: 775-787

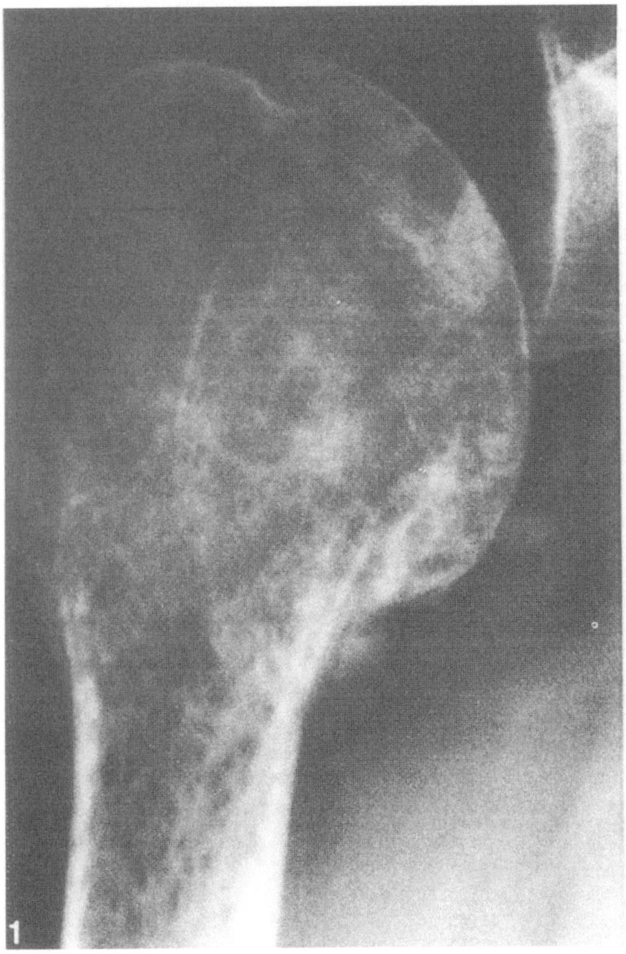

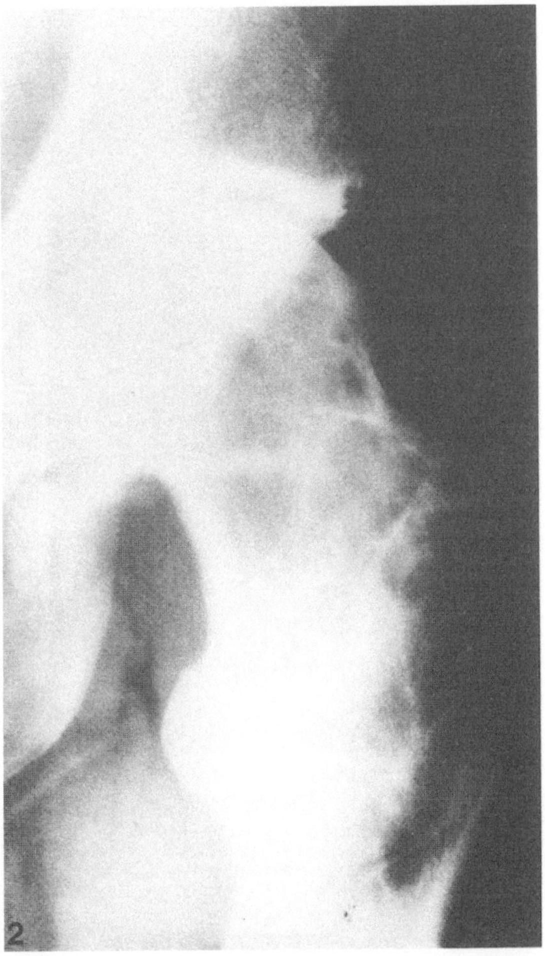

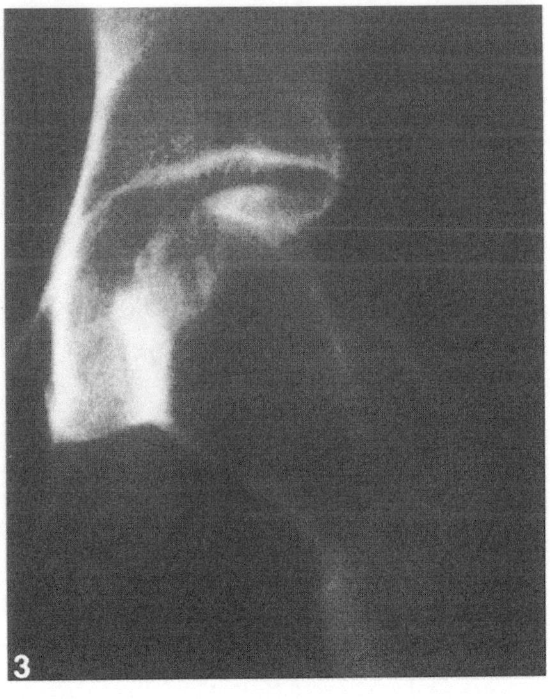

Fig. 1. Upper end of humerus: osteolysis of alveolar appearance, speckled with some zones of calcification. There are also calcifications in the soft tissues, particularly adjacent to the lower pole of the head

Fig. 2. Clear-cell chondrosarcoma of upper end of femur. Areolar osteolysis of the neck and great trochanter is seen

Fig. 3. Clear-cell sarcoma of femoral head and neck. Vast zone of osteolysis, apparently well-circumscribed in this standard film

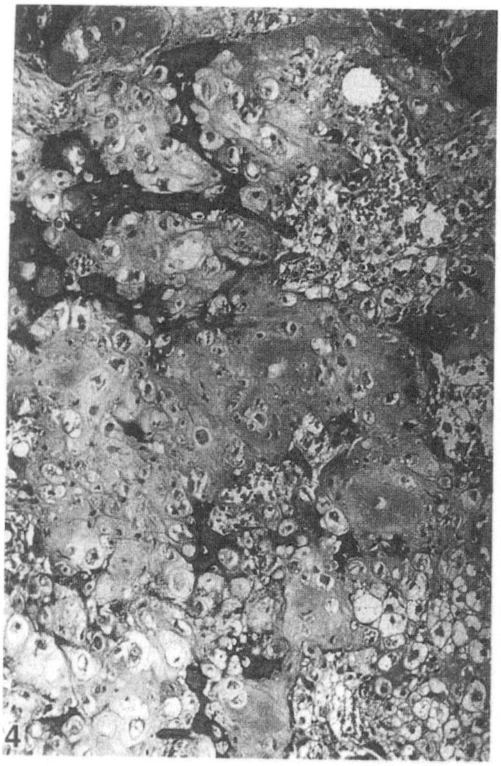

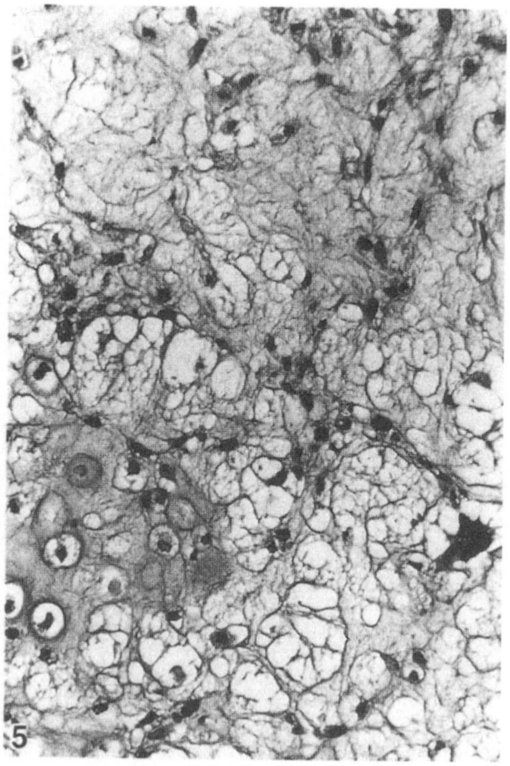

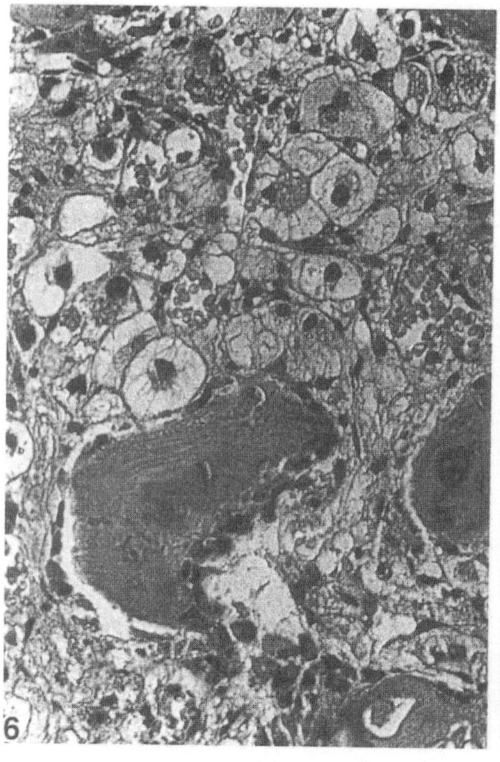

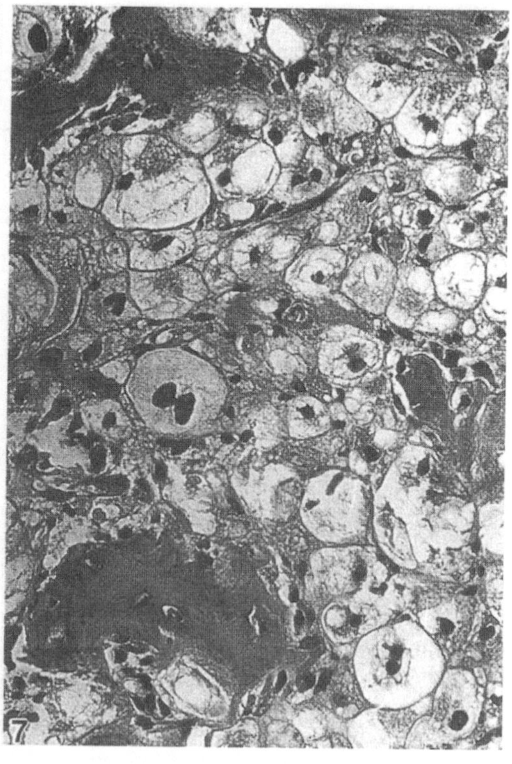

Fig. 4. General view of chondrosarcomatous tissue. The tumour lobules are surrounded by blackish borders of calcification

Fig. 5. Numerous clear cells, many in course of necrosis; their membranes are clearly visualised. These ballooned cells are grouped together into small islets

Figs. 6, 7. Bulky cells with clear cytoplasm, sometimes partitioned by a fine plexus centered on the nucleus. Obvious anisocytosis. Some chondrocytes have a double nucleus. The nuclei are dense and very chromophil. Ground substance is rare between the cells. Small slightly calcified osteoid plaques, partly surrounded by osteoblasts

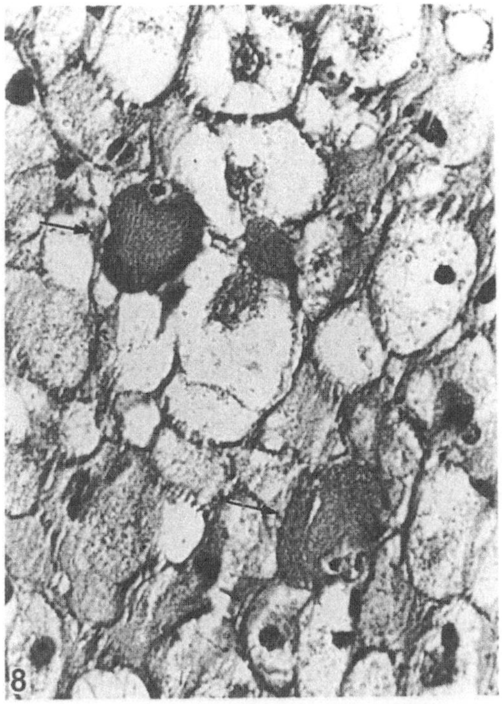

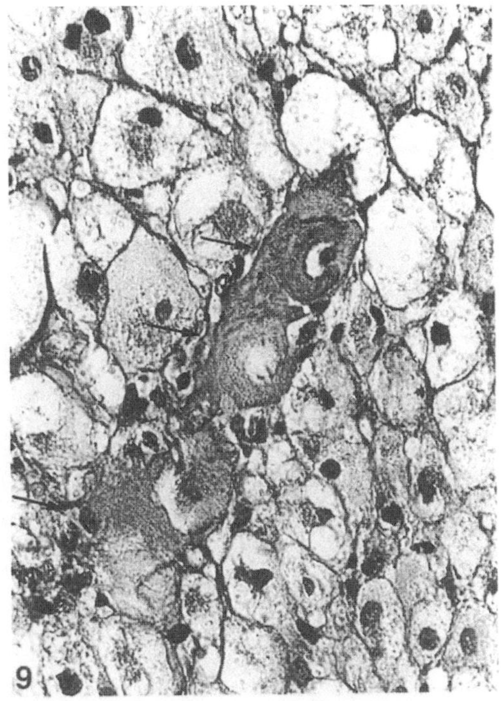

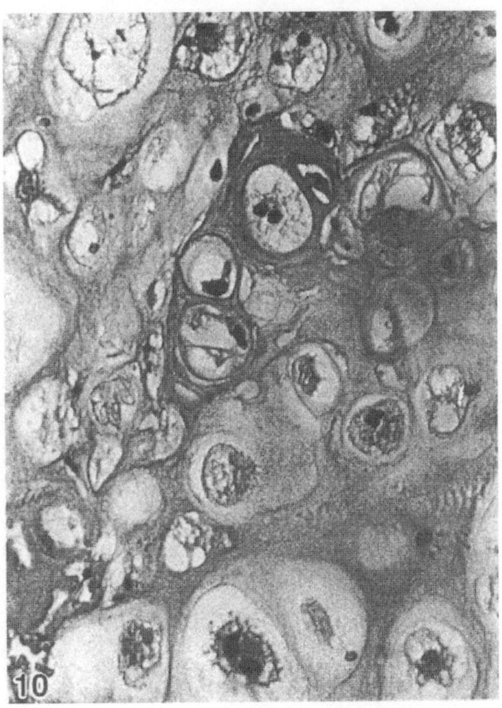

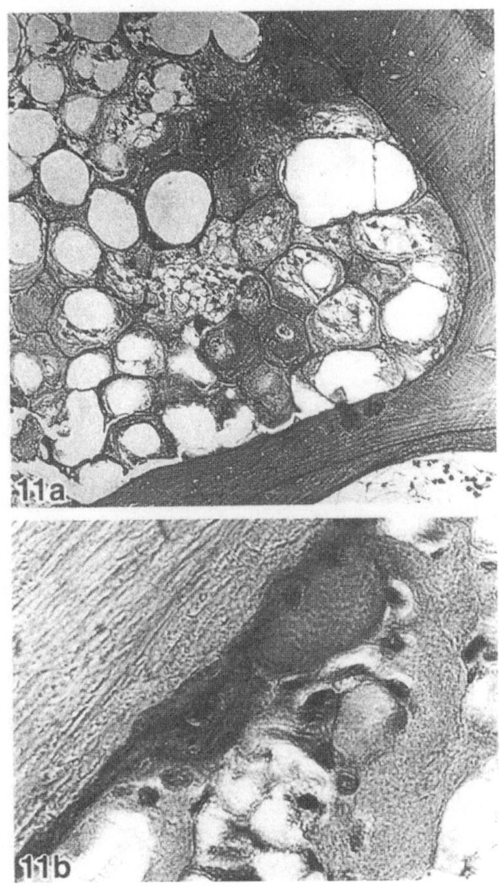

Figs. 8, 9. The cells are in contact with each other. "Gelification" of the cytoplasm, which changes from clear to dense safranophil and displaces the nucleus at the periphery (*arrows*)

Fig. 10. Elaboration of a scanty ground substance between the chondrocytes. Several chondrocytes have a double nucleus

Fig. 11 a, b. The cytoplasmic "gelification" appears here in tumour chondrocytes situated in the fatty marrow (**a**) or in contact with a bony trabecula (**b**)

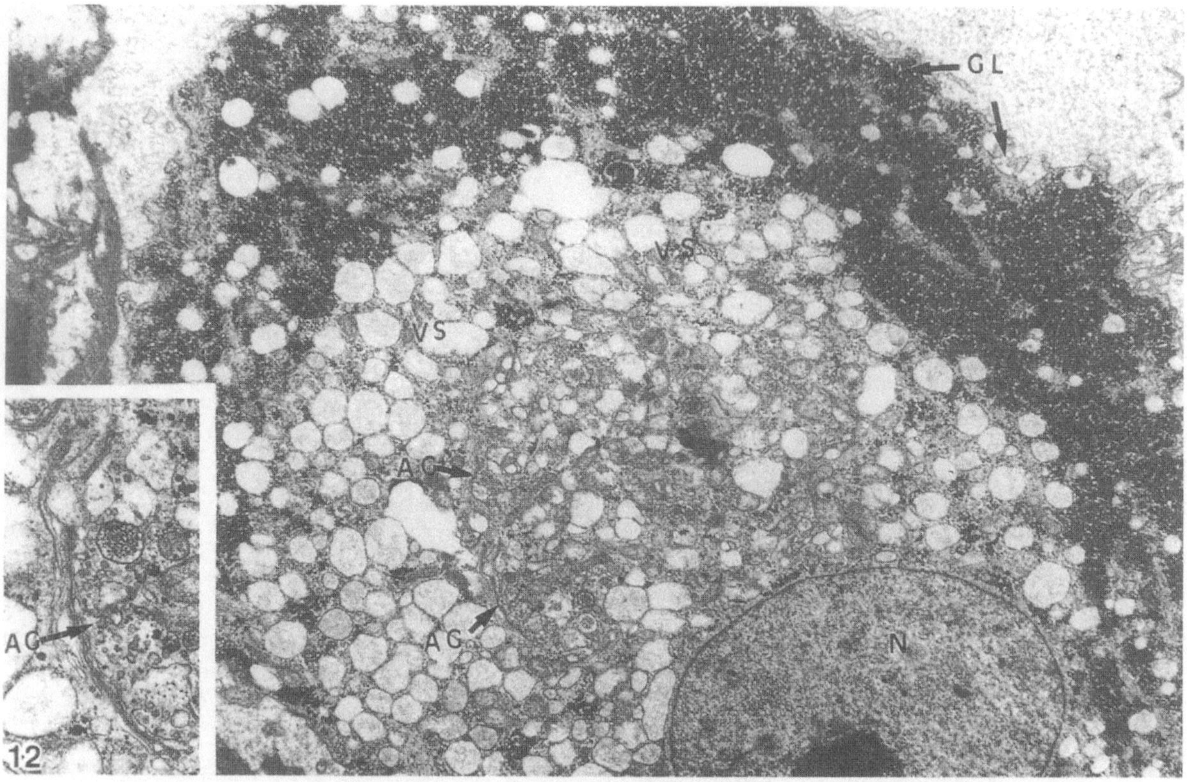

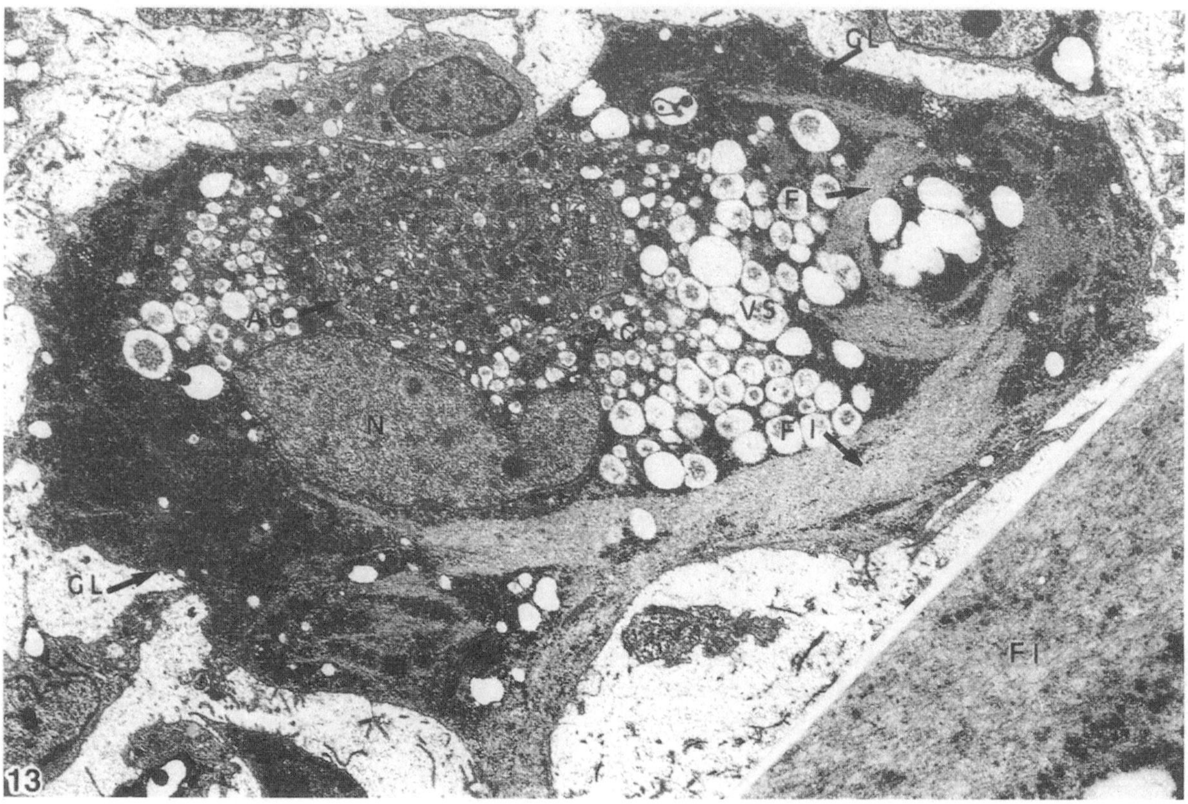

Figs. 12, 13. Ultrastructure (JP Thiery). Two microphotographs with magnifications of 6000 and 4000 respectively. *GL*, glycogen; *VS*, secretory vacuole; *FI*, bundle of intermediate filaments; *N*, nucleus and its nucleolus. Inset (13): enlargement of bundles of intermediate filaments

4. Mesenchymal chondrosarcoma

This is one of the most astonishing tumours in pathology. Its singular characteristics include its origin, bony in only 2 cases out of 3, its histology, a collection of cartilaginous and cellular areas, its unpredictable course and the poor response to current antimitotic agents despite its quota of undifferentiated cells.

Case history

In January 1986, a female patient aged 70 attended the orthopaedic clinic, referred by a general practitioner for a tumour elevating the right scapula and extending from the summit of the hemithorax to the 6th rib (fig. 1b). This patient already had a case record in this hospital, where, nine years previously, she had been treated in the department of orthopaedic surgery for a juxta-articular tumour of the supero-medial aspect of the left thigh (fig. 1a) which had developed slowly and insidiously over 2 years; it was easily palpable and fixed to the femur. On the radiographs it appeared to extend widely into the soft tissues, had a rounded form, marbled with calcifications. At the level of its point of femoral attachment there was a dense zone of calcification which extended towards the femoral neck, and which substituted for the partly destroyed cortex. Complementary investigations performed in January 1986 showed no other lesion.

The surgical procedure removed a bulky subscapular tumour, ovoid and apparently encapsulated, without bony attachment. Its histological appearance, characteristic of a mesenchymal chondrosarcoma, was identical to that of the tumour removed nine years earlier. One year later, and 10 years after removal of the first tumour, multiple metastatic lesions, particularly hilar and pulmonary, failed to respond to chemotherapy and brought about her death.

General considerations

Mesenchymal chondrosarcoma was defined as an entity in 1959 by Lichtenstein and Bernstein. Its incidence is of the order of 0.5% of malignant tumours of bone and both sexes may be regarded as equally affected, although some statistics indicate a slight female predominance. The tumour is encountered from the 1st to the 8th decades, but the majority of cases are diagnosed between the 2nd and 5th, and in 111 cases at the Mayo Clinic [Nakashima et al 1986] 60% were diagnosed in the 2nd and 3rd decades.

Two-thirds of the cases have a bony origin; in a third of the cases the tumour develops in the soft tissues, in a juxtaosseous and more especially a juxta-articular position. The flat bones of the limb-girdles, the vertebrae, ribs, mandible (a frequent site, 12 mandibular lesions out of 86 skeletal sites in Nakashima's report), clavicle and sternum are the bones most often affected, more rarely the long bones of the limbs are involved. Twelve meningeal, cranial or spinal cases were reported by Scheithauer et al (1978) and the localisation is usually epiphyseal or metaphyseo-epiphyseal.

Clinical features and course

The clinical features are those of dysfunction, dull pain, and progressively enlarging swelling or signs of compression. The disquiet produced by these symptoms, determined by the site of the tumour and the psychological state of the patient, determines the time between the earliest symptoms and the first consultation, an interval varying from a few months to a few years, (10 years in a case I reported in 1974).

Table 1. Mesenchymal chondrosarcoma

The tumour site is:
- intraosseous, or
- juxtaosseous with invasion of the soft tissues, or
- exclusively extraosseous (a third of cases)

Histological diagnosis:
- coexistence of cartilaginous areas and small anaplastic cells. Major vascularisation, appearances of angiopericytoma. There are no mesenchymal chondrosarcomas of low grade malignancy.

Differential diagnosis:
- dedifferentiated chondrosarcoma
- a "selective" biopsy with a fine aspiration needle may suggest: small-cell sarcoma, Ewing's tumour, lymphosarcoma. These diagnoses are usually easy to exclude. In case of doubt it is essential to request a second and more representative biopsy.

On clinical examination, the tumour may or may not be adherent to the bony plane, as a firm lumpy painless structure.

The course is that of a sarcoma, but the rapidity of this course is unpredictable. In patients in their 2nd decade, I have noted rapid progress in sternomediastinal or pelvic tumours, sites which do not allow of satisfactory surgical excision. Telecobalt therapy only arrests progress temporarily and death supervenes in less than 2 years from local progressive recurrence, visceral compression and pulmonary metastasis. In adults, the course of mesenchymal chondrosarcoma of the limbs seems slower, but after excision of the primary tumour other lesions develop at various sites remote from the original localisation. For this reason, some authors consider that these are not metastases but tumours developing de novo. Despite repeated surgical intervention, what we shall continue to call metastases, whether pulmonary, bony or in the soft tissues destroy the patient after 8-10 years or more, interrupted by apparent "cures". In other patients metastases develop after several local recurrences [Salvador et al 1971]. In 23 patients admitted to the Mayo Clinic, 5-year survival was 54.6% and 10-year survival 27.3%. In the 12 patients followed up by Dowling (1964), the mean survival was 8 years, ranging between 11 months and 24 years. Huvos et al (1983) found a 10-year survival of 28% in 35 patients. Currently, the statistics vary around 50% survival at 5 years and 30% at 10 years.

Patients who have really benefited from irradiation and chemotherapy are quite rare. Early surgical intervention with wide removal of the tumour appears to be the best treatment pending the arrival of a truly effective antimitotic therapy for the undifferentiated chondrocytic proliferation.

Imaging

Within the bone, the tumour is evidenced in radiographs by a zone of osteolysis speckled by calcification (fig. 2) or by a markedly calcified irregular zone, much denser than the surrounding bony tissue (fig. 3). Even at its intraosseous origin, the often bulky tumour develops widely in the soft tissues as an ovoid, polycyclic, partly calcified shadow.

Pathological anatomy and histopathology

At macroscopic examination, the tumour may or may not adhere to the underlying bone; it is ovoid, 4-10 cm in diameter, multilobular, grayish-white in colour and of firm consistency. Tendinous and musculo-aponeurotic fibers adhere to its surface.

On section, the cut surface has a glistening bluish-white fibrocartilaginous appearance. Between the cartilaginous islets there are zones of haemorrhage and there are multiple foci calcification in the cartilage. At low magnification, the sections exhibit chondroid areas, calcified in places, surrounded by a proliferation of small round or ovoid cells which may resemble a lymphomatous proliferation or a Ewing's sarcoma (fig. 4). The cartilaginous islets consist of a usually hyaline matrix in which the irregularly distributed chondrocytes are often more numerous peripherally. These chondrocytes are poorly differentiated; sometimes they are of uniform appearance (fig. 9) but sometimes anomalies and deformities are evident (figs. 6, 7). Different cartilaginous zones are traversed by zones of necrosis and calcification (fig. 13), sometimes by osteoid or bony strands (fig. 16). The vessels are well-marked, possibly surrounded by a chondrohyaline cuff (fig. 5). The cellular zones are composed of undifferentiated cells, of small size, rounded or ovoid, with a very evident nucleolus (fig. 8). These cells proliferate in a dense reticular plexus. The frequency of mitoses varies widely in different cases.

The abundance of vessels may give the tumour an endocrinoid appearance, or else suggest a haemangiopericytoma, but the reticular plexus is not at all characteristic of this latter tumour (figs. 14, 15).

Ultrastructural examination [Steiner et al 1973, Chomette et al 1987] demonstrates the presence of glycogen, some intercellular junctions of primitive type, immature cells and differentiated cells of a fibroblastic and chondroblastic nature.

Metastatic lesions sometimes faithfully reproduce the primary tumour, but sometimes depart from this widely enough to suggest a diagnosis of ordinary chondrosarcoma in process of calcification. The biphasic appearance is less definite; the chondrocytes are more numerous in the cartilaginous areas and the anaplastic cellular zones; a rudimentary chondroid substance tends to separate the cells from one another. The histological modifications that hamper recognition of the origin of the primary tumour may correspond to a true progression of mesenchymal chondrosarcoma.

Differential diagnosis

The diagnosis of mesenchymal chondrosarcoma is easily made; nevertheless, it is useful to make some remarks regarding this composite tumour.

There are wide variations from one tumour to another in the proportion of cartilaginous tissue to cellular proliferation and the pericytic arrangement of the cells may suggest an angiopericytoma, particularly in cases where the cartilaginous content is small; within the same tumour, there may be a definite boundary between the cellular areas and the cartilaginous tissue, or a more gradual transition may occur.

One diagnosis to be excluded may be that of a chondrosarcoma with a peripheral undifferentiated cellular proliferation. The cells of an undifferentiated chondrosarcoma are much more polymorphic than those of mesenchymal chondrosarcoma. Anisocytosis, cytonuclear anomalies, fusiform or stellate cells together with obvious atypical cartilaginous cells, all aid in the diagnosis. Both these tumours are chondrosarcomas for which no specific treatment is currently available. Assuming, (which is unlikely), that a single cellular component is involved at biopsy, a chondroblastoma may be considered when cartilaginous areas, calcified in places, are seen. This diagnosis is not defensible in the absence of chondroblastic proliferation with scattered giant cells.

The clinical course and radiographic appearances of the two tumours are quite different. Note that the immunological anti-protein S100 test, while positive in cartilaginous tissues, is only so in cells from cartilaginous zones of mature appearance and is negative in the proliferation of undifferentiated cells which form the greater part of mesenchymal chondrosarcoma. In chondroblastoma, cells from the cartilaginous areas and mononuclear cells (chondroblasts) are positive reactors.

A predominant cellular proliferation may suggest a diagnosis of small round-cell tumours (Ewing, neuroblastoma). Actually, the cells of a mesenchymal chondrosarcoma are much less uniform than those of a Ewing's sarcoma; moreover, the rudimentary formation of chondroid material separating the cells from one another, is a critical finding and the elaboration of reticular fibers is a further major argument for this diagnosis (figs. 15, 16).

Treatment

Treatment is surgical. The prognosis is largely determined by the possibilities of intervention; we have seen that the 5-year survival is of the order of 50%.

References

Chomette G, Vaillant JM, Auriol M (1987) Chondrosarcome mésenchymateux. Etude anatomoclinique, immunohistochimique et ultrastructurale. A propos d'une observation. Rev Stomatol Chir Maxillofac 88: 350-355

Dahlin DC, Henderson ED (1962) Mesenchymal chondrosarcoma. Further observations on a new entity. Cancer 15: 410-417

Dowling EA, (1964) Mesenchymal chondrosarcoma. J Bone Joint Surg 46A: 747-754

Goldman RL (1967) Mesenchymal chondrosarcoma, a rare malignant chondroid tumor usually primary in bone. Report of a case arising in extraskeletal soft tissue. Cancer 20: 1494-1498

Hollins RR, Lydiatt DD, Markin RS, Davis LF (1987) Mesenchymal chondrosarcoma: a case report. J Oral Maxillofac Surg 45: 72-75

Huvos AG, Rosen G, Dabska M, Marcove RC (1983) Mesenchymal chondrosarcoma. A clinicopathologic analysis of 35 patients with emphasis on treatment. Cancer 51: 1230-1237

Louret C, de Gramont A, Krulik M, Jagueux M, Hubert D, Brissaud L, Simelli A, Augereau B, Tubiana JM, Debray J (1985) Extraskeletal mesenchymal chondrosarcoma: case report and review of the literature. J Clin Oncol 3: 858-863

Mainwaring BL, Khoury MB, Khodadoust K (1988) Mesenchymal chondrosarcoma of the left fifth rib. Skeletal Radiol 17: 295-297

Mazabraud A (1974) Le chondrosarcome mésenchymateux. A propos de six observations. Rev Chir Orthop 60: 197-203

Nakashima Y, Unni KK, Shives TC, Swee RG, Dahlin DC (1986) Mesenchymal chondrosarcoma of bone and soft tissue. A review of 111 cases. Cancer 57: 2444-2453

Nezelof C, Mazabraud A, Meary R (1965) Le chondrosarcome mésenchymateux. A propos d'un cas de localisation pararachidienne. Arch Anat Pathol 13: 26-28

Pepe AJ, Kuhlmann RF, Miller DB, (1977) MesencLymal chondrosarcoma. A case report. J Bone Joint Surg 59A: 256-258

Salvador AH, Beabout JW, Dahlin DC (1971) Mesenchymal chondrosarcoma observations on 30 new cases. Cancer 28: 605-615

Scheithauer BW, Rubinstein LJ (1978) Meningeal mesenchymal chondrosarcoma. Report of 8 cases with review of the literature. Cancer 42: 2744-2752

Steiner GC, Mirra JM, Bullough PG (1973) Mesenchymal chondrosarcoma. A study of the ultrastructure. Cancer 32: 926-939

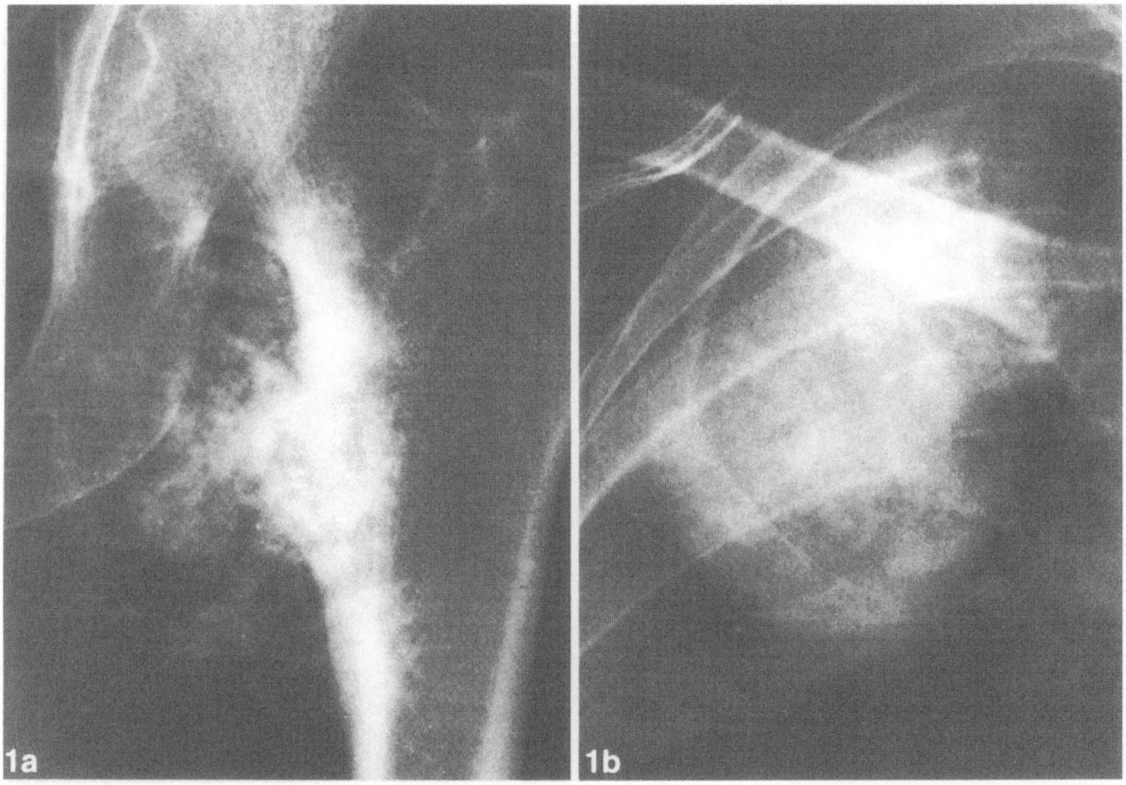

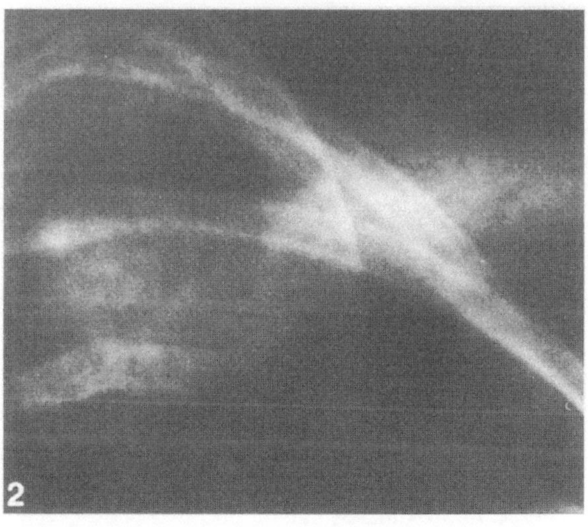

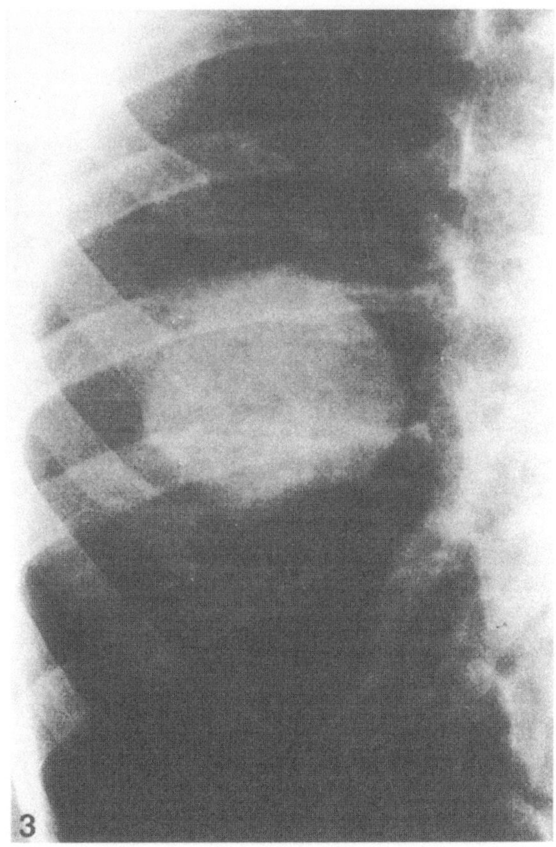

Fig. 1 a, b. Tumour of the inner aspect of the upper end of the femur in a woman aged 61. The inner boundary is poorly visualised. The calcified zones are diffuse and abundant, particularly in the vicinity of the femur (**a**). Nine years after resection a second, subscapular tumour histologically identical to the femoral tumour, is shown at the apex of the right lung (**b**)

Fig. 2. Speckled appearance of the inner half of a thickened clavicle; there was rapid spread into the antero-superior mediastinum

Fig. 3. Mesenchymal chondrosarcoma of 4th rib in man of 20

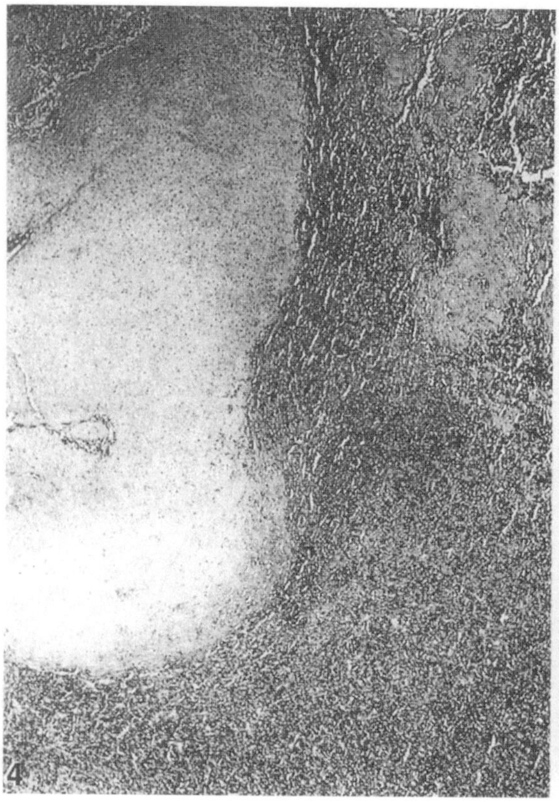

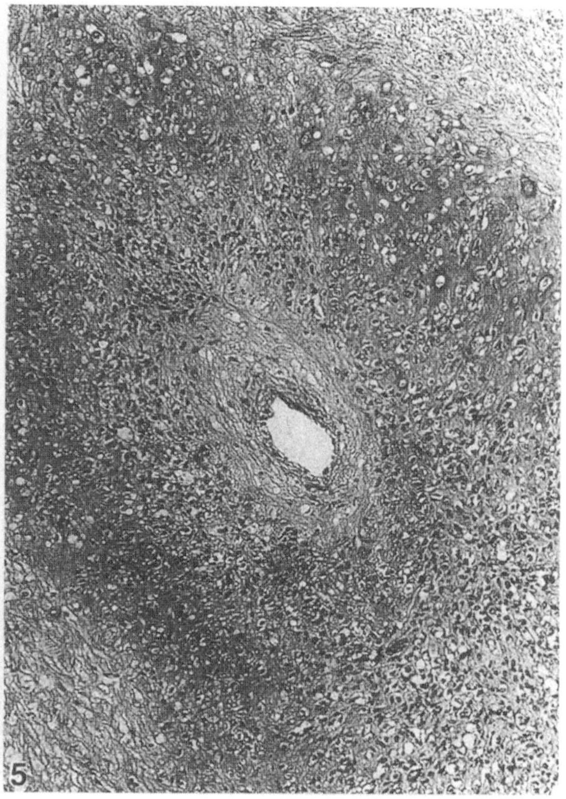

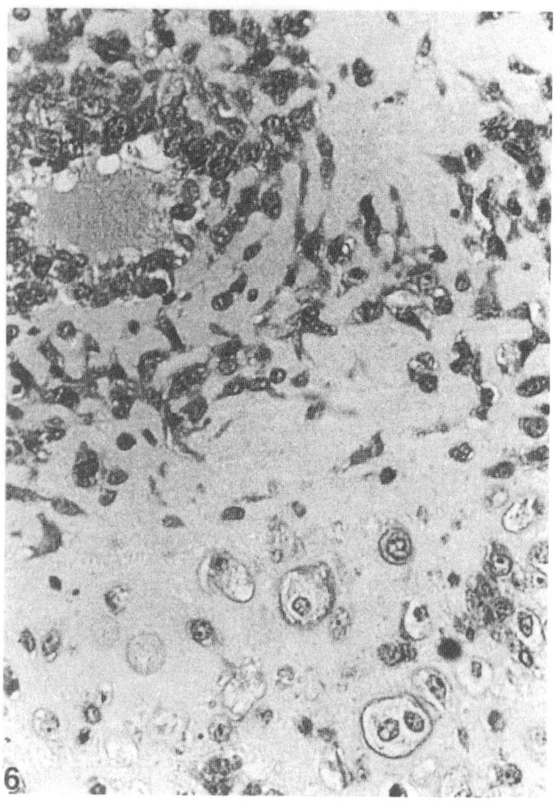

Fig. 4. Approximately half of this microphotograph is occupied by a clear cartilaginous area which seems well demarcated from the tumour cell proliferation

Fig. 5. Inequality of cellular distribution in a chondroid matrix, in which a zone of a deeper grey shade indicates the onset of calcification. At the center is a vessel surrounded by a paucicellular cartilaginous sheath

Fig. 6. It is common to observe, as in this case, a degree of cellular irregularity with round and fusiform cells, cells with dense nuclei and binucleate cells

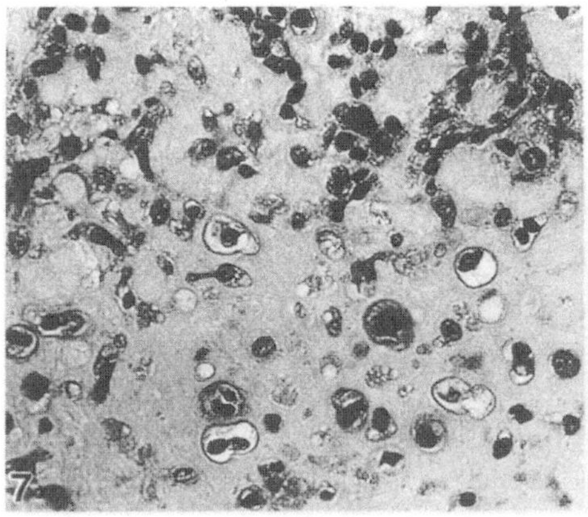

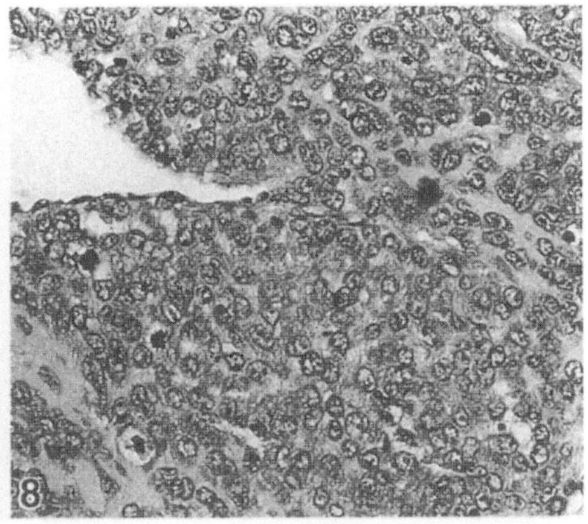

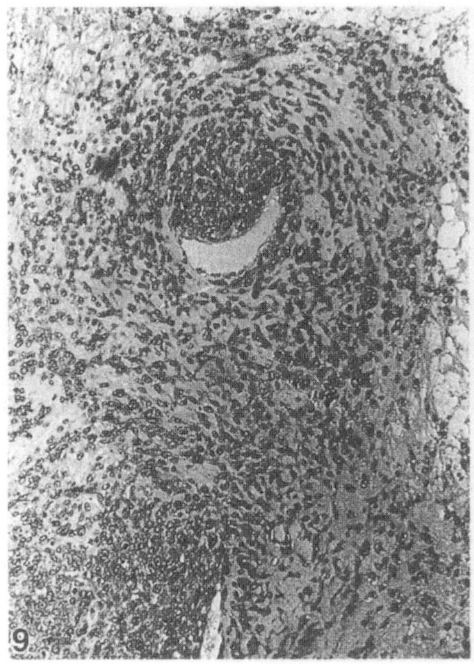

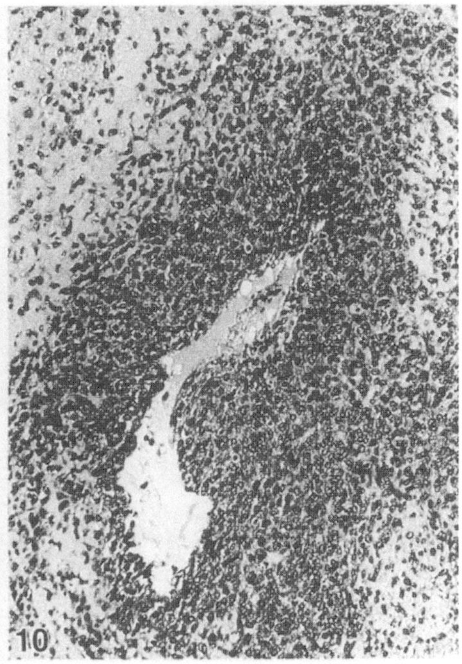

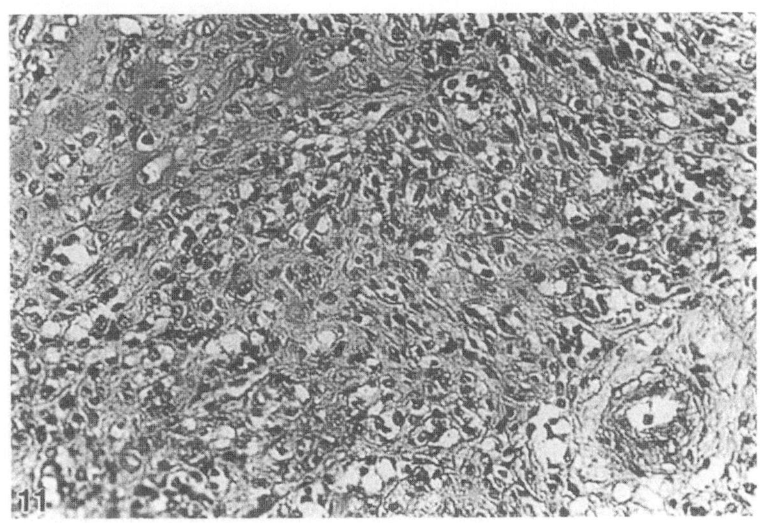

Fig. 7. Cellular abnormalities are evident in this mesenchymal chondrosarcoma of the pelvis. Girl aged 17 years. Death occurred in 2 years due to multiple visceral and bony metastases

Fig. 8. Dense cellular zone composed of cells with a large clear nucleus and a prominent nucleolus

Figs. 9, 10. Zone of cellular proliferation closely related to the vessels: angiopericytic appearances are sufficiently suggestive to compel a search for frankly cartilaginous zones

Fig. 11. Many nuclei are eccentric and displaced to the periphery of the cell by clear cytoplasm. Under low magnification such appearances are not highly suggestive of a mesenchymal chondrosarcoma

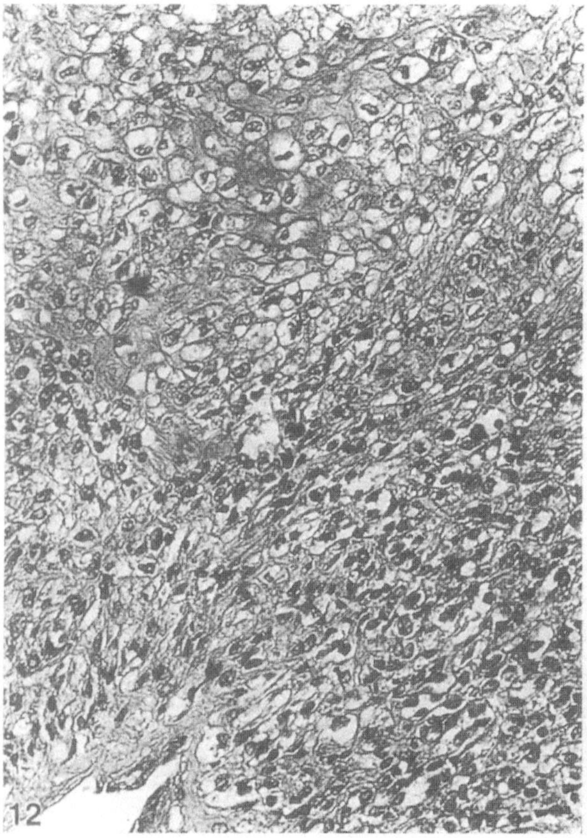

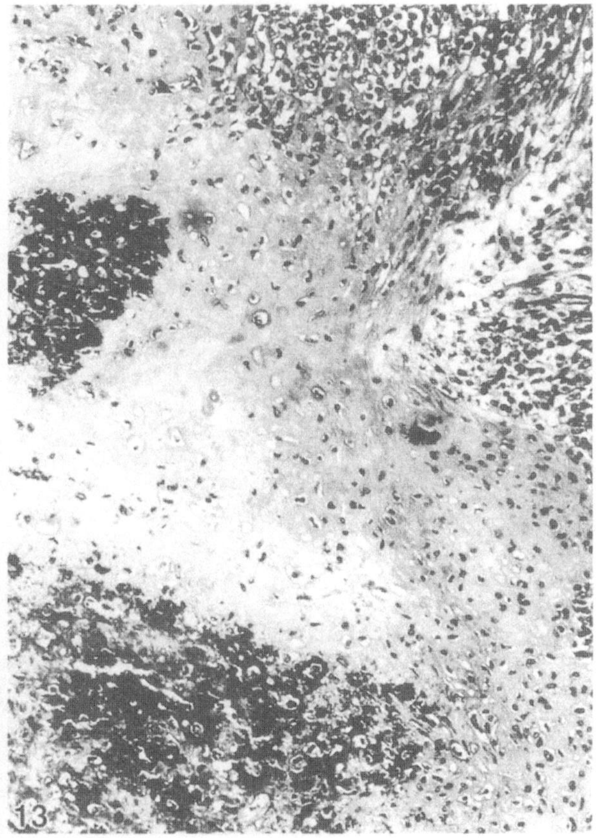

Fig. 12. Tumour zone composed of cells with clear cytoplasm, separated from each other only by a thick membrane

Fig. 13. Zones of calcified cartilage with irregular outlines

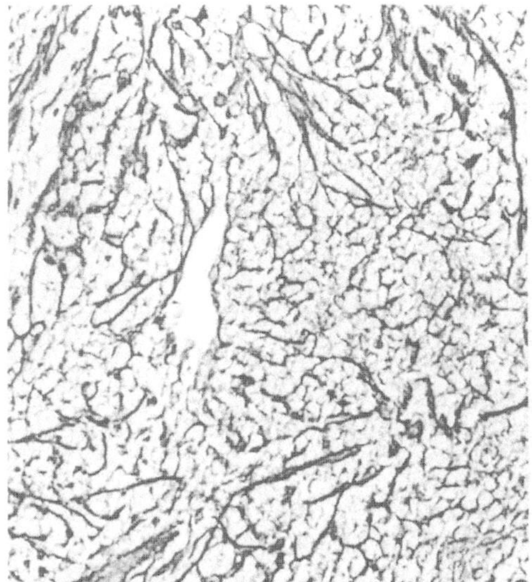

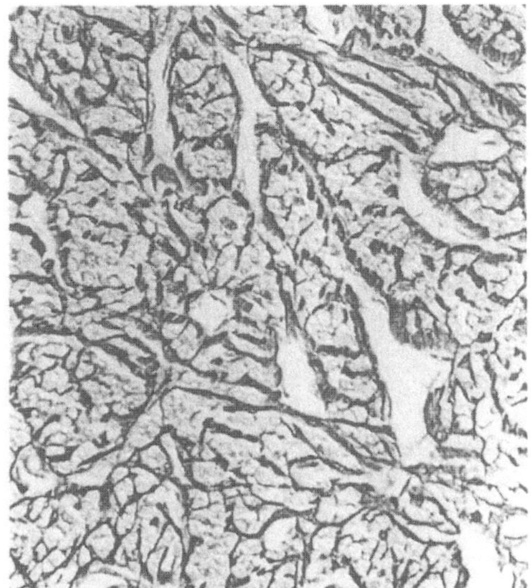

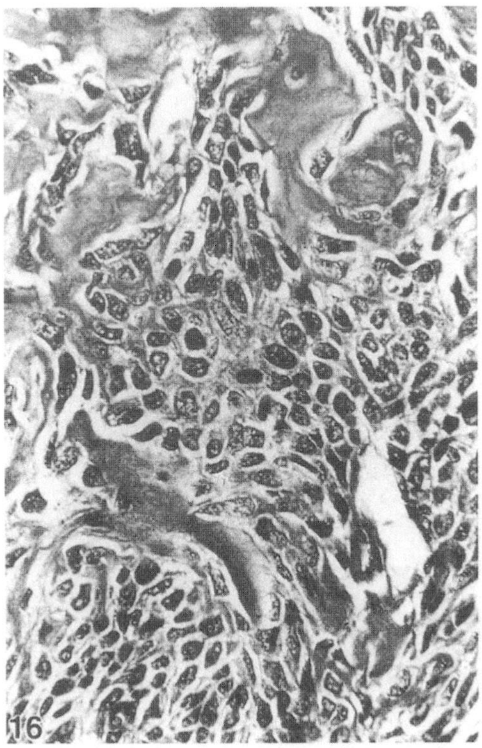

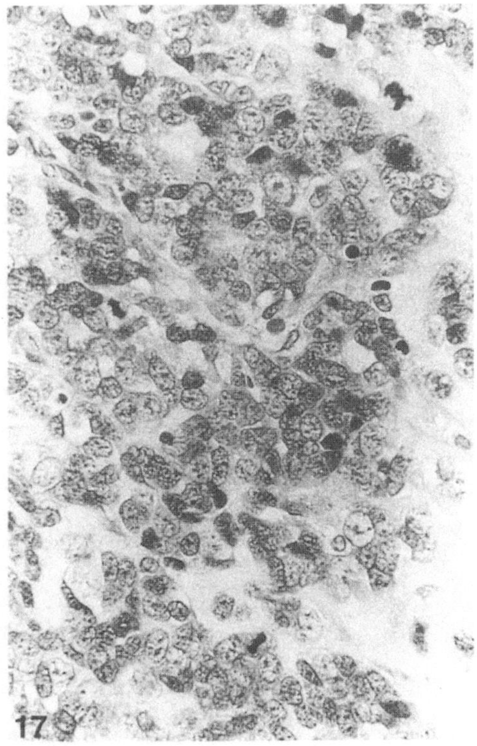

Figs. 14, 15. The rich reticular plexus and major vascularisation resemble an angiopericytoma, but the perivascular aggregations characteristic of angiopericytoma are not present

Fig. 16. Zone of osteoid reaction in a mesenchymal chondrosarcoma of the mandible, otherwise histologically typical

Fig. 17. Temporal metastasis from a mesenchymal chondrosarcoma; the mitoses and undifferentiated appearance of the cells argue in favour of a progressive lesion

5. Chondroblastoma

Pathologists have an instinctive distrust of the term "blasts", founded on the assiduous but inadvisable association of this term with that of sarcoma, but it is important to remember that there are normal blasts and pathological blasts, with greater or lesser features of malignancy. It may have been to avoid any such difficulty that Jaffe and Lichtenstein, in 1942, originally defined the benign chondroblastoma.

Benign chondroblastoma

Case history

At the end of September a young man of 20 attended the orthopaedic department, complaining of pain in the left hip. This pain had commenced during the second term of the academic year. Of moderate severity, it was attributed to fatigue, overstrain and strenuous but intermittent athletic exertion. Dull at the onset, it had increased during the holiday period.

On examination, mobility of the hip was limited by pain evoked by forced movement. General and local clinical examination revealed no palpable tumour formation, the lymph nodes were not enlarged, and the skin of the left lower limb showed no special lesion. The history revealed no notable previous pathology, and the skin reactions were positive to BCG vaccination.

Radiography of the hips, an ESR and blood-count were requested; the results some hours later were as follows: ESR normal for the first two hours, blood count normal. The radiographs showed a zone of osteolysis in the femoral head, relatively well circumscribed. There was no narrowing of the joint-space and the acetabulum was normal (fig. 4).

Under these conditions, a relatively well-defined epiphyseal osteolysis in an apparently healthy adolescent or young man suggests an initial diagnosis of chondroblastoma. However, neither the unlikely possibility of histiocytosis X, nor an aneurysmal cyst in course of development could be formally excluded, nor could a cyst of indeterminate nature.

During the following days, surgical approach to this lesion disclosed a reddish granular formation with a cystic center, an appearance very characteristic of chondroblastoma. The diagnosis was confirmed by histological examination.

General considerations

Chondroblastoma was for long confused with giant-cell tumour. This epiphyseal tumour, calcified and with giant cells, was defined by Codman in 1931 and termed benign chondroblastoma by Jaffe et al eleven years later. Its incidence is of the order of 1% of tumours of bone. Male predominance is given as 63% in the 69 cases of Schajowicz and Gallardo (1970) and the same percentage in the 30 cases in the series of the Hôpital Cochin [Corsat et al 1989]. This is a tumour of young persons, the maximum incidence being between 10 and 25 years of age; 70% of cases are seen in the second decade, but the tumour may occur at any age. Its site is epiphyseal and apophyseal.

It has been suggested that it develops from the epiphyseal aspect of the growth cartilage. The commonest sites are the humeral head (figs. 1-3) and the femoral head (fig. 4) as confirmed by a review of 30 cases [Corsat et al 1989]. Next comes the great trochanter, then lesions in the cranium, ribs, iliac bones, os calcis (fig. 9), and so on. In absolute terms, a patellar site (fig. 10) is relatively rare, but if patellar tumours only are considered, chondroblastoma is in a leading position, Kransdorf et al (1989) having collected 16 cases among 38 benign patellar neoplasms. Mercuri et al (1991) report 16.6% of chondroblastomas in 210 tumours of the patella collected from the literature.

Clinical features and course

The index symptom was pain in 86% of the patients of Turcotte et al (1993). Initially moderate, it often goes back to a year or more before the first consultation. The course of chondroblastoma is benign, in the sense that life is not threatened, but the risk of joint complications is considerable. Local recurrences after curettage are of the order of 20%. However perfect prostheses may be, their use in young patients is nonetheless a handicap (we shall see later that 0.5-25% of chondroblastic chondrosarcomas are confused with a chondroblastoma).

Imaging

In the radiographs, the osteolysis is often quite well circumscribed towards its inner border, but the tumour may extend into the joint across the epiphyseal plate (fig. 3), as in the case reported by Sotelo-Avila (1986), and is speckled by opacities representing small foci of calcification. In other cases it is frankly cystic. MRI and CT define these different appearances and allow assessment of possible spread into the soft tissues.

Chondroblastoma of the bones of the true pelvis combines an image of acetabular lysis and an intrapelvic mass, which may or may not be calcified, very suggestive of chondrosarcoma [McLaughlin et al 1975]. At the site, the tumour is often discovered only after considerable development.

As for any bony tumour, a chest X-ray is made routinely and shows the lung-fields to be clear. In some cases, the clinical data and radiological appearances together with the gross appearance of the tumour affirm the diagnosis, and if the pathologist is well acquainted with this lesion, a spot diagnosis will permit immediate curettage.

Pathological anatomy and histopathology

Macroscopically, curettage removes soft reddish haemorrhagic tissue containing small granules of a gelatinous consistency whose centers may be calcified. The whole recalls the structure of a raspberry, composed of an assembly of small drupes.

Microscopically, a review of the sections at low magnification demonstrates zones of small round, very eosinophil cells scattered irregularly, giant cells and some cartilaginous islets of variable size (figs. 11, 12). At higher magnification, these round mononuclear cells with strongly eosinophil cytoplasm and a rounded chromatophil nucleus, appear separated from each other by a fine clear border (figs. 13, 16). This is doubtless an artefact but is a constant finding. There are also inequalities of size and shape that break the monotony of these areas of chondroblasts (fig. 16). Some nuclei are notched, rather like histiocytic cells [Dahlin & Unni 1986]. Mitoses are not numerous, but are always present in some chondroblastic cells (fig. 14). More obvious against this cellular background are the giant cells and cartilaginous islets. The multinucleate giant cells are usually less numerous and of smaller size than those of giant-cell tumours (figs. 12, 14), but I have seen some of monstrous dimensions. They are irregularly distributed and irregular in shape. Their cytoplasm is as eosinophilic as that of the mononucleate chondroblasts, and their markedly chromatophil nuclei have no tendency to group in any particular manner. The cartilaginous or often fibrocartilaginous islets are of metaplastic origin, the result of elaboration of a ground substance and cellular metamorphosis; hence the generally gradual transition between the streaks of mononucleate cells and the chondroid islets which depart markedly from the familiar types of physiological cartilage (figs. 17, 18, 19a). In places there is rudimentary perichondrocytic calcification and sometimes a relatively major zone of calcification (fig. 19b), more rarely of ossification. These deposits of calcium salts thus become radiologically detectable.

In some cases, the tissue for examination consists of fibrous septa bounding a central cystic zone, rather like the wall of an aneurysmal cyst (fig. 20). Silver impregnation shows abundant reticulin fibers, which surround the mononuclear cells and are interrupted by the cartilaginous islets. The immunoreaction to antiprotein S100 is positive. The divergences observed in the ultrastructural studies may be related to different stages of cell maturation [Méary et al 1975, Monda & Wick 1985, Brecher & Simon 1988].

It is necessary to familiarise oneself with the great variability of the relationships between cell proliferation and chondroid tissue, as a consequence of which some sections may consist only of plaques of chondroblasts. Sufficient sections are required to find a rudiment of chondroid metamorphosis in some fields of comparable appearance to that which may be seen at the periphery of differentiated cartilaginous foci. With some luck, and in some cases much perseverance, one may find a small but typical cartilaginous islet. Conversely, the cartilaginous islets may predominate; this situation will be considered in relation to the differential diagnosis.

Differential diagnosis

From the purely radiological viewpoint the differential diagnosis of villonodular synovitis sometimes arises.

From the histological aspect , confusion may occur with giant-cell tumour, aneurysmal cyst, chondromyxoid fibroma and osteoblastoma. Chondrosarcoma and osteosarcoma may also be difficult to exclude.

A diagnosis of haemopigmented villonodular synovitis is often possible at gross inspection. In the sections, the cellular polymorphism, foamy histiocytes, and macrophages laden with haemosiderin leave no doubt, even if there are some hyaline plaques of chondroid appearance.

In a giant-cell tumour, the cytoplasm is amphophil and not strongly eosinophil as in chondroblastoma. Fine extensions connect the cells together. There is no formation of cartilaginous substance and the immune reaction to anti-protein S100 is negative. The localisation is metaphyseo-epiphyseal. It is exceptional before 15 years of age and rare between 15 and 20 years.

Aneurysmal cyst is haemorrhagic and cystic, as may also be the case in chondroblastoma, and is found at the same age. If we add the possibility of repair cartilage in a fracture, which is relatively common in aneurysmal cysts, the diagnostic difficulties may be imagined. The diagnosis then rests on cell morphology: rounded in chondroblastoma, markedly more varied in aneurysmal cyst, and on the immune reaction to anti-protein S100, which is negative.

Chondromyxoid fibroma differs from chondroblastoma in its tissue polymorphism and metaphyseal localisation, but it is accepted that there are intermediate forms between one tumour and the other. Advanced chondroblastomas and chondromyxoid fibromas destroy the epiphyseal plate and the tumour is then metaphyso-epiphyseal. Here again, the immune reaction to anti-protein S100 is negative.

When the curettage material for examination is that of a recurrence of a genuine chondroblastoma, the tissue observed is usually much more like that of a chondromyxoid fibroma than that of a chondroblastoma, a probable consequence of the development of regenerative tissue of fibromyxoid appearance following the original curettage.

Table 1.

Benign tumour; maximum incidence between 10 and 25 years; site: epiphyses and apophyses. Cells independent, very eosinophil.

Differential diagnosis:
- giant-cell tumour
- aneurysmal cyst
- osteoblastoma

Two rare and difficult diagnoses:
- chondrosarcoma of chondroblastic type with epiphyseal localisation
- epiphyseal osteosarcoma

A pitfall (harmless):
- recurrence of a chondroblastoma simulating a chondromyxoid fibroma

Osteoblastoma may be considered in cases where the intercellular matrix is scanty and insufficiently characterised. In these conditions, it is difficult to distinguish osteoid from chondroid tissue. In osteoblastoma there are nests of well-differentiated osteoblasts, often even exaggeratedly so with their peripherally displaced nuclei and abundant cytoplasm.

A chondrosarcoma may possibly be suspected when the cartilaginous component is clearly dominant. It is true that some chondrosarcomatous nodules are surrounded by a cellular proliferation of chondroblastic appearance, but often these cells are bulkier and much more irregular than the chondroblasts of chondroblastomas. Moreover, atypical cells may be seen in both the cartilaginous islets and the peripheral zones of cellular proliferation. A chondrosarcoma of chondroblastic epiphyseal type may be virtually impossible to distinguish from a chondroblastoma (cf Chapter 2).

Another serious pitfall is the coexistence of typical chondroblastic areas with the presence on some rare sections of a tumour. It is important to have the radiographs at hand and to examine the widest possible sectional surfaces so as not to miss an exceptional osteosarcoma of epiphyseal origin.

Treatment

The treatment of chondroblastoma is surgical. The procedures employed will depend on the site of the tumour mass, with a view to securing both complete excision and a functional joint.

Metastasising chondroblastoma and aggressive chondroblastoma

It is quite remarkable that these labels are applied after the event and not on the initial histological appearances. If a femoral head is seen to be destroyed in a man aged 18, either originally or after recurrence of chondroblastoma, we speak of aggressive chondroblastoma. Recurrences are unfortunately commonplace in cartilaginous tumours. If pulmonary metastases develop subsequently, then it is a metastasising chondroblastoma: it is all very simple!

Case history

In April 1969, a boy of 14 was referred for pain in the left elbow. The radiographs showed a well-circumscribed lytic image of the lower humeral epiphysis. In the chest X-ray, there were several nodular opacities regarded as metastases from the elbow tumour. Any intervention directed towards the lung lesions was declined. Biopsy of the humeral tumour led to a diagnosis of chondroblastoma; the histological sections were discussed at a slide conference without any other diagnosis being suggested. Our clinical colleagues, impressed by the presence of pulmonary nodules, and despite the results of the pathological examination, prudently prescribed a single course of antimitotics. This solitary course was not followed by any modification of the lesions. In view of this apparent failure, the child was sent home, he resumed his work and led a normal life for 18 months.

In November 1987, after 18 years of apparently perfect health, the patient was admitted to a cancer center for a fulminating aggressive recurrence of both the pulmonary and humeral sites. Antimitotics were ineffective against this progressive flare-up.

General considerations

The percentage of tumours diagnosed as chondroblastoma which give rise to metastases is of the order of 0.5 to 2% [Kahn et al 1969, Reyes & Kathuria 1979, Kyriakos et al 1985]. The metastases are either of chondroblastic type or chondrosarcoma grades 2 and 3.

Are there any doubts as to the interpretation of the sections at the first examination when the sarcomatous course is virtually immediate, or follows one or two local recurrences after a short interval? In some cases progress is very slow and this fact justifies prolonged surveillance. It is difficult to concede in the case reported above that a single course of antimitotics (this was in 1969) could have led to a remission of 18 years.

Diagnosis

In my view, the problem posed by these metastasising "chondroblastomas" is identical with that of malignant "osteoblastomas". Chondroblastoma is a benign tumour, as clearly established by Jaffe and Lichtenstein. It is better to admit that, with the classical methods of histological examination, we are incapable of recognising the rare form of slowly evolving chondrosarcoma which is the chondrosarcoma of chondroblastic type. An abnormal abundance of atypical cells in a "chondroblastoma" should justify resection rather than curettage; and current high-technology imaging must be given its full due, perhaps also, in the not so remote future, study of the DNA.

Chondroblastoma at atypical sites

These account for about 2% of cases. Though localisation is usually metaphyseal or metaphyseo-epiphyseal, Dahlin and Unni (Bone Tumors 1986), Kurt et al (1989), Brien et al (1995) report cases at craniofacial and metatarsal sites. Dahlin believes that these heterotopic chondroblastomas may develop from secondary centers of ossification. Brien suggests a possible origin from tissue fragments derived from the tendon sheaths.

Figure 21 is that of a cortico-metaphyseal chondroblastoma. The diagnosis of benign chondroblastoma at an atypical site remains suspect. It is best to study further sections to confirm the homogeneity of the tumour and formally to exclude a chondroblastic type of chondrosarcoma.

References

Brecher ME, Simon MA (1988) Chondroblastoma: an immunohistochemical study. Hum Pathol 19: 1043-1047

Brien EW, Mirra JM, Ippolito (1995) Chondroblastoma arising from a non-epiphyseal site. Skeletal Radiol 24: 220-222

Codman (1931) Epiphyseal chondromatous giant cell tumors of the upper end of humerus. Surg Gynecol Obstet 52: 543-548

Corsat JP, Tomeno B, Forest M, Vinh TS (1989) Chondroblastomes bénins: une revue de 30 cas. Rev Chir Orthop 75: 179-187

Dahlin DC, Ivins JC (1972) Benign chondroblastoma. A study of 125 cases. Cancer 30: 401-413

Fanning CV, Sneige NS, Carrasco CH, Ayala AG, Murray JA, Raymond AK (1990) Fine needle aspiration cytology of chondroblastoma of bone. Cancer 65: 1847-1863

Fontaine R, Muller JN, Le Gal Y (1960) Un cas de chondroblastome bénin épiphysaire. Presse Med 68: 154-160

Gardner DJ, Azouz EM(1988) Solitary lucent epiphyseal lesion in children. Skeletal Radiol 17: 497-504

Green P, Whittaker RP (1975) Benign chondroblastoma. Case report with pulmonary metastasis. J Bone Joint Surg 57A: 418-420

Huvos AG, Marcove RC, Erlandson RA, Mike V (1972) Chondroblastoma of bone. A clinicopathologic and electron microscopy study. Cancer 29: 760-771

Jaffe HL, Lichtenstein M (1942) Benign chondroblastoma of bone. Reinterpretation of so called calcifying or chondromatous giant cell tumour. Am J Pathol 18: 969-991

Kahn LB, Wood FM, Ackerman LV (1969) Malignant chondroblastoma. Report of two cases and review of literature. Arch Pathol 68: 371-376

Kransdorf MJ, Moser RP, Vinh N, Aoki J, Callaghan JJ (1989) Primary tumors of the patella. Skeletal Radiol 18: 365-371

Kurt AM, Unni KK, Sim FH (1989) Chondroblastoma of bone. Hum Pathol 20: 965-976

Kyriakos M, Land VJ, Penning H, Parker G (1985) Metastatic chondroblastoma report of a fatal case with a review of the literature on atypical, aggressive and malignant chondroblastoma. Cancer 55: 1770-1789

Lesec G (1974) Les chondroblastomes bénins des os. Etude anatomaclinique (à propos de 11 observations). Thèse, Clermond-Ferrand

Levine GD, Bensch KG (1972) Chondroblastoma. The nature of the basic cell. A study by means of histochemistry, tissue culture, electron microscopy and autoradiography. Cancer 9: 1546-1562

Matsuno T, Hasegawa I, Masuda T (1987) Chondroblastoma arising in the triradiate cartilage report of two cases with review of the literature. Skeletal Radiol 16: 216-222

McLaughlin RE, Swect DE, Webster T, Merritt WM (1975) Chondroblastoma of the pelvis suggestive of malignancy report of an unusual case treated by wide excision. J Bone Joint Surg 57A: 549-551

Méary R, Abelanet R, Forest M, Le Charpentier Y, Tomeno B, Languepin A, Nezelof C, Lesec G (1975) Les chondroblastomes bénins. Etude anatomoclinique et ultrastructurale, à propos de 11 observations. Rev Chir Orthop 61: 717-734

Mercuri M, Casadei R, Ferraro A, Cristofaro R, Balladelli A, Picci P (1991) Tumours of the patella. Int Orthop 15: 115-120

Monda L, Wick R (1985) S-100 protein immunostaining in the differential diagnosis of chondroblastoma. Hum Pathol 16: 287-293

Moser RP, Brochimole DM, Vinh TN, Kransdorf MJ, Aoki J (1988) Chondroblastoma of the patella. Skeletal Radiol 17: 413-419

Nezelof C, Mazabraud A, Jobard P (1962) Le chondroblastome bénin des os à propos de 4 observations. Arch Anat Pathol 10: 111-117

Pignati G, Nigrisoli M (1989) Chondroblastoma. Skeletal Radiol 18: 225-227

Reyes CV, Kathuria S (1979) Recurrent and aggressive chondroblastoma of the pelvis with late malignant neoplastic changes. Am J Surg Pathol 3: 449-455

Roberts PF, Taylor JG (1980) Multifocal benign chondroblastoma: report of a case. Hum Pathol 11: 296-298

Schajowicz F, Gallardo H (1970) Epiphyseal chondroblastoma of bone. J Bone Joint Surg 52B: 205-226

Sirsat MV, Vatsala M (1970) Benign chondroblastoma of bone. Report of a case of malignant transformation. J Bone Joint Surg 52B: 741-745

Sotelo-Avila C, Sundaram M, Kyriakos M, Graviss ER, Tayob AA (1986) Diagonsis: diametaphyseal chondroblastoma of the upper portion of the left femur. Skeletal Radiol 15: 387-390

Springfield DS, Capanna R, Gherlinzoni F, Picci P, Campanacci M (1985) Chondroblastoma A review of seventy cases J Bone Joint Surg 67A: 748-755

Turcotte RE, Kurt AM, Sim FH, Unni KK, McLeod RA (1993) Chondroblastoma. Hum Pathol 24: 944-949

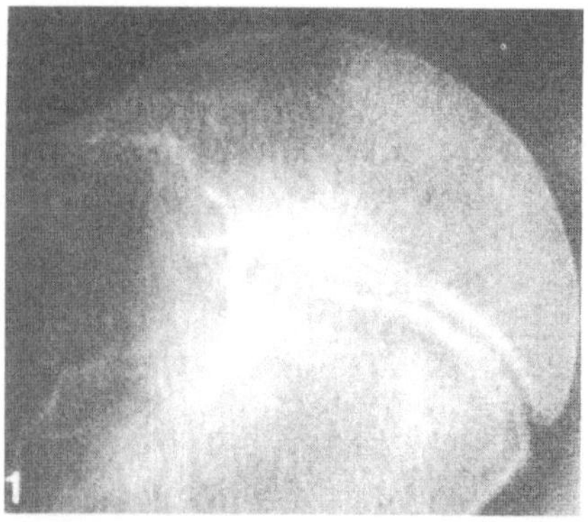
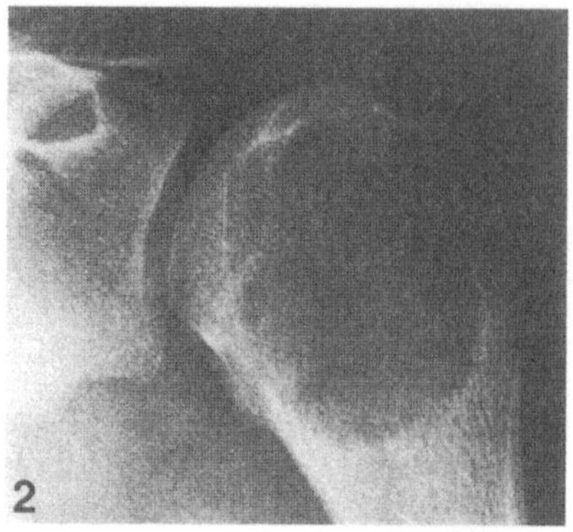
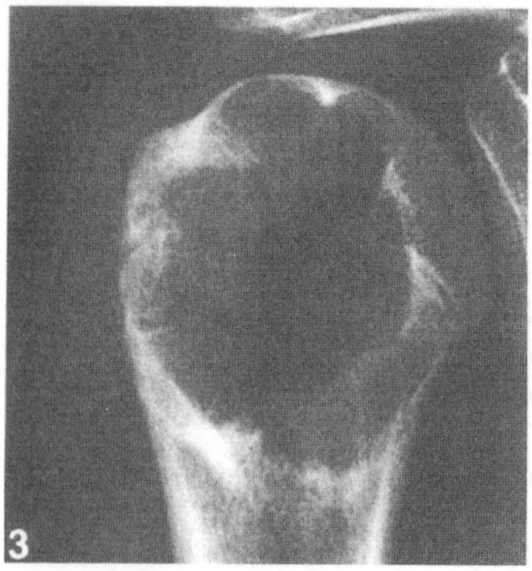
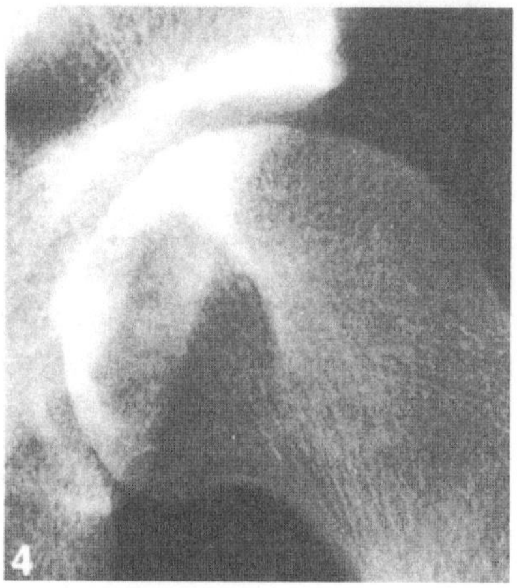
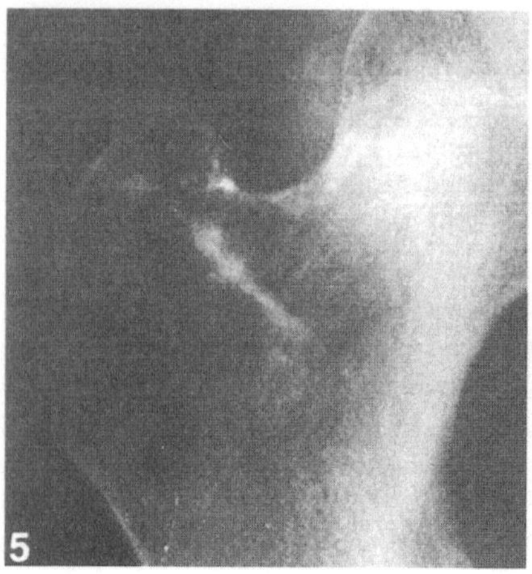
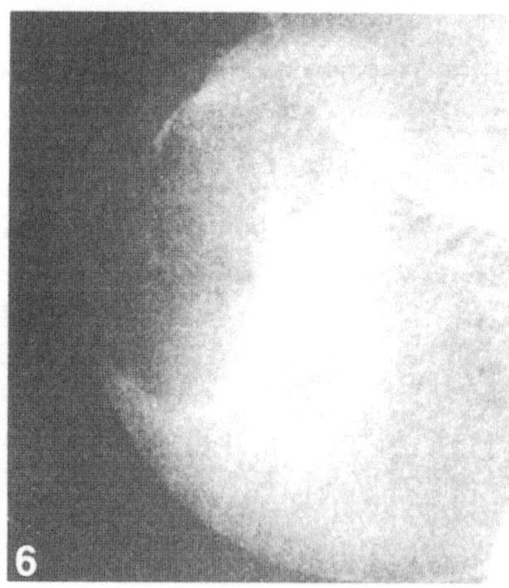

Fig. 1. Chondroblastoma of greater tubercle of humerus, osteolytic image circumscribed at its inner border and speckled with opacities due to calcification of cartilaginous islands (child of 13)

Fig. 2. Chondroblastoma of greater tubercle of humerus, more extensive than in previous case (child of 15)

Fig. 3. Large chondroblastoma of upper end of humerus destroying the growth plate and extending towards the metaphysis (girl aged 16)

Fig. 4. Clear circumscribed osteolysis of femoral head transgressing on the neck (boy of 20)

Fig. 5. Chondroblastoma of great trochanter, whose outer border is not visible in the film. The inner limit of the tumour cannot be identified in this standard radiograph (girl of 8 years)

Fig. 6. Chondroblastoma of anterolateral portion of femoral condyle (boy aged 20). The boundaries of these tumours can be defined by CT examination, but these conventional radiographs allow initial assessment of the magnitude of the therapeutic problem and the effects of development of this benign tumour on an often immature articular epiphysis

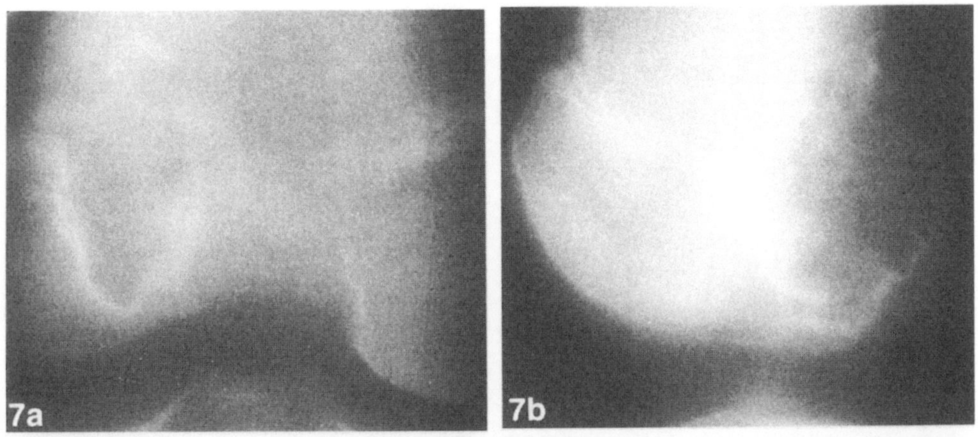

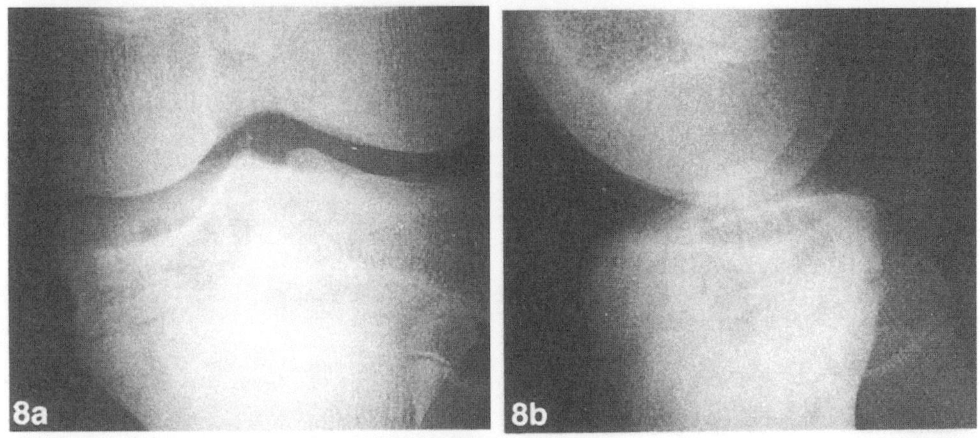

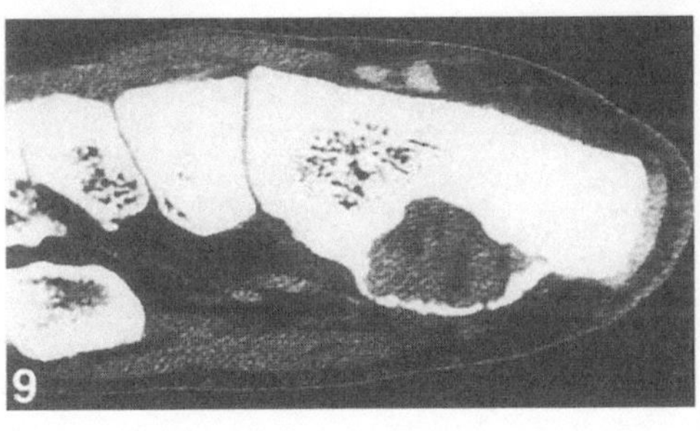

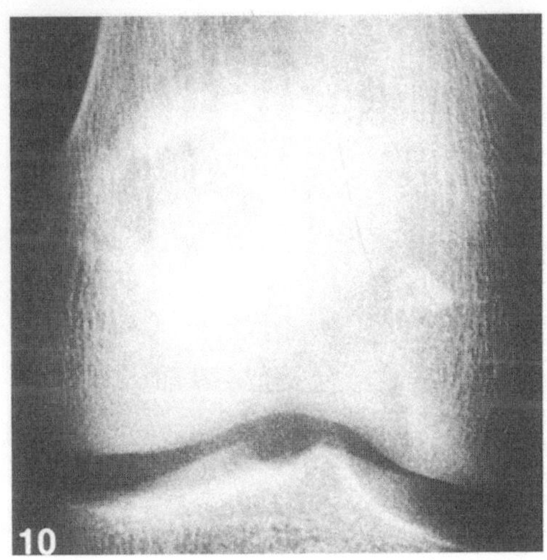

Fig. 7 a, b. Chondroblastoma of posteromedial part of medial femoral condyle, bounded by a sclerotic border (boy aged 14)

Fig. 8 a, b. Chondroblastoma of upper epiphysis of tibia. The growth plate is still clearly visible (boy aged 14)

Fig. 9. Chondroblastoma of calcaneum. The CT image precisely defines the limits of bone destruction

Fig. 10. Relatively rare patellar site of chondroblastoma (radiograph kindly lent by Dr Houngbadji)

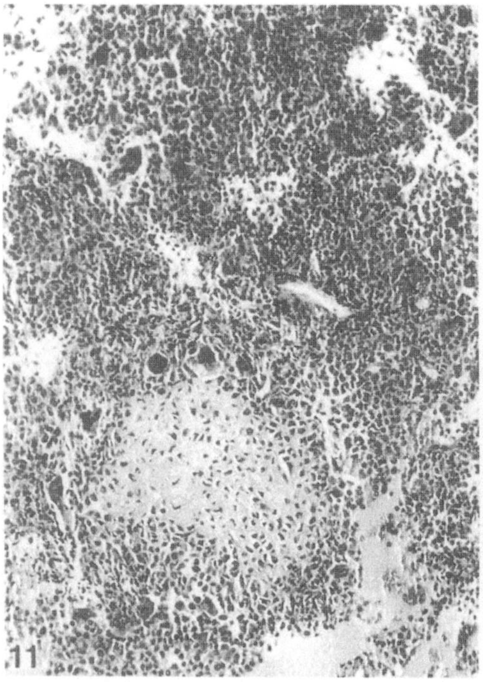

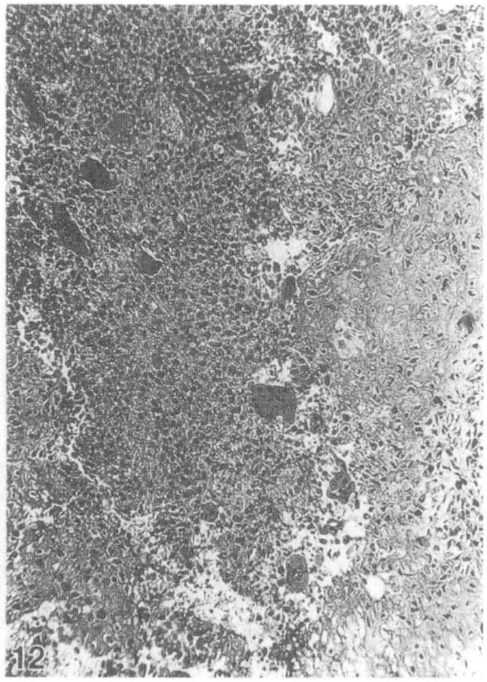

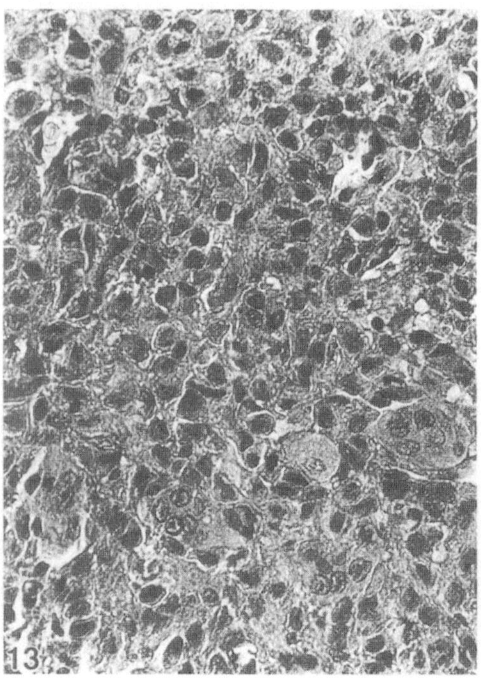

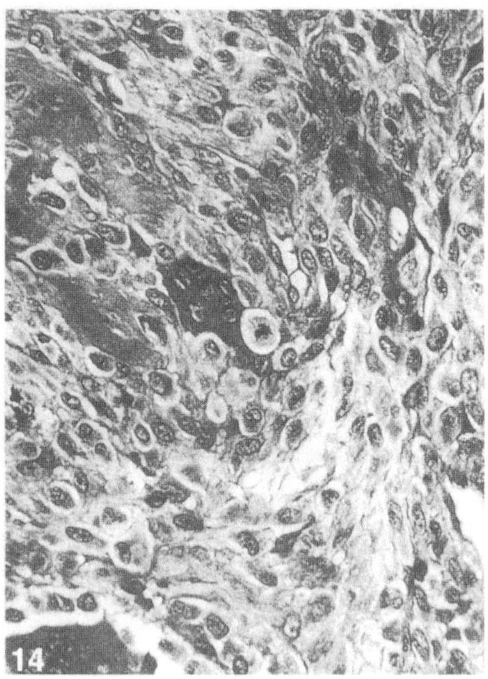

Figs. 11, 12. A cartilaginous zone and a zone of cell proliferation with scattered giant cells. This low magnification shows the irregular arrangement of chondrocytes in the cartilaginous area

Fig. 13. A rudimentary matrix separates the cells from each other; this appearance calls for a search for better characterised cartilaginous areas

Fig. 14. In the upper left quadrant of this microphotograph, the ground substance appears more definitely chondroid

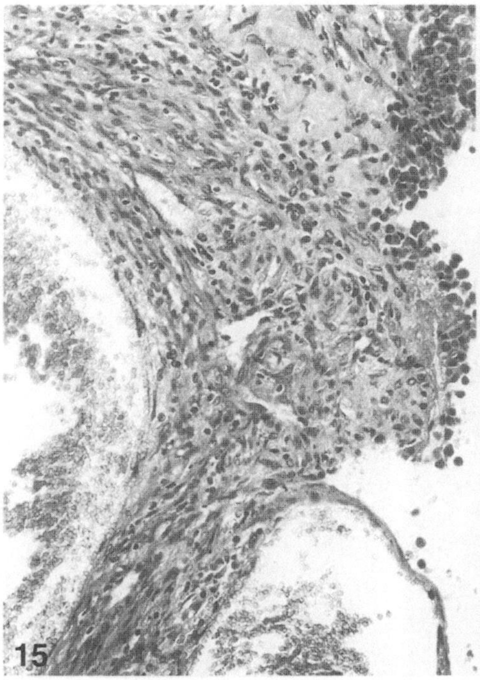

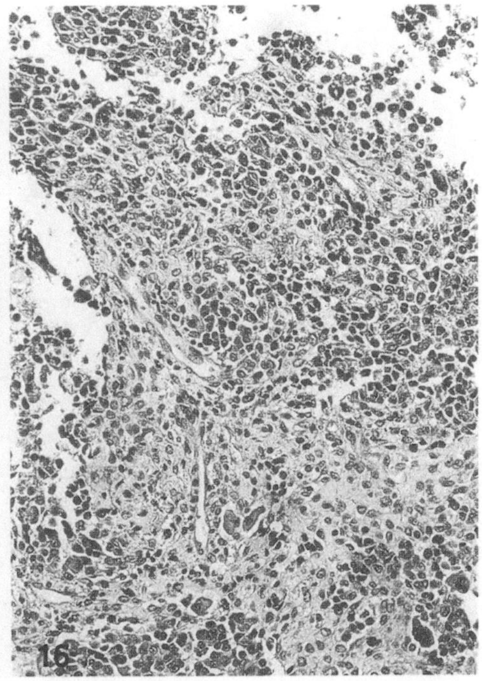

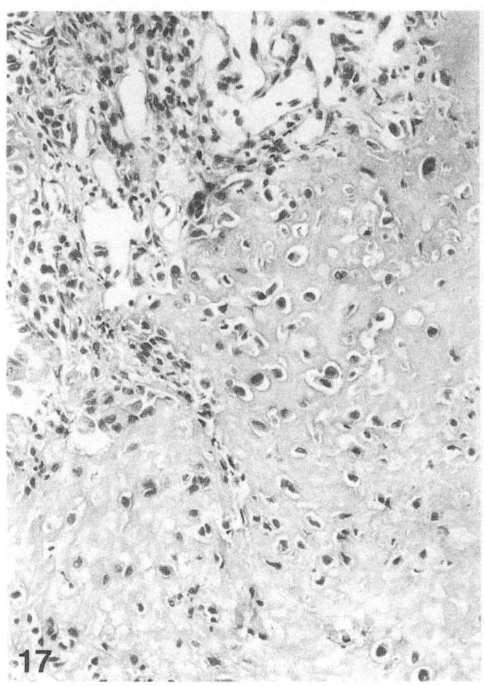

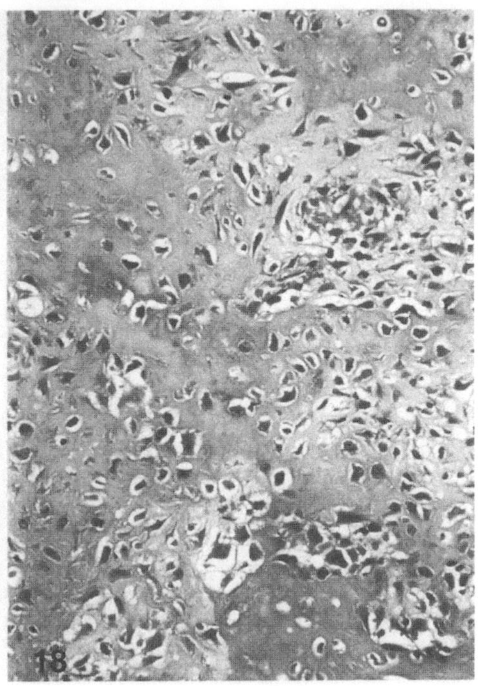

Fig. 15. The chondroblastic proliferation develops adjacent to large vessels, which may be the origin of the cystic formations

Fig. 16. In the zones of purely chondroblastic proliferation the cells, which are not mutually adherent but slightly retracted, are surrounded by an optically empty border

Figs. 17, 18. The chondrocytes of these cartilaginous areas are irregularly shaped and distributed; the general pattern is not that of a growth cartilage or of hyaline articular cartilage

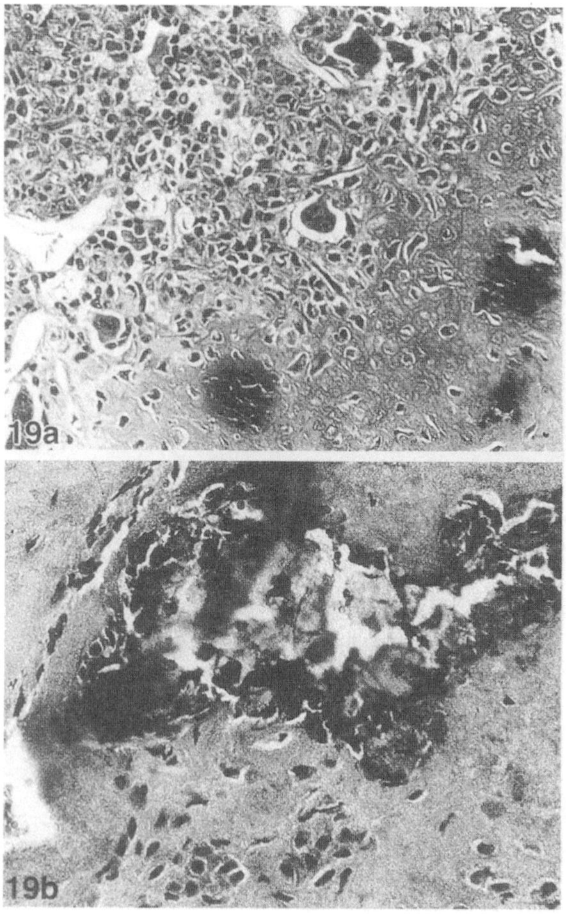

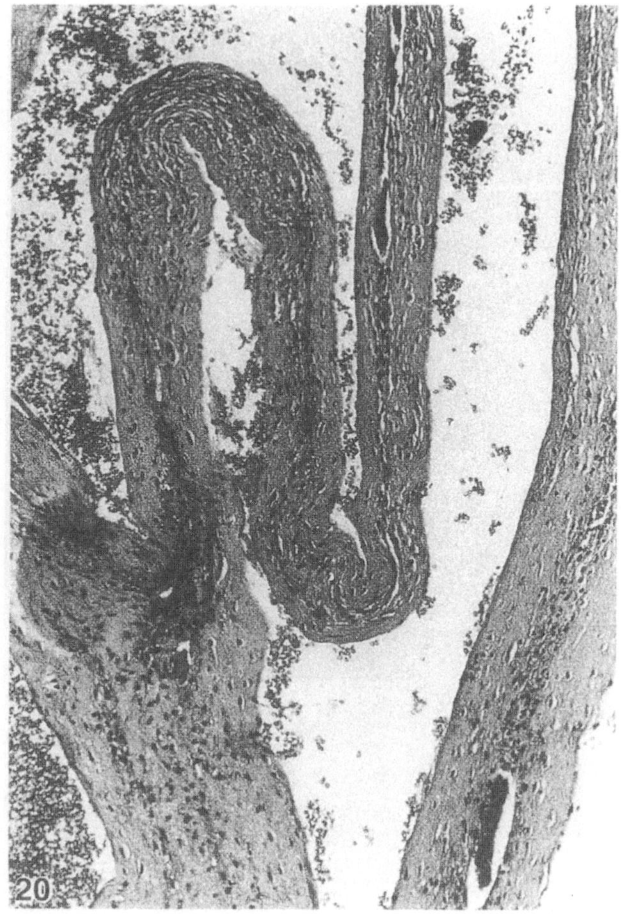

Fig. 19 a, b. Zones of calcification in the fibrocartilage at low and high magnifications

Fig. 20. Fibrous membrane surrounding a cystic cavity in a chondroblastoma

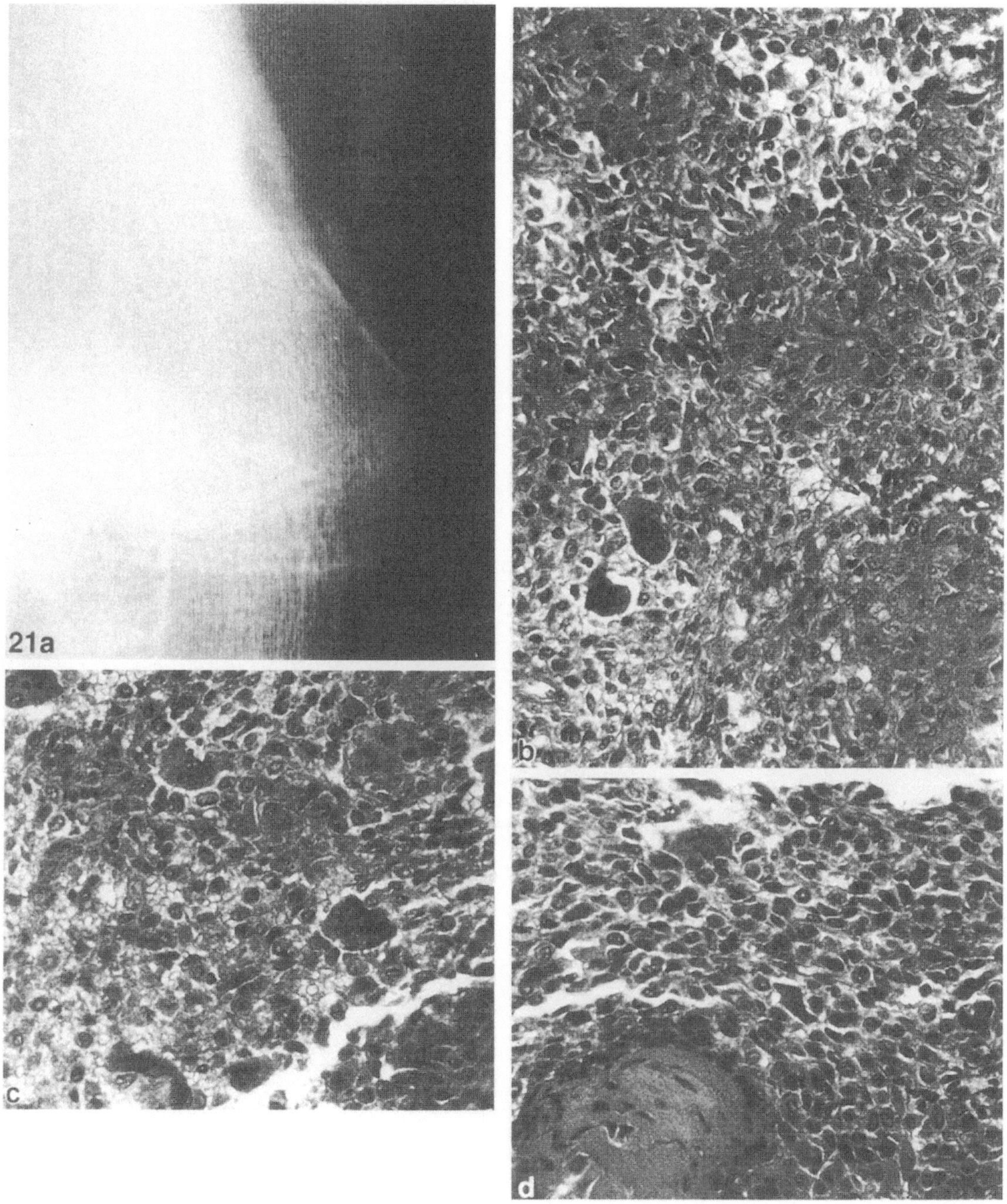

Fig. 21 a-d. Chondroblastoma at aberrant cortico-metaphyseal site in a boy of 14 (case of Dr Gubler, Hôpital Saint-Vincent-de-Paul, Paris)

6. Osteogenic exostosis (osteochondroma), multiple exostoses, subungual exostosis, metachondromatosis

Osteogenic exostosis and multiple exostoses

If we exclude fibrous structures such as non-ossifying fibroma and cortico-metaphyseal detect, the exostosis is the commonest of benign tumours: 40% of the total according to Dahlin and 10% of all tumours of bone.

Multiple exostoses is a familial and hereditary disorder of dominant mode [Maroteaux 1982] in which the prognosis must be more guarded.

Case history

Here is a case report which time may duplicate.

In 1980, Dr H., an orthopaedic surgeon, sent me for examination a typical exostosis developed on the inner aspect of the inferior right tibial malleolus. Two and a half years later, at the outer aspect of the lower end of the tibia, this adolescent young man developed an osteogenic sarcoma. This is one reason why it seemed wise to end the report with the advice to monitor the zone from which the exostosis had developed for at least 2 years, without causing the patient or parents too much concern.

Some have suggested that an osteosarcoma "always" develops on a preexisting lesion, but this is uncertain.

General considerations

Exostoses are commonest in males and are detected before the age of 10 years in multiple exostoses and before 20 in isolated cases. The elective sites are the metaphyses, at which they develop during the growth period: the metaphyses of the long bones are involved (lower end of femur, figs. 1, 2, upper end of tibia, but also the upper metaphysis of the humerus). The flat bones of the limb-girdles, ribs and vertebrae may be affected.

Clinical features

When solitary and painless, the lesion is often discovered by palpation as a hard mass attached to the bone in the vicinity of a joint. More rarely it is revealed by signs of compression of vessels or nerves or by interference with joint movements. The multiple form is often associated with deformities of the limbs and shortening (fig. 10). In most cases a solitary exostosis of moderate size, whose growth has ceased with that of the skeleton, remains "silent".

Maroteaux (1982) stresses the fact that it is impossible to predict the course of multiple exostoses in a young child with several exostoses of small size. At the end of development the number of exostoses may reach several dozen. It is obvious that the risks of complications are greater than in cases of solitary exostosis: deformities requiring corrective procedures, fracture of the pedicle, aneurysm [Stevenson & Zuska 1957, Clark & Koekarnt 1965, Schoene et al 1973], cord compression [Madignan et al 1974, Rosset et al 1990].

A rare developmental complication, but one to which the multiple disorder is more often exposed, is sarcomatous transformation. This is usually chondrosarcomatous rather than osteosarcomatous. The indicative features are recent increase in size and appearance of pain, and these features, which are by no means pathognomonic, make biopsy imperative or, better, should lead to immediate excision guided by imaging.

Imaging

The radiological appearances are varied (figs. 1-11). The tumour pedicle is of varying length and its base nar-

Table 1. Osteogenic exostosis

Exclude: - a juxtaosseous chondroma, which makes an impression on the cortex but only communicates with the medullary canal at a very late stage
Determine whether or not it forms part of: - a multiple exostosis or other dystrophic syndrome
Look for: - possible sarcomatous transformation, commoner in multiple exostoses

row or wide. The distal end is either part of a sphere or multilobular. In a view in the long axis, the base of the exostosis forms a rounded or oval image bordered by osteosclerosis. Radiography easily distinguishes between a sessile exostosis and a juxtacortical chondroma.

CT and radio-isotope scans are variously credited with the information they provide about malignant transformation. Both inflammation of the serious bursa which sometimes covers the exostosis and sarcomatous transformation are associated with an increased take-up of radio-isotopes (^{99m}Tc).

Pathological anatomy and histopathology

Macroscopically, the exostosis is formed by a body of spongy bone in continuity with the medullary cavity of the bone on which it is implanted. This spongy bone is bounded by a cortex continuous with that of the parent bone (fig. 9). Its distal extremity, at maturity, is covered with a bony layer overlaid by periosteum but at earlier stages by cartilage whose deep part undergoes ossification (figs. 16-18). In very young children, the thickness of this cartilaginous cap is often considerable.

The discovery of an exostosis calls for a skeletal survey to exclude any multiple disorder.

Histologically, the body of the exostosis consists of often porotic spongy bone; the marrow is of the same type as that of the parent bone. Superficially, the growth cartilage is covered by a fibrous perichondrium (fig. 15). The existence of immature cells in a thick cartilaginous cap is commonplace in young patients. The periphery of this cartilage cap, at its junction with the periosteum and bony tissue, is sometimes the site of a degree of cellular activity (fig. 22). The persistence of cartilaginous islands in the spongy bone at some distance from the growth zone is common (fig. 21).

The extremity of the exostosis may be covered with a newly-formed serous bursa (fig. 23).

In those cases, where I have observed transformation into a chondrosarcoma, the diagnosis was simple, even in cases of commencing malignant transformation and was characterised by a focus of cell proliferation with atypical cells while the overall morphology remained unchanged (figs. 24, 25).

Diagnosis

The diagnosis of exostosis is usually obvious macroscopically and microscopically. The main reasons for excising an exostosis only rarely involve the pathologist. Excision is usually a routine to protect the patient from possible malignant transformation, especially if there is a bulky exostosis or multiple lesions; for cosmetic reasons; following fracture; or when compression of organs, vessels or nerves develops.

Despite its relative frequency on the first rib, (18 out of 40 cases according to Rosset et al 1990), the exostosis is rarely incriminated in the syndrome of thoracic outlet compression, only once in 116 operations according to the same authors. The essential feature of the diagnosis is the continuity that exists between the parent bone and the exostosis. The exostosis develops like an accessory abortive epiphysis, and is connected to the parent bone like the appendix to the cecum.

The differential diagnosis of sessile exostosis (fig. 15 b) is juxtaosseous chondroma, adherent to the outer aspect of the cortex, which it tends to erode (fig. 13). In the vicinity of a small articulation, distinction may possibly be from an osteophyte, at least macroscopically.

When an exostosis is present, the main problems are to recognise whether it is a solitary lesion or part of a syndrome, a disorder of dominant transmission. (Maroteaux states that some apparently unaffected women may transmit the defect) and to detect malignant transformation originating from the cartilaginous cap. Here, cell proliferation and cells with large nuclei are indicative of this malignant transformation. Excision must be complete as persistence of a cartilaginous zone may lead to recurrence (fig. 12).

Subungual exostosis

General considerations

Described by Dupuytren, this lesion is specified not only by its site but also by its mode of development.

Usually solitary, it is primarily a fibroblastic lesion in its early stages (fig. 6 a, b).

It is localised on a phalanx of the hands or feet, in 77% of cases at the great toe; 10% occur in other toes and 13% on the fingers [Ganzhorn et al 1981, Muse & Rayan 1986, Miller-Breslow & Dorfman 1988]. It is slightly commoner in women (52%). It occurs at all ages, but is usually discovered during the third decade.

Clinical features

These are quite specific. Sometimes frankly subungual, it elevates the nail, which becomes perpendicular to the bony plane; sometimes it grows out laterally from the bone in contact with which it develops (figs. 6, 7). The diagnosis is often made at the outset, but in some cases the lesion is pigmented and suggests a melanoma; or, if ulcerated and infected, the diagnosis of malignant tumour or osteitis may be initially considered.

Imaging

At onset the radiological appearance is limited to a dense zone elevating the nail; at a later stage, calcified osteogenesis fused to the ungual phalanx is more characteristic.

Pathological anatomy and histopathology

From the histological angle, this curious lesion seems to develop as a fibroblastic or myofibroblastic proliferation which undergoes first cartilaginous and then osseous metaplasia. Some authors find a traumatic origin in 25% of cases; others deny this aetiology, while others still favour chronic irritation. However this may be, the presence of large chondrocytic nuclei in this type of lesion is not of serious import.

Metachondromatosis

This disorder, identified by Pierre Maroteaux in 1970, is listed here because under certain circumstances its diagnosis may be confused with that of osteogenic exostosis.

The lesions are polymorphous, sited mainly on the bones of the hand or foot, frequently associated with deformities of the metacarpals or phalanges of the fingers and toes. They may closely resemble exostoses developing at the epiphyseo-metaphyseal junction. Others assume bizarre forms and some ossifications or calcifications appear unrelated to the subjacent bone, from which they are separated by a clear border (fig. 14). One of the important points is the labile character of some lesions, which means that they should not be treated hastily; even a biopsy may give rise to complications.

Dominant transmission may be claimed but it seems that the expression of the gene may be variable [Maroteaux 1971].

References

Basset GS, Cowell HR, Delaware W (1985) Metachondromatosis. Report of four cases. J Bone Joint Surg 67A: 811-814

Beals RK (1982) Metachondromatosis. Clin Orthop 169: 167170

Clark PM, Keokarnt T (1965) Popliteal aneurysm complicating benign osteocartilaginous exostosis. J Bone Joint Surg 47A: 1386-1388

Dahlin DC, Unni KK (1986) Bone tumors. Charles C Thomas, Springfield

Deparis M, Manigand G, Manigand C, Guedon J (1959) La maladie exostosante. Sem Hop Paris 6: 400-405

Fanney D, Tehranzadeh J, Quencer RM, Nadji M (1987) Osteochondroma of the cervical spine. Skeletal Radiol 16: 170-174

Ganzhorn RW, Bahri G, Horowitz M (1981) Osteochondroma of the distal phalanx. J Hand Surg 6: 625-626

Kennedy LA (1983) Metachondromatosis. Radiol 148: 117-118

Landon RC, Johuson KA, Dahlin DC (1979) Subungual exostoses. J Bone Joint Surg 61A: 256-259

Madigan R, Worral TH, McClain EJ (1974) Cervical cord compression in hereditary exostosis. Review of the literature and report of a case. J Bone Joint Surg 56A: 401-404

Maroteaux P (1971) La métachondromatose. Kinderheilkunde 109: 246-261

Maroteaux P (1982) La maladie exostosante: maladies osseuses de l'enfant. Flammarion Médecine-Sciences, Paris, pp 110-120

Miller-Breslow A, Dorfman HD (1988) Dupuytrens (subungual) exostosis. Am J Surg Pathol 12: 368-378

Muse G, Rayan G (1986) Subungual exostosis. Orthopedics 9: 997-998

Perera S (1936) Recherches expérimentales sur la pathogénie des exostoses ostéogéniques à l'aide de greffes de cartilage de conjugaison. Presse Med 8: 162-166

Puigrenier P (1988) La métachondromatose (à propos d'un nouveau cas et revue de la littérature). Thèse, Limoges

Rosset P, Martinat H, Barsotti J, Gaisne E (1990) Exostose ostéogénique de la première côte: une étiologie rare de syndrome de traversée thoracobrachiale. A propos d'une observation. Rev Chir Orthop 76: 62-65

Schoene HR, Berthelsen S, Ahn C (1973) Aneurysm of femoral artery secondary to osteochondroma. J Bone Joint Surg 55A: 847-849
Stevenson CA, Zuska JJ (1957) Aneurysm of the popliteal artery from perforation by a solitary exostosis of the femur. A case report. J Bone Joint Surg 39A: 431-434
Unger EC, Gilula LA, Kyriakos M (1987) Ischemic necrosis of osteochondroma of tibia. Skeletal Radiol 16: 416-421

Fig. 1. Exostosis of lower end of femur. The trunk (or pedicle) of the exostosis supports a cap of lobulated outline. The cortices of exostosis and femur are continuous

Fig. 2. Unusual appearance of exostosis located in popliteal region

Fig. 3. Sessile exostosis of upper end of humerus in boy of 14 accompanied by deformation of the axis of the humerus

Fig. 4. Bulky lobulated exostosis of upper end of fibula in a man of 30. The extreme opacity suggests the presence of numerous islands of calcified cartilage. Such appearances usually pertain to multiple exostoses

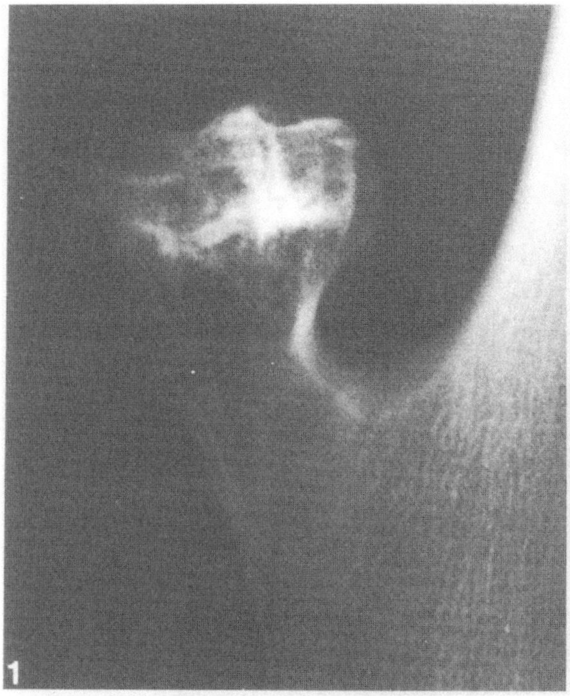
1

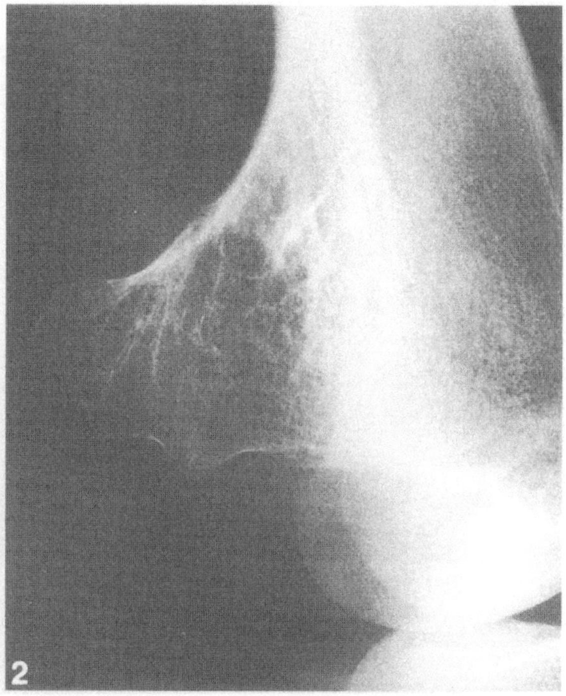
2

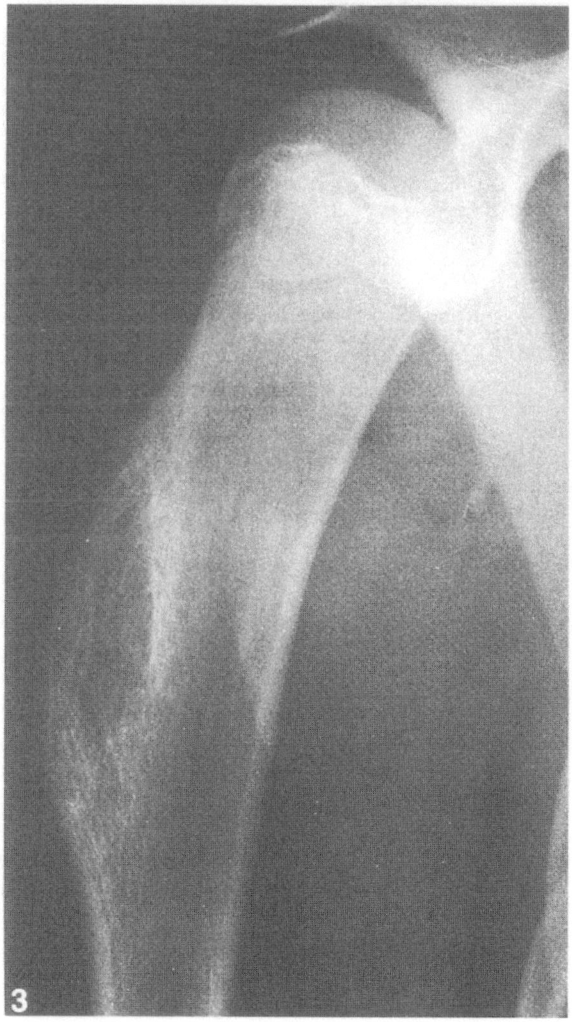
3

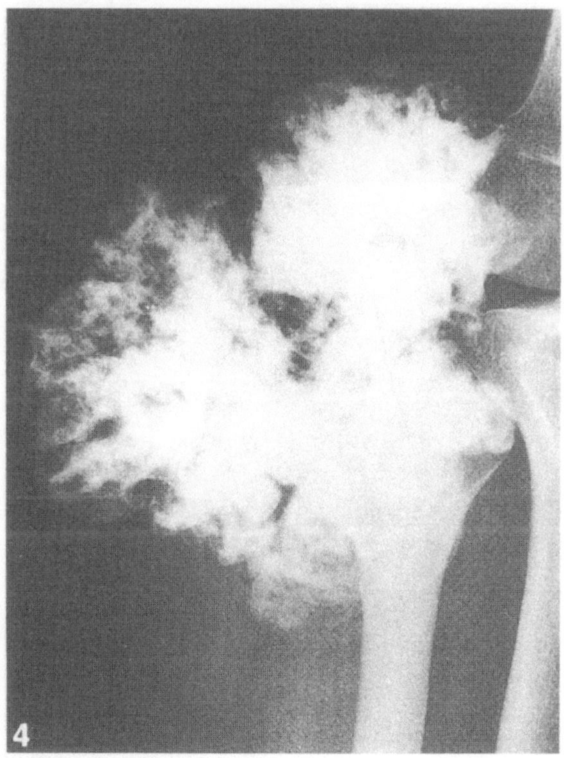
4

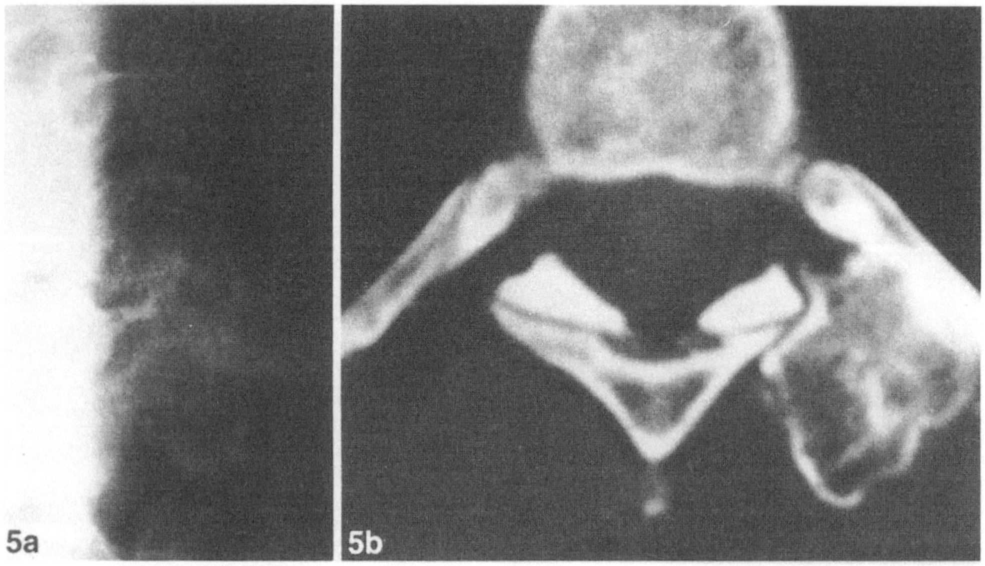

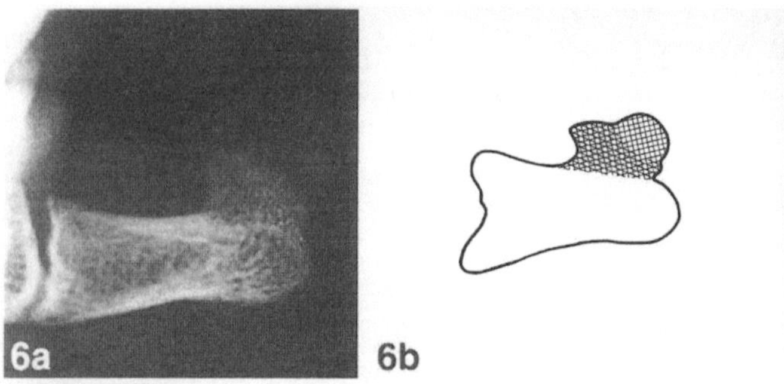

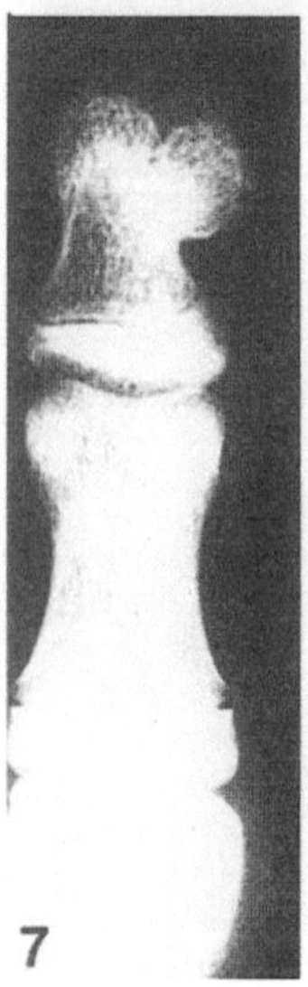

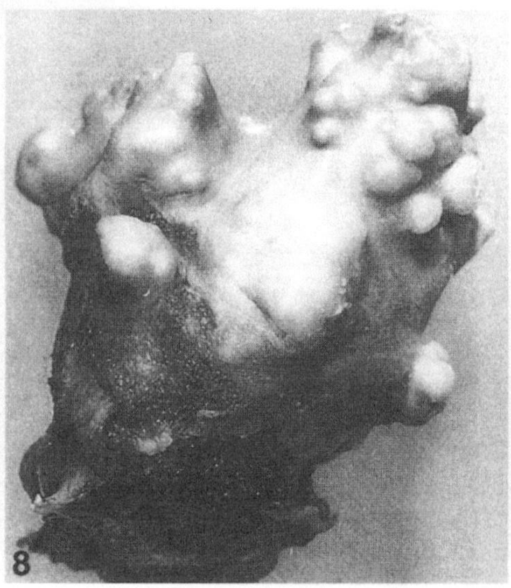

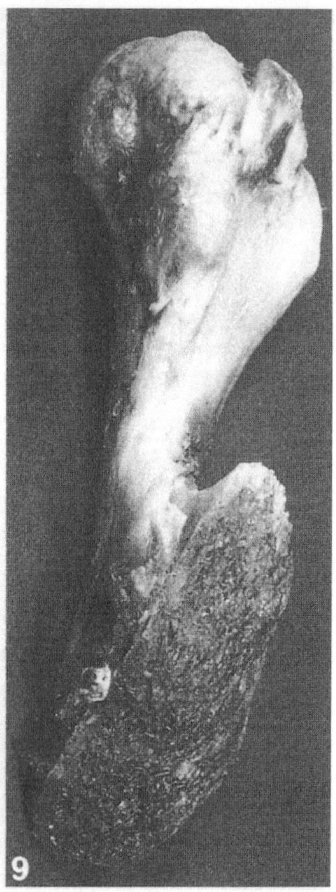

Fig. 5 a, b. Large exostosis developing in posterior vertebral groove in a girl aged 15

Fig. 6 a, b. Subungual exostosis. **a** Subungual exostosis covered by extensive cartilage elevating the nail almost perpendicular to the skin plane. **b** Diagram of this subungual exostosis: the deep part is ossified, the superficial part is a sort of ball of cartilage

Fig. 7. Exostosis developing at outer border of an ungual phalanx

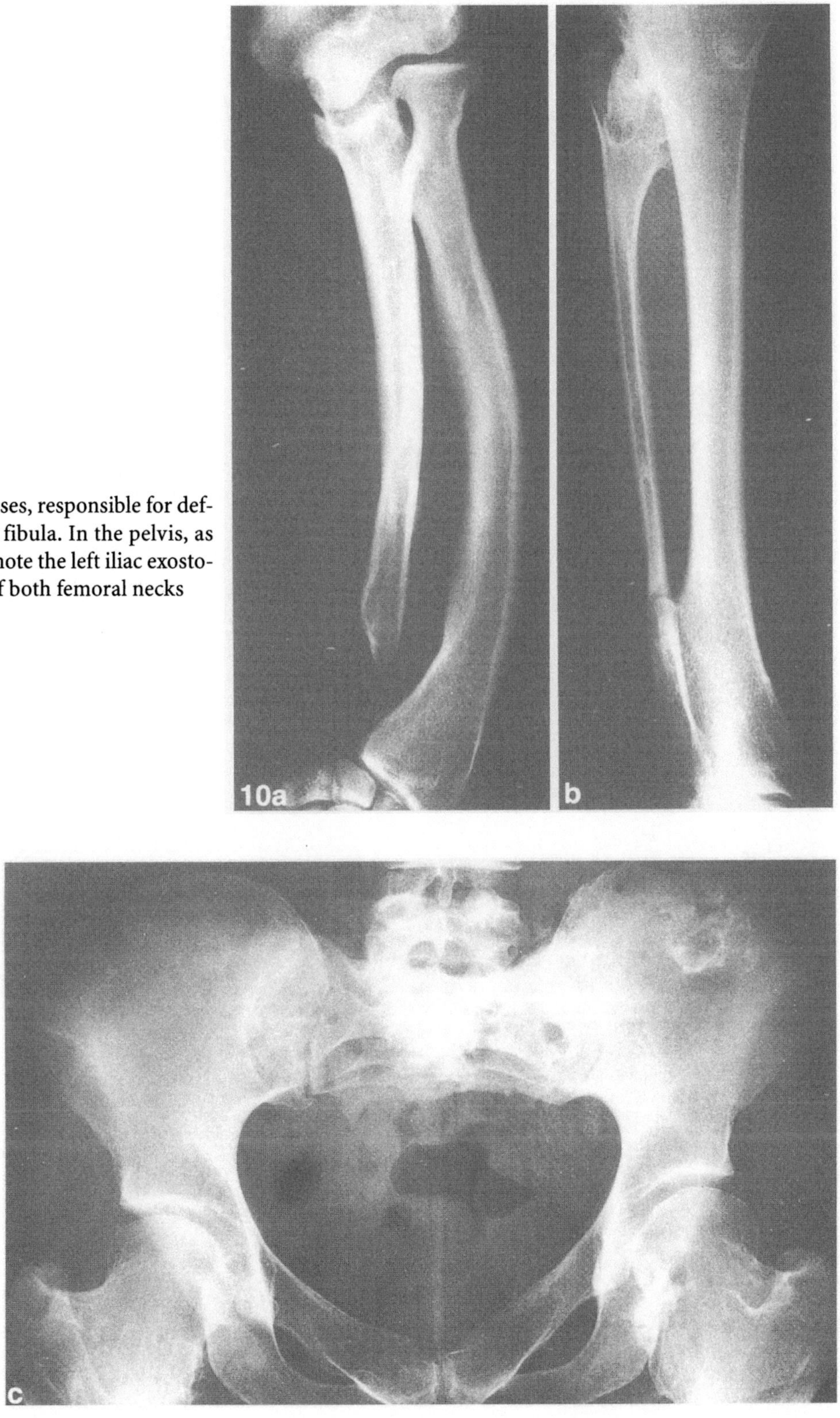

Fig 10 a-c. Multiple exostoses, responsible for deformation of forearm and fibula. In the pelvis, as well as the sacral lesions, note the left iliac exostosis and the hypertrophy of both femoral necks

Fig. 8. Large globular exostosis, covered with cartilage over much of surface. The possibilities of proliferation of this irregularly distributed cartilage lead to this appearance, which may suggest exostoses of the second generation

Fig. 9. Gross "hat-peg" appearance of pedicled exostosis. Excision, which has widely removed its base of implantation, inevitably opens into the medullary canal of the parent bone

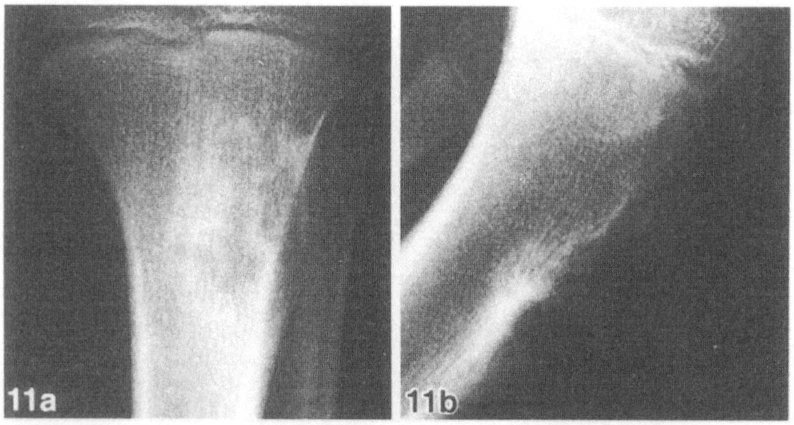

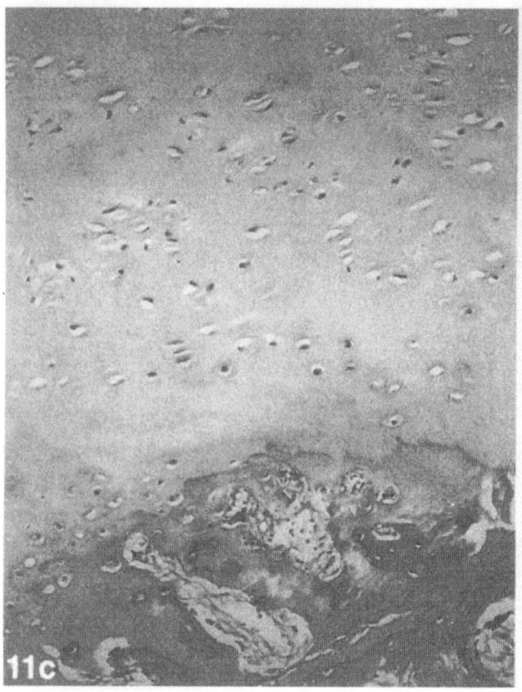

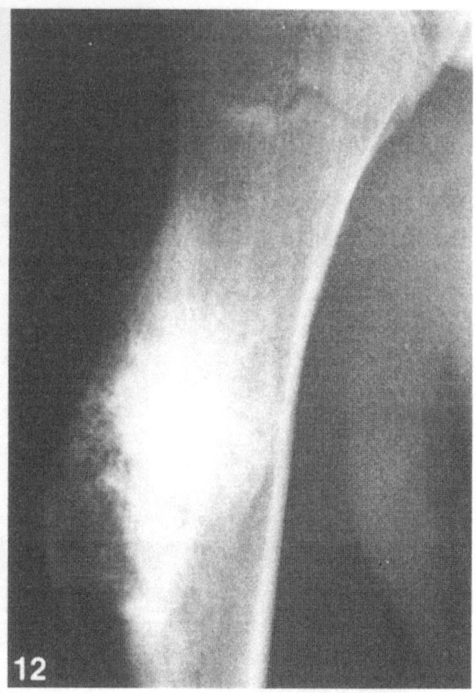

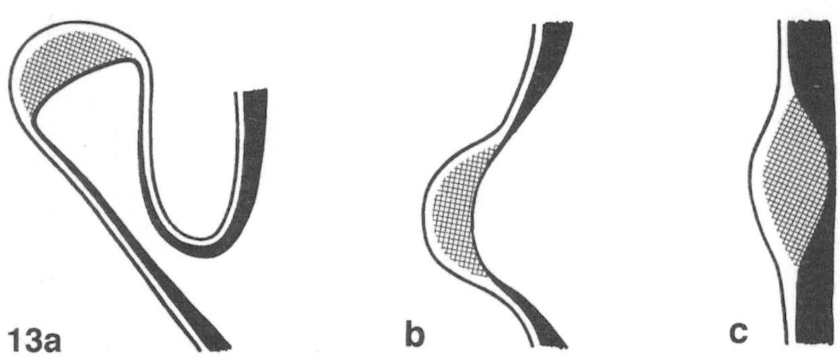

Fig. 11 a, b. Frontal and lateral radiographs of large cartilaginous "tumour" developing at the anterior tibial tuberosity in a girl of 7. **c** The histological sections reveal hyaline cartilage in which the relatively numerous chondrocytes, with small round nuclei, are embedded in well-defined chondroplasts

Fig. 12. Recurrence of sessile exostosis of humerus 4 years after operation (youth aged 15)

Fig. 13 a-c. Diagram showing types of (**a**) pedicled and (**b**) sessile exostoses; in both cases there is continuous communication with the marrow of the parent bone, contrasting with a periosteal chondroma (**c**) which makes a concave indentation on the cortex

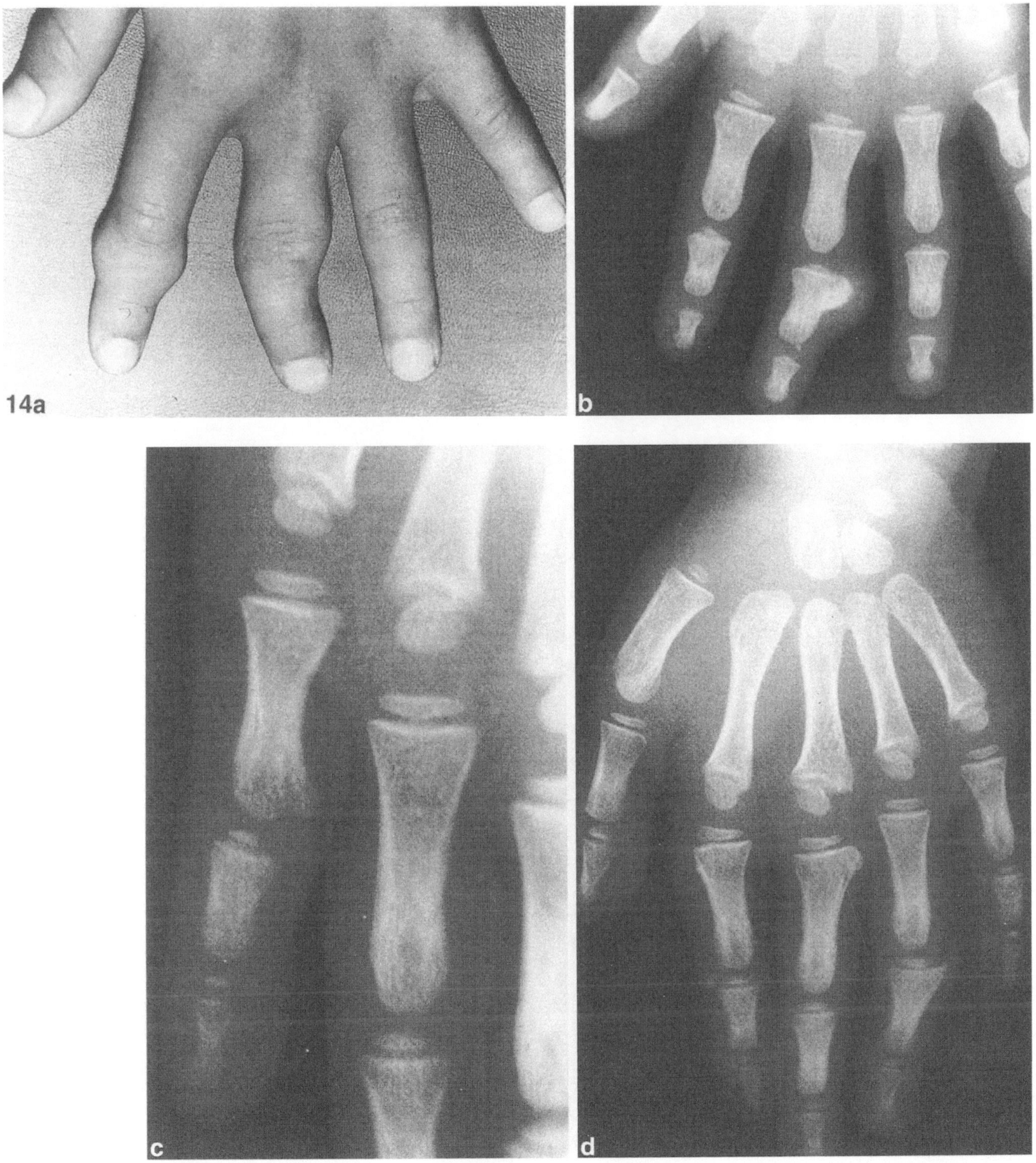

Fig. 14 a-d. Metachondromatosis. The multiple bony excrescences (**a, b**) visible in the radiographs are associated with deformities of the fingers (records kindly supplied by Dr Mouliès, Limoges, described in thesis of Dr Puigrenier, Limoges, October 1988). The radiographs (**c, d**) demonstrate juxta-articular bony excrescences at the origin of the angulation of the fingers (Case supplied by Dr Maroteaux, Hôpital des Enfants Malades, Paris)

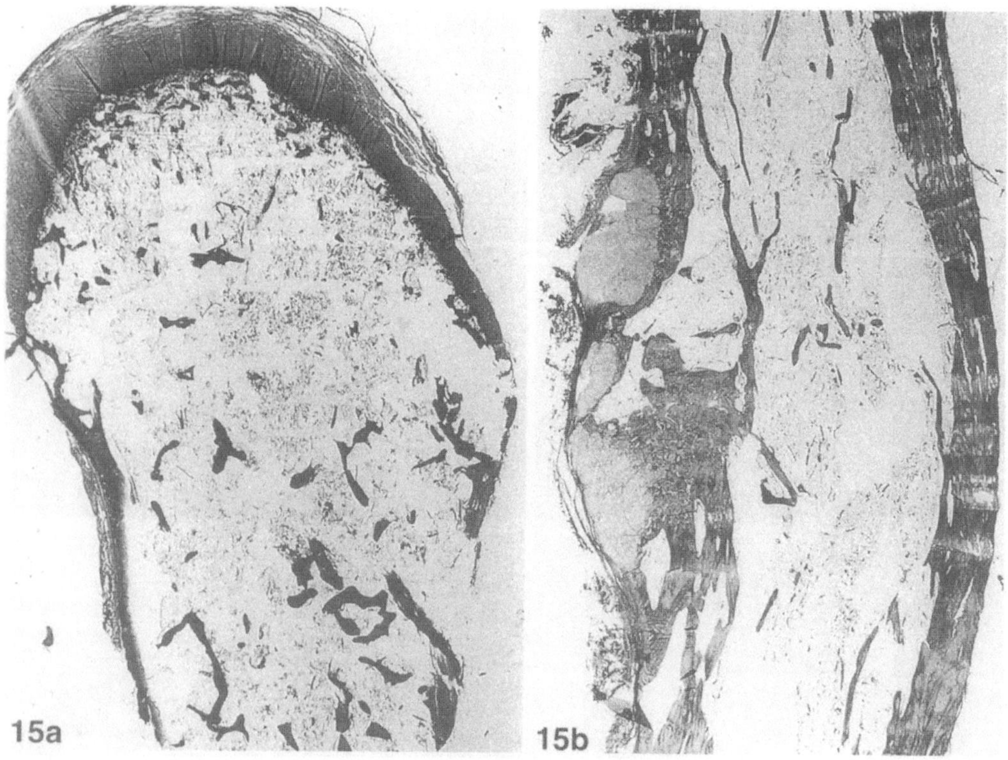

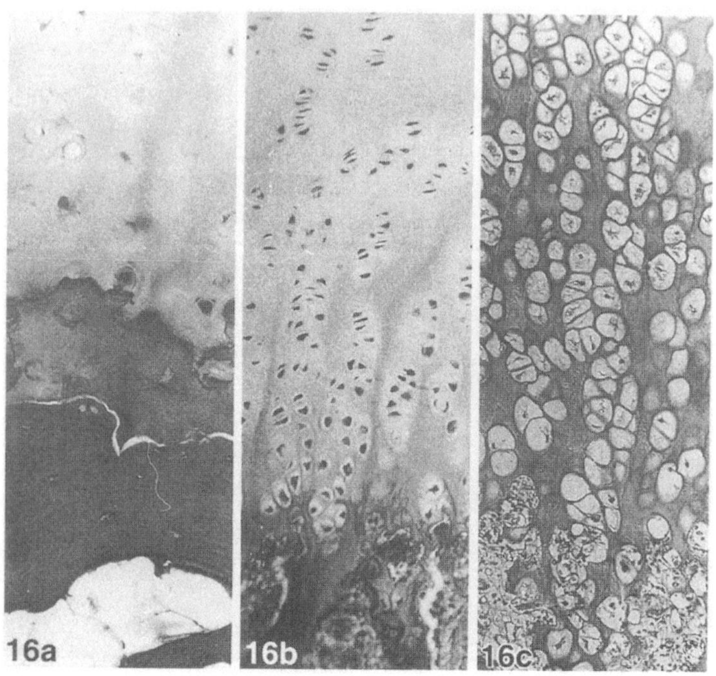

Fig. 15. **a** Low magnification of section of pedicled exostosis; the exostosis is covered by a thick smooth cartilage shell. The marrow of the spongy bone is fatty. **b** Sessile exostosis developed on a markedly curved ulna. Each is covered with a fibrous perichondrium

Fig. 16. **a** The cartilage is comparable to that of mature articular cartilage. Its deep calcified portion rests on a subchondral plaque of mature lamellar bone. **b, c** The arrangement of the chondrocytes in irregular small columns resembles that of growing articular cartilage. There is no subchondral bony plaque, the cartilage being in direct contact with a hypervascular medullary zone (figs. 17, 18)

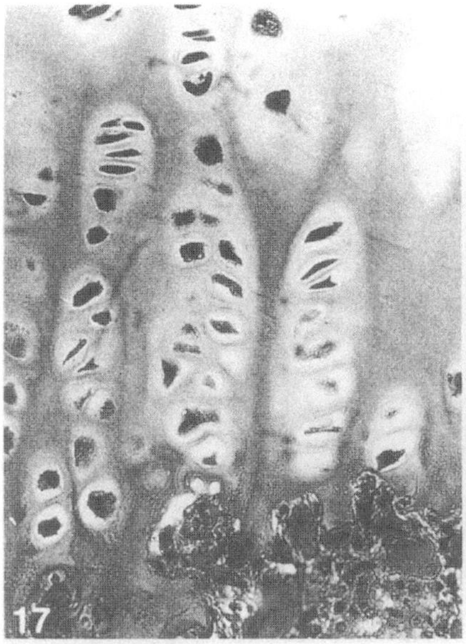

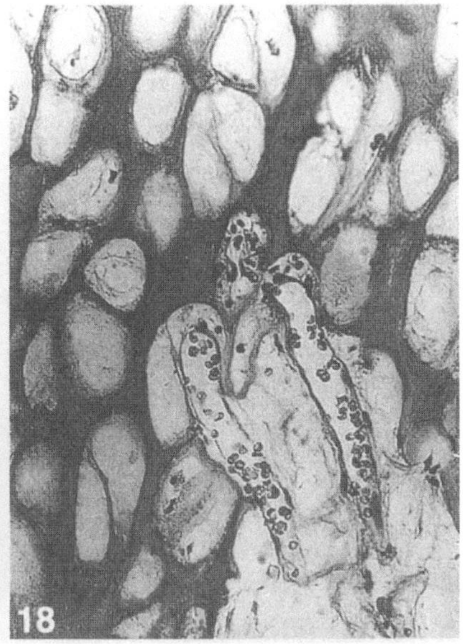

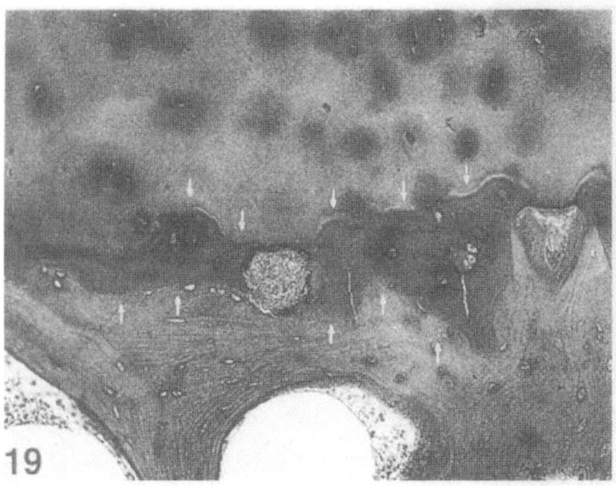

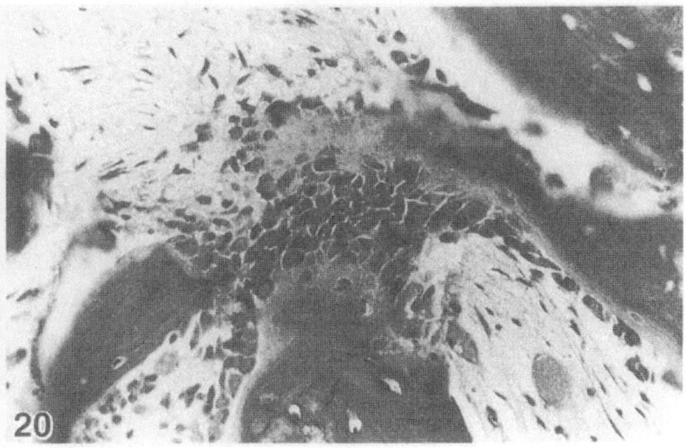

Fig. 17. Small chondrocyte columns of the cartilage of an exostosis, entirely comparable to those of articular cartilage; irregular hyperchromatic nuclei. At its base the cartilage is destroyed by the vascular proliferation

Fig. 18. Ballooned chondrocytes in a cartilage devitalised and invaded by bone marrow capillaries, in a phase preceding bone metaplasia

Fig. 19. For comparison: the zone of bone-cartilage junction in a femoral head, virtually identical to that observed in a mature exostosis. Arrows: zone of calcified cartilage

Fig. 20. Body of growing exostosis in a youth of 15. Considerable osteoblastic activity

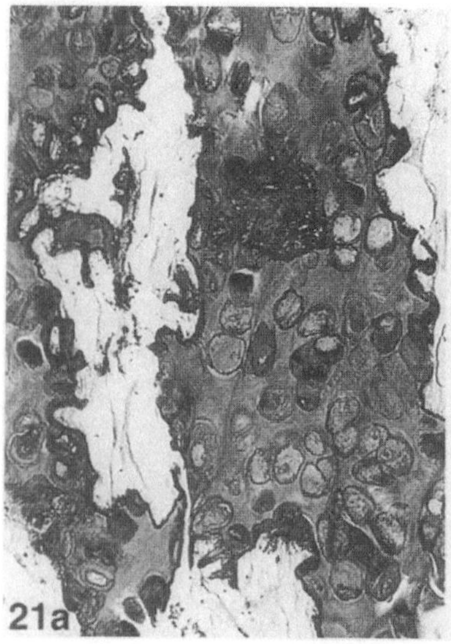

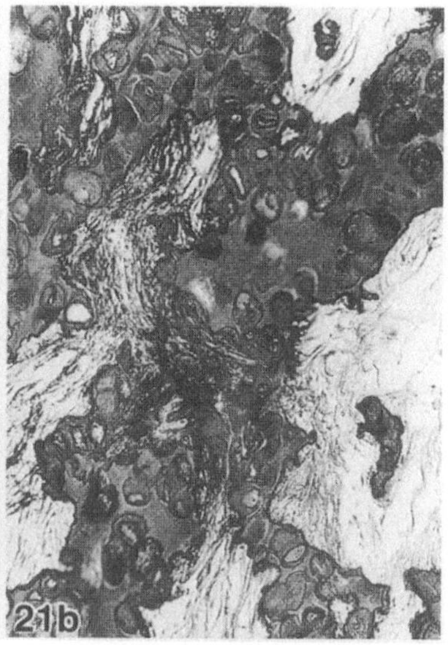

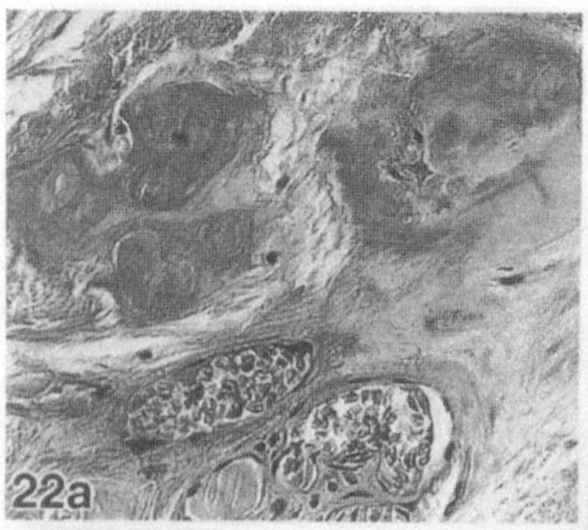

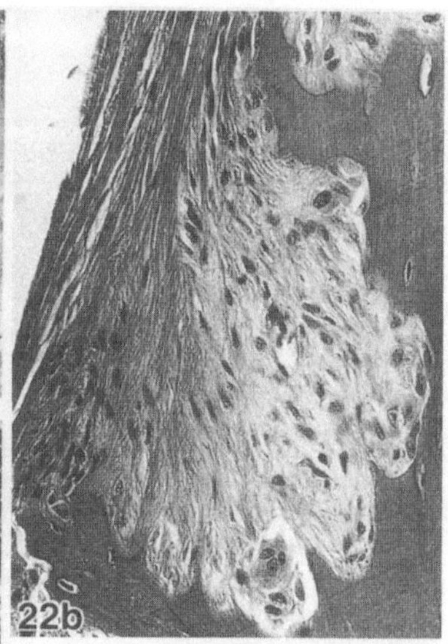

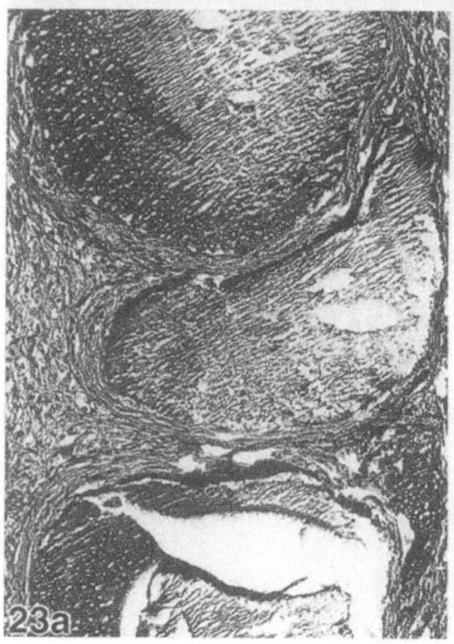

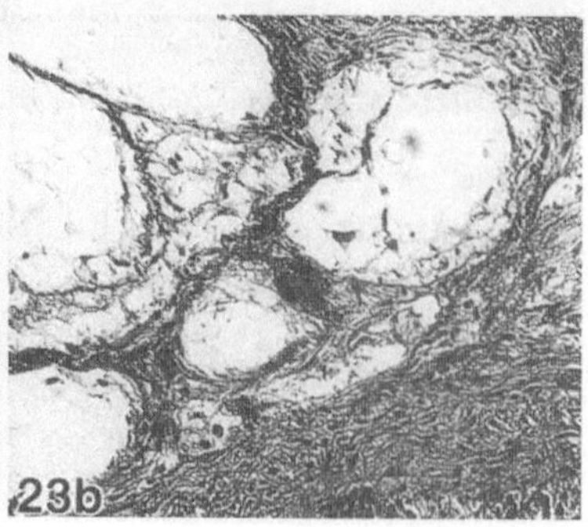

Fig. 21 a, b. The young bony strands often contain cartilaginous islands, sometimes numerous and relatively deep, remote from the superficial cartilage. This is seen especially in large exostoses, in a fibrous medulla (**a**). In the fibrous medulla there are also evident calcified deposits which resemble those of bone infarction (**b**)

Fig. 22 a, b. In growing exostoses, at the periphery of the cartilage, there is a zone of remodelling variably rich in osteoclasts. This resorption-remodelling may lead to the formation of an exostosis with a thin smooth "trunk" rather than a bulky "head"

Fig. 23 a, b. Degenerative changes in the compact tissues covering the exostosis sometimes lead to the formation of a serous bursa

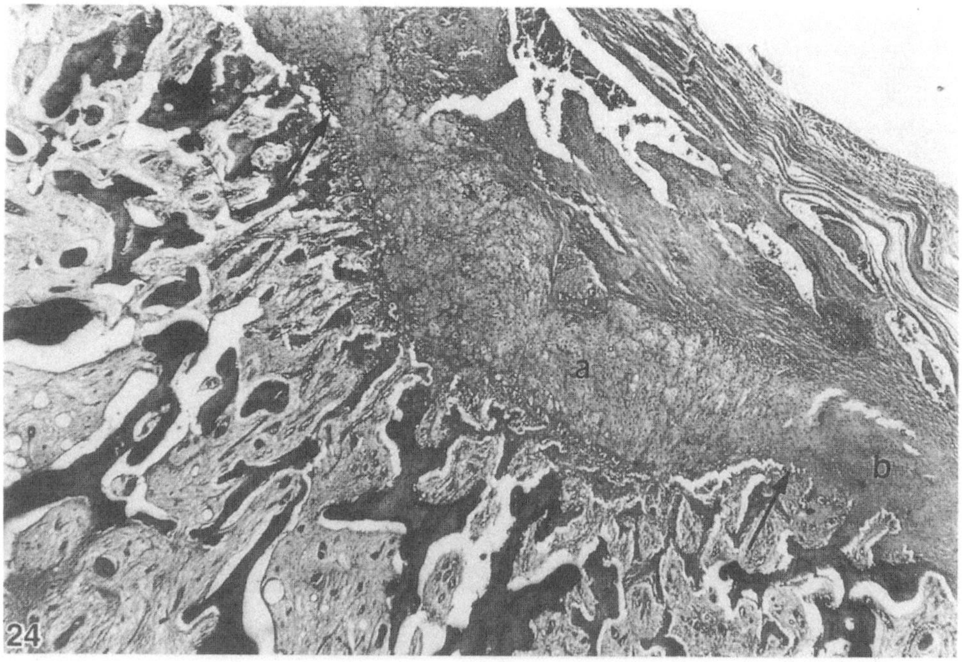

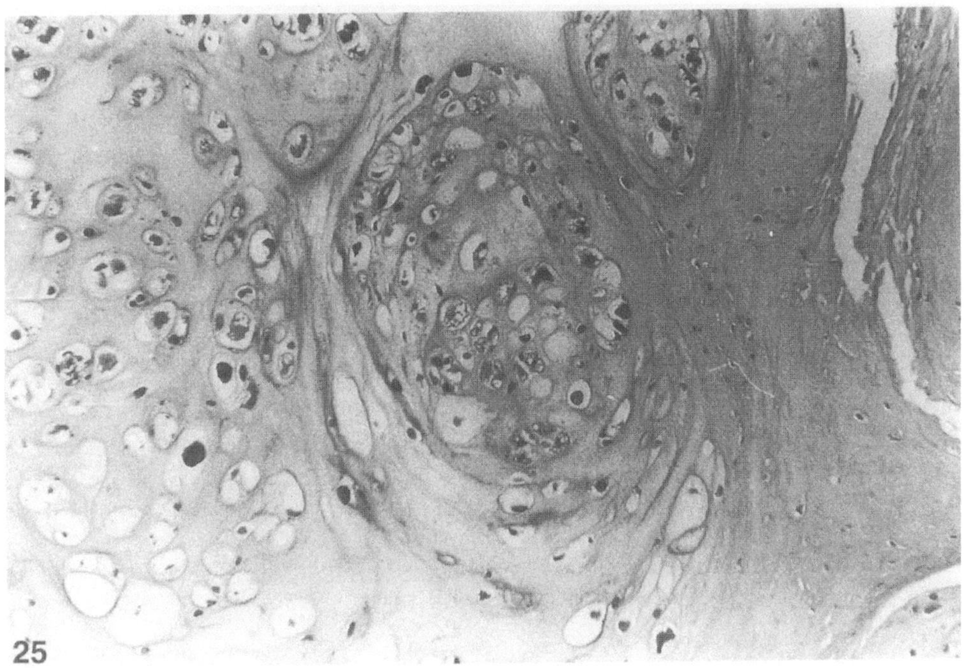

Fig. 24. At the surface of this exostosis, note an abrupt thickening of the cartilaginous cap (*arrows*). In this zone (a) the cells are more numerous and less differentiated and the ground substance takes up the stain unequally, giving a "flamed" appearance between the cell islands, an appearance very different from that of zone (b) where the hyaline matrix stains more uniformly and cellularity is less marked. These architectural and cellular changes may indicate the onset of malignant degeneration

Fig. 25. Here, the cell proliferation, anisocytosis, anisonucleosis and especially the presence of bulky nuclei, leave no doubt as to the malignant transformation of the cartilage of this exostosis

7. Osteoid osteoma and osteoblastoma

General considerations

In these two lesions, so often compared with one another, the cause is obscure, but the vascular component plays an essential part, in their pathological appearance if not in their genesis.

At its outset, the nidus of the osteoid osteoma, which is actually the entire lesion, is represented on radiographs by a round, clear, uncalcified image. The first stages of a superficial osteoid osteoma are very significant. The radiological image of an osteoid osteoma of the neck of the talus, for example, is only a simple notch hollowed out on the superficial aspect of the neck. During the following months, the development of an opaque zone at the center of the clear image is evidence of the calcium content of the osteoid strands of the nidus. At this stage, the nidus has the shape of a small reddish ball, easily enucleable from the cavity in which it is embedded. If operation is deferred, the image of the nidus continues to opacify.

Considered individually, the bony trabeculae are atypical, but the whole, on the contrary, suggests an organoid structure. On examining a mature osteoid osteoma, it is remarkable for its organoid appearance, which contrasts with the irregular angioid and osteoblastic proliferation of an osteoblastoma. As I wrote in 1971 in the Annales d'Anatomie Pathologique: "The osteoid osteoma is organoid, and its osteogenesis, particularly at the periphery of the nidus, is relatively regular, often like the spokes of a wheel... In contrast, the diffuse lesion of an osteoblastoma does not lend itself to any systematisation; it is evidently a non-organoid lesion". This distinction of architectural organisation seems more important than one depending on measurements of the diameter of the nidus.

The characteristic appearance of a mature nidus is quite different from that of an osteoblastoma, where clumps of osteoblasts, associated or not with an osteoid deposit, are distributed at random in a loose tissue traversed by numerous vessels and angiectases suggesting a diagnosis of angioma or aneurysmal cyst. But at their onset it is, even histologically, probably impossible to differentiate, between these two lesions, whose first radiological manifestation is only a small rounded translucent image.

However, it is useful to distinguish these two entities from the clinical, radiological and pathological aspects. This does not mean that we should ignore their resemblances, which may support the hypothesis that both tumours represent a sort of angio-osteoblastoma, one finite and organoid, the other diffuse.

Should a role in the morphogenesis of the osteoid osteoma be accorded to the unmyelinated nerve fibers which accompany the vascular axis and disappear into the nidus, whereas their absence in osteoblastoma may explain its architectural disorder and diffuseness? One may perhaps hazard this comparison; that the osteoid osteoma is to the osteoblastoma what, before antibiotics, the furuncle was to anthrax. Thus, starting from a probably common base, each tumour retains its specific anatomo-clinical expression.

References

Amari H (1972) Ostéome ostéoide et ostéoblastome bénin. A propos de 9 cas personnels. Thèse, Alger

Byers PD (1968) Solitary benign ostéoblastic lesions of bone. Osteoid osteoma and benign osteoblastoma. Cancer 22: 43-57

Campanna R, Vanhorn JR, Ayala A, Picci P, Betteli G (1986)

Osteoid osteoma and osteoblastoma of the talus. Skeletal Radiol 15: 360-364
Healey JH, Ghelman B (1986) Osteoid osteoma and osteoblastoma. Current concepts and recent advances. Clin Orthop 204: 78-85
Mazabraud A (1972) Remarques à propos de l'ostéome ostéoide et de l'ostéoblastome. Ann Anat Pathol 17: 177-186
Schajowicz F, Lemos C (1970) Osteoid osteoma and osteoblastoma. Closely related entities of osteoblastic derivation. Acta Orthop 41: 272-291

8. Osteoid osteoma

This lesion was described by Bergstrand in 1930 and then by Milch in 1934. In 1935, Jaffe reported 5 cases and termed it osteoid osteoma. Jaffe and Lichtenstein reported 30 cases in 1940. At certain sites, osteoid osteoma raised, and still raises, difficult problems of differentiation from osteoblastoma. The hyperalgic nature of the osteoid osteoma is related to its over-vascularity [Lindblom et al 1960] and to the presence of nerve filaments [Sherman & McFarland 1965], easier to follow in the vascular pedicle than in the tumour itself.

Case histories

Case 1. A man of 35, a woodcutter by trade, sought advice for neck pain, worse at night and partly relieved by aspirin. There was no relevant history, apart from the falls and strains common to this occupation. Pressure over C3 was painful, and the radiograph showed a rosette image at the base of the right apophysis of C3. The clinical history and radiographs were typical. Surgical intervention was followed by disappearance of the pain on the very day of operation.

Epilogue: two years later the patient was quite cured, and his father asked me if the miracle could not be repeated for his own arthritic hip.

Case 2. Miss X, aged 16, had suffered for 10-15 days from a pain located in the left ankle. This was worsened by fatigue, but not at night. The attentive and solicitous mother took her daughter to an orthopaedic surgeon; there was no time to lose, so they took a short-cut. The radiographs were negative. Clinical examination revealed slight pain on movement of the ankle joint. The laboratory work-up was negative. I received a biopsy of the ankle-joint synovium. There was a manifest inflammatory condition, with oedema, much vascularisation, and some perivascular lymphoplasmacytic infiltration; none of which did much to account for the aetiology of this arthritis.

The pain persisted, became more characteristic, and some months later I received the cause of this joint disorder: a nidus from the medial malleolus.

Epilogue: the mother of the young patient wanted to sue this incompetent pathologist who had not made a diagnosis of osteoid osteoma 3 months earlier from an inflammatory synovium; my surgical colleague dissuaded her.

Case 3. An adult required to lift heavy weights daily complained of uncharacteristic pain at the outer aspect of the lower third of his leg. In this patient, whose intervertebral disks showed obvious signs of damage, the rheumatologist consulted had thought first of sciatica. The radiographs of the leg were negative. Failure of medical treatment allowed the nidus to make an impression on the lower third of the fibula.

General considerations

Despite the fact that nearly half the patients describe a history of initial trauma, the aetiology of this lesion remains unknown. Osteoid osteoma is classed by most authors among benign tumours of bone [Dahlin & Unni 1986], of which it represents 10% of cases. Male predominance is of the order of 3: 1 or 3: 2; the statistics vary. The tumour emerges mainly between the ages of 5 and 25 years, but some cases have been reported as late as the 7th decade.

The femur and tibia share nearly equally in half the cases, as confirmed by the study of 26 cases by Furnes et al (1995). Sites in the long bones of the hands and feet, carpus and tarsus, are common. The neck of the talus (subperiosteal localisation), calcaneum (subperiosteal or intraosseous) are rarer but quite typical sites.

Clinical features and course

Pain as a symptom is sufficiently typical in the majority of cases to point to an initial diagnosis. It begins abruptly, first at night, and increases as the weeks pass to become both diurnal and nocturnal with the latter predominating. This pain is relieved by aspirin, and when the patient first attends it is not unusual for him to be taking several grams a day. Sometimes this classical pattern is absent and the pain may be moderate but some "giant" osteoid osteomas with little or no pain are probably osteoblastomas. In children, a vertebral lesion is often revealed by a stiff and painful scoliosis [Dubousset et al 1971].

Whether it is metaphyseal or epiphyseal [Blair & Kobe 1977, Seitz & Dick 1983, Fassier et al 1986, Damsin et al 1987], the development of osteoid osteoma often poses a diagnostic and therapeutic problem in preventing axial deviation (valgus, varus or recurvatum) in young patients. When the lesion is superficial, as at the inner aspect of the tibia, there is a palpable swelling and this zone may be tender on pressure, warmer and redder than the opposite side. In the vicinity of a joint the lesion is generally accompanied by a non-specific synovitis [Seruzier et al 1976, Moser et al 1990].

Cases are known with a typical radio-clinical diagnosis in which there is a spontaneous course towards cessation of pain after several years. One case to my own knowledge had two lesions, of which only one was treated surgically. Current medical treatments shorten the long delays before spontaneous cure [Kneisl et al 1992]. Precise location of the nidus is essential to successful management; complete excision leads to cure, with disappearance of the pain on the day of operation.

Osteoid osteoma does not undergo malignant change and a reported case of malignant transformation of a lesion treated surgically 7 years previously, without radiotherapy, does not constitute adequate proof.

Imaging

Some preliminary comments are helpful. Firstly, the appearance of the radiological image in a standard film is delayed in relation to the painful phenomena. If the lesion is juxta-articular, failure to resort to more efficient imaging will lead the clinician to suspect a joint disorder justifying synovial biopsy. Secondly, in the immature skeleton the development of an osteoid osteoma on a limb bone acts as if the tumour accelerated bony maturation. In the femoral neck, for instance, the increase in length and thickness is evident on comparison with the sound side.

Image of the early nidus

This is a rounded translucency of some millimeters in diameter.

Fully developed nidus

Some months after onset, the central portion of the nidus opacifies, giving the image of a little spherical ball (figs. 1, 3, 4). The bone around the nidus is the site of major secondary remodelling. The manifestations of this remodelling are determined by the site of the nidus in the bone and the skeletal age.

The image of an osteoid osteoma (that is of the nidus) is merely a simple notch hollowed out in the subjacent cortex in a superficial site, for example at the upper part of the neck of the talus (fig. 8a). In an intracortical situation on the shaft of a long bone, there is a major periosteal reaction forming a spindle aligned in the long axis and surrounding the shaft over two-thirds of its periphery. The cortical bone itself in contact with the nidus is spongy. Radiologically, the dominant feature is the diaphyseal hypertrophy, referred to as osteosclerosis (fig. 5). The opacity resulting from the superimposition of the spongified cortex and the apposed periosteal new bone is a density that may obscure the osteolysis of the nidus in a standard film. When the nidus is deeply embedded in the spongy bone, the hyperplastic bone reaction is much more discrete. I have noted the acceleration of bony maturation in an immature metaphyseal zone.

In cases where the standard radiological image is doubtful, scintigraphy and/or CT allow good location of the nidus.

In the metacarpals and metatarsals, the hyperplastic bone reaction may be considerable, suggestive of spino ventosa or even osteogenic sarcoma. In the digits, the tissue hypertrophy may involve the soft tissues, as seen in some angiomas.

The presence of a double nidus in one and the same zone of opacification has been reported as have double lesions in the same patient [Gkynn & Fichtenstein 1973, Nelson et al 1994].

Pathological anatomy and histopathology

Macroscopically, the nidus presents in the form of a little compartment containing a small spherical "ball", reddish and more granular than smooth in consistency and more elastic than bony (fig. 8 b). This small ball, surrounded by a fine layer of reddish connective tissue, is easily separable from its bony compartment. If the nidus is hollowed out in a bony cortex, the latter is spongified and thickened by periosteal apposition.

At the neck of the talus, the nidus is often intra-articular, at the junction with the articular cartilage. It elevates the synovium in the form of a small "raspberry", whose upper part is within the joint and lower half in the bony cavity. There is an associated inflammatory synovial hypertrophy.

At histological examination, the central zone of the nidus is immature atypical bony tissue, made up of strands of unequal thickness joined in an irregular network (fig. 11). The most central part is often a small partly calcified osteoid zone (fig. 17 a). In some niduses, there may be a small markedly calcified area of pagetoid appearance in the central part or at the periphery of the ossified zone (fig. 21). This central part of the nidus is surrounded by osteoid strands of more regular arrangement, often radial (fig. 14). Between the bony strands there develops a loose and very vascular connective tissue. Numerous osteoclasts and osteoblasts surround the bony web. The osteophytes are irregularly distributed (fig. 17 a, b).

One osteoid osteoma may vary greatly from another; in some the nidus is very calcified, in others the difference between the central and peripheral zones is minimal.

It is an important to note that the nidus itself typically contains no necrosis, inflammatory infiltration or atypical mitoses. It is surrounded by bone with wide interlacing strands within a fibrous and highly vascularised marrow. With a cortical diaphyseal lesion, as in the femur, the haversian canals are markedly enlarged (fig. 11), and this spongified cortex is continuous with the periosteal apposed bone on the one hand and with a medullary osteogenesis on the other; this latter may be absent and is usually less well developed than the superficial osteogenesis. Lastly, the spongified cortex, periosteal bone and newly-formed medullary bone exhibit great architectural similarity. In the spongy bone, the remodelling surrounding the nidus is evidenced by a more or less marked thickening of the bony strands (fig. 12). It is apparent that these changes in the bony tissue around the nidus are contingent, and depend on local conditions.

Table 1. Osteoid osteoma: differential diagnosis

Early osteosarcoma. The diagnosis is based on the cytology, irregular osteogenesis, sometimes plexiform. The overall architecture of an osteoid osteoma is destroyed by curettage or aspiration.
Brodie's abscess: there is no necrosis or leukocytosis in the nidus; if need be, look for micro-organisms
Early osteoblastoma: small rounded structure, impossible to distinguish from osteoid osteoma

When removal is performed by block resection of the tumour, examination of serial sections reveals a vascular pedicle in almost every case. When the nidus is superficial, this pedicle is directly connected to the capsulo-synovial tissues (figs. 14, 15). In cortical osteoid osteomas, sections in a favourable plane make it possible to follow the course of a thick-walled artery in a bony canal through the periosteal and cortical bone (fig. 16 a, b). Unmyelinated nerve fibers accompany these vessels, to be distributed in the connective tissue in and around the nidus [Schulman et al 1970].

It is impossible to avoid comparison with Masson's glomus tumour, of which osteoid osteomas seems to be the bony homologue: the angio-leio-neural components of the glomus have become angio-osteo-neural. As with the glomus tumour, osteoid osteoma may be either hyperalgic or almost painless. Lastly, if some fragments of synovium accompany the excised nidus, it is commonplace to observe therein perivascular lymphoplasmocytic infiltrates, more rarely true lymphoid aggregations [Seruzier & Dorfman 1976].

Diagnosis

The diagnosis is obvious in well-characterised forms; alerted by the clinical features and imaging, the histological examination readily reveals the features described above. The absence of necrosis, atypical mitoses and cytonuclear anomalies is an important negative feature. When block resection is made, the overall appearance is organoid. This resolves a problem of a nosologic nature, as was stressed in the introduction to the chapters on osteoid osteoma and osteoblastoma. Given this distinction, it is quite certain that it is not always possible to differentiate between these two lesions in the histological sections. Vertebral or metacarpal lesions readily depart from the standard pattern. The important fact remains recognition of the benign nature of a lesion, which can be cured if correctly treated.

Another problem, rare in the light of recent progress in imaging and peroperative location of the nidus by radioactive isotopes using mini-probes [Vigorita & Ghelman 1983, Augereau et al 1988, Pernot et al 1991], used to be the histological demonstration of the nidus in a zone of painful osteosclerosis suspected of harbouring an osteoid osteoma.

There is one problem which may always confront every pathologist, and our rheumatologists and orthopaedists colleagues: the examination of a synovial biopsy for "arthritis" of unknown origin. The synovitis is certainly present, clinically and histologically; there is hypervascularity, oedema, lymphocytic and lymphoplasmocytic perivascular infiltration. The report must allow for the possibility, among other causes, of a nonspecific synovitis associated with an underlying bony lesion [Jaffrès et al 1970, Cronemeyer et al 1981].

In cases where the clinical features are not clearly specific, other diagnoses are necessarily suggested by the radiological appearances. A "hailstone" image surrounded by bony sclerosis at the lower end of the femur may suggest a Brodie's abscess, while in a phalanx a poorly circumscribed round translucent image may evoke a chondroma, glomangioma or spherical cyst, lesions which present no problems in histological recognition. A Brodie's abscess is not difficult to exclude, bearing in mind that there is neither necrosis nor leukocytic infiltration in the nidus of an osteoid osteoma.

The really important differential diagnosis is from well-differentiated osteoblastic osteosarcoma. Current techniques of removal of the nidus, fortunately increasingly less traumatic for the patient [Kohler et al 1990] do not allow recognition of the organoid nature of osteoid osteoma and consequent confirmation that removal has been complete. Moreover, even when removed by curettage, small bony fragments of atypical osteogenesis from the nidus do not bear the stamp of a benign lesion beyond all dispute. Thus it is imperative to examine multiple sections to ensure the absence of cytonuclear monstrosities, atypical mitoses and necrosis. Despite every care, it is very probable that the histological report may only mention in its conclusions the absence of histological signs of malignancy and the possible compatibility of the removed fragments with a nidus, to the extent that the clinical and radiological findings support this hypothesis.

Treatment

Current treatment is well discussed in the article by Kohler (1996). It is to be feared that minimal techniques of ablation of the nidus may be followed by a certain number of "recurrences". The various possibilities include the continuing development of an incompletely removed nidus. In this context, it should be realised that it is easier to make a firm diagnosis from the first intervention than from a recurrence, since the resumption of tumour development occurs in a setting modified by the first operation. One must also consider an osteoblastoma, whose initial radio-clinical and histological features reproduce the morphology of an osteoid osteoma, and an osteosarcoma undiagnosed at the first ablation.

Hyperalgic osteoma

Before concluding this section, we should remember that every painful osteosclerosis is not an osteoid osteoma. In some cases, although resection of a thickened densified bony region may have completely eliminated the painful phenomena, radiography of the specimen and even serial sections every 5 mm do not reveal the nidus. These cases of undiscovered nidus may be interpreted as representing the progress towards healing of a lesion which, oddly enough, has remained painful, unless this is an osteoma or osteoangioma that may be labelled a hyperalgic osteoma (cf Chapter 10).

In other circumstances this may relate to post-traumatic Paget's disease, as in a case of Paget's disease of the upper third of the tibia in a male patient aged 38. The orthopaedist, after long hesitation, was finally convinced of the propriety of operation by the patient's eloquent expression of intolerable pain persisting for over a year.

References

Augereau B, Wioland M, De Labriolle-Vaylet C, Padovani JP, Martin TH, Verneret C, Apoil A, Milhaud G (1988) Le repérage isotopique per-opératoire des ostéomes ostéoides et autres lésions hyperfixantes à la scintigraphie. Rev Chir Orthop 74: 764-770

Bergstrand H (1930) Über eine eigenartige, wahrscheinlinch bisher nicht beschriebene osteoblastiche Krankheit in den langen Knochen der Hand und des Fusses. Acta Radiol 2: 597-613

Blair WF, Kube WJ (1977) Osteoid osteoma in a distal radial epiphysis. Clin Orthop 126: 160-161

Brailsford JF (1944) Radiology of bones and joints. Williams & Wilkins, Baltimore

Bulas RV, Hayes CW, Conway WF, Loughran T (1992) Osteoid osteoma of the patella. Skeletal Radiol 21: 326-329

Cronemeyer RL, Kirchmer NA, De Smet AA, Neff JR (1981) Intra-articular osteoid osteoma of the humerus simulating synovitis of the elbow. A case report. J Bone Joint Surg 63A: 1172-1174

Dahan PH (1962) Etude d'un cas d'ostéome ostéoide du col de l'astragale. Thèse, Paris

Dahlin DC, Unni KK (1986) Bone tumors. 4th edn. General aspects and data on 8,542 cases, pp. 88-101

Damsin JP, Aufaure P, Sirinelli D, Carlioz H (1987) Un cas d'ostéome ostéoide épiphysaire. Rev Chir Orthop 73: 63-65

Dockerty MB, Ghomerley RK, Jackson AE (1951) Osteoid osteoma; a clinico-pathologic study of 20 cases. Ann Surg 133: 77-89

Dubousset J, Queneau P, Lacheretz M (1971) Problèmes diagnostiques posés par les scolioses raides douloureuses chez l'enfant. Rev Chir Orthop 57: 215-226

Fassier F, Duhaime M, Marton D, Brochu P (1986) Un cas d'ostéome ostéoide de l'épiphyse de la tête fémorale chez un enfant de 9 ans. Rev Chir Orthop 72: 215-217

Gille P, Nachin P, Laurian IM, Aubert D (1985) Le repérage isotopique per-opératoire dans la chirugie de l'ostéome ostéoide. Rev Chir Orthop 75: 123-126

Gkynn JJ, Lichtenstein L (1973) Osteoid osteoma with multicentric nidus. A report of two cases. J Bone Joint Surg 55A: 855-858

Israeli A, Zwas S, Horoszowski H, Farine I (1983) Use of radionucleid method on pre-operative and intra-operative diagnosis of osteoid osteoma of the spine. Clin Orthop 175: 194-196

Jaffe HL (1935) A benign osteoblastic tumor composed of osteoid and atypical bone. Arch Surg 31: 709-728

Jaffrès R, Courtois B, Mazabraud A (1970) Ostéome ostéoide avec réaction articulaire de voisinage. Rev Rhum Mal Osteoartic 37: 394-396

Kneisl JS, Simon MA (1992) Medical management compared with operative treatment of osteoid osteoma. J Bone Joint Surg 74 A: 179-185

Kohler R, Mazoyer JF, Besse JL, Bascoulergue Y (1990) Traitement de l'ostéome ostéoide par résection percutanée sous contrôle tomodensitométrique. A propos de 5 cas. Rev Chir Orthop 76: 284-287

Kohler R (1996) Ostéome ostéoïde in: Les tumeurs osseuses bénignes de l'enfant. Sauramps Medical, Montpellier

Lindblom A, Lindval PN, Sodergerg G, Spjut HJ (1960) Angiography in osteoid osteoma. Acta Radiol 54: 327-333

Milch H (1934) Osteoid-tissus-forming tumor simulating annular sequestrum. J Bone Joint Surg 16: 681-688

Moser RP, Kransdorf MJ, Brower AC, Hudson T, Aoki J, Hudson Berrey B, Sweet DE (1990) Osteoid osteoma of the elbow a review of six cases. Skeletal Radiol 19: 181-186

Nelson MC, Brower AC, Ragsdale BD (1987) Osteoid osteoma of left 6th rib with inflammatory reaction in the adjacent pleura and hyperostosis of the adjacent ribs. Skeletal Radiol 16: 601-603

Nelson MC, Lack EE, Freedman MT (1994) Multifocal osteoid osteoma in a 26 years old child (case report). Skeletal Radiol 23: 465-467

Pernot PH, Rigal S, Yedeas M, Gaillard JF, Wioland M, Desgeorges M (1991) Exérèse des ostéomes ostéoides rachidiens sous contrôle isotopique. Rachis 3: 455459

Piatkowski S, Warda E (1973) L'ostéome ostéoïde localisé au niveau du calcanécum. Rev Chir Orthop 59: 609-613

Rinsky LA, Goris M, Bleck EE, Halpern A, Hirschman P (1980) Intraoperative skeletal scintigraphy for localization of osteoid osteoma on the spine. J Bone Joint Surg 62: 143-144

Schulman L, Dorfman H (1970) Nerve fibers in osteoid osteoma. J Bone Joint Surg 52A: 1351-1356

Seitz WH, Dick HM (1983) Intra-epiphyseal osteoid osteoma of the distal femur in a 8 year old girl. J Pediatr Orthop 3: 505-507

Seruzier E, Simonin JL, Ducastelle C, Hemet J, Biga N, Thomine JP, Deshayes P (1976) Ostéome ostéoïde avec synovite. A propos de 2 observations. Rev Rhum Mal Osteoartic 43: 521-526

Seze S, Debeyre J, Ordonneau P, Djian A, Mazabraud A (1955) L'ostéome ostéoide. Sem Hôp Paris 30: 1-7

Sherman MS (1947) Osteoid osteoma. Review of the literature and report of 30 cases. J Bone Joint Surg 29: 918-930

Sherman MS, McFarland G (1965) Mechanism of pain in osteoid osteoma. Southern Med J 58: 163-166

Vigorita VJ, Ghelman B (1983) Localization of osteoid osteomas use of radionuclide scanning and autoimaging on identifying the nidus. Am J Clin Pathol 79: 223-225

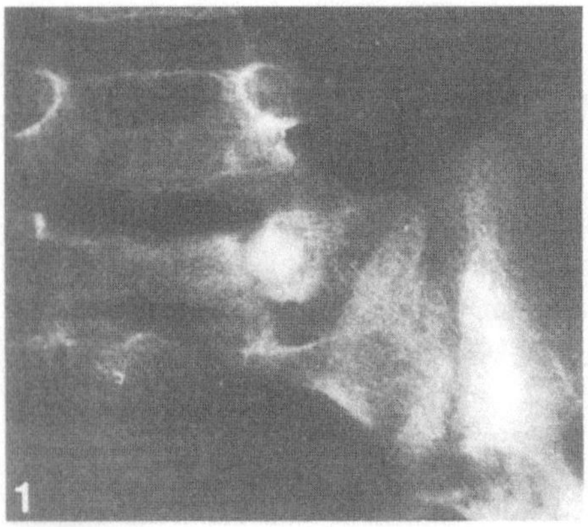

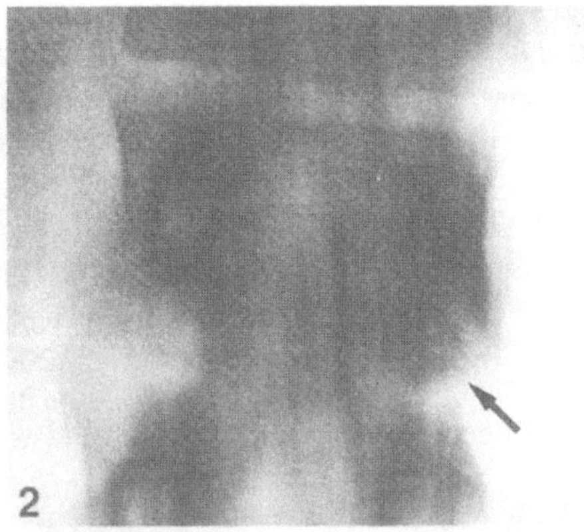

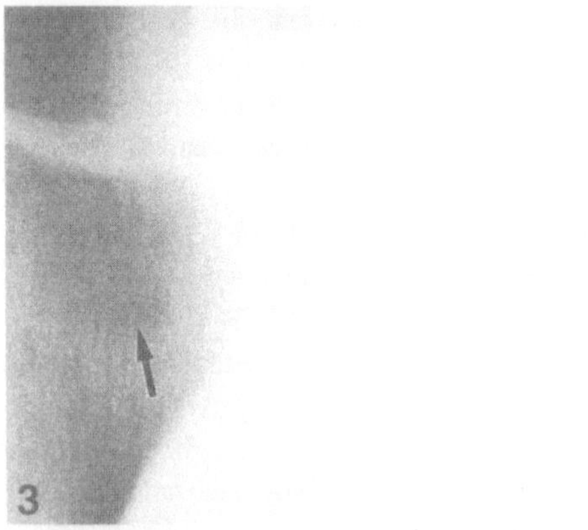

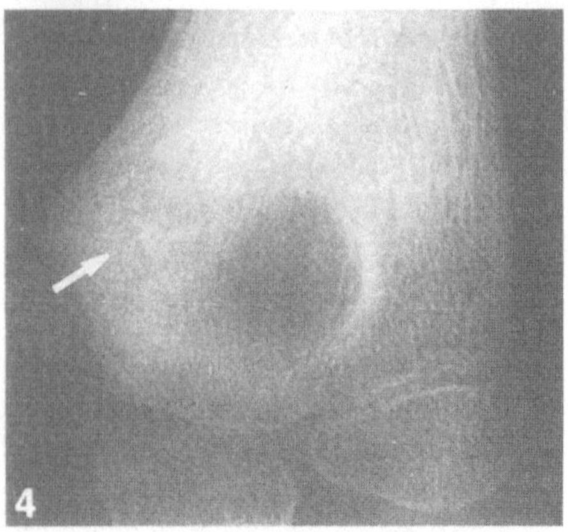

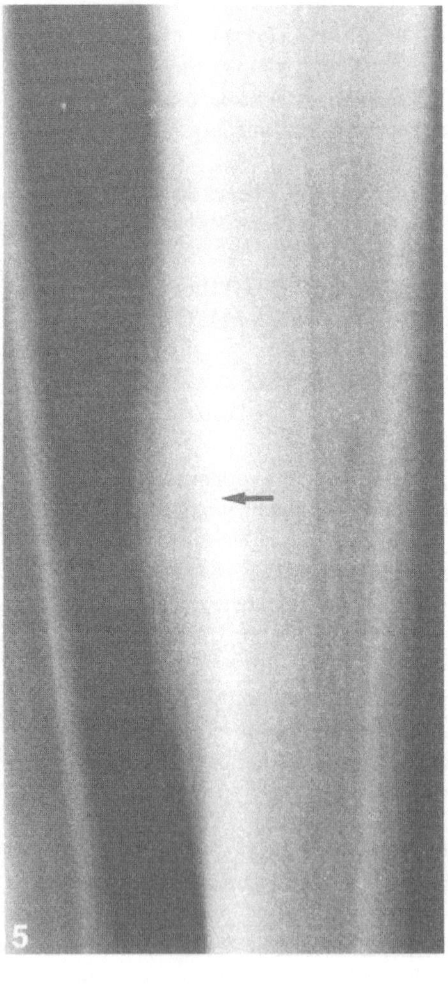

Fig. 1. Osteoid osteoma of first sacral segment. The nidus is particularly opaque, and seen as a disk surrounded by a radiolucent halo. In contrast with the marked calcification of the nidus, the peripheral osteosclerosis is relatively minor

Fig. 2. Osteoid osteoma of first lumbar vertebra. The calcified nidus is plainly visible, as is the clear halo (*arrow*). The opacity of the osteosclerosis partly conceals the attachment of the pedicle on the vertebral body

Fig. 3. Osteoid osteoma of lateral tibial plateau. The central calcification, the clear halo and the peripheral osteosclerosis give the so-called "rosette" image (*arrow*)

Fig. 4. Osteoid osteoma of lower end of humerus. Typical rosette image: the peripheral sclerosis is moderate

Fig. 5. Osteoid osteoma of tibial shaft. The superficial tumour is surrounded by a spindle of bony sclerosis developed along the axis of the bone; this bony sclerosis tends to ensheath the cortex. At the center of this extensive periosteal osteogenesis the translucent image of the nidus is visible even in this standard film (*arrow*)

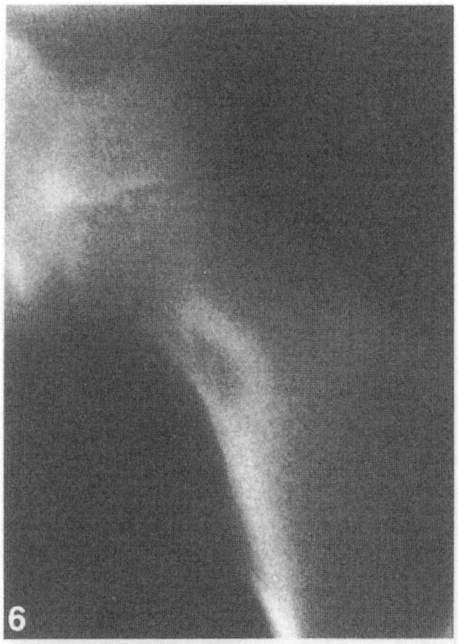

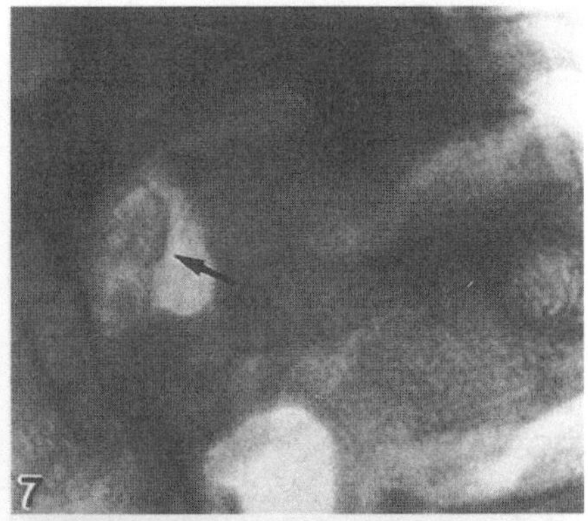

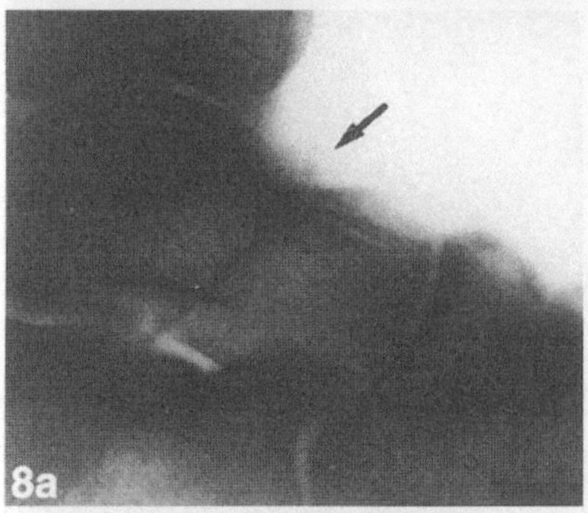

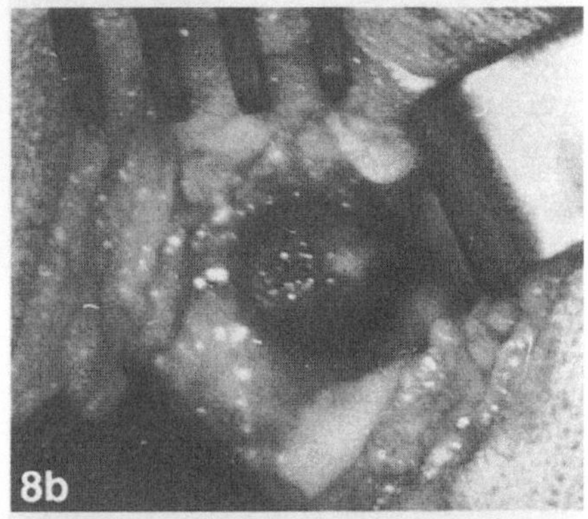

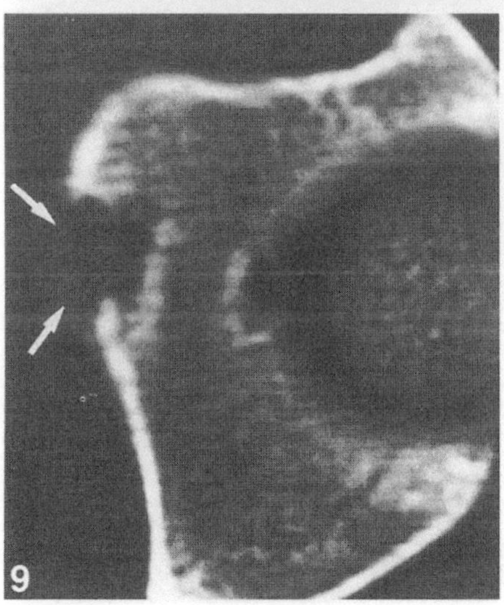

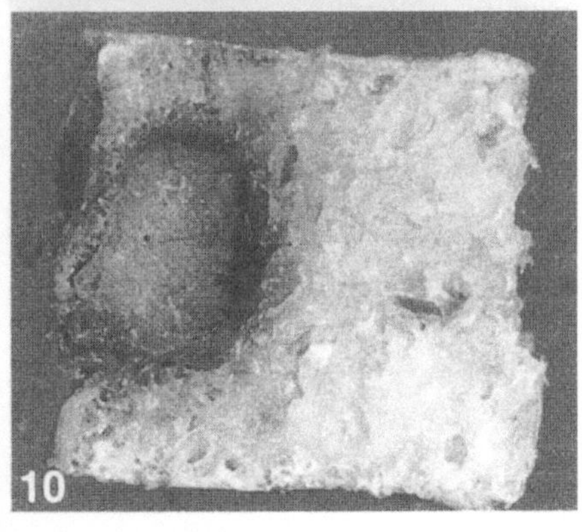

Fig. 6. Osteoid osteoma of inferior border of femoral neck. Typical appearance; however, the sclerosis has developed mainly below the tumour

Fig. 7. Osteoid osteoma of upper articular apophysis of C3. The typical rosette image is located at the base of the articular apophysis. This hypertrophied apophysis partly obstructs the intervertebral foramen (*arrow*). Case history 1

Fig. 8 a, b. Osteoid osteoma of upper aspect of neck of talus [Thesis of Dr Dahan 1962)]. In this radiograph taken several months after onset of clinical features, there is seen (**a**) a minuscule round slightly densified "patch" above the neck (*arrow*). At operation, the incision led to a reddish "sphere" (**b**) which seemed to be applied to the neck of the talus. Its removal was followed by immediate and permanent cure

Fig. 9. CT image of osteoid osteoma of acetabulum

Fig. 10. Resection specimen (femur) The central ossified part of the nidus is separated from the reactive bone by a zone of hypervascular connective tissue (blackish in this photograph)

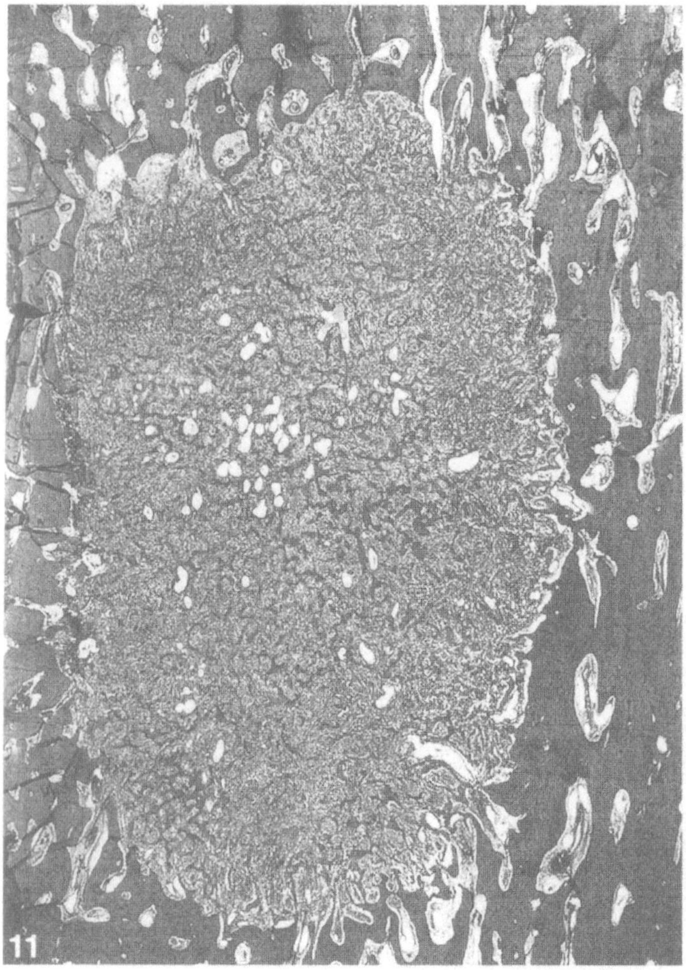

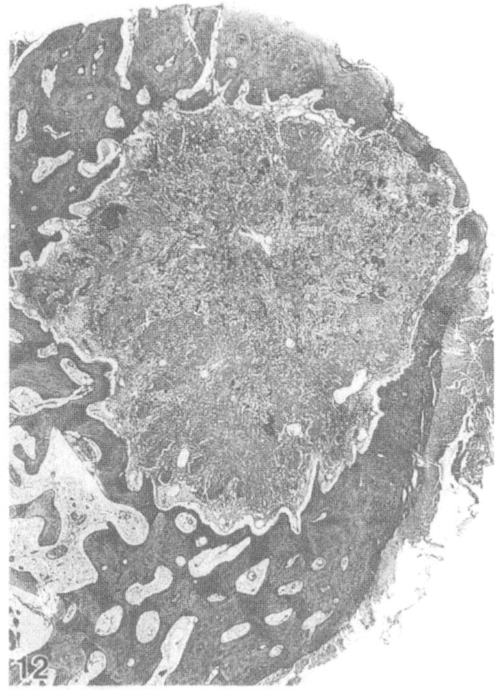

Fig. 11. Osteoid osteoma of femur, low magnification: the nidus is ovoid, its long axis parallel to that of the femur. The osteoid strands form a relatively regular plexus. Around the nidus, the enlarged haversian canals are traversed by wide vessels. The nidus is well circumscribed and the whole has an organoid appearance (-archive specimen)

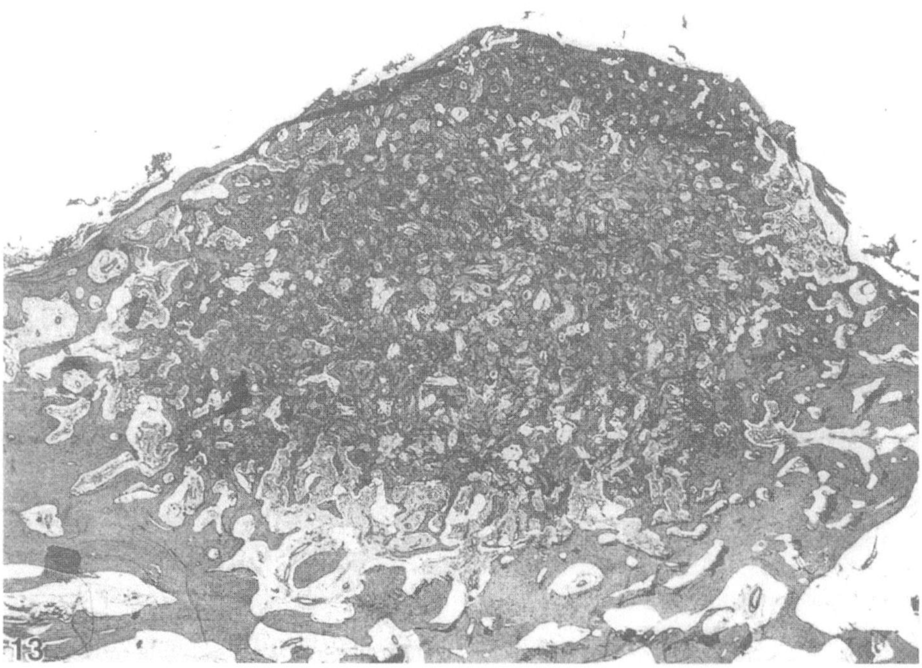

Fig. 12. Osteoid osteoma of metatarsal. The section is perpendicular to the axis of the bone and shows thickening of the trabeculae of spongy bone and destruction of the cortex

Fig. 13. This superficial nidus developing subperiosteally has partly destroyed the cortex, which is spongified. The nidus is virtually completely ossified. There is no appreciable periosteal reaction

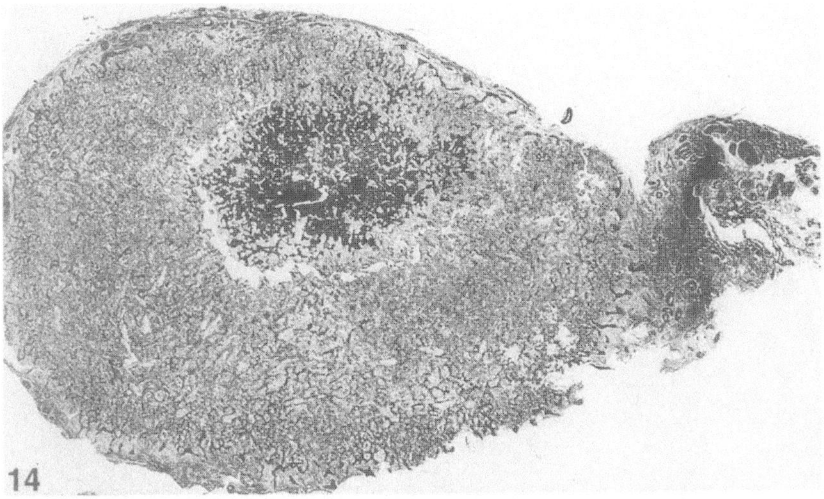

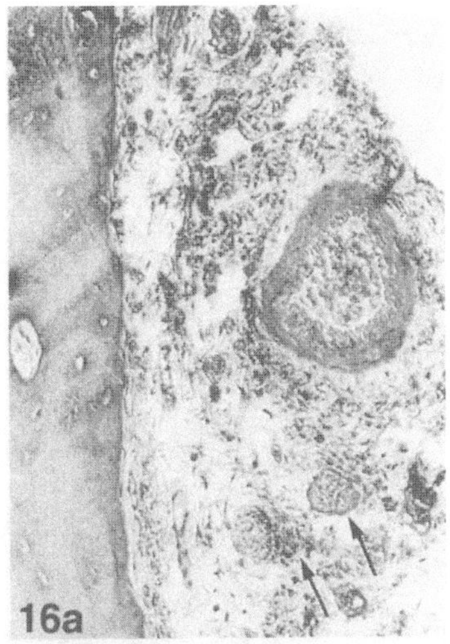

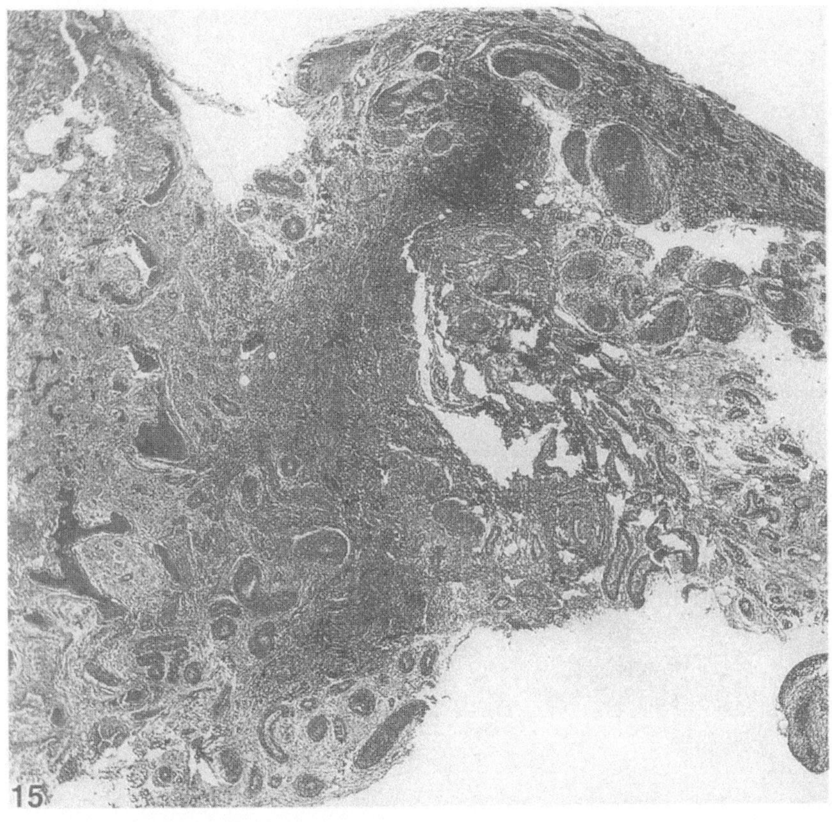

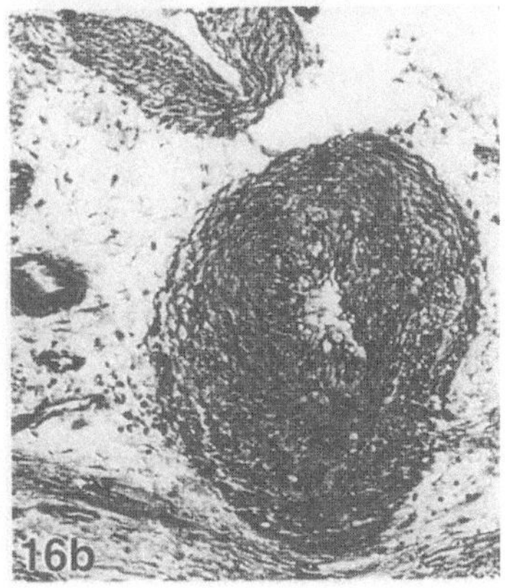

Fig. 14. Osteoid osteoma of neck of talus (radiograph fig. 8). Around the nidus, partly calcified centrally, has developed a relatively regular trabecular osteogenesis. The center of the lesion is organoid, which we consider an essential feature and is the major anatomical feature distinguishing osteoid osteoma from osteoblastoma

Fig. 15. Pedicle of nidus traversed by large vessels with thick muscular walls, accompanied by some nerve fibers which cannot be followed by standard staining where they enter the nidus

Fig. 16 a, b. Artery and nerves (*arrows*) of pedicle of nidus (**a**). Large artery with muscular wall in pedicle (**b**). Nocturnal exacerbation of pain is related to circulatory changes in decubitus

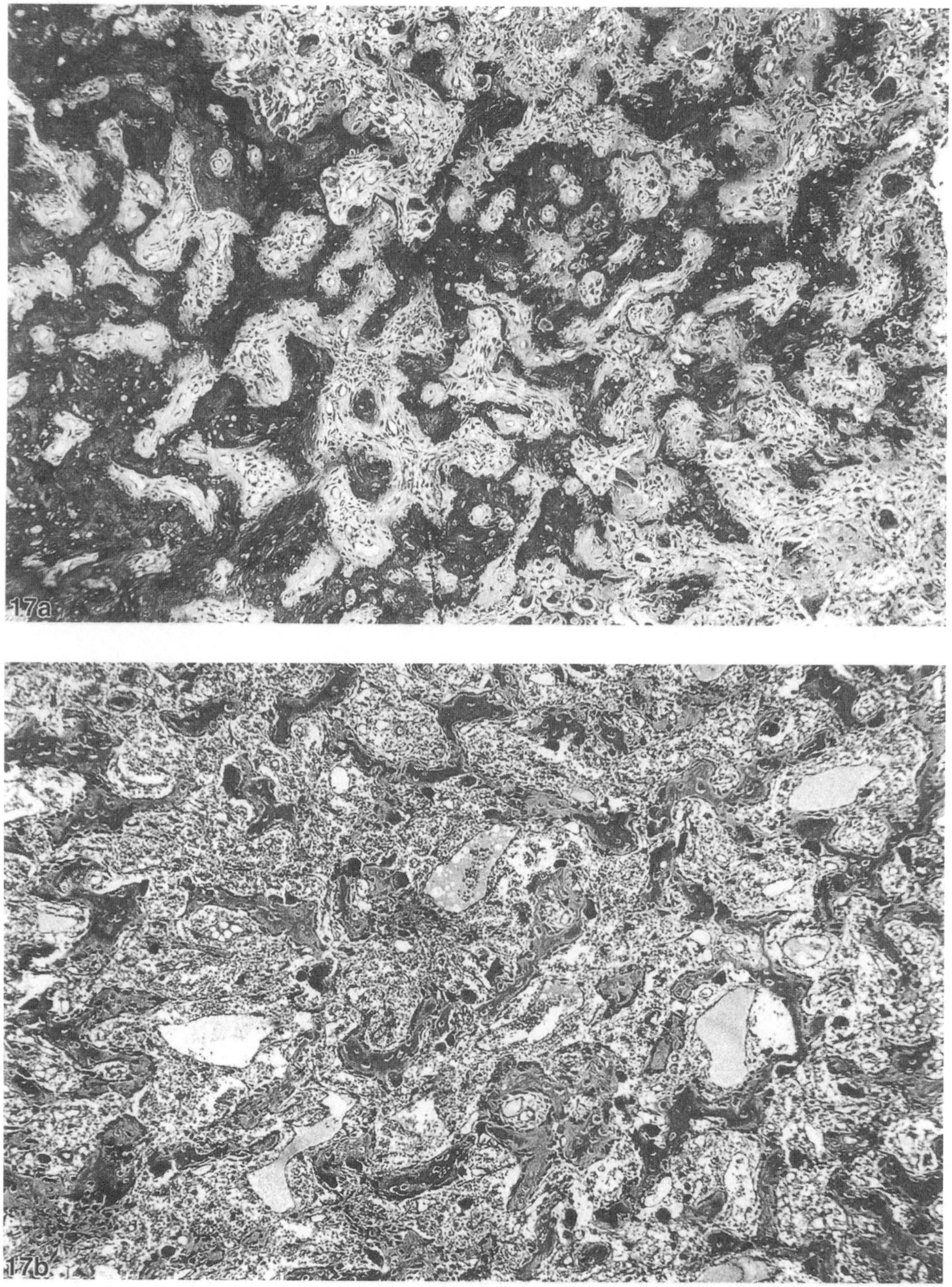

Fig. 17 a, b. Metatarsal nidus. This microphotograph (**a**) is taken in the central zone of the nidus; bone formation is very irregular and markedly calcified. In a peripheral zone of the nidus (**b**), the osteogenesis is less calcified and more regular. The osteoid strands are bordered by osteoblasts and osteoclasts. The vascularisation is abundant, with numerous capillaries, some widely dilated

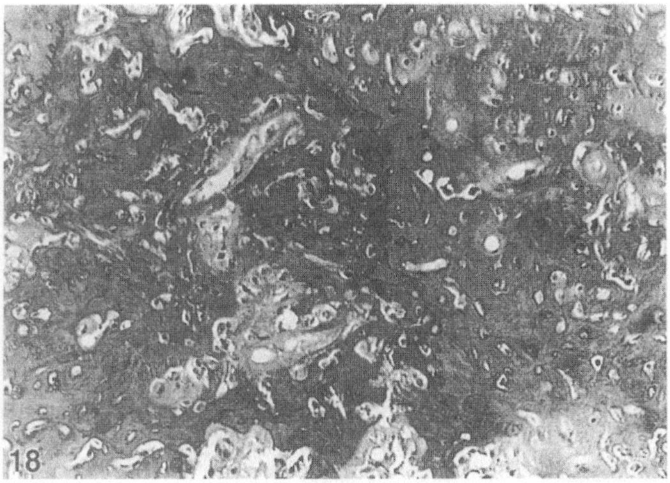

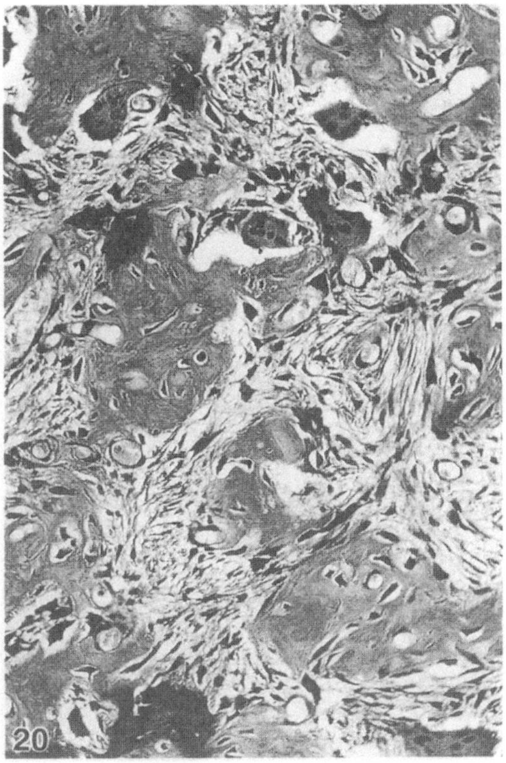

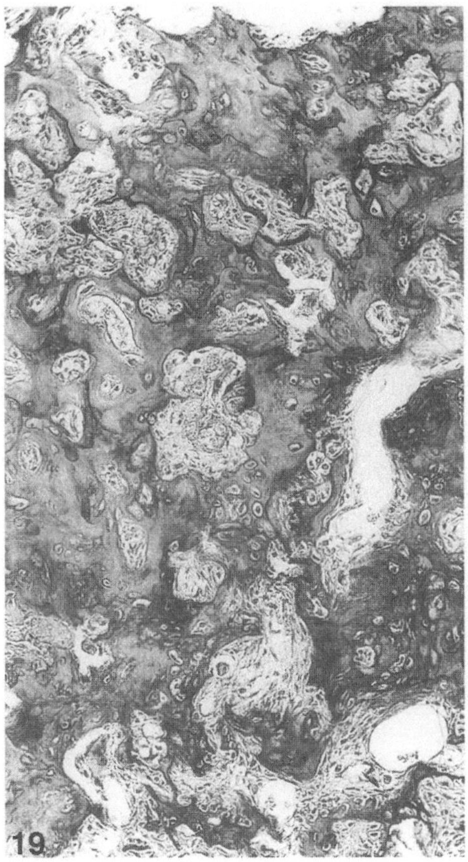

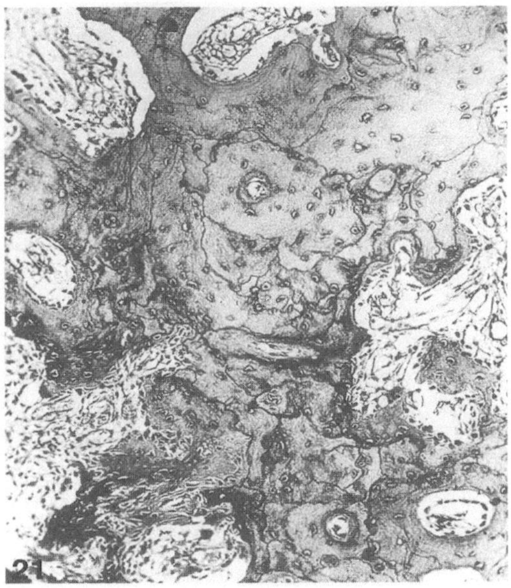

Fig. 18. In this central zone of a nidus, the bony tissue formed is quite special, characteristic of neither haversian nor spongy bone

Fig. 19. Central zone of a nidus. The calcification is not uniform and the distribution of the osteocytes very irregular. The loose fibrous marrow is traversed by dilated capillaries

Fig. 20. In a fibrous, well-vascularised marrow at the center of the nidus there is a struggle between the absorptive osteoclasts and the bone-forming osteoblasts

Fig. 21. In this old nidus, calm has been restored. The osteoblasts are the victors, but the osteoclasts have left their mark in the form of numerous calcified irregular lines of arrested growth. Overall, the appearance is pagetoid

9. Benign osteoblastoma

In 1956, Jaffe and Lichtenstein separately suggested the term benign osteoblastoma for this lesion. This non-organoid angio-osteoblastic tumour had previously been described by the terms of osteogenic fibroma or giant osteoid osteoma [Dahlin & Johnson 1954].

Case history

In May 1968, the only clinical manifestation in this young girl of 21 was to exhibit, in the orthopaedic department of the Hôpital Foch (Paris), a linear scar on her leg which she regarded as disfiguring as the bathing season approached. The history was that, at the age of 9, she had been referred to the orthopaedic surgery department for an "osteoarthritis" of the knee which coincided with taking her tuberculin skin test.

On examination, there was a palpable, firm, slightly painful swelling of the upper half of the leg. In the radiographs, there was a non-uniform opacity extending to the upper half of the tibial shaft; the tibia was thickened quite regularly by a periosteal reaction (fig. 1a). The blood count was normal, but the ESR was 43 mm in the first hour. A biopsy was done, the histological report was descriptive and concluded that there was no histological evidence of malignancy.

The pain intensified and the radiographic appearances deteriorated. Convinced that this was an osteosarcoma, the orthopedist assumed that the biopsy was not representative, but a second biopsy gave the same result. The general condition worsened and the ESR remained raised. There was total discordance between the clinical picture and the histology, between orthopaedist and pathologist, each very competent and properly respectful of the other's opinion.

Amputation of the thigh or resection? No pulmonary lesion was detectable, nor any atypical mitoses. A third biopsy: same report; the pathologist took the responsibility, resection, and grafting was carried out (fig. 1b). Twelve years later (fig. 1c), were it not for the fine scar parallel to the reconstructed tibia, no-one would suspect "that anything had happened" [Rainaut et al 1970].

General considerations

This is a rare tumour, representing about 3% of benign tumours of bone. It is approximately twice as common in males as in females. The tumour usually manifests in the first 3 decades of life, but has been seen up to the 8th decade. It may involve any of the bones of the skeleton. A third of the cases are located in the vertebral column, often on the posterior arch. In a national enquiry carried out by the neurology departments [Fuentes et al 1990], osteoid osteoma and osteoblastomas represented 32.5% of benign primary tumours of the spine. Next commonest are the long bones: femur and tibia.

Some authors believe that the cementoma of the mandible is a particular expression of osteoblastoma in this flat bone. It is open to anyone to decide. But it is imperative in every general article on osteoblastoma to specify the exact sites of the reported cases. We know that the bones of the skull and face "react" differently to other parts of the skeleton.

Clinical features and course

In children, a painful rigid scoliosis is very suggestive of a vertebral localisation of osteoblastoma (fig. 4). At this site, neurological signs are often informative (3 out

Table 1. Osteoblastoma

Non-organoid angio-osteoid-osteoblastic structure
Large swollen bizarre "lazy" osteoblasts, reluctantly secreting some osteoid zones
Differential diagnosis: very well differentiated osteoblastic osteosarcoma. A difficult or even impossible diagnosis by optical microscopy alone, requiring a perfect technique for cytological study

of 4 patients in the department of paediatric orthopaedics at the Hôpital Saint-Vincent-de-Paul). If they are not quite obvious, they should be carefully sought for: root pain, amyotrophy, disturbance of gait are often detected, at least while they are still minor [Lepage et al 1984, Clement et al 1990]. In osteoblastoma, at whatever site, pain is generally less severe than in osteoid osteoma and the nocturnal exacerbation is less marked. Apart from the spinal localisation, pain is almost invariably the main feature. Spontaneous fracture has been reported in the lower limbs, but is exceptional. Superficially, a tumour may be palpable; if deep, it is tender on gentle pressure. At the outset, the pain is very moderate, which explains the long months of symptoms which precede the first consultation (unlike osteoid osteoma, it should be noted that nerve fibers are not demonstrable in osteoblastoma).

The supplementary investigations supply little information. The blood count is usually found to be normal, though I should stress the fact that in the cases of osteoblastoma I have seen the sedimentation rate was abnormally increased.

The spontaneous course is towards extension of the lesion. Complete excision of an osteoblastoma, without useless mutilation, is followed by cure. If incompletely removed, the tumour recurs, or more exactly continues to progress, requiring a second operation [Lerat & Rebouillard 1977].

When the resumption of growth is rapid and massive, the interpretation of further biopsies may lead to a diagnosis of osteoblastic osteosarcoma or, in the absence of cytological signs of malignancy, of aggressive osteoblastoma [Kenan et al 1985]. It is accepted that the term "aggressive" is in no way synonymous with malignant. I have seen such tumours assume considerable local development, without giving rise to metastatic lesions and without demonstrable evidence of malignancy in the histological sections.

Imaging

If observed at the outset, which is rare, the radiological appearance of osteoblastoma is that of a translucent round image which initially suggests an osteoid osteoma. If the patient refuses any intervention for some months, the tumour develops and it is usually at this advanced stage that osteoblastoma is detected. This fact in no way denies that an osteoblastoma may be the outcome of an osteoid osteoma; many lesions (infective or neoplastic) begin as a small rounded focus of osteolysis.

At the stage when usually detected, the radiological image of an osteoblastoma is heterogeneous, with alternating clear and dense zones, some predominating over the others. A periosteal apposition, in lamellae or spicules, covers the entirety of the tumour. In a quarter of the cases this appearance obviously suggests a malignant lesion, especially as the cortex may be breached (fig. 2). In the metatarsals and metacarpals, there is usually ballooning of the bone, a sort of spina ventosa, which reveals the entire lesion (fig. 3). In the spine, this may be the hypertrophy of an articular apophysis, a lamina or a spinous process. Sometimes the lesion extends to the body and posterior arch, but more often involvement of the vertebral body remains confined to this site and may lead to vertebral collapse with dramatic consequences in the case of a cervical vertebra, if treatment is misguided.

In some exceptional cases two adjacent vertebrae are affected. It is useless to attempt to portray the frequency of involvement of the different segments of the vertebral column, since the figures reported in different publications are variable. However, there seems to be some lumbar predominance.

CT clearly demonstrates the relations of the tumour and the marrow, and angiography is an essential prerequisite to operation in many cases, allowing selective preoperative embolisation.

Pathological anatomy and histopathology

Macroscopically, the appearance is relatively characteristic, but the major vascularisation of this zone of osteolysis may suggest an angioma or aneurysmal cyst

[Tehranzadeh et al 1983]. However, the presence of dark-red calcified granular structures may suggest the diagnosis of osteoblastoma. The boundaries of the lesion are irregular but sharp.

Histologically, it is rare to have an overall view of this tumour. Around the vascular lakes and numerous vessels, osteoblastic cell proliferation produces more or less calcified osteoid islands (figs. 5, 6). These osteoblasts are grouped in dense clumps, true cell nests (figs. 7, 8) at the center of which there may or may not be a minuscule osteoid rudiment. These osteoblasts are large, even to the point of caricature; the very developed Golgi apparatus displaces the nucleus (figs. 9-11).

Differential diagnosis

In its typical form the diagnosis of osteoblastoma is relatively easy. However, confusion between osteoid osteoma and osteoblastoma is inevitable in some cases, the tumour architecture being rarely definitive; this is particularly the case for the metacarpals and metatarsals.

In the biopsy, osteogenesis being virtually nil and vascularisation considerable, the diagnoses of angioma or aneurysmal cyst may be suggested (figs. 12, 13).

The only major differential diagnosis is from well-differentiated osteoblastic osteosarcoma. Therefore it is important to verify, when studying numerous sections, the absence not only of atypical mitoses, necrosis and inflammatory phenomena, but also of a fine plexus of osteogenesis, a sort of osteoid filigree, commoner in osteosarcoma than in osteoblastoma. Lastly, a diffuse osteoblastic proliferation not grouped in clumps or cell nests, but scattered among the osteoid formations, should raise the alarm and lead to the consideration of a cellular polymorphism not to be embraced by the term "benign osteoblastoma".

A recurrence with local extension should be examined with special care to discover any signs of malignancy; however, if the numerous mitoses are not identifiably atypical, and if the cells retain their characteristic osteoblastic appearance, and even if the boundary is less defined than is usually observed, one can do no more than mention the aggressive nature of the tumour in the report. It is obvious that recurrences are more to be feared when complete excision of the tumour is particularly difficult, for example at vertebral and sacral sites [Lerat & Rebouillard 1977, Bisset et al 1987].

Treatment

Treatment of osteoblastoma is surgical; the problems posed depend on the extent and site of the lesion.

The angiomatous nature of the tumour has been noted, and is particularly to be feared in vertebral lesions. This risk of haemorrhage usually calls for selective embolisation 24-48 hours before the operative procedure. As for the rare neurological complications of a static nature, related to the magnitude of the operative procedure, these, in some cases, justify preventive treatment by stabilisation of the spine [Dubousset 1992].

Radiotherapy should be rejected because of the major risk of irradiation-induced sarcoma.

So-called "malignant osteoblastoma"

While we may concede, a priori, as for the majority of benign lesions, that malignant transformation of an osteoblastoma is possible, the term "malignant osteoblastoma", which can only add to the confusion, must be rejected. The so-called malignant osteoblastoma is a very well differentiated osteoblastic sarcoma. Its diagnosis very difficult to assert, and sometimes impossible [Bertoni et al 1985, and cf Chapter 11). We adopt the wise remark of Dahlin, who considers that the concept of malignant osteoblastoma represents a group of debatable and certainly controversial tumours.

It is difficult to accept certain cases reported under the label of aggressive osteoblastoma when the architectural and cytological characteristics are quite clearly those of a well differentiated osteoblastic osteosarcoma. The therapeutic argument of cure after amputation is invalid, since a sarcoma of such feeble malignancy is completely curable by amputation. We are aware - and the reports of earlier decades are very clear on this - of a rate of around 20% of long-term (definitive) cures of the common forms of osteogenic sarcoma (grade 2 or 3) of the long bones of the limbs following amputation; all the more reason why cure of a well-differentiated osteoblastic sarcoma is possible after a correct surgical procedure. A tumour is properly considered aggressive which tends to local extension and invasion and such a tumour is generally cured by local intervention. The cure of an osteoblastic osteosarcoma of low malignancy by amputation or wide resection does not give it the right to be included in the category of "aggressive osteoblastomas".

References

Aparisi T, Arborgh B, Ericsson JLE (1978) Studies on the fine structure of osteoblastoma with notes on the localization of nonspecific acid and alkaline phosphatase. Cancer 41: 1811-1822

Bertoni F, Unni KK, McLeod RA, Dahlin DC (1985) Osteosarcoma resembling osteoblastoma. Cancer 55: 416-426

Bisset GS, Kaufman RA, Towgin R, Bove KE (1987) Recurrent sacral osteoblastoma (case report). Skeletal Radiol 16: 666-669

Clement JL, Cahuzac JP, Roger D, Sabatie J, Bergoin JM, Onimus M (1990) Problèmes diagnostiques et thérapeutiques des ostéoblastomes rachidiens. Rachis 2: 127-136

Dahlin DC, Johnson EW jr (1954) Giant osteoid osteoma. J Bone Joint Surg 36A: 559-572

Dubousset J (1992) Abstracts of the eighth annual stonwin medical conference. Spinal instability. J Spinal Disorders 5: 141

Fuentes JM, Benezech J, Iborra F, Many M, Monthieu JY (1990) Les tumeurs rachidiennes primitives résultat d'une enquête nationale. Rachis 2: 301-310

Gentry JF, Schechter JJ, Mirra JM (1989) Periostal osteoblastoma of rib (case report). Skeletal Radiol 18: 551-555

Jaffe HL (1956) Benign osteoblastoma. Bull Hosp Jt Dis Orthop Inst 17: 141-151

Jaffrès R, Wargnier M, Mazabraud A (1968) Un nouveau cas d'ostéoblastome bénin. Ouest Medical 14: 1105-1109

Kenan S, Floman Y, Robin GC, Laufer A (1985) Aggressive osteoblastoma. A case report and review of the literature. Clin Orthop 195: 294-298

Kevin RA, Raymon PG, Edeikon J (1989) Epiphyseal osteoblastoma end of femur. Skeletal Radiol 18: 143-146

Lepage J, Rigault P, Nezelof C, Padovani JP, Pierre-Kahn A, Guyonvarc'h G (1984) Ostéoblastome bénin chez l'enfant. Rev Chir Orthop 70: 117-127

Lerat DL, Rebouillard J (1977) Problèmes diagnostiques et thérapeutiques posés par les ostéoblastomes du rachis. Rev Chir Orthop 63: 483-489

Lichtenstein L (1956) Benign osteoblastoma. Cancer 2: 1044-1052

Lichtenstein L, Sawyer WR (1964) Benign osteoblastoma. Further observations and report of twenty additional cases. J Bone Joint Surg 46A: 755-765

Marsh BW, Bonfiglio M, Brady LP, Enneking WF (1975) Benign osteoblastoma: range of manifestations. J Bone Joint Surg 57A: 1-9

Meary R, Merle d'Aubigné R, Mazabraud A (1965) Ostéoblastomes bénins. Mém Acad Chir 91: 91 1-925

Mitchell ML, Ackerman LV (1986) Metastatic and pseudomalignant osteoblastoma: a report of two unusual cases. Skeletal Radiol 15: 213-2318

Miyayama H, Sakamoto K, Ide M, Ise K, Hirota K, Yasunaga T, Ishihara A (1993) Aggressive osteoblastoma of the calcaneus. Cancer 71: 346-353

Rainaut JJ, Mazabraud A, Robinet L (1970) A propos d'un cas d'ostéoblastome bénin d'un os long. Mém Acad Chir 96: 309-315

Ramadier JO, Buard J, Seguy E (1982) Ostéoblastome de la 4e vertèbre cervicale. Un cas avec hypertrophie des arcs postérieurs à 3 niveaux. Rev Chir Orthop 68: 407-413

Schajowicz F, Lemos C (1976) Malignant osteoblastoma. J Bone Joint Surg 58B: 202-211

Tehranzadeh J, Jeukins JJ, Horton JA (1983) Osteoblastoma with secondary aneuvrysmal bone cyst of the frontal bone (case report). Skeletal Radiol 10: 276-280

Tonai M, Campbell CJ, Ahn GH, Schiller AL, Mankin HJ (1982) Osteoblastoma: classification and report of 16 patients. Clin Orthop 167: 222-235

Trifaud A, Payan H, Bureau H, Argenson C (1965) Les ostéoblastomes bénins à propos de 5 observations. Mém Acad Chir 91: 890-895

Vilain A (1963) L'ostéoblastome bénin. Revue générale à propos de quatre observations. Thèse, Bordeaux, n° 196

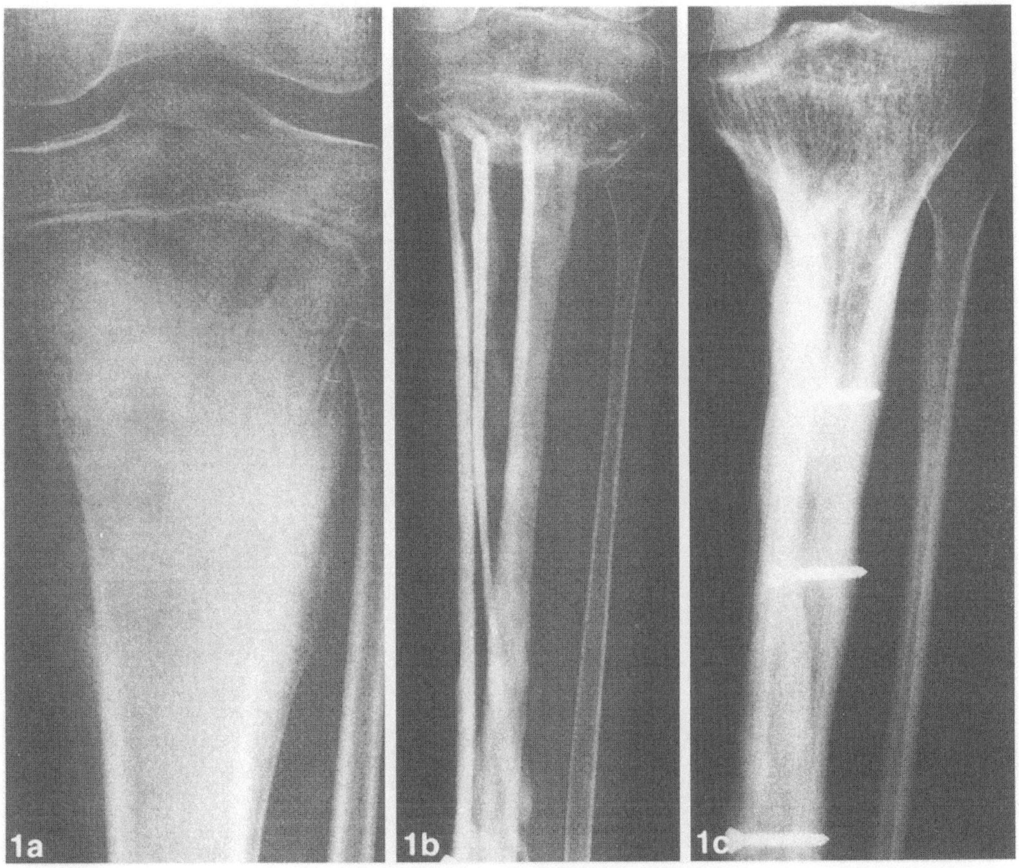

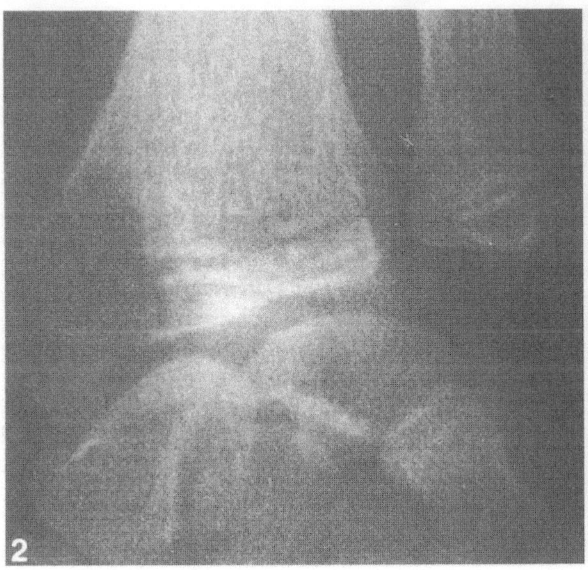

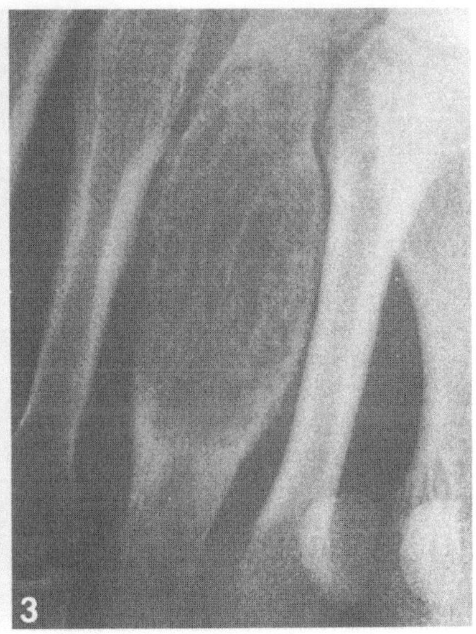

Fig. 1 a-c. Osteoblastoma of tibia from the case history reported at the beginning of this chapter. The lesion at the age of 9 years (**a**), resection and grafting (**b**), radiological appearance 13 years after operation (**c**)

Fig. 2. Girl aged 13. Osteolytic remodelling of radial styloid. Rupture of cortex and growth plate, absence of osteosclerosis

Fig. 3. Shaft of third metatarsal is ballooned; the lesion is diffuse without reactive osteosclerosis

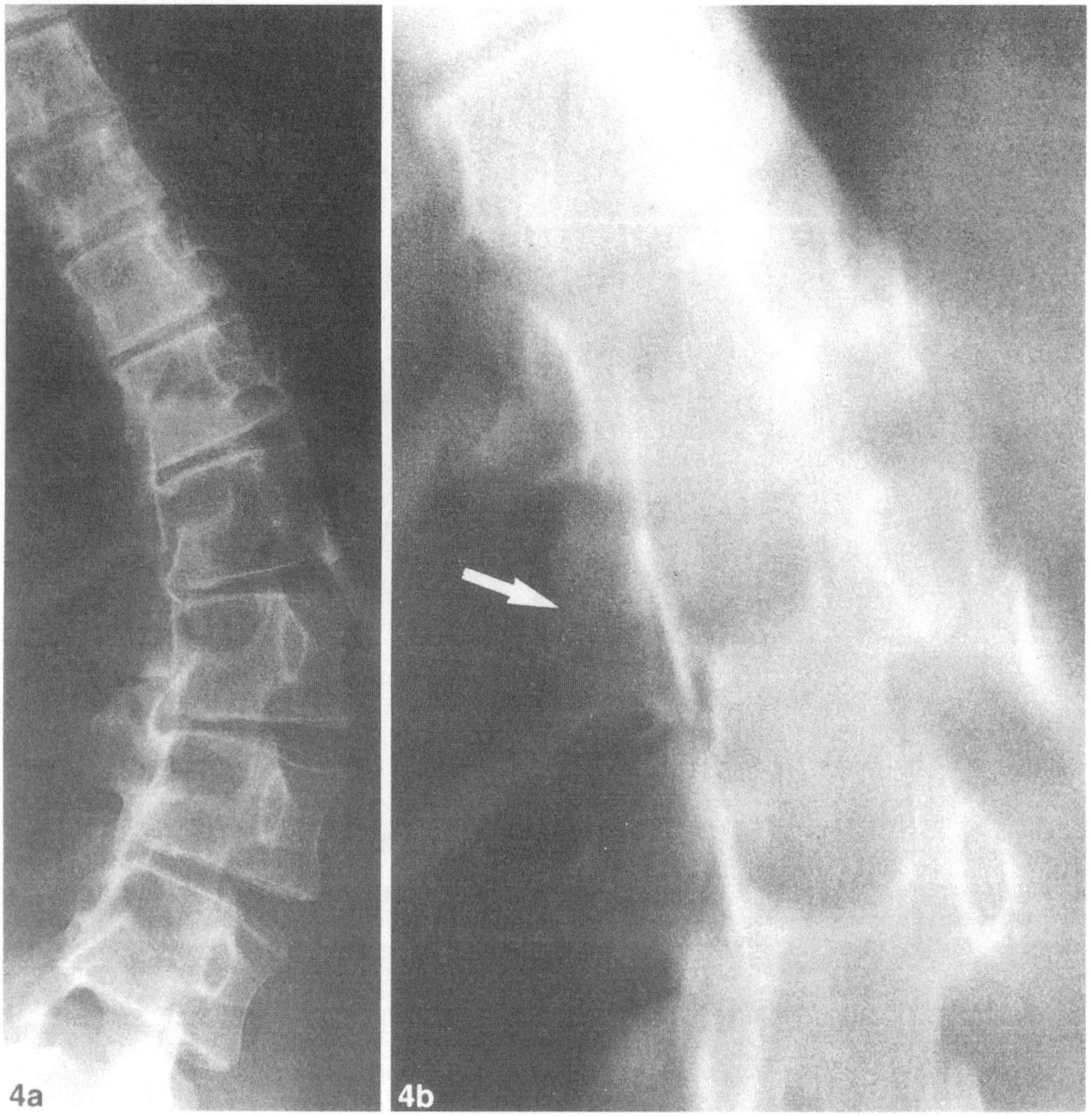

Fig. 4. a Vertebral osteoblastoma, scoliotic deformity with vertebral rotation. **b** The lesion is better shown (*arrow*) in a tomograph of the dorsolumbar junction

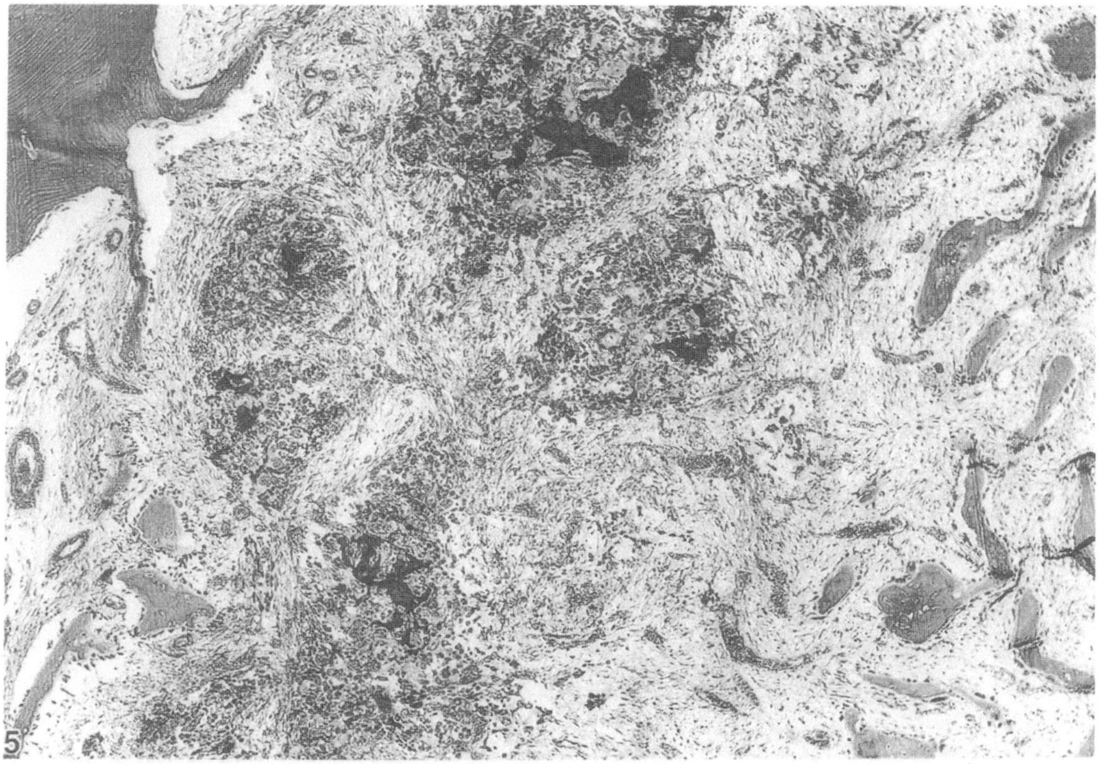

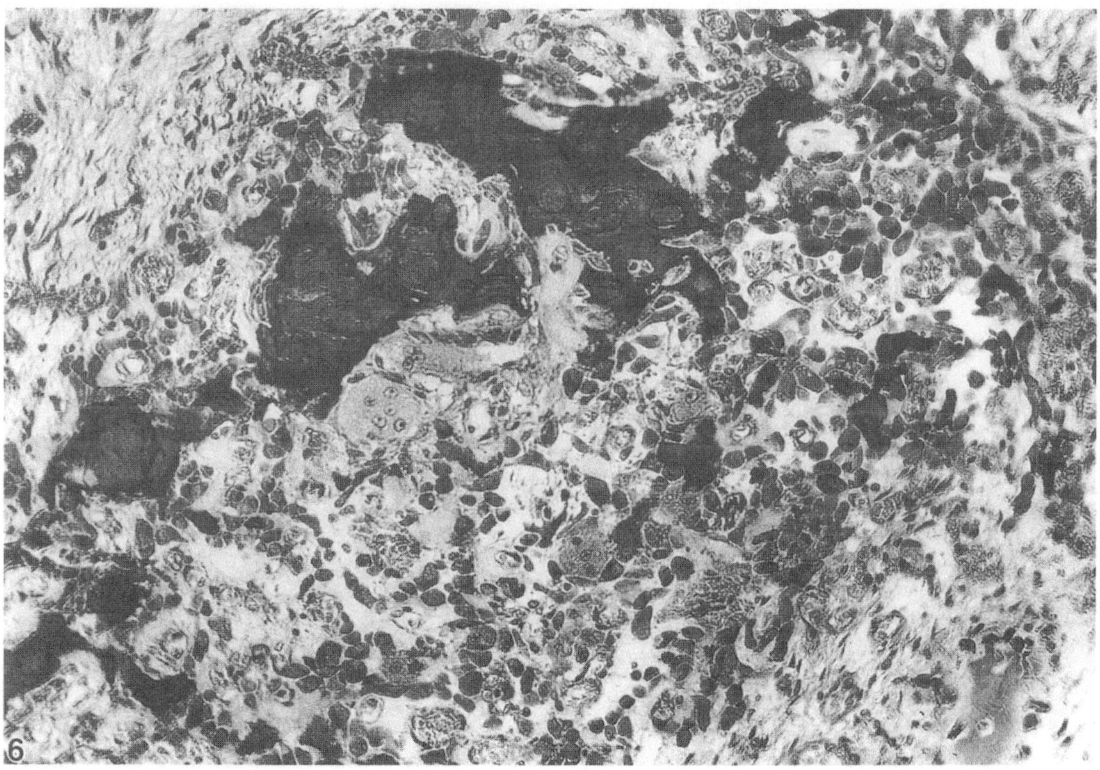

Fig. 5. Osteoblastic foci in a zone of osteolysis. Some foci have a center of calcified osteoid tissue (low magnification)

Fig. 6. In this osteoblastic focus the osteoid islands are virtually acellular, markedly calcified, and their margins are scalloped by osteoclastic lacunae

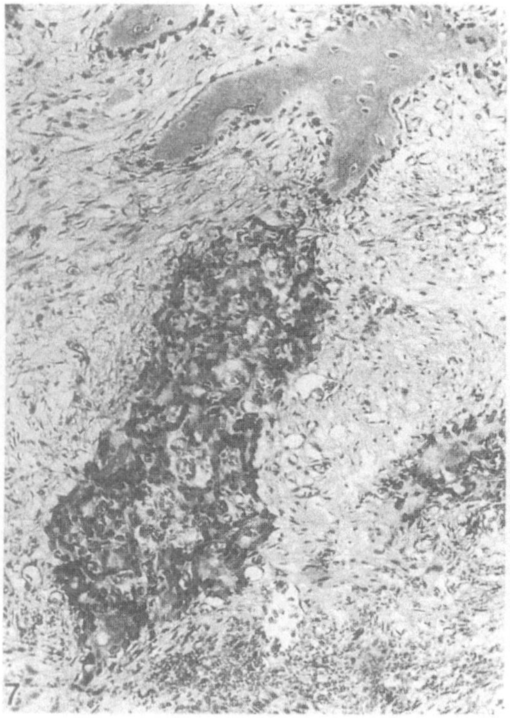

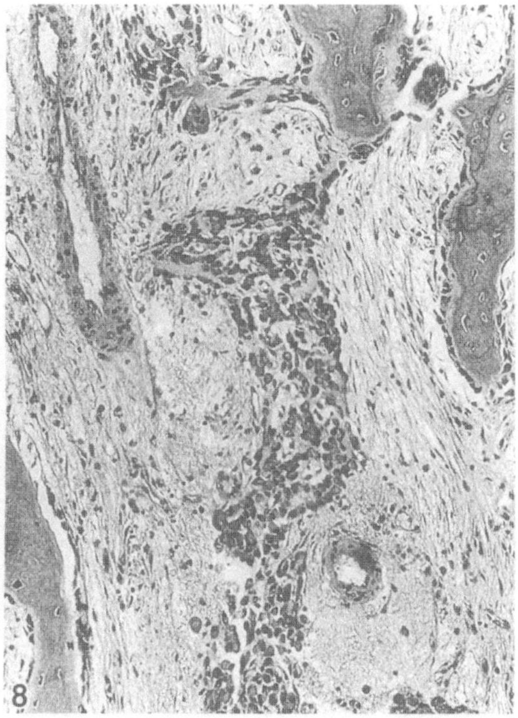

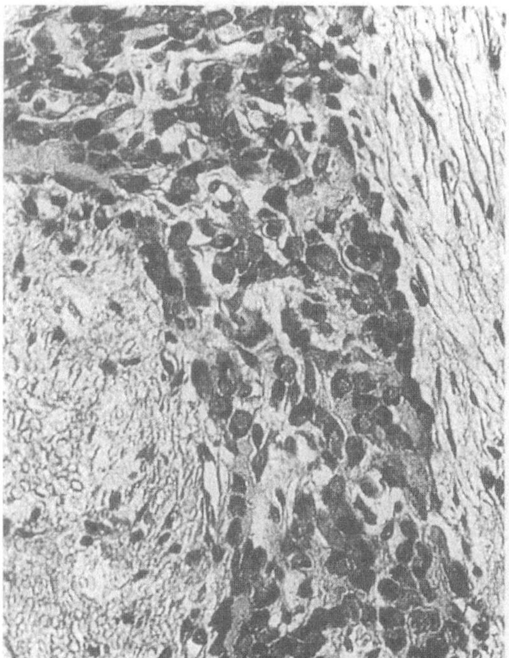

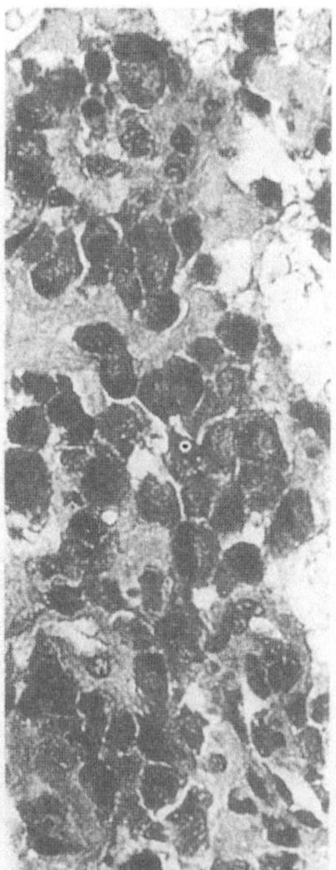

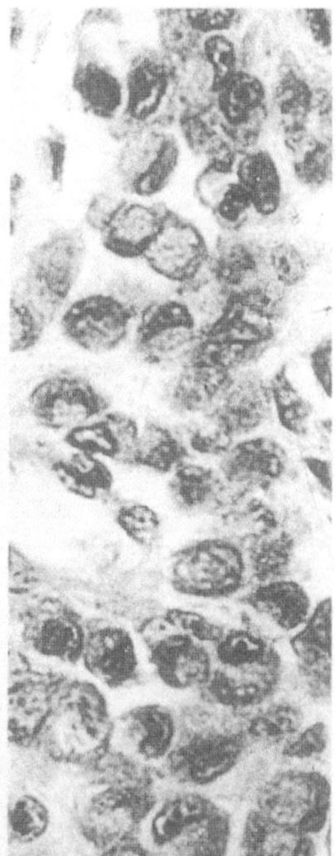

Fig. 7. In the upper third of the figure the osteoid strands are surrounded by osteoblasts. The subjacent osteoblastic focus, surrounded by fibrous marrow, secretes only small amounts of osteoid tissue

Fig. 8. This osteoblastic streak is in continuity with a bony strand bordered by osteoblasts and osteoclasts

Fig. 9. A nest of osteoblasts which secrete only minimal amounts of osteoid tissue in a fibrous marrow

Figs. 10, 11. High magnification, bizarre appearance of osteoblasts: the voluminous archoplasm displaces the nucleus, which is eccentric and bow-shaped

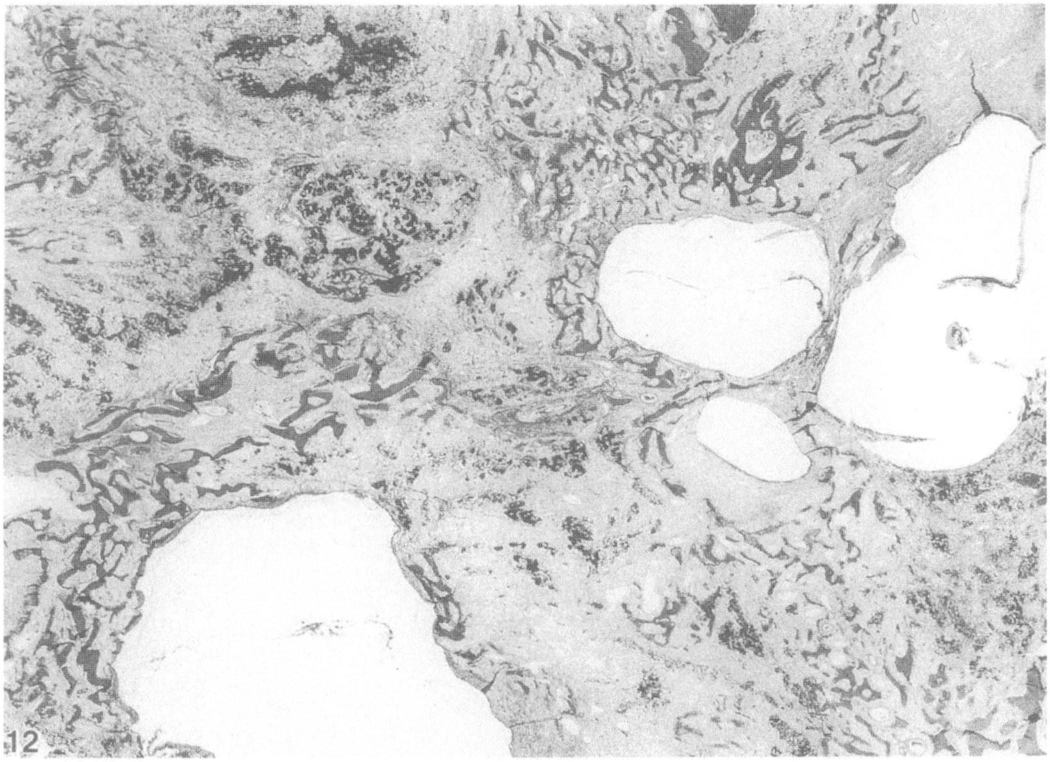

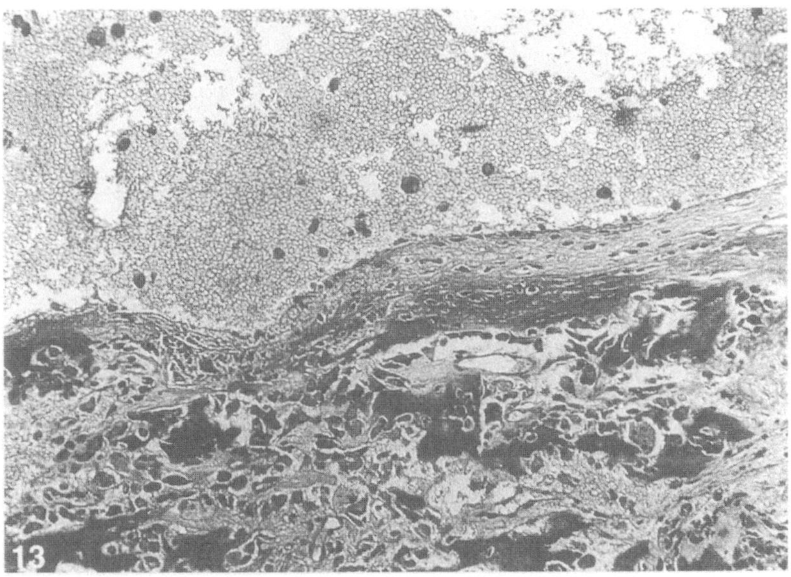

Fig. 12. Angiomatous appearance in an overall view: a biopsy from such a lesion may suggest an angioma

Fig. 13. Wall of a vascular lacuna (or of a true vessel) bordered by a partly calcified osteoid band. Some pathologists would consider this to be "an associated aneurysmal cyst", here related to an osteoblastoma; but this interpretation would be defensible only if the specificity of this parietal appearance were proven, which is certainly not the case (cf Chapter 31)

10. Osteoma

Osteoma is not a definite pathological entity; the term covers a radiological and clinical concept. Thus only a very general definition can be attempted, such as: a benign limited pseudotumoural osseous formation, variable in its location, architecture and mode of elaboration. This excludes the small, and generally trabecular ossifications that develop in the soft tissues and viscera, as well the highly osteosclerosing bony disorders.

Clinical types

Osteoma may be found as a rounded solitary densification of the iliac wing, discovered unexpectedly in a radiograph of the pelvis, or a hard bony structure developing rapidly on the frontal bone following an injury, or a joint restricted by a bony proliferation after trauma, or a hard and mobile "tumour" of the inner aspect of the thigh.

General considerations

This is a rare lesion resulting from multiple causes: trauma, infection or neoplastic growth. Cranial osteomas are the commonest: cranial vault (fig. 2), sinuses, mandible (cf Chapter 38); then come the flat bones (fig. 13) and the long bones of the limbs (fig. 7).

Clinical features and course

When the osteoma consists of a localised densification of the femoral neck or iliac wing, it is usually asymptomatic. The classic example is the osteoma of the iliac wing, a solitary benign island [Attali & Lièvre 1957] detected during a radiological examination performed for another reason (fig. 1). The site plays a determining part in the likelihood of detection of an osteoma. An osteoma-excrescence of a bone of the skull is frequently recognised by the patient. This also applies to the detection of the numerous osteomas of the soft tissues.

The presence of multiple osteomas associated with sebaceous cysts, desmoid fibromas and intestinal polyps characterises Gardner's syndrome (1952, 1953). Lièvre, reporting a disorder combining multiple bony and soft tissue osteomas, has described an endocranial osteoma and a histiocytofibroma in a woman of 28 who also presented with bony anomalies of the skull and tarsus.

Solitary, so-called "pure", osteomas of no known aetiology, have been attributed to various categories; they have been variously thought to be a variety of osteoblastoma, the terminal stage of fibrous dysplasia and even simple hamartoma.

The following lesions should not be regarded as osteomas: firm mass, painful or not, of the sternoclavicular region, which often leads to biopsy. Arthritis, arthrosis and Tietze's syndrome are the principal causes [Resnick 1980]; Sonozaki's syndrome (1974) characterised by costoclavicular hyperostosis together with ossification of the adjacent tissues; and lastly, I believe it would be an abuse of language to consider as osteoma a sclerotic form of Paget's disease, myeloma or a metastasis.

When there is an indication for surgical excision of an osteoma, this is normally followed by definitive cure.

Imaging

The diagnosis of osteoma is usually made from a radiographic image of a dense, round or ovoid opacity in the

Table 1. Osteomas

Schematically three types: - dense - spongy - angio-osteoma (telangiectatic bony outgrowth)
Seek an aetiology: - inflammatory, neoplastic, traumatic, etc.
Differential diagnosis: - juxtacortical or extraskeletal osteosarcoma in its osteogenic form. The mildly atypical bony strands develop on a sarcomatous background, usually fusiform. An osteoma is in part mature, with an adipose or mixed marrow - myositis ossificans adherent to the periosteum at its onset - hamartoma, habitually pluritissular and without histological signs of malignancy

spongy bone (or soft tissues), extending from the surface of a long bone along its long axis. The contour is regular or slightly sinuous.

Pathological anatomy and histopathology

Histological examination confirms excessive bone formation, either simple or associated with an obvious swelling.

One may distinguish osteomas of dense type, which may properly be called petrified and spongy osteomas which correspond to a mature stage and whose appearance is virtually that of a sesamoid, with a cortex and spongy bone containing fatty or mixed marrow. Angio-osteoma is a sort of telangiectatic bony outgrowth, homologous to a fleshy telangiectatic outgrowth. The lesions may be isolated or may occur in association with a causative factor.

Modes of formation of osteomas

These vary with the tissue in which they develop.

-*Type 1:* densification of the spongy bone by regular lamellar apposition. Osteoblasts of endosteal origin deposit osteoid tissue which calcifies and eventually gives the spongy bone an almost haversian appearance: atypical haversian bone is produced by excessive lamellar apposition (fig. 8).

- *Type 2:* densification of the cortical bone by abnormally abundant lamellar apposition in haversian canals (fig. 9). This apposition leads to a strangulation of the vascular axis, an appearance designated osteopetrosis (fig. 10). This petrifaction is inevitably followed by necrosis of all the osteocytes of the haversian system (figs. 9, 10). The dead bone is in its turn destroyed by a vascular outgrowth which engenders the same process of osteopetrosis.

- *Type 3:* formation of atypical metaplastic bone. This metaplastic bone may fill the medullary spaces or develop from tendino-aponeurotic structures attached to the bony segment (figs. 12-14). It is this process that appears most commonly in the formation of the osteomas of paraplegics. It is only secondarily that these osteomas extend and invade the muscle bundles adjacent to the attachments.

- *Type 4:* osteogenesis of periosteal origin. Numerous pathological processes can exhibit ossification in reaction to necrosis, a tumour, a neuroma or without detectable cause (fig. 7).

- *Type 5:* osteogenesis in muscle tissue. In its first stages, this is a myositis ossificans (cf Chapter 41) and at the end of its course an osteoma is formed of spongy bone with a fatty marrow, bounded by a narrow cortex.

-*Type 6:* imaging sometimes reports as "calcification" the relatively common micro-osteomas of the viscera.

In practice, at least two criteria are necessary for the lesion to qualify as an osteoma: there must be a tumour swelling visible radiologically and/or macroscopically, and a bony architecture which produces hyperplasia of the preexisting bony system in a flat or long bone, or a mass bounded by a bony cortex whose center is spongy bone, with marrow, in the juxtaosseous or soft tissues.

Differential diagnosis

From the diagnostic viewpoint it is important to recognise that this entity is a pseudotumour and to confirm that it is a pure osteoma. Recognition of an osteoma is not particularly difficult. Osteomas develop in spongy bone, typically as benign solitary islands [Lagier 1983, Greenspan 1991], as in an iliac wing for example (fig. 1), presenting as a particularly dense bony island without cytological anomalies. In cases with densification of the osteopetrosis type, it is always wise to ensure that the osteoma is not the consequence of an underlying pathological process.

Metaplastic bone developed from tendino-aponeurotic tissues may be of considerable density, giving rise to virtual pathological arthrodesis (fig, 4), but it may also exist as a bone in miniature, with cortex and spongiosa.

If periosteal, the osteoma calls for a search for an infective or neoplastic cause or a fatigue fracture, for example. Local vascular disorders or neurofibromatosis (cf Chapter 41) tend to cause periostoses rather than true osteomas. But a juxtacortical osteoma of a long bone (more so if its site is popliteal) raises the possibility of a juxtacortical sarcoma. Basically, three findings of a histopathological nature may help to resolve this problem :

- the new bone formation, despite its calm and quasi-organoid appearance, develops in a variably dense connective tissue with fusiform cells (and not in medullary tissue);

- the presence of atypical cells, to be carefully sought for in the connective tissue;

- the possible existence of cartilaginous islands, provided it is certain that this is not a mature callus, in which atypical cells may be observed.

It is to be noted that hypertrophic callus is common in injured persons with a history of loss of consciousness, even of very short duration. The rapidity of development of such a callus virtually excludes the diagnosis of a malignant tumour.

Various problems are discussed in Chapter 38 in relationship to craniofacial lesions. We mention here only that the presence of osteomas whose location is mainly mandibular and maxillary, often multiple, should promote a search for other manifestations of Gardner's syndrome [Gardner & Plenk 1952, Gardner & Richards 1953, Gorlin & Chaudhry 1960].

The histological aspects that have been reviewed may also be seen in specific sclerosing bone dysplasias. Isolated from its context, it is altogether unlikely that the pathologist will be able to recognise the causal disease in these cases. It is for clinicians and radiodiagnosticians to suggest the disorder in the information that accompanies their examination request. It goes without saying that these diverse dysplasias have no part in the framework of osteomas; usually, the pathologist will only be able to recognise the compatibility of the lesions with the dysplasia suggested. The soft tissue osteoma, which may come into contact with adjacent bony tissue as it develops, often retains the secret of its aetiology.

Osteosarcoma of the soft tissues (cf Chapter 39) develops within a sarcomatous connective tissue.

Hamartoma is relatively common in the young but rare in adults; its diagnosis rests on the benign characteristics of a pluritissular structure.

Hyperalgic osteoma or hyperalgic periostosis

The lesion is found on the long bones of the limbs, more often in young adults than in children. The presenting feature is pain, whose rhythm is less definite than that of osteoid osteoma. The radiographs show a periosteal "osteoma" adherent to the diaphysis. There is no nidus. Radiography of a specimen which includes the periosteal reaction and the subjacent cortex shows no translucence.

For histological examination, the specimen should be cut in slices 5 mm thick in the search for a possible nidus; multiple sections are made from the embedded blocks. The histology is that of a dense periostosis covering a slightly remodelled cortex. The marrow is fibrous and very vascularised, but there is no nidus. Surgical excision is followed by cure.

It may be that a surgical error or an inadequate histological examination may be responsible for non-discovery of a nidus, but current methods of location make failure of detection very unlikely.

The existence of hyperalgic periostosis is sometimes doubled but just as post-traumatic Paget's disease may be the cause of intolerable pain, this possibility should be accepted. We may also hypothesise the persistence of the painful symptoms in an anatomically cured osteoid osteoma In every case, one must ensure that the changes are not a periosteal reaction overlying a subjacent unidentified lesion, not been included in the surgical biopsy.

References

Attali P, Lièvre JA (1957) L'îlot osseux bénin solitaire. Rev Rhum 24: 641-646

Baum PA, Nelson MC, Lack EE, Bogumill GP (1989) Parosteal osteoma of tibia. Skeletal Radiol 18: 406-409

Cervilla V, Haghighi P, Resoick D, Sartoris DJ (1990) Parosteal osteoma of the acetabulum. Skeletal Radiol 19: 135-137

Gardner EJ, Plenk HP (1952) Hereditary patterm for multiple osteomas in a family group. Am J Hum Genet 4: 31-36

Gardner EJ, Richards RC (]953) Multiple cutaneous and subcutaneous lesions occuring simultaneously with hereditary polyposis and osteomatosis. Am J Hum Genet 5: 139-147

Gorlin RJ, Chaudhry AP (1960) Multiple osteomatosis, fibromas, lipomas and fibrosarcomas of the skin and mesentery, epidermoid inclusion cysts of the skin, leiomyomas and multiple intestinal polyposis. A heritable disorder of connective tissue. New Engl J Med 263: 1151-1158

Greenspan A (1991) Sclerosing bone dysplasia; a target-site approach. Skeletal Radiol 20: 561-583

Greenspan A, Steiner G, Knutzon R (1991) Bone island (enostosis): clinical significance and radiologic and pathologic correlations. Skeletal Radiol 20: 85-90

Ihmeidan H, Tehrauzadeh J, Oldham SA, Mnaymneh W, Ghandur Mnaymneh L (1987) Florid cortical and periosteal reactions due to stress fractures of the right femur and left calcaneus in a "break dancer". Skeletal Radiol 16: 581-583

Lagier R (1983) L'îlot osseux bénin solitaire. Etude anatomoradiologique d'un cas. Radiologie J CEPUR 3: 125-127

Lièvre JA (1958) Nouveau syndrome: ostéome endocrânien, ostéomes du squelette, ostéomes des parties molles périphériques, histiocyto-fibrome. Presse Med 66: 1143-1146

Resnick D (1980) Sternocostoclavicular hyperostosis. AJR 135: 1278-1280

Sonozaki H, Furusawas, Seki H, Kurokawa T, Tateishi A, Kabata K (1974) Four cases with symmetrical ossifications between the clavicles and the first ribs of both sides. Kanso J Orthop Traum 5: 244-247

Stern PJ, Lim EV, Krieg JK (1985) Giant metacarpal osteoma. J Bone Joint Surg 67A: 487

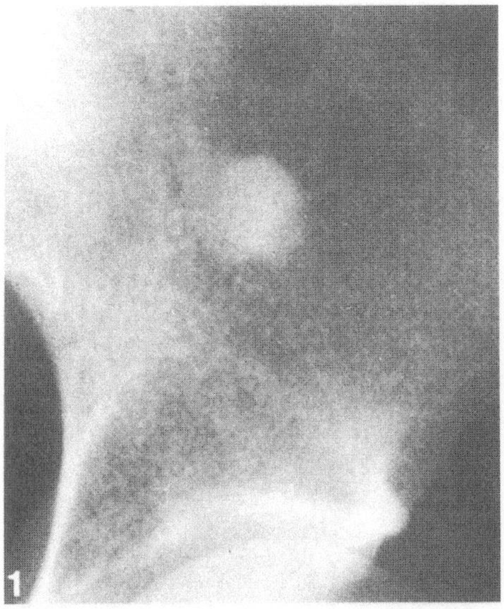

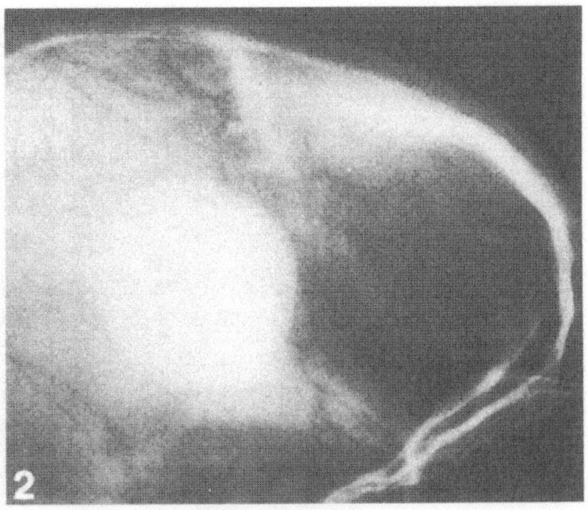

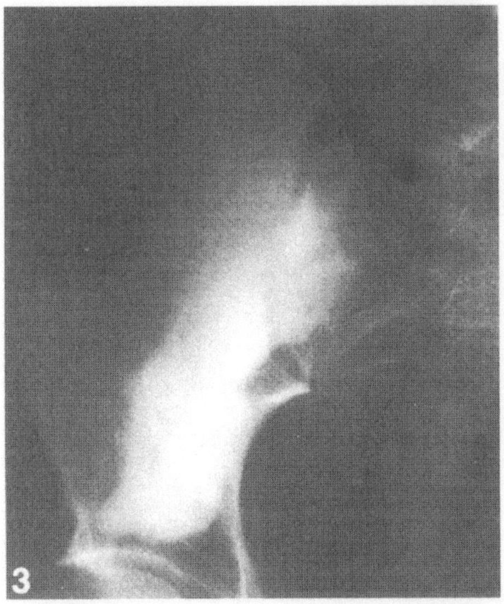

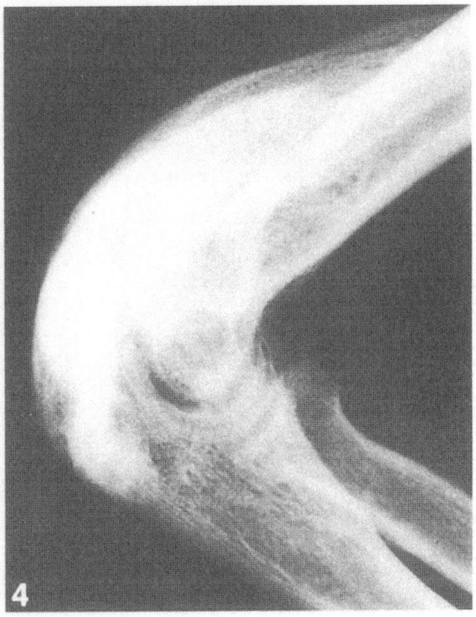

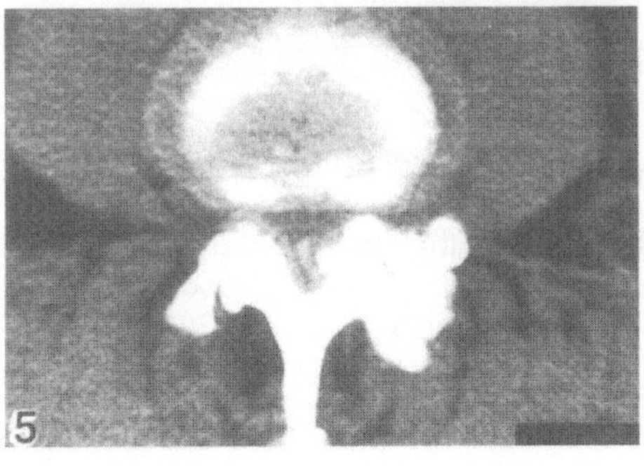

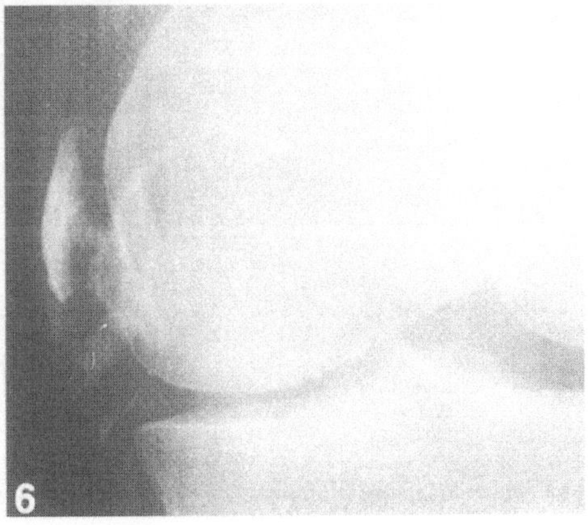

Fig. 1. Solitary benign island in iliac wing: radiological discovery in a woman of 27

Fig. 2. Dense rounded temporal opacity. Woman aged 22

Fig. 3. Iliac osteoma present since age of 8 years, slowly developing in an adolescent of 17

Fig. 4. Osteoma of elbow in a paraplegic

Fig. 5. Juxta-articular osteoma at level of L4

Fig. 6. Para-articular osteoma after injury (with coma)

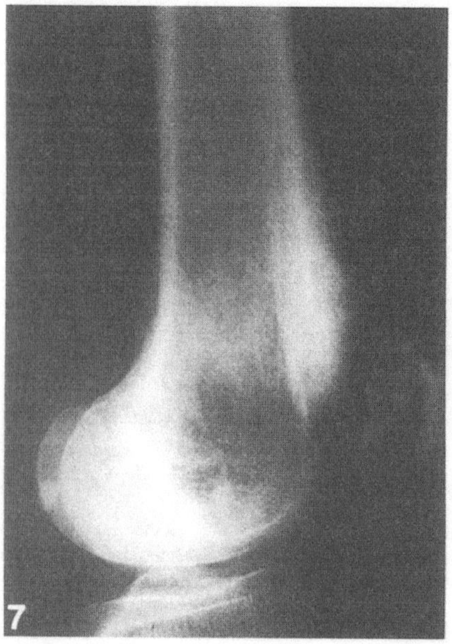

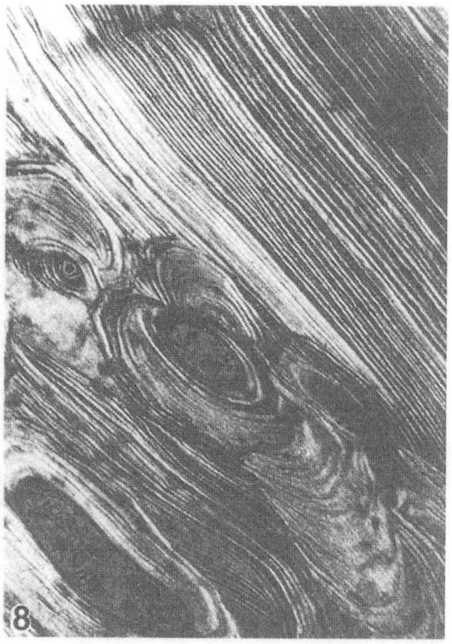

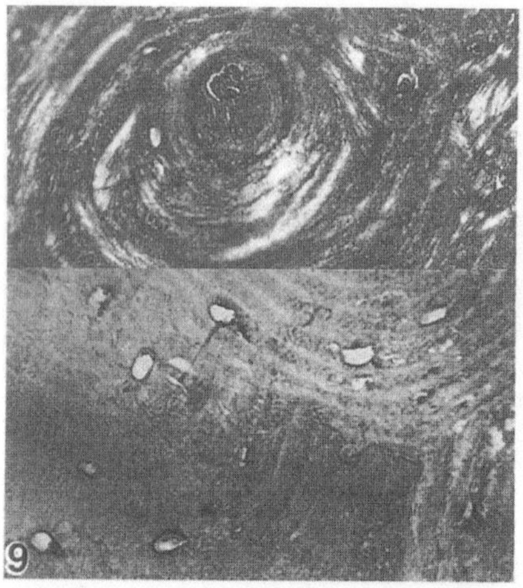

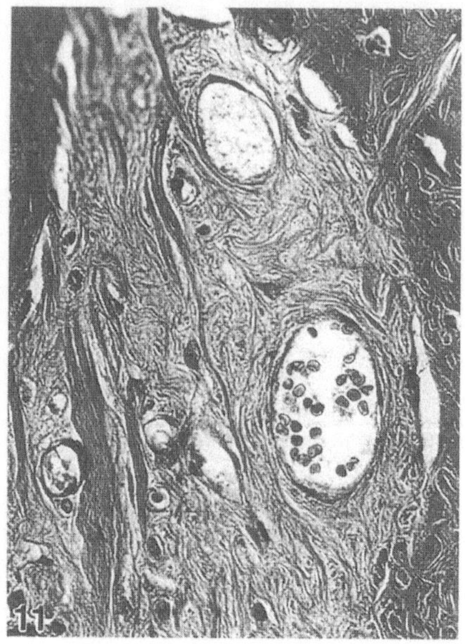

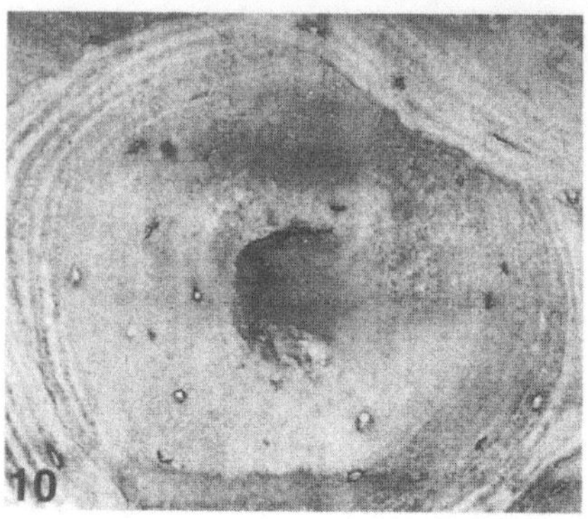

Fig. 7. Juxta-osseous osteoma of anterior aspect of femur, aetiology unknown

Fig. 8. Organisation in haversian bone, abundance of regularly arranged bony lamellae

Fig. 9. "Petrifed" haversian system (polarised light); at higher magnification, large uninhabited osteocytic cavities are seen (osteocytic oncosis)

Fig. 10. Haversian canal with a completely obstructed lumen. This petrifaction provokes osteocytic necrosis

Fig. 11. Rudimentary chondroid metaplasia of collagen fibers

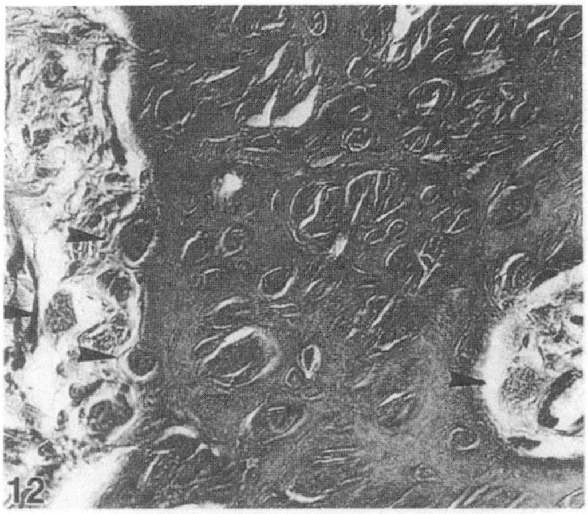

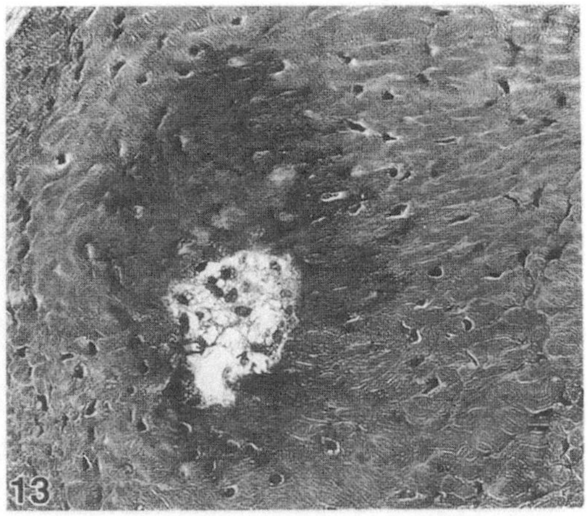

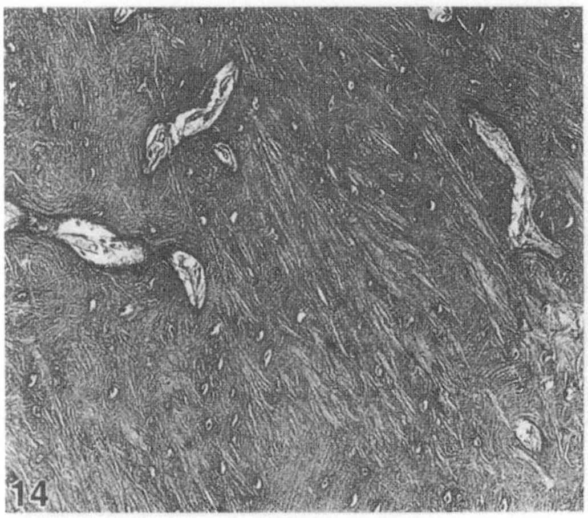

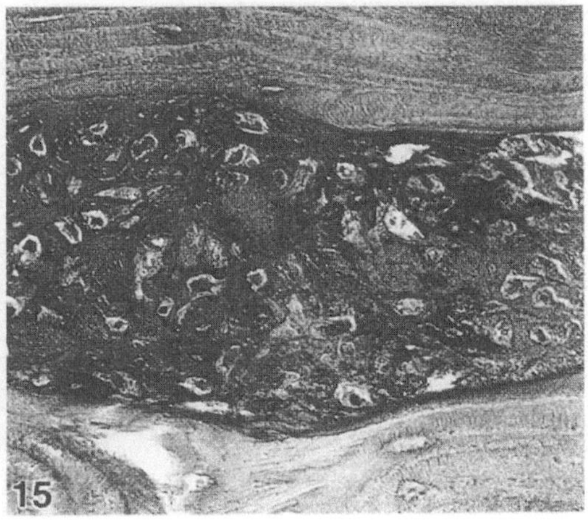

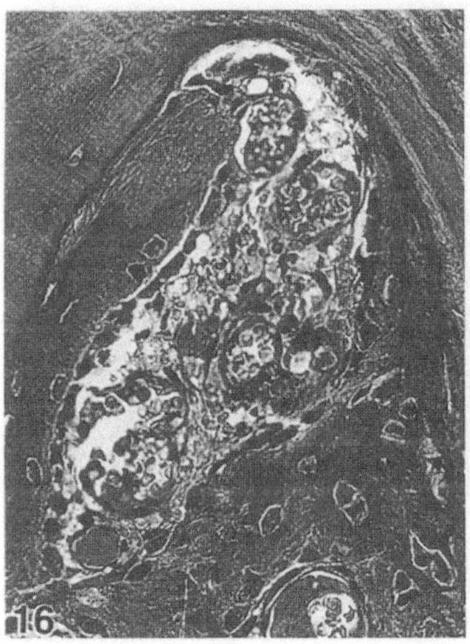

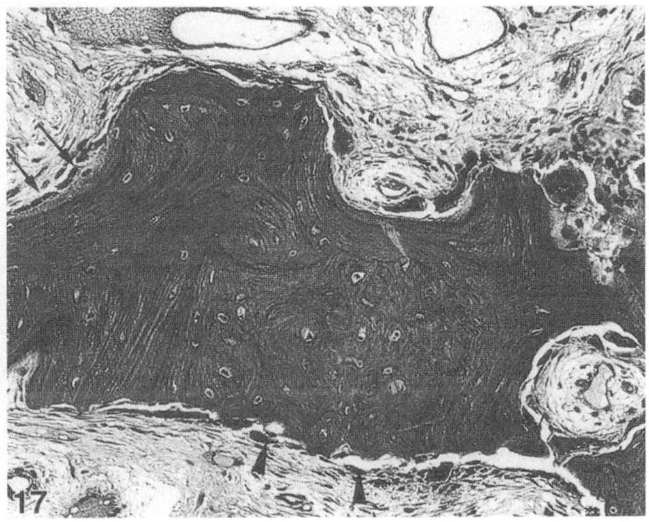

Fig. 12. Osteoid metamorphosis of large collagen fibers (*arrow-heads*)

Fig. 13. Thickening and hyalinisation of partly calcified aponeurotic fibers

Fig. 14. Osteoma formed by metaplastic ossification in tendino-aponeurotic tissue

Fig. 15. Osseous densification due to metaplasia and calcification of marrow spaces

Fig. 16. Lamellar osteoblastic deposition

Fig. 17. Resorption of primary large-fibered metaplastic bone (*arrow-heads*). Above and to left of the bony strand in course of remodelling, a row of osteoblasts apposes lamellar bone (*arrows*)

11. Osteogenic sarcoma

Osteogenic sarcoma is a tumour formed by the proliferation of sarcomatous cells giving rise to osteoid or bony tissue (figs. 25-28). This definition excludes any sarcomatous tumour accompanied by the formation of benign reactive osteoid or osseous tissue.

Among osteogenic sarcomas, cases at the ends of the spectrum of malignancy give rise to some objections in nomenclature. The first of these objections is often formulated thus: How can a sarcoma which is anaplastic be classifed among "osteogenic" sarcomas? To this question counsel for the defense might perhaps reply: This bony tumour, of which we have examined a small biopsy fragment, resembles in its type of cell proliferation what is observable in the anaplastic areas of sarcomas which otherwise are genuinely osteogenic. Moreover, the clinical findings and imaging are not inconsistent with this classification. Lastly and especially, we know that the ultrastructural study of such biopsies reveals the presence of fine fibers on which crystals of hydroxyapatite are deposited.

The second objection relates to well-differentiated osteoblastic sarcomas of slow evolution, rich in osteoid and bony material, and whose components osteoblastic cells are so poor in mitoses that the diagnosis between sarcoma and osteoblastoma is tentative. How can one combine "osteoblastic", which implies a young cell, and "well-differentiated", which suggests a mature process.

One possibility would be to qualify these tumours as "malignant osteoblastomas", but osteoblastoma has been described as a benign tumour and we support this view.

Is it not necessary to distinguish a fibroblastic sarcoma, a liposarcoma and a chondrosarcoma of low grades of malignancy from a fibroma, a lipoma or a chondroma? Despite the difficulties, this pattern of thought also applies to the well-differentiated osteoblastic osteogenic sarcoma.

Case histories

Case 1. In September, after the school holidays, a young girl of 15 attended for vague pain in the left knee. The history mentioned the presence of some fugitive pain in June which did not stimulate any special investigation. The standard radiographs made in September showed an already extensive metaphyseal lesion of the femur, with a breach of the cortex. The boundaries of the osteolysis were imprecise (fig. 1).

Case 2. In this active young girl of 20, there had appeared, some weeks previously, a submalleolar swelling which was much more alarming than the vague ankle pains she had felt for some months. This swelling increased progressively. It was below and behind the malleolus at the time of the first consultation.

On examination there was no fluctuant swelling that might suggest a synovial effusion, but a sort of ill-defined doughy mass. In the standard film the remodeling of the bone structure of the calcaneum, added to the clinical findings, led to the diagnosis.

Examination of the biopsy posed no problems; there was no synovitis or synovial sarcoma, but a predominantly cartilaginous osteosarcoma.

In the resection specimen invasion of the soft tissues was considerable, and the tumour was also developing between the anterior aspect of the Achilles tendon and the tibiotarsal joint. The effect of preoperative antimitotic treatment on this osteosarcoma was very limited, because of the abundance of cartilaginous tissue (fig. 10).

Case 3. One morning, the pathologist was asked for a frozen section of a femoral biopsy in a lad of 18. Pain which had been present for some months had led to clinical and radiological examination. The proximal part of the right thigh was very slightly increased in volume, as shown by comparative measurement. There was no detectable adenopathy, the general condition was excellent and there were no remarkable pathological antecedents. But in the radiographs a lytic image slightly ballooned the upper femoral metaphysis

Biopsy revealed a soft friable, very haemorrhagic tumour. The diagnosis of aneurysmal cyst made from the radiographs was confirmed at operation ... and unfortunately in the frozen section.

Happily, our experience is limited. In 50 million inhabitants, new cases of osteosarcoma are rather fewer than 200 annually. Therefore, in marginal cases of juxtacortical, periosteal, anaplastic and telangiectatic sarcomas where error is very costly, a "delay" of 48 hours for the reading of paraffin sections is less harmful than the curettage of a sarcoma. If need be, a course of antimitotic treatment embarked on because of the radiological and clinical findings can always be interrupted.

General considerations

Osteogenic sarcoma accounts for some 20% of bone sarcomas: 1274 cases in the statistics of the Mayo Clinic (excluding parosteal sarcoma), that is 19.6% of all bone sarcomas.

It is twice as common in males as in females.

The tumour maximum incidence occurs in the second decade, and is rare after the age of 35.

The elective site is the metaphysis of the long bones of the limbs, particularly the lower end of the femur and the upper end of the tibia; 50% develop around the knee, followed by the upper end of the femur and the upper end of the fibula. Any bone may be affected, except, or only very rarely, the sesamoids. About 10% of sarcomas are situated in the bones of the skull and face and 10% in the flat bones of the limb-girdles. According to Ikada et al (1995), whose statistics related to 26 cases of osteosarcoma of a high grade of malignancy, the femur is affected in 45% of cases, then the humerus in 15% of cases. The mortality in 21 cases was 57%.

Clinical features

In the common form the symptomatology is not specific. Pain, swelling, perhaps particularly after exertions such as gymnastics, deserve attention. A presentation after fracture is exceptional. The symptoms usually go back for some months, more rarely a few weeks, as initially the pain is often intermittent and consultation is deferred.

Examination may reveal increased visiblity of veins on the affected limb at the level of the swelling and a slight increase in local warmth. Comparative measurements of the perimeter of the limb at the level of the lesion and at the same level on the sound side, repeated regularly during the first chemotherapy courses, allow assessment of their effect to some extent [Huvos et al 1977]. Careful palpation of the nodal areas reveals an adenopathy in about 5% of cases.

While pulmonary metastases are found in 95% of autopsies of osteogenic sarcoma, they are sometimes detected at the first examination. Study of the lung fields during the course of the disease is an essential feature of surveillance of these patients.

Imaging

The supplementary investigations, particularly imaging, specify:
- the topography and dimensions of the tumour;
- its local extent and relationships to adjacent organs (vessels, nerves, joints);
- the presence or absence of adjacent tumour foci and more remote lesions (scintigraphy).

In the common form with metaphyseal localisation, the image of the tumour, rarely median, shows both sclerosis and lysis. The cortex is destroyed and the soft tissues are invaded. Around this cortical breach the periosteum reacts by forming new bony layers parallel to the cortex. This periosteal neoformation is known by the name of Codman's triangle (fig. 1 a). This bony reaction is in no way specific. The neoplastic osteogenic proliferation sometimes develops in strands perpendicular to the long axis of the bone. This type of proliferation has been described under the names of "grass fire" and "sunburst" (fig. 3), etc.

This appearance of invasion of the soft tissues is only seen in already advanced forms.

It is important to measure the dimensions of the tumour on the CT image in the three planes of space (fig. 8). MRI will also show (fig. 2) its extension into the medullary canal on the one hand and towards the growth plate and the epiphysis on the other. These examinations will permit assessment of the circumferential extension towards muscle, skin and neuro-vascular structures.

Angiography is of no diagnostic value but is often necessary before operative resection. It shows the position of the vessels, which may be displaced or invaded by the tumour, but also the presence of newly-formed peripheral vessels which argues in favor of major involvement of the principal vessels.

Scintigraphy, besides providing an image of the lesion, allows detection of other possible skeletal lesions (fig. 23 a, b), and also evaluation of the tumour capture of a radio-labelled antimitotic agent, such as interferon (fig. 24). Compared with the healthy limb, there is usually an increase of labelling at the distal and proximal extremities of the long bones of the affected limb. These phenomena are associated with the hypervascularisation of the limb (or with its effects) and are not usually of practical importance, but in one of our cases this hyperfixation to an epiphysis opposite to the tumour, regarded as normal, corresponded to a genuine metastasis.

Tumour lesions near the primary focus have been described by the name of "skip metastases" [Enneking & Kagan 1965, Anani et al 1987].

Lymphography will be indicated if the clinical examination discloses superficial adenopathies.

During resection performed after the first courses of chemotherapy, the pathologist must verify the absence of tumour in the medullary canal and the integrity of the soft tissues covering the tumour by frozen section.

Subsequently, after paraffin embedding, he will assess the efficacy of the therapeutic program from a section of the tumour through its widest diameters. The prognosis, though transformed by the administration of chemical agents, remains grave: 20-30% of patients, the statistics show, die in the first five years from metastatic spread, particularly pulmonary, but bony or visceral metastases are not uncommon.

Biopsy

It is essential that the biopsy, of limited dimensions, be performed:
- from the center of the tumour as located by the imaging;
- through as short an incision as possible, allowing for the access route that will be used for the resection if this is envisaged.

The biopsy may involve only one of the histological aspects of a polymorphic sarcoma and thus lead to a false classification.

Frozen section

Immediate examination by pathologists who have to deal with this type of tumour fairly often may be justified. While it may not provide a firm diagnosis, it at least ensures that the fragment removed is neoplastic, and not necrotic, and sections can be placed on slides under the best conditions.

Other and more daring pathological units are satisfied with a cytological examination, which usually does no more than confirm a diagnosis obvious from the clinical features and imaging, but which does not permit strict classification of the tumour.

Assessment of the efficacy of the treatment program

Before the era of chemotherapy, macroscopic examination of the amputation specimen showed the polymorphism of the sarcoma, the alternation of chondroid, bony, necrotic and haemorrhagic zones and the fleshy reddish areas of cell proliferation.

Nowadays, resection or amputation are performed after several courses of antimitotic agents. The difficult problem for the pathologist is to assess the percentage of visible cells in a section passing through the main axes of the tumour (diagram 1).

It is useful to recall the classification of Rosen (1982):

I	viable cells:	95%
IIa	viable cells:	50-94%
IIb	viable cells:	6-49%
III	viable cells:	1-5%
IV	viable cells:	0%

Classes III and IV respond well to treatment.

In the study of Valenty (1989), based on this scale of classification, only 42% of patients were classed as good responders.

This numerical reckoning does not exclude the need for a general description or a diagram indicating the sites of breaching of the cortex or growth-plate, or invasion of the soft tissues. It is also useful to define the distance between the tumour and the level of surgical section, in both the bony and soft tissues.

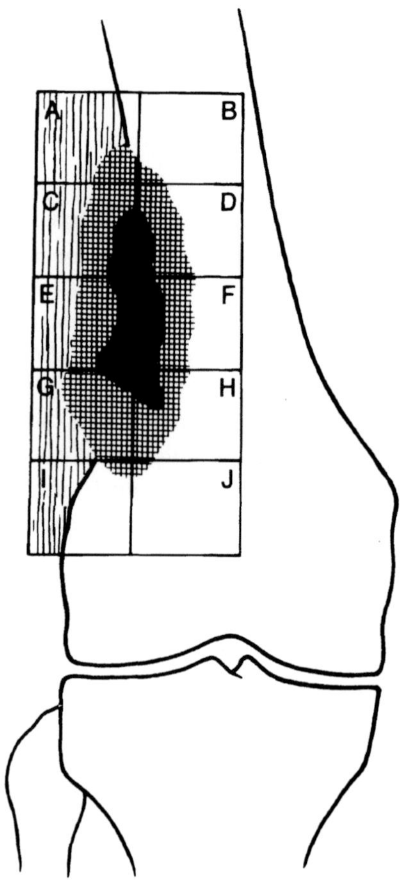

Diagram 1. Diagram to show the percentage of necrosis after the first courses of antimitotic agents. From the resection specimen submitted to the pathologist, he must choose the greatest sectional areas of the tumour for sampling. He takes as many samples as necessary to study the entirety of the sarcoma and its immediate bony and possibly musculo-aponeurotic environment. In the diagram above, ten blocks for embedding are necessary to assess on each surface the percentage of necrotic tissue in relation to healthy tissue. It is also useful to study the distal and proximal extremities of the resection. In the case of a poor responder seen here, only the central zone is necrotic (black). This represents 17% of the total surface of the tumour section (which corresponds to about 7% in volume). Figures of 95% of the surface would need to be reached to estimate at around 90-92% the true amount of necrotic tissue. Currently, some teams estimate that 80% of necrotic surface justifies classification among the "good responders".

Histological grade of malignancy

An attempt to give the numerical value to the histological grade of malignancy may be attempted for the ordinary type of skeletogenic sarcoma. Knowledge of this factor is of value in assessing the prognosis, and may consequently affect the treatment program. Most of the other forms have their own special prognosis, wich contributes to their classification. Currently, in most cases, the statistics do not take into account either the pathological type or the histological grade of malignancy. At least two reasons may be cited for this deficiency; first, the small number of cases in each subgroup, of both common and anaplastic forms and, second, a degree of imprecision in the histological diagnosis. It is obvious also that fine-needle biopsy cannot provide classification in a precise subgroup.

Nevertheless, some clinicians find it frustrating not to be able to refer to a numerical code for histological malignancy. In these conditions one may try to apply one of the systems recommended for tumours of the soft tissues; some rely solely on the number of cells in division, others consider mitoses, differentiation and necrosis [Broders, Myrrhe-Jensen, cancer centers, etc.]. The degree of malignancy can also be measured using the grading developed by the teams of cancer centers such as the Institut Gustave-Roussy and the Bergonié center (table 1).

Whatever the option of the pathologist, one important fact remains: one must be able to compare the histological appearance of the biopsy with that of the tumour after the first courses of preoperative chemotherapy, so as to assess the efficacy of the treatment program instituted.

After some years, and experience based on examination of resection specimens, it appears that:
- anaplastic sarcomas are very sensitive to chemical agents, including, according to several reports, telangiectatic sarcoma (this needs to be confirmed on a greater number);
- skeletogenic sacomas are less sensitive to antimitotics when they are richer in cartilaginous tissue.

These fundamental findings influence the formulation of the pathologist's report, but it should not be forgotten, as every oncologist can confirm, that two tumours of identical localisation and histology in patients of the same age may have a very different outcome.

Course

It may be of some value to assess the modification of the clinical course over the last 15 years and to note some statistics.

Dun and Dehner (1977), studying pulmonary metastases, remarked on their resemblance to the primary tumour (60%), but deduced no prognostic feature from their observations in 15 patients whose 5-year survival was 33%. In the same year, Shrikhande and Rao (1977) studied the local and regional lymph nodes removed during amputation. A sinus histiocytosis seemed to be a favorable prognostic factor, but the 5-year survival rate in their 77 patients was less than 20%.

Prognosis

The prognosis of osteogenic sarcoma has been transformed by the introduction of antimitotic agents. Although there are some divergences between the statistics presenting the overall results, probably due in large part to the recruitment of the patients, the incidence of "good responders" based on 80% necrosis (and not 95% as Rosen proposes) is of the order of 80%.

The 3-year survival after chemotherapy and resection, supplemented if need by irradiation, is around 80-85%. Before the antimitotic era, many prognostic factors were analysed. Among all the variables considered, three appear determinant:

- the presence of metastases noted at the first examination;
- the size of the tumour;
- a "non-surgical" location, pelvic or thoracic, that is one not allowing wide resectional surgery in good conditions.

Valenty (1989) studied the prognostic factors in osteosarcoma based on 139 case histories from the Institut Gustave-Roussy, excluding osteosarcomas of the pelvis and craniofacial region. In monofactorial analysis among the 19 variables studied, 7 had prognostic value for long-term survival.

Unfavorable prognostic factors were:

- the presence of metastases;
- breaching of the epiphyseal growth-plate;
- tumour extent exceeding 33% of the bone;
- ossification of the tumour and soft parts unchanged or less than that observed in the initial radiographs;
- increase in size under chemotherapy;
- necrosis less than 95% according to Rosen in the resection specimen (this figure is probably too high);
- absence of complete remission at the end of treatment.

However, the development of a metastasis or local and regional recurrence was not associated with any of the variables studied (clinical, radiological or histological). The value of statistical studies is to confirm and quantify ideas for the most part already known to clinicians, even though there are sometimes considerable variations between the figures provided by different statistics.

Table 1.

Grade 1:	undifferentiated portion differentiated	0-25%, 75%
Grade 2:	undifferentiated differentiated	25-50%, 75-50%
Grade 3:	undifferentiated differentiated	50-75%, 50-25%
Grade 4:	undifferentiated differentiated	75-100%, 25%

Grading of Broders established for epitheliomas (Archives of Pathology and Laboratory Medicine 1926, 2; 376-381)

Grade 1:	well-differentiated tumour, 2 mitoses per 20 fields of 250 cells
Grade 2:	moderately differentiated tumour, 10 mitoses per 20 fields
Grade 3:	10 mitoses or more per 20 fields

Netherlands Committee

Necrosis	0	
	1	less than 50% of sectional surface
	2	50% and more of sectional surface
Mitoses	1	0-9 per 10 fields at magn. 40 x 10
	2	10-19 per 10 fields
	3	20 or more per 10 fields
Differentiation	1	sarcoma reproducing a near-normal tissue appearance
	2	of certain histological type
	3	undifferentiated sarcoma
Total:		2 and 3: grade 1; 4 and 5: grade 2; 6, 7, 8: grade 3

Established for sarcomas of soft tissues, adopted by the majority of French cancer centers

Grade 1:	minimal anaplasia
Grade 2:	moderate anaplasia
Grade 3:	severe anaplasia
Biologic grades of malignancy:	
Grade 1:	slow growth, less than 10% with metastases in 5 years
Grade 2:	rather rapid growth
Grade 3:	very rapid growth, more than 50% with metastases in 5 years

From Mirra JM, Picci P, Gold RH (1989) In: Bone Tumours

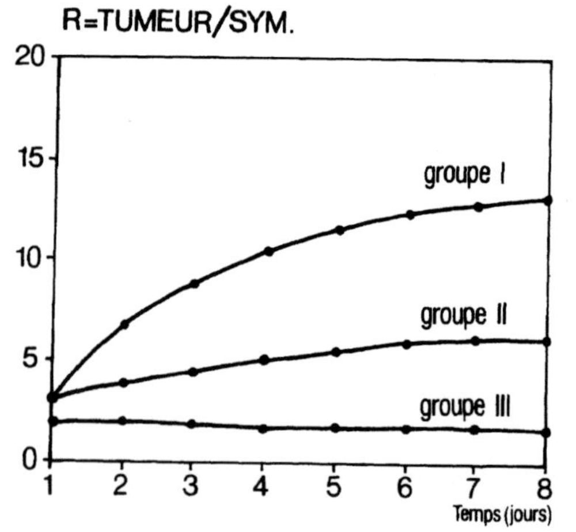

Diagram 2. Kinetic curves of fixation of $^{85}SrCl_2$ by "common types" of osteogenic sarcoma

Group I: osteoblastic: 25% of observed cases

Group Ii: mixed: 50% of cases studied

Group III: anaplastic: 25% of cases studied

Principle of method: after intravenous administration of a dose of $^{85}SrCl_2$ related to patient age, external measurements are made daily of the gamma radiation of ^{85}Sr at the level of the tumour and over the symmetric healthy zone. These measurements are simple and quick to perform (60 s). The curve drawn over a week is representative of the tumour capture of the osteotrope for each patient.
Ordinate: ratio R of clicks per second = tumour zone / symmetric healthy zone.
Abscissa: time in days.

groupe = group
temps (jours) = time in days

It is even more serious for the pathologist to note the impossibility of harmonising the data emanating from different centers. For example: Price (1961, 1966) diagnosed four times as many chondroblastic as fibroblastic sarcomas, whereas Dahlin (1977, 1986), in 650 cases, diagnosed 155 chondroblastic and 152 fibroblastic lesions. In the Danish statistics [Bentzen et al 1988] osteoblastic sarcomas (102) were 5 times as numerous as fibroblastic lesions (20); Dahlin found osteoblastic lesions occur twice as often (333 against 152). In some reports, the majority of tumours are described as of the "ordinary" type. Such discordant pathological data renders their inclusion in a unified statistical study illusory.

Supplementary investigations

Many authors have endeavored to obtain supplementary information to aid in diagnosis and prognosis.

Enzymatic studies demonstrate a high activity of alkaline phosphatase in the intra- and extracellular vesicles [Thorpe et al 1979]. An increased blood-level of alkaline phosphatase seems to be correlated with the prognosis, but allowance must be made for the size of the tumour, which is also known to be so correlated. Carbohydrate metabolism is disturbed in around 75% of cases. An increased blood level of lacto-dehydrogenase above 200 IU/ml indicates a poor prognosis [McMaster 1977, Goodman et al 1978]. DNA studies have not yet provided sufficiently convincing results for incorporation into current practice.

Nevertheless, for Mankin et al (1991) the study of the nuclear concentration of DNA by flow cytometry, employing some technical improvements, may supply information of prognostic value and also allow assessment of the efficacy of treatment.

Another supplementary examination, using radioisotopic markers, has allowed us to validate the classification into skeletogenic and anaplastic sarcomas in a study of over 100 cases of common forms of sarcoma at the Institut Curie; the latter group represent 25% of common types of sarcoma (diagram 2).

In fact, there is available an ideal marker for the functional differentiation of sarcoma cells: their ability to produce osteoid. The identification of osteoid tissue by means of a radioactive agent to obtain an overall functional estimation of the tumour metabolism, unlike histological examinations which study the tumour process is only carried out in a small sample. Because its metabolism resembles that of calcium and its ease of use, $^{85}Sr\ Cl_2$ was chosen for this study [Mazabraud et al 1986]. The measurements carried out allowed distinction of three functional isotopic groups among the ordinary types of sarcoma:

- group 1: osteogenic sarcomas which produce major amounts of virtually pure osteoid tissue;
- group II: mixed sarcomas which produce both osteoid and chondroid material;
- group III: anaplastic sarcomas.

These isotopic results were compared with imaging and pathological examination, biopsies and resection specimens.

CT and MRI form part of routine imaging. Angiography is often indispensable as a preoperative inestigation. Scintigrapy with ^{99m}Tc-labeled diphosphonates is an excellent technique, not only for studying the extent of the lesion and later for the very early detection of possible metastases, but also for recognising anaplastic telangiectatic sarcomas.

Aetiology

Numerous hypotheses have been advanced and a role for irradiation has been demonstrated many times.

A viral origin, suggested as possible or even probable in a certain number of cases, has not been demonstrated formally [Finkel et al 1966, 1967].

In their study of 91 secondary sarcomas, where 68 osteosarcomas developed in children treated for various tumours, Newton et al (1991) attempt to identify the roles of irradiation, antimitotic agents and genetic factors. It is interesting to note that 48 osteosarcomas developed in the irradiation field, while 20 appeared outside this field and in non-irradiated children

In these 68 cases of osteosarcoma, the primary tumour was a retinoblastoma in 26; in the other cases, it was Ewing's sarcoma, neuroblastoma, Hodgkin's disease, rhabdomyosarcoma, and so on. The authors consider that they had confirmed the importance of genetic factors, irradiation and the mutagenicity of the anthracyclines.

Molecular analyses [Araki et al 1991, Yamaguchi et al 1992, Scholz et al 1992] have demonstrated loss of heterozygosity (LOH) at the retinoblastoma locus (RB) in more than 50% of primary osteosarcomas. This RB LOH seems to be correlated with an unfavourable outcome [Feugeas et al 1996]. Hansen states (1991) that the association of at least two molecular modifications is necessary: that of the retinoblastoma gene and the p53 gene (chromosome 17).

The Rothmund-Thomson syndrome is regarded as an aetiological factor. Sim et al (1992) reported a case of multicentric osteosarcoma in a girl of 15 and four other cases have been reported previously, of which that of Rebaud et al (1985) is a familial manifestation of this syndrome.

The role of trauma, so often discussed, sometimes poses a difficult medicolegal problem. Every pathologist at some time in his career has examined cases of a tumour developing at the exact site of an injury sustained some months or years previously. While the facts may be beyond dispute, it is difficult to demonstrate a cause and effect relationship with any degree of certainty. Apart from the great variability of the latent period, it is necessary to be able to observe the radiographs showing integrity of the bone either just before the injury or in the hours following. The presence of a haemorrhage often followed by a large hematoma with local over-production of platelets (platelet growth factor), possibly associated with a genetic factor, may be invoked hypothetically. To deny the fact on the basis of its rarity would be an error of judgment.

Several cases of malignant tumours have been reported in bone infarctions and in contact with prosthetic material, particularly at the hip-joint. In such cases one should perhaps take into account, beside the surgical trauma as a factor in haemorrhage and infarction, the presence of metallic foreign bodies which might induce sarcoma by chemical induction.

Common histopathological types

Skeletogenic sarcomas

Mixed osteogenic and chondrogenic

The essential nature of this common type is its polymorphism.

Within the sarcomatous cellular proliferation, rich in mitoses and anomalous forms, there is atypical osteogenesis consisting of unequal strands with large fibers, without regular lamellar organisation. Zones of denser osteogenesis alternate with looser zones. There is an infinite range of modalities of this osteogenesis. Sometimes it is a plexus, packed with fine osteoid strands, sometimes there are small osteoid patches isolated from one another whose haematinophil centers are partly calcified. Sometimes the frayed apppearance of the osteogenesis and its marked calcification suggest bone infarction (fig. 32). Between these osteoid or bony areas, the tumour cells proliferate in a loose and very vascular connective tissue.

The chondroid sarcomatous zones are irregularly distributed and vary in their profusion. Usually commoner in young children, they risk being the only zone involved in the biopsy.

It is important to mention in the pathological report the existence of these chondrosarcomatous zones, which are less sensitive to chemotherapy than the poorly differentiated osteoblastic areas. Tumour zones may be observed with fusiform cells and especially anaplastic areas (fig. 26 c). It is customary to assess the extent of the zones of haemorrhage and necrosis in the biopsy, and the degree of vascularisation, and presence or absence of intravascular tumour cells. The presence of some giant cells, macrophages and inflammatory cells is commonplace.

Table 2. System of differential diagnosis (Dd): "common type" of sarcoma

a) Skeletogenic sarcomas
- correct biopsy, no differential diagnosis
- biopsy too small, only one aspect of mixed forms available
- search for anaplastic areas
- mention presence or even predominance of chondroid tissue

b) Anaplastic sarcomas
- telangiectatic sarcoma, a major problem: exclude aneurysmal cyst by minute study of cytology
- cytological variants:
  - small-cell sarcoma: differentiate from Ewing's tumour, neuroepithlioma, lymphoma, resort to histochemistry and histoimmunology
  - sarcoma with giant cells: in adults consider: giant-cell tumour, malignant fibrous histiocytoma

In some polymorphous sarcomas of the common type, vascularisation may become considerably overdeveloped. These sarcomas are very likely to cause metastases through the bloodstream but must not be confused with telangiectatic sarcomas of anaplastic type.

Predominantly osteogenic

This again is a mixed type of sarcoma, but the osteogenesis occupies 75% or more of the surface area of the sections, the remainder being represented by chondroid tissue and small patches of poorly differentiated cells.

Predominantly chondrogenic

Some osteogenic sarcomas, with typical cytonuclear monstrosities, are particularly rich in chondroid tissue (fig. 33), which occupies at least 75% of the sectional surface. The radiological image is both lytic and sclerotic. The report should mention the presence of abundant cartilaginous tissue, which suggests that surgical treatment of this chondroid subgroup of ordinary sarcoma should not be too long deferred. In this case, the differential diagnosis from a chondrosarcoma does not arise; the problem arises in the other direction, with a partly ossified chondrosarcoma. Another difficulty, posed by a biopsy which has involved only the periphery of a cartilaginous lobule surrounded by undifferentiated cells, is to distinguish this tumour from a mesenchymal chondrosarcoma. In this chondroid osteosarcoma the differentiated cells which show the tumour activity are more atypical than the small round or fusiform mesenchymal cells of mesenchymal chondrosarcoma.

Purely osteoid and osteogenic

Examination of the radiographs attracts attention to the density of the tumour opacity, which may suggest a sclerosing osteosarcomatosis or a very differentiated osteoblastic sarcoma. The histological examination shows a tight plexus of largely calcified osteoid tissue within a sarcomatous stroma.

Diagnosis of skeletogenic sarcoma

By definition, a differential diagnosis only arises for variants from the typical mixed form.

A predominantly osteoblastic sarcomatous tumour may be associated with major osteoclastic proliferation. With a little - or a lot - of bad luck, if the biopsy removes virtually only a very cellular zone, one may then suspect a sarcomatous giant-cell tumour.

When presentation has been with fracture, a reparative cartilaginous reaction must be distinguished from a predominantly cartilaginous sarcoma.

In some tumours, the predominance of osteoblasts of fusiform appearance in a biopsy may suggest a non-osteogenic sarcoma, such as fibroblastic sarcoma, malignant fibrous histiocytoma or leiomyosarcoma.

The major problems arise either from an inadequate or unsatisfactory biopsy, coupled with failure to forward the clinical and radiological records. In these circumstances, the pathologist need not give an opinion. If the biopsy is inadequate, he should request a second, and if despite his request he does not receive the clinical and radiological data, he cannot be expected to give a categoric response.

Anaplastic sarcomas

Within the infinite variety of cellular anaplasia, several types of sarcoma have been distinguished, some by their histological characteristics, others by their cellular morphology. This systematisation allows a classification of these rare tumours, whose radiological appearance is essentially lytic (fig. 4).

Telangiectatic

This tumour has been the subject of numerous publications [Huvos et al 1982, Pignatti et al 1991, Mervak et al 1991].

- General considerations

Telangiectatic forms represent around 6-9% of osteogenic sarcomas. Male predominance is of the order of 2 :1. The maximum incidence occurs in the second decade. The preferential localisation is classically metaphyseal, but I have seen several cases of diaphyseal and diaphyso-metaphyseal lesions.

- Symptomatology and course

In this type, the cortex is rapidly destroyed and fracture is the presenting feature more often than in the common type.

The history should convey the notion that the injury described could not have accounted for fracture of the femur in an adolescent without previous pathology. In other cases, it is swelling and/or pain that attract attention.

The cases currently reported are few, though the statistics of Pignatti et al (1991) and Mervak et al (1991), of 17 and 19 cases respectively, seem to confirm the sensitivity of this anaplastic sarcoma to chemotherapy.

- Imaging

The radiological image, essentially lytic (fig. 7), sometimes suggests a diagnosis of aneurysmal cyst or giant-cell tumour. If there has been a fracture, the displacement of the fragments may mask the cortical lysis.

If there is the slightest suspicion, and if the imaging does not allow of unequivocal interpretation, the fracture site must be accessed for the purpose of diagnosis with biopsy through the least damaging approach in a territory which will be removed during a possible resection.

- Pathological anatomy and histopathology

The radiological and clinical diagnosis of aneurysmal cyst or giant-cell tumour will not necessarily be corrected by the macroscopic appearance when accessing the lesion: a haemorrhagic cystic cavity fragments of whose wall are removed. Such findings may "wrong foot" the pathologist.

Histological examination (figs. 35, 36) shows a very cellular cyst wall in which some narrow osteoid or bony bands border a haemorrhagic cavity, an appearance completely identical with that of an aneurysmal cyst.

It is the close study of cells in technically perfect sections that will allow the diagnosis by identifying some frankly atypical monstrous cells.

In cases where the pathologist is requested to identify this "aneurysmal cyst" or "giant-cell tumour" from a frozen section, if he cannot be certain, surgical treatment should be deferred until after the examination of paraffin sections. Inappropriate treatment (curettage of this "cyst-sarcoma" or nailing of a "fracture-sarcoma") will make resection definitely impracticable, thus compelling amputation.

In a giant-cell tumour, the cells are more regular in their form and dimensions. There is no increase in the nuclear-cytoplasmic ratio in a benign giant-cell tumour.

Osteoblastoma is easier to exclude because of the presence of patches of well-differentiated bizarre osteoblasts, without atypical mitoses.

At low magnification a haemangio-endothelioma may be suggested. Apart from the fact that there is no tumour related osteogenesis in endothelioma, the turgescent endothelial cells, the formation of cells of different sizes and, if necessary, the immunohistochemistry, provide arguments separating the lesion completely from telangiectatic anaplastic sarcoma with its areas of atypical cells and cavities devoid of endothelium.

Confusion of this anaplastic sarcoma with a hypervascular osteogenic sarcoma is less serious, particularly since the same treatment program is currently applied to both lesions. However, it is important to diagnose anaplastic telangiectatic sarcoma, whose prognosis before the chemotherapy era was particularly grave, so as to monitor the efficacy of treatment in a greater number of cases.

- The value of dynamic vascular tests

Current imaging techniques, especially when supplemented by dynamic vascular tests, prove capable of identifying the effective extent of tumour vascularisation.

The technique published by Perdereau et al (1993) imposes no additional constraint on the patient. It is based on the study of the kinetic bio-distribution of a radioactive isotope (^{99m}Tc-MDP) used routinely during assessment of the extent of primary bone tumours. Information can thus be gathered directly, derived in real time from the blood circulation in the tumour. These data are sufficient to identify unambiguously the hypervascularisation characteristic of telangiectatic forms. A study made at the Institut Curie on 20 patients affected by anaplastic osteogenic sarcoma showed that the initial vascular distribution of the radio-technetium tracer can be analysed from the kinetic curves of the passage of the radioactive embolus in the dynamic scintigrams. Of the various variables considered, the most significant are the height and breadth of the first peak

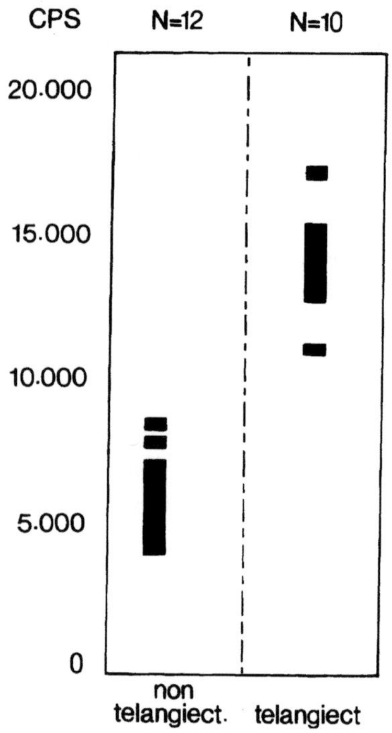

Diagram 3. Vascularisation of anaplastic sarcomas. Tumour vascular distribution of 99mTc-MDP (peak value of first passage of radioactive total). Rapid kinetic analysis by sequential scintigraphy (SSK): clicks per second. The number of clicks per second clearly separates telangiectatic anaplastic sarcoma from non-telangiectatic varieties

(diagram 3). The 20 cases analysed were divided into two groups in terms of tumour vascularity.

- hypervascularised forms
  ratio vasc T/vasc sym = 7.01 ± 0.67 (8 cases)
- non-hypervascularised forms
  ratio vasc T/vasc sym = 2.73 ± 0.25 (12 cases)

Analysis of the curves of passage allow the sharp distinction of a functional vascularisation from simple circulatory stasis, based on the breadth of the first peak of transit. A transit time greater than 30 seconds is evidence of stasis. The eight cases studied all exhibited a transit time of less than 30 seconds (mean 22.4 ± 2.1). Histological confirmation was made fom the biopsy in five cases and from the resection specimen in the other three cases. This technique allows improvement of the diagnosis of telangiectatic forms of anaplastic sarcomas and more generally the assessment of the global effective vascular status of any tumour lesion.

Cytological variants

Small celled (figs. 4-6, 13, 39, 40)

- General considerations

This is a very rare type of anaplastic osteogenic sarcoma, about 4-5% of total osteosarcomas.

It is equally distributed in both sexes, and affects children and adults.

The lesion sometimes has a metaphyseal site, sometimes diaphyseal, extending rapidly to virtually the entire diaphysis.

- Clinical features and course

The clinical features are those of anaplastic sarcoma; it is lytic and is more often revealed by spontaneous fracture than the common type. It responds well to chemotherapy.

- Imaging and diagnosis

Both radiologically and at low magnification in histological examination, the tumour may suggest a lymphosarcoma or a Ewing's sarcoma [Sim et al 1979, Ayala et al 1989].

Lymphosarcoma is easily excluded by the immunohistological reactions, and Ewing's sarcoma by the monotonous morphology of cells with fine fragmented chromatin, a barely visible nucleolus, and complete absence of osteoid formation. However, the presence of intracytoplasmic glycogen was demonstrable in 10 of the 27 cases of small-celled osteosarcomas studied by Ayala et al (1989). I have often noted the fact that the presence of intracytoplasmic glycogen in a small-cell sarcoma in no way signifies that it is a Ewing's sarcoma.

However anaplastic they may be, these sarcomas are osteogenic and study of the surfaces of sufficient sections reveals the presence of fine osteoid strands, a fundamental feature which also excludes the diagnoses of neuroepithelioma and metastases from neuroblastoma. But Dickersin and Rosenberg (1991) stress the difficulty of ultrastructural diagnosis in Ewing's sarcoma and mesenchymal chondrosarcoma if the biopsy contains no osteoid tissue.

Polymorphic celled

- General considerations, clinical features

This is a rare form of osteogenic sarcoma. Its site is electively metaphyseal. Pain is the usual presenting symptom.

- Imaging

Radiologically, there is a rounded translucent area with fuzzy outlines, and minimal or no periosteal reaction.

- Pathological anatomy and histology

A fleshy haemorrhagic mass replaces the destroyed bony tissue.

At histological examination the tumour consists of polyhedral cells of varying shape. Mitoses are numerous and cytonuclear anomalies abound.

The presence of some fine osteoid strands excludes any diagnosis other than that of osteogenic sarcoma, but such anaplastic polymorphous zones may also coexist with frankly osteogenic zones as found in osteo-sarcomatosis (fig. 41b).

Giant celled

- General considerations

This is a very rare type of anaplastic osteogenic sarcoma but its histology poses particular problems. The few cases I have observed affected young adults.

- Imaging

In the radiographs the tumour presents as a metaphyseal or metaphyseo-epiphyseal lytic image without definite boundaries.

- Pathological anatomy and histopathology

The proliferation of poorly differentiated polyhedral sarcomatous cells is somewhat reminiscent of an osteoblastic proliferation. The whole is strewn with giant cells of unequal size; monstrosities and atypical cells are numerous (fig. 38).

Though osteoid formation is particularly scanty, it does allow the tumour to be classed with the osteogenic sarcomas.

- Diagnosis

In its typical form the diagnosis of sarcoma is obvious.

However, if a zone of active osteoclastic resorption happens to be the only one removed in the biopsy of a common type of sarcoma, it should not be confused with an anaplastic sarcoma with giant cells. The imaging is incompatible with this diagnosis.

The diagnosis of a possible giant-cell tumour may arise, and be countered by the observation in the resection specimen of a typical tumour zone with benign giant cells: hypothesis and observation are at odds.

A malignant fibrous histiocytoma with giant cells is to be considered if there are frankly overlapping ("tiled") appearances and if the osteogenesis is in fact only a minor elaboration of a few reactive osteoid strands.

The diagnosis of sarcoma supervening in Paget's disease does not arise in this solitary tumour in a young adult.

Once these various possibilities are excluded, the existence of an anaplastic sarcoma with giant cells must be accepted.

Fusiform celled

This may pose a difficult problem of differentiation from malignant fibrous histiocytoma, which may elaborate some minuscule osteoid areas (fig. 37). According to Naka et al (1995) the percentage of "malignant fibrous pseudo-histiocytomas" in patients over 40 is 29.2%, but only 5.4% before that age.

If the biopsy technique provides very small samples, there is a risk that the pathologist may consider a diagnosis of fibroblastic sarcoma.

In this subsection on the anaplastic osteogenic sarcomas, the errors in histological interpretation of the different variants listed have been mentioned.

These sarcomas share a destructive lytic nature and a sparse osteogenesis, due to the functional non-differentiation of the cells, but also a sensitivity to chemotherapy as noted in the resection specimens. Just as, in our view, it is useful to distinguish between functional and morphological differentiation, so it is useful to distinguish between sensitivity and curability. Unfortunately, probably because of the small number of cases, the statistics usually ignore these anatomo-pathologic variants.

Anatomo-clinical types

Besides these common anatomo-pathological types, which may be classed in two subgroups, skeletogenic and anaplastic, clinical and pathological types have been distinguished which cause the pathologist more specific problems.

Onset type

Presenting early with pain, an osteosarcoma at its very onset appears in the radiographs only as a small rounded lytic lesion, variably studded with fine opacities [de Santos & Edeiken 1985].

Diagnosis

In these circumstances, the diagnosis of osteoid osteoma or osteoblastoma may have to be considered (fig. 11).

At low magnification, examination of the sections is not incompatible with the hypothesis of an osteoid osteoma (fig. 44) or an osteoblastoma (fig. 45). Examination at higher magnification reveals anisocytosis and an increased ratio of nucleus to cytoplasm, which is sufficient, even if mitoses are rare, to indicate a cell proliferation which conceals its malignancy behind a benign architecture.

Conversely, in other circumstances, the radiological and histological appearances wrongly suggest a diagnosis of early osteosarcoma, particularly in the case of insertional tendinitis. The demonstration of its very common bilateral nature suffices to dispel the anxiety provoked by the radiological image of "breach of the cortex and ossification in the soft tissues with subjacent lysis". Despite the architectural derangement, the sections do not show any cytonuclear monstrosities.

Table 3. System of differential diagnosis (Dd): clinical-morphological types

Early forms
Differential diagnosis: osteoid osteoma, osteoblastoma suggested by imaging. Conversely, distinguish between insertional tendinitis and osteosarcoma

Four entities of low malignancy
Juxtacortical sarcoma
Differential diagnosis: osteoma (medullary tissue), fibroma (no malignant cells)
Periosteal sarcoma
Differential diagnosis: chondroma, fibroma
Intramedullary fusiform-cell sarcoma
Differential diagnosis: fibrous dysplasia, fibromatosis, fibrosis secondary to inflammation or a treated tumour, fibroblastic sarcoma of low grade malignancy
Well-differentiated osteoblastic sarcoma
Differential diagnosis: osteoblastoma (bizarre osteoblasts)

Common form of sarcoma of grades I, II or III malignancy, deceptive from their localisation:
Juxta-osseous, intracortical, epiphyseal, intramedullary. The site does not necessarily determine the histology
Synchronic osteosarcomatosis: young patients
Diachronic osteosarcomatosis: adults, axial predominance
Differential diagnosis: osteosclerotic metastases, sarcomatous transformation at multiple foci of Paget's disease, metastases from osteosarcoma

Four entities of low grade malignancy

Juxtacortical osteosarcoma

- General considerations

This represents around 4% of osteogenic sarcomas. It is as common, or even commoner, in women than in men. Its maximum incidence is in the third and fourth decades and the site is the popliteal surface of the femur. It may affect the diaphyseal or metaphyseal regions of any of the long bones.

- Clinical features

Pain is minimal or absent and the only sign is the tumour, which is discovered by the patient or during a medical examination performed for some other reason.

- Imaging

Imaging reveals a dense well-circumscribed mass implanted on the metaphyseal or diaphyseal cortex by a relatively wide base, but above and below this there persists a clear space between tumour and cortex. This clear space is easily demonstrable, even in standard films, when the tumour is not too bulky. During its course the tumour "rolls itself up" around the cortex; the CT sections are then very important, for this rather characteristic clear space differentiates this tumour from periosteal sarcoma (figs. 15-18).

- Pathological anatomy and histopathology

Macroscopically, this is a smooth, apparently well-circumscribed tumour, plastered with tendino-aponeurotic fibers. On section, its consistency is either that of a dense fibroma of whitish surface or that of a markedly ossified tumour, the base of which is continuous with the cortex. These appearances are very different from the spongy architecture of an osteoma, whose medullary spaces are occupied by fatty, sometimes even mildly haematopoietic, marrow.

The histological appearances vary with cases, but also in different parts of the same tumour (figs. 42, 43):

- a dense appearance of fusiform cells crowded together;
- collagenous plaques in which the elongated cells are difficult to analyse and with a varying degree of bone formation;
- anastomosed bony strands or densely marbled zones.

The fusiform cells are regular and quiescent; mitoses are very rare. A search of large areas of the section under high magnification is necessary to detect mitoses and rare anomalies. Peripherally, the tumour infiltrates the tendino-aponeurotic tissues and the boundary between tumour and healthy tissue is often difficult to detect.

If diagnosis is delayed, the tumour will have destroyed the cortex and invaded the medullary canal. If treated without undue delay, wide resection is followed in the great majority of cases by definitive cure, but too "economical" a procedure is invariably followed by local recurrence. These recurrences sometimes exhibit a marked deterioration in histological appearances. Metastases may finally develop.

- Differential diagnosis

The most serious diagnostic error is to think in terms of a benign lesion of the nature of an osteoma, myositis ossificans or ossifying tendinitis, in view of the cellular density in which the osteogenesis develops. Osteoma, myositis and ossifying tendinitis do not develop in a sarcomatous stroma.

An error with equally grave consequences is failure to recognise a sarcoma of the ordinary type developing at a juxacortical site (figs. 9, 30), whose prognosis is quite different from that of the entity of "juxtacortical sarcoma". But genuine sarcomas of juxtacortical type have been reported which showed a zone of "dedifferentiation" from the outset [Pintado et al 1989].

Periosteal sarcoma

- General considerations

This rare tumour accounts for around 1% of osteogenic sarcomas. It is commoner in men. Its age distribution is more extensive than in the common form. Its localisation is most frequently at the diaphyseal or metaphyseo-diaphyseal regions of the long bones: tibia, femur, humerus, but it has also been found in flat bones.

- Clinical features and course

The tumour presents with dull pain or swelling. Its prognosis is relatively favorable, though in some series the mortality was of the order of 15%, due to pulmonary metastases, after an average period of 6 years and 7 - months [Hall et al 1985].

- Imaging

The origin of the tumour is supposedly periosteal. The important fact is its adhesion to the underlying cortex throughout its extent. In the radiographs there is no clear space between tumour and cortex. Some opaque spots and some bony spicules at right angles to the cortex stand out against the radiolucent background of the tumour (figs. 10, 12, 14).

- Pathologic anatomy and histopathology

Macroscopically, the tumour adheres to the bone and is apparently well demarcated from the superficial planes. On section it is glistening, of cartilaginous consistency and appearance, with some grayish-white spicules of ossification.

If the tumour is advanced, it destroys the cortex and invades the cancellous bone.

In view of the predominance of cartilaginous tissue shown at histological examination, some authors class this tumour with the juxtacortical chondrosarcomas, but the formation of new tumoural bone justifies the label of osteosarcoma. Hall et al (1985) , reviewing 55 cases from the literature and 6 personal cases, stress the essential distinction between periosteal chondrosarcoma and periosteal osteosarcoma.

Well-differentiated fusiform-cell intramedullary sarcoma

- General considerations

This rare form represents 1.25% of the osteosarcomas in the Mayo Clinic series [Dahlin & Unni 1986]. It is of slow growth and a low grade of malignancy.

In the series of Kurt et al (1990), there are listed 41 men and 39 women, with a maximum incidence in the third decade and a mean age of 28.2 years in these 80 patients aged from 9 to 83 years.

Half of the cases are sited in the metaphyseal or metaphyso-diaphyseal regions of the femur, and the distribution in the bones of the skeleton as a whole is identical to that of the common form of sarcoma.

- Clinical features and course

The symptomatology is very minor - pain is not severe and late in onset - in keeping with the sluggish course. Sometimes there is a painless or slightly painful swelling, or the discovery of the bony lesion in a radiograph performed for pain in an adjacent joint may stimulate investigation and biopsy [Unni et al 1977, Sim et al 1990].

In the absence of proper treatment, the course is followd by local recurrence with possible increase in the histological grade of malignancy, noted in 15% of cases in the report of Kurt et al (1990).

- Imaging

The imaging demonstrates an osteolysis within the bone with reactive periosteal apposition. In very advanced forms, the cortex may be partly destroyed.

- Pathologic anatomy and histopathology

In the resection specimen, the firm whitish tumour occupies a more or less major part of the medullary canal; the inner aspect of the cortex is eroded. Some small hard grayish plaques represent small islands of osteogenesis. Superficially, the cortex is covered with several layers of periosteal bone.

Histologically, the medullary cavity is partly filled with bundles of fusiform cells of fibroblastic appearance. The nuclei are relatively large but without monstrosities; mitoses are rare. The whole is traversed by thin-walled vessels of large caliber. Osteogenesis is represented only by rare, small, slightly calcified zones or by fine osteoid strands sometimes reminiscent of "Chinese" letters or calligraphy, classical in fibrous dysplasia. Rarely, there are also some cartilaginous islands. The inner aspect of the cortex is irregular, partly absorbed, and the tumour as a whole is poorly demarcated.

- Diagnosis

Because of its deceptively slow course, two benign conditions may be suggested by the radiograph: fibrous dysplasia and ossifying fibroma.

The closely packed long fusiform cells, sometimes forming collagen which in places suggests a desmoid fibroma, are quite different from the short squat fusiform cells of fibrous dysplasia, regularly dispersed in a fibrillary matrix.

As for ossifying fibroma, this is quite exceptional in the long bones, apart from a tibial localisation where it is confused with osteofibrous dyslasia, in all probability a minor form of adamantinoma (cf Chapter 20).

Less serious is confusion with a fibroblastic sarcoma or a fibrous form of admantinoma justifying a wide resection. This would rectify the mistake made in interpretation of the biopsy.

Well-differentiated osteogenic sarcoma of osteoblastic type

This is a very rare type, of relatively slow development.

- Clinical features and course

The presenting feature is pain. Before the antimitotic era, this form of osteogenic sarcoma was curable by amputation in a high proportion of cases, provided that the diagnosis had been made before the onset of metastases.

- Imaging

The dense radiological image recalls that of an osteoblastoma, more rarely of an osteoma or even a local lesion of sarcomatosis.

- Pathologic anatomy and histopathology

From the histological aspect, it may be very difficult to distinguish this tumour from an osteoblastoma [Bertoni et al 1985]. But if large sectional surfaces are examined, it is very unlikely that there will not be found, less differentiated zones at the cellular level and osteoid and bony strands whose intermingling or fine plexiform appearances are incompatible with the bony production of an osteoblastoma. Small plaques of osteogenesis impossible to distinguish from those of an osteoblastoma are also found.

Examination at high magnification shows an obviously increased nuclear-cytoplasmic ratio in some cells, major variations in size and shape, and possibly one or two atypical mitoses.

The relationship of this tumour to malignant osteoblastoma is considerd in the chapter devoted to osteoblastoma (Chapter 9).

Sarcomas of common anatomo-pathological types but with unusual and deceptive localisations

Juxta-osseous, juxtacortical

The cautious terminology of the WHO - "high-grade surface osteosarcoma" - stresses the possibility of sarcomas of a high grade of malignancy located juxtacortically. Prudently, the WHO does not repeat the term "juxtacortical", a possible source of confusion. The tumour shares the characteristiscs of common types of sarcoma: higher incidence in men, involvement of the same bony sites, even their severity. While both clinicians and radiologists are inclined to speak of a "juxtacortical" sarcoma, it is wiser not to use this term in the pathological report, but on the contrary to stress the high grade of malignancy of the tumour.

It must be realised that all skeletogenic sarcomas may develop in a juxta-osseous position, whatever their histological grade of malignancy [Ahuja et al 1977, Wold et al 1984, Schajowicz et al 1988]. It has therefore been suggested [Raymond 1991] that true juxtacortical sarcomas, periosteal lesions, tumours of the common type, and those juxtacortical lesions which are dedifferentiated from the outset or subsequently, should all be listed under the heading of "surface sarcomas".

It is just as important to remember that all of these may invade the cortex and then the medullary canal, slowly in those of low-grade malignancy, more rapidly in the others. Treatment must necessarily allow for these both histological grading of malignancy and the extent of the invasion.

Intracortical

General considerations

This is a very rare type, described by Jaffe in 1960 in relation to two patients. Kyriakos (1980) reported a third case in a patient aged 24; the imaging showed a tumour developing in the tibial diaphysis and was suggestive of a benign lesion. In 1984, Vigorita et al reported another case in the lower third of the tibia. Anderson et al (1989) reported a cortical osteosarcoma of the tibia developing in a girl of 10; the radiographs were suggestive of osteoid osteoma.

This sarcoma seems to arise from the mesenchyme of the haversian canals.

Clinical features and course

The tumour presents with pain felt for 2-12 months before the first consultation. The few cases reported which were treated by resection, whether or not followed by the administration of antimitotics, were apparently cured after 7-10 months observation.

Imaging

In the radiographs the lesion is purely cortical, composed of a central lytic zone of irregular outline surrounded by a reactive osteosclerosis of varying extent, both endosteal and peri-osteal. This appearance usually suggests the hypotheses of non-ossifying fibroma, osteoid osteoma, Brodie's abscess, even adamantinoma.

Pathological anatomy and histopathology

The anatomical lesion may correspond to an ordinary type of sarcoma or a well-differentiated osteoblastic sarcoma, posing a difficult diagnosis from an osteoid osteoma or osteoblastoma.

Confronted with some radiographs, when the periosteal reaction is considerable and the cortical surface is barely eroded, the intracortical origin of the tumour may be questionable. However, it is useful, as Kyriakos suggests (1980), to distinguish two entities: periosteal sarcoma and intracortical sarcoma.

Intra-epiphyseal

General considerations

This form, localised to the epiphysis, with or without persistence of the growth plate, is very rare. Of 286 osteosarcomas, Tsuneyoshi et al (1987) collected only four cases. Paltiel et al (1988) reported another case and listed less than 10 cases reported in the English-language literature. The five cases reported by the authors cited above were localised to the lower femoral epiphysis in patients aged 15 to 34 years, four of them male.

Clinical features and course

The symptom is pain in a joint. From its epiphyseal origin, the tumour may destroy the cortex and extend towards the metaphysis and/or into the joint. It is one of the objectives of advanced imaging to define the tumour extension before a surgical procedure.

Imaging

The image shows a lytic lesion, possibly wih a small central opacity.

Pathological anatomy

Usually the examination reveals a common type of sarcoma.

Diagnosis

The diagnosis is generally simple for the pathologist who must exclude other diagnoses that need logically to be considered because of their site: chondroblastoma, eosinophil granuloma, enchondroma, clear-cell chondrosarcoma. Only the last diagnosis may raise some difficulties from that of a predominantly chondroid osteosarcoma, but in clear-cell chondrosarcoma one must be strict on "clear cells" as an entity; the bony strands are of a reactive nature.

It is evident that this sarcoma, of strictly epiphyseal origin, must be distinguished from the extension of a sarcoma of metaphyseal origin to the epiphysis through the growth plate [Enneking & Kagan 1978, Norton et al 1991].

Osteosarcomas at multiple sites

Definition

These present in two different ways, as simultaneous development of multiple lesions (synchronic osteosarcomatosis) or successive development at several locations (diachronic ostesarcomatosis).

Synchronic osteosarcomatosis

- General considerations

Osteosarcomatosis is characterised by the simultaneous development, ie synchronic development or at least at a very short interval, of multiple skeletal lesions (6, 8, 10 or more). Very often, the tumour locations are symmetrical and predominantly at the metaphyses of the long bones.

In the great majority of cases the disease is found in young patients with an average age of the order of 10-12 years. In the dozen cases collected by Mahoney et al (1979) the youngest patient was 5 and the oldest 17.

- Clinical features and cou...

Pain is the essential symptom, often associated with impairment of general condition. The course is particularly grave, survival not exceeding several months in most reported cases. The survival of 24 months [Hopper et al 1990] of a girl aged 14 years is a rarity. Another girl, also aged 14 years, whose case is reported by Gherlinzoni et al (1983) survived only 9 months. The 9 - patients, with a mean age of 11 years, studied by Parham et al (1985) died between 6 and 37 months after diagnosis, with a median survival of 12 months.

- Imaging

Imaging reveals the presence of bony opacities with indefinite outlines (figs. 19-21).

The symmetry of the lesions is often remarkable, and affects the lower metaphyses of the femora, the upper metaphyses of the tibiae and fibulae, the elbows, wrists and shoulders [Hopper et al 1990].

- Pathological anatomy and histopathology

The bone biopsies demonstrate plaques of anaplastic cell proliferation, zones of osteosclerosis (fig. 41) and other zones with a dense network of bony strands of irregular mesh. There are also osteoid islands containing very chromophil cells of bizarre shapes and osteoblastic appearance. Mitoses are few, and some nuclei are abnormally large.

Diachronic osteosarcomatosis at successive sites

The disorder is characterised by the successive development, usually in an adult, of sarcomatous lesions. The tumour sites are less numerous than in synchronous osteosarcomatosis. After the initial treatment followed by apparent cure, a second and then a third lesion appear within 5 to 10 years.

The distribution of the tumours is predominantly axial: skull, vertebrae, pelvis, ribs, with a tendance to spare the long bones of the limbs.

In the long term the prognosis is remarkable. Dahlin and Unni (Bone Tumours 1986, p. 281) mention the case of a patient who survived for 26 years after the first amputation and 12 years after the second.

While it is the case that synchronous osteosarcomatosis affects mainly young persons and the diachronic form mainly adults, from my fortunately limited experience, I do not believe that age is an inviolable parameter. It seems more important to take account of the rapidity of the course and perhaps of the number of lesions when classifying the disorder.

- Diagnosis

In the presence of multiple osteosarcomatous foci it is proper to eliminate sclerosing metastatic foci from an as yet unidentified tumour, bony metastases arising from a primary osteosarcoma (or skip metastases), and sarcomatous degeneration in multiple foci in Paget's disase.

Aetiopathogenic hypotheses and classification

The complexity of these observations has given rise to differing interpretations.

In favor of the lesions being multicentric from the outset, there is the possible action of an unknown carcinogenic agent; the virtually symmetric distribution of the tumours might the be explained by the special sensitivity of the growth sites adjacent to the joints. The absence of pulmonary metastases in some 50% of cases also argues in favor of a multicentric origin.

Conversely, the proponents of metastatic dissemination have not failed to note the greater development of one of the tumours, which is supposed to be the origin of the dissemination. The histological similarity of the different lesions may also argue in favor of this view. This is also the opinion of Guy et al (1956), based on two cases they observed. These were two girls aged 10 and 12 years, in whom the course, with bony and pulmonary lesions, did not exceed 3 months. These two cases were considered to be an acute, rapidly metastasising form. It is also certain that, in the case of unfavorable evolution of the common form of osteosarcoma, bony metastases are detected in more than 15% of persons. Lastly, while an osteosarcomatous focus of sclerotic type may raise the hypothesis of osteosarcomatosis, it may remain solitary (fig. 22).

As for the proposed classifications, three by Amstutz (1969), two by McCarthy et al (1987), it seems that classification into two groups (or two entities) is sufficient if we are not to have an infinity of variants.

It is inevitable that certain "cases" should be classed arbitrarily. Thus, Mahoney et al (1979) reported a case with essentially axial development in a patient of 23 which had a course of 5 months. If we consider the age and tumour distribution, as do these authours, it is classed as an atypical case of diachronic osteosarcomatosis. But if we consider the extreme rapidity of the clinical course it belongs to the synchronic type.

The case reported by Tillotson et al (1988), is not really either of these two "entities", although there were multiple lesions. This was a child of 8 years whose leg had been irradiated for an embryonal rhabdomyosarcoma at the age of 23 months and who developed four ostesarcomatous lesions in the tibia and fibula.The father of this child had died at the age of 22 from an osteosarcoma.

Table 4. System of differential diagnosis (Dd): special types

Sarcoma in children. Often predominantly cartilaginous; risk of confusion with chondrosarcoma in biopsy; compare with imaging. Prognostic importance of breaching of growth plate (MRI). In very young children the immature reactive bone may resemble tumour osteogenesis
Sarcoma in adults. Appears on a preexisting lesion in 25% of cases: Paget's disease, fibrous dysplasia, irradiated bone, etc. Craniofacial and pelvic locations relatively common. Quite often of cartilaginous type
Sarcoma on preexisting lesion. Beware remodelling of recent appearance in: infarction, exostosis, Paget's disease, contact with prosthesis, osteomyelitis, etc.
Sarcoma with craniofacial location. Likely to have fusiform cells, particularly in the mandible; differentiate from fibroma. In well-differentiated osteoblastic forms, diagnose from osteoblastoma
Sarcoma with associated epithliomatous component. Rare type. Consider epithelial metastasis in a preexisting sarcoma. In the tibia, exclude an adamantinoma
Radiation-induced osteogenic sarcomas. Diagnostic difficulties vary with circumstances
Primary extraskeletal skeletogenic sarcoma. Not to be confused with osteoma or myositis ossificans. Also exclude periosteal or juxtacortical sarcoma

Special types

The developmental circumstances of osteogenic sarcomas allow us to envisage different clinical types.

Osteogenic sarcoma in childhood

General considerations

Before 15 years of age there is a very minor masculine predominance (51-52%).

There is a high incidence in the long bones of the limbs: 96% in the 125 cases studied by Price at al (1975).

Pathological anatomy and histopathology

Histologically, these are usually sarcomas of the ordinary type but there is a greater incidence of the chondroid variety than in young adults.

It was for long thought that the epiphyseal growth plate was a barrier to extension of the tumour. But the work of Enneking and Kagan (1978) showed that this plate was breached 21 times in 28 patients studied, and Norton et al (1991), studying 15 cases of osteosarcoma in patients with a persistent growth plate, found it breached by the tumour in 12 cases. In this context, the authors therefore stress the importance of MRI in detecting such extension.

Diagnosis

In the very young child, before 10 years and particularly around 4-5 years, osteogenic sarcoma is very rare and the pathologist must bear in mind that the samples he examines come from an immature bone, rich in large fibers. The least lesion will give rise to formation of primary bone which may possibly suggest tumour. As for cellular activity, for example in the vicinity of a fractured cyst, this may be considerable, but the bulky nuclei are surrounded by a no less bulky cytoplasm, and mononuclear osteoclasts are also present. The diagnosis can only be made in the presence of atypical mitoses.

Treatment

In the young child, resection followed by a prosthesis is not feasible. Even if cured, the child with a reconstruction-prosthesis is left with unpleasant sequelae, both physical (atrophy, limb shortening) and mental (problems of relating to schoolmates). After some years a further procedure is required to change the now too small prosthesis. Lastly, in children treated by antimitotics and irradiation the development of a radiation induced sarcoma, though rare, is more to be feared if the child was very young at the time of irradiation.

Osteosarcoma in adults

General considerations

After 30-35 years, primary osteosarcoma is rare and its election for the growth zones has disappeared. In 25-50% of cases it develops on a preexisting lesion (Paget's disease, an irradiated bone, fibrous dysplasia).
An analysis of 117 cases of osteogenic sarcoma [Huvos 1986] of which 101 were skeletal and 16 extraskeletal, revealed a slight male predominance of 68/49.

In the same study the sites were mainly in the bones of the axial skeleton (27%) and craniofacial skeleton (13%).

Pathological anatomy and histopathology

From the histological aspect, Fahey et al (1992) confirm the great frequency of the chondroblastic type. Dahlin and Unni (Bone Tumours 1986) found their adult osteosarcomas to be essentially fibroblastic and chondroblastic. The frequency of the chondroblastic type is probably related to the presence of a preexisting cartilaginous tumour.

Prognosis

Despite good response to antimitotics, the prognosis of adult sarcomas is poor [Siegel et al 1987].

This may be partly due to the problems of surgical access to an axial tumour, but also to the development of the tumour in a preexisting lesion. Pregnancy seems not to influence tumour development [Huvos et al 1985]. These authors, who studied 18 cases of osteosarcoma in pregnant women compared with 18 cases in women with histologically identical osteosarcomas at the same sites, noted no effect of the pregnancy on the tumour or reciprocally, of the tumour on the pregnancy.

Sarcomas developing in a preexisting lesion

Precancerous bony lesions include Paget's disease in its extended form, chondromatosis (Ollier's disease), multiple exostoses and, less clearly, fibrous dysplasia.

Particular attention must be devoted to the difficult problems sometimes posed to the pathologist by sarcomatous transformation in Paget's disease.

The frequency of such malignant change is unknown. Too many localised forms of Paget's disease pass unnoticed for any great value to be attributed to statistics which relate only to cases of Paget's disease diagnosed because of clinical signs or complications.

It is probable that the incidence of this malignant degeneration is less than 1%. Hadjipavlou et al (1992) suggest a figure of 0.7%. What seems more definite is that after the age of 45 about 25% of osteogenic sarcomas develop in this disease.

Men are affected twice as often as women, except for cranial lesions, when this proportion is reversed.

Sarcoma in Paget's disease develops after the age of 40, with a maximum incidence (36% of cases) between the ages of 61 and 70 in the 82 cases studied by Haibach et al (1985).

Any bone may be affected, but the commonest are the femur, humerus, pelvis and tibia, rarely also the vertebrae. In patients affected by polyostotic Paget's disease, several tumours may develop simultaneously.

The tumour presents with the appearance or exacerbation of pain or with spontaneous fracture.

Given the importance of active remodelling in progressive Paget's disease, interpretation of the imaging may be difficult, particularly as there is also a fracture. However, extensive lysis with cortical destruction is strongly suggestive and calls for biopsy.

Diagnosis

Every pathological type of sarcoma has been described. There may be osteogenic sarcomas of the common type, often with fibroblastic predominance, fusiform-cell sarcomas, histiocyto-fibrosarcomas, giant-cell sarcoma which may or may not be osteogenic, and other forms. Among all these differing appearances, often complicated by fracture with reactive osteogenesis and chondrogenesis, the pathologist has to distinguish:

- an osteogenic sarcoma from hyperactive pagetoid remodeling (cf Pagetoid remodelling, p. 40)
- a fusiform-cell sarcoma from medullary fibrosis;
- an ostesarcoma from a benign giant-cell tumour;
- a simple post-fracture remodelling from a true sarcoma.

The diagnosis of malignancy in these different types is based on the certain finding of cytonuclear anomalies and monstrosities; in practice, haemorrhage and necrosis are inseparable, this architectural anarchy being quite typical of fracture in active Paget's disease. However, some tumours are easy to diagnose, as for instance in the case of a small-cell osteogenic sarcoma.

But though the clinical features and the imaging suggest some form of malignant tumour, Haibach et al (1985) list 77 osteoarcomas, 3 fibrosarcomas, 1 chondrosarcoma and 1 giant-cell tumour in 82 cases of tumours developing in Paget's disease. In the 8 cases collected by Hadjipavlou et al (1992), in patients with an average age of 67 years, 5 were osteogenic sarcomas and the other 3 were a lymphoma, a malignant histio-cytofibroma and an epithelioid sarcoma. I have twice observed adenoarcinomatous metastases in a pagetic vertebra.

Apart from Paget's disease, other predisposing disorders are more likely to give rise to chondosarcoma than to osteogenic sarcoma.

The malignant changes developing in Ollier's disease or in an exostosis are rare, but may justify preventive treatment such as ablation of the larger cartilaginous lesions and exostoses. Sarcoma developing in fibrous dysplasia is commoner if there are cartilaginous islands in this dysplasia. Since these disorders have a tendency to spontaneous "degeneration", any irradiation must be avoided.

Cases have also been reported of osteogenic sarcoma developing in an old focus of osteomyelitis or bone infarction, etc. [Mirra et al 1974, Resnick et al 1990]. Some of these sarcomas may pose a medicolegal problem in the current state of our knowledge, since pathological anatomy cannot demonstrate a cause and effect relationship even though this may be probable in certain circumstances.

The development of an osteogenic sarcoma in patients suffering from disorders combining often complex cutaneous, vascular, visceral and bony lesions, whether the latter predominate or not, raises the problem of a possible relationship between the disorder in question and the tumour. This is the case, for instance, in the development of an osteogenic sarcoma in a patient with the Rothmund-Thomson syndrome; a syndrome that may be associated with an immune deficiency. To my knowledge, only 5 cases have been reported of the coexistence of the two lesions [Kozlowski et al 1980, Baro et al 1989]. In such cases, where a rare syndrome and an osteogenic sarcoma, itself a rare tumour, coexist, it is for the statisticians to verify if such a disease predisposes to the development of an osteosarcoma or not.

In cases where the diagnosis of osteogenic sarcoma is under consideration in patients aged 50, 60 or over, the pathologist must be completely informed as to the history and the current radiological and clinical appearances.

Sarcomas of axial and craniofacial localisation

(cf Chapter 38)

Vertebral osteosarcomas

Vertebral osteosarcomas are rare, less than 2% of all osteogenic sarcomas [Patel et al 1984]; however, 70% of these have developed in a Paget's disease affected bone or have been induced by irradiation. The same remarks apply to osteosarcomas developing in the pelvic bones [Fahey et al 1992], though at this site an exostosis is sometimes incriminated.

Sarcomas at craniofacial sites

Sarcomas of craniofacial localisation are rare, but sarcomas induced by irradiation of "non-surgical" craniofacial tumours may complicate primary lesions.

General considerations

It is accepted that the totality of craniofacial sarcomas represent no more than 4% of all osteosarcomas. The statistics show a female predominance and the mean age is slightly higher than that of sarcoma of the long bones.

Pathological anatomy and histopathology

Sarcomas are found with osteogenic, chondrogenic or fusiform cell predominance. We have found the fibroblastic type to be commoner in the mandible, where it may be compared with some juxtacortical sarcomas of the long bones. Its prognosis is relatively better than that of ethmoidal sarcoma, which is particularly grave.

Differential diagnosis

The first difficulty concerns fibroblastic sarcomas of the mandible, which must be distinguished from simple fibroma, often very dense at this site but devoid of cell abnormalities. But even minor osteogenesis, if frankly neoplastic, suffices to change the diagnosis of fibroblastic sarcoma into one of osteogenic sarcoma.

The second difficulty relates to certain tumours of the base of the skull, rich in cartilage. These osteosarcomas are to be distinguished from chondrosarcomas by their polymorphism and the presence of sarcomatous osteoid strands.

Osteogenic sarcoma associated with an epitheliomatous component

Tumours of the soft tissues provide us with numerous examples of the coexistence of sarcomatous and carcinomatous tissue. Numerous hypotheses have been advanced to explain this bipotentiality.

In the context of bone sarcoma, cases have been reported of the coexistence of an osteogenic sarcoma and malpighian or glandular carcinomatous plaques, with sometimes even a combination of both these latter appearances.

I have an instinctive distrust for cases developing in the tibia, but I have never observed such a linkage between an adamantinoma and an evidently malignant osteogenic sarcoma.

I also have some suspicion of cases affecting adults; an epithelial metastasis in an osteosarcoma is, perhaps, no rarer and no commoner than a putative "osteogenic carcino-sarcoma".

Given these reservations, it is probably useful to acknowledge the existence of such tumours; immunohistochemical and genetic studies provide grounds for their existence.

In their study, Kramer et al (1993), who report a case in a child aged 13 years, proposed the term "epithelioid osteosarcoma". It seems to me that such a label suggests a particular appearance of the sarcoma, as for example in the well-recognised epithelioid sarcoma of the soft tissues, and not merely the coexistence of two components differing in their morphology and topography.

Radiation-induced osteogenic sarcoma

It is generally accepted that the risk of provoking a sarcoma by irradiation increases with the dose, but "a single irradiation is sufficient" according to Professor Lacassagne. It is also agreed that the growing skeleton of children is more vulnerable than that of adults.

The latent period between irradiation and development of the osteosarcoma is variable. In the 25 cases reported by Varela-Duran & Dehmer (1980) the latent period ranged from 3 to 14 years, and for Huvos et al (1985), who studied 66 cases of radiation-induced osteosarcoma, 7 of these extraskeletal, the latent period varied from 3.5 to 33 years. In 24 cases the irradiation was for a bony tumour or pseudotumour.

Of the total of radiation-induced sarcomas, bone tumours represented only 10 cases out of 133 in the paper of Wiklund et al (1991). Four were extraskeletal, which puts at 18% the incidence of skeletal osteogenic sarcomas in relation to the generality of radiation-induced sarcomas.

In this context, the only osteosarcomas to be included are those which develop in the irradiation field, occur in a bone known to be radiographically normal before irradiation and after a latent period (which has strangely become shorter during recent decades).

Cases have been reported of sarcoma of the ribs after irradiation of the breast or nodes, of iliac sarcoma after irradiation of an ovarian tumour, of sarcomas of the face after irradiation of an epithelioma or retinoblastoma, and so on. Accidental irradiation, with a succession of acute episodes, may also be complicated by osteogenic sarcoma after some years of latency. The radiation-induced sarcomas I have observed were usually of fibroblastic type.

The pathologist is often supposed to be capable of answering the following questions:

- Is this a malignant lesion?
- Is this an osteogenic sarcoma?
- Is this a tumour related to the lesion previously irradiated?
- Is this a radiation-induced tumour?

It is sometimes very difficult to recognise the onset of sarcomatous transformation in bony territory remodelled by irradiation. It is important to note any mitotic activity, even more to record any abnormal mitoses in the area suspect of malignant transformation. A search must be made for any discontinuity between the tumour and the remodelling of the irradiated bone, an important architectural feature.

The osteogenic nature of the tumour may not be evident in the midst of radiotherapeutic sclerosis. If the irradiated tumour was an osteogenic sarcoma one or more adjacent bones may have been irradiated, (in the leg, forearm or face). If an osteogenic sarcoma develops in one of these bones, originally healthy, it is hazardous to try to distinguish a metastasis from a radiation-induced sarcoma from the histology alone. The interval between the appearance of the sarcoma and irradiation is of relative value. Metastatic proliferation in fibro-sclerotic tissue does not have the same appearance as the original tumour, which arises in a well-vascularised metaphysis.

There is no histological evidence that allows a definitive conclusion that osteogenic sarcoma is radiation-induced to be drawn.

Primary extraskeletal skeletogenic sarcoma

This is a rare tumour. In some cases an injury is invoked as its origin. The main differential diagnosis is from myositis ossificans. The problems posed by this sarcoma are considered in Chapter 39.

References

Ackerman AJ (1948) Multiple osteogenic sarcoma. Am J Roentgenol 60: 623-632.

Ahuja SC, Villacin AB, Smith G, Bullough PG, Huvos AG, Marcove R (1977) Juxtacortical (parosteal) osteogenic sarcoma, histological grading and prognosis. J Bone Joint Surg 59A: 632-647

Amstutz HC (1969) Multiple osteogenic sarcoma metastatic or multicentric? Report of two cases and review of literature. Cancer 24: 923-931

Anani AP, Costa J, Remagen W (1987) L'échappement métastatique dans la moelle osseuse (skip métastase) de l'ostéosarcome. Ann Pathol 7: 193-197

Anderson RB, McAlister JA, Wrenn RN (1989) Intracortical osteosarcoma of tibia. Skeletal Radiol 18: 627-630

Araki N, Uchida A, Kimura T, Yoshikawa H, Aoki Y, Ueda T, Takai S, Miki T, Ono K (1991) Involvement of the retinoblastoma gene in primary osteosarcomas and other bone and soft-tissue tumors. Clin Orthop 270: 271-277

Ayala AG, Rojy Raymond AK, Jaffe N, Chawla S, Carrasco H, Link M, Jimenez J, Edeiken J, Wallace S, Murray JA, Benjamin R (1989) Small cell osteosarcoma. A clinicopathologic study of 27 cases. Cancer 64: 2162-2173

Ballance WA, Mendelsohn G, Carter JR, Abdul-Karim FW, Jacobs G, Makley JT (1988) Osteogenic sarcoma malignant fibrous histiocytoma subtype. Cancer 62: 763-771

Baro PR, Bastart FM, Bartrina JR, Mateo JM, Vidal MTR (1989) Osteosarcoma of calcaneus with Rothmund-Thompson syndrome. Case report. Skeletal Radiol 18: 136-139

Benedikt RA, Kransdorf MJ, Jelinek JS, Moser RP (1992) Osteosarcomatosis in a skeletal immature girl. Skeletal Radiol 21: 187-189

Bentzen SM, Poulsen HS Kaae S, Myhre-Jensen O, Johansen H, Mouridsen HT, Daugaard S, Arnoldi C (1988) Prognostic factors in osteosarcomas. Cancer 62: 194-202

Bertoni F, Boriani S, Laus M, Campanacci M (1982) Periosteal chondrosarcoma and periosteal osteosarcoma: two distinct entities. J Bone Joint Surg 64B: 370-376

Bertoni F, Unni KK, McLeod RA, Dahlin DC (1985) Osteosarcoma resembling osteoblastoma. Cancer 55: 416-426

Catanese J, Dutcher JP Dorfman HD, André DF, Wiemil PH (1988) Mediastinal osteosarcoma with extension to lungs in a patient treated for Hodgkin's disease. Cancer 62: 2252-2257

Charig MJ, Golding SJ, Lindsell DRM (1990) Osteosarcoma: an unusual thoracic metastasis. Br J Radiol April: 304-306

Dahlin DC, Unni KK (1977) Osteosarcoma of bone and its important recognizable varieties. Am J Surg Path 1: 61-72

Dahlin DC, Unni KK, (1986) General aspects and data on 8,542 cases; 4th edn, Charles Thomas, Springfield, pp. 269-307

De Santos LA, Edeiken B (1982) Purely lytic osteosarcoma. Skeletal Radiol 9: 1-7

De Santos LA, Edeiken BS, (1985) Subtle early osteosarcoma. Skeletal Radiol 13: 44-48

Dickersin GR, Rosenberg AE (1991) The ultrastructure of small cell osteosarcoma with a review of the light microscopy and differential diagnosis. Hum Pathol 22: 267-275

Dubousset J, Missenard G, Kalifa CH (1991) Management of osteogenic sarcoma in children and adolescents. Clin Ortop 270: 52-59

Dun D, Dehner P (1977) Metastatic osteosarcoma to lung. A clinicopathologic study of surgical and resections. Cancer 40: 3054-3064

Dwinnell LA, Dahlin DC, Ghormley RK (1954) Parosteal (juxtacortical) osteogenic sarcoma. J Bone Joint Surg 36A: 732-744

Enneking WF, Kagan A (1975) "Skip" metastases in osteosarcoma. Cancer 36: 2192-2205

Enneking WF, Kagan A (1978) Transepiphyseal extension of osteosarcoma: incidence, mechanism and implications. Cancer 41: 1526-1537

Fahey M, Spanier SS, Vander Griend RA (1992) Osteosarcoma of the pelvis. A clinical and histopathological study of twenty-five patients. J Bone Joint Surg 74A: 320-330

Feugeas O, Guriec N, Babin-Boilletot A, Marcellin L, Simon P, Babin S, Thyss A, Hofman P, Terrier P, Kalifa C, Brunat-Mentigny M, Patricot L-M, Oberling F (1996) Loss of heterozygosity of the RB gene is a poor prognostic factor in patients with osteosarcoma. J Clin Oncol 14: 467-472

Finkel MP, Biskis BO, Farell C (1967) Pathogenic effects of extracts of human osteosarcomas in hamsters and mice. Arch Path 84: 425-428

Finkel MP, Biskis BO, Jinkins PB (1966) Virus induction of osteosarcomas in mice. Science 151: 698-701

Fitzgerald RH, Dablin DC, Sim FH (1973) Multiple metachronous osteogenic sarcoma. J Bone Joint Surg 55A: 595-605

Forest M, Abelanet R, Daudet-Monsac M (1981) L'étude morphologique d'une tumeur osseuse. Notions pratiques macroscopiques, radiographiques et cytologiques. Ann Pathol 1: 86-89

Garbe LR, Monges GM, Paregrin EM, Payan HL (1981) Ultrastructural study of osteosarcoma. Hum Pathol 12: 891-896

Gherlinzoni F, Antoci B, Canale V (1983) Multicentric osteosarcomata (osteosarcomatosis). Skeletal Radiol 10: 281-285

Glasser DB, Lane JM, Huvos AG, Marcove RC, Rosen G (1992) Survival, prognosis and therapeutic response in osteogenic sarcoma. Cancer 69: 698-708

Goodman MA, McMaster JH, Drash AL, Diamond PE, Kappakas GS, Scranton PE (1978) Metabolic and endocrine alterations in osteosarcoma patients. Cancer 42: 603-610

Guy EP, Hourtoule FG, Loisillier F (1956) Ostéosarcomes ossifiants muticentriques des os. Bull Cancer (Paris) 43: 258-265

Hadjipavlou A, Lander P, Srolovitz H, Enker P (1992) Malignant transformation in Paget disease of bone. Cancer 70: 2802-2808

Haibach H, Farrel C, Dittrich F (1985) Neoplasms arising in Paget's disease of bone: a study of 82 cases. Am J Clin Pathol 83: 594-600

Hall RB, Robinson LH, Malawar MM, Dunham WK (1985) Periosteal osteosarcoma. Cancer 55: 165-171

Hansen MF (1991) Molecular considerations in osteosarcoma. Clin Orthop 270: 237-246

Haye C (1981) A propos de la survenue d'un ostéosarcome primitif chez une enfant traitée pour tumeur de la rétine. Bull Soc Ophtal Fr I: 99-100

Healy JH, Buss D (1991) Radiation and pagetic osteogenic sarcoma. Clin Orthop 270: 120-127

Hopper KD, Haseman DB, Moser RP, Sweet DE, Madewell DE (1990) Osteosarcomatosis (case report). Skeletal Radiol 19: 535-537

Hopper KD, Moser RP, Haseman DB. Sweet DE. Madewell JF, Kransdorf MJ (1990) Osteosarcomatosis. Radiol 175: 233-239

Huvos AG (1986) Osteogenic sarcoma of bones and soft tissues in older persons. A clinicopathologic analysis of 117 patients older than 60 years. Cancer 57: 1447-1449

Huvos AG, Butler A, Bretsky SS (1983) Osteogenic sarcoma associated with Paget's disease of bone. A clinicopathology study of 65 patients. Cancer 52: 1489-1495

Huvos AG, Butler A, Bretsky SS (1985) Osteogenic sarcoma in pregnant women, pronostic, therapeutic implications, and literature review. Cancer 56: 2326-2331

Huvos AG, Rosen G, Bretsky SS, Butler A (1982) Telangiectatic osteogenic sarcoma: a clinicopathologic study of 124 patients. Cancer 49: 1679-1689

Huvos AG, Rosen G, Marcove RC (1977) Primary osteogenic sarcoma. Pathologic aspects in 20 patients after treatment with chemotherapy en bloc resection, and prosthetic bone replacement. Arch Path Lab Med 101: 14-18

Huvos AG, Woodard HQ, Cahan WG, Higinbotham NL, Steward FW, Butler A, Bretsky SS (1985) Postradiation osteogenic sarcoma of bone and soft tissues. A clinicopathologic study of 66 patients. Cancer 55: 1244-1255

Jeffree GM, Price CHG, Sissons HA (1975) The metastatic spread of osteosarcoma. Br J Cancer 32: 87-107

Kevin Raymond A (1992) Osteosarcoma: perspectives. Am J Surg Pathol 16: 193-194

Knudson AG, Meadows AT, Nichols WN (1976) Chromosomal deletion and retinoblastoma. N Engl J Med 295: 1120-1123

Kozlowski K, Scougall JS, Oates RK (1980) Osteosarcoma in a boy with Rothmund-Thomson syndrome. Pediatr Radiol 10: 42-45

Kramer K, Hicks DG, Palis J, Rosier RN, Oppenheimer J, Fallon MD, Cohen HJ (1993) Epithelioid osteosarcoma of bone immunocytochemical evidence suggesting divergent epithelial and mesenchymal differenciation in a primary osseous neoplasm. Cancer 71: 2977-2982

Kurt AM, Unni KK, Mcleod RA, Pritchard DJ (1990) Low-grade intraosseous osteosarcoma. Cancer 65: 1418-1428

Kyriakos M (1980) Intracortical osteosarcoma. Cancer 46: 2525-2533

Lacassagne A, Gricourouff G (1966) Effets cancérigènes des rayonnements ionisants. Radiobiologie appliquée. Gauthier-Villars, Paris, pp 584-646

Lee WR, Laurie J, Townsend AL (1975) Fine structure of a radiation-induced osteogenic sarcoma. Cancer 76: 1414-1425

Lichtenstein L (1955) Tumors of periosteal origin. Cancer 8: 1060-1069

Mahoney JP, Spanier SS, Morris JL (1979) Multifocal osteosarcoma. A case report with review of the literature. Cancer 44: 1897-1907

Malawer MM, Dunham WK (1983) Skip metastases in osteosarcoma: recent experience. J Bone Onc 22: 236-245

Mankin HJ, Gebhardt MC, Springfield DS, Litwat GJ, Kusazaki K, Rosenberg AE (1991) Flow cytometric studies of human osteosarcoma. Clin Orthop 270: 169180

Matsuno T, Unni KK, McLeod RA, Dahlin DC (1976) Telangiectatic osteogenic sarcoma. Cancer 38: 2538-2547

Mazabraud A, Perdereau B, Contesso G (1992) Réflexions sur la validation de la classification des formes les plus fréquentes des sarcomes ostéogènes par des méthodes fonctionnelles isotopiques. Bull Cancer 79: 759-765

Mazabraud A, Perdereau B, Gongora R (1986) Classification of osteosarcoma by 85Sr scintimetry. Arch Orthop Scan 57: 74-77

McCarthy EF, Tolo VT, Dorfman HD (1987) Multicentric, metachronous, low-grade, sclerosing osteogenic sarcoma. Case report. Skeletal Radiol 16: 592-596

McMaster JH (1977) Carbohydrate metabolism in osteosarcoma. Int Orthop 1: 19-21

Meadows AT, Strong LC, Lif P (1980) Bone sarcoma as a second malignant neoplasm in children. Influence of radiation and genetic predisposition. Cancer 46: 2603-2606

Merle d'Aubigné R, Thomine JM (1970) A propos de 9 cas de sarcomes juxtacorticaux. Mém Acad Chir 96: 4549

Mervak TR, Unni KK, Pritchard DJ, McLeod RA (1991) Telangiectatic osteosarcoma. Clin Orthop 270: 135-139

Mirra JM, Bullough PG, Marcove RC, Jacobs B, Huvos AG (1974) Malignant fibrous histiocytoma and osteosarcoma in association with bone infarcts. Report of four cases, two in caisson workers. J Bone Joint Surg 56A: 932-940

Mirra JM, Dodd L, Johnston W, Frost DB, Barton D (1991) Primary intracortical osteosarcoma of femur, sclerosing variant, grade I to 2 anaplasia. Skeletal Radiol 20: 613-616

Mirra JM, Kameda N, Rosen G, Eckardt J (1988) Primary osteosarcoma of toe phalanx: first documented case. Review of osteosarcoma of short tubular bones. Am J Surg Pathol 12: 300-307

Newton WA, Meadows AT, Shimada HS, Bunin GR, Vawter GF (1991) Bone sarcomas as second malignant neoplasms following childhood cancer. Cancer 67: 193-201

Naka T, Fukuda T, Shinohara N, Iwamoto Y, Sugioka Y, Tsuneyoshi M (1995) Osteosarcoma versus malignant fibrous histiocytoma of bone in patients older than 40 years. Cancer 76: 972-984

Noguera R, Navarro S, Triche TJ (1990) Translocation (11; 22) in small cell osteosarcoma. Cancer Genet Cytogenet 45: 121-124

Norton KI, Hermann G, Abdelwahab IF, Kein MJ, Granometter LM, Rabinowitz JG (1991) Epiphyseal involvement in osteosarcoma. Radiology 180: 813-816

Olson PL, Prewitt L, Griffiths HJ, Cherkna B (1991) Multifocal osteosarcoma. Skeletal Radiol 20: 624-627

Paltiel HJ, Wilkinson RH, Kozakewich HPW (1988) Osteosarcoma of the distal femoral epiphysis. SkeJetal Radiol 17: 527-530

Pappo A, Schneider NR, Sanders JM, Buchanan GR (1991) secondary myelodysplastic syndrome complicating therapy for osteogenic sarcoma. Cancer 68: 1373-1375

Parham DM, Pratt CB, Parvey LS, Webber BL, Champion J (1985) Chidhood multifocal osteosarcoma clinicopathologic and radiologic correlates. Cancer 55: 2653-2658

Patel DV, Hammer RA, Levin B, Fisher MA (1984) Primary osteogenic sarcoma of the spine. Skeletal Radiol 12: 276-279

Perdereau B. Mazabraud A, Gongora R (1993) Contribution de la scintigraphie dynamique à l'aide de 99Tc-MDP à la classification nosologique des sarcomes ostéogènes anaplasiques. J Med Nucl Biophys 17: 212-217

Pignatti G, Bacci G, Picci P, Dallari D, Bertoni F, Bacchini P, Capanna R (1991) Telangiectatic osteosarcoma of the extremities. Results in 17 patients treated with neoadjuvant chemotherapy. Clin Orthop 270: 99-106

Pintado SO, Lane J, Huvos AG (1989) Parosteal osteogenic sarcoma of bone with coexistent low and high-grade sarcomatous components. Hum Pathol 20: 488-491

Porter DE, Holden ST, Cohen BB, Wallace MR, Reid R (1992) A significant proportion of patients with osteosarcoma may belong to Li-Fraumeni cancer families. J Bone Joint Surg 74B: 883-892

Price CHG (1961) Osteogenic sarcoma. An analysis of survival and its relationship to histological grading and structure. J Bone Joint Surg. 43B: 300-313

Price CHG (1966) The prognosis of osteosarcoma. An analytical study. Br J Radiol 39: 181-188

Price CHG, Zhuber K, Salzer-Kuntschik M, Salzer M, Willert HG, Immenkamp M, Groh P, Matejorsky Z, Keyl W (1975) Osteosarcoma in children a study of 125 cases. J Bone Joint Surg 57B: 341-345

Raymond AK (1991) Surface osteosarcoma. Clin Orthop 270: 140-148

Rebaud P, David L, Plauchu H, Chatelain P, Moulin G, François R (1985) Observation familiale de syndrome de Rothmund-Thonson. Pediatrie 40: 487-

Reddick RL, Michelitch H, Levine AM, Triche TJ (1980) Osteogenic sarcoma. A study of the ultrastructure. Cancer 45: 64-71

Remagen W, Jani L, Luthi A, Schuman L (1981) Atypical (dedifferentiated) chondrosarcoma or osteosarcoma with preponderant chondrobastic differentiation? J Cancer Res Clin Oncol 101: 177-182

Resnik CS, Aisner SC, Young JWR, Levine A (1993) Osteosarcoma arising in bone infarction. Case report. Skeletal Radiol 22: 58-61

Rosen G, Caparos B, Huvos AG, Kosloff C, Nirenberg A, Cacavio A, Marcove RC, Lane JM, MeRta B, Urban C (1982) Pre-operative chemotherapy for osteogenic sarcoma: selection of post-operative chemotherapy. Cancer 49: 1221-1230

Schajowicz F, McCuire MH, Araujo ES, Muscolo DL, Giletis S (1988) Osteosarcomas arising on the surfaces of long bones. J Bone Joint Surg 70A: 555-564

Schlienger P, Calle R, Haye C, Vilcoq P (1985) Sarcomes osseux et tumeurs malignes de la rétine. Bull Cancer (Paris) 72: 16-24

Scholz RB, Kabish H, Weber B, Röser K, Delling G, Winkler K (1992) Studies of the RB1 gene and p53 gene in human osteosarcoma. Pediatr Hematol Oncol 9: 125-137

Seeger LL, Gold RH, Chandnani VP (1991) Diagnostic imaging of osteosarcoma. Clin Orthop 270: 254-263

Shrikhande SS, Rao RS (1977) Histopathological study of regional lymph nodes in osteosarcoma. J Surg Oncol 9: 371 -377

Siegel RD, Ryan LM, Antman KH (1989) Osteosarcoma in adults. One institution's experience. Clin Orthop 240: 261-269

Sim FH, Kurt AM, McLeod RA, Unni KK (1990) Low-grade central osteosarcoma. Skeletal Radiol 19: 457-460

Sim FH, Unni KK, Beabout JW, Dahlin DC (1979) Osteosarcoma with small cells simulating Ewing's tumor. J Bone Joint Surg 61A: 207-215

Sim FH, De Vries EMG, Miser JS, Unnik K (1992) Osteoblastic osteosarcoma (grade 4) with Rothmund-Thomson syndrome (case report). Skeletal Radiol 21: 543-545

Thorpe WP, Reilly IJ, Rosenberg SA (1979) Prognostic significance of alkaline phosphatase measurements in patients with osteogenic sarcoma receiving chemotherapy. Cancer 43: 2178-2181

Tillotson C, Rosenberg A, Gebhardt M, Rosenthal Dl (1988) Postradiation multicentric osteosarcoma. Cancer 62: 67-71

Tomeno B, Languepin A (1982) Sarcome juxtacortical. Rev Prat (Paris) 32: 3515-3520

Tsuneyoshi M, Dorfman HD (1987) Epiphyseal osteosarcoma: distinguishing features from clear cell chondrosarcoma, chondroblastoma and epiphyseal enchondroma. Hum Pathol 18: 644-651

Unni KK, Dahlin DC, Beabout JW, Ivins JC (1976) Parosteal osteogenic sarcoma. Cancer 37: 2466-2475

Unni KK, Dahlin DC, McLeod RA, Pritchard DJ (1977) Intraosseous well-differentiated osteosarcoma. Cancer 40: 1337-1347

Valenty M (1989) Facteurs pronostiques de l'ostéosarcome à propos d'une série de 130 malades traités à 1'institut Gustave-Roussy entre 1981 et 1988. Mémoire (diplôme d'études approfondies, statistique et santé) Université Paris Sud (UFR Kremlin Bicêtre)

Valenty M, Bendjaballah F, Vanel D, Terrier PH, Henry-Amar M (1990) Facteurs pronostiques de l'ostéosarcome. Bull Cancer (Paris) 77: 545 (summary)

Van Der Heul RO, Von Ronnen JR (1967) Juxtacortical osteosarcoma. Diagnosis, differential diagnosis, treatment and an analysis of eighty cases. J Bone Joint Surg 49A: 415-439

Van Rijssel TG (1980) Classification and prognosis of osteosarcoma. In: Therapeutic progress in ovarian cancer,testicular cancer and the sarcomas. AT Van Oosterom edn

Varela-Duran J, Dehner LP (1980) Postirradiation osteosarcoma in childhood a clinicopathologic study of three cases and review of the literature. Am J Pediatr Hematol Oncol 2: 263-271

Vigorita VJ, Ghelman B, Jones JK, Marcove RC (1984) Intracortical osteosarcoma. Am J Surg Pathol 8: 65-71

Wiklund TA, Blomvist CP, Raty J, Elomaa J, Rissanen P, Miettinen M (1991) Postirradiation sarcoma. Analysis of a nationwide cancer registry material. Cancer 68: 524-531

Wold LE, Unni KK, Beabout JW, Pritchard DJ (1984) Highgrade surface osteosarcomas. Am J Surg Pathol 8: 181-186

Wold LE, Unni KK, Beabout JW, Sim FM, Dablin DC (1984) Dedifferentiated parosteal osteosarcoma. J Bone Joint Surg 66A: 53-59

Yamaguchi H, Nojima T, Matsuno T, Sasaki T, Isu K, Ubayama Y, Yamawaki S, Gotoh M (1988) The alteration in the pattern of pulmonary metastasis with adjuvant chemotherapy in osteosarcoma. International Orthopaedics (SICOT) 12: 305-308

Yamaguchi H, Ioguchida G, Yamamuro I, Koloura Y, Iakada N, Kawaguchi N, Kanekoy Y, Nakamura Y, Sasaki MS, Ishizaki K (1992) Allelotype analysis in osteosarcomas: Frequent allele loss on 3q, 13q, 17 p and 18 q. Cancer Res 52: 2419-2423

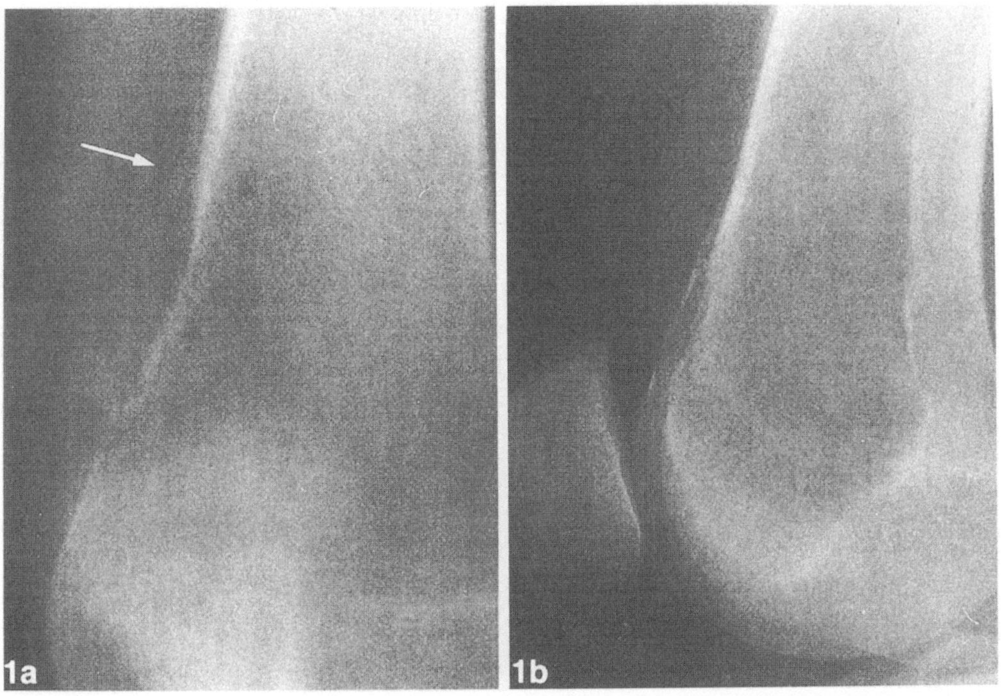

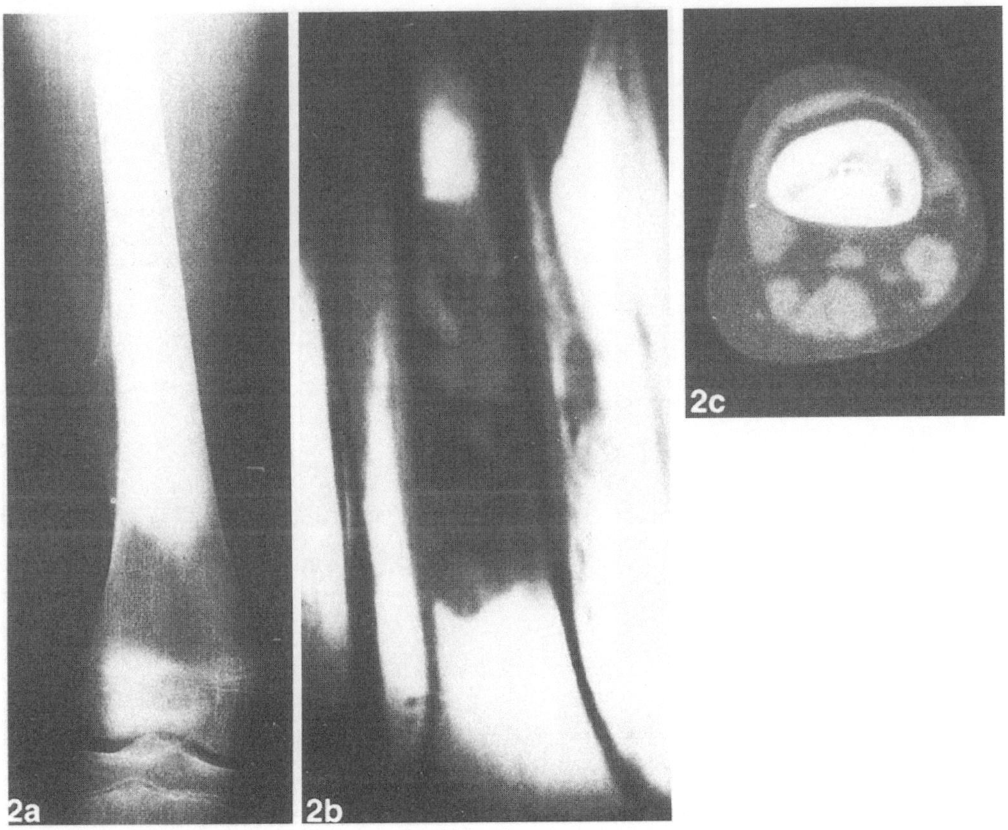

Fig. 1 a, b. Osteolysis of lower metaphysis of femur with ill-defined boundaries. The tumour is invading the soft tissues. Major periosteal reaction forming a Codman's triangle (*arrow*). Girl of 15 (case-history 1)

Fig. 2. a The standard film demonstrates a sclerotic sarcoma of the femur. **b** MRI, frontal section in T1: the tumour lesion in hyposignal is well contrasted with the medullary tissue in hypersignal. **c** In axial section, the tumour hyperdensity extends at the expense of the inner aspect of the cortex, invading the medullary canal

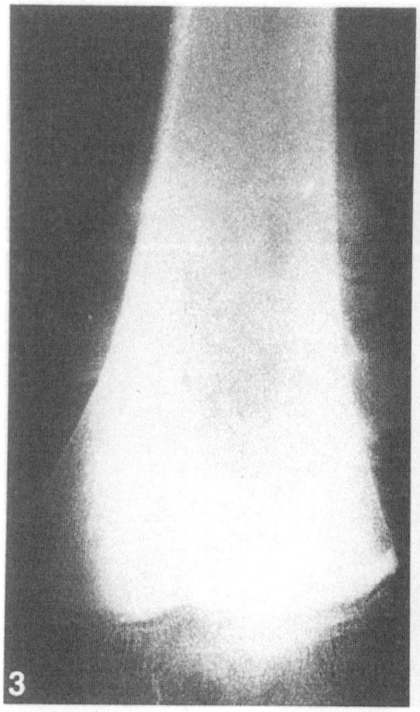

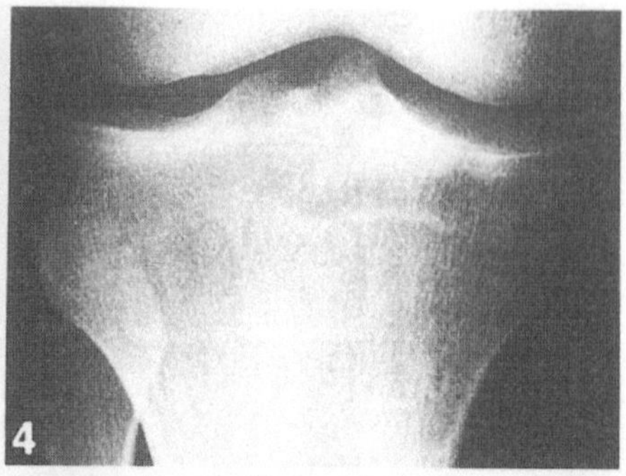

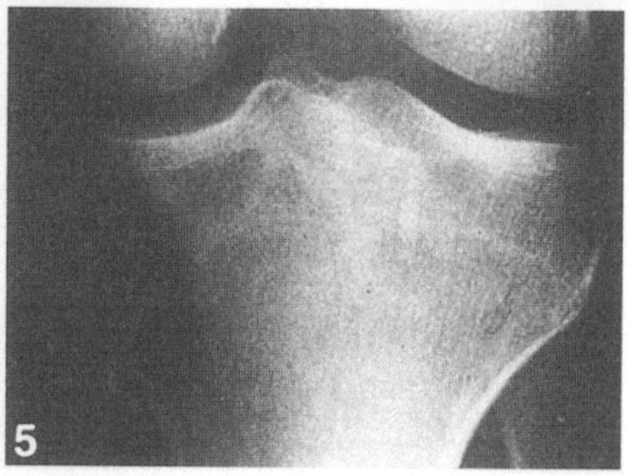

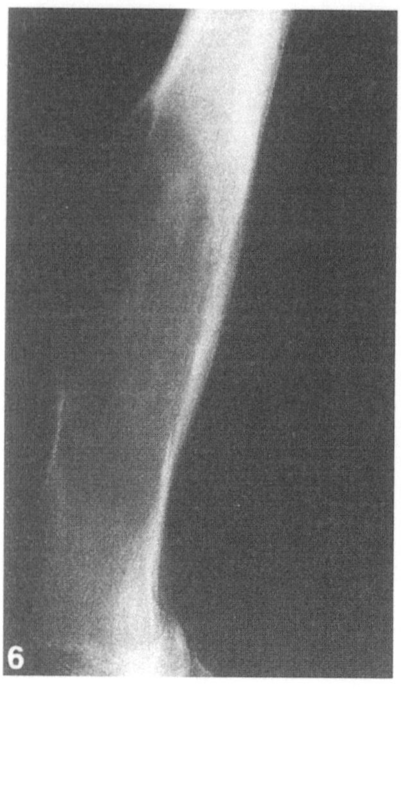

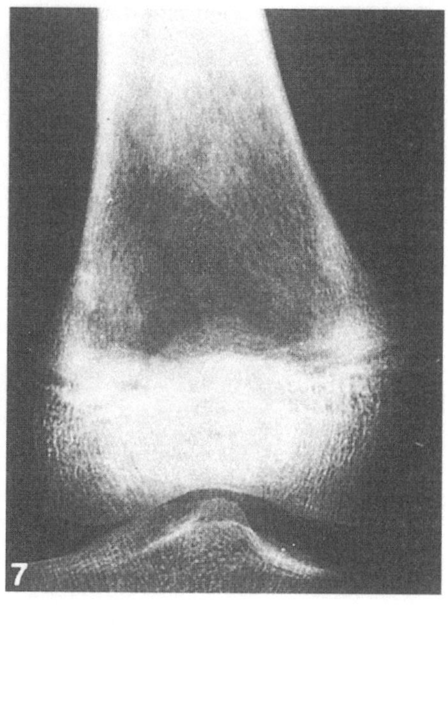

Fig. 3. Boy of 15, complaining of increasing size of thigh. Large tumour invading the soft tissues, osteogenesis of "grass fire" type (histology: osteoblastic type)

Fig. 4. Superomedial osteolysis of tibia with virtually no periosteal reaction (histology: anaplastic sarcoma, predominantly of osteoblastic type, abundant mitoses). Boy aged 19

Fig. 5. Lytic metaphyseo-epiphyseal lesion with clear-cut margins, no periosteal reaction (small-cell anaplastic sarcoma). Boy aged 17

Fig. 7. Lytic metaphyseal tumour (histology: anaplastic telangiectatic sarcoma). Girl aged 9

Fig. 8. **a** Standard frontal radiograph; osteosarcoma of knee in man of 35. Ill-defined sclerosing metaphyseal tumour of right femur, periosteal apposition. **b** The CT image illustrates the sclerosis, cortical lysis and periosteal apposition. **c** Axial section, MRI, T1-weighted (TR600, TE20). The involvement of the medulla, invasion of the soft parts and relations with the vessels are clearly shown; the cortical destruction and periosteal apposition are best studied in CT. **d** MRI, frontal section, T1-weighted (TR600, TE 20). The medullary involvement in the shaft (which determines the level of resection) and the relations with the joint are readily studied (Kindly supplied by Dr Vanel, Institut Gustave-Roussy)

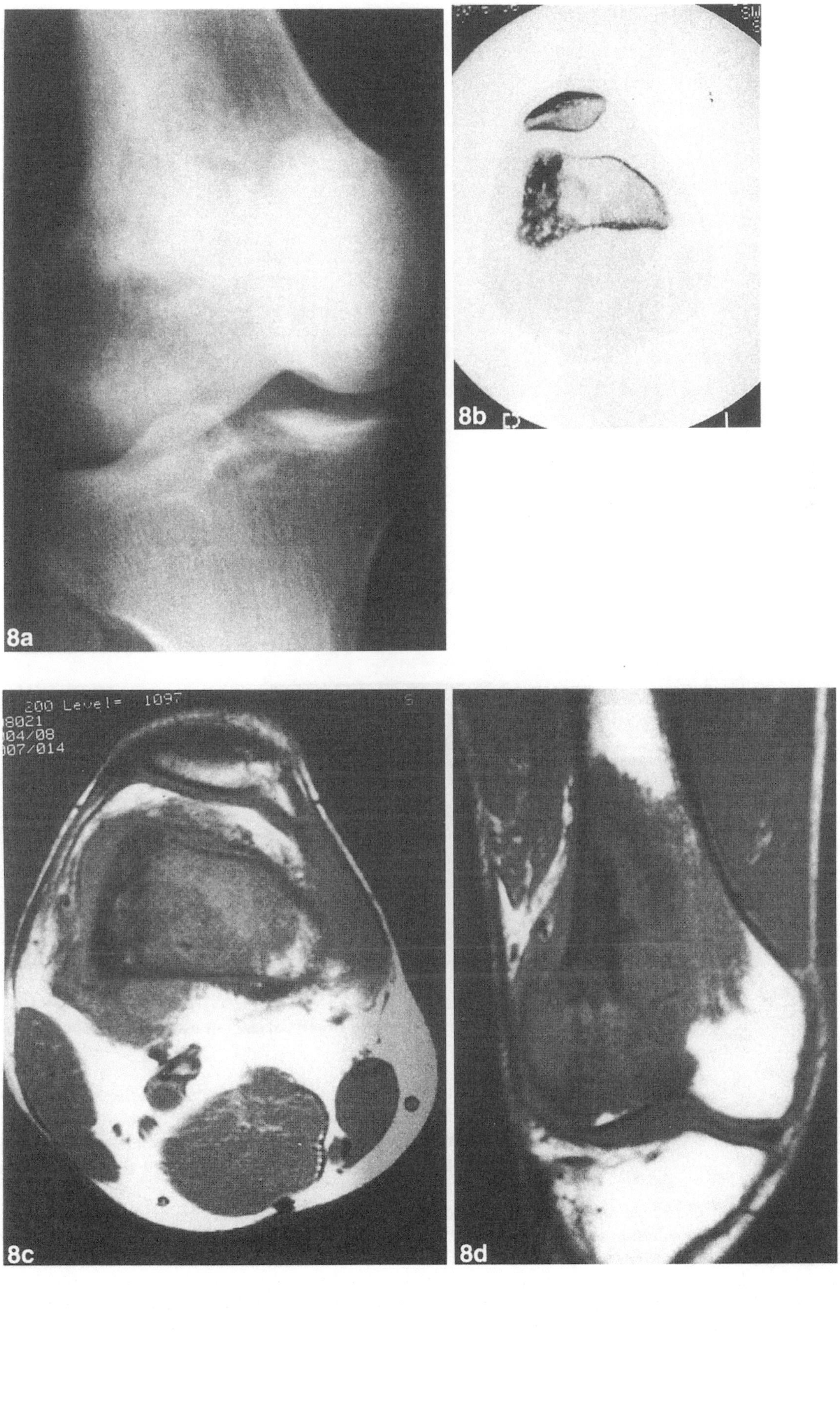
8a
8b
200 Level= 1097
8021
04/08
07/014
8c
8d

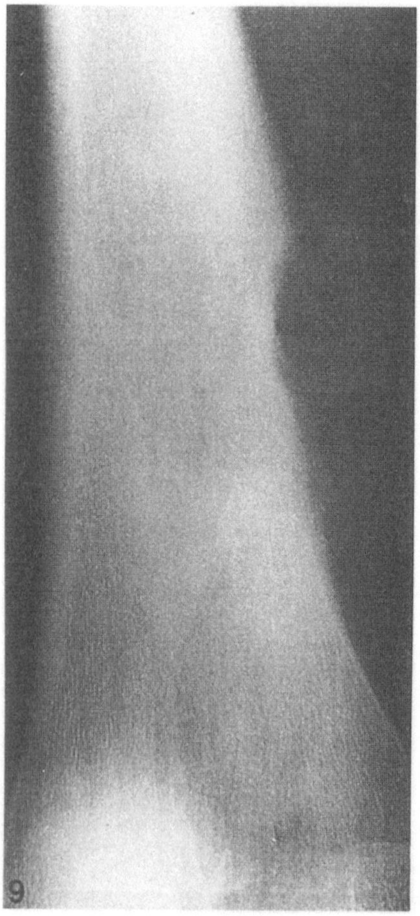

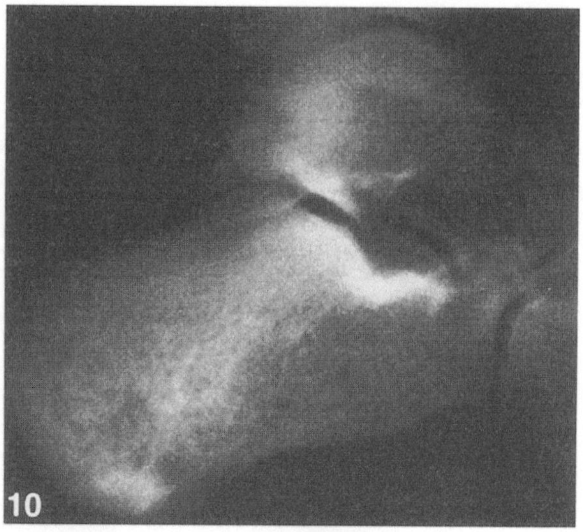

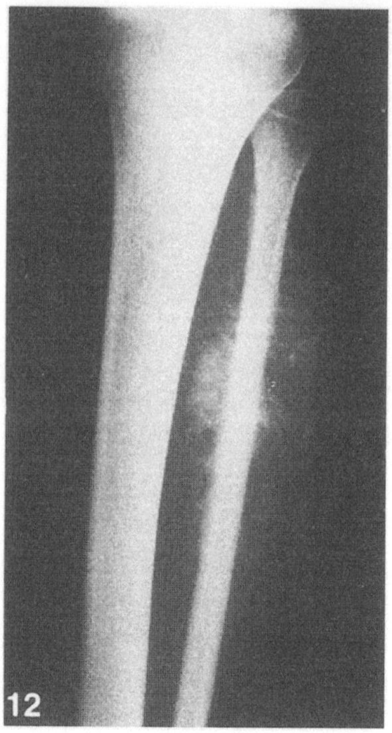

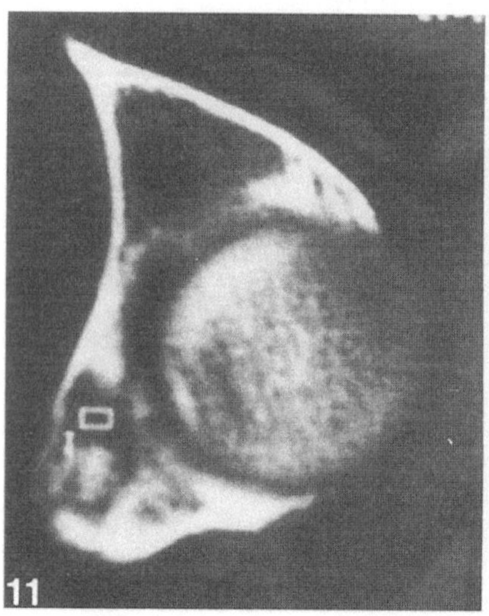

Fig. 9. Osteosarcoma in superfical site but histologically of common type (fig. 30)

Fig. 10. Osteosarcoma of calcaneum. Tumour invading soft tissues above and behind malleolus and proliferating behind between lower end of tibia and anterior aspect of Achilles tendon, widely penetrating the spongy bone. However, its periosteal origin is visible (histology: fig. 34 a, b). Girl of 20

Fig. 11. Lesion in depth of acetabulum, poorly defined, consisting of dense central island surrounded by zone of osteolysis. This radiological appearance, and an "ambiguous" histology, may suggest an osteoblastoma but it was in fact a genuine osteogenic sarcoma (fig. 45 a, b)

Fig. 12. Osteosarcoma of fibula developing superficially, histologically predominantly cartilaginous, probable origin periosteal

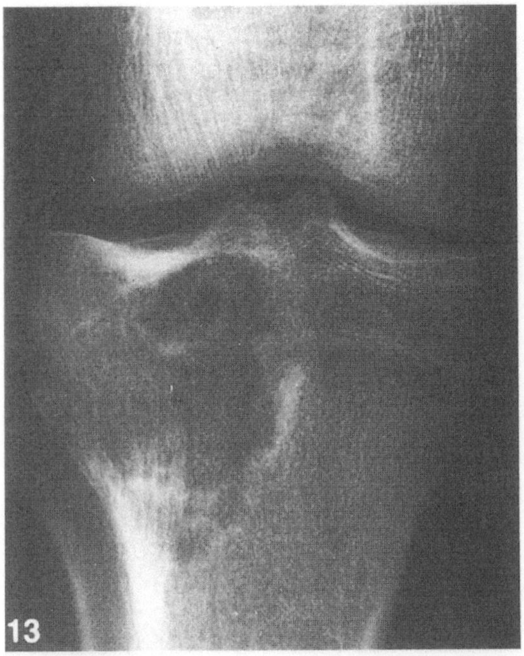

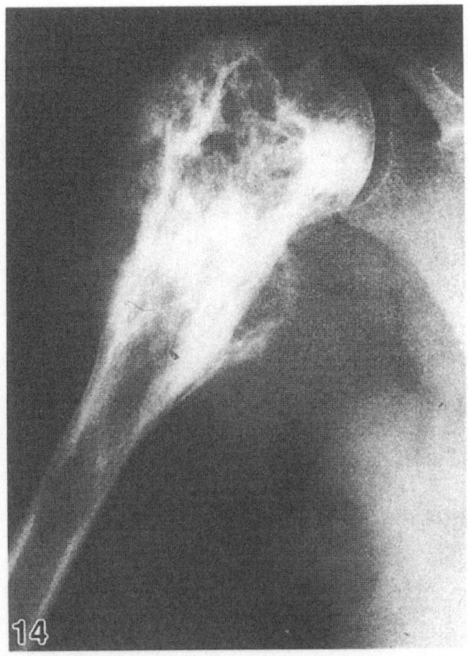

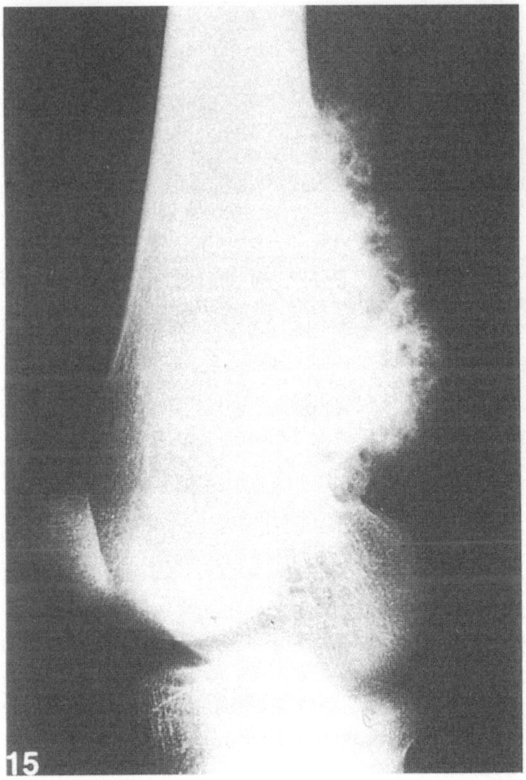

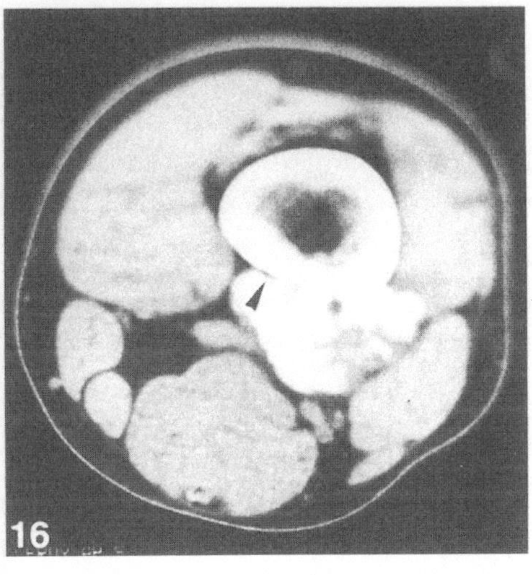

Fig. 13. Lytic metaphyso-epiphyseal tumour of tibia: anaplastic round-cell sarcoma (fig. 40). Man of 30

Fig. 14. Large slowly-growing sarcoma probably originating from periosteum at upper end of humerus and invading the spongy bone: osteosarcoma with a major cartilaginous component

Fig. 15. The slow painless growth of this highly ossific juxtacortical sarcoma caused much delay in diagnosis; the posterior femoral cortex is invaded. In these circumstances it is impossible to demonstrate in a stardard film the clear line that separates the femoral shaft from the tumour osteogenesis (fig. 42)

Fig. 16. In a very advanced juxtacortical sarcoma, CT examination is more explicit (*arrow-head*), revealing the presence of a clear zone between the tumour and the bony cortex

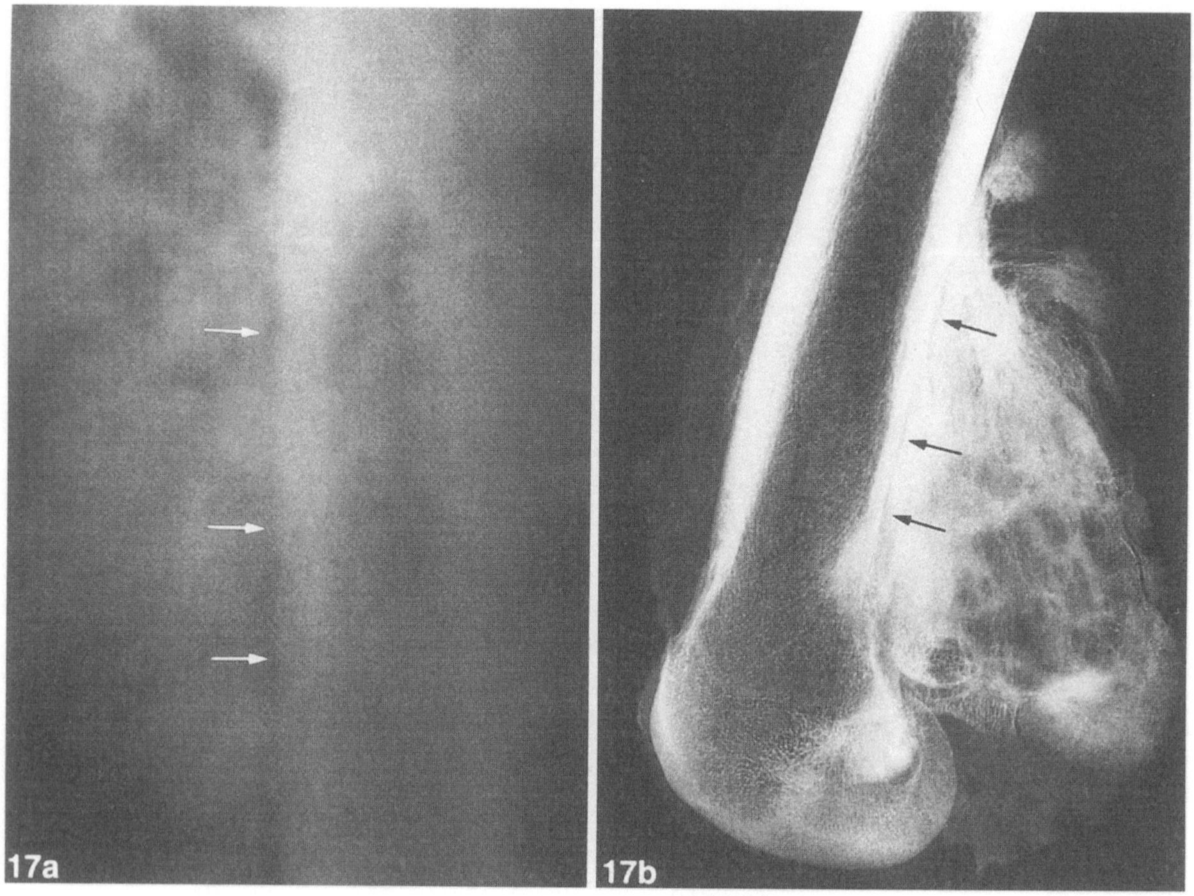

Fig. 17. a Very advanced juxtacortical sarcoma of femur; the clear line persists between cortex and tumour but is barely visible (arrows). **b** The clear line is more apparent in the radiograph of a longitudinal section (*arrows*)

→

Fig. 18 a-e. Juxtacortical osteosarcoma. **a** Standard film of left femoral shaft, surrounded by ossified mass. The clear border corresponding to the uninvaded periosteum is not visible CT after contrast injection (**b**) "soft tissue" and (**c**) "osseous" windows. The partly ossified mass surrounds the femur; the cortex is partly destroyed and limited invasion of the medulla is seen. **d** MRI, frontal section, T1-weighted (TR600, TE20) after injection of contrast. The extension into the bony marrow is perfectly defined. **e** MRI, axial section, T1-weighted (TR600, TE20) after injection of contrast, The ossifications (in black) are less analysable, but the extension into the soft parts and medulla are much easier to study because of the better contrast (Kindly supplied by Dr Vanel, Institut Gustave-Roussy)

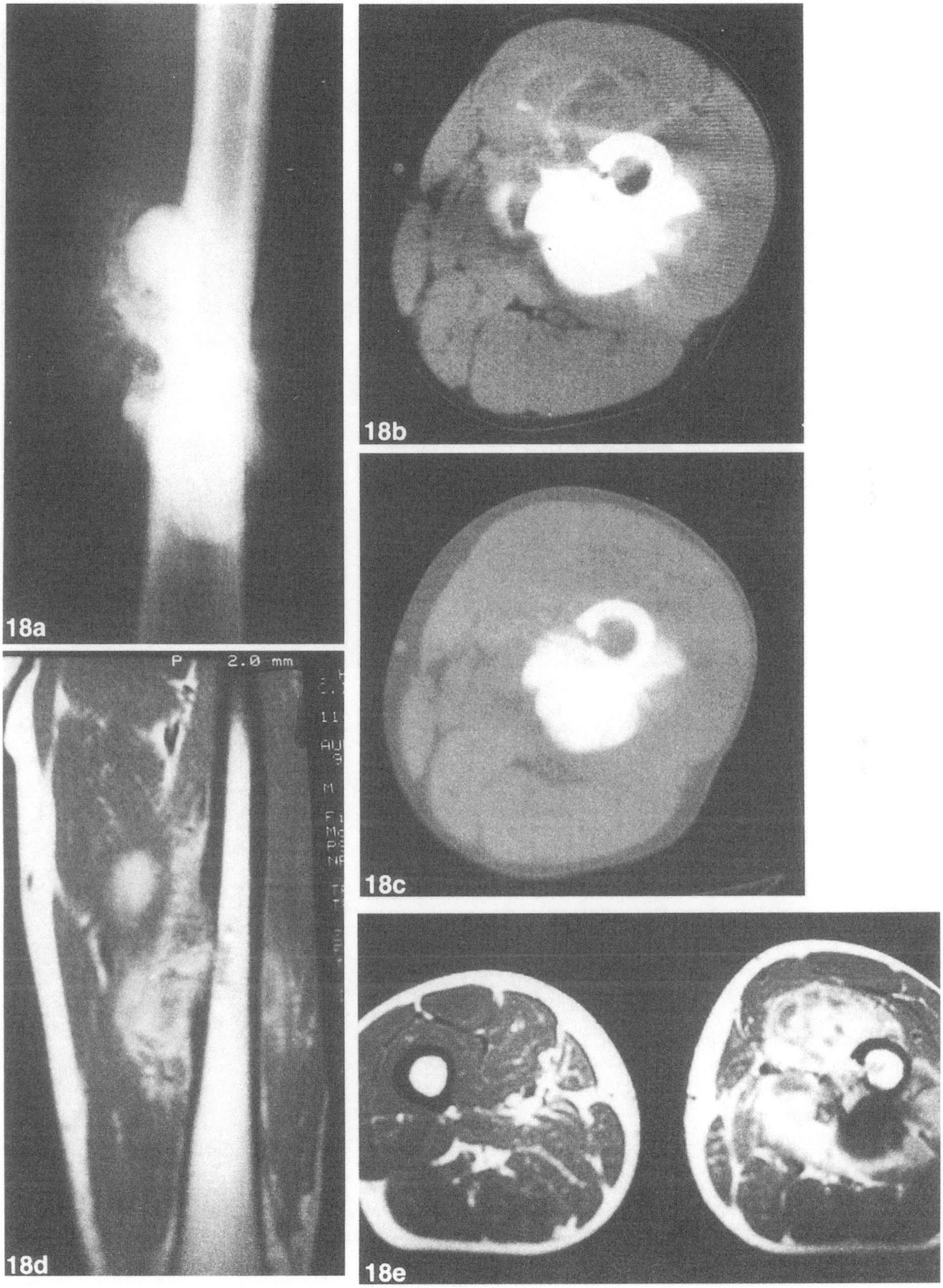
18a
18b
18c
P 2.0 mm
18d
18e

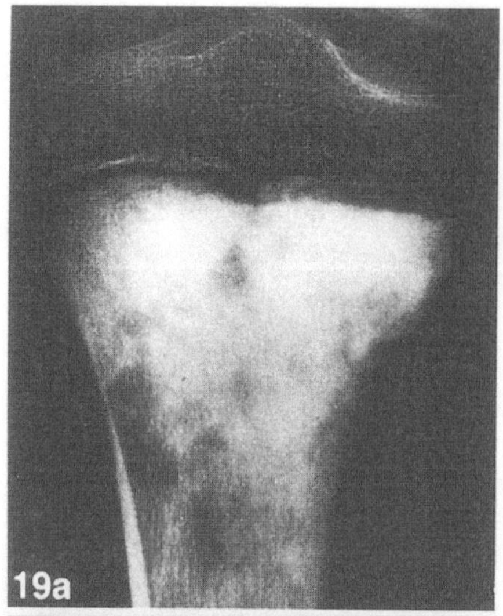

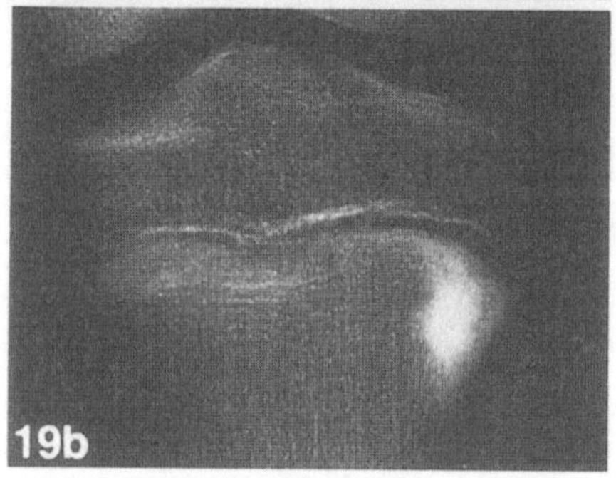

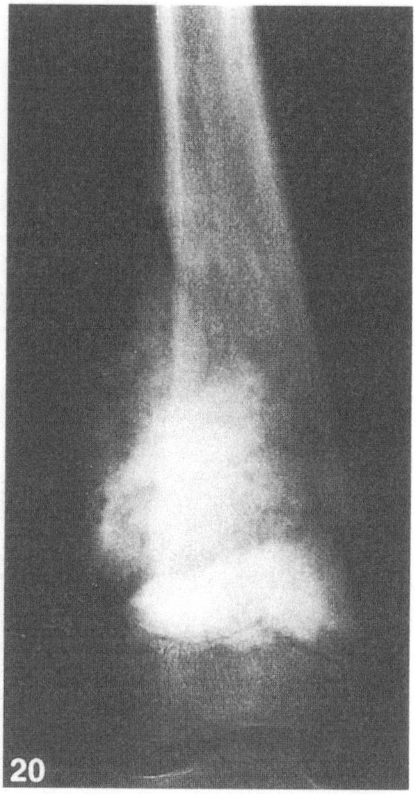

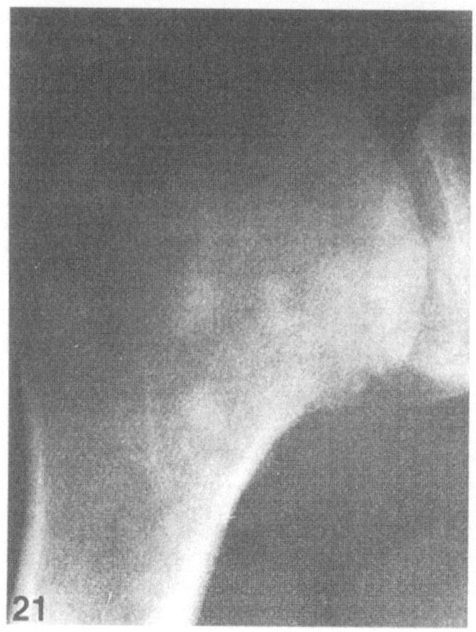

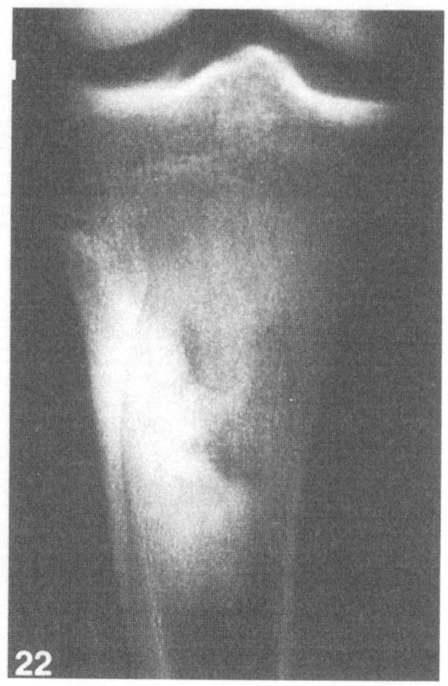

Fig. 19 a, b. Synchronic osteosarcomatosis in a child of 11 whose epiphyseal cartilages are clearly visible. Radiographs **a** and **b** show the upper metaphyseal localisations in the tibia. These osteoblastic tumours are dense on X-ray

Fig. 20. Advanced stage of osteosarcomatosis in an adolescent. The tumour, highly opaque in radiography, has invaded the soft tissues widely, but invasion of the epiphyseal cartilage is not evident

Fig. 21. This 23 year old patient presented 5 months after pain started in his right shoulder. Examination of the skeleton revealed 4 other localisations

Fig. 22. Solitary localisation of an radiodense sarcoma in the upper 1/3 of the tibia. Boy of 17

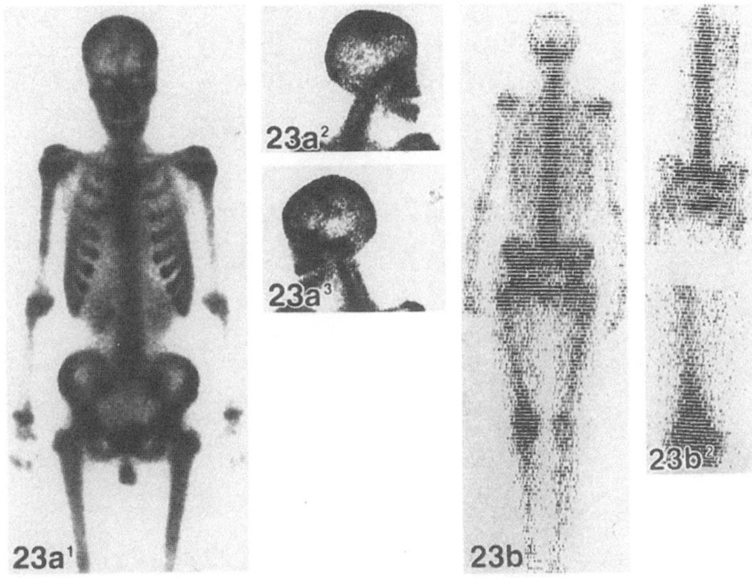

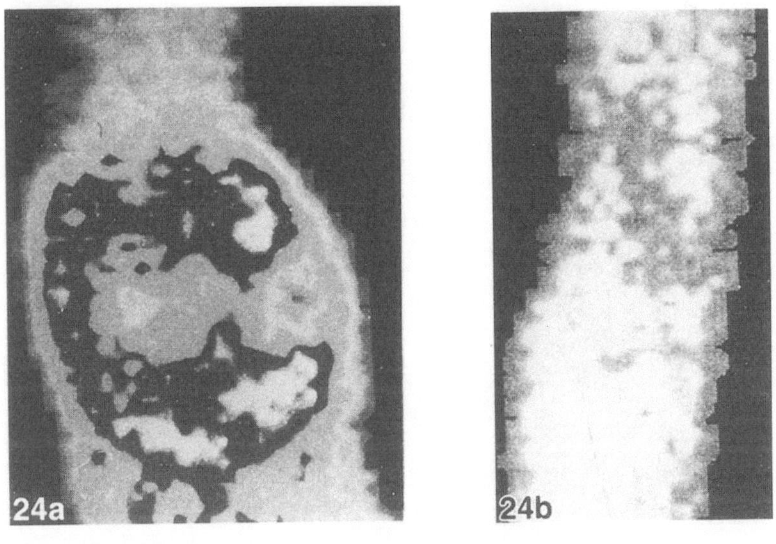

Fig. 23. **a** Girl of 14 with an osteogenic sarcoma of upper end of right humerus. Bone scintigraphy (^{99m}Tc-MDP) 15 months after treatment by radiation and chemotherapy. The survey demonstrates significant anomalies of the cranial vault which were confirmed radiologically 3 months later. **b** Scintigraphy of fixation of an organophosphorous osteotrope (^{99m}Tc-MDP) in a woman of 22 affected by an osteogenic sarcoma of the lower end of the right femur. Scintigraphy reveals a left iliac metastatic lesion

Fig. 24 a, b. Osteogenic sarcoma of upper third of tibia, man of 26. **a** Scintigraphy of biodistribution one hour after intravenous administration of interferon alpha^{121}I. This record demonstrates the precocity and extent of tumour capture of radio-labelled interferon as well as its relative heterogeneity. The greatest fixation is essentially peripheral, in crescent shape here in black (red in the original film), the white areas correspond to zones of saturation. Comparison of fixation by the tumoral zone (T) with (**b**) the symmetric healthy zone (Sym) gives the ratio T/Sym = 4.3

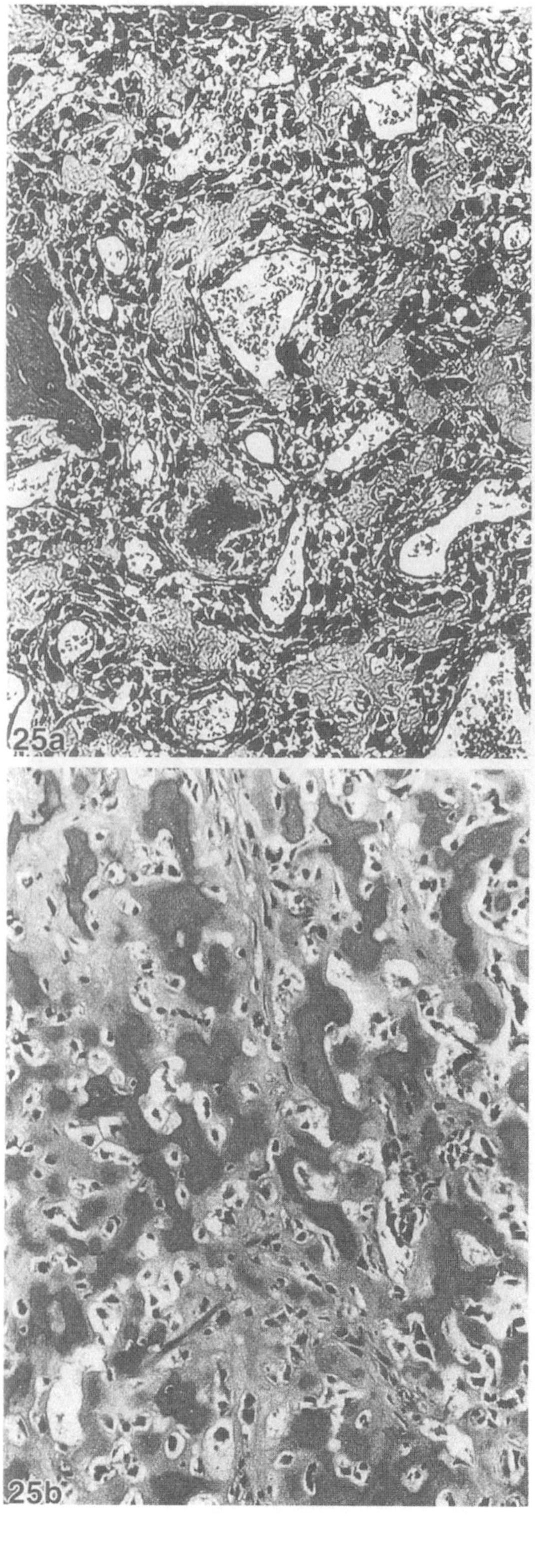

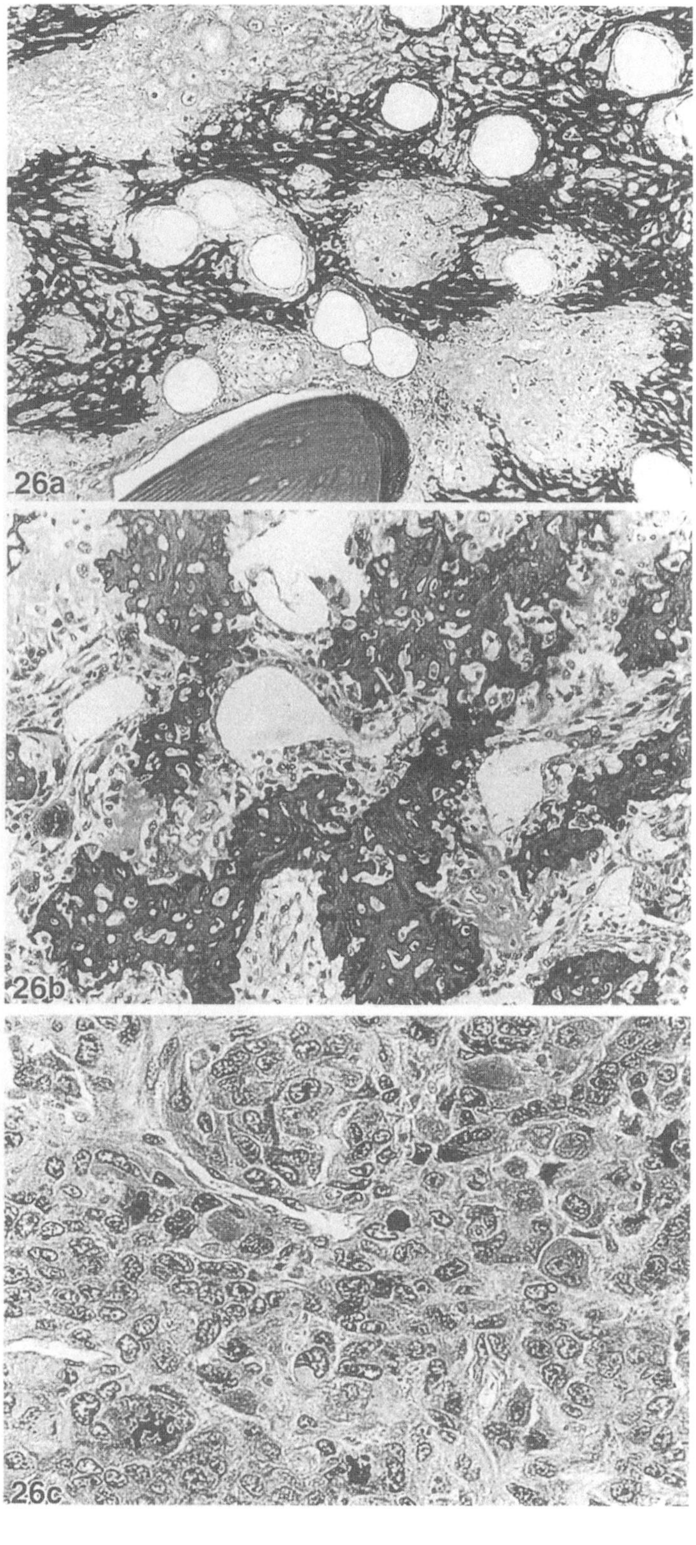

Figures 25-28 illustrate the histological polymorphism of the common form of sarcoma

Fig. 25. a Anarchic elaboration of partly calcified osteoid tissue, abundant vascularisation. **b** In the osteoid tissue are tumour cells of irregular size and shape with densely staining nuclei

Fig. 26 a-c. "Osteochondroid" tissue with plexiform calcification surrounding a strand of old necrosed bone (**a**). Irregular calcification of osteoid tissue in vicinity of wide vascular lacunae (**b**). Another zone of this osteosarcoma: a very cellular anaplastic area devoid of osteogenesis (**c**)

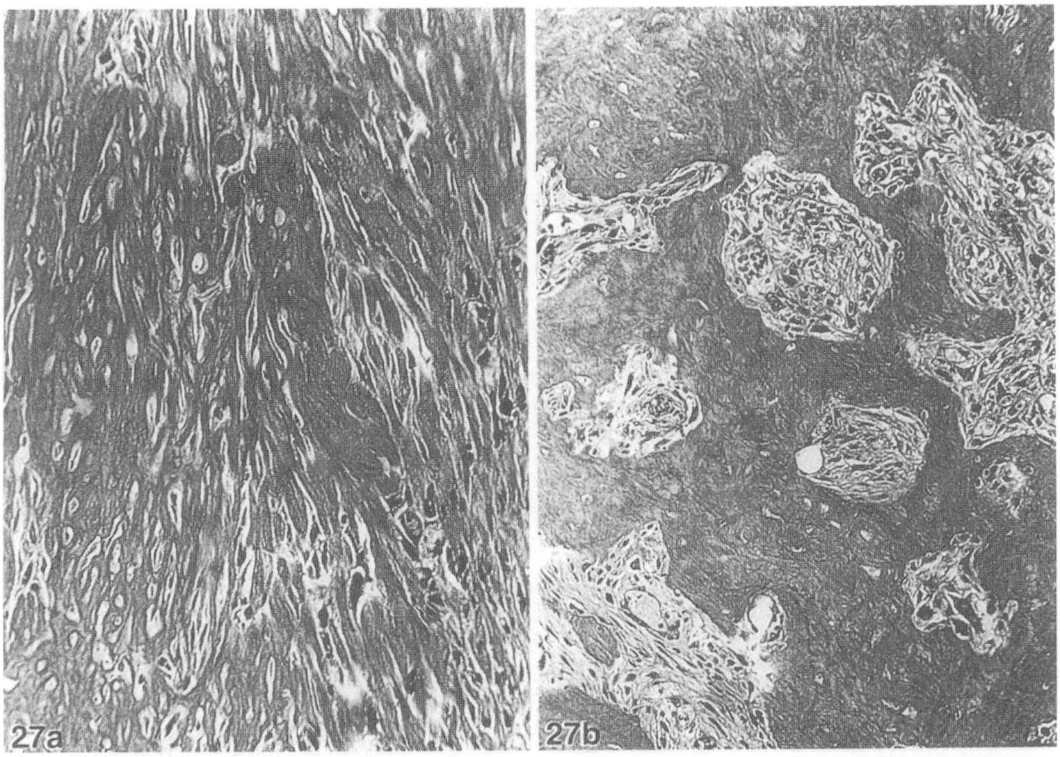

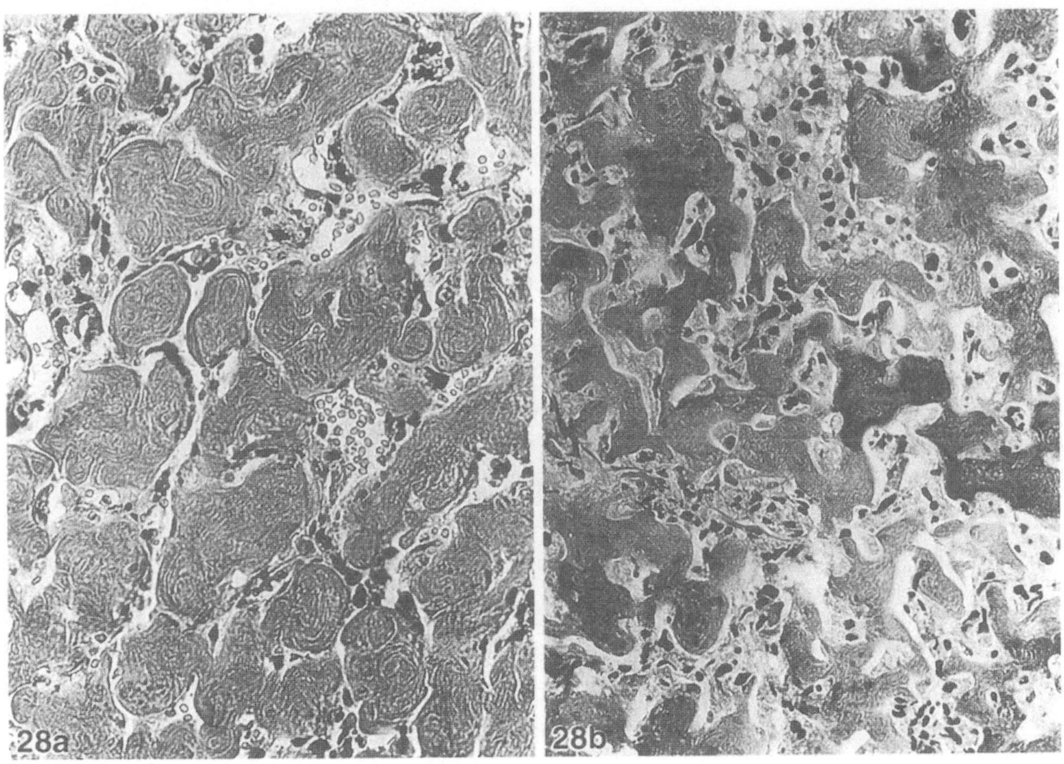

Fig. 27 a, b. Two different aspects of osteogenesis in an osteosarcoma of the tibia in a man of 19. **a** Patterned arrangement of osteoid lamellae with interposed cells. **b** Sparsely cellular osteoid areas with inter-anastomosis

Fig. 28 a, b. Other appearances of osteogenesis: sarcoma of femoral neck, child of 12. **a** Virtually acellular fibro-osteoid islands arranged like wreaths of smoke. **b** Osteoid deposits of anarchic arrangement, unequally calcified, a sort of jigsaw puzzle with proliferation of tumour cells between the pieces

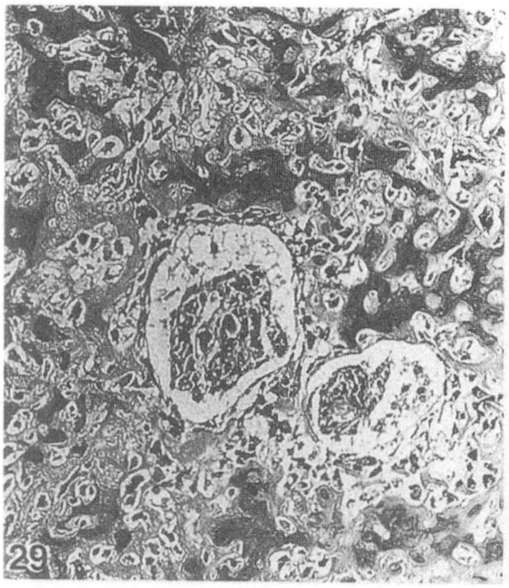

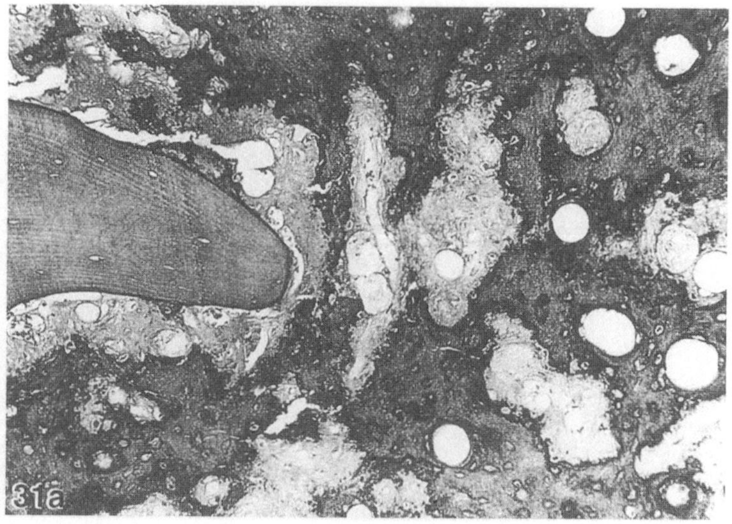

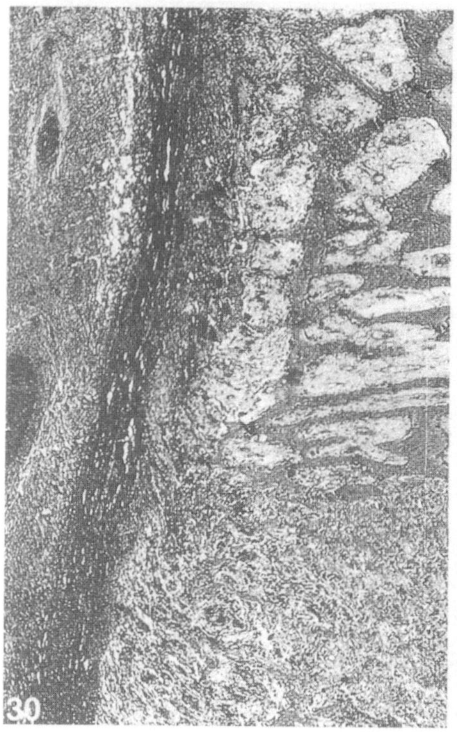

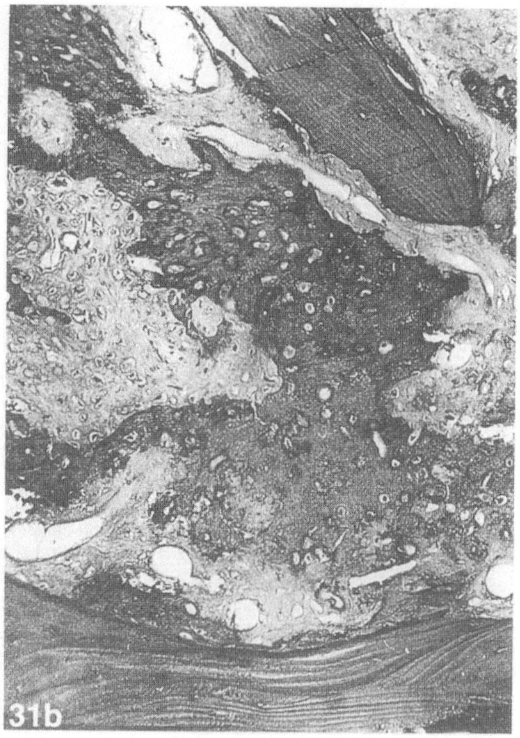

Fig. 29. Tumour tissue is quite often present in the vascular lumina of osteosarcomas

Fig. 30. Left: connective tissue covering a thickened fibrous periosteum. Right: upper 2/3, reactive periosteal osteogenesis; lower 1/3, tumour proliferation destroying the periosteal osteogenesis (common type of sarcoma developing superficially, fig. 9)

Fig. 31 a, b. Sclerosing sarcoma of tibia: diffuse calcification in the chondro-osteoid tissue, which occupies the medullary spaces of the spongy bone

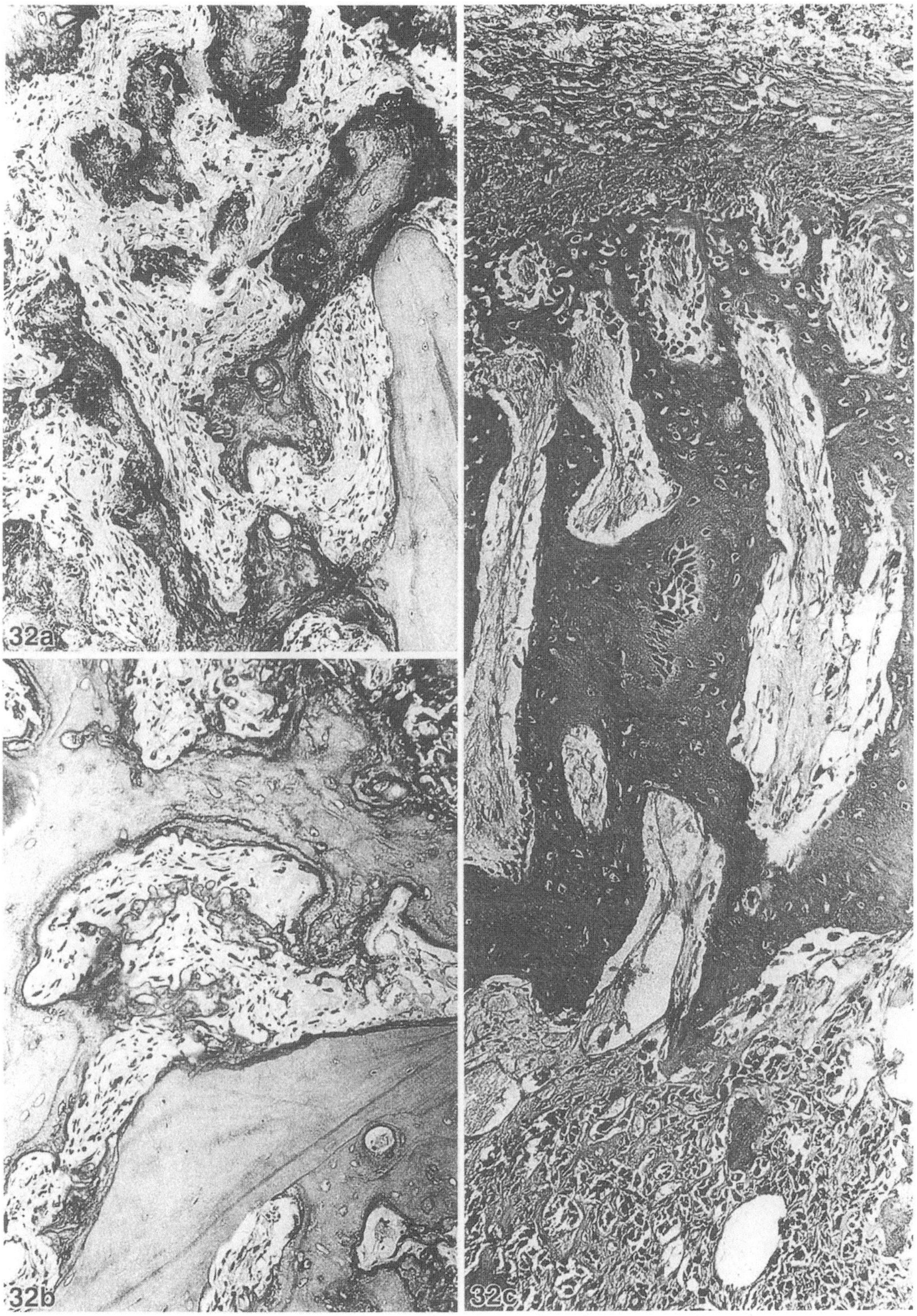

Fig. 32. a, b At low magnification, this appearance may suggest a bone infarction, a hypothesis refuted by examination of the cells. **c** In the lower part, the sarcomatous cell proliferation encounters the illusory barrier of immature bone elaborated by the periosteum

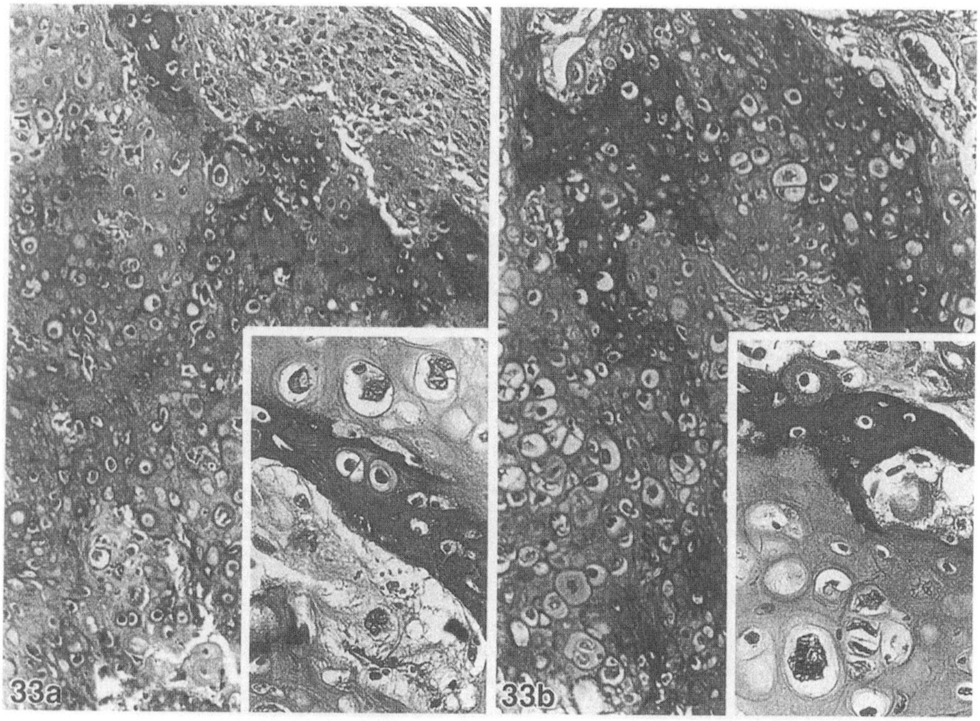

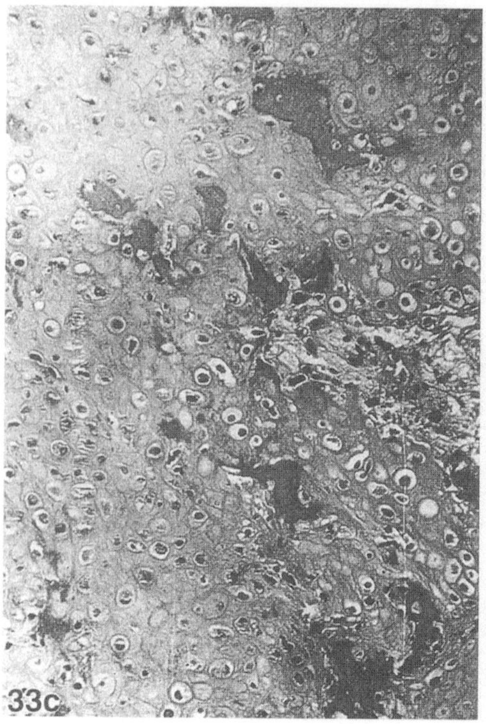

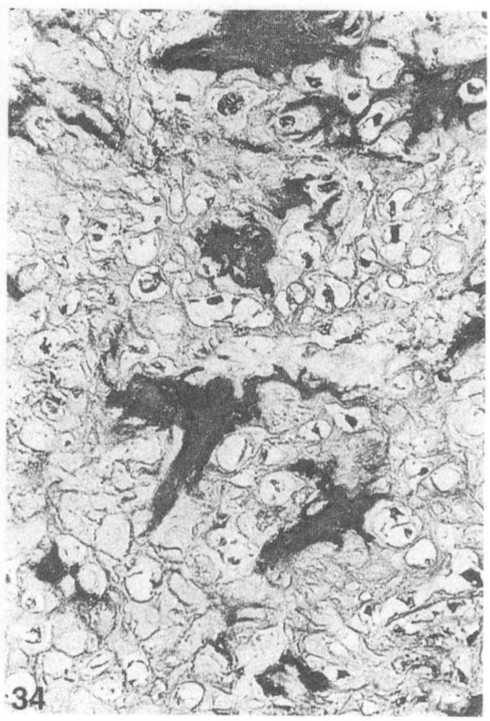

Fig. 33. a, b Predominantly cartilaginous intraosseous osteosarcoma, some areas with strands of tumour osteogenesis. Calcaneum, girl of 20, possibly of periosteal origin (fig. 10). **c** The same problem in the femur: osteosarcoma or chondrosarcoma? Requires study of large sectional surfaces. Adolescent boy of 15

Fig. 34. Periosteal osteosarcoma, essentially cartilaginous: some rudiments of tumour osteogenesis in this microphotograph

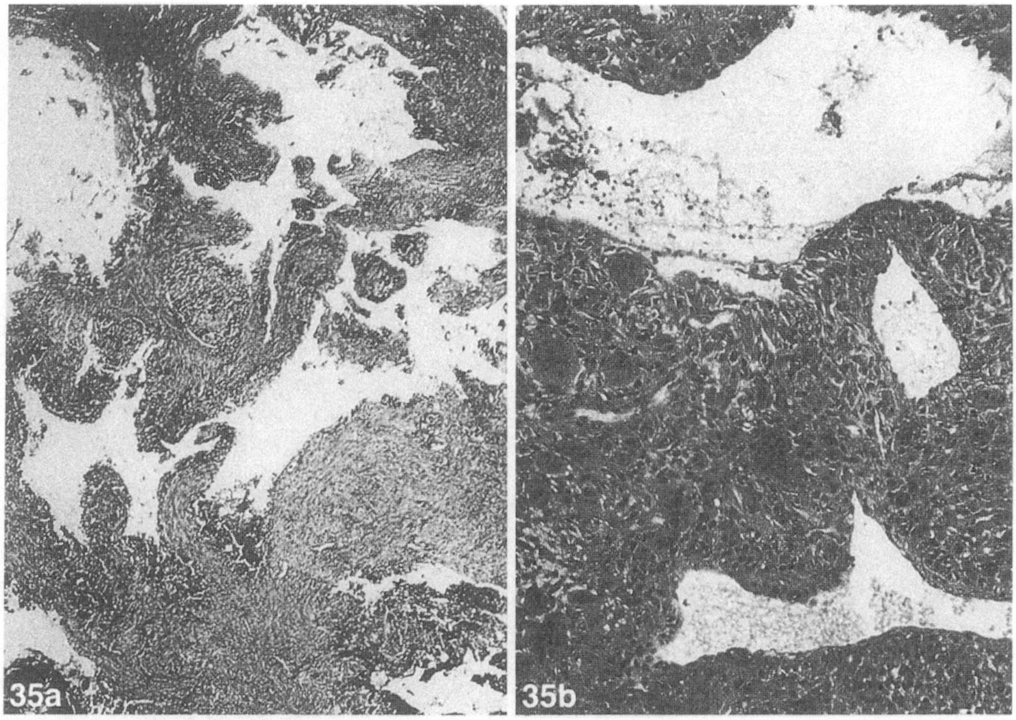

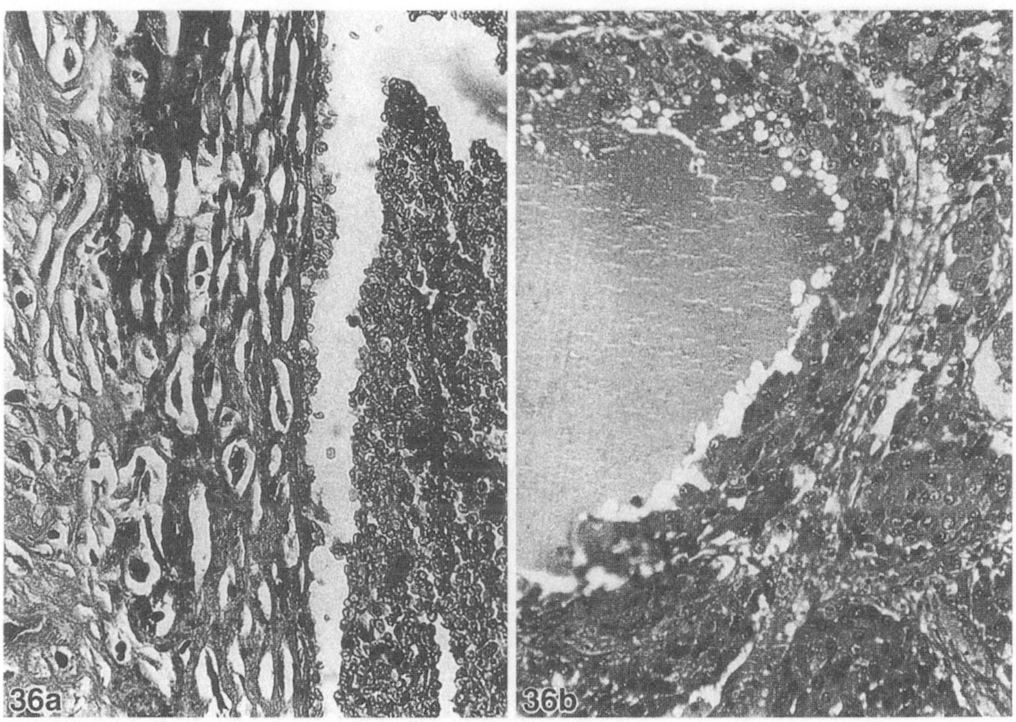

Fig. 35 a, b. At low magnification, the large vascular lacunae and the giant cells may suggest an aneurysmal cyst. The presence of atypical anaplastic cells permits the diagnosis of anaplastic telangiectatic sarcoma. Boy of 17

Fig. 36 a, b. In another case, the vascular lacuna (**a**) is bordered by tumour osteogenesis (unlike the osteoid or osseous margins of aneurysmal cysts). **b** In this zone too small a sample might lead to a wrong diagnosis of angioendothelioma

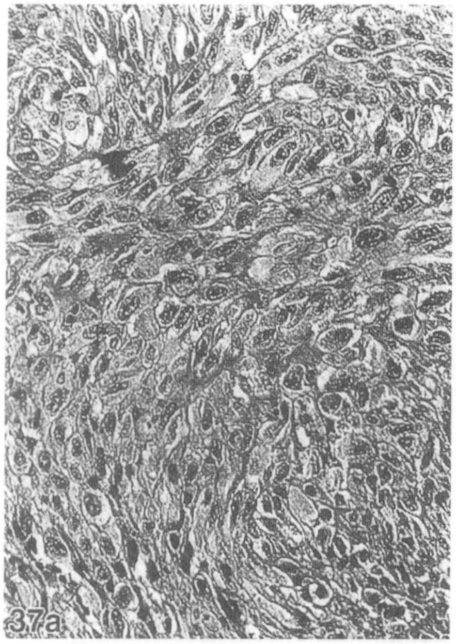

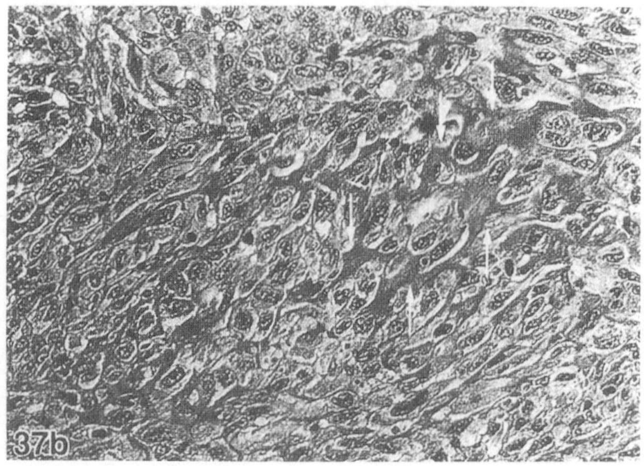

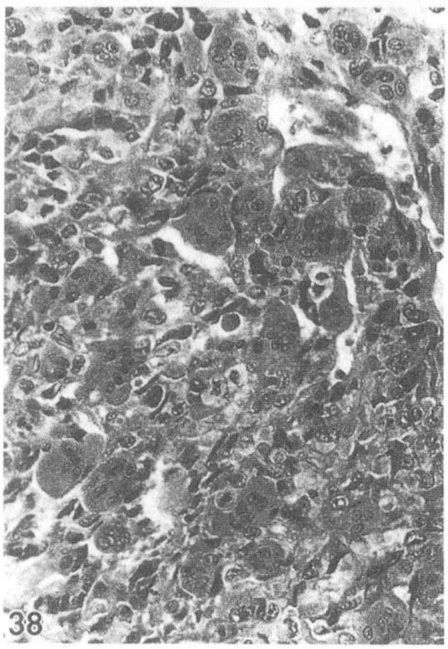

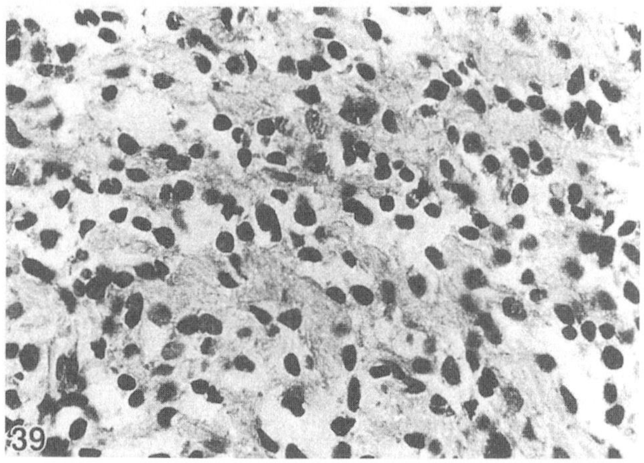

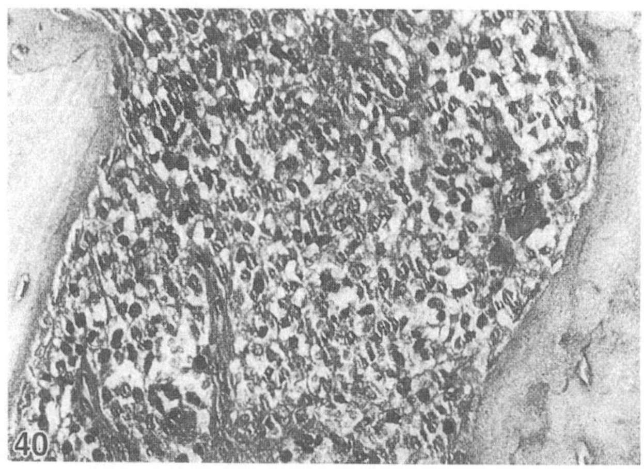

Fig. 37. a Anaplastic osteosarcoma of femur with fusiform cells. **b** In some zones there is some minor osteoid formation. Girl of 13 years

Fig. 38. This osteosarcoma with giant cells in an adolescent boy of 16 is unrelated to a giant-cell tumour or Paget's disease or parathyroid osteosis, disorders to be considered in older patients. Anaplastic osteoarcoma of femur containing giant cells

Fig. 39. Lytic metaphyseo-epiphyseal sarcoma of tibia (fig. 13): proliferation of undifferentiated cells with hyperchromatic nuclei, rare osteoid strands. Round-celled anaplastic osteosarcoma. Man of 30

Fig. 40. Another case of small-celled anaplastic sarcoma. Man of 37 (fig. 5)

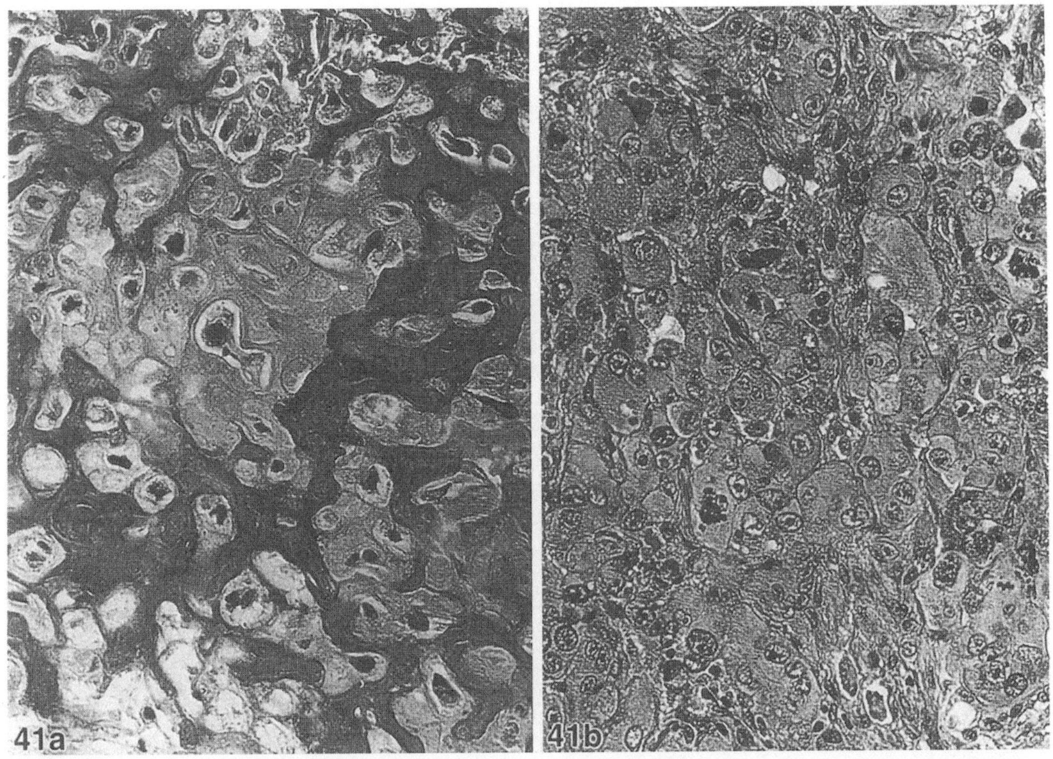

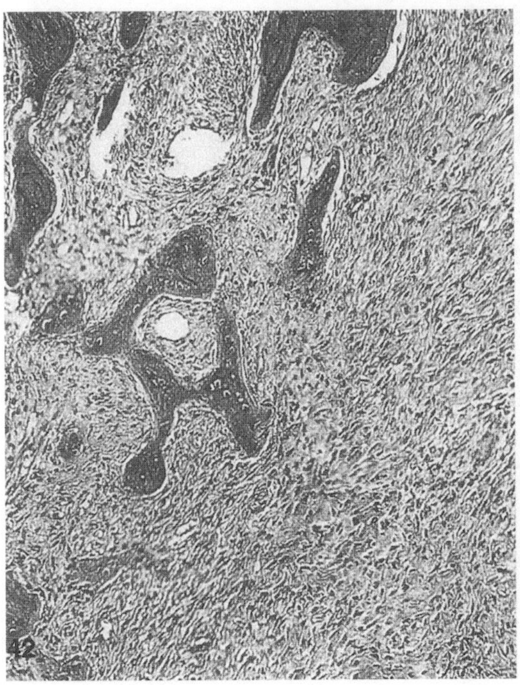

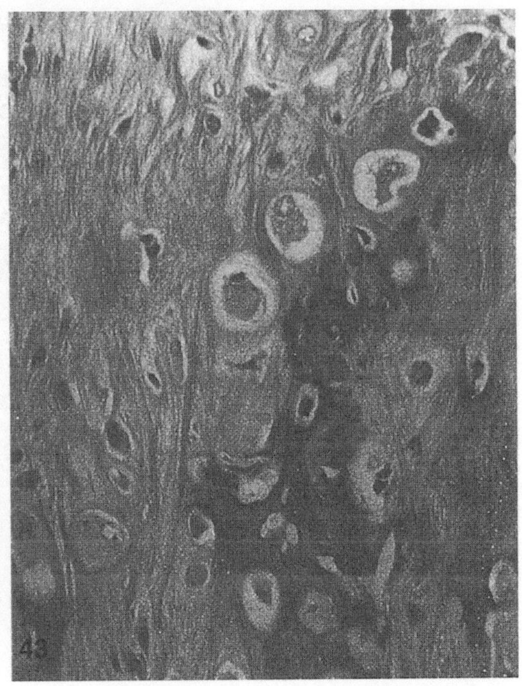

Fig. 41 a, b. Osteosarcomatosis. These two microphotographs show the polymorphous nature of the osteoid evolution and cell proliferation, in places (**b**) devoid of osteoid tissue, in contrast with the radiological density of this tumour (fig. 19)

Fig. 42. Juxtaortical sarcoma of popliteal fossa, radiologically typical (woman of 35). Osteogenesis is reduced to a few small bony strands appearing in the midst of a proliferating sarcomatous connective tissue with rare cytological anomalies. Overall, this is quite different from the structure and architecture of an osteoma, in which there is a differentiated, usually fatty, marrow tissue

Fig. 43. Another case of juxtacortical sarcoma (fig. 15). The fusiform cell proliferation was quite obviously sarcomatous, unlike the preceding case (fig. 42). The patchy, partly calcified chondro-osteoid formation allocates the tumour to the skeletogenic sarcomas

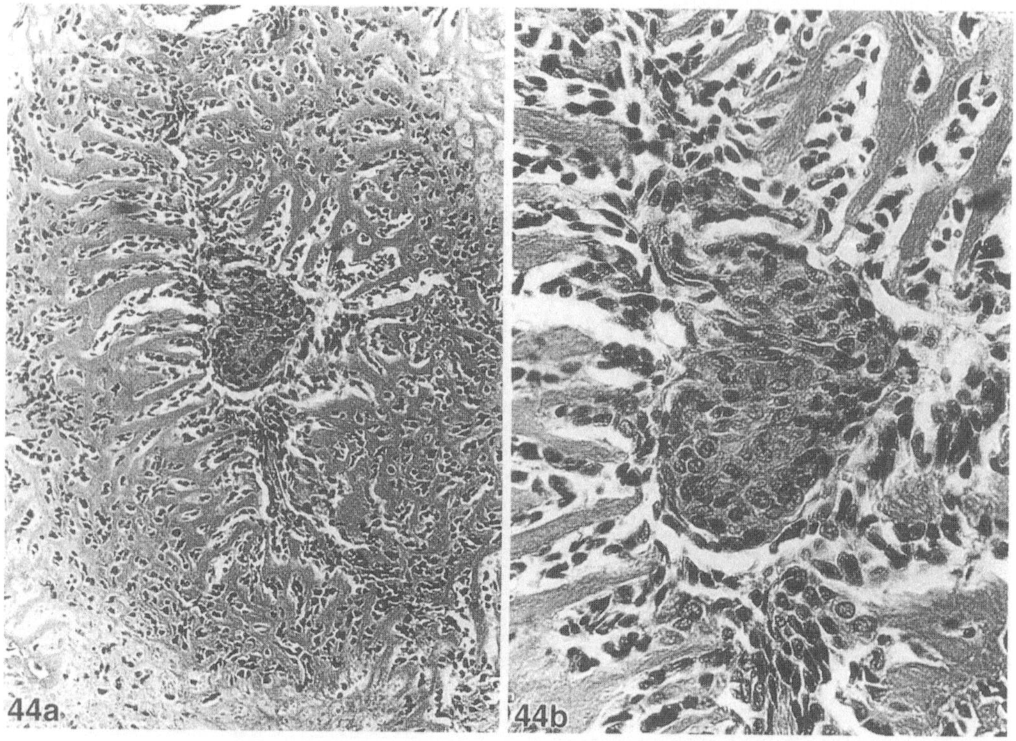

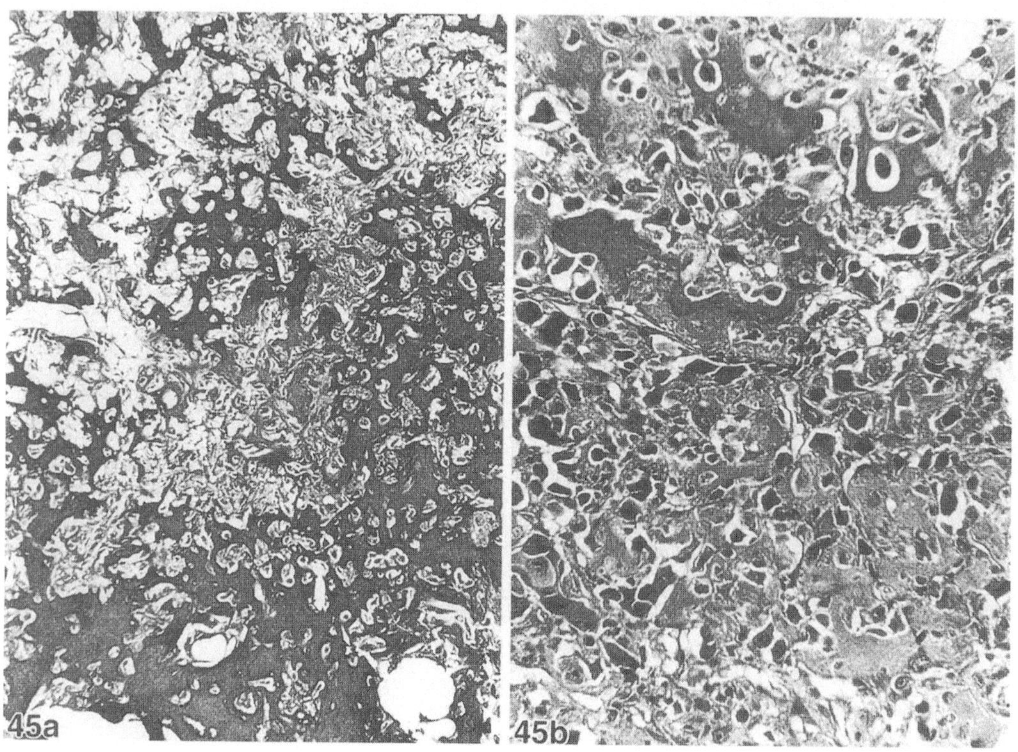

Fig. 44 a, b. Around this cellular center the bony lamellae have a radiating pattern. At low magnification this organoid appearance may suggest an osteoid osteoma (**a**). In fact, it is an osteoblastic osteosarcoma of the 5th rib (**b**). Death ensued after 5 years

Fig. 45 a, b. The radiograph of this tumour in the depth of the acetabulum (fig. 11), and the low magnification sections (**a**) suggest an osteoblastoma. At higher magnification (**b**) the cellular morphology is unlike the classical appearance of osteoblasts in osteoblastoma. The matrix, which is sometimes chondroid, fibrous or osteoid and the cell anomalies, led to a diagnosis of osteosarcoma in this woman aged 61. (Material kindly supplied by Dr Françoise Collin, CAC, Dijon)

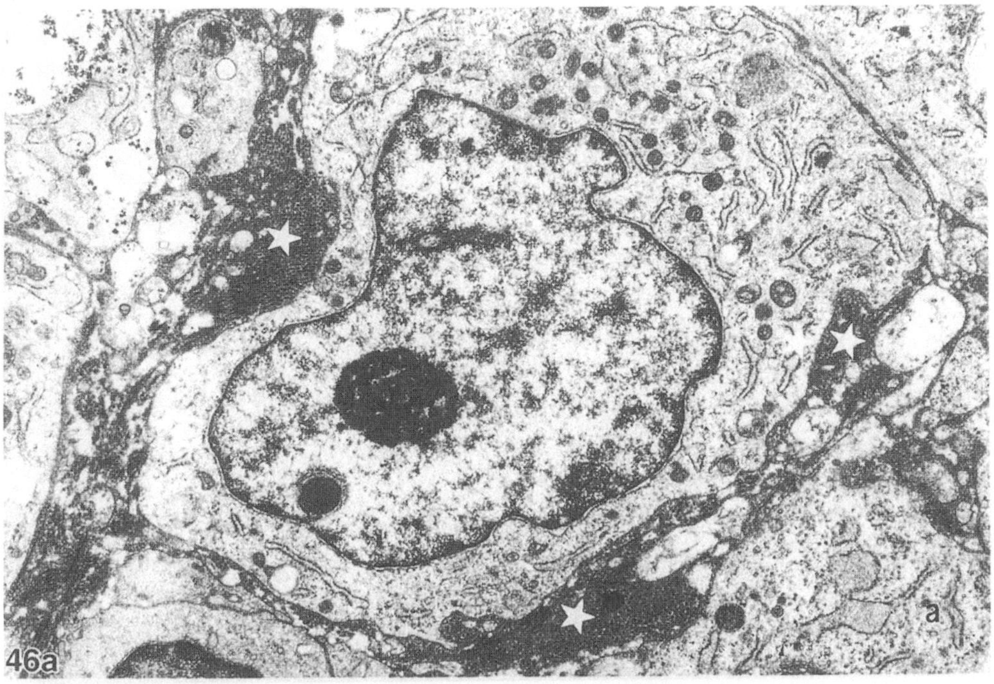

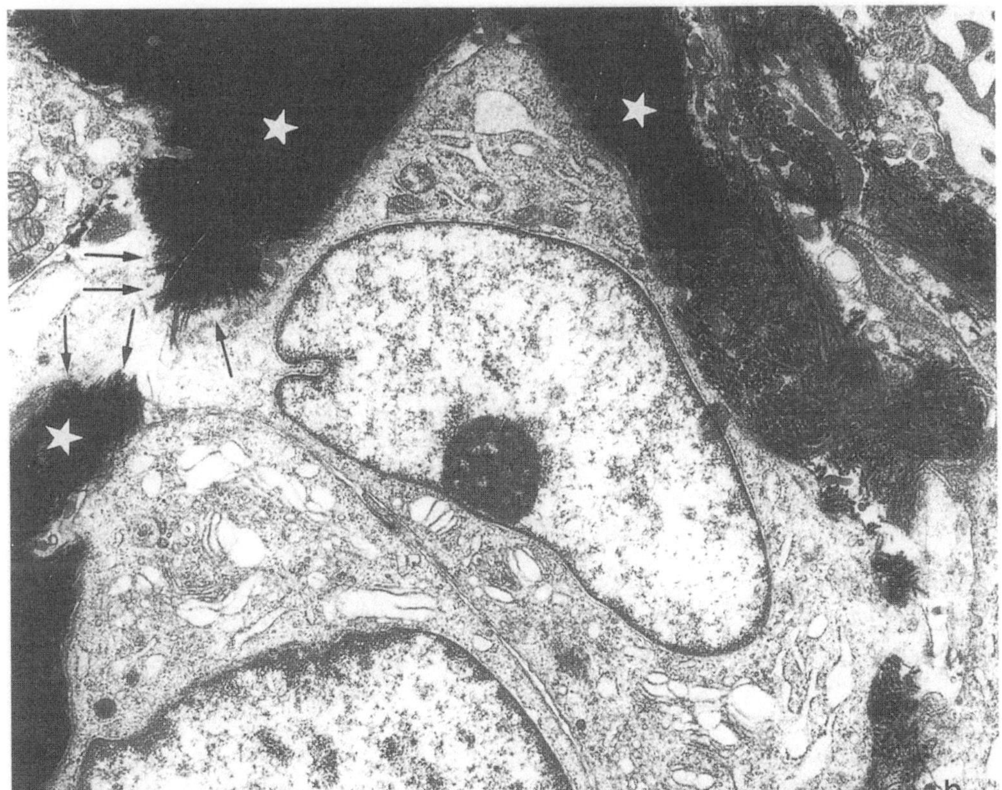

Fig. 46 a, b. Comparison of ultrastructural cytology between (**a**) an anaplastic osteogenic sarcoma fixing very little ^{85}Sr and (**b**) a well-differentiated osteogenic sarcoma strongly fixing ^{85}Sr. The strands of osteoid material (*starred*) are thin and very little calcified in (**a**); on the contrary, they are thick and markedly calcified in (**b**) with apatite crystals visible at the periphery (*arrows*). Fig. **a** x 9200; fig. **b**, x 10200 (illustration JP Thiery)

12. Cortico-metaphyseal fibrous defect, non-ossifying fibroma, multiple fibromas, benign fibrous histiocytoma

The numerous common features of these lesions justify their inclusion in the same chapter.

Case histories

Case 1. A boy, aged 6, was examined at the Clinique d'Orthopédie Infantile for a minor degree of scoliosis. Examination of the lower limb showed perfect equality of the tibiae, but in one of them a small enclosed clear image at the lower metaphysis was diagnosed as a fibrous defect. The child was regularly reviewed and in a few years the cortical lacunar image in the tibia lessened and disappeared.

Case 2. Near the Hôpital des Enfants-Assistés, Delphine, aged 9, was skipping like a model little girl and suddenly fractured her tibia. Half-an-hour later the radiograph suggested a diagnosis of spontaneous fracture at an osteolytic lesion with polycyclic outlines bordered by a narrow margin of sclerosis. The diagnosis was easily made and treatment was designed to terminate the development of this non-ossifying fibroma and ensure union of the fracture in good position.

Case 3. Moderate but persistent pain in the right thigh in a young girl of 16 led to the discovery of an extensive lesion in the lower third of the femur. In the radiographs the well-defined polycyclic osteolysis was characteristic of a benign lesion. The diagnosis of non-ossifying fibroma seemed most likely. Spontaneous disappearance of the lesion was not probable given the patient's age and the size of the tumour, but the risk of spontaneous fracture was considerable. Therefore surgical treatment was indicated, which also allowed the pathologist to confirm the diagnosis.

Cortico-metaphyseal fibrous defect in adolescents

General considerations

In radiographs of the limbs of children and adolescents there is very often observed a clear, lacunar cortico-metaphyseal image which moves away from the epiphyseal plate during growth. This zone of osteolysis disappears spontaneously in the majority of cases. It was described by Sontag and Pyle (1941), in 101 cases in femoral metaphyses in children, as a zone of cystic appearance. Later, Jaffe & Lichtenstein termed it "fibrous cortical defect".

In children followed from birth to the age of 18, it is found that these defects are not present at birth and do not appear before the end of the first year [Nezelof et al 1956]. Their number then reaches a maximum; up to 30% of children are said to exhibit this lesion. The minute percentage of such defects found in the routine examination of the femur in older adults and young adults argues in favor of their spontaneous absorption. There is a familial factor. Certain series indicate a slight male predominance, though Maroteaux (1982) found no gender difference in this lesion.

The site of the defects is metaphyseal and cortical. They progressively move away from the growth plate as the child grows. Multiple foci may be found in the same child. The bones electively affected are the long bones of the limbs, particularly the lower metaphyses of the femur and tibia.

Clinical features and course

A fibrous defect of small size often has no clinical expression and is only discovered during a radiographic examination performed for some other reason. Some transient pain may attract attention. Rarely, examination may reveal slight palpable swelling. In other cases, it is the radiological examination of a fracture that reveals a cortical defect that has hitherto been asymptomatic.

The spontaneous course is unpredictable. The defect may regress and disappear, or it may persist unchanged, moving away from the growth plate during growth. It may disappear and reappear several times at the same site [Nezelof et al 1956]. The essential feature is its benign nature, which excludes routine surgical intervention. However, when it tends to extend, its preferential site in the lower limbs carries a risk of fracture, a fracture which leads to a surgical procedure treating at once both the benign "tumour" and the fracture.

Imaging

The radiological appearance, though variable with the age of the patient and the specific evolution of the tumour, is still sufficiently characteristic to permit diagnosis in the majority of cases (figs. 1-6). Ritschk et al (1989) distinguish four progressive stages: A, B, C and D.

Stage A. A small round or oval intracortical image situated near the growth plate, with defined margins but no sclerosis.

Stage B. The clear image is at some distance from the growth plate, round or polycyclic, its margins enclosed in a discrete sclerotic border. Although always cortical in site, there is little or no periosteal reaction with a minor protrusion.

Stage C. Sclerosis is more marked and expansion is also towards the diaphysis.

Stage D. The sclerosis affects virtually the entire lesion; the radiological image then disappears gradually to give way to a normal bone structure.

Pathological anatomy and histopathology

Curettage yields a tissue of fibrous consistency, of a whitish, yellow or rusty color. The walls of the cavity, made of a narrow smooth bony layer, surround the lesion.

The dominant cellular element is a fusiform cell (fig. 9) of fibroblastic or histiocyto-fibroblastic appearance. The cells are grouped in whirled, intermingled, sometimes braided bundles. The whole is strewn with multinucleate cells. These giant cells (figs. 11, 12) are however only moderate in size. They vary in abundance in different cases and in different parts of the same tumour. In some tumours they are rare, while in others they may be so many as to resemble a giant-cell tumour. Areas of foamy fibrohistiocytic cells (fig. 10), often containing haemosiderin pigment and fatty acid crystals, are often seen but without justifying a diagnosis of xanthoma.

The presence of small perivascular lymphocytic infiltrations is not uncommon, but there are no true inflammatory foci with necrosis and polynuclear cells. The elaboration of collagen and reticulin fibers is the rule, but the tumour is much more cellular than collagenous. Some fine osteoid strands at the periphery of the lesion, or even a rare small osteoid island, in no way alter the diagnosis. Lastly, it is essential to note the absence of nuclear monstrosities and atypical mitoses. The mitoses are of normal appearance and few in number.

Electron microscope studies [Steiner 1974] have confirmed the fibroblastic nature of the cells, including some loaded with haemosiderin pigment and droplets of fatty acids. Ultrastructural study does not explain the presence of osteoclastic cells which resemble those in giant-cell tumours but all their margins are smooth and no "brush border" can be demonstrated.

Diagnosis

The radiological features usually suffice to make the diagnosis and prevent unnecessary surgery. A small well-defined lacuna or, better, several lacunae may suggest a cartilaginous lesion. However, if the diagnosis is uncertain, a biopsy will remove any doubts.

Some fibrous defects rich in giant cells may simulate a giant-cell tumour (though this will hardly be compatible with the radiographic appearances). Giant-cell tumour is virtually non-existent before the age of 15 and rare before 20 and its background is totally different, made up of ovoid cells and not of bundles of fusiform cells (cf Chapter 21).

In fibrous dysplasia, the cells are fusiform, short and slender, and the matrix relatively abundant. Elaboration of cartilaginous areas and specially of bony strands is the rule.

In the radiographs, confusion is possible with a lesion of the tendon attachments, but the histological appearance is quite different. Some osteoclasts in contact with bony fragments in course of necrosis and a fibro-fatty marrow should not produce confusion with adolescent fibrous defect (cf Chapter 40).

Following a fracture and during consolidation, the radiographs may show the development of a small rounded translucent lytic cortical image, usually nonmetaphyseal. This has been variously explained by absorption of a subperiosteal haematoma or, more likely, as the imaging seems to demonstrate, as an adipose medullary inclusion. The course is towards absorption of this fatty inclusion, which becomes undetectable only 3-4 weeks after the fracture in adolescents followed by regular radiography. The rarity of such a lesion must be borne in mind and, if it is biopsied, its difference from a fibrous defect is evident (cf Chapter 29).

The most important differential diagnosis is from a fusiform-cell sarcoma of intracortical onset. The complete absence of cytological anomalies, the rarity of mitoses and the absence of abnormal mitoses militate against this diagnosis.

Special problems

This pseudo-tumour raises unresolved problems. Ritschk et al (1988) note that it often arises at a zone of attachment of muscle tendons or ligaments. This may be interesting, but throws no light on its true origin, for which a vascular anomaly has been suggested. Its course, during which the fibrous defect increases, develops, and is then enclosed in a sclerotic wall is unusual; its disappearance without apparent reason and without leaving traces is remarkable. However, it may not disappear but may extend, producing the non-ossifying fibroma. One wonders about the significance of the giant cells of osteoclastic appearance, sometimes numerous, which are seen far from any histologically identifiable bony contact.

If the fibrous defect is left untreated, its sometimes atypical appearance, extension, and major complication by fracture, may all lead to a surgical approach to this "failure" of ossification.

Non-ossifying fibroma

From the clinical viewpoint it seems reasonable to reserve the term of fibroma for extensive lesions which considerably weaken the bone in which they develop and therefore call for surgical intervention. In 23 pathological fractures associated with this condition, treated at the Mayo Clinic [Arata et al 1981], 10 were located at the lower end of the tibia. The fibroma occupied over 50% of the transverse plane in the frontal and lateral films. The mean age of the patients at the time of fracture was 12 years; whereas the maximum incidence of fibroblastic sarcoma is around the 4th and 5th decades.

Histologically, this lesion cannot be distinguished from the cortico-metaphyseal fibrous defect. The absence of cellular anomalies and the well-defined boundaries of the lesion exclude the diagnosis of fibrosarcoma.

The histogenesis of these fibromas, large but benign lesions, is as unknown as is that of the cortical defects.

Multiple non-ossifying fibromas

The histological appearance is no different from that of solitary fibroma. Fusiform cells grouped in bundles, foamy histiocytes and giant cells are the fundamental components; the foamy and giant cells vary greatly in amount.

The histological problems raised are those accompanying fibromas: the lesions must be distinguished from fibrous dysplasia, giant-cell tumour, and certain lesions of neurofibromatosis. But one of the more important questions is whether or not to link them to pathological conditions whose manifestations are primarily clinical, including fibromas or fibroxanthomas with no pathological associations, the familial multiple fibromatosis of Evans and Park (1978) and of Blau and Zwick (1988), the latter being a radioclinical entity with dominant transmission, and the fibromas associated with Gardner's syndrome.

Three entities cause real difficulty: fibrous dysplasia and Albright's syndrome, neurofibromatosis in its well-individualised form, with the presence of intraosseous neurofibromas (cf Chapter 41), and multiple fibromatosis of infancy associated with muscular tumours which are very firm and whose number, site and size are very variable [Maroteaux 1982].

Benign fibrous histiocytoma (histiocytoxanthoma, fibrohistiocyto-xanthoma, also non-osteogenic fibroma, non-ossifying fibroma) (figs. 7, 8, 12)

Histologically, both benign fibrous histiocytoma and non-osteogenic fibroma consist of cells of fibroblastic and histiocytic appearance, areas of foamy cells and multinucleate giant cells; the fusiform cells are grouped in bundles arranged in a braided overlapping pattern. Based on this histological resemblance, two views may be taken.

The first recognises that the multiple terms employed, particularly "fibrous histiocytoma" and "non-osteogenic fibroma" cover a single entity.

The second, while admitting the histological resemblance, argues that the clinical picture encourages a distinction between the two entities [Clarke et al 1985]. The arguments are that non-ossifying fibroma or cortico-metaphyseal defect develops in children and adolescents and benign fibrous histiocytoma is more often diagnosed in adults; that non-ossifying fibroma is essentially metaphyseal and fibrous histiocytoma develops in any bone in the skeleton (iliac bones, ribs, vertebrae and long bones, where it is usually metaphyseo-epiphyseal). It is also true that non-ossifying fibroma is often a chance radiological discovery, that fibrous histiocytoma is more likely to present with pain, that the course of cortico-metaphyseal defect is quite often to spontaneous regression and that fibrous histiocytoma may recur after curettage.

In this context, fibrous histiocytoma is the benign tumour as opposed to the malignant fibrous histiocytoma, first described in the soft tissues and later in bone. Fibrous defect and non-ossifying fibroma are non-tumour dysplasias.

In conclusion, the term "fibrohistiocytic proliferation" covers the generality of these formations, just as "histiocytosis X" covers well-differentiated radiological and clinical entities. Let us recall once more that, to judge from the publications I have been able to read, the distinction between these diverse entities - cortico-metaphyseal fibrous defect, non-ossifying fibroma, benign fibrous histiocytoma and their varying labels - is based in a large part on their radiological and clinical appearances.

References

Cortico-metaphyseal fibrous defect

Arata MA, Peterson HA, Dahlin DC (1981) Pathological fractures through non-ossifying fibromas. Review of the Mayo Clinic experience. J Bone Joint Surg 63A: 980-988

Brower AC, Culver JE, Keats TE (1971) Histological nature of the cortical irregularity of the medial posterior distal femoral metaphysis in children. Radiology 99: 389-392

Hatcher H (1945) The pathogenesis of localized fibrous lesions in the metaphyses of long bones. Am J Surg 122: 1016-1030

Malghem J, Maldague B (1986) Transient fatty cortical defects following fractures in children. Skeletal Radiol 15: 368-371

Maroteaux P (1982) Maladies osseuses de l'enfant. Flammarion, p. 124

Morton KS (1964) Bone production in non-osteogenic fibroma. An attempt to clarify nomenclature in fibrous lesions of bone. J Bone Joint Surg 46B: 233-243

Nezelof C, Faure C, Huc M, Guy E, Errera A (1956) Les lacunes corticales fibreuses des os longs des enfants et des adolescents. Arch Anat Path 4: 1451-1458

Ritschk P, Hajek PC, Pechmann U (1989) Fibrous metaphyscal defects. Magnetic resonance imaging appearances. Skeletal Radiol 18: 253-259

Ritschk P, Karnel F, Hajek PC (1988) Fibrous metaphyseal defects; determination of their origin and natural history using a radiomorphological study. Skeletal Radiol 17: 8-15

Sontag LW, Pyle Sl (1941) The appearance and nature of cyst like areas in the distal femoral metaphyses of children. Amer J Roentg 46: 185-188

Steiner GC (1974) Fibrous cortical defect and nonossifying fibroma of bone. A study of ultrastructure. Arch Pathol 97: 205-210

Wellinger CL, Mazabraud A (1962) Les lacunes cortico-métaphysaires fibreuses des enfants et des adolescents. Ouest Med 9: 449-456

Benign fibrous histiocytoma

Bertoni F, Unni KK, McLeod RA, Sim FH (1988) Xanthoma of bone. Am J Clin Pathol 90: 377-384

Clarke BE, Xipell JM, Thomas DP (1985) Bening fibrous histocytoma of bone. Am J Surg Pathol 9, 11: 806-815

Destouet JM, Kyriakos M, Gilula LA (1980) Fibrous histiocytoma (fibroxanthoma) of a cervical vertebra. A report with a review of the literature. Skeletal Radiol 5: 241-246

Herman G, Steiner GC, Sherry HH (1988) Benign fibrous histiocytoma (BFH). Skeletal Radiol 17: 195-197

Houke MME, Razmon JP, Leclair HP (1961) A propos de deux nouvelles observations de xanthome solitaire de l'os. Lille Chir XVI: 177-194

Matsuno T (1990) Benign fibrous histiocytoma involving the ends of long bone. Skeletal Radiol 19: 561-566

Moser RP, Sweet DE, Haseman DB, Madewell JE (1987) Multiple skeletal fibroxanthomas: radiologic-pathologic correlation of 72 cases. Skeletal Radiol 16: 353-359

Roessner A, Immenkamp M, Weidner A, Hobik HP, Grundmann E (1981) Benign fibrous histiocytoma of bone. Light and electron-microscopic observations. J Cancer Res Oncol 101: 192-202

Non-ossifying fibroma

Blau RA, Zwick DL (1988) Multiple non-ossifying fibromas. A case report. J Bone Joint Surg 70: 299-304

Campanacci M, Laus M, Boriani S (1983) Multiple non-ossifying fibromata with extraskeletal anomalies: a new syndrome? J Bone Joint Surg 65B: 627-632

Evans GA, Park WM (1978) Familial multiple non-osteogenic fibromata. J Bone Joint Surg 60B: 416-419

Gross ML, Soberman N, Dorfman HD, Seimon LP (1989) Multiple non-ossifying fibromas of long bones in a patient with neurofibromatosis. Skeletal Radiol 18: 389-391

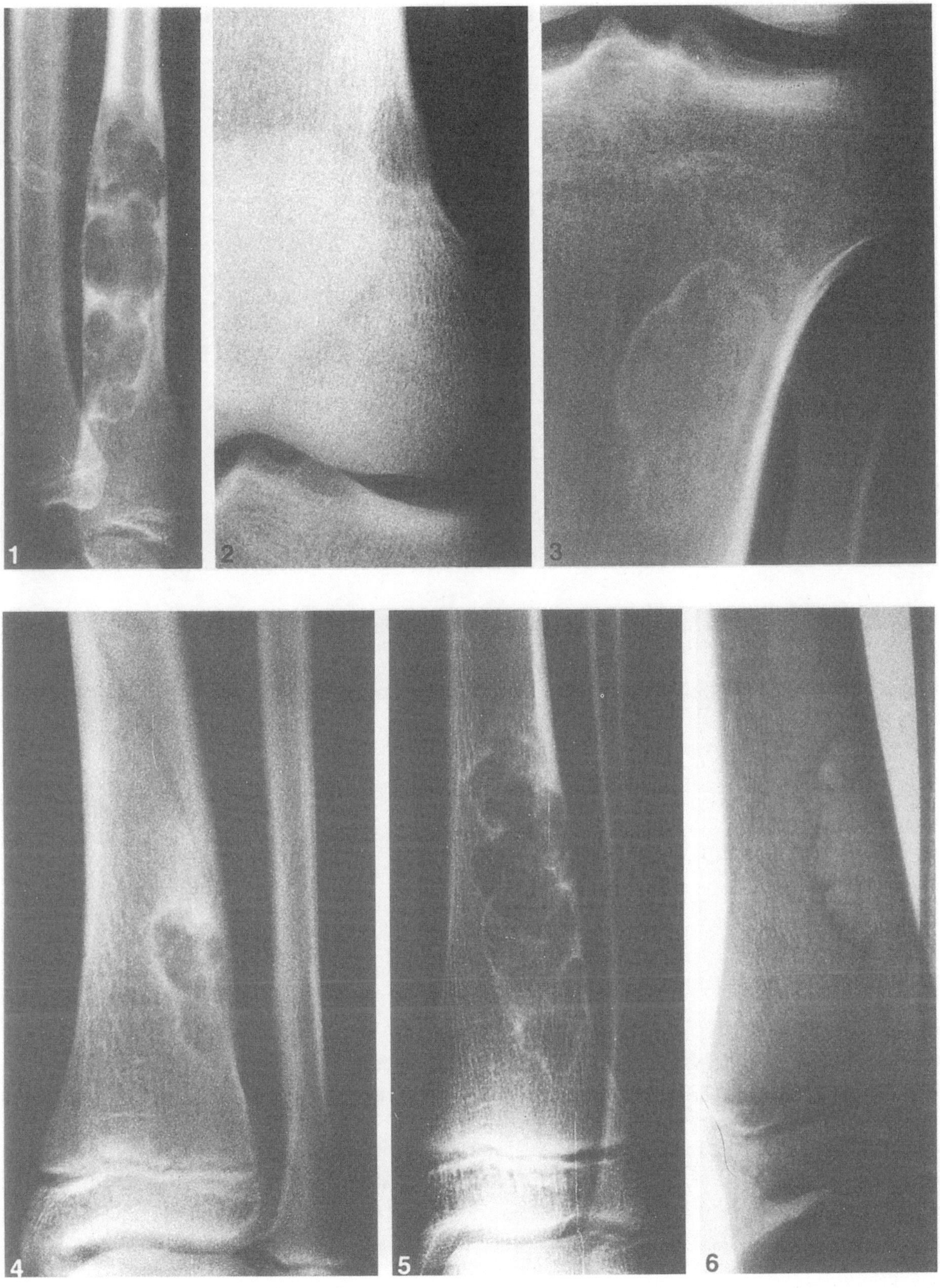

See legends next page

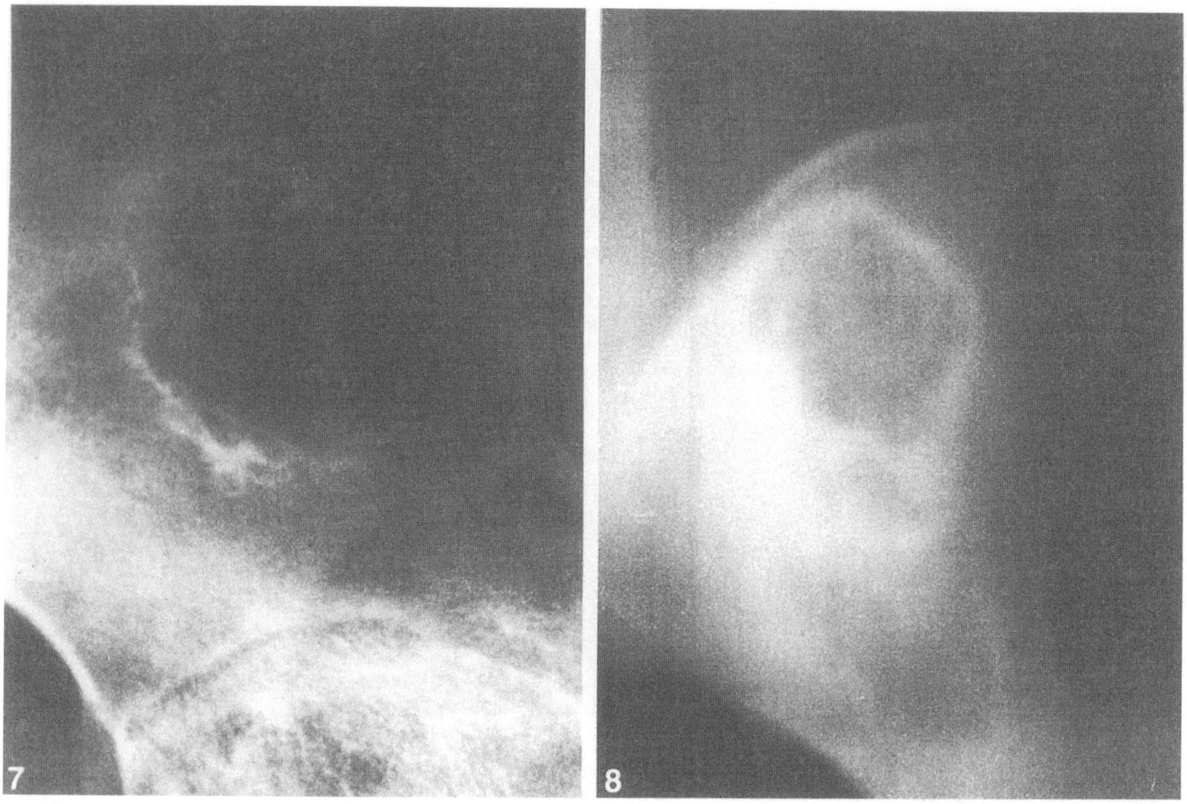

Figs. 7, 8. Non-ossifying fibromas, or rather benign fibrous histiocytomas, of iliac wing, well defined by a fine sclerotic scalloped border

←

Fig. 1. Non-ossifying fibroma: polycystic image and swelling of lower third of radius. Adolescent boy of 14

Fig. 2. Cortico-metaphyseal fibrous defect: cavity hollowed out in posteromedial cortex of femur, surrounded by fine osteosclerotic border. Adolescent boy of 17

Fig. 3. Non-ossifying fibroma with sharp polycyclic outlines in upper metaphysis of tibia. Man of 24

Fig. 4. Non-ossifying fibroma of tibia presenting with pathological fracture. Boy of 15

Fig. 5. Non-ossifying fibroma with multilocular outlines in lower third of tibia. Boy of 14

Fig. 6. Characteristic appearance of cortico-metaphyseal defect of lower metaphysis of tibia: well-demarcated polycyclic outline

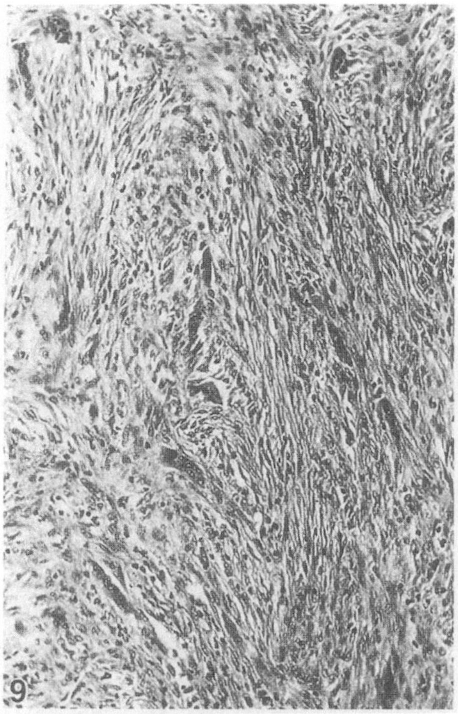

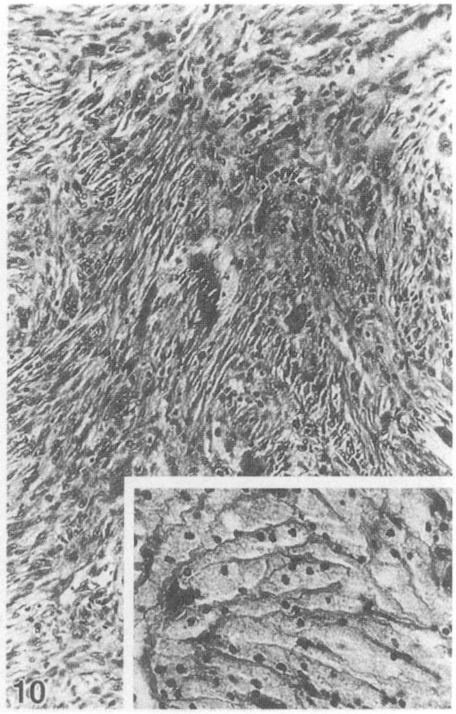

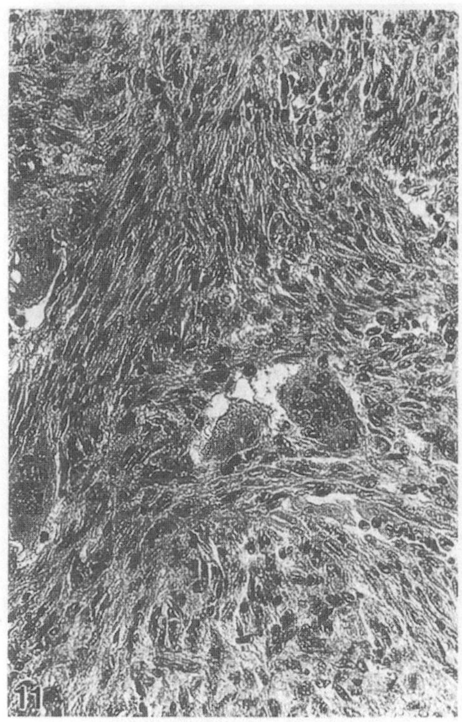

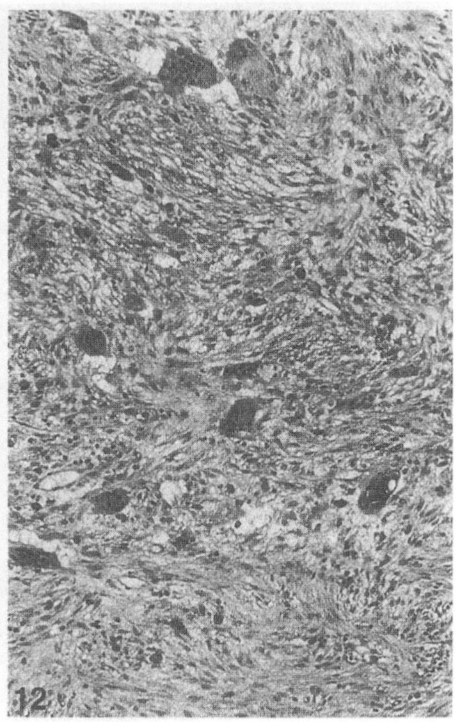

Fig. 9. Cortico-metaphyseal fibrous defect: bundles of fusiform cells with irregularly distributed multinucleate giant cells

Fig. 10. Same case, islands of foamy histiocytes, large clear cells with small round, central, very chromophil nuclei. These xanthelasmic cells are a virtually constant feature of fibrous defects

Fig. 11. Some giant cells break the monotony of the fusiform areas

Fig. 12. Benign fibrous histiocytoma of iliac wing (fig. 7). Inflammatory cells and intermingled braided bundles of fusiform cells. Woman of 41. (Courtesy of Prof. Payen, Poitiers)

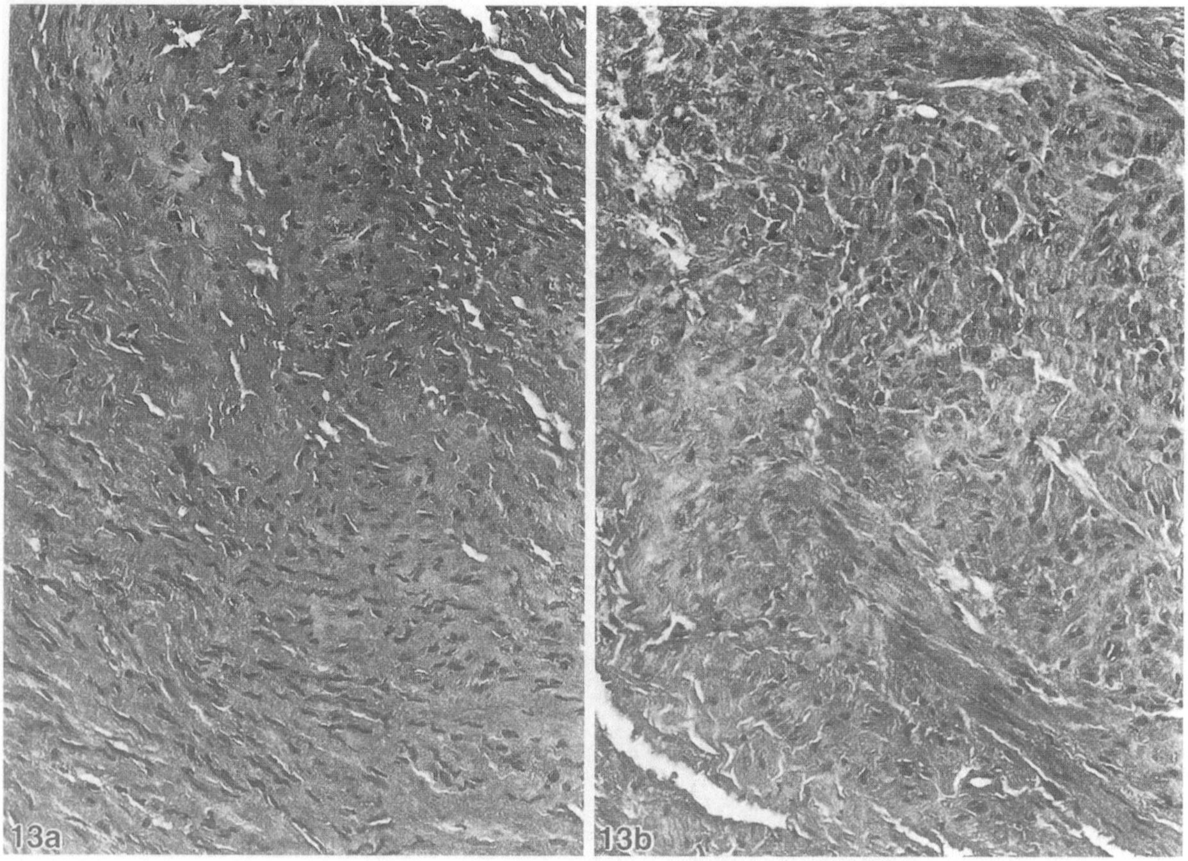

Fig. 13 a, b. Multiple fibromas in woman of 40, apparently with no other pathological lesions. In this case the very abundant collagen gives a desmoid appearance in places

13. Xanthoma

Solitary xanthoma of bone is a rare lesion and probably the progressive form of a preexisting lesion(non-ossifying fibroma, giant-cell tumour, aneurysmal cyst, fibrous dysplasia, simple cyst).

General considerations

Only 21 cases were collected at the Mayo Clinic between 1919 and 1986 [Bertoni et al 1986]. In this series men were twice as numerous as women and the ages ranged between 7 and 60 years. It seems that any bone may be affected: the flat bones of the limb-girdles and skull but also the limb bones.

Clinical features and course

The commonest presenting feature is pain, 61% in the Mayo Clinic statistics, rarely a pathological fracture. The lesion may be asymptomatic and discovered by chance, for instance in a radiograph performed for injury.

The course of this benign lesion is towards healing following simple curettage, supplemented by grafting if the xanthoma is very large, as in one of the cases reported by Houcke et al (1961).

Imaging

The radiological appearances may suggest a benign tumour or pseudo-tumour (fig. 1), but the irregular outline may sometimes suggest a diagnosis of malignancy including lymphoma and plasmocytoma.

Pathological anatomy and histopathology

On macroscopic examination the lesion is embedded in a bony cavity with sclerotic margins. The xanthoma consists of soft tissue of a rusty yellowish colour. It may be cystic and the cavity may then contain an amber or even haemorrhagic fluid. The lesion may also be partitioned by fibrous septa.

The histological appearance is characteristic. The bony tissue is replaced by a proliferation of foamy cells associated with clumps of cholesterol crystals (figs. 3, 4). In places, giant cells (fig. 4a) are adherent to the crystals, actually to the crystalline casts of fatty acids dissolved during the preparation.

Diagnosis

When the primary lesion, whether tumour or pseudo-tumour, is identifiable, and the xanthoma occupies only part of the sample removed, it is the denomination of the primary lesion that should be applied. It is more logical to make a diagnosis of fibroma with zones of xanthelasma rather than that of fibroxanthoma since while fibroma may be regarded as a tumour, xanthoma cannot. However, it is important to report the presence of giant cells [Schajowicz 1981] which argue in favor of a benign course. Thus it is only in cases where the primary lesion is not identifiable that the diagnosis of xanthoma is legitimate.

The bony lesions are often multiple, a manifestation of hyperlipoproteinaemia, often associated with tendinous sites (particularly the Achilles tendon); the diagnosis is usually made before biopsy from the clinical features and the laboratory tests. Actually, bony involvement in the hyperlipidaemias is much rarer than involvement of the viscera, skin and tendons [Hamilton et al 1975].

A combination of unfavourable circumstances may lead to the biopsy suggesting a bony lesion of the sinus histiocytosis of Destombes, Dorfman and Rosaï, a metastasis from a clear-cell cancer, or the multiple systemic granulomatosis of Erdheim-Chester, a bony lesion associated with a storage disease.

References

Bertoni F, Unni kk, McLeod RA, Sim FH (1988) Xanthoma of bone. Am J Clin Pathol 90: 377-384

Blostein SH, Caldwell D, Carter DM (1985) Bone lesions in xanthoma disseminatum. Arch Dermatol 121: 1313- 1317

Hamilton WC, Ramsey PL, Hanson SM, Schiff DC (1975) Osseous xanthoma and multiple hand tumors as a complaction of hyperlipidemia. J Bone Joint Surg 57A: 551-553

Houcke E, Razemon JP, Leclair HP (1961) A propos de deux nouvelles observations de xanthome solitaire de l'os. Lille Chirurgical XVI: 187-194

Schajowicz F (1981) Tumors and tumorlike lesions of bone and joints. Springer-Verlag, New York, Heidelberg, Berlin

Yokoyama K, Shinohara N, Wada K (1988) Osseous xanthomatosis and a pathologic fracture in a patient with hyperlipidemia. A case report. Clin Orthop 236: 307-310

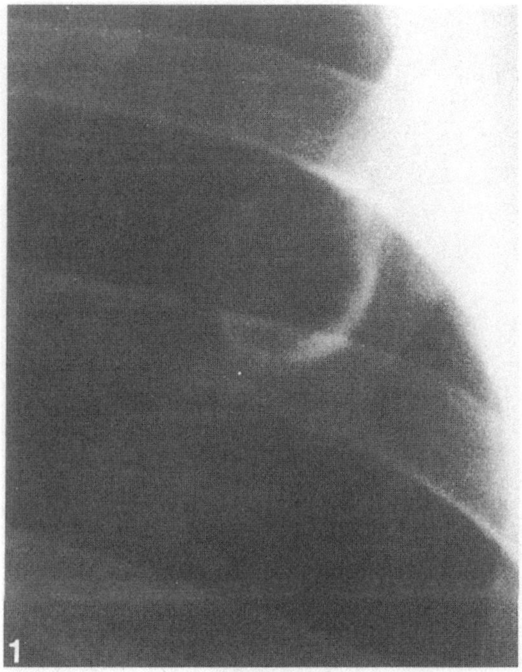

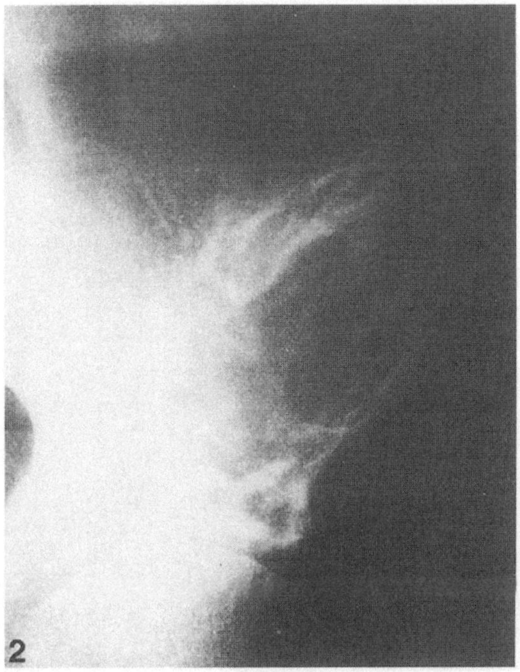

Fig. 1. Xanthoma of rib in a man of 47. A round image enclosed in a sclerotic margin

Fig. 2. Xanthoma of ilium, ill-defined lesion of irregular "density"

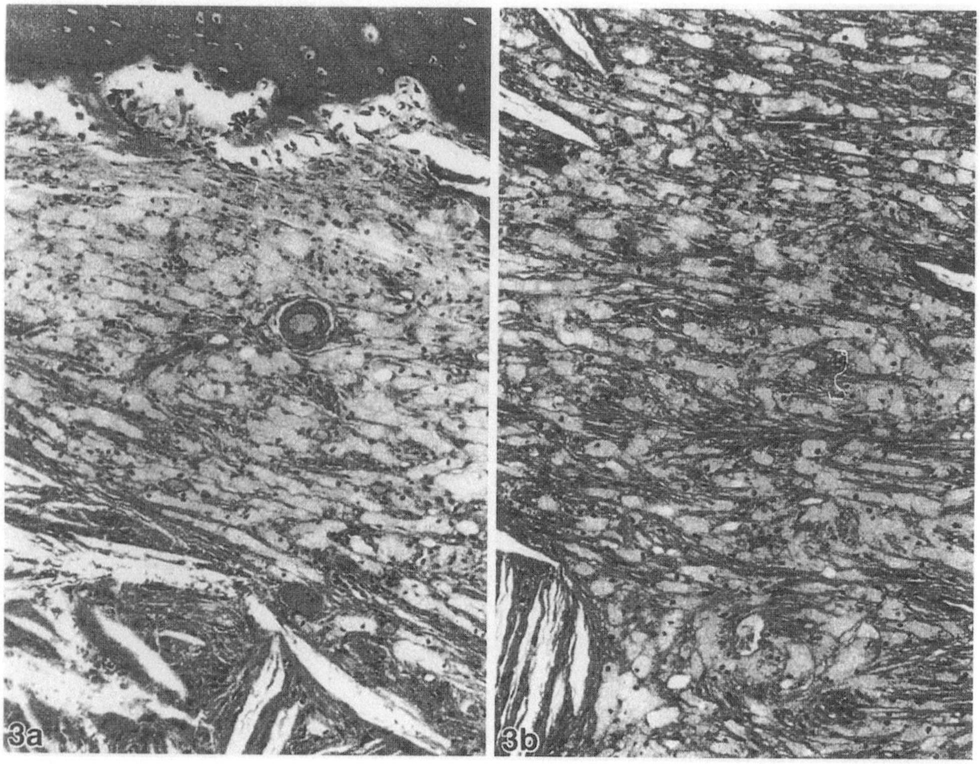

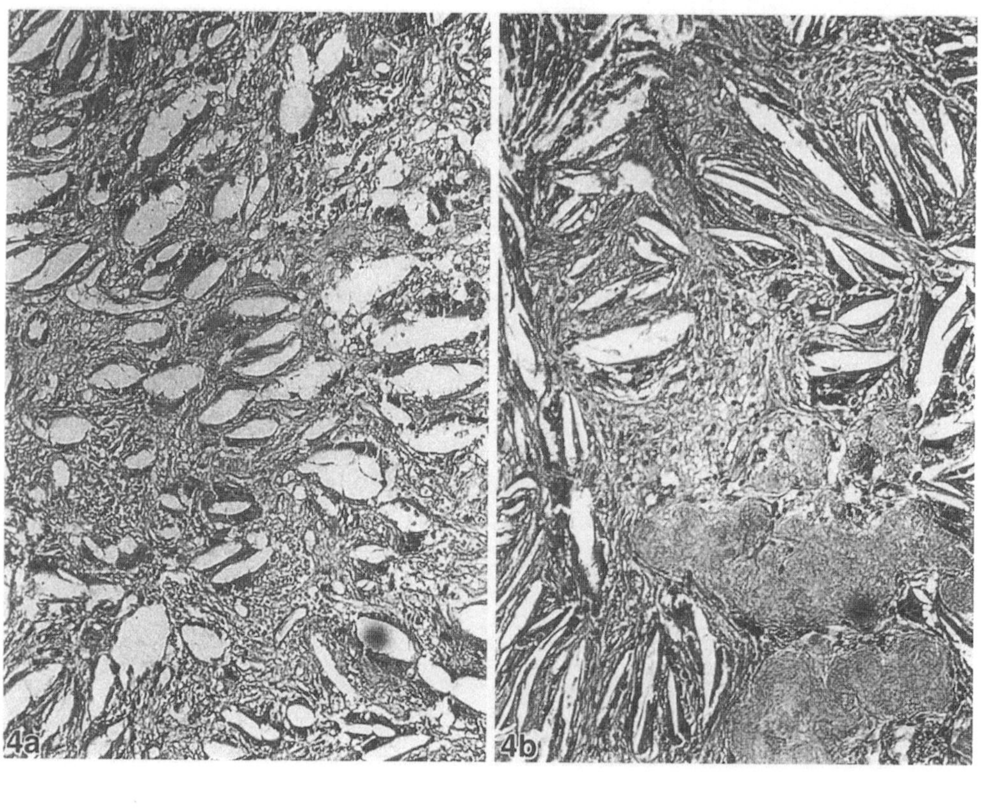

Fig. 3 a, b. Large histiocytic areas surround numerous crystalline casts. In the microphotograph (**a**), transverse section of thick-walled vessel. **b** Presence of some lymphocytes in the histiocytic zones

Fig. 4 a, b. Content of a "cyst" of the fibular malleolus. **a** The tissue contains numerous crystalline casts with adherent giant cells. **b** In the lower third, scrolled casts as observed in the wall of numerous cysts and whose histological appearance is either ordinary collagen or osteoid

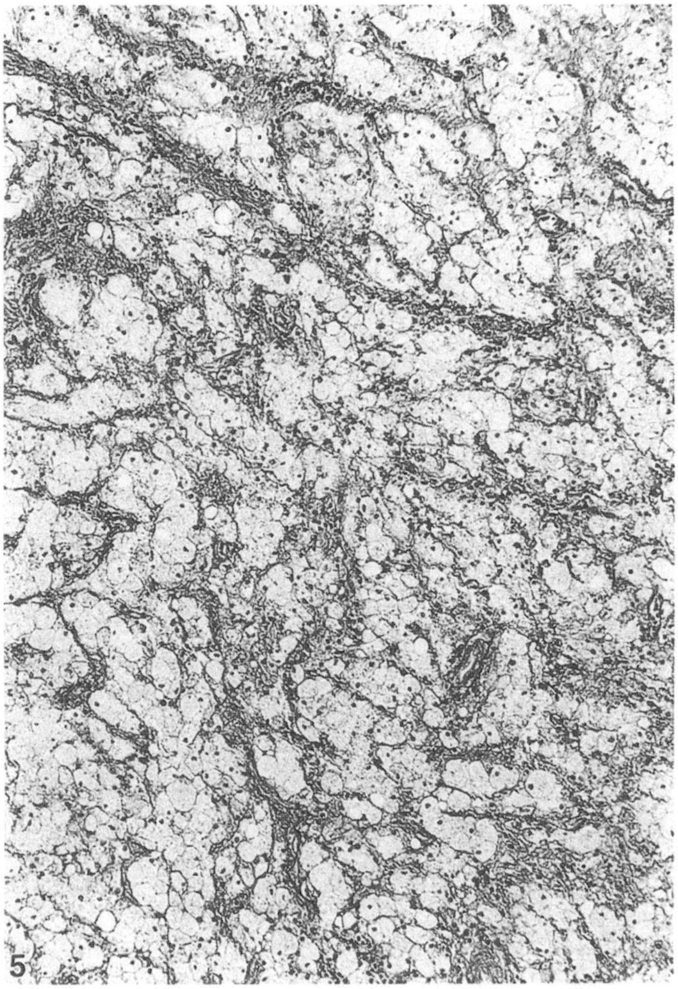

Fig. 5. Cystic lesion of ilium. The proliferation of foamy histiocytes is intersected by a fine connective-vascular network

14. Desmoid fibroma

This tumour was defined by Jaffe in 1958. The essential problem confronted by the pathologist is that of distinguishing it from a fibroblastic sarcoma of low grade malignancy. However, whether central or periosteal, it is a tumour which several recent publications have shown to possess an aggressive nature.

General considerations

This is a rare tumour; less than 100 cases have been reported. It affects both sexes, apparently equally or with a slight masculine predominance. Its age distribution is very extensive. It has been reported in very young children, but its maximum incidence is in the 2nd and 3rd decades; 74% of the 27 Mayo Clinic cases [Inward et al 1991] were in the 3rd decade. Of the 18 cases reported by Taconis et al (1994), two were under 15. The ultrastructural study of Lagacé et al (1979) was of three patients aged 3, 9 and 13 years.

The chief sites are the long bones of the limbs, but the flat bones of the limb-girdles, clavicles, mandible and even certain tarsal bones may be affected. In the long bones the lesion is usually deep-seated in the metaphysis or diaphysis, but it may be superficial in the cortex. In fact, virtually any bone may be affected, including the vertebrae, raising problems of radiological differentiation from a chordoma [Sammy et al 1992].

Clinical features and course

The tumour presents with mild pain which has often been present for over a year before the patient attends. More rarely, attention is attracted by swelling or fracture. In certain sites the tumour develops following a local injury.

The spontaneous course is slow, and as it is asymptomatic for so long the tumour may attain a considerable size before being diagnosed. Such cases may lead to a wide resection requiring reconstruction by prosthesis, as in the case reported by Thirupathi et al (1983). The desmoid fibroma of the shoulder examined by our colleague Dr Pastricot [cf Nourissat et al 1989] is one of the rare reported cases of a lethal course with pulmonary metastases.

Imaging

From the radiographic aspect (figs. 1-3), this is usually a lytic expanding metaphyseal tumour [Young et al 1988] which may invade the soft tissues after having destroyed the cortex, well shown by imaging. Often, however, there are sharp boundaries and more rarely a transitional zone [Lichtman et al 1985].

Pathological anatomy and histopathology

In resection specimens the tumour is firm, whitish, fasciculated and occupies the central part of the bone, eroding the cortex to a varying degree. Its boundaries are definite but irregular. In the flat bones or when juxtacortical the tumour volume in the soft tissues is often greater than its intraosseous portion.

In histological sections, the tumour tissue consists of bundles of thick collagen fibers and slender fusiform cells layered between the collagen fibers (fig. 4 a, b).

Table 1. Differential diagnosis

	Cell anomalies	Collagen character	Invasive
Non-ossifying fibroma	o	+	+
Desmoid fibroma	o	+++	++
Fibrosarcoma of low-grade malignancy	+	++	++

Pitfall: to report a desmoid fibroma in a genuine tumour from a relatively superficial sample. Examination of the specimen will show the central part of the tumour to be a fibroblastic sarcoma of low-grade but indisputable malignancy.
The pathologist can only describe what he sees

The fusiform nuclei are sometimes very chromophil (fig. 5 a, b), sometimes pale. Mitoses are very rare and there are no atypical mitoses or cell monstrosities. Overall, cellularity is sparse. At the microscopic level, the boundaries of the lesion are imprecise; at its periphery, the tumour infiltrates the medullary spaces. To sum up, this is the appearance of a fibroma with few cells whose collagen density resembles that of a tendon (desmoid) and whose cells are rare, slender and quiescent, without chondrogenesis or osteogenesis, but with the possible persistence at the periphery of some bone spicules undergoing necrosis.(fig. 6 a, b). More rarely, there is an oedematous state which separates the collagen fibers (fig. 7a).

Ultrastructural examination shows that the tumour is composed of myofibroblasts and primitive mesenchymal cells [Lagacé et al 1979]. The relative abundance of fibroblasts and myofibroblasts varies with the tumour studied, possibly in relation to its evolutional stage [Jouvin et al 1984]. In a lesion at the lower end of the ulna, reported by Thirupathi et al (1983) the authors noted a greater content of myofibroblasts towards the center of the tumour.

Differential diagnosis

The diagnosis of desmoid fibroma is based on the clinical, radiological and pathological anatomy findings, but in terms of the histology it may have to be distinguished from a genuinely malignant fibroblastic tumour.

The following circumstances may give rise to particular problems.

When a biopsy is from a peripheral part of a fibroblastic sarcoma, it may contain only collagen-rich tissue, suggestive of a desmoid fibroma. The diagnosis of desmoid fibroma from a tumour biopsy known to be very peripheral is worthless. The right course is to request a deeper and more central biopsy.

Other difficulties may arise from a fibroblastic sarcoma of low grade malignancy. The solution rests with scrupulous observation of numerous sections in the search for cell anomalies including fibroblasts with large hyperchromatic nuclei and abnormal mitoses.

A fusiform-cell intramedullary sarcoma of low malignancy may be difficult to identify, but the poorly demarcated nature of the tumour, its much greater cellularity and some cytonuclear anomalies invalidate the diagnosis of desmoid fibroma. However, it must be realised that cytonuclear anomalies are rare, that the progress of this tumour is slow, and that it may be confused with fibrous dysplasia. Fibrous dysplasia itself consists of small cells dispersed in a fibrillary matrix but here and there some islands of chondroid tissue and especially of metaplastic bone stand out against this fibrillary background. Further, in most of cases the appearances on imaging are markedly different.

In non-ossifying fibroma, which is more a histiocytofibroma than a fibroma, the mass consists of intermingled collagen and cellular bundles. Some xanthomatous areas and giant cells usually complete the histological picture (cf Chapter 12). The diagnosis of non-ossifying fibroma carries the risk of a tendency to inadequate treatment, favouring recurrences [Gebhard et al 1985].

References

Dahlin DC, Unni KK (1986) Bone tumors. General aspects and data on 8542 cases, 4th edn. Charles Thomas, Springfield, p. 375

Gebhardt MC, Campbell CJ, Schiller AL, Mankin HJ (1985) Desmoplastic fibroma of bone. Report of eight cases and review of the literature. J Bone Joint Surg 67A: 732-746

Greenspan A, Unni KK (1993) Desmoplastic fibroma. Case report. Skeletal Radiol 22: 296-299

Hilimann JS, Mesgarzadeh M, Tang CK, Bonakdarpour A, Reyes TG (1988) Desmoplatic fibroma of the proximal end of the left femur. Skeletal Radiol 17: 356-360

Inwards CY, Unni KK, Beabout JW, Sim FH (1991) Desmoplastic fibroma of bone. Cancer 68: 1978-1983

Jaffe HL (1985) Tumors and tumorous conditions of the bones and joints. Lea & Febiger, Philadelphia, pp. 298-303

Jouvin MH, Tomeno B, Carlioz A, Forest M, Abelanet R (1984) Fibrome desmoïde osseux des os longs. Revue de la littérature et problèmes diagnostiques. A propos de deux observations dont une avec étude ultrastructurale. Sem Hop Paris 41: 2887-2892

Lagacé R, Delage C, Bouchard HL, Seemayer TA (1979) Desmoplastic fibroma of bone. An ultrastructural study. Am J Surg Pathol 3: 423-430

Lichtman EA, Klein MJ (1985) Desmoplastic fibroma of the proximal end of the left femur. Skeletal Radiol 13: 160-163

Meary R, Danan J, Tomeno B, Forest M, Cirotteaux (1978) Fibromes desmoïdes des membres. Rev Chir Orthop 64: 195-204

Nilsonne U, Gothlin G (1969) Desmoplastic fibroma of bone. Acta Orthop Scand 40: 205-215

Nourissat C, Patricot LM, Brunat-Mentigoy M, Tachon G Manoukian A (1989) Fibrome desmoïde de l'omoplate. Récidive avec métastases pulmonaires. Rev Chir Orthop 75: 569-572

Savy JM, Laredo JD, Prier A, Jagueux M, Apoil A, Kaplan G (1992) Desmoplastic fibroma. Skeletal Radiol 21: 388-391

Taconis WK, Schütte HE, Van der Heul RO (1994) Desmoplastic fibroma of bone: a report of 18 cases. Skeletal Radiol 23: 283-288

Thirupathi RG, Vuletin JC, Wadwa R, Ballah S (1983) Desmoplastic fibroma of the ulna. Clin Orthop 179: 231-238

Young JWR, Aisner SC, Levine AM, Resnik CS, Dorfman HD (1988) Computed tomagraphy desmoid tumors of bone: desmoplastic fibroma. Skeletal Radiol 17: 333-337

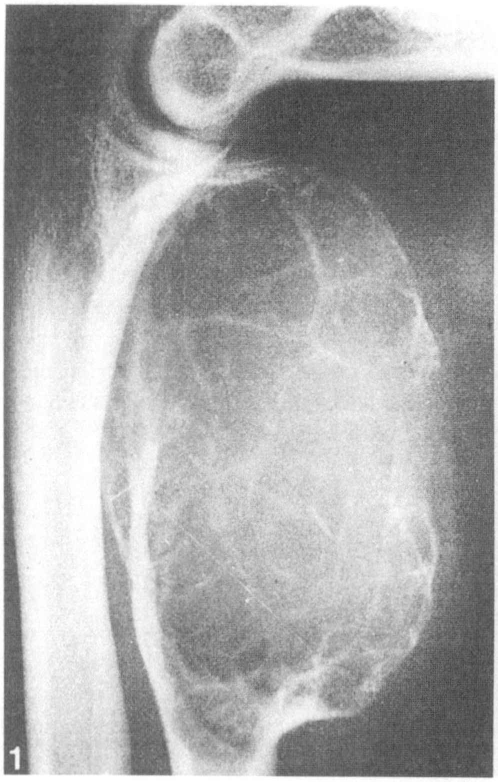

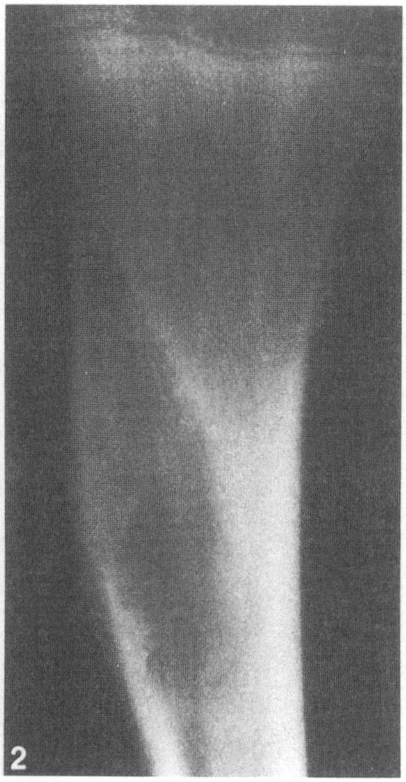

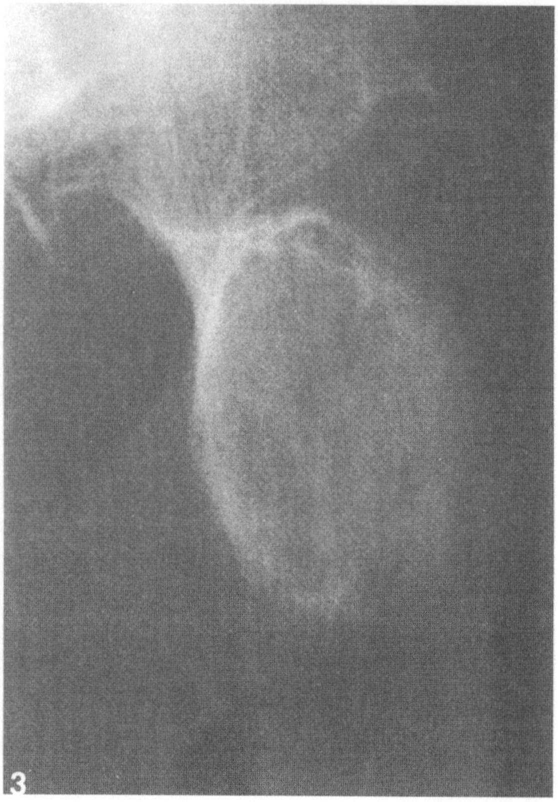

Fig. 1. Large desmoid fibroma of ulna in a boy of 17. The persistence of some bony ridges gives a false appearance of compartmentalisation of the tumour

Fig. 2. The tomogram of this slightly ballooned desmoid fibroma of the left tibia in a girl of 12 demonstrates a translucent image bounded by the cortex and sclerosed bone

Fig. 3. This intertrochanteric desmoid fibroma has developed in a man aged 68. It forms an ovoid, well-circumscribed mass with a boundary of dense bone

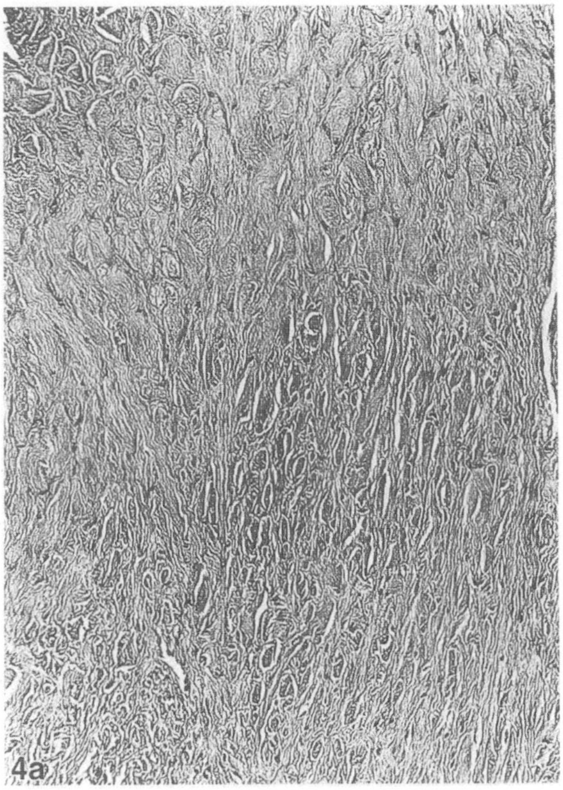

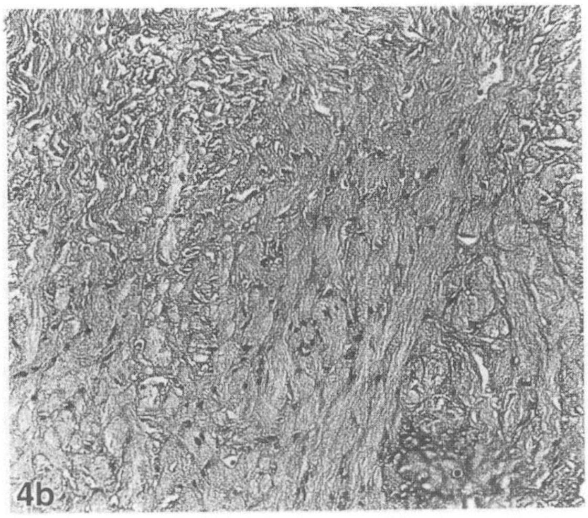

Fig. 4 a, b. The microphotographs at low and medium magnification show the uniform appearance of this tumour, with abundant collagen and few cells

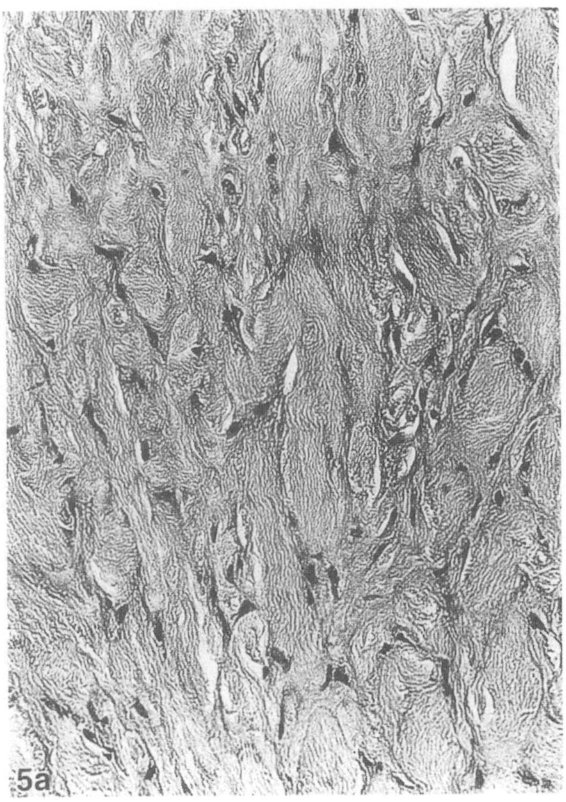

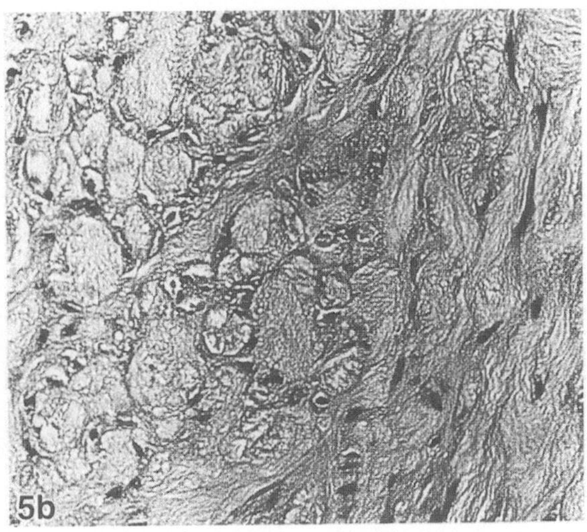

Fig. 5 a, b. At higher magnification, only the nuclei of the fibroblasts are visible between the bundles of collagen fibers; these nuclei are very chromophil, without monstrosities. The rare mitoses are difficult to detect in these cells, layered by production of collagen fibers

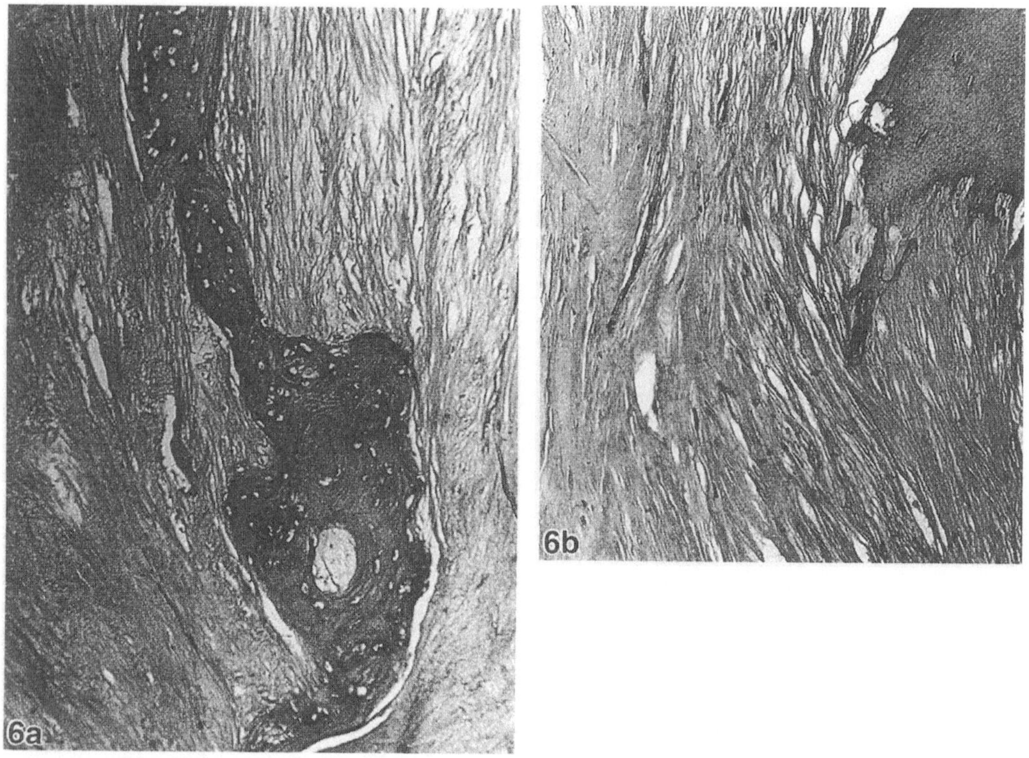

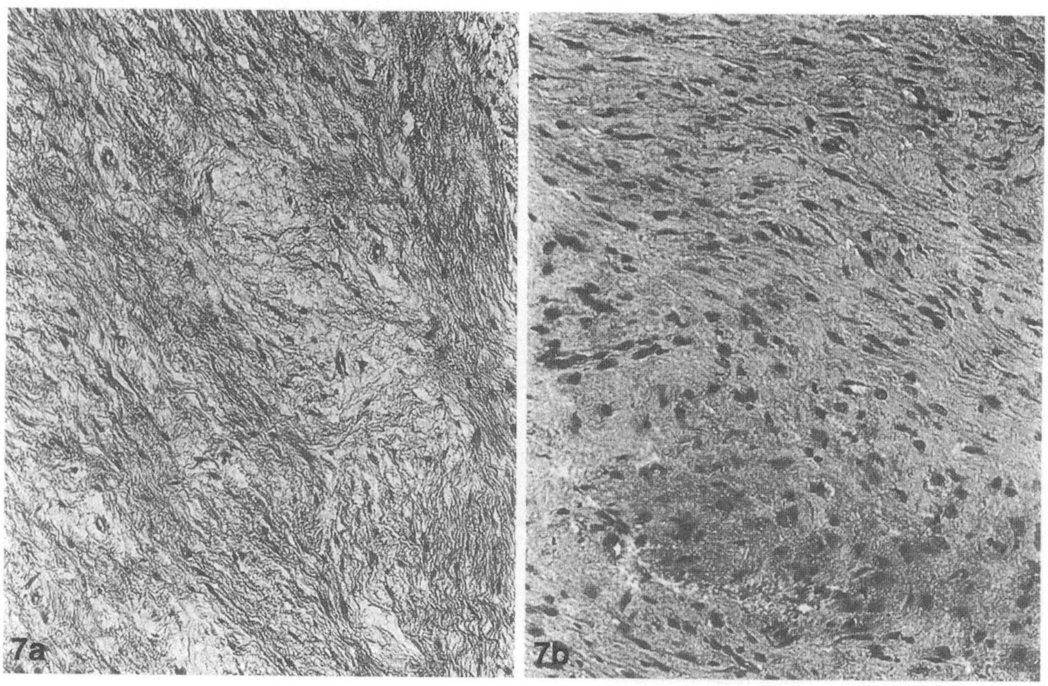

Fig. 6 a, b. In this desmoid fibroma of the femur, the regular orientation of the collagen fibers, arranged in parallel bundles, completely resembles the texture of a tendon. Some areas of lamellar bone belonging to the cortex can be seen in these microphotographs

Fig. 7 a, b. Two slightly different aspects of the same tumour (fig. 3). In the greater part of the sections, an oedematous condition slightly separates the fibers from one another (**a**). In the other zones, the fibroma is dense and traversed by rare vessels of very unequal diameter (**b**). The fibroblasts with very chromophil nuclei are sometimes sectioned parallel to their long axis and sometimes at right angles to this, depending on the orientation of the collagen fibers

15. Chondromyxoid fibroma

In the past this benign cartilaginous tumour was probably often confused with a chondrosarcoma before its definition by Jaffe and Lichtenstein in 1948. It is generally accepted that the tumour develops from the diaphyseal aspect of the cartilaginous growth plate.

Case history

J.M., aged 25, was referred to a treatment center for a tumour of the upper metaphysis of the right tibia. The history showed that the patient had complained of moderate pain which he located slightly below the knee-joint but whose onset was 15-16 months previously. There was no remarkable antecedent and in particular no history of injury. Comparison of both metaphyseal regions revealed slight vaulting of the right tibial metaphysis. In the standard radiograph, there was a translucent well-circumscribed image with hardly any border, measuring 2.5 cm in its main diameter.

The slow course of over a year, the minor symptomatology, the good demarcation of the clear lacuna and its metaphyseal position were the features leading to the consideration, among other possible diagnoses, of that of chondromyxoid fibroma.

General considerations

This is one of the rarest benign tumours of bone (less than 1% of the total in most series). Some statistics mention a male predominance, the lesion is seen at almost any age, but mainly in the 2nd or 3rd decade. Major review is given by Lefort (1996).

The tumour develops in the metaphyseal region of the long bones, its elective sites being the upper tibial and lower femoral metaphyses. When it becomes extensive, it is usually metaphyseo-epiphyseal. It is rarer in the short bones [Peeters 1974, Mitchell et al 1992] and the flat bones, though rare cases have been diagnosed in the bones of the skull and face. A case has even been reported in a sesamoid of the metatarsophalangeal joint of the great toe [Ribalta et al 1990].

Clinical features and course

The usual presenting feature is moderate pain, sometimes swelling, but many months or even years may elapse between the appearance of symptoms and the first consultation. The course is benign; cure is the rule after excision of the entire tumour. Curettage may be followed by recurrence [Rahimi et al 1972]. Dahlin (1956) reports a case of malignant transformation of a non-irradiated tumour several years after treatment.

Imaging

An osteolytic metaphyseal image, eccentric and ovoid, with its long axis parallel to that of the bone and surrounded by a fine sclerotic border, is the usual appearance of the tumour in the long bones of the limbs (figs. 1-4). When the tumour is large, it deforms the metaphysis and may breach the cortex [Turcotte et al 1962, Wilson et al 1991]. In the short and flat bones (fig. 5), the bone may appear ballooned by a lesion which sometimes occupies the whole of a phalanx, for example (fig. 7); in such cases, a pathological fracture, possibly the presenting feature, may be the source of diagnostic difficulties.

Table 1. Differential diagnosis

A trap: chondrosarcoma, especially if: - the patient is an adult male - the radiographic boundaries are less definite than usual - the biopsy contains only cartilaginous and myxoid tissue
The solution: normally, if it is a poorly differentiated sarcoma, atypical cells will be evident. If doubt persists, a second biopsy should be requested

Pathological anatomy and histopathology

The most characteristic macroscopic feature is the lobulation of this tumour, embedded in a completely circumscribed bony cavity. On section it is often firm, fibrous and grayish; the cartilaginous component is variable [Schajowicz et al 1971, Zillmer & Dorfman 1989]. The sections include chondroid, fibrous and myxoid zones in very variable proportions. The lobular nature of the tumour is difficult to deduce from fragments removed by curettage. The medley of such different appearances of the matrix and cells, whose considerable polymorphism is necessarily related to their environment, renders formal portrayal of the lesion somewhat artificial. At low magnification some zones of great cell density may suggest the cellular areas of a chondroblastoma (figs. 8, 9).

The fibrous zones (fig. 10) are characterised by a proliferation of fusiform cells surrounded by saffron-staining collagen fibers.

When there is no sharp transition (fig. 15), the cells abound in an increasingly abundant hyaline or fibrohyaline matrix (fig. 11) while their shape undergoes change from polyhedral to stellate, the whole assuming a myxoid appearance (figs. 12, 13).

In other zones, in contrast, the transition between the tumour nodule and the internodular connective tissue is definite (fig. 16). In places the chondroid metamorphosis of the matrix keeps pace with the chondrocytic metamorphosis of the cells producing fibrochondroid areas in which the cells are very irregularly distributed. Rarely, small haematinophil islands suggest commencing calcification of the chondroid material (fig. 18).

In the myxoid and chondroid areas the presence of cells with a large nucleus is common and of no prognostic significance (fig. 10). Giant cells and macrophages containing haemosiderin are also seen, and the cell population is denser at the periphery of the lobules, between which the connective tissue is very vascular (fig. 17).

Silver impregnation reveals a rich reticulin network and staining with alcian blue is positive in the cartilaginous zones.

Some variants of this pattern should be recognised: there are cases where chondromyxoid fibromas are strewn with frankly calcified zones, at times even with osteoid or bony strands. Some tumours have the cystic appearance of aneurysmal cysts, others have "chondroblastomatous" zones and some may represent genuine transitional forms between chondroblastoma and chondromyxoid fibroma [Dahlin 1956].

Diagnosis

Diagnosis depends on recognition of the simultaneous fibrous, myxoid and cartilaginous nature of the lesion. The rarity of mitoses, the absence of necrosis despite some large-nucleated cells dispersed here and there in the cartilaginous and myxoid zones, are all in favor of a benign prognosis. But this triple pattern is also a trap if only a small sample is available, the more so if this is from a fine-needle biopsy, as the case of Iwata et al (1958).

The diagnosis of chondromyxoid fibroma is difficult, as evidenced by Kreicbergs et al (1985). Of 9 cases considered to be chondromyxoid fibromas from curettage material, a further examination of the sections confirmed only 2 cases. Six of the cases were classed as benign tumours and one proved to be a chondrosarcoma. The rarity of the tumour and the honesty of such reports arouses some reservations about series grouping hundreds of cases collected from the literature, as well as cases of atypical location.

In practice, the radiological image is often very suggestive. If in such cases a first biopsy demonstrates only fibrous and myxoid tissue further sections should be made and, when the specimen is excised, a further study will detect small foci of cartilaginous tissue. Too hasty a diagnosis of non-ossifying fibroma or myxoma will not then prove to have serious consequences.

The serious error is to make a diagnosis of chondrosarcoma. In a chondrosarcoma, which so poorly differentiated, cellular anomalies are evident and further, the boundaries between bone and tumour are much sharper in chondromyxoid fibroma.

In an intraosseous mesenchymal chondrosarcoma, the cell proliferation around the cartilaginous islands is represented by small irregular formations, markedly haematinophil and heaped together. The reticulin forms a network resembling that of haemangiopericytoma.

We have mentioned the possibility of a quasi-association of chondroblastoma and chondromyxoid fibroma and the possibility of cyst formation, which some - though this is not my own opinion - regard as a combination of the tumour with aneurysmal cyst (cf Chapters 5 and 30).

Lastly, bear in mind that the histological appearance of a recurrence of a previously curetted chondroblastoma is much more like that of a chondromyxoid fibroma than that of the initial chondroblastoma.

References

Dahlin DC (1956) Chondromyxoid fibroma of bone, with amphasis on its morphological relationship to benign chondroblastoma. Cancer 9: 195-203

Feldman F, Hecht HL, Johnston AD (1970) Chondromyxoid fibroma of bone. Radiol 94: 249-260

Iwata S, Coley BL (1958) Report of six cases of chondromyxoid fibroma of bone. Surg Gyneco Obst 107: 571-576

Jaffe HL, Lichtenstein L (1948) Chondromyxoid fibroma of bone: a distinctive benign tumor likely to be mistaken especially for chondrosarcoma. Arch Path 45: 541-551

Kreicbergs A, Lonnguist PA, Willems J (1985) Chondromyxoid fibroma. A review of the literature and a report on our own experience. Acta Path Microbiol Immunol Scand Seut 93A: 189-197

Lefort G (1996) Fibrome chondromyxoïde in: Les tumeurs osseuses bénignes de l'enfant. Sauramps Medical edn

Mitchell M, Sartoris DJ, Resnick D (1992) Chondromyxoid fibroma of the third metatarsal. Skeletal Radiol 21: 252-255

Peeters EG (1974) Chondrome fibro-myxoïde ou fibrome chondromyxoïde à propos de deux localisations phalangiennes. Med (Biologie) Environ mars-mai: 100-109

Rahimi A, Beabout JW, Ivins JC. Dahlin DC (1972) Chondromyxoid fibroma: a clinico-pathologic study of 76 cases. Cancer 30: 726-736

Ribalta T, Ro JY, Carrasco H, Heffelman C, Ayala AG (1990) Chondromyxoid fibroma of sesamoid bone. Case report. Skeletal Radiol 19: 549-551

Schajowicz F, Gallardo H (1971) Chondomyxoid fibroma (fibromyxoid chondroma) of bone. A clinico-pathological study of thirty-two cases. J Bone Joint Surg 53B: 198-216

Turcotte B, Pugh DG, Dahlin DC (1962) The roentgenologic aspects of chondromyxoid fibroma of bone. Am J Roentgenol 87: 1085-1095

Wilson AJ, Kyriakos M, Ackerman LV (1991) Chondromyxoid fibroma: radiographic appearance in 38 cases and in a review of the literature. Radiol 179: 513-518

Zillmer DA, Dorfman HD (1989) Chondromyxoid fibroma of bone. Thirty-six cases with clinico-pathologic correlation. Hum Pathol 20: 952-964

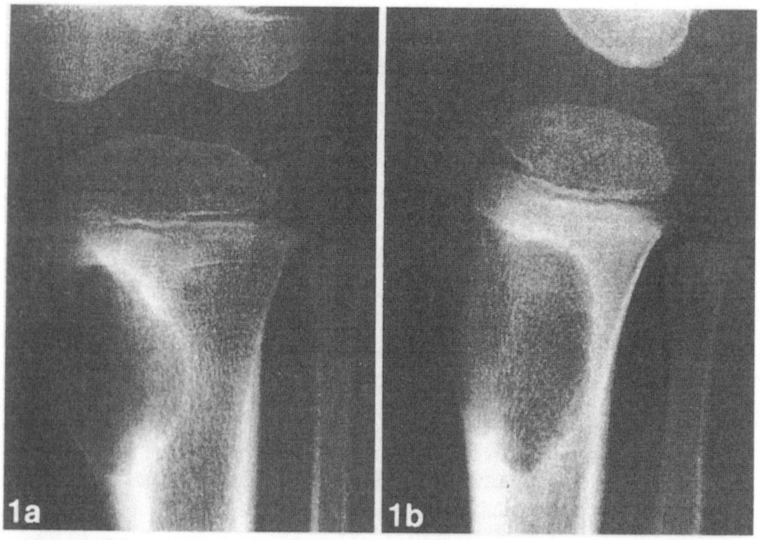

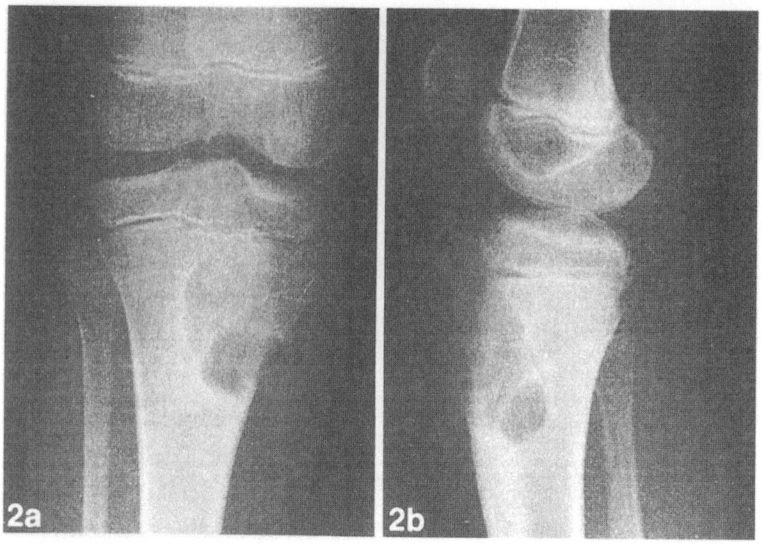

Fig. 1 a, b. The osteolysis of the upper metaphysis of the tibia in this chondromyxoid fibroma is bounded by a sclerotic border separating it from the adjacent bone. In the medial periosteal zone, the bone is slightly ballooned

Fig. 2 a, b. Lytic metaphyseal image of well-circumscribed lateralised osteolysis of chondromyxoid fibroma

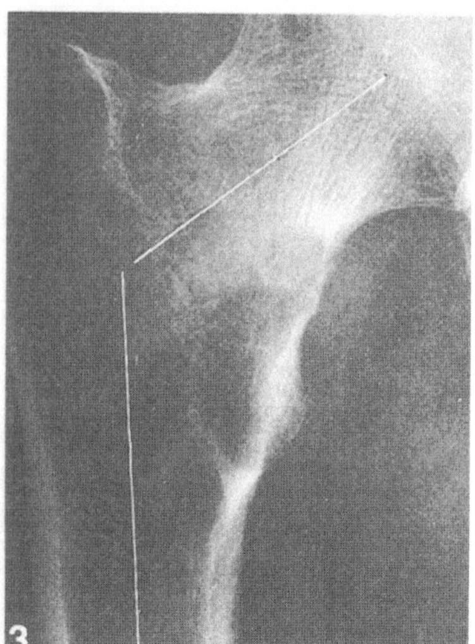

Fig. 3. Chondromyxoid fibroma in region of lesser trochanter. The boundary between tumour and spongy bone is somewhat less definite

→

Fig. 4. Tumour located at lower end of tibia in a young man of 15. The ovoid lesion is very well demarcated

Fig. 5. Chondromyxoid fibroma in woman of 57. Compartmental osteolysis of iliac wing, apparently benign. The osteolysis balloons the inner cortex

Fig. 6. Chondromyxoid fibroma of 5th rib in a woman of 28: ballooned appearance involving entire thickness of bone

Fig. 7. Enormous cavity with irregular outlines but bounded by a sclerotic border: chondromyxoid fibroma of terminal phalanx of great toe

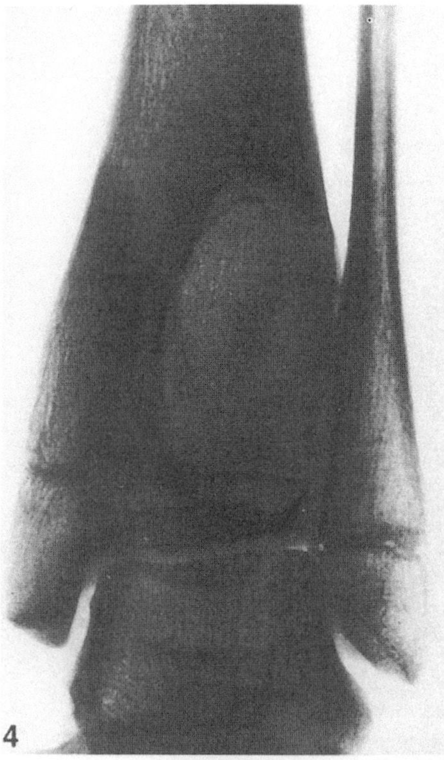
4

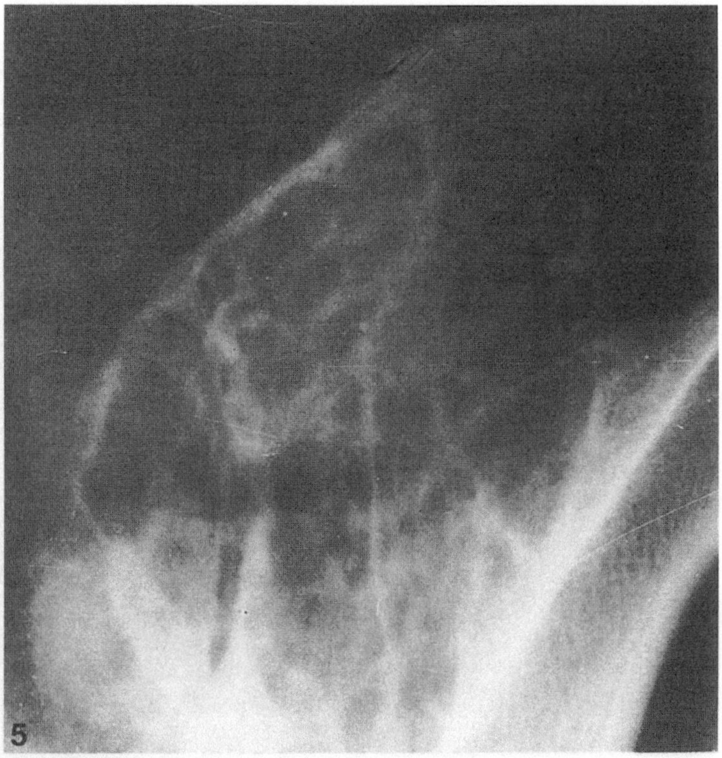
5

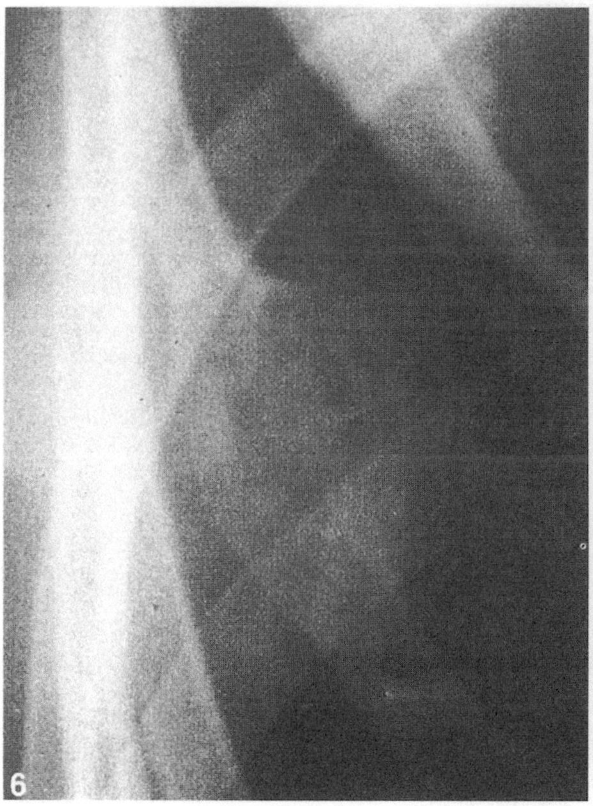
6

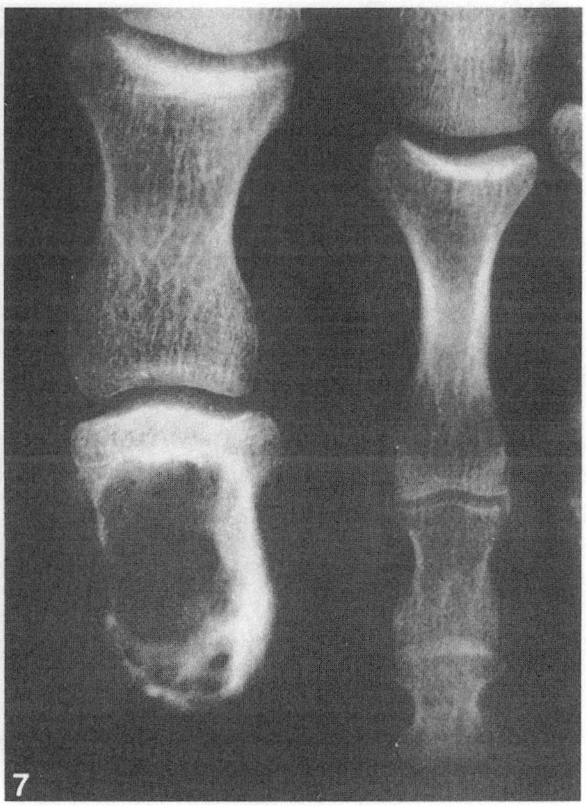
7

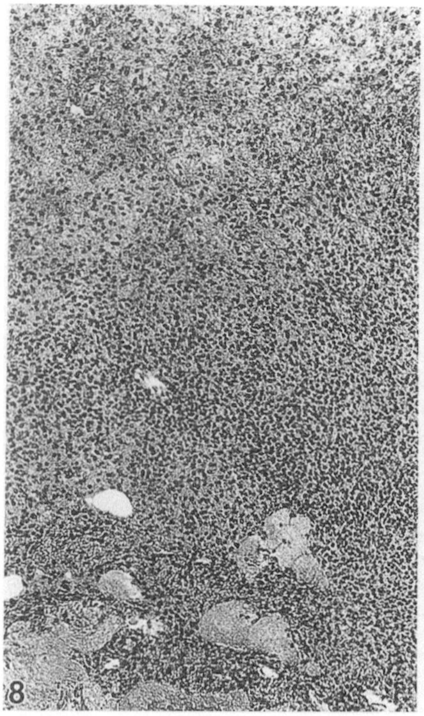

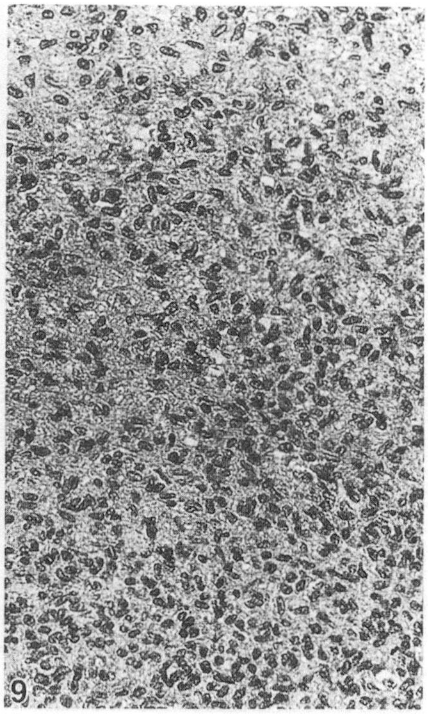

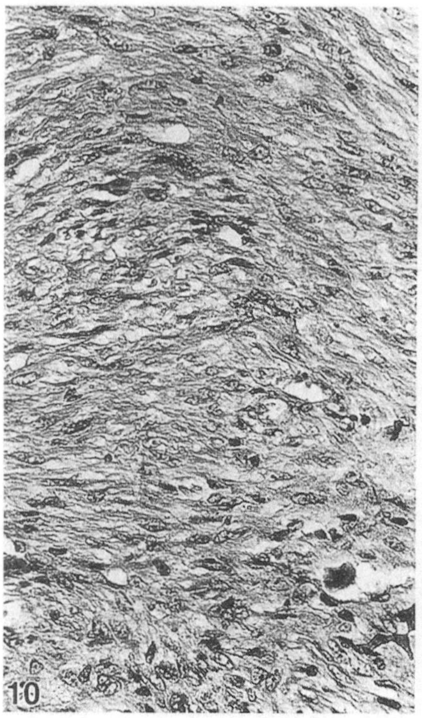

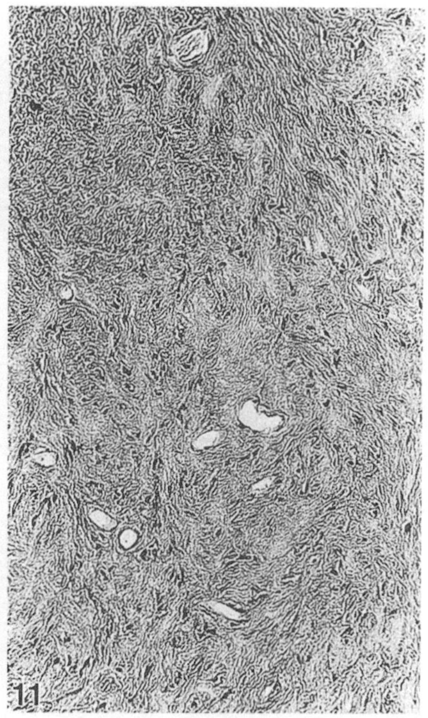

Figs. 8, 9. Low magnification: a zone of major cell density, but with a rudimentary matrix separating the cells from one another, may suggest a chondroblastoma

Fig. 10. In this fibrous area, the fusiform cells contain very unequal and sometimes bulky nuclei

Fig. 11. The matrix is more abundant and fibrohyaline, the cells are elongated, some vascular lumina of unequal size are irregularly distributed

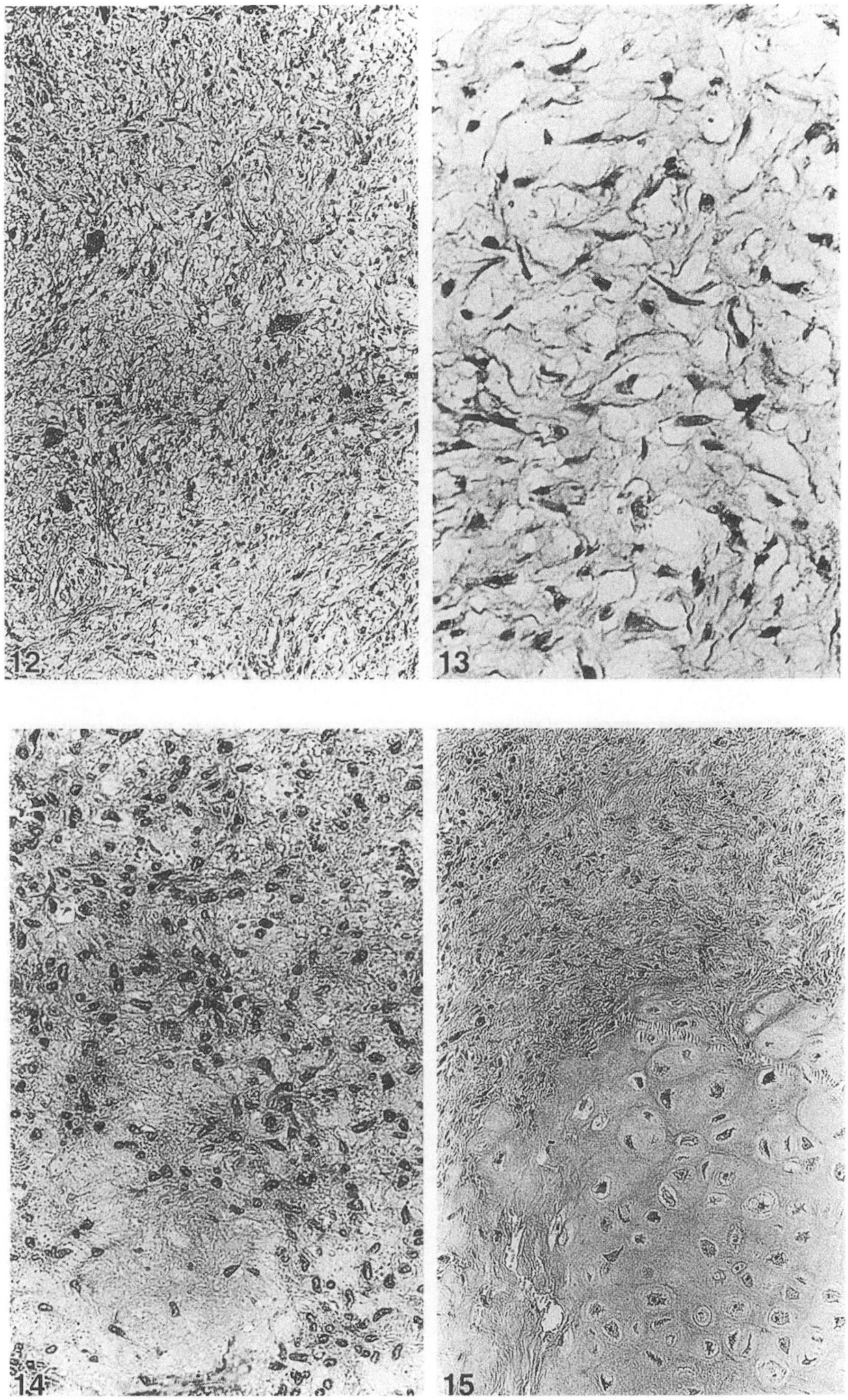

Figs. 12, 13. Myxoid zone at low and higher magnifications. Cells and nuclei of bizarre shape; the clear cytoplasm may suggest the lipoblasts of liposarcoma

Figs. 14, 15. In microphotograph 14 the matrix is more abundant in the lower half. In 15, the cartilaginous metaplasia is marked. Here again, the size and shape of the chondrocytes are very unequal

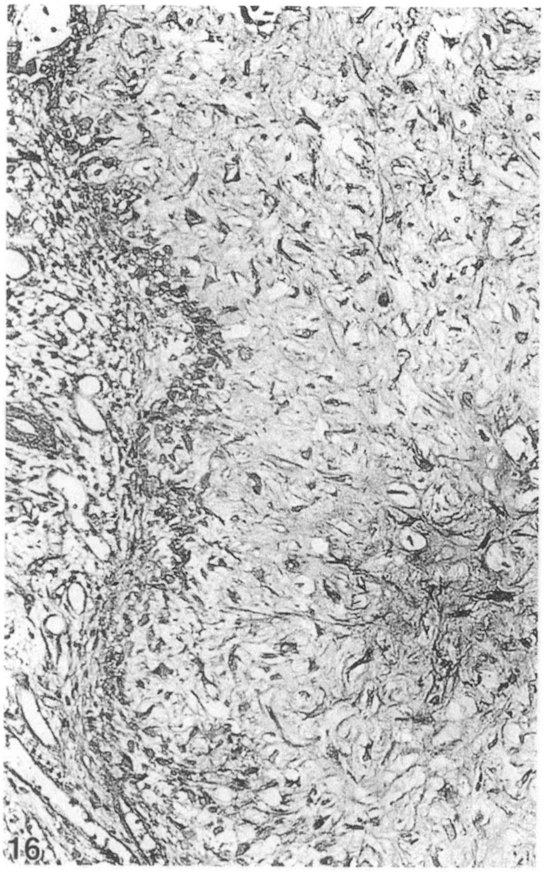

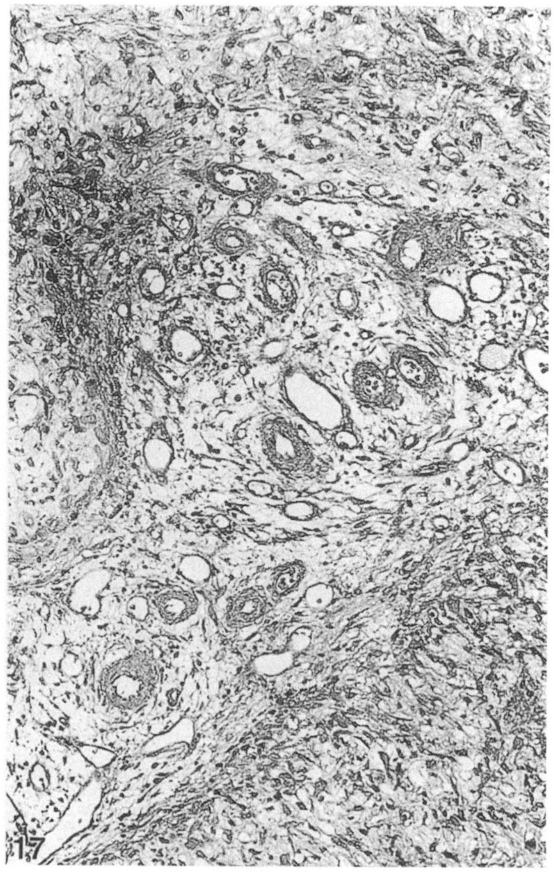

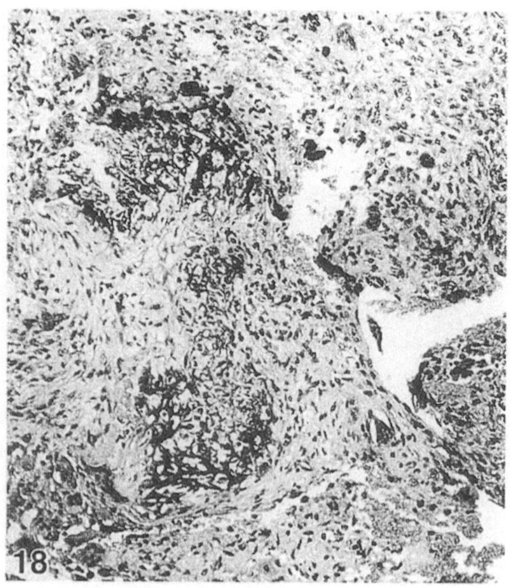

Fig. 16. Chondromyxoid nodule with bizarre cellular morphology. On the left, the boundary between this nodule and the internodular connective tissue is clearly seen

Fig. 17. Hypervascular connective tissue between the fibrochondroid nodules

Fig. 18. In some chondromyxoid fibromas, calcification and even ossification may be seen. In this microphotograph, the calcified zones appear as dense black

16. Malignant fibrous histiocytoma

This entity was defined following the studies of Ozzello, Stout and Murray (1963), O'Brien and Stout (1964) and by the report of Feldman and Norman in 1972 of 9 cases of malignant intraosseous histiocytoma. But while malignant fibrous histiocytoma is a common tumour of the soft tissues in adults and the elderly, the primary bone tumour is much more rare. However, a review of bone tumours previously classed under the diagnosis of fibroblastic sarcoma has allowed the listing of several hundred: Demol collected 535 cases from the literature in his thesis (1987).

It is generally accepted that the tumour derives from a mesenchymal cell expressing a dual potential: fibroblastic and histiocytic. This view is supported by tissue culture where Ozzello et al (1963) secured the transformation of neoplastic histiocytes into fibroblasts in vitro, by ultrastructural studies [Katenkamp & Stiller 1981, Nakashima et al 1985] and by immunohistological studies. Hirose et al (1989) studied 34 cases and found reactions with anti-vimentin antibodies positive in 80%, and reactions with anti-desmin and anti-alpha smooth muscle actin were also positive. More important is the demonstration of positivity to the monoclonal antibody KP-1 (CD 68), used to label histiocytes and macrophages. In 25 cases studied the reaction with KP-1 was positive in 18 (72% of cases) but the percentage of positive cells varied greatly. Alpha-1-antitrypsin and alpha-1-antichymotrypsin give a positive reaction in 92% of cases but these tests are less specific [Binder et al 1992].

Iwasaki et al (1992) stress the heterogeneity of the histiocytic proliferation, which they see as partly tumour-like and partly reactive. Dahlin and some other authors consider that the term "fibrous" is not essential in denominating this histiocytofibroblastic sarcoma, given the considerable variations in collagen formation. Other workers [Taconis & Van Rijssel 1985] opine that this tumour should be regarded as a simple but variant form of fibroblastic sarcoma, in view of the clinical and evolutional resemblance found between the two tumours. It seems logical to accept that most of the remarks made on malignant fibrous histiocytoma of the soft tissues are applicable to the tumour in its bony situation.

Case history

This man of 56 was already known in the orthopaedic department; his first attendance at the age of 29 was for pain located below the right hip. The imaging revealed several foci of bone infarction, one of which was biopsied. The history was that 7 years earlier he had been diving daily for a year off the African coast when installing telephone cables. Currently, he complained of persistent pain in the upper part of the left leg, probably related to a known infarct of the upper third of the tibia. Imaging demonstrated a poorly demarcated lytic lesion which almost completely surrounded the dense zone of the infarction. Histological examination of the lesion revealed the presence of a malignant fibrous histiocytoma developing in contact with the focus of infarction.

General considerations

This is a rare tumour, 10 times less frequent than osteogenic sarcoma. It accounts for about 1-2% of all tumours of bone. There is a slight male predominance, of the order of 2 or 1.5/1. It is seen mainly around the age of 35 to 40, a little later for tumours developing after irradiation of a preexisting bony lesion.

The commonest sites are the metaphyses of the long bones, particularly at the upper end of the tibia and the lower end of the femur; of the 511 cases in which Demol

(1987) reported the site, 197 involved the knee (38%). In the 13 patients studied by Nakashima et al (1985), 7 tumours were in the knee region, but the tumour also affects the bones of the pelvis, skull and face [Chikhani et al 1995]. These are followed by the bones of the thoracic skeleton and the vertebrae.

Clinical features and course

Advice is sought for pain, peritumour swelling, rarely for spontaneous fracture. Pain may precede the consultation by some months to 2 years.

In some 25% of cases the tumour develops in a preexisting lesion: infarction [Mirra et al 1977, Galli et al 1978, Abrahams & Hull 1986, Gaucher et al 1991], Paget's disease, fibrous dysplasia, but also in contact with a hip prosthesis [Vives et al 1987], or in an irradiated bone [Hardy et al 1978, Vanel et al 1983]. Among 130 malignant fibrous histiocytomas [Huvos et al 1986], 20 were due to irradiation, but only 7 of these 20 cases had been irradiated for a preexisting bony lesion. The latent period ranged from 4 to 47 years; most of the patients were in their 5th decade, and 3-year survival was 58%.

The course of the generality of malignant fibrous histiocytomas is grave; local recurrences and pulmonary metastases limit the 10-year survival rate to around 30-45% [Campana 1984, Huvos 1985]. Nodal metastases are relatively rare, though their involvement was detected in 3 of the 13 patients studied by Nakashima et al (1985) and in 5 of the 8 patients reported by Yuen and Saw (1985).

Bad prognostic factors include a high histological grade of malignancy, advanced patient age, but also development on a preexisting lesion, though this last point is not confirmed by all the statistics.

Imaging

The radiological appearances observed vary considerably from one case to another. The most typical image is that of a solitary clear lytic zone, but there may be a confluence of several adjacent zones of osteolysis or even the appearance of microcavities or a "moth-eaten" appearance (figs. 1-3). The margins of the lesion are ill-defined (fig. 4). There is endosteal erosion but the cortex is often spared (fig. 3). Usually there is no periosteal reaction. A subperiosteal form has been described [Kemp & Byers 1987] and Castillo et al (1987) have reported a case with lesions in both ilium and femur.

The appearances seen when the tumour develops in contact with a preexisting lesion tend to have their own special features (fig. 4).

Pathological anatomy and histopathology

Macroscopically, the tumour is firm and whitish, with brownish-yellow zones related to necrosis and haemorrhage.

Low magnification shows the plaited, overlapping arrangement of dense bundles of cells of histiocytofibroblastic appearance (figs. 7-9). The fusiform cells have abundant eosinophil cytoplasm. The bizarrely shaped nuclei are notched, sectioned or are even perforated; sometimes multiple, they are surrounded by voluminous cytoplasm. These giant cells have irregular serrated margins (fig. 6). Macrophages are often evident (lipids, iron) but this phagocytosis is quite ordinary and does not amount to a firm factor in making a diagnosis. The mitoses vary in number and are sometimes very numerous; some are atypical. In addition to these histiocytofibroblastic cells, there are inflammatory cells, sometimes rare and sometimes abundant, possibly coexisting with areas of foamy histiocytes (figs. 5, 6).

Some tumours are particularly rich in cellular monstrosities; the large cells suggest a muscle tumour, or what might be termed a primary malignant giant-cell tumour (fig. 11). Haemorrhagic zones are not rare. Some cellular appearances may suggest liposarcoma, muscle tumours or a giant-cell tumour [Kahn 1978]. Collagen is usually scanty, but areas rich in collagen may be found in a very cellular tumour (figs. 10, 12). The reticulin network is moderately developed. Small areas of metaplastic bone or cartilage occur in authentic malignant fibrous histiocytomas [Dorfman & Bhagavan 1982].

A few metaplastic bony lamellae are unimportant, but it is necessary to distinguish a network of large collagen fibers from osteoid tissue, which may be particularly difficult [McCarthy et al 1979]. Confusion with osteoid tissue or tumour bone may suggest a diagnosis of osteosarcoma.

The contribution of immunohistological reactions to the demonstration of the dual histiocytic and fibroblastic potential, justifying the naming of the tumour, was discussed at the start of this chapter. Obviously, a percentage of positivity to the monoclonal antibody KP-1 (CD 68) of the order of 70-75% is not enough for absolute reliability in diagnosis; and the nonspecificity of the antibodies alpha-1-antitrypsin and alpha-1-antichymotrypsin fails in guarantee certainty. Lastly, some studies report positivity to antikeratin antibodies; the cellular anarchy of the tumour allows for free expression of this protein [Weiss et al 1988, Hirose et al 1989].

Ultrastructural studies describe fibroblasts, histiocytes, giant cells and undifferentiated cells in some variants. Nakashima et al (1985) found the histiocytic element predominant. The cell is furnished with an oval or lobed nucleus; the cytoplasm contains numerous lipid droplets and lysosomes. There are also fibroblasts and small undifferentiated mesenchymal cells. Martinez-Tello et al (1981) recorded 6 cell types: stem cells, histiocytes, fibroblasts, myofibroblasts, foamy cells and giant cells. Katenkamp and Stiller (1981) report the presence of myofibroblasts and myoblastic cells.

Differential diagnosis

It seems that the histological features by light microscopy are more reliable than clinical and radiological findings in this tumour. In its typical form, the differential diagnosis suggested is fibroblastic sarcoma. We have mentioned the view of some authors for whom this tumour is only a variant of fibroblastic sarcoma. However, the plaited stellate appearance though not pathognomonic, is not the rule in fibroblastic sarcoma. The addition of bizarre multinucleate cells, histiocytes and inflammatory cells and the absence of any "fishbone" organisation are sufficient to confirm the diagnosis.

Certain aspects - which have been specified in malignant fibrous histiocytomas of the soft tissues - may in particular suggest a giant-cell tumour or a muscle sarcoma. But can one differentiate a primary malignant giant-cell tumour from a malignant fibrous histiocytoma now that the latter entity has been recognised as having a form rich in giant cells?

Leiomyosarcoma and rhabdomyosarcoma have been reported in the bony tissue; these are quite rare tumours and the presence of a few large eosinophil cells are rather weak evidence to support this diagnosis. The immunological reactions, cautiously interpreted, are of appreciable assistance.

References

Abrahams TG, Hull M (1986) Malignant fibrous histiocytoma (MFH) arising in an infarct of bone. Skeletal Radiol 15: 578-583

Bayer Kristensen I, Myhre Jensen O (1984) Malignant fibrous histiocytoma of bone. A clinico-pathologic study of 9 cases. Acta Path Microbiol Immunol Sect 92A: 205-210

Bednar B (1957) Storiform neurofibromas of skin, pigmented and non pigmented. Cancer 10: 368-376

Binder SW, Said JW, Shintaku IP, Pinkus G (1992) A histiocyte-specific marker in the diagnosis of malignant fibrous histiocytoma. Use of monoclonal antibody KP-I (CD 68). Am J Clin Pathol 97: 759-763

Boland PJ, Huvos AG (1986) Malignant fibrous histiocytoma of bone. Clin Orthop 204: 130-134

Capanna R, Bertoni F, Bacchini P, Bacci G, Guerra A, Campanacci M (1984) Malignant fibrous histiocytoma of bone. The experience at the Rizzoli institute: report of 90 cases. Cancer 54: 177-187

Castillo M, Tehranzadeh J, Becerra J, Mnaymneh W (1987) Malignant fibrous histiocytoma of innominate bones and femur (multicentric). Skeletal Radiol 16: 74-77

Chikhani L, Favre d'Auvergne E, Fleuridas G, Bertrand JCh, Guilbert F, Auriol M, Le Charpentier Y (1995) Xanthogranulome malin de la mandibule. Présentation d'un cas et revue de la littérature. Rev Stomatol Chir Maxillofac 96: 83-87

Demol B (1987) L'histiocytome fibreux malin osseux. Etude anatomoclinique de 6 observations et revue de la littérature. Thèse de Doctorat en Médecine, Lille II

Den Heeten GJ, Koops HS, Kamps WA, Oosterhuis JW, Sleijfer DT, Oldhoff J (1985) Treaument of malignant fibrous histiocytoma of bone. A plea for primary chemotherapy. Cancer 56: 37-40

Dorfman HD, Bhagavan BS (1982) Malignant fibrous histiocytoma of soft tissue with metaplastic bone and cartilage formation: a new radiologic sign. Skeletal Radiol 8: 145-150

Feldman F, Norman D (1972) Intra and extraosseous malignant histiocytoma (malignant fibrous xanthoma). Radiol 104: 497-508

Fletcher CDR (1992) Pleomorphic malignant fibrous histiocytoma fact or fiction? A critical reappraisal on 159 tumors diagnosed as pleomorphic sarcoma. Am J Surg Pathol 16: 213-228

Frierson HF, Fechner RE, Stallings RG, Wang GJ (1987) Malignant fibrous histiocytoma in bone infarct. Association with sickle cell trait and alcohol abuse. Cancer 59: 496-500

Galli SJ, Weintraub HP, Proppe KH (1978) Malignant fibrous histiocytoma and pleomorphic sarcoma in association with medullary bone infarcts. Cancer 41: 607-609

Gaucher AA, Regent DM, Gillet PM, Pere PG, Aymard BM, Clement V (1991) Malignant fibrous histiocytoma in a previous bone infarct. Skeletal Radiol 20: 137-140

Ghandur-Mnaymneh L, Zych G, Mnaymneh W (1982) Primary malignant fibrous histiocytoma of bone: report of six cases with ultrastructural study and analysis of the literature. Cancer 49: 698-707

Hirose T, Kudo E, Hasegawa T, Abe Jl, Hizawa K (1989) Expression of intermediate filaments in malignant fibrous histiocytomas. Hum Pathol 20: 871-877

Huvos AG, Heilweil M, Bretsky SS (1985) The pathology of malignant fibrous histiocytoma of bone. A study of 130 patients. Am J Surg Pathol 9: 853-871

Huvos AG, Woodard HG, Heilweil M (1986) Postradiation malignant fibrous histiocytoma of bone. A clinicopathologic study of 20 patients. Am J Surg Pathol 10: 9-18

Iwasaki H, Kenzo Y, Ohjimi Y, Kikuchi M, Isayama T, Yoh S, Shinohara N, Enjoji M (1992) Malignant fibrous histiocytoma. Proliferative comportment and heterogeneity of "histiocytic" cells. Am J Surg Pathol 16: 735-745

Katenkamp D, Stiller D (1981) Malignant fibrous histiocytoma of bone: light microscopic and electron microscopic examination of four cases. Virchows Arch 391: 323-335

Kemp HBS, Byers PD (1987) Subperiosteal malignant fibrous histiocytoma (MFH) of thigh, with involvement of femur. Skeletal Radiol 16: 584-588

Kindblom LG, Jacobsen GK, Jacobsen M (1982) Immunnohistochemical investigations of tumors of supposed fibroblastic-histiocytic origin. Hum Pathol 13: 834-840

Lecomte-Houcke M, Parent M (1987) L'histiocytome malin fibreux osseux. Rev Chir Orthop 73: 81-86

Lideman G, McKay MJ, Taubman KL, Bilous AM (1990) Malignant fibrous histiocytoma developing in bone 44 years after shrapnel trauma. Cancer 66: 2229-2232

Martinez-Tello FJ, Navas-Palacios JJ, Calvo-Asensio M, Loizaga-lriondo JM (1981) Malignant fibrous histiocytoma of bone. A clinico-pathological and electronmicroscopical study. Pathol Res Pract 173: 141-158

McCarthy EF, Matsuno T, Dorfman HD (1979) Malignant fibrous histiocytoma of bone: a study of 35 cases. Hum Pathol 10: 57-70

Mirra JM, Gold RH, Marafiote R (1977) Malignant (fibrous) histiocytoma arising in association with a bone infarct in sickle-cell disease: coincidence or cause and effect? Cancer 39: 186-194

Nakashima Y, Morishita S, Kotoura Y, Yamamuro T, Tamura K, Onomura T, Sudo Y, Awaya G, Hamashima Y (1985) Malignant fibrous histiocytoma of bone. A review of 13 cases and an ultrastructural study. Cancer 55: 2804-2811

O'Brien JE, Stout AP (1964) Malignant fibrous xanthomas. Cancer 17: 1445-1455

Ozzello L, Stout AP, Murray MR (1963) Cultural characteristics of malignant histiocytomas and fibrous xanthomas. Cancer 16: 331-344

Pere P, Adolphe J, Delgoffe C, Froment N, Gaucher A (1984) Ostéonécroses épiphysaires, infarctus osseux multiples et histiocytome fibreux malin. Rev Rhum 51: 427-430

Pezzi CM, Rawlings MS, Esgro JJ, Pollock RE, Romsdahl MM (1992) Prognostic factors in 227 patients with malignant fibrous histiocytoma. Cancer 69: 2098-2103

Spanier SS, Enneking WF, Enriquez P (1975) Primary histiocytoma of bone. Cancer 36: 2084-2098

Spector DB, Miller JO, Villoria J (1979) Malignant fibrous histiocytoma, an unusual lesion of interest to the orthopaedic sungeon. J Bone Joint Surg 61B: 190-193

Taconis WK, Van Rijssel THG (1985) Fibrosarcoma of long bones, a study of the significance of area of malignant fibrous histiocytoma. J Bone Joint Surg 67B: 111-116

Urban C, Rosen G, Huvos AG, Caparros B, Cavavio A, Nierenberg A (1983) Chemotherapy of malignant fibrous histiocytoma of bone: a report of five cases. Cancer 51: 795-802

Vanel D, Hagay C, Rebibo G, Oberlin O, Masselot J (1983) Study of three radio-induced malignant fibrohistiocytomas of bone. Skeletal Radiol 9: 174-178

Vives P, Sevestre H, Grodet H, Marie F (1987) Histiocytome fibreux malin du fémur après prothèse totale de hanche. A propos d'un cas. Rev Chir Orthop 73: 407-409

Weiss SW, Bratthauer GL, Morris P (1988) Postirradiation malignant fibrous histiocytoma expressing cytokeratin. Implications for the immunodiagnosis of sarcomas. Am J Surg Pathol 12: 554-558

Weiss SW, Enzinger (1978) Malignant fibrous histiocytoma. Cancer 41: 2250-2266

Yuen WH, Saw D (1985) Malignant fibrous histiocytoma of bone. J Bone Joint Surg 67A: 482-486

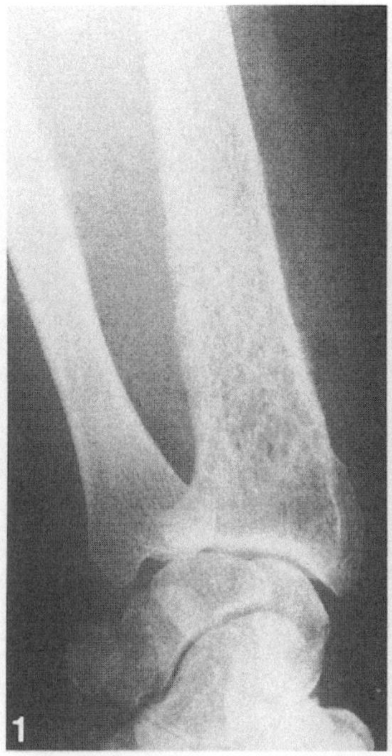

Fig. 1. The tumour occupies the lower part of the radius. The cortex penetrated by the tumour assumes a moth-eaten microcavitary appearance. This phenomenon of "permeation" is associated with invasion of the surrounding soft tissues

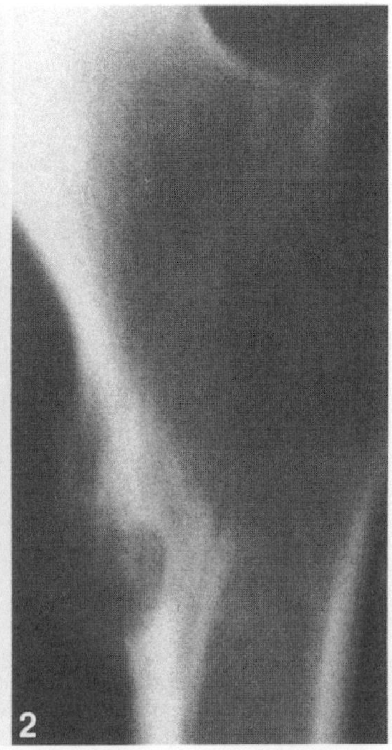

Fig. 2. The tumour has developed in the cortical zone of the upper third of the femur, forming a sort of nodule covered by periosteum but infiltrating the subjacent bone. Man of 61

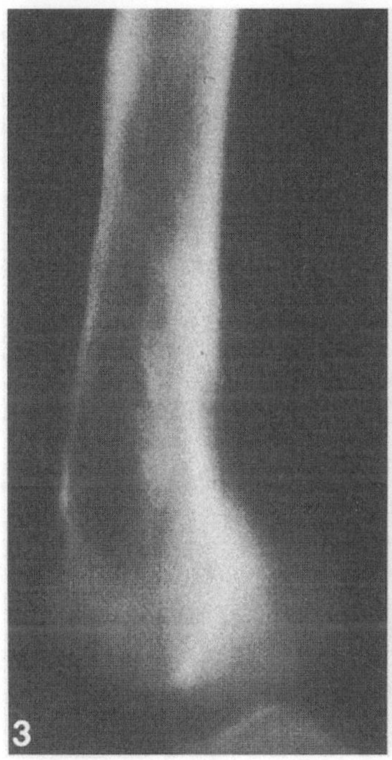

Fig. 3. The tumour is central and has destroyed all of the deep part of the anterior femoral cortex. Woman aged 21

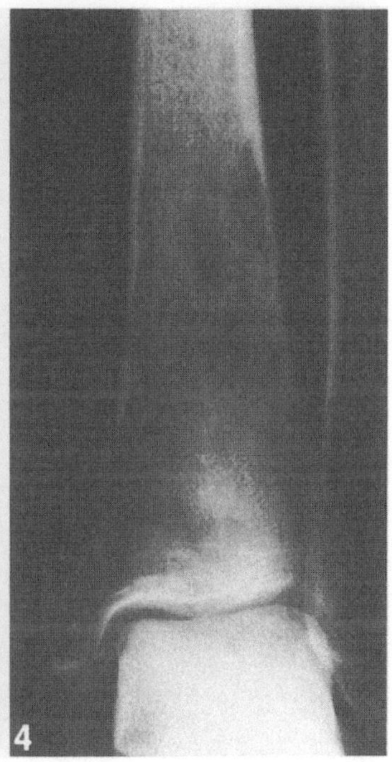

Fig. 4. A skeletal survey showed the presence of multiple bone infarctions in this patient. In contact with one of these, located at the lower end of the left tibia, a malignant fibrous histiocytoma has developed, whose lytic image surrounds a small dense area corresponding to the infarct, known to have been present for 5 years (courtesy of Pr Gaucher and our colleague Bernadette Aymard; this case was published in Skeletal Radiology in 1991, see references)

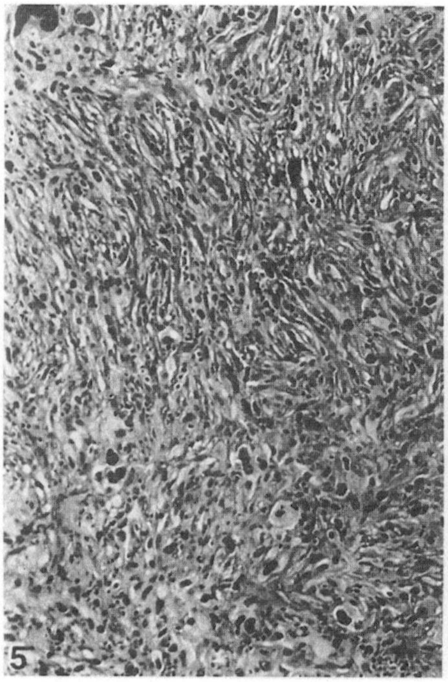
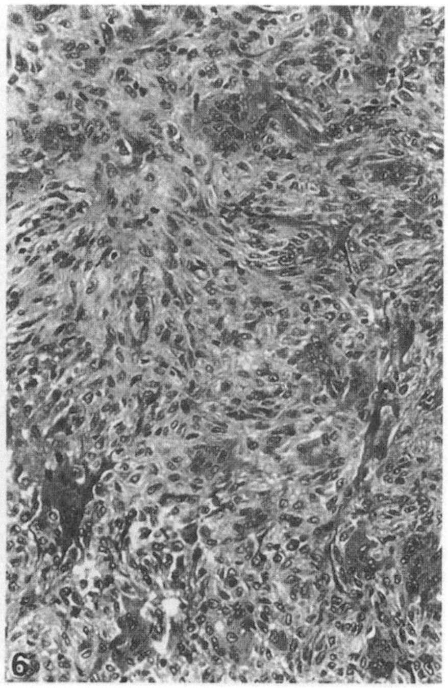
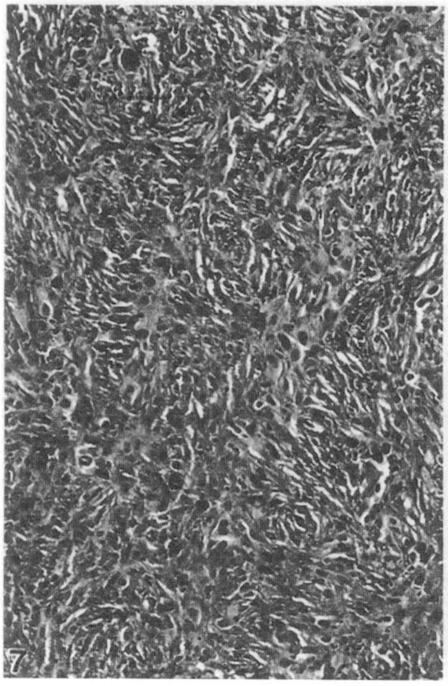
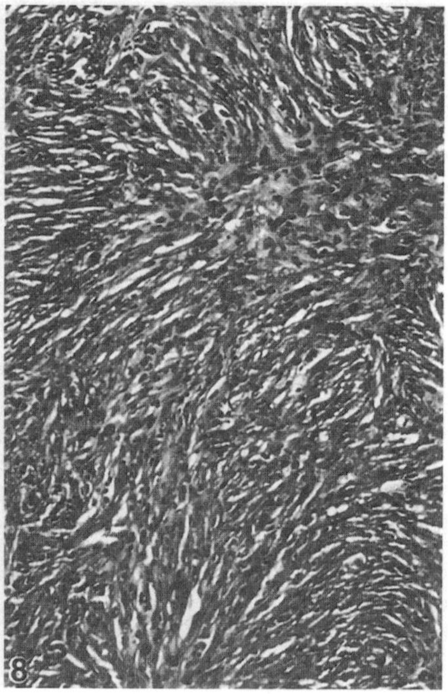

Fig 5. Multinucleate cells with atypical nuclei. Cellular polymorphism: clear foamy cells of histiocytic appearance, giant cells, a majority of fusiform cells grouped in bundles should arouse some suspicion

Fig. 6. At higher magnification, there appear lymphocytic inflammatory cells, as well as the cellular anomalies. The giant cells have scalloped margins

Figs. 7, 8. In reviewing the sections, some zones of fusiform cells give this plaited storiform appearance, described by Bednar in malignant fibrous histiocytoma of the soft tissues

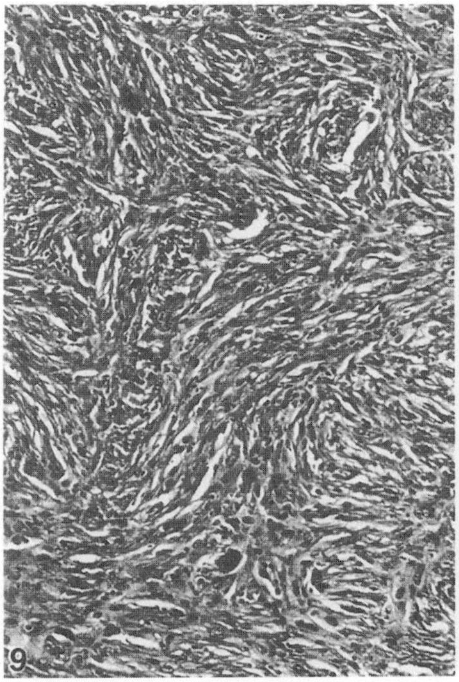

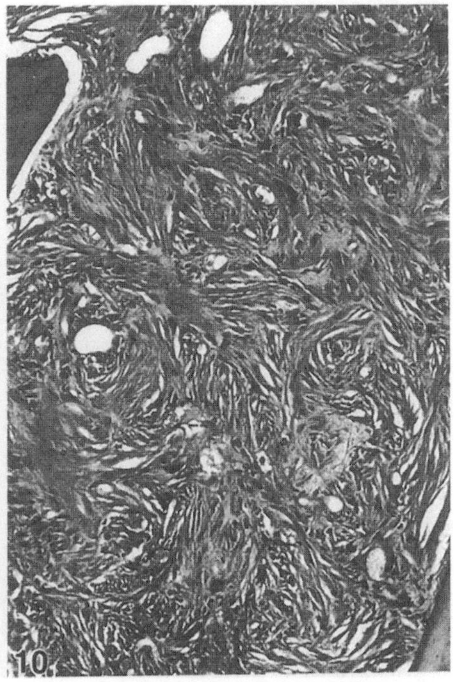

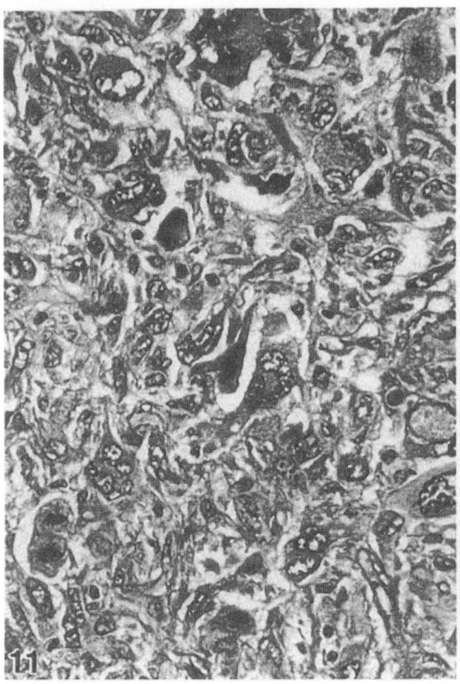

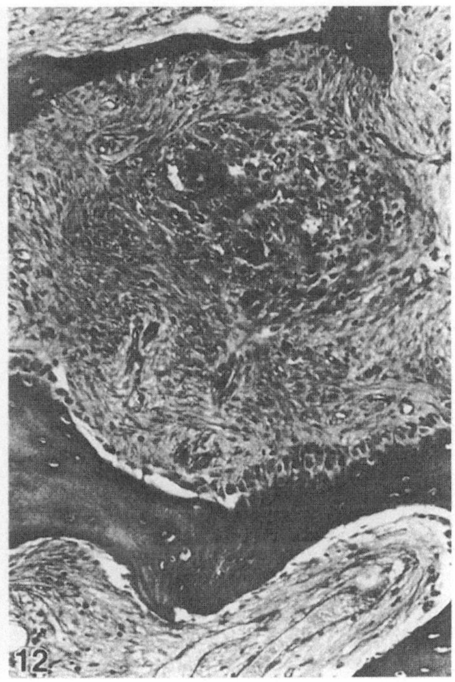

Fig. 9. Whorled appearance of fusiform cells and atypical giant cells

Fig. 10. In some cases, there coexist zones particularly rich in collagen which preserve this storiform appearance

Fig. 11. Polymorphism and cell monstrosities are sometimes considerable; such appearances were probably considered to respect a malignant giant-cell tumour

Fig. 12. In the medullary spaces, a cellular tumour island stands out against a dense fibrous background

17. Fibroblastic sarcoma

This tumour is represented by a proliferation of fibroblastic cells which do not elaborate osteoid or chondroid tissue but a varying amount of collagen, related of the functional differentiation of the tumour cells. It may be primary, or secondary to irradiation or to a pre-existing benign or malignant tumour, or perhaps even a chronic osteitis.

In primary sarcomas every degree of malignancy exists between slowly growing tumours rich in collagen and anaplastic lesions.

Primary fibroblastic sarcoma

Case histories

Case 1. A man of 40 had suffered from moderate pain for 3-4 months, increasing in recent weeks. The radiological image was that of osteolysis of the lower femoral metaphysis with blurred boundaries. The biopsy gave the pathologist a tumour tissue in which the diagnosis of fibroblastic sarcoma of grade 3 malignancy was obvious. There was no formation of osteoid or bony tissue.

Case 2. A woman of 25 complained of pain in the left arm. A standard radiograph revealed a moth-eaten appearance extending to the upper part of the humeral shaft. A first biopsy was too distal and mainly involved osteoporotic cortex and some small fragments of dense collagen, giving rise to a discussion of desmoid fibroma or fibrosarcoma of low grade of malignancy as differential diagnoses. The inconsistency of this finding with the radiological appearances justified a second biopsy. This, taken from the middle part of the shaft, showed the presence of a very cellular fibroblastic sarcoma, virtually devoid of collagen.

General considerations

The incidence of fibrosarcoma in relation to primary malignant tumours of bone is of the order of 3-6% in the series of the Mayo Clinic [Dahlin & Ivins 1969], and 5% in that of Huvos & Higginbotham (1975) dealing with 130 cases of primary fibrosarcomas. But its incidence has decreased in recent years in proportion to the increasing (or hypertrophying) diagnosis of malignant fibrous histiocytoma. Fibroblastic sarcoma is 5-10 times less common than osteosarcoma. There is a slight male predominance. The age distribution of fibroblastic sarcoma is very wide, with maximal incidence towards the 4th and 5th decades. But the diagnosis is sometimes made in paediatric departments, and in some rare cases the lesion is congenital; note that in the first 6 months of life the correlation between histology and prognosis is far from being rigorous in this type of tumour.

Location in the long bones exceeds 50%, and is essentially metaphyseal and metaphyseo-diaphyseal. However, the flat bones of the skeleton, the vertebrae and craniofacial bones as well as the ribs are responsible for some 40% of cases. In the long bones, the upper end of the tibia and lower end of the femur are most often affected.

Some cases of multiple lesions have been reported [Hernandez et al 1993].

In a study of 130 cases of fibroblastic sarcoma, Kenan et al (1993) found 89 tumours of medullary origin and 41 of periosteal origin. The periosteal form has a better prognosis, but this may be because it is diagnosed earlier than the intramedullary form.

Table 1. Diagnostic problems

Desmoid fibroma (low histological malignancy)
Reactive fibrosis to metastasis from a primary tumour
Fusiform-cell primary or metastatic tumour: - fusiform-cell carcinoma - sarcoma - malignant melanoma - malignant schwannoma - malignant fibrous histiocytoma
Two pitfalls: 1) The zone of osteoporosis often extends widely beyond the tumour and thus a peripheral bony biopsy may show only osteoporosis of unknown origin 2) The peripheral tumour zone may be of low malignancy, unlike the central zone

Clinical features and course

Presentation is with pain in over 50% of cases. The duration of symptoms is related to the progress of the tumour: it is of the order of 12 months in differentiated forms but of less than 6 months in anaplastic forms. Rarely, a fracture is the presenting feature. In over half the cases, the tumour is palpable at the first consultation.

Depending on the histological grade of malignancy and the possibilities of treatment (chemotherapy and surgery), the 5-year survival rate varies from 30 to 70%. When the course is unfavourable, death supervenes following pulmonary and bony metastases. Nodal metastases are rare.

Imaging

The radiological aspects are varied and these too depend on the rapidity of the course of the tumour. The commonest image is an area of metaphyseal osteolysis with fuzzy borders, sometimes more sharply bounded but without sclerosis (figs. 4, 5). This osteolytic zone may exceed the tumour zone widely. If progress is slow, a minor periosteal reaction may develop; the cortex is destroyed on its deep, medullary aspect and the whole lesion may assume a slightly ballooned appearance. The most rapidly growing forms are evidenced by moth-eaten, permeative, areolar appearances (fig. 1) which extend throughout the metaphysis without precise boundaries. Usually there is no periosteal reaction, but in the case reported by Lysko et al (1986) the intra- and extraosseous spread of the tumour was associated with a rudimentary Codman's triangle. Some very rapidly growing tumours destroy the cortex. However, particularly slowly growing lesions may be associated with extensive osteoporosis which spreads widely beyond the tumour. Biopsies made from these pathological but not tumour areas do not permit a correct diagnosis. When located juxtacortically, the tumour destroys the outer aspect of the cortex and infiltrates the soft tissues, accompanied by a periosteal reaction.

Pathological anatomy and histopathology

The macroscopic appearance is variable, depending on the abundance or otherwise of collagen. Sometimes the tumour is grayish-white and firm, sometimes softer and strewn with haemorrhagic and necrotic zones. In the long bones it occupies the medullary canal and the metaphysis.

Periosteal reaction is minor, whether it involves a long bone of a limb or a rib. In the metaphyseal region, this periosteal reaction offers only a feeble barrier to the tumour, which destroys it to infiltrate the soft tissues. In the diaphyseal region, where the cortical tissue persists, the tumour infiltrates and enlarges the haversian spaces. When juxtacortical, the tumour is usually firm, richer in collagen and ovoid, and makes a marked impression on the adjacent bone.

The relatively monotonous histology of the tumour is more characteristic than the radiological appearance. The fusiform cells are grouped in intermingled bundles, and here and there are arranged in "fish-bone" pattern (fig. 6 a, b). These cells of fibroblastic appearance have a large and nucleolated nucleus with coarsely distributed chromatin. Their cytoplasm is eosinophil but quite often there is a cytoplasmic "clarification" (fig. 7). Between the cells there are collagen fibers in an abundance determined by the degree of cell differentiation. The frequency of mitoses varies with cases. Also, in very undifferentiated forms, necrotic zones are the rule. There is an abundant reticulin network. Every intermediate form exists between the cellular anaplastic types and forms very rich in collagen whose appearance resembles that of a desmoid fibroma. The cells are rare and attenuated and layered between the collagen fibres, but if numerous sections are studied it is rare not to find some more evolved and much more cellular areas.

It is important to emphasise that in the infant before 6 months the biological malignancy does not always correspond to the histological appearance.

Taconis and Van Rijsell (1985) mention the presence of atypical zones of malignant fibrous histiocytoma in

46% of 102 fibroblastic sarcomas of the long bones studied. This fact had no influence on the course of the tumour; therefore these authors suggest that malignant fibrous histiocytoma should be regarded as a variant of fibroblastic sarcoma of bone.

Diagnosis

Diagnosis is simple in the majority of cases. However, depending on their site and histological appearance, fibroblastic sarcomas may suggest other possibilities. Two major difficulties occur at both ends of the continuum of fibroblastic tumours. A sarcoma with very abundant collagen may be confused with a fibroma and conversely, an anaplastic sarcoma will pose no problem as to its malignancy but its origin remains uncertain.

In either case it is helpful to study many sections in the search for more significant zones. A tumour with fusiform cells as well as an anaplastic tumour totally devoid of collagen may be a metastasis from a carcinoma; in such cases the immunological reactions (antivimentin, antikeratin) will help to make a firm diagnosis. Another problem is that posed by storiform groupings; according to Bednar (personal communication) these appearances are not pathognomonic. In malignant fibrous histiocytoma cellular pleomorphism is a major feature (cf Chapter 16).

A fibroblastic sarcoma rich in cells may suggest a diagnosis of giant-cell tumour. In the latter the giant cells retain their benign nature, unlike those of fibroblastic sarcoma: a subtle distinction but one which argues in favor of the existence of malignant giant-cell tumours. The localisations are somewhat different; giant-cell tumour is metaphyseo-epiphyseal and fibroblastic sarcoma metaphyseal, but this observation is of less value in advanced lesions (cf Chapter 21).

Other diagnoses may be considered: malignant schwannoma, metastasis from a malignant melanoma, bony invasion by a fibroblastic sarcoma of the soft tissues or, in quite exceptional circumstances, metastasis from a missed or previously treated sarcoma. Lastly, the biopsy may be from the fusiform cell proliferation or undifferentiated zone of a preexisting tumour.

The possibility of an osteosarcoma is to be considered if the biopsy is from a tumour developing in an adolescent. The imaging is particularly important here. Although fibroblastic sarcoma affects patients of all ages, it is imperative in these conditions to study numerous sections to seek out even minimal tumour osteogenesis, which is sometimes more obvious only in the resection specimen.

In every case it is important to specify the histological grade of malignancy of these fibroblastic sarcomas (cf p. 113).

Secondary fibroblastic sarcoma

This sarcoma may develop in preexisting dystrophies or tumours. Some are related to irradiation performed for a tumour of quite a different nature, often epithelial. The tumour may also develop in contact with a hip prosthesis, for instance. The relevant dystrophies and tumours include: fibrous dysplasia, Paget's disease, bone infarction, progressive dedifferentiation of a chondrosarcoma and chronic osteomyelitis.

References

Akbarnia BA, Wirth CR, Colman N (1976) Fibrosarcoma arising from chronic osteomyelitis. Case report and review of the literature. J Bone Joint Surg 58A: 123-125

André S, Tomeno B, Forest M, Carlioz A (1983) Fibrosarcomes des os. Rev Chir Orthop 69: 107-116

Dahlin DC, Ivins JC (1969) Fibrosarcoam of bone: a study of 114 cases. Cancer 23: 35-41

Frassica FJ, Sim FH, Wold LE (1988) Grade 2 myxoid fibrosarcoma of femur. Skeletal Radiol 17: 77-80

Hernandez FJ, Fernandez BB (1976) Multiple diffuse fibrosarcoma of bone. Cancer 37: 939-945

Huvos AG, Higginbotham NL (1975) Primary fibrosarcoma of bone: a clinicopathologic study of 130 patients. Cancer 35: 837-847

Jeffree GM, Price CHG (1976) Metastatic sprend of fibrosarcoma of bone: a report on forty-nine cases and a comparison with osteosarcoma. J Bone Joint Surg 58B: 418-425

Kenan S, Abdel Wahab IF, Klein MG, Hermann G, Lewis MM (1993) Lesions of juxtacortical origin (surface lesions of bone). Skeletal Radiol 22: 337-357

Larson SE, Lorentzon R, Boquist L (1976) Fibrosarcoma of bone. A demographic, clinical and histopathological study of all cases recorded in the swedish cancer registry from 1958 to 1968. J Bone Joint Surg 58B: 412-417

Lysko JE, Guilford B, Siegal GP (1986) Primary fibrosarcoma of the right femur (case report). Skeletal Radiol 15: 268-272

Pritchard DJ, Soule EH, Taylor WF,lvins JC (1974) Fibrosarcoma: a clinicopathologic and statistical study of 119 tumors of the soft tissues of the extremities and trunk. Cancer 33: 888-897

Taconis WK, Van Rijssel THG (1985) Fibrosarcoma of long bones . A study of the significance of areas of malignant fibrous histiocytoma. J Bone Joint Surg 67B: 111-116

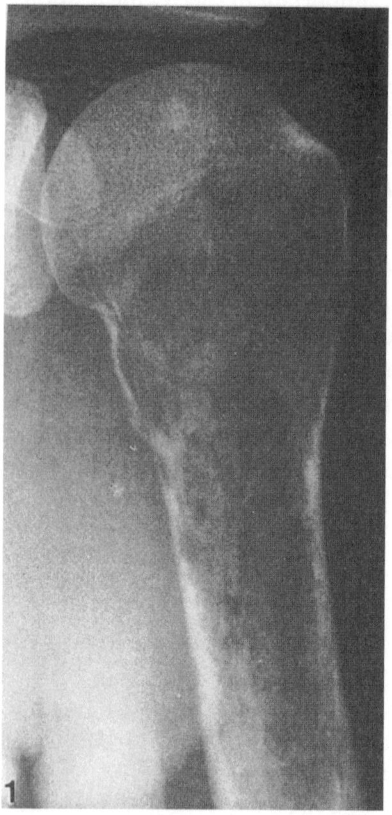

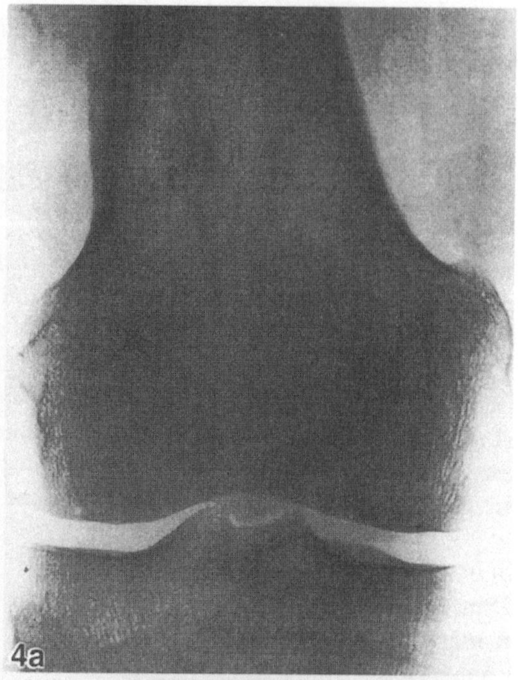

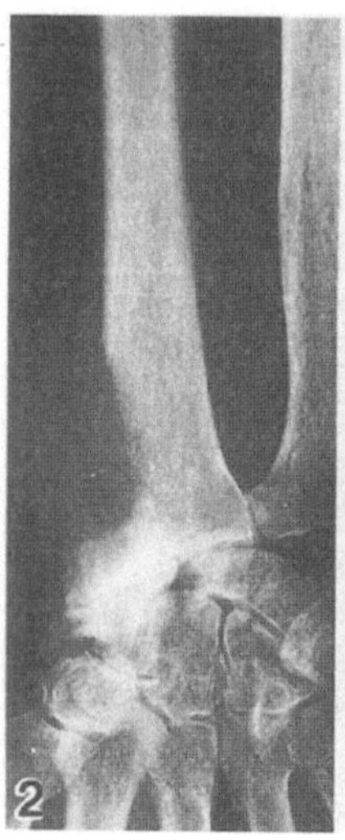

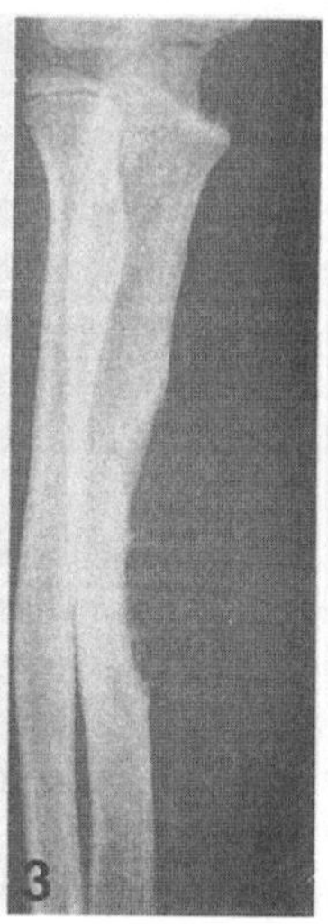

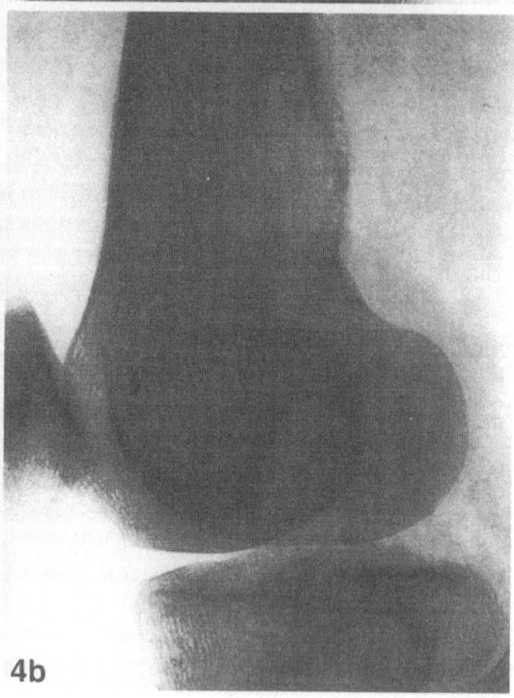

Fig. 1. Moth-eaten micro-areolar appearance of upper end of humerus. Too peripheral a biopsy had been mistaken for an "ordinary" osteoporosis. Case history 2, woman aged 25

Fig. 2. Sarcoma of superficial periosteal origin: infero-lateral third of radius. Circumscribed lysis but no sclerosis and without periosteal reaction. Man of 70

Fig. 3. Periosteal sarcoma: two recurrences after excision. Wide resection followed by cure. Child of 10 years (fig. 6 a, b)

Fig. 4 a, b. Clear ill-defined image of lower end of femur, extending transversely and axially. Man of 50

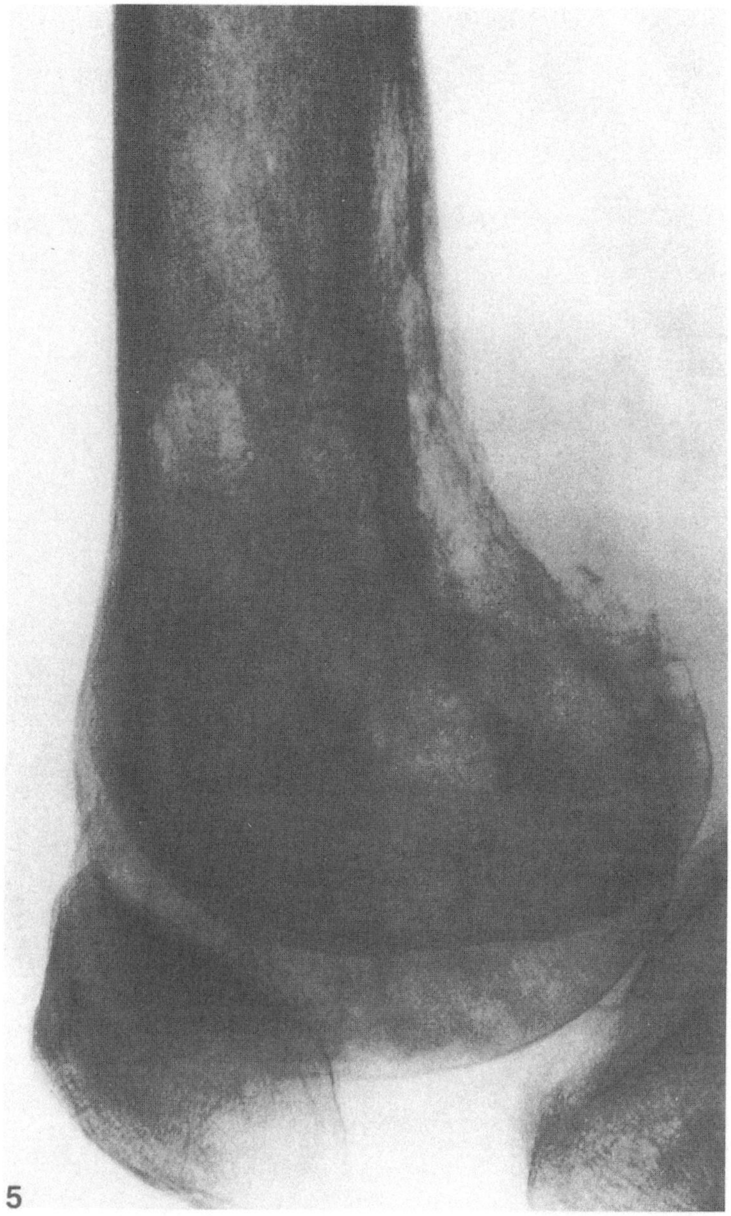

5

Fig. 5. Sarcoma invading entire lower end of femur, extending to articular cartilage and destroying posterior cortex. Man of 30

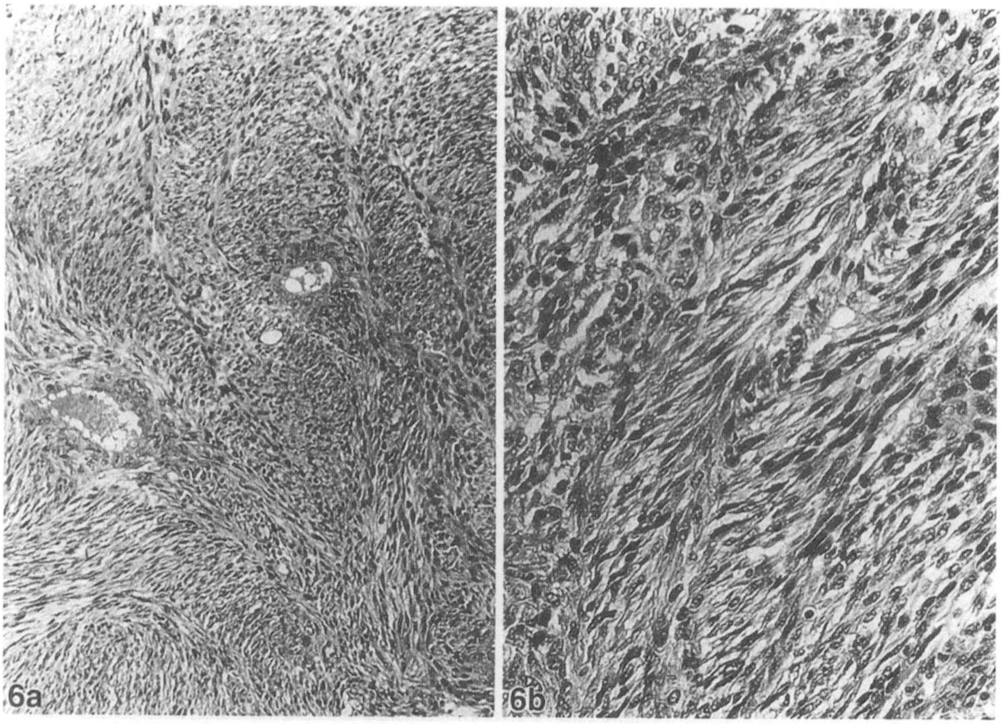

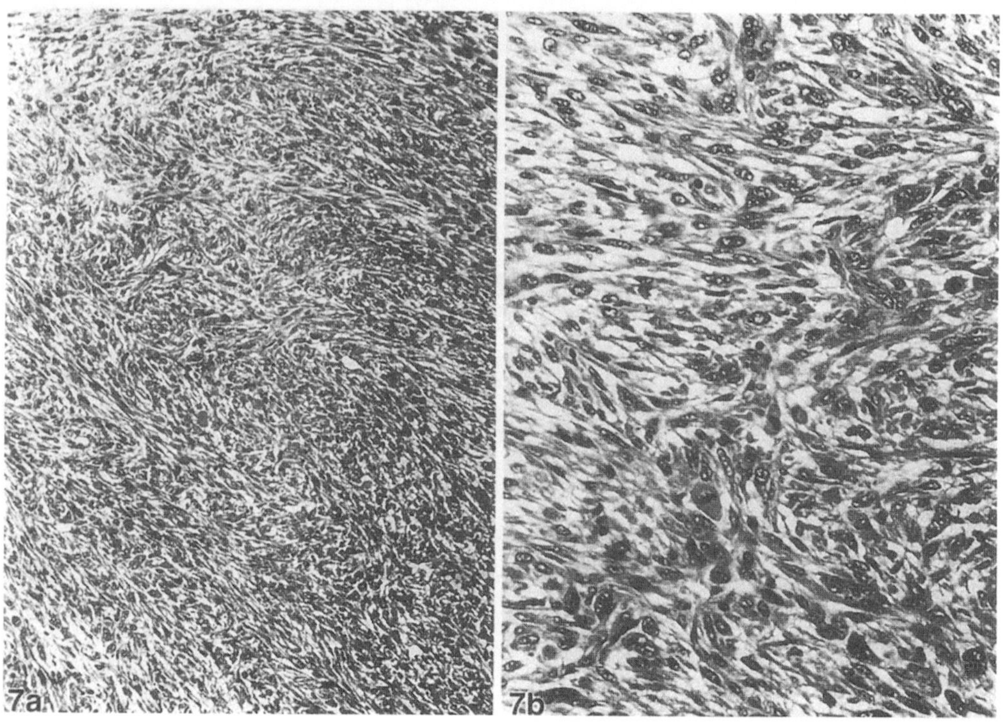

Fig. 6 a, b. Proliferation of fusiform cells. The so-called "fish-bone" pattern, clearly visible (**b**), is relatively characteristic of these sarcomatous fibroblastic groupings

Fig. 7. a Low magnification: uniformity of grouping in bundles of fusiform cells. **b** Higher magnification: anisocytosis, anisokaryosis and some mitoses are evident. The clear appearance of the cytoplasm is quite common in fusiform-cell sarcoma; its importance in the cytoplasmic component and the role of the method of fixation remain to be assessed

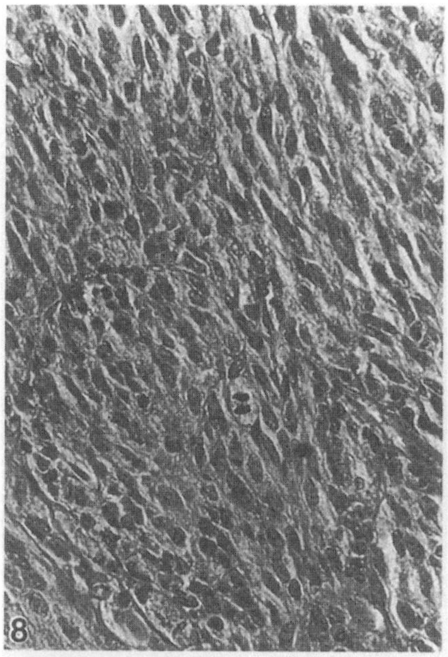

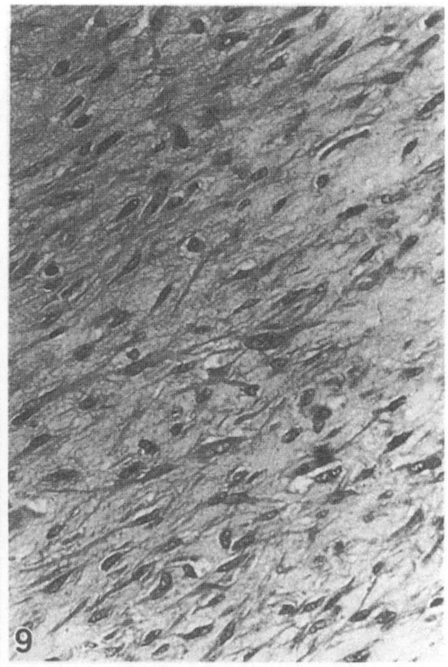

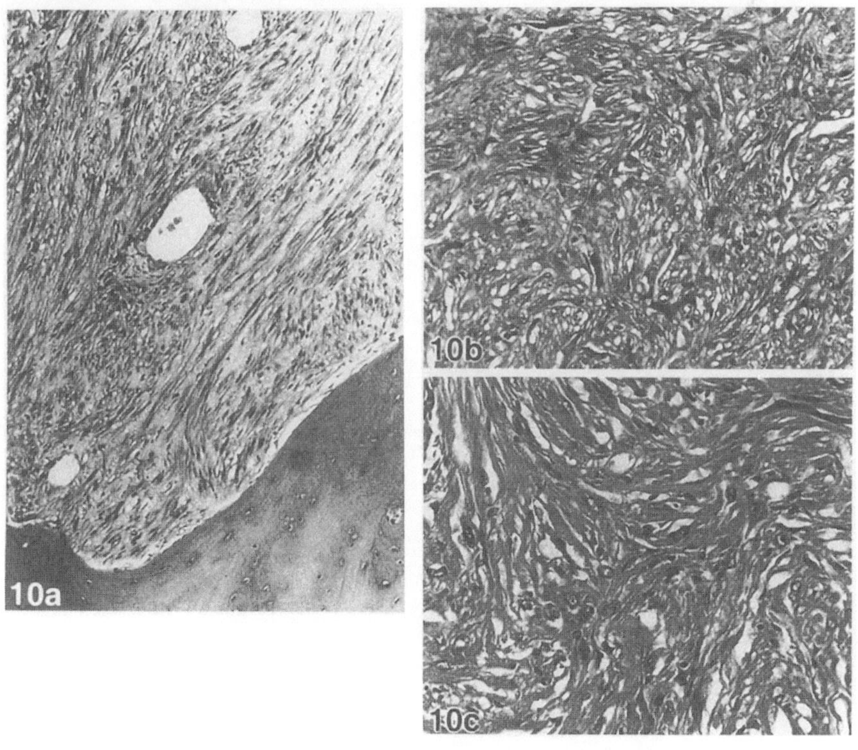

Fig. 8. Parallel cells grouped in bundles, irregular large nuclei; as in the two previous cases the collagen is abundant

Fig. 9. Separated from one another by some collagen fibers, the cells preserve their fusiform appearance despite anomalies (anisocytosis, anisokaryosis)

Fig. 10 a, b, c. At low magnification (**a**) reactive fibrosis is evident: small cells of lymphocytic appearance are scattered throughout the section; but this is a peripheral zone of a collagen-rich sarcoma in which obvious cytological anomalies exclude fibromatosis and desmoid fibroma. **b, c** Fibrous storiform zones suggest a possible diagnosis of malignant fibrous histiocytoma. The appearance is very similar to that of a malignant fibrous histiocytoma (Chapter 16, figs. 9, 10)

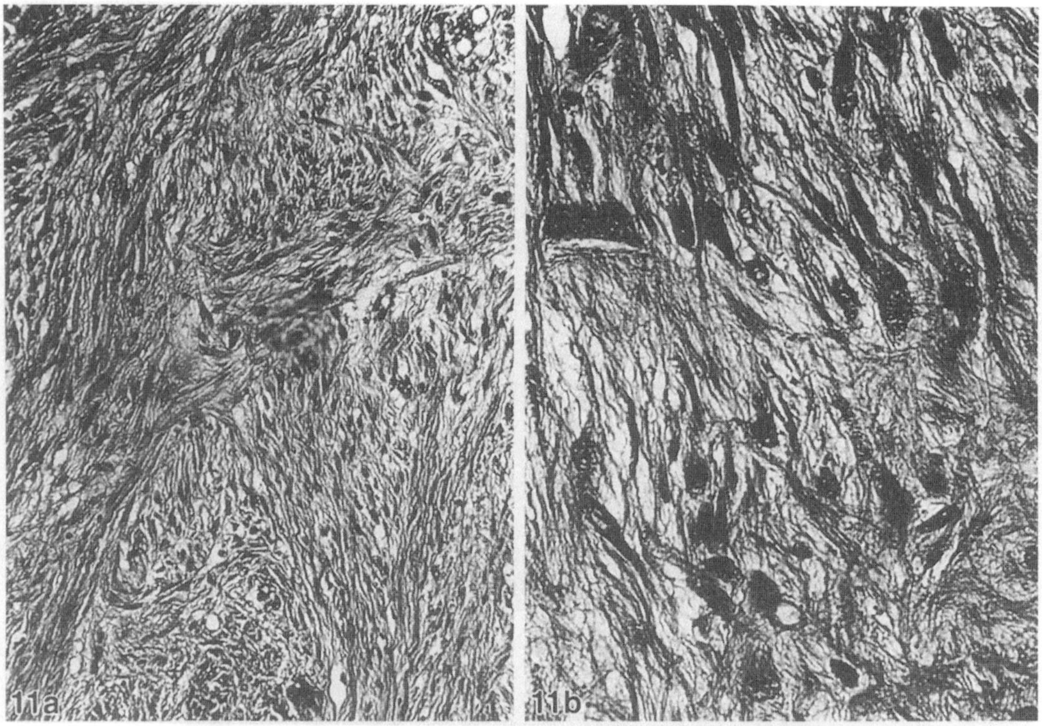

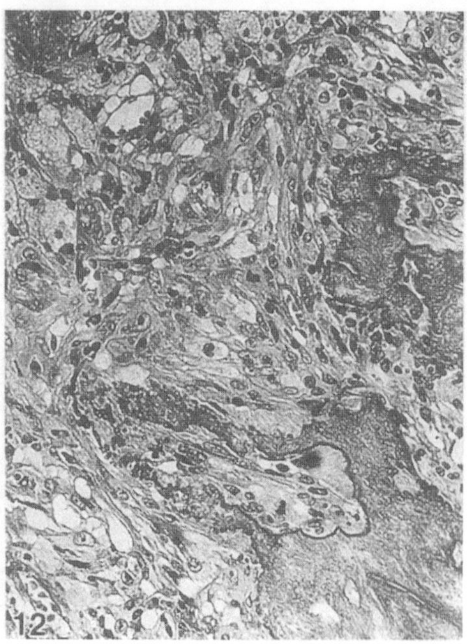

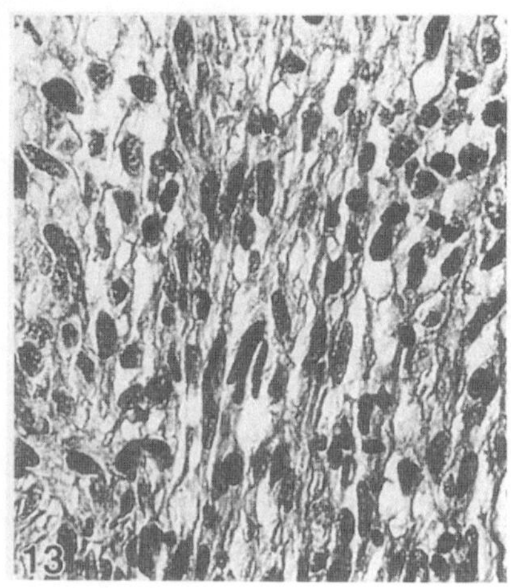

Fig. 11 a, b. Periosteal fibroblastic sarcoma: the cell anomalies increase between the first operation and the second recurrence (fig. 3)

Fig. 12. Fibroblastic sarcoma in contact with old infarct

Fig. 13. The clear aspect of the cytoplasm in this fusiform-cell sarcoma may at first sight suggest a lipoblastic origin

18. Ewing's sarcoma, neuroepithelioma and Askin's tumour

In 1921, Ewing distinguished among round-cell sarcomas a tumour of particularly grave prognosis which he regarded as an endothelioma of bone. Over the decades, discussions on the histiogenesis of this tumour have not provided an unequivocal answer to its origin, and the term "Ewing's sarcoma" without reference to the origin of the cell, has been generally accepted.

Ewing's sarcoma

In 1983, both Aurias et al and Turc-Carel et al discovered a translocation t(11;22)(q24;q12) characteristic for the tumour cells of this sarcoma (fig. 25). In 1975, Angervall and Enzinger had described 39 cases of "a tumour of the soft tissues which cannot be distinguished from Ewing's sarcoma". The validity of this observation was confirmed by the demonstration of the same translocation in this (Ewing's) sarcoma of the soft tissues by Becroft et al in 1984, in a tumour of the postero-superior aspect of the right arm in a child of 9 years, this lesion having no relationship to the underlying bone. In 1969, Lagerkvist et al reported three cases of malignant neuroepithelioma in children aged 4 months, 6 months and 7 years. Two of these tumours were located in the axillary fossa, the third in the paravertebral mediastinal region. Two of them originated from the nerves of the brachial plexus, the other from a thoracic nerve. Ten years later, in 1979, Askin et al described 20 cases of a small-celled thoracic tumour developing in parietal nodules in children and adolescents. Electron microscopy of three of these cases suggested a neuroepithelial origin. In 1981, de Chadarevian et al demonstrated the translocation t(11;22)(q24;q12) in a soft tissue tumour of the left hemithorax and the 5th rib in a girl aged 11.

Since then, cases of malignant neuroepitheliomas of bone have been reported, the first by Jaffe et al in 1984. Jacqueline Whang-Peng et al (1984) found the same chromosomal translocation as that of Ewing's sarcoma in the peripheral cells of these neuroepitheliomas. Ewing's sarcoma possibly represent the most undifferentiated of these primary malignant tumours of neuroectodermal origin.

Case history

In November, Sylvain, aged 10, came for consultation, mainly for pain located just above the right knee. This had been present for some 5-6 weeks, especially in the evenings after returning from school. Fatigue and rowdy games were thought responsible; but for 8-10 days he was more easily tired, rather pale and had lost his usual liveliness. He was slightly febrile at night. The history mentioned a rhinopharyngitis present since his return to school at the beginning of October.

On examination, the lower part of the right thigh was slightly bulkier than the left and a little warmer. In view of the history the diagnosis of osteomyelitis was considered. But though there was slight anaemia and a minor leukocytosis, the standard radiograph was more alarming because of a moth-eaten appearance of the lower third of the femur and a marked lamellar periosteal reaction.

During operation for biopsy of a representative fragment, smears were made on slides and a bacteriological culture. Fragments of fresh tissue were kept for cytogenetic study and also for possible phase-contrast examination and/or tissue culture. Immediate examination of the smears and the cells in phase-contrast made it possible to undertake Sylvain's treatment very quickly. The diagnosis of Ewing's sarcoma was confirmed by study of the paraffin sections and by the pres-

Table 1.

	Ewing	Neuroepithelioma (Askin) pPNETs	Small-celled anaplastic sarcoma
Cellular monomorphism	+	+	±
Rosettes	0	0 or ++	0
Glycogen	++	+ or ±	± or +
HBA71	+ 95%	?	0
NSE	+ 50%	+	0
Dense neurosecretory bodies	0 or very rare	+ or ++	+
Karyotype	t(11;22)(q24;q12)	t(11;22)(q24;q12)	

Reminder:

Embryonal rhabdomyosarcoma	Polyhedral cells Unequal size Eosinophils ++
Neuroblastoma metastases	Estimation of catecholamines and their derivatives ++
Lymphosarcoma	Immunohistology (very rarely intracellular glycogen)

ence of the translocation t(11;22)(q24;q12). Cultures remained sterile.

General considerations

Ewing's sarcomas of bone represent 6-10% of malignant tumours of bone. The black race seems to be virtually spared. There is a slight male predominance of the order of 55-60%. The maximum incidence is between 5 and 15 years of age, after which cases decrease rapidly and the tumour is rare after 30. As with osteogenic sarcoma, the peak incidence is earlier in girls, between 5 and 10 years, and for boys between 10 and 15.

The elective sites are the long bones of the limbs, of which 25-30% of cases are in the femur; next come the tibia and fibula (the two together equally share 15% of cases), the humerus, then the flat bones (pelvis, scapula) and ribs. Except for the sesamoids (at least, to my knowledge), no bone is immune: vertebrae, skull, face, bones of the feet and hands, may all be affected. In the long bones the site is usually metaphyseo-diaphyseal.

Clinical features and course

There is nothing remarkable about the presenting features; usually there is pain, possibly accompanied by a palpable swelling. The general condition often deteriorates. Increase in the ESR, minor fever, anaemia with leukocytosis are all considered to be bad prognostic signs. Very rarely, the regional lymph nodes are invaded and palpable. Such a clinical picture, more or less complete, readily suggests a diagnosis of osteomyelitis.

Rib localisation is deceptive because of the pleuropulmonary symptoms [Voog et al 1964]. A minor rib lesion easily goes unnoticed in standard radiographs. Pleural aspiration withdraws a yellowish or haemorrhagic effusion.

A vertebral lesion may present with dorsal or lumbar pain. Here again, the standard films are not always explicit. Sometimes indirect signs are noted, such as a slight scoliotic posture or, in some cases, a narrowed disk space.

The course of Ewing's sarcoma, the most serious of the bony tumours of childhood, has been transformed by chemotherapy. Before this treatment the 5-year survival rate was of the order of 5%; currently, it is around 50%. This improvement in survival has allowed a better evaluation of prognostic factors. Apart from evident metastatic lesions, the main aggravating factors are location in the trunk, early age at presentation and the presence of fever. In a statistical study of 140 cases from the Mayo Clinic [Wilkins et al 1986], the only significant prognostic factors were elevation of the sedimentation rate, a pelvic location and the presence of metastases.

Imaging

The techniques of modern imaging (CT, MRI, radioisotopes) are capable of detecting an early lesion and define invasion by an already developed tumour; all too often radiological lesions are apparent when the young patient first comes for consultation.

The radiological image of tumour osteolysis is characterised by multiple zones of rarefaction, often extending widely in the metaphysis and diaphysis (figs. 1, 2, 3, 6). This irregular lysis is usually associated with an osteogenic periosteal reaction which lays down multiple concentric layers of newly-formed bone. This reactive osteogenesis thickens the shaft to give a layered or "onion skin" appearance (fig. 4). In the sacral wing, a less common site, an early lesion which merely blurs the bone structure may be missed in a standard film. A rib lesion is also difficult to interpret and the pleural reaction which often accompanies it may lead to a misdiagnosis of a pleuropulmonary disorder.

In many cases, there is extensive osteolysis at the first consultation and, depending on the associated periosteal reaction, differential diagnoses may include osteosarcoma, osteomyelitis, lymphosarcoma and even histiocytosis X (figs. 7-10).

The CT images are therefore of the greatest importance. They demonstrate lesions which are usually much more extensive than the standard films suggest and reveal their extension into the soft tissues. At the first examination, a study supplemented by modern imaging procedures will verify the presence or absence of secondary lesions.

Pathological anatomy and histopathology

The macroscopic appearance is very special; like the hero of Marcel Aymé's novel, *Le Passe-muraille*, Ewing's sarcoma has the ability to traverse the femoral or tibial cortex with astonishing ease. A minimal enlargement of the Volkmann and Haversian canals readily brings the periosteum and medullary cavity into communication. This well known fact accounts for the reluctance of pathologists who refuse to acknowledge the existence of a Ewing's sarcoma developing entirely in the soft tissues.

At operation the surgeon discovers, under a taut deep fascia, if this has not already been breached, a soft friable whitish-gray tumour, in places haemorrhagic and sometimes frankly necrotic. This tissue is removed more easily with the curette than the knife and allows immediate distribution for routine bacteriological examination, smears, various fixations and cytogenetic study. In other cases the bone surface has merely lost its smoothness and a proper biopsy requires bone trephining, so that tumour fragments can be obtained by curettage of the medullary cavity.

It is interesting to add to this account the few published cases of "*subperiosteal*" Ewing's sarcoma. At this site the tumour erodes the surface of the cortex, whose moth-eaten appearance is very disturbing. Wuisman et al (1992) report three cases. However, as I have observed during biopsies at the Hôpital Saint-Vincent-de-Paul (Dr Dubousset), it is important that the greatest caution is called for before asserting that the tumour is entirely subperiosteal (or periosteal) and that the medullary canal is uninvolved.

Whenever possible, phase-contrast examination of the living cells, as performed by us at the Institut Curie with J.-P Thiery, is very important in the context of cytonuclear monomorphism, the disintegrated condition of the chromatin and the punctiform appearance of the nucleoli. In the perinuclear cytoplasmic ring, glycogen forms small gray areas adherent to fine clear lipid droplets. Overall, the appearances are relatively characteristic for a trained pathologist informed of the clinical and imaging findings. In the right conditions, slide smears allow the demonstration of glycogen (Best's carmine, PAS). The study of sections of 2-4 microns in paraffin or of semifine sections leads to findings described for the most part by Ewing in 1921. The tumour consists of cellular areas demarcated by some thick fibrous septa (figs. 13-16), but between the cells there exists neither collagen nor reticulin fibers. The cells, packed together, reproduce no identifiable architecture; their boundaries are visible to a degree depending on the excellence of the fixation. In the absence of spontaneous cell degradation, the rounded or oval cells have nuclei of similar shape but often indented by a deep notch. The finely distributed chromatin predominates at the periphery. One or two nucleoli are clearly visible but are always small compared with the nucleus. As Schajowicz (1959) has shown, the cytoplasm contains fine droplets of glycogen. It is not always possible to demonstrate this glycogen in paraffin sections, especially when the pathologist is not well-versed in fixation; but in every case where fresh tissue is available the glycogen is easily demonstrated in smears and in ultrafine sections (figs. 18, 19) fixed in glutaraldehyde.

Under the electron microscope (figs. 26-29) the cytoplasmic membrane is clearly visible, the nucleolus is small, and the chromatin finely distributed. There are no true cell junctions; mitoses are equally scarce and have only a few ridges. The endoplasmic reticulum is poorly developed. The Golgi apparatus is sometimes quite abundant. In the cytoplasm, areas of glycogen (type alpha) usually jostle against small areas of lipids. Certain special features should be familiar to the pathologist. The abundance of vessels and the arrangement of the cells in concentric rings around the capillaries may at first sight suggest an haemangiopericytoma.

In some cases the tumour cells appear more bulky than usual, hence the term "large-celled Ewing's sarcoma". Rosette appearances may also be seen which may suggest a metastasis from a neuroblastoma or neuroepithelioma. These are in fact pseudo-rosettes, whose centers, devoid of fibrils, are occupied by a cell undergoing necrobiosis.

In optical microscopy, but also in electron microscopy, two cellular appearances may be recognised. Apart from the cells described above there is a second type represented by small cells with dense nuclei, whose interpretation is not unequivocal. Either there is really a second variety of cell or else this is only a degenerative change; the former hypothesis would favor the heterogeneity of Ewing's sarcoma. The coexpression of vimentin and cytokeratin [Moll et al 1987] and the demonstration of monofilaments on ultrastructural examination may possibly support the hypothesis of the heterogeneity of Ewing's tumour. This may be the case in a tumour of the humerus reported by Steiner et al (1995) as a Ewing's sarcoma with epithelial differentiation. These reports should not be allowed to obscure the totipotent nature of the tumour cells and still less the possibility of a continuum ranging from Ewing's sarcoma to neuroepithelioma.

It is important to realise that necrosis may be a considerable hindrance to histological interpretation, hence the justification for immediate frozen section to ensure the validity of the sample.

The cells of Ewing's sarcoma do not produce reticulin fibers. However, when the biopsy has been made on soft tissues outside the bone, silver impregnation often reveals a quite abundant reticulin network. It is easy to recognise the non-tumour origin of this reticulin weave from the patterned nature of its fibers (fig. 17). Lastly, the immunohistological reaction with antibody HBA71 is positive in a high proportion of Ewing's sarcomas, though it is not specific.

In the rare cases of local nodal lesions which I have observed and in the very numerous cases of pulmonary lesions examined, the cell proliferation was pure in type without any trend to osteogenesis or chondrogenesis.

It is to be remembered that the assessment of histological malignancy remains unconvincing in this disease. Mitoses vary greatly in number; their abundance and the sometimes major degree of necrosis constitute unfavourable factors. Invasion of the muscle fibers has also been reported to be a sinister feature [Stratton et al 1982].

Differential diagnosis

In many cases the pathologist has available only a fixed specimen to make his diagnosis. Apart from the diagnosis of osteomyelitis, suggested by the radiographs but easy to exclude, it is the diagnosis from round-cell sarcoma that is posed by biopsy of a Ewing's tumour. In particular, differentiation from lymphosarcoma is important: not the lymphosarcoma with polymorphous cells and irregular nuclei, a large nucleolus and no intracellular glycogen, but the monomorphous lymphosarcoma in which the presence of glycogen droplets may be detectable. Certain features however refute the diagnosis of Ewing's sarcoma: the cells are larger and more irregular, the chromatin is less fine, in particular the nucleoli are not so large. If there is the least doubt, a series of immunocytochemical tests will confirm the diagnosis of lymphosarcoma and specify its variety.

Anaplastic osteogenic sarcoma in its small-celled form has an astonishing resemblance to Ewing's sarcoma. The formation of reticulin fibers is negligible. The same applies to the formation of a few very rare and particularly attenuated osteoid strands, best demonstrated in semifine sections or by electron microscopy [Llombart-Bosch 1987]. These immature cells contain glycogen (PAS +, Best's carmine +). However, the reaction with the antibody anti-ostonectin is positive in osteosarcoma, and negative in Ewing's tumour. Conversely, the demonstration of surface glycoprotein p30/32 M1C2 [Kovar et al 1990, Fellinger et al 1991, 1992, Ambros et al 1991] by the monoclonal antibody HBA71 (or 12E7 for Perlman et al 1994) is positive in around 95% of Ewing's sarcomas and (malignant) PNETs (peripheral neuroectodermal tumours) and negative in osteosarcoma and other small round-cell tumours. Further, according to Roessner and Jürgens (1993) the positivity of the reaction is of real importance in assessing the percentage of viable cells in a tumour biopsy after chemotherapy.

Lee et al (1995) reported two cases of sudoriparous carcinoma which expressed the antigen MIC2 and genetic study of one of these showed the translocation t(11;22) (924;912). The patients were followed annually for 16 years after ablation of the tumour without recurrence or other lesions. The authors suggest that these tumours are forms of Ewing's or PNE tumours of a low grade of malignancy, curable by local surgery. Merkel's tumour, in an as yet undefined proportion of cases, is positive with antibody 12E7 (Perlman et al 1995). However interesting it may be to demonstrate the antibody p30/32MIC2, it seems essential in tumours of the skin and subcutaneous tissue to supplement the examinations with a cytogenetic analysis.

In young children, metastasis from a neuroblastoma must be excluded. The absence of fibrils within the pseudo-rosettes is a very important feature. The diagnosis is confirmed or vitiated by estimation of the catecholamines and their metabolites.

The haemangiopericytic appearance possible in certain Ewing's sarcomas has been mentioned. In haemangiopericytoma the cells are ovoid and larger, and the abundant reticulin around the vessels forms images of encorbellment (successive overlapping from above downwards) (cf Chapter 23). A more important fact to report is the presence of some reticulin fibers around the vessels in Ewing's sarcoma.

In the various diagnoses we have listed, the cellular distribution in compact plaques often intersected by bands of collagen in Ewing's sarcoma is not found.

Neuroepithelioma, like Ewing's tumour is a representative of the primary peripheral neuroectodermal tumours (pPNETs). Its more chromophil cells and the presence of rosettes with a neurofibrillary center allow this classification. As in Ewing's tumour there is the same chromosomal translocation. Ultrastructural examination demonstrates cellular prolongations between the cells, microfilaments at the centers of the rosettes and neurosecretory granules in the cell prolongations.

Apart from the differential diagnoses mentioned above, those of mesenchymal chondrosarcoma, histiocytosis X and embryonal rhabdomyosarcoma may pose serious problems in fine-needle aspiration. However, phase-contrast examination - by pathologists trained in this type of examination - and immunological tests on small cell islands are valuable aids. However this may be, while cytological study by fine-needle aspiration of a metastasis is perfectly logical, the same procedure on a primary tumour requires serious training and caution - humility, even at the expense of our pride, if the patient is to be safeguarded from inadequate treatment.

Cell aspiration allows immediate study in phase-contrast, if the pathologist is adequately trained, and the demonstration within 24 hours by the techniques of molecular biology of the translocation t(11;22), allowing certain classification of the tumour in the group of pPNETs.

Another approach to the detection of translocation has been worked out by Desmaze et al (1992). This consists of hybridising the specific molecular probes of chromosome 22; the proximal probes at the breakpoint are revealed by a green fluorescence and the distal probes by a red fluorescence. In cases of specific remodelling of chromosome 22, the green and red parts of one of the chromosomes 22 are found dissociated in the nucleus, confirming the translocation. The Ewing family of tumours is characterised by a highly recurrent t(11;22)(q24;q12) translocation [Aurias et al 1983, Turc-Carel et al 1983], encountered in about 85% of the tumours [Turc-Carel et al 1988]. Cloning of the breakpoints of the t(11;22) translocation has shown that this rearrangement generates two fusion genes involving the EWS gene, located in band 22q12, and a member of the ETS gene family, the human FLI1 gene, located in band 11q24 [Delattre et al 1992, 1994, Zucman et al 1992]. Fluorescence in situ hybridisation (FISH) with cosmid probes corresponding to loci flanking or overlapping both the 11 and 22 breakpoints is an efficient tool for precise analysis of the classic t(11;22) translocation [Desmaze et al 1992].

In Ewing's sarcoma and peripheral neuroepithelioma (ES/PNE), in which neither classic nor variant or complex t(11;22) translocations have been found, a molecular rearrangement has been demonstrated in most cases. This rearrangement consists of the fusion of the EWS gene with other members of the ETS gene family: the ERG gene, located in band 21q22.2 [Zucman et al 1993], the ETVI gene, located in band 7p22 [Jeon et al 1995], or the E1AF gene, located in band 17q12 [Urano et al 1996].

Neuroepithelioma and Askin's tumour

Case history

A small girl of 5 was admitted as an emergency to the paediatric oncology department of the Institut Curie (Dr Zucker) for serious dyspnoea with chest pain. The child was pale and febrile, and examination showed a slight deformity of the left hemithorax. A standard film showed an ovoid opacity projecting into the chest cavity and involving the mid-portions of the 5th and 6th ribs. There was a haemorrhagic pleural effusion. This child's general condition was poor, so as a first step only needle aspiration was done. The cellular features and the clinical picture, with its costal location in a girl of 5, suggested the possibility of an Askin's tumour, a diagnosis which was subsequently confirmed.

General considerations

In its thoracic location, there seems to exist a marked female predominance, but this finding seems not to be the case in neuroepithelioma of the limbs. The ages of the patients are more spread out than those of patients with Ewing's sarcoma. Lesions of the long bones of the limbs and the pelvic bones have been reported.

Clinical features and course

Pain and swelling are the features that usually attract attention. Fever of above 38° C is also common. In 13 cases reported by Rousselin et al (1989), four cases presented with fracture.

The course of this tumour is grave: recurrences and metastases in the lungs, bones and liver appear rapidly (over three years in the case we describe). Metastases are sometimes detected at the first examination.

Imaging

This shows a lytic tumour which may or may not have destroyed the cortex, depending on the stage of the disease at the time of its recognition. The extensive, poorly defined lysis is predictive of a highly malignant tumour, without its being possible to distinguish it clearly from a Ewing's sarcoma.

Pathological anatomy and histopathology

At operation the tumour is whitish-gray; on section it has scattered small areas of necrosis and haemorrhage. The displaced tissues form a pseudo-capsule at the periphery.

In optical microscopy the tumour consists of small round cells of 10-15 μm, grouped in patches or bands separated by a fibrovascular stroma. The nuclei are round, the chromatin dispersed; they are surrounded by a ring of moderately chromophil cytoplasm. In some zones the cells are grouped in rosettes with a neurofibrillary center but, depending on the case, these abundant rosettes may form a veritable swarm or, in contrast, be rare and difficult to identify. At ultrastructural examination, the nuclei are generally rounded, but some are notched with deep clefts. The mitochondria are moderate in number.

The presence of Homer-Wright rosettes, the cytoplasmic prolongations, the presence of dense neurosecretory bodies and the positive immunohistological reaction to the anti-neuron-specific-enolase of some cells all argue in favor of a neuroectodermal origin.

Differential diagnosis

The differential diagnoses to be considered are largely dependent on the age of the patient. In certain cases in young persons, the most difficult diagnosis to exclude is Ewing's sarcoma. Abundant neurosecretory granules in electron microscopy argue in favor of a neuroepithelioma; the distinction is important as the treatment programs currently used for Ewing's sarcoma are less effective in neuroepithelioma.

Embryonal rhabdomyosarcoma and lymphosarcoma are relatively easy to eliminate.

A metastasis from a poorly differentiated neuroblastoma in a very young child may be very difficult to diagnose without the aid of ultrastructural examination and estimation of catecholamines and their metabolites.

Review of the clinical entity: Askin's tumour

In 1979, Askin distinguished 20 cases of a tumour of thoracic localisation for which he suggested a neuroectodermal origin. Fifteen of the patients were female, all children or adolescents.

Clinical features

Consultation is usually for swelling, but may also be for dyspnoea and chest pain. Examination reveals one or more nodules of 2-4 cm in diameter, whose origin is difficult to pinpoint exactly in view of the virtually constant involvement of the adjacent pleura, diaphragm and ribs. The severe dyspnoea is related to a haemorrhagic pleural effusion and is accompanied by fever. The course is particularly grave.

Imaging

This defines the extent of the tumour, the rib involvement, spread to the pleura and possibly the diaphragm and the extent of the pleural effusion. It does not usually show metastatic lesions at the onset.

Pathological anatomy and histopathology

The macroscopic and microscopic appearances are identical with those described in the previous pages in relation to neuroepithelioma. The pleura is invaded and the osteolysis often affects several ribs.

Secondary bony lesions are very rare, but pulmonary lesions are the rule.

Chadarevian et al (1984) have demonstrated a translocation t(11;22) identical with that of Ewing's sarcoma and neuroepithelioma. However, the cases reported in the literature and those I have observed at the Institut Curie display such a distinctive clinical picture that it is justifiable to single it out as a clinical form within the group of neuroepitheliomas, the "entity" described by Askin.

Continuum or discontinuity of primary peripheral tumours of neuroectodermal origin?

The demonstration of the translocation t(11;22)(q24;q12) by Aurias (team of B. Dutrillaux, Paris) and by Turc-Carel (Dijon) in Ewing's sarcoma, and the subsequent identification of the same translocation in neuro-epithelioma, Askin's tumour and extraskeletal Ewing's tumour, has led many authors to group all these primary peripheral tumours of neuroectodermal origin (pPNETs) under a common heading.

This concept is supported by the immunological test proposed by Ambros et al (1991). The monoclonal antibody HBA71 demonstrates a membrane protein in 95% of pPNETs tested (49/51). This immune reaction, which stains the cell membranes strongly, is applicable to paraffin-embedded material. The reaction is weakly positive in alveolar rhabdomyosarcoma but negative in other small round-celled tumours of children and adolescents (lymphosarcoma, small-celled osteosarcoma, neuroblastoma, retinoblastoma, the blastemic type of nephroblastoma, nonalveolar rhabdomyosarcoma).

Fellinger et al (1992) have confirmed the lack of specificity of the surface antigen recognised by the antibody HBA71 (p30/32 MIC2), which produced a strongly positive immunological reaction in 42 out of 43 Ewing's sarcomas tested. According to Roessner and Jürgens (1993), the positivity of the reaction is of real importance in assessing the percentage of viable cells in a biopsy following chemotherapy. From a somewhat different point of view, the study of Moll et al (1987) of 11 cases of Ewing's sarcoma by immunofluorescence, immuno-ultrastructure and electrophoresis confirm the heterogeneity of Ewing's sarcoma, which may then represent a cellular mosaic at different stages of evolution.

The isotopic kinetic study presented by Perdereau at the Cancerology Forum in Paris (1985) may perhaps be interpreted in the same sense. Multifactorial analysis of the significant variables in the distribution of two osteotropic isotopic tracers ($^{85}SrCl_2$ and ^{99m}Tc MDP) led to the isolation of three groups among 56 patients in whom the diagnosis of Ewing's sarcoma had been established by optical microscopy. The largest group (60%) possibly represents Ewing's sarcoma in the strict sense; the second group (25%) may perhaps concern neuroepitheliomas, the third (15%) concerns other patients.

Hartman et al (1991) distinguish histologically typical Ewing's sarcomas (57%) and atypical sarcomas. The histologically typical sarcomas (all PAS-positive) have a survival rate markedly superior to that of atypical sarcomas and neuroepitheliomas.

Lastly, the same research teams at the Institut Curie (Gilles Thomas and Bernard Dutrillaux) have isolated the genes involved in the translocation t(11;22) and demonstrated a translocation t(21;22) in 10% of Ewing's sarcomas. It is also the same gene of chromosome 22 which is involved in the translocation t(12;22) in clear-cell sarcoma identified as malignant melanoma of the soft tissues [Zucman et al 1993]. It is again chromosome 22 which is incriminated in type 2 neurofibromatosis [Rouleau et al 1993].

It seems wise to refrain from entrenched attitudes which would formally separate or unite Ewing's tumour and PNET [Dehmer 1993]; but it is possible that there is actually a continuum ranging from Ewing's sarcoma to the most differentiated form (neuroepithelioma). However this may be, our paediatric oncology colleagues are well aware that the prognosis of neuroepithelioma is currently graver than that of Ewing's sarcoma.

References

Ambros IM, Ambros PF, Strehl S, Kovar H, Gadner H, Salzer-Kuntschik M (1991) MIC2 is a specific marker for Ewing's sarcoma and peripheral primitive neuroectodermal tumors: evidence for a common histogenesis of Ewing's sarcoma and peripheral primitive neuroectodermal tumors from MIC2 expression and specific chromosome aberration. Cancer 67: 1886-1893

Angervall L, Enzinger FM (1975) Extraskeletal neoplasm resembling Ewing's sarcoma. Cancer 36: 240-251

Askin FB, Rosai J, Sibley RK, Dehmer LP, McAlister HW (1979) Malignant small cell tumor of the thoracopulmonary region in childhood. A distinctive clinicopathologic entity of uncertain histogenesis. Cancer 43: 2438-2451

Aurias A (1988) Données cytogénétiques dans les sarcomes des os et des tissus mous. Bull Cancer 75: 423-429

Aurias A, Rimbaud C, Buffe d, Zucker IM, Mazabraud A (1984) Translocation involving chromosome 22 in Ewing's sarcoma. A cytogenetic study of four fresh tumors. Cancer Genet Cyto 12: 21-25

Aurias A, Rimbaut C, Buffe D, Dubousset J, Mazabraud A (1983) Translocation du chromosome 22 dans le sarcome d'Ewing. CR Acad Sc Paris 296: 1105-1107

Aurias A, Rimbaut C, Buffe D, Dubousset J, Mazabraud A (1983) Chromosomal translocation in Ewing's sarcoma. N Engl J Med 309, 8: 496-498

Bator SM, Bauer TW, Marks KE, Norris DG (1986) Periosteal Ewing's sarcoma. Cancer 58: 1781-1784

Becroft DMO, Pearson A, Shaw RL, Zwi LG (1984) Chomosomal translocation in extraskeletal Ewing's tumor. Lancet 8399, 2: 400

Bolen JW, Thorning D (1980) Peripheral neuroepithelioma: a light and electron microscopic study. Cancer 46: 2456-2462

Bouziani A, Ben Rejeb A, Mazabraud A, Jagueux M, Orcel L (1987) Le sarcome Ewing. Etude rétrospective de 108 cas avec revue de la littérature. Arch Inst Pasteur Tunis 64, 3: 327-340

Carey PJ, Malcom AJ, Pearson ADJ, Kemshead TK, Reid MM (1988) Immunocytochemical detection of tumors of neuroectodermal origin. J Clin Pathol 41: 586-589

Carter RL, Al-Sam SZ, Corbett RP, Clinton S (1990) A comparative study of immunohistochemical staining for neuronspecific enolase, protein gene product 9.5 and S-100 protein in neuroblastoma, Ewing's sarcoma and other round cell tumours in children. Histopathology 16: 461-467

Cavazzana AO, Miser JS, Jefferson J, Triche TJ (1987) Experimental evidence for a neural origin of Ewing's sarcoma of bone. Am J Pathol 127: 507-518

Chadarevian JP, Vekemans M, Seemayer T (1984) Reciprocal translocation in small-cell sarcomas (letter). N Engl J Med 311: 1702

Dehmer LP (1993) Primitive neuroectodermal tumors and Ewing's sarcomas. Am J Surg Pathol 16: 192-193

Delattre O, AzambuJa JC, Aurias A, Zucman J, Peter M, Zhang F, Hors-Cayla MC, Rouleau G, THomas G (1991) Mapping of human chromosome 22 with a panel of somatic cell hybrids. Genomics 9: 721-727

Delattre O, Zucman J, Plougastel B, Desmaze C, Melot T, Peter M, Kovar H, Joubert I, Dejong P, Rouleau G, Rouleua G, Aurias A, Thomas G (1992) Gene fusion with an ETS DNA-binding domain caused by chromosome translocation in human tumors. Nature 359: 162-165

Delattre O, Zucman J, Melot T, Sastre X, Zucker JM, Lenoir G, Ambros P, Sheer D, Turc-Carel C, Triche T, Aurias A, Thomas G (1994) The Ewing family of tumours: a subgroup of small round cell tumours defined by specific chimeric transcripts. New Engl J Med 331: 294-299

Desmaze C, Zucman J, Delattre O, Thomas G, Aurias A (1992) Unicolor and bicolor in situ hybridization in the diagnosis of peripheral neuroepithelioma and related tumors. Genes Chromosomes Cancer 5: 1-5

Dickman PS, Triche TJ (1986) Extraosseous Ewing's sarcoma versus primitive rhadomyosarcoma. Diagnostic criteria and clinical correlation. Hum Pathol 17: 881-893

Ehara S, Kattapuram SV, Egglin TK (1991) Ewing sarcoma. Radiographic pattern of healing and bony complications in patients with long-term survival. Cancer 68: 1531-1535

Ewing J (1921) Diffuse endothelioma of bone. Proc New York. Path Soc 21: 17-24

Fellinger EJ, Garin-Chesa P, Glasser DB, Huvos AG, Rettig WG (1992) Comparison of cell surface antigen HBA71 (p30/32MIC2), neuron-specific enolase, and vimentin in the immunohistochemical analysis of Ewing's sarcoma of bone. Am J Surg Pathol 16: 746-755

Frouge C, Vanel D, Coffre C, Couanet D, Contesso G, Sarrazin D (1988) The role of magnetic resonance imaging in the evaluation of Ewing's sarcoma. A report of 27 cases. Skeletal Radiol 17: 387-392

Garand R, Nomballais F, Lemevel A, Mouraud E, Lemevel B (1981) Leucémie aiguë myéloblastique après sarcome d'Ewing: complication iatrogène? Bull Cancer (Paris) 68: 25-31

Gonzalez Crussi F, Wolfson SL, Migusi K, Nakajima T (1984) Peripheral neuroectodermal tumor (neuroepithelioma) of the chest wall. Cancer 54: 2519-2527

Haas OA, Chott A, Ladenstein R, Gardner H (1987) Poorly differentiated, neuron-specific enolase positive round cell tumor with two translocations t(11; 22) and t(21; 22). Cancer 60: 2219-2223

Haimoto H, Tkahashi Y, Koshikawa T, Nagura H, Kato K (1985) Immuno-histochemical localization of enolase in normal human tissues other than nervous and neuroendocrine tissues. Lab Invest 52: 257-263

Hartman KR, Triche TJ, Kinsella TJ, Miser JS (1991) Prognostic value of histopathology in Ewing's sarcoma. Long-term follow-up of distal extremity primary tumors. Cancer 67: 163-171

Isayama T, Iwasaki H, Kikuchi M, Yoh S, Tkagishi N (1990) Neuroectodermal tumor of bone. Evidence for neural differentiation in a cultured cell line. Cancer 65: 1771-1781

Jaffe R, Santamaria M, Yunis EJ, Agastini RM, Medina J, Goodman H (1984) The neurocctodermal tumor of bone. Am J Surg Pathol 8: 885-898

Jeon IS, Davis JN, Braun BS, Sublett JE, Roussel MF, Denny CT, Shapiro DN (1995) A variant Ewing's sarcoma translocation (7; 22) fuses the EWS gene to the ETS gene ETV1. Oncogene 10: 1229-1234

Jürgens H, Bier V, Harms D, Beck G, Brandeis W, Etsptiler G, Gardner H, Schmidt D, Treuner J, Wilkler K, Gôbel V (1988) Malignant peripheral neuroectodermal tumors. A retrospective analysis of 42 patients. Cancer 61: 349-357

Kahn HJ, Thorner PS (1989) Monoclonal antibody MB2: a potential marker for Ewing's sarcoma and primitive neuroectodermal tumor. Pediatric Pathol 9: 153-162

Kontozoglou T, Krakauer K, Qilzilbash AH (1986) Ewing's sarcoma cytologic features in fine needle aspirates in two cases. Acta Cytol 30: 513-518

Kovar H, Dworzak M, Strehl S, Schnell E, Ambros IM, Ambros PF, Gardner H (1990) Over expression of the pseudoautosomal gene M1C2 in Ewing's sarcoma and peripheral primitive ectodermal tumor. Oncogene 5: 1067-1070

Ladanyi M, Heinemann FS, Huvos AG, Rao PH, Chen Q, Jhanwar SC (1990) Neural differentiation in small round cell tumors of bone and soft tissue with the translocation t(ll; 22)(q24; q12): an immunohistochemical study of 11 cases. Hum Pathol 21: 1245-1251

Lagerkvist B, Ivemark B, Sylven B (1969) Malignant neuroepithelioma in childhood. A report of three cases. Acta Chir Scand 135: 641-645

Lee CS, Southey MC, Slater H, Auldist AW, Chow CW, Venter DJ (1995) Primary cutaneous Ewing's sarcoma peripheral primitive neuroectodermal tumors in childhood. A molecular, cytogenetic and immunohistochemical study. Diagn Mol Pathol 4: 174-181

Leroy JP, Volant A, Mazabraud A (1984) Les sarcomes d'origine nerveuse. Sem Hôp Paris 60, 29: 2081-2086

Linnoila RI, Tsokos M, Triche TJ, Marangos PJ, Chandra RS (1986) Evidence for neural origin and PAS-positive variants of the malignant small cell tumor of thoracopulmonary region (Askin tumor). Am J Surg Pathol 10: 124-133

Lipinski M, Braham K, Caillaud JM, Carlu C, Tursz T (1983) HNK-I antibody detects and antigen expressed on neuroectodermal cells. J Exp Med 158: 1775-1780

Lipinski M, Braham K, Philip I, Wiels J, Philip T, Dellagi K, Goridis C, Lenoir GM, Tursz T (1986) Phenotypic characterization of Ewing sarcoma cell lines with monoclonal antibodies. J Cell Biochem 31: 289-296

Lipinski M, Braham K, Philip I, Wiels J, Philip T, Goridis C, Lenoir GM, Tursz T (1987) Neuroectodermal-associated antigens on Ewing's sarcoma cell lines. Cancer Res 47: 183-187

Lipinski M, Tursz T (1982) Tumeur d'Ewing: origine neuroectodermique? Analyse à l'aide d'anticorps monoclonaux. Research 42: 706-711

Lipinski M, Turzs T (1988) Apports de l'immunologie et de la biologie moléculaire. Bull Cancer 75: 417-421

Llombart-Bosch A, Lacombe JT, Olaya AP, Contesso G (1989) Peripheral neuroectodermal sarcoma of soft tissue (peripheral neuroepithelioma): a pathologic study of ten cases with differential diagnosis regarding other small, round-cell sarcomas. Hum Pathol 20: 273-280

Llombart-Bosch A, Lacombe MJ, Contesso G, Peydro-Olaya A (1987) Small round blue cell sarcoma of bone mimicking atypical Ewing's sarcoma with neuroectodermal features. An analysis of five cases with immunohistochemical and electron microscopical support. Cancer 60: 1570-1582

Lloreta J, Tusquets I, Prieto V, Serrano S, Prat J (1990) Primary neuroectodermal tumor of bone. Report of a case in an adult. Surg Pathol 3: 325-331

Mark A, Israel MA, Thiele C, Whang-Peng J, Koa-Shan CS, Triche TJ, Miser J (1985) Peripheral neuroepithelioma: genetic analysis of tumor derived cell lines. Advances in neuroblastoma research, pp. 161-170

Moll R, Lee I, Gould VE, Berndt R, Franke WW (1987) Immunocytochemical analysis of Ewing's tumors patterns of expression of intermediate filaments and desmosomal proteins indicate cell type heterogeneity and pluripotential differentiation. Am J Pathol 127: 288-304

Nesbitt KA, Vidone RA (1976) Primitive neuroectodermal tumor (neuroblastome) arising in sciatic nerve of a child. Cancer 37: 1562-1570

Oberling CH (1928) Le réticulo-sarcome et le réticulo-endothélio-sarcome de la moelle osseuse (sarcomes d'Ewing). Bull Cancer 17: 259-296

Oberling CH, Raileaou C (1932) Nouvelles recherches sur les réticulosarcomes de la moelle osseuse (sarcomes d'Ewing). Bull Cancer 21: 333-345

Pagès A (1981) Pathologie de la crête neurale. Ann Pathol 1: 109-119

Parham DM, Thompson E, Fletcher B, Meyer WH (1991) Metastatic small cell tumor of bone with true rosettes and glial fibrillary acidic protein positivity. Am J Clin Pathol 95: 166-171

Perlman EJ, Dickman PS, Askin FB, Grier HE, Miser JS, Link MP (1994) Ewing sarcoma-routine diagnostic utilisation of M1C2 analysis: A pediatric oncology group-/ Childrens cancer group intergroup study. Hum Pathol 25: 304-307

Perlman EJ, Lumadue JA, Hawkins AL, Cohen K, Colombani P, Griffin CA (1995) Primary cutaneous neuroendocrine tumors. Diagnostic use of cytogenetic and M1C2 analysis. Cancer Genet Cytogenet 82: 30-34

Rettig WJ, Garin-Chesa P, Huvos AG (1992) Ewing's sarcoma: new approaches to histogenesis and molecular plasticity. Editorial Lab Invest 66: 133-137

Reynolds CP, Smith RG, Frenkel EP (1981) The diagnostic dilemma of the "small round cell neoplasm" catecholamine fluorescence and tissue culture morphology as markers for neuroblastoma. Cancer 48: 2088-2094

Rimbaud C, Mazabraud A, Aurias A, Thiery JP, Buffe D (1983) Ewing's sarcoma graft on nude rat. Typing of cytological and cytogenetic characteristics. 11th meeting of the Int Soc Onco-developmental Biol, Stockholm

Roessner A, Jürgens H (1993) Round cell tumors of bone. Path Res Pract 189: 1111-1136

Rouleau GA, Merel P, Lutchman M, Sanson M, Zucman J, Marineau C, Hoang-Xuant K, Demczuk S, Desmaze C, Plougastel B, Pulst S, Lenoir G, Bijlsma E, Fashold R, Dumanski J, deJong P, Parry D, Eldrige R, Aurias A, Delattre O, Thomas G (1993) Alteration in a new gene encoding a putative membrane-organizing causes neuro-fibromatosis type 2. Nature 363: 515-521

Rousselin B, Vanel D, Lacombe MJT, Istria BJM, Spielman M, Masselot J (1989) Clinical and radiologic analysis of 13 cases of primary neuroectodermal tumors of bone. Skeletal Radiol 18: 115-120

Rud NP, Reiman HM, Pritchard DJ, Frassica FJ, Smithson WA (1989) Extraosseous Ewing's sarcoma. A study of 42 cases. Cancer 64: 1548-1553

Schajowicz F (1959) Ewing's sarcoma and reticulum cell sarcoma of bone, with special reference to the histochemical demonstration of glycogen as an aid to differential diagnosis. J Bone Joint Surg 41A: 349-356

Siegal GP, Oliver WR, Reinus WR, Gilula LA, Foulkes MA, Kissane JM, Askin FB (1987) Primary Ewing's sarcoma involving the bones of the head and neck. For the intergroup Ewing's sarcoma study. Cancer 60: 2829-2840

Stéfani (de) E, Carzoglio J, Deneo Pellegrini H, Olivera L, Cendan M, Kasdorf H (1984) Ewing's sarcoma: value of tumor necrosis as a predictive factor. Bull Cancer (Paris) 71: 16-21

Steiner GC, Matano S, Present D (1995) Ewing sarcoma of humerus with epithelial differentiation. Skeletal Radiol 24: 379-382

Stephenson CF, Bridge JH, Sandberg AA (1992) Cytogenetic and pathologic aspects of Ewing's sarcoma and neuroectodermal tumors. Hum Pathol 23: 1270-1277

Stout AP (1918) A tumor of the ulnar nerve. Proc NY Pathol Soc 18: 2-12

Stratton B, Askin FB, Kissane JM (1982) Intramyofiber skeletal muscle invasion in Ewing's sarcoma of bone. Clinicopathologic observation from the intergroup Ewing's sarcoma study. Am J Pediatr Hematol Oncol 4: 231

Tayton KJJ (1980) Ewing's sarcoma at the site of a metal plate. Cancer 45: 413-415

Thomas G (1992) Identification des gènes impliqués dans la translocation t(11;-22) caractéristique du sarcome d'Ewing. Médecine-Sciences 8: 994-995

Triche TJ (1988) Diagnosis of small round cell tumors of childhood. Bull Cancer 75: 297-310

Triche TJ, Askin FB (1983) Neuroblastoma and the differential diagnosis of small-, round-, blue-cell tumors. Hum Pathol 14: 569-595

Turc-Carel C, Aurias A, Mugneret F, Lizard S, Sidaner I, Volk C, Thiery JP, Olschwzan S, Philip I, Berger MP, Philip T, Lenoir GM, Mazabraud A (1988) Chromosomes in Ewing's sarcoma. An evaluation of 85 cases and remarkable consistency of t(11;-22)(q24;-q12). Cancer Genet Cytogenet 32: 229-238

Turc-Carel C, Philip I, Berger MP, Philip T, Lenoir GM (1983) Chromosomal translocation in Ewing's sarcoma. N Engl J Med 309: 497-498

Turc-Carel C, Philip I, Berger MP, Philip T, Lenoir GM (1984) Chromosome study of Ewing's sarcoma (ES) cell lines: consistency of a reciprocal translocation t(ll;-22)(q24;-ql2). Cancer Genet Cytogenet 12: 1-19

Urano F, Umezawa A, Hong W, Kikuchi H, Hata J (1996) A novel chimera gene between EWS and E1AF, encoding the adenovirus E1A enhancer-binding protein, in extaosseus Ewing's sarcoma. Biochem Biophys Res Commun 219: 608-612

Vecchio G, Cavazzana AO, Triche TJ, Ron D, Reynolds CP, Eva A (1989) Expression of the dbl proto-oncogene in Ewing's sarcomas. Oncogene 4: 897-900

Voog R, Couderc P, Barrie J (1964) Sarcome d'Ewing costal révélé par un hémothorax spontané. J Fr Med Chir Thor 18: 449-456

Wang-Peng J, Triche TJ, Knutsen T, Miser J, Kao-Shan S, Tsai S, Israel MA (1986) Cytogenetic characterization of selected small round cell tumor of childhood. Cancer 21: 185-208

Whang-Peng J, Triche TJ, Knutsen T, Miser J, Douglass EC, Israel MA (1984) Chromosome translocation in peripheral neuroepithelioma. N Engl J Med 311: 584-585

Wilkins RM, Pritchard DJ, Burget EO, Unni KK (1986) Ewing's sarcoma of bone. Experience with 140 patients. Cancer 58: 2551-2555

Wuisman P, Roesner A, Blasius S, Erlemann R, Winkelmann W, Ritter J (1992) (Sub) periosteal Ewing's sarcoma of bone. J Cancer Res Clin Oncol 118, 1: 72-74

Zucker JM, Michon J, Mazabraud A, Quintana E, Bataini JP (1983) Sarcome d'Ewing. Rev Prat 33: 1169-1183

Zucman G, Delattre O, Desmaze C, Epstein AL, Stenman G, Speleman F, Fletchers CDM, Aurias A, Thomas G (1993) EWS and ATF-I gene fusion induced by t(l2;-22) translocation in malignant melanoma of soft parts. Nature Genetics 4: 341-345

Zucman J, Delattre O, Desmaze C, Plougastel B, Joubert I, Melot T, Peter M, Dejang P, Rouleau G, Aurias A, Thomas G (1992) Cloning and characterization of the Ewing's sarcoma and peripheral neuroepthelioma t(11;-22) translocation breakpoints. Genes Chromosomes and Cancer 5: 271-277

Zucman J, Melot T, Desmaze C, Ghysdael J, Plougastel B, Peter M, Zucker JM, Triche T, Sheer D, Turc-Carel C, Ambros P, Combaret V, Lenoir G, Aurias A, Thomas G, Delattre O (1993) Combinatorial generation of variable fusion proteins in peripheral primitive neuroectodermal tumors. EMBO 12: 4481-4487

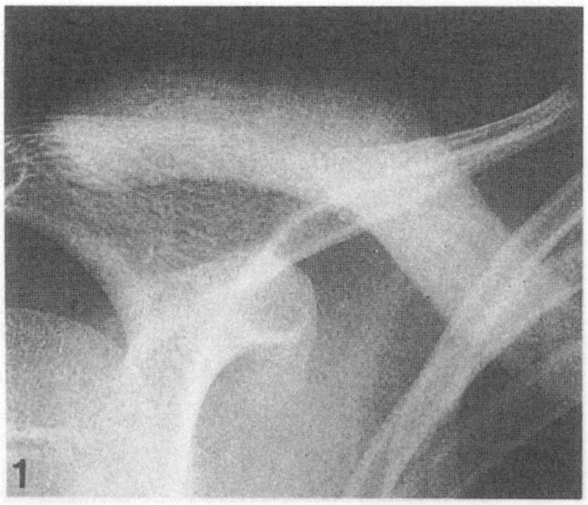

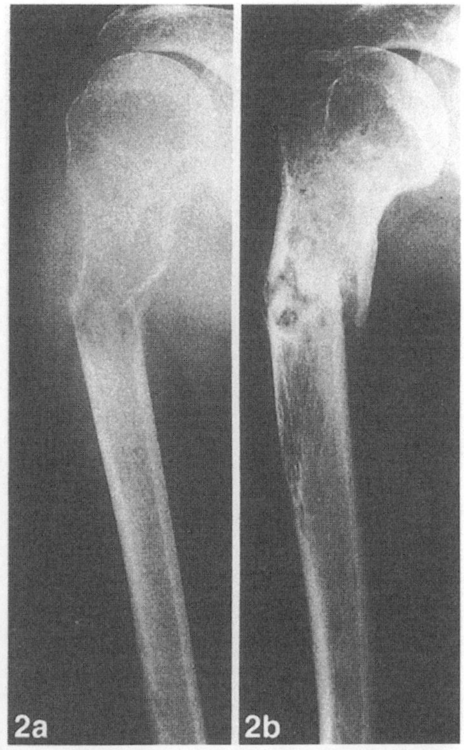

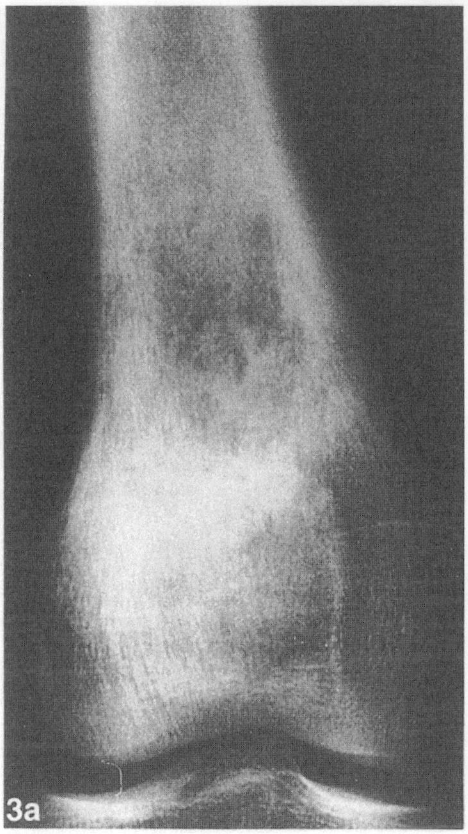

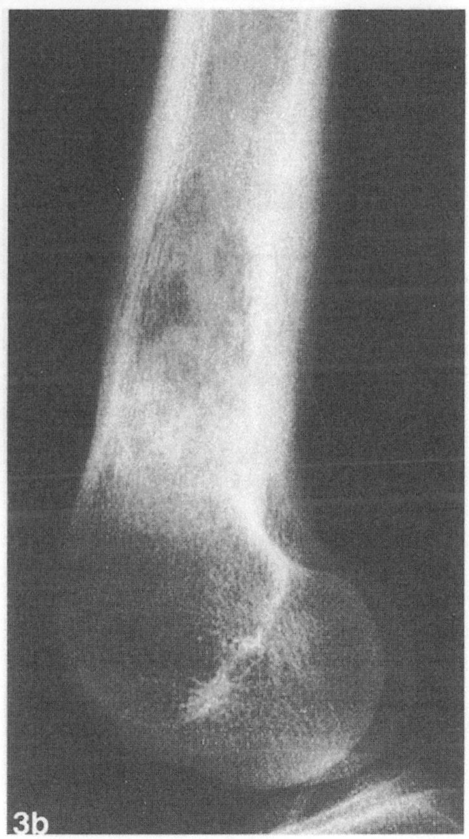

Fig. 1. Slightly thickened outer third of clavicle: the definition of the cortices is replaced by a finely moth-eaten blurred spongiosa

Fig. 2. a Ewing's sarcoma of upper third of humerus complicated by fracture, treated at the time by irradiation (cobalt). **b** 10 months later: some recalcification, fracture ununited. Woman aged 23

Fig. 3 a, b. Ill-defined osteolytic tumour of lower end of femur: innumerable small erosions of the cortex give a finely areolar moth-eaten appearance. The benign lamellar periosteal apposition is barely visible in these films

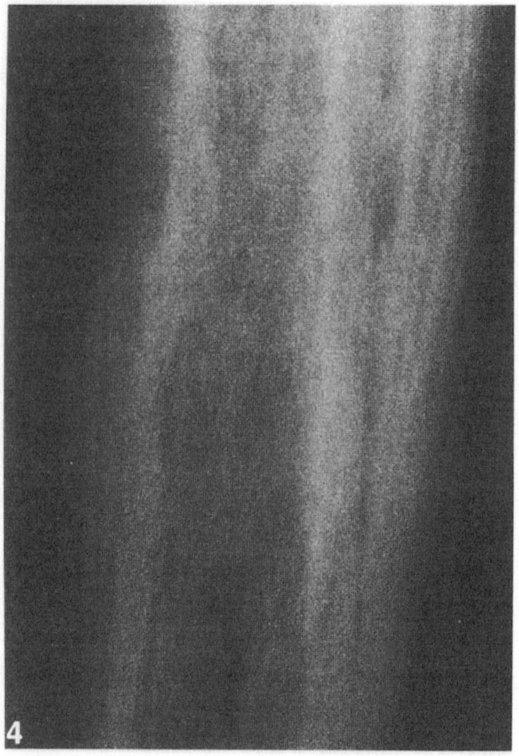

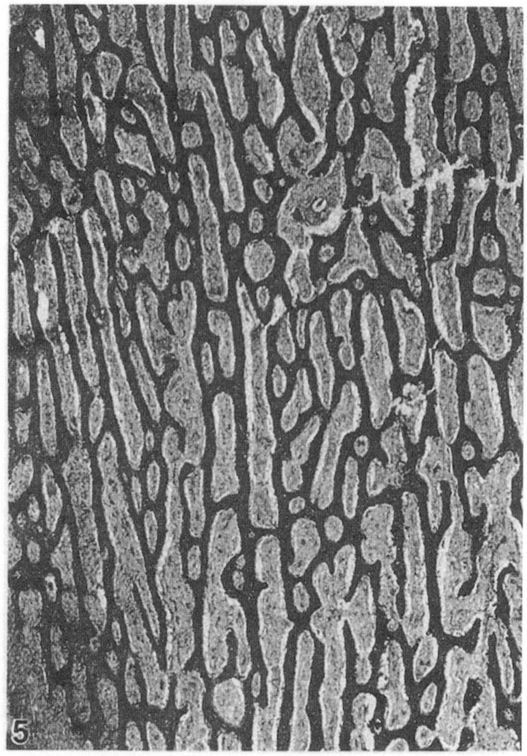

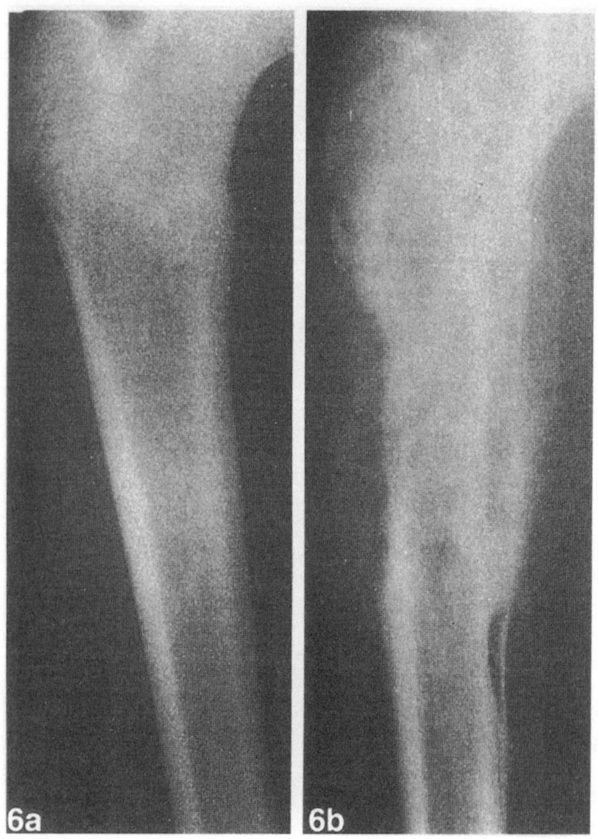

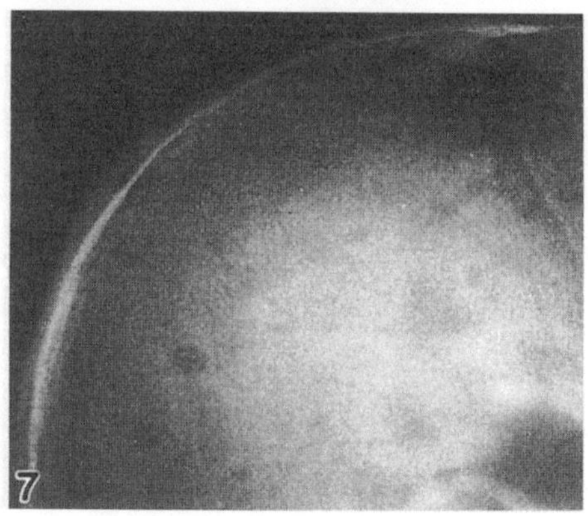

Fig. 4. Sarcoma of diaphyseal region of femur. The bone is thickened and the virtually destroyed original cortex is replaced by a lamellar periosteal osteogenesis, thickening the diaphysis and visible in the lateral and medial tangential zones. Girl aged 11

Fig. 5. Histological appearance of benign periosteal apposition

Fig. 6. a The blurred appearance of the upper third of the femur did not attract attention for lack of an ordinary comparative film of the other limb. **b** Seven months later the film shows the rapid advance of this Ewing's sarcoma. Boy of 13

Fig. 7. "Punched-out" zones of cranial osteolysis: metastatic lesions of Ewing's sarcoma (fig. 6 a, b)

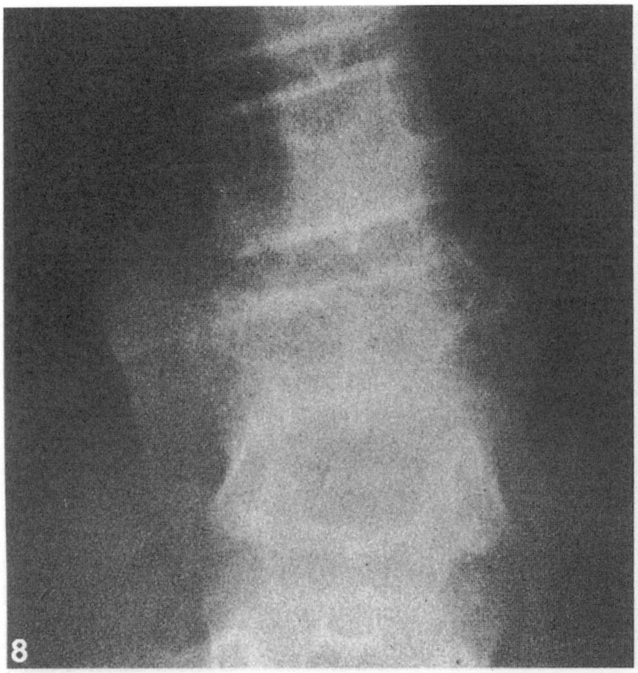

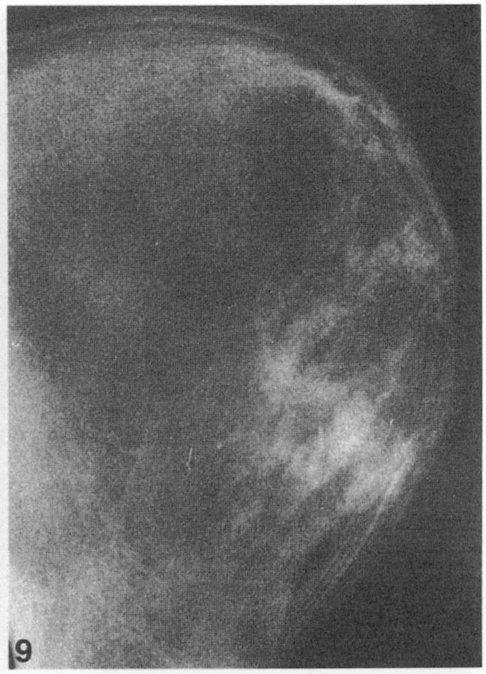

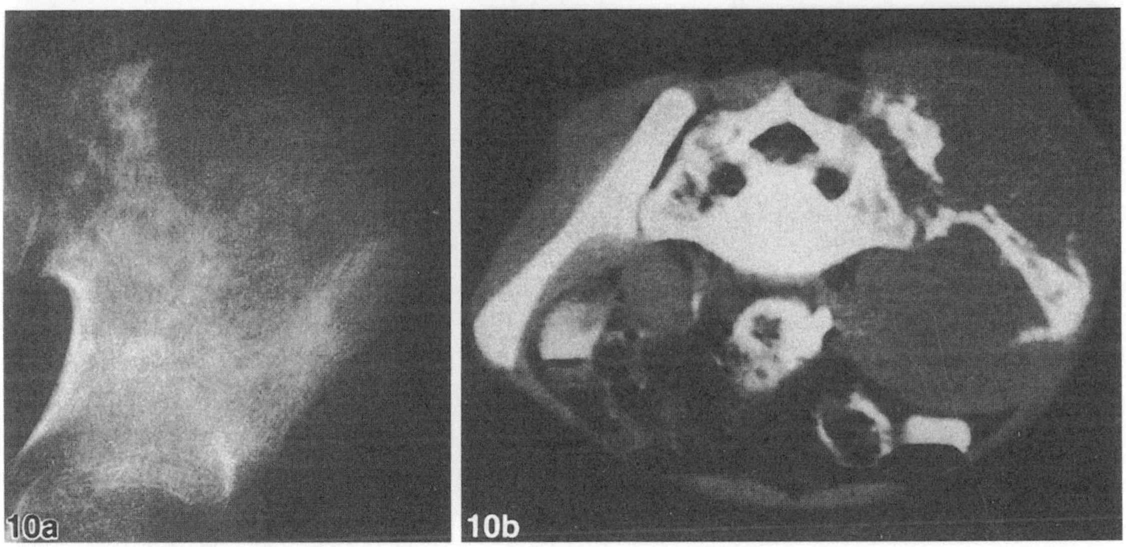

Fig. 8. Almost total destruction by Ewing's sarcoma of the body of vertebra T11

Fig. 9. Extensive zones of osteolytic remodelling of ilium. The sarcoma widely invades the soft tissues. Young girl of 15

Fig. 10 a, b. Ewing's sarcoma of left ilium. **a** In this standard radiograph, there is the image of both a lytic and a sclerosing tumour, ill-defined, destroying the cortex of the left ilium. **b** This CT image readily allows study of the bony lesions: lysis, sclerosis, cortical destruction and periosteal reactions, and the involvement of soft parts

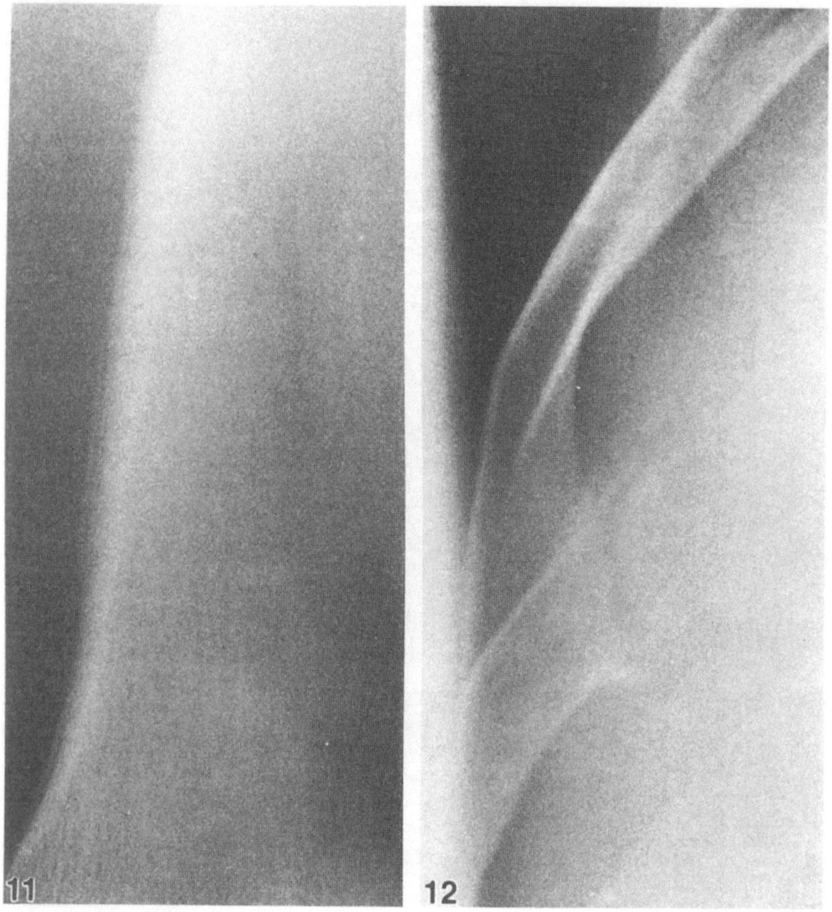

Fig. 11. Neuroepithelioma of lower end of femur in a boy of 13. Mild pain led to this radiograph, which shows slight thickening of the outer border by apposition of periosteal bony lamellae, as well as osteolysis and a roughened appearance of the bony tissue

Fig. 12. This Askin tumour is evidenced by a localised lysis of the 8th rib

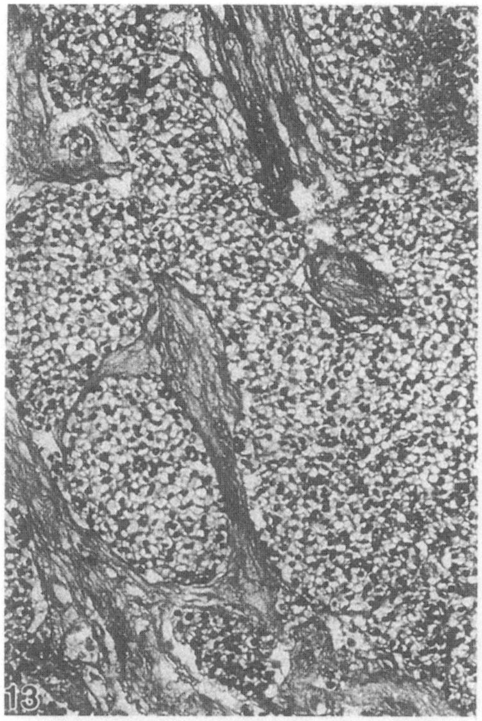

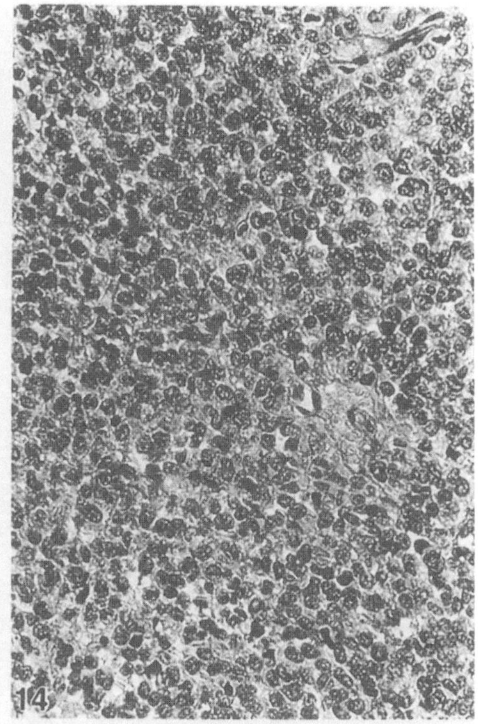

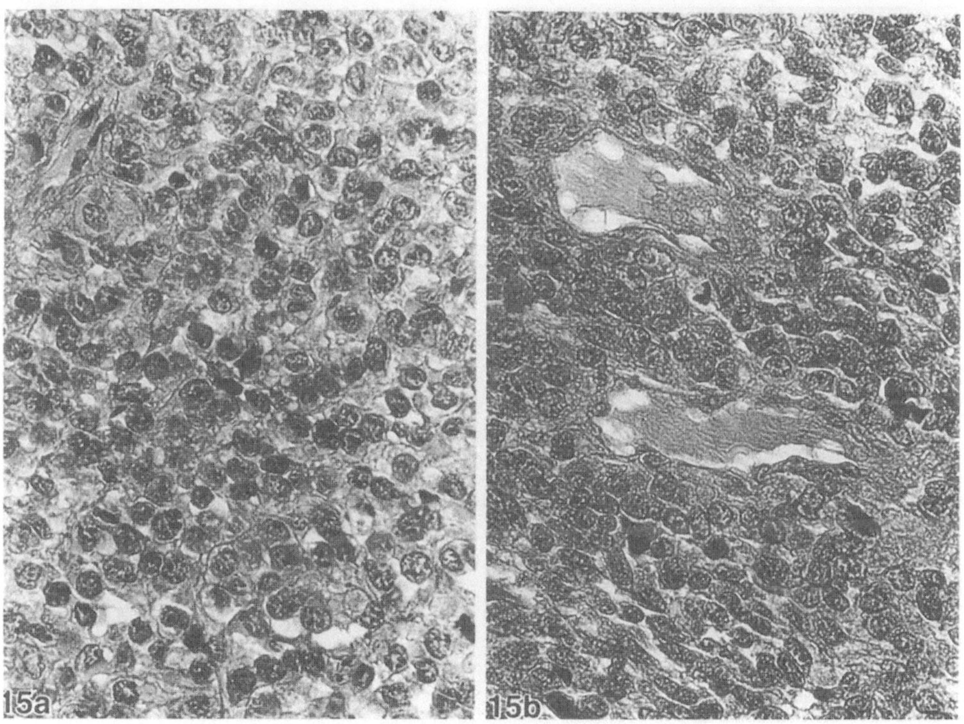

Fig. 13. Biopsy of sarcoma of clavicle (fig. 1). The cell proliferation between the fibrous septa that partition it consists of units of uniform size with clear cytoplasm. Some biopsies of Ewing's sarcomas have this clear appearance of the glycogen-rich cells, probably largely due to the method of fixation

Fig. 14. Sarcomatous proliferation appearing monomorphous. Nuclei are round or slightly ovoid; some appear dense

Fig. 15 a, b. At this magnification, cytonuclear inequalities are seen and some nuclei are notched. The chromatin is dispersed in fine granules, the cytoplasm is pale, but the cell boundaries are clearly visible. Mitoses are rare, the vessels are clearly seen

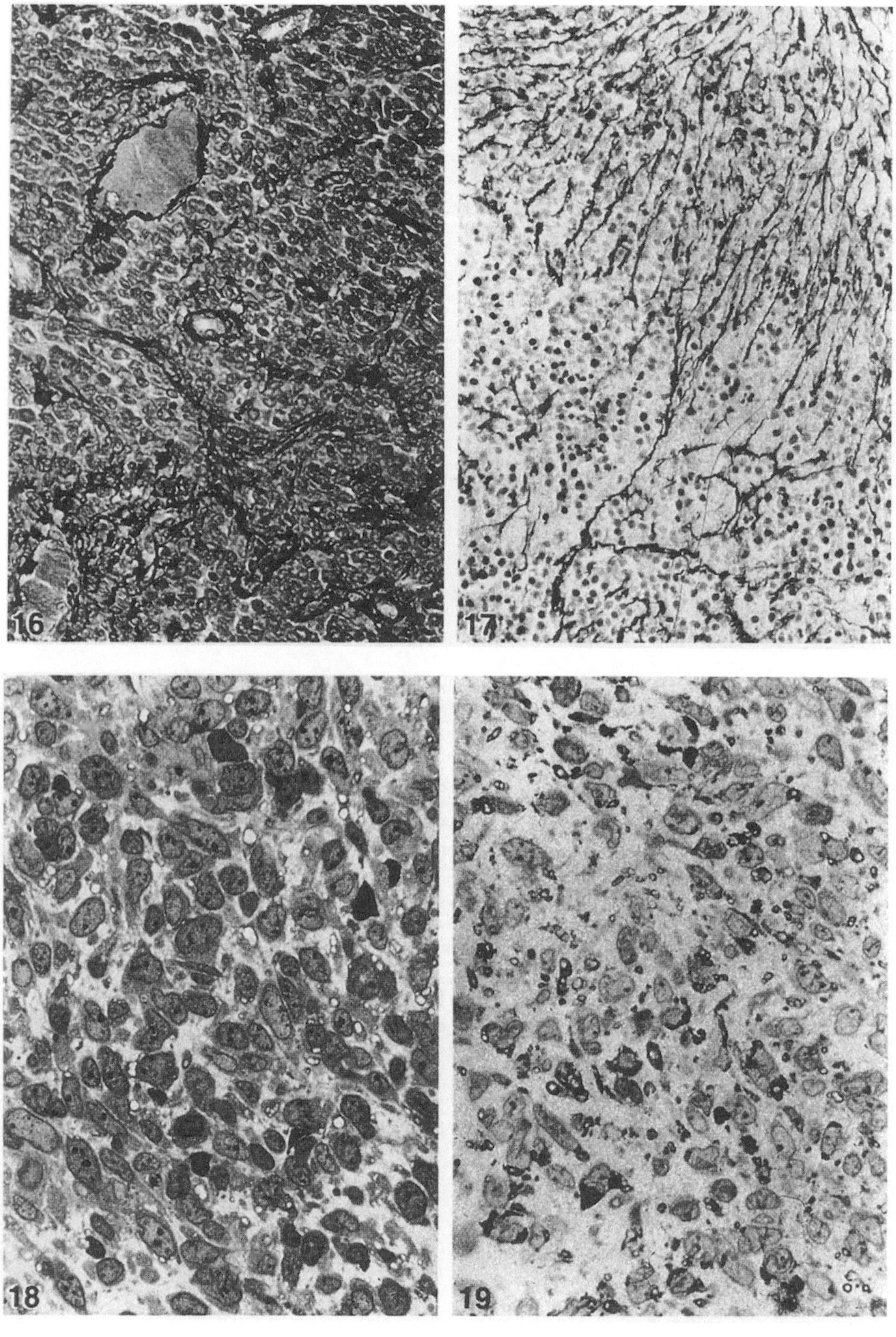

Fig. 16. Silver impregnation. Reticulin fibers are present only around the vessels. The tumour areas are devoid of reticulin

Fig. 17. In the upper right part of the microphotograph, it is easy to recognise that there is a network of well-oriented and therefore preexisting reticulin fibers, belonging to the tissue invaded by the Ewing's sarcoma

Fig. 18. Microphotograph of semifine section (J.-P. Thiery), showing the irregular outline of some nuclei and their clearly visible punctiform nucleoli

Fig. 19. In this semifine section the glycogen, stained with PAS, appears intensely black, and is often in contact with a small clear lipid droplet

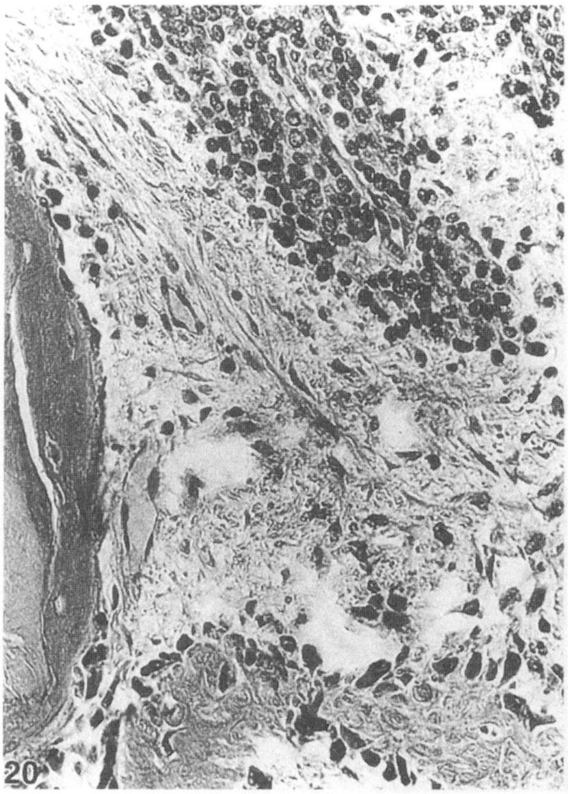

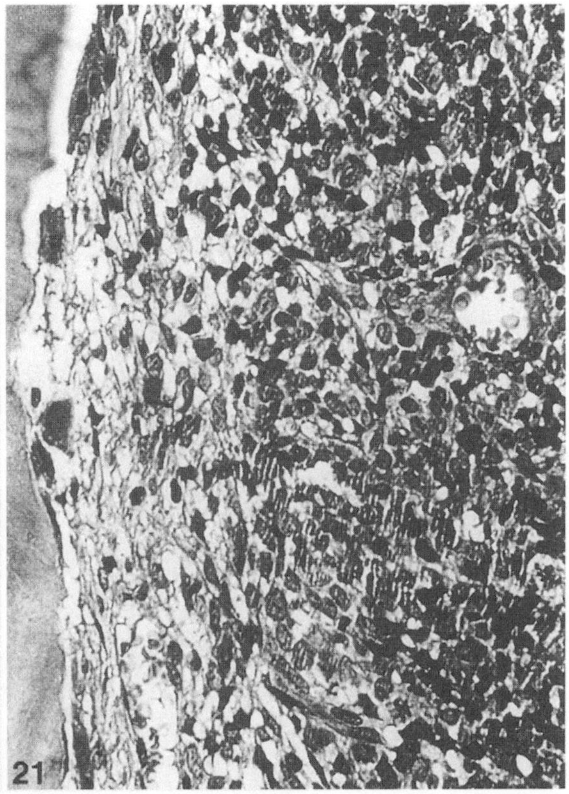

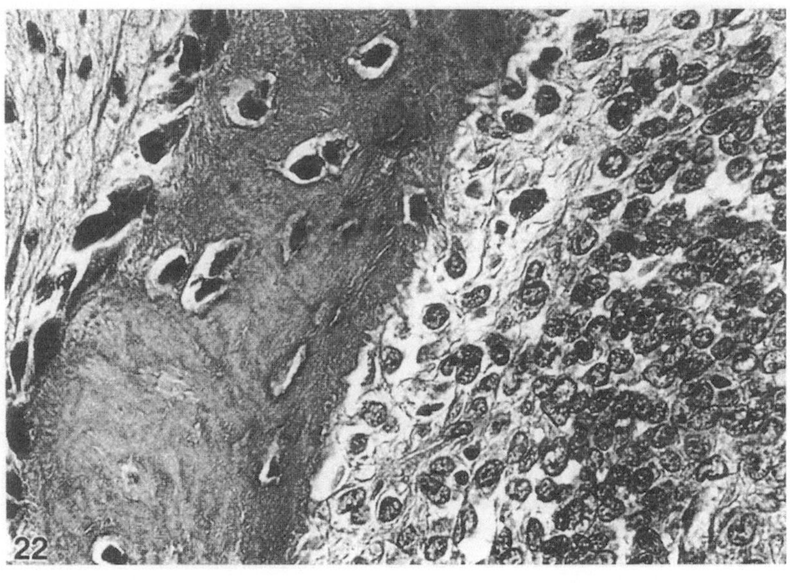

Fig. 20. At the margin of the microphotograph, is a necrotic bony lamella, as shown by the uninhabited osteoplasts. Osteogenesis remains active and covers this bony lamella with new bone. In the lower part of the figure, rows of osteoblasts secrete immature bone with large fibers, a last effort which will be overwhelmed by the osteoclastic advance heralding the sarcomatous proliferation

Fig. 21. On the left, the dead bone is the site of osteoclastic absorption in the immediate vicinity of the sarcoma which occupies the right side of the microphotograph

Fig. 22. In this strand of primary bone laid down by osteoblasts (left margin), a conflict is in process with the Ewing's sarcoma which occupies the right third of the microphotograph. The right margin of the bony strand is jagged, evidence of absorption by small-sized osteoclasts with few (or only one) nuclei

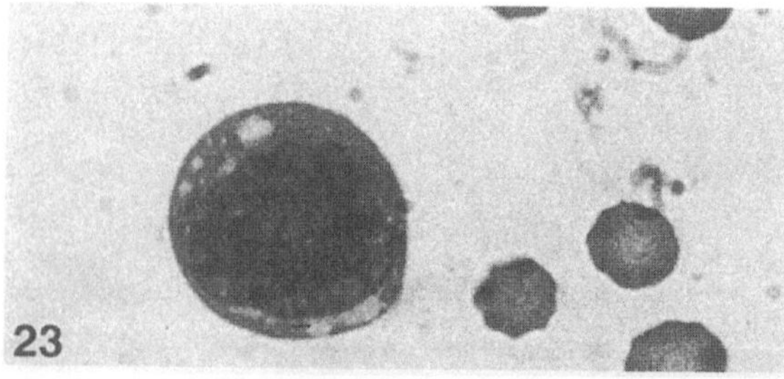

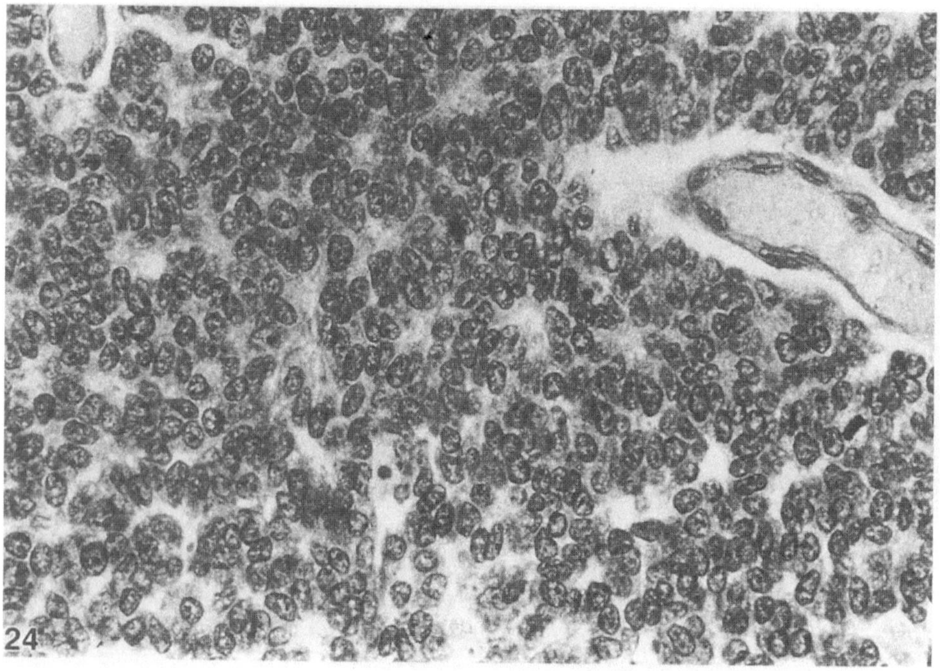

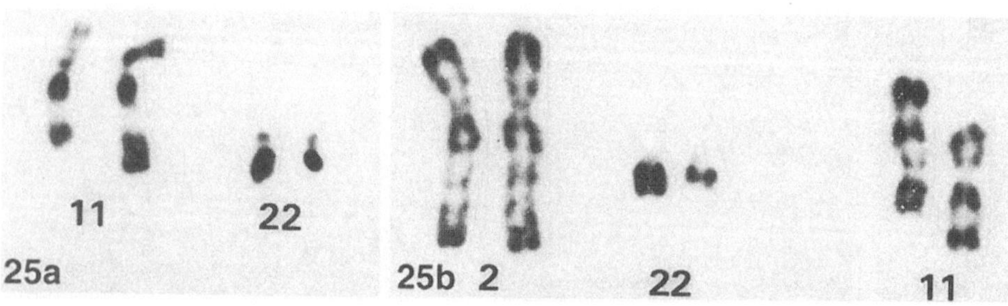

Fig. 23. Cell biopsy by needle aspiration in sarcoma. The cytoplasm contains multiple rounded clear droplets of glycogen. The chromatin of the nucleus is dispersed, the nucleoli barely visible

Fig. 24. Rosette formation is commonplace in many small round-cell proliferations. The neuroepithelioma present in this microphotograph has been confirmed by ultrastructural study, but the presence of neurofibrils in this standard staining is more suspect than proven. The multiplicity of these rosette appearances is one of the factors which favours the diagnosis of neuroepithelioma in a monomorphous proliferation of small cells with round or ovoid nuclei

Fig. 25. a Simple translocation t(11;22) observed in most Ewing's sarcomas. **b** An example of complex translocation t(2;11;22) [Aurias 1983]

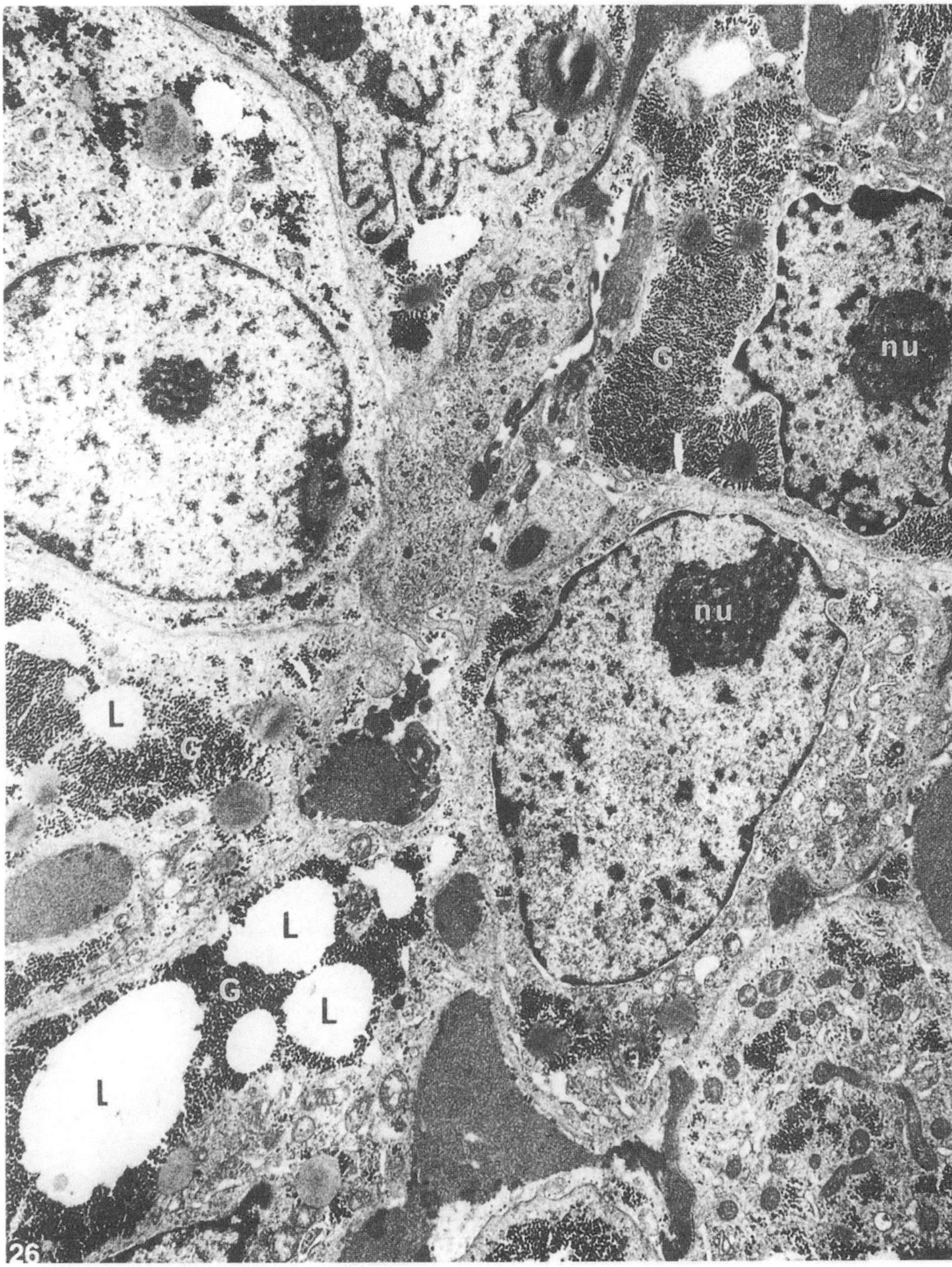

Fig. 26. Overall view showing several cells piled against one another, whose rounded nuclei contain large nucleoli (*nu*). In the cytoplasm there are large dense zones stuffed with glycogen (*g*). Some clumps of glycogen contain clear lipid inclusions (*l*). (x 8000)

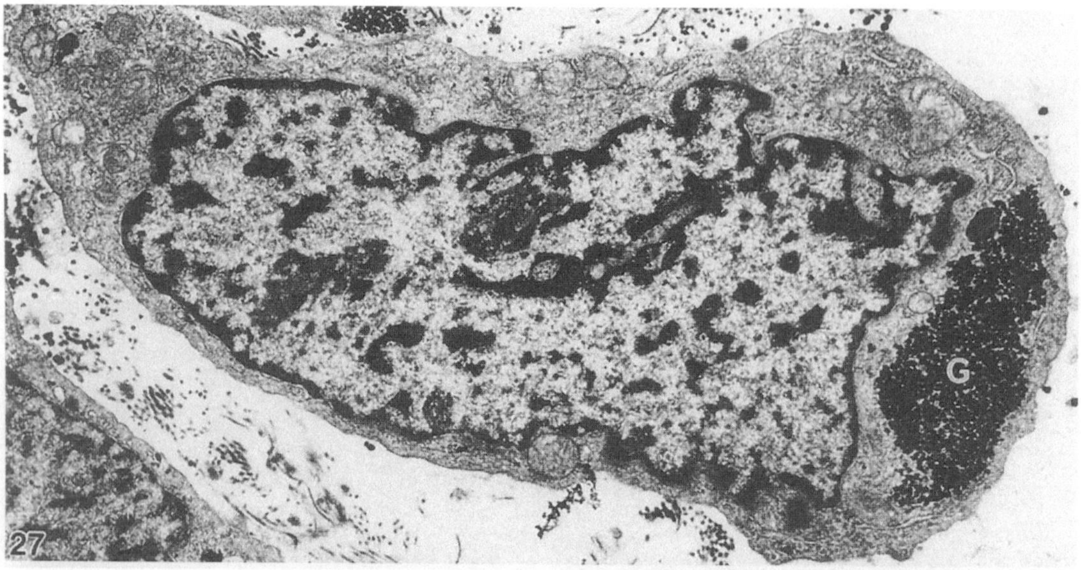

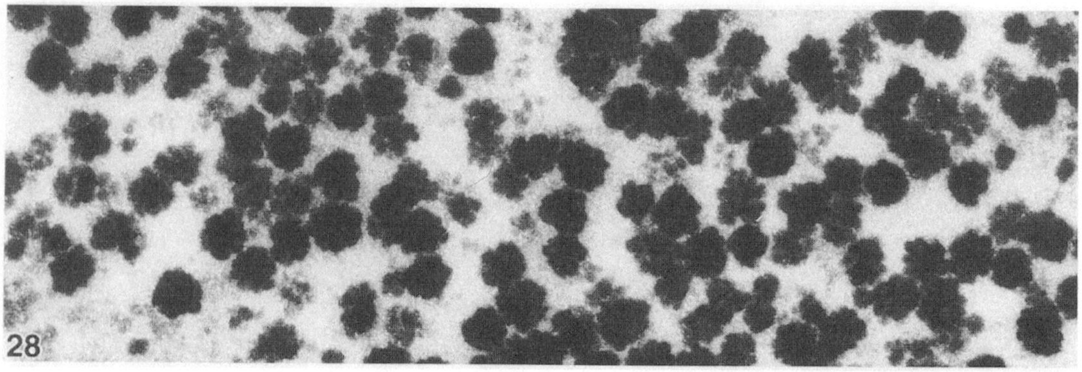

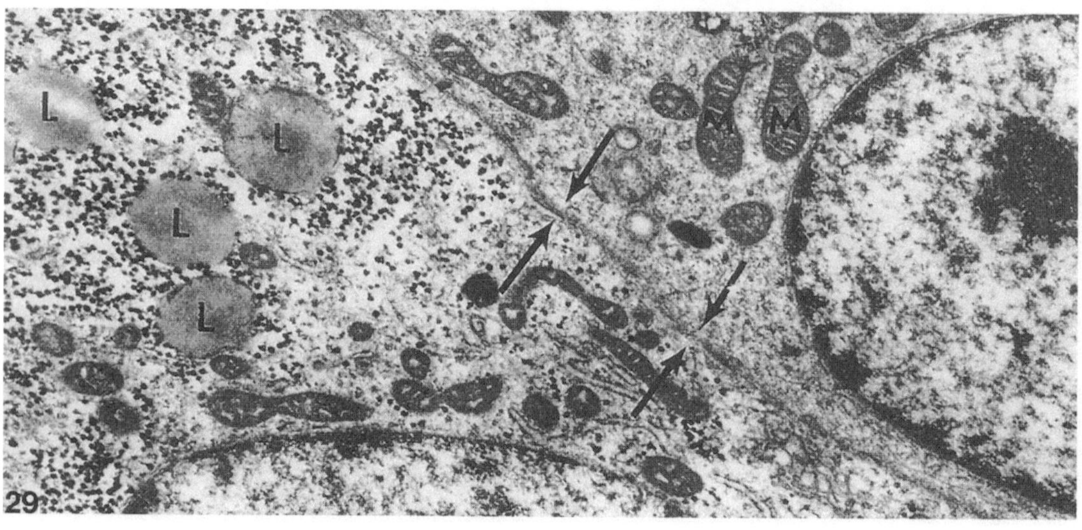

Fig. 27. Cells of Ewing's sarcoma with a dense mass of glycogen (*g*) situated at the pole of the cell, a characteristic arrangement (x 11,000)

Fig. 28. High magnification view of a mass of glycogen in a cell of Ewing's sarcoma. This glycogen consists of beta particles in rosettes formed by the association of alpha subunits. (x 100,000)

Fig. 29. Zone of contact between two cells at different stages: the one above on the right (young stage) does not yet contain glycogen but has large mitochondria (*m*); the other, below, (later stage) contains dispersed particles of glycogen and gray lipid vacuoles (*l*); the mitochondria are long and fine. The cells are closely packed (*arrows*) and their membranes are in contact but well individualised (ultrastructural photographs, x 15,000, by courtesy of J.-P. Thiery)

19. Adamantinoma of the long bones

This is one of the rarest of tumours of bone. It was described by Fischer in 1913, and before him by Billroth in 1869 and Thevenot in 1900, by the name of primary epithelioma of bone. These diverse denominations reflect its histological polymorphism; despite its resemblance to the enamel organ which gained it the name of adamantinoma given it by Fischer, there is no enamel formation in this tumour.

Case history

Jacques W. a 20-year-old student whose favourite sport was football, was worried by a slight change in his left tibia which had begun about 18 months previously. The swelling of the inner aspect of the tibia had slowly developed together with some dull aching, at first intermittent and then increasingly persistent. General examination, a chest X-ray and routine checks furnished no guidance. A periosteal reaction following several local injuries might have been considered if the standard radiograph made at the first consultation had not shown more alarming lesions. The internal cortex of the tibia was displaced by lysis with a "bullous" appearance which occupied the diaphysis over a length of 5 cm. It was this irregular ballooning of the bone which finally disturbed this young patient. Of the suggested diagnoses of fibroma, chondroma and adamantinoma, it was the last which was confirmed by study of the biopsy, an easy confirmation given on the recognition of some paucicellular structures of epithelial appearance in the midst of extensive fibrous areas, the majority situated in contact with a vessel (fig. 7 a-d).

General considerations

The tumour is commoner in men than in women. In the 85 cases of the Mayo Clinic reported by Keeney et al (1989), masculine predominance was 45:39. Adamantinoma is found at all ages, but with a marked predominance in the 2nd and 3rd decades.

The elective site is in the tibial diaphysis; rare cases have been reported in the other long bones: femur, humerus, radius, ulna, fibula and in the pretibial soft tissues, or periosteal [Bambira & Miranda 1983, Mills & Rosai 1985, Bertoni et al 1988, Ishida et al 1992].

Clinical features and course

The usual presenting feature is pain, which is dull and intermittent, so that consultation is delayed. More rarely, the patient attends for a virtually painless palpable tumour. Some rare cases present with spontaneous fracture. The course is slow and the tumour has sometimes been recognised for over 10 years at first consultation [Braud et al 1987].

In the absence of proper treatment, death may ensue due to local haemorrhage or pulmonary and nodal metastases, usually after a long course. The possibility of spontaneous cure by a fibrotic process exists in certain particular forms. Overall, the prognosis is worse in men than in women. Recent symptoms (less than 5 years) and severe pain are ominous features, but the quality of the treatment is a cardinal factor. Collective studies suggest that about 30% of cases show local recurrences, 15% pulmonary metastases and 7% nodal metas-

Table 1. Differential diagnosis

1) Epithelial form. Exclude:
   - bone invasion by a cutaneous endothelioma
   - metastasis, especially in forms with glandular appearance
   - synovial sarcoma in the case of a superficial subperiosteal adamantinoma. The development of synovial sarcoma is mainly extraosseous and in the vicinity of the joints
   - haemangioendothelioma in its angiomatous form
2) Fibrous form:
   - further sections, identify the often juxtavascular paucicellular epithelial islands
   - immunohistology: antikeratins
3) Degraded (cryptic) forms:
   - numerous sections
   - immunohistology essential

tases. In the series of Hazelbag et al (1994), deaths due to metastases totalled 29% with a mean survival period of 12 years and 8 months.

Imaging

The imaging shows a lytic, often eccentric, lesion, either uni- or multilocular, well-defined, slightly "ballooning" the diaphysis. The tumour is often surrounded by an irregularly distributed and discrete sclerosis (figs. 1-3). It tends to invade the diaphysis, forming a series of superimposed bubbles; the progressively thinned cortex is then breached and the adamantinoma develops in both the bone and the soft tissues.

Pathological anatomy and histopathology

The macroscopic appearance is very variable in different cases: relatively firm and grayish-white, or mucoid, cystic or even haemorrhagic and of soft gelatinous consistency. The tumour is embedded in a cavity with polycyclic outlines, and macroscopically well circumscribed. The periosteal bony appositions form a regular swelling.

The microscopic appearance is dominated by the abundance and organisation of two cell-types: fusiform cells on the one hand, and cells of epithelial appearance on the other. This allows an initial distinction of two types of adamantinoma: a typical or epithelial form and a fibrous form in which the detection of rare paucicellular epithelial islands, often in the immediate vicinity of the vessels, requires a search of numerous sections. In recent years, adamantinoma has been enriched by a minor, degraded, almost exclusively fibrous form, in which the presence of rare paucicellular epithelial formations or simply solitary (antikeratin positive) cells, scattered in the fibrous stroma, passed unnoticed before the introduction of the immunohistological reactions.

Lechevallier and Muller (1996) stress the contrast between the apparently benign histology and the gravity of the prognosis in the absence of correct surgical treatment.

Typical epithelial form

The epithelial cells are grouped in strands, or more often in islands whose dimensions vary from one case to another, suggesting in some cases, a basocellular epithelioma, but in other cases, the appearance of a malpighian epithelioma, sometimes with strongly eosinophil formations and the appearances of keratin pearls (figs. 8, 9). Epithelial areas are seen which may be hollowed out into numerous small cavities filled with mucus (fig. 5 b). In the majority of cases, various appearances are associated in the same tumour, with intermediate transitional zones.

Some variants show appearances which do not fit this scheme. The epithelial cells may simulate an adenocarcinomatous metastasis in their arrangement and morphology and areas of fusiform cells may suggest a fusiform-cell sarcoma according to Czerniak et al (1989). The extent of the vascularisation may arouse suspicion of an angioma. Before Fischer, the tumour had been described by the name of endothelioma, and then by Changus et al (1957) by that of angioblastoma. The immunohistological reactions make it impossible to overlook the epithelial component, but the presence of these angiomatous forms is incontestable.

The fibrous tissue may be loose or dense. In samples from the peripheral zones of the tumour, zones of fibroblastic appearance are often seen in which strands of newly-formed bone are differentiated. Hazelbag et al (1993) demonstrated the presence of keratins 14 and 19 in 4 specimens studied, and of keratins 5 and 17 in 74% and 50% of cases respectively. These reactions, independent of the histological type, are different from those of synovial sarcomas, chordomas, and epithelioid sarcomas, the reactions to antikeratins 8 and 18 being negative in 34 and 33 of the specimens.

Two negative points are of value in diagnosis. In biopsies of these "florid" epithelial forms, there is normally neither osteogenesis nor chondrogenesis (apart from the cases presenting with fracture, in which a histiocytic reaction can be seen). In addition, at the periphery of the sample, the tumour invades the medullary canal on the one hand and infiltrates the partly destroyed cortex on the other.

Usually, the histological grade of malignancy is low. The presence of marked cell atypia and of numerous mitoses should arouse the fear of a more guarded prognosis than is usually the case in this tumour with the appearance of pulmonary metastases, often after local recurrences.

Table 2. Immunohistological reactions

Anatomo-pathological forms	Cytokeratin (14 and 19)	Vimentin	Epithelial membrane antigens
Typical epithelial form	+ In numerous epithelial areas	+	-
Fibrous form	+ In small epithelial islands	+	-
Degraded form	+ In scattered cells	+	-

Fibrous form

The epithelial form may be formally contrasted with the fibrous form, which is not easily diagnosed judging by the requests for a second opinion it evokes from young pathologists. Despite a virtually certain clinical diagnosis, based on the clinical and imaging findings, the pathologist observes only fibrous tissue. But if he examines some supplementary sections he will detect some small cell groupings, often adjacent to the vessels (fig. 7 a-d), which will stimulate him to further increase the number of sections. In the sections as a whole it is then possible to detect some rare epithelial areas of very limited dimensions but sufficiently characteristic to prevent any discord between clinician and pathologist. The immunohistological reaction (antikeratin) is positive not only in the small epithelial areas, but also in the paucicellular perivascular zones and in the scanty cells, in the fibrous tissue.

Degraded form

Before the use of immunohistological reactions the lesion was described by the name of ossifying fibroma by Kempson in 1966. The existence of these ossifying fibromas, outside the craniofacial territory, has always been disputed. The lesion was reviewed in 1976 and 1981 by Campanacci et al under the term of osteofibrous dysplasia. The clinical features and imaging of this tibial (rarely fibular) lesion are identical with those of adamantinoma, but the site is essentially cortical and the mean age younger. Campanacci found the course was either towards regression or to extension and local recurrences. The studies of Czerniak et al (1989) and those of Ueda et al (1992) clearly demonstrated that osteofibrous dysplasia and adamantinoma were one and the same entity. Using two monoclonal antibodies, KL-1 and MNF-116 (specific to keratins of 53-57 kDa and 45-56.5 kDa) Ueda et al (1992) demonstrated small epithelial islands (2 cases of 11 KL-1+) and sparse cells (MNF-116+) in 8 cases of lesions previously diagnosed as osteofibrous dysplasia. The authors state that 9 of these cases had progressed to typical adamantinoma over observation periods with a maximum of 10 years. They added that prolonged observation is essential, given the slow course of this lesion. The important fact is clearly the slow evolution of this form and, to some extent, its benign nature and curability.

The case reported by Durroux et al (1993) is particularly instructive. The diagnosis of typical adamantinoma was made in a young man of 25, some 18 years after that of ossifying fibroma had been made from the biopsy of a fibrous lesion of the tibia at the age of 7 years. Immunohistological study of sections of this ossifying fibroma showed no cells positive to the antikeratin antibody, but the progress towards adamantinoma after several local recurrences is convincing. Two other cases are reported in the very well documented study of Hazelbag et al (1994) in patients of 13 and 16 years. The diagnosis had initially been one of fibrous dysplasia, but revision of the sections showed the presence of scattered keratin-positive cells. The course towards adamantinoma was confirmed by block resection performed 5 and 8 years after the first curettage. Currently, no-one would regard a diagnosis of osteofibrous dysplasia as valid if it was based on a radiological image and an anatomical-pathological study which failed to report explicitly a determined search with appropriate antibodies for epithelial cells scattered in the fibrous tissue.

Table 3. Adamantinoma of tibia

Age	Adolescents and young adults	Children
Site	Medullary and cortico-medullary	Cortical (shaft)
Histological forms	Typical epithelial Predominantly fibrous	Cryptic Regressive (?), immuno histology needed

Diagnosis

The diagnosis is often easily made from the totality of the clinical, radiological and anatomical-pathological findings. But the slow course and relatively well circumscribed lytic appearance may raise the possibility of fibroma, cyst or chondroma, possibilities readily excluded by examination of the biopsy specimen.

The epithelial form, however, may raise some differential diagnostic difficulties with a synovial sarcoma, an angiosarcoma or a metastasis. Synovial sarcoma is extraosseous and juxta-articular, so that secondary bone invasion would have to be assumed. The epithelial clumps and cordons are usually frankly demarcated. The immunohistological reaction to the antikeratin antibody in the epithelial cells and numerous fusiform cells is positive. Some authors, well before the introduction of immunology into histological techniques, had described adamantinoma of the long bones as an intraosseous synovial sarcoma.

Malignant haemangioendothelioma may be considered in the differential diagnosis of the hypervascular forms of adamantinoma, but the endothelial proliferation should not obscure the presence of epithelial islands.

The sometimes striking glandular appearance may suggest a diagnosis of metastases from an adenocarcinoma, but the absence of atypical cells and the absence or poverty of reactive sclerosis in adamantinoma militate against this.

The fibrous form requires examination of a relatively large number of slides. The aid of immunology is considerable and allows exclusion of a possible fibrous dysplasia (the clinical picture and imaging of which are different). In cases of fibrous dysplasia the reaction to antikeratin is totally negative.

Some publications have reported an association of fibrous dysplasia and adamantinoma, but I have never found this to be the case in more than 30 specimens I have had the opportunity to examine, even when the tumour had a double tibial and fibular location [Levack et al 1986, Mirra 1989]. It is evident, as stressed by Laucirica et al (1992), that the diagnosis of such a predominantly fibrous lesion by fine-needle aspiration calls for the greatest caution. The risks of interpreting the structures as being part of a fibrous dysplasia, a non-ossifying fibroma or a cortico-metaphyseal fibrous defect are considerable.

The prognosis depends on early diagnosis and adequate treatment. Of 32 patients studied by Hazelbag et al (1994) 28 were followed up for a mean period of 122 - months. Of the 9 patients treated by curettage or marginal resection, 8 developed metastases and their mean survival was 12 years and 8 months.

In the degraded form the diagnosis is even more difficult. It is necessary to examine a large number of sections and to carry out immunological reactions addressed to keratins of different molecular weights.

The presence of even a few cells in which the reaction to the antikeratin antibody is positive, unidentifiable by morphology alone, seems to me a sufficient argument for classifying this lytic lesion of the tibial cortex with the adamantinomas. The same phenomenon of functional differentiation of sparse cells in the fusiform cellular component of a synovial sarcoma seems not to pose any problem to pathologists. In these conditions it seems logical to admit the existence of a continuum between these degraded, cryptic, possibly regressive forms and the more epithelial forms. I have had no experience of adamantinoma of the soft tissues, but only of adamantinoma of periosteal origin which "licks" the bone and develops mainly in the soft tissues.

Histogenesis

It may be worthwhile reviewing some of the histogenetic interpretations of this tumour, which is so special in its site and course. The following hypotheses have been advanced:

- inclusion of epithelial tissue during the fetal period (dysembryoplastic theory), [Fischer 1913];
- a late post-traumatic epithelial inclusion [Ryrie 1932];
- propagation of a cutaneous epithelioma, spinocellular for some, basocellular for others;
- a synovial origin, evoked by the slits and mucoid appearances [Lauke 1947];

- an endothelial origin [Changus 1957, but also Thevenot 1900];
- a reticular origin with malpighian metaplasia [Mandard 1971].

References

Alguacil-Garcia A, Alonso A, Pettigrew NM (1984) Osteofibrous dysplasia (ossifying fibroma) of the tibia and fibula and adamantinoma. Am J Clin Pathol 82: 470-474

Baker PL, Dockerty MB, Coventry MB (1954) Adamantinoma (so-called) of the long bones: review of the literature and a report of three new cases. J Bone Joint Surg. 36A: 704-720

Bambirra EA, Miranda D (1983) Adamantinoma of the soft tissue of the leg. Arch Pathol Lab Med 107: 500

Baux S, Apoil A, Orcel L (1971) Adamantinome du tibia traité par résection large suivie de greffe. Rev Chir Orthop 57: 479-484

Bertoni F, Zucchi V, Mapelli S, Bacchini P (1988) Adamantinoma of the soft tissues of leg. Skeletal Radiol 17: 522-526

Braud P, Tomeno B, Courpied JP, Ramadier JO, Forest M, Merle d'Aubigné R (1987) Une tumeur singulière. L'adamantinome des os longs. A propos de 7 cas consécutifs suivis après résection. Rev Chir Orthop 73: 3-13

Campanacci M, Giunti A, Bertoni F, Laus M, Gitelis S (1981) Adamantinoma of long bones. The experience of the Istituto orthopedico Rizzoli. Am J Surg Pathol 5: 533-542

Campanacci M, Laus M (1981) Osteofibrous dysplasia of the tibia and fibula. J Bone Joint Surg 63A: 367-375

Campbell CJ, Hawk T (1982) A variant of fibrous dysplasia (osteofibrous dysplasia). J Bone Joint Surg 64A: 231-236

Castellote A, Garcia-Pena P, Luaaya J, Lorenzo J (1988) Osteofibrous dysplasia. Skeletal Radiol 17: 483-486

Changus GW, Speed JS, Stewart FW (1957) Malignant angioblastoma of bone; a reappraisal of adamantinoma of long bone. Cancer 10: 540-559

Cohen DM, Dahlin DC, Pugh DG (1962) Fibrous dysplasia associated with adamantinoma of the long bones. Cancer 15: 515-521

Czerniak B, Rojas-Corona RR, Dorfman HD (1989) Morphologic diversity of long bone adamantinoma. The concept of differentiated (regressing) adamantinoma and its relationship to osteofibrous dysplasia. Cancer 64: 2319-2334

Delarue J, Chomette G, Bousquet M (1960) Les "adamantinomes" du tibia. A propos de deux observations. Ann Ant Path 5: 336-351

Durroux R, Ducoin H, Gaubert J (1993) Adamantinome du tibia et ostéo-fibro-dysplasie. Ann Pathol 13, 5: 336-340

Fischer B (1913) Uber ein primares Adamantinom der Tibia. Frankfurt Ztschr Path 12 :422-441

Fontaine R, Warter P, Muller JN, Bridher JJ, Mandard JC (1968) Les adamantinomes des os longs. J Radio-Electr 44: 114-118

Gouttallier D, Debeyre J (1972) Une observation d'adamantinome du tibia. J Chir (Paris) 103: 231-236

Hazelbag HM, Fleuren GJ, Van Den Broek LGCM, Taminiau AHM, Hogendoorm PCW (1993) Adamantinoma of the long bones: keratin subclass immunoreactivity pattern with reference to its histogenesis. Am J Surg Pathol 17, 12: 1225-1233

Hazelbag HM, Taminiau AHM, Fleuren GJ, Hogendoorn PCW (1994) Adamentinoma of the long bones. A clinicopathological study of thirty-two patients with emphasis on histological subtype. Precursor lesion and biological behavior. J Bone & Joint Surg 76A: 1482-1499

Huvos AH, Marcove RC (1975) Adamantinoma of long bones. A clinicopathological study of fourteen cases with vascular origin suggested. J Bone Joint Surg 57A: 148-154

Ishida T, Kikuchi F, Oka T, Machinami R, Kojima T, Iijima T, Higaki S, Imamura T (1992) Juxtacortical adamantinoma of humerus (simulating Ewing tumor). Skeletal Radiol 21: 205-209

Ishida T, Iijima T, Kikuchi T, Kitagawa T, Tanida T, Imamara T, Machinami R (1992) A clinicopathological and immunohistochemical study of osteofibrous dysplasia, differentiated adamantinoma and adamantinoma of long bones. Skeletal Radiol 21: 493-502

Keeney GL, Unni KK, Beabout JW, Pritchard DJ (1989) Adamantinoma of long bones. A clinicopathologic study of 85 cases. Cancer 64: 730-737

Kempson RL (1966) Ossifying fibroma of the long bones. A light and electron microscopic study. Arch Pathol 82: 218-233

Lauke H (1947) Zur Kenntnis von Pathologie und Klinik der geschwalste mit synovialmenbranartigem Bau (Synovialome, oder synoviale Endotheliofibrome und Sarkome). Frankfurt. Ztschr Path 59: 2-29

Lauricia R, Mody D, Mac Lean L, Kearns R, Ramzy I (1992) Acta Cytol 36: 951-956

Lechevallier J, Muller Ch (1996) Adamantinome in: Les tumeurs bénignes de l'enfant. Sauramps Medical edn

Levack B, Revell PA, Roper BA (1986) Adamantinoma associated with fibrous dysplasia. Int Orthop 10: 253-259

Mandard JC, Le Gal Y, Fievez M (1971) L'adamaninome des os longs. Ann Anat Path 16: 483-497

Markel Sheldon F (1978) Ossifying fibroma of long bone. Its distinction from fibrous dysplasia and its association with adamantinoma of long bone. Am J Clin Pathol 69: 91-97

Merle d'Aubigné R (1966) Adamantinome du tibia. 2 cas. Rev Chir Orthop 52: 182-189

Mills SE, Rosai J (1985) Adamantinoma of the pretibial soft tissue. Clinicopathologic features, differential diagnosis, and possible relationship to intraosseous disease. Am J Clin Pathol 83: 108-114

Mirra JM (1989) Adamantinoma and osteofibrous dyplasia. In: Bone tumors. Clinical, radiologic and pathologic correlations. Lea & Febiger, Philadelphia, pp 1203-1231

Nakashima Y, Yamamuro T, Fujiwara Y, Kotoura Y, Mori E, Hamashima Y (1983) Osteofibrous dysplasia (ossifying fibroma of long bones): a study of 12 cases. Cancer 52: 909-914

Oberling CH, Vermes E, Chevereau J (1938) Adamantinome du tibia. Bull Assoc Cancer 27: 373-382

Rosai J (1969) Adamantinoma of tibia. Electron microscopic evidence of its epithelial origin. Am J Clin Pathol 51: 786-792

Rosai J, Pinkus GS (1982) Immunohistochemical demonstration of epithelial-differentiation in adamantinoma of the tibia. Am J Surg Pathol 6: 427-434

Salmon M, Payan H, Titaud A (1956) Les adamantinomes du tibia. Adamantinomes des os longs. A propos d'une observation. Arch Anat Pathol 1: 281-285

Schajowicz F, Santini-Araujo E (1989) Adamantinoma of the tibia masked by fibrous dysplasia. Report of three cases. Clin Orthop 238: 294-301

Unni KK, Dablin DC, Beabout JW, Ivins JC (1974) Adamantinomas of long bones. Cancer 34: 1796-1805

Ueda Y, Blasius S, Edel G, Wuisman P, Bocker W, Roessner A (1992) Osteofibrous dysplasia of long bones: a reactive process to adamantinomatous tissue. J Cancer Res Clin Oncol 118: 152-156

Ueda Y, Roessner A, Bosse A, Edel G, Bocker W, Wuisman P (1991) Juvenile intracortical adamantinoma of the tibia with predominant osteofibrous dysplasia-like features. Pathol Res Pract 187: 1039-1043

Volpe R, Mazabraud A (1984) Adamantinoma of long bones. Pathologica 76: 313-322

Weiss SW, Dorfman HD (1977) Adamantinoma of long bone. An analysis of nine new cases with emphasis on metastasizing lesions and fibrous dysplasia-like changes. Hum Pathol 8: 141-153

Yoneyama T, Winter WG, Milsow L (1977) Tibial adamantinoma: its histogenesis from ultrastructural studies. Cancer 40: 1138-1142

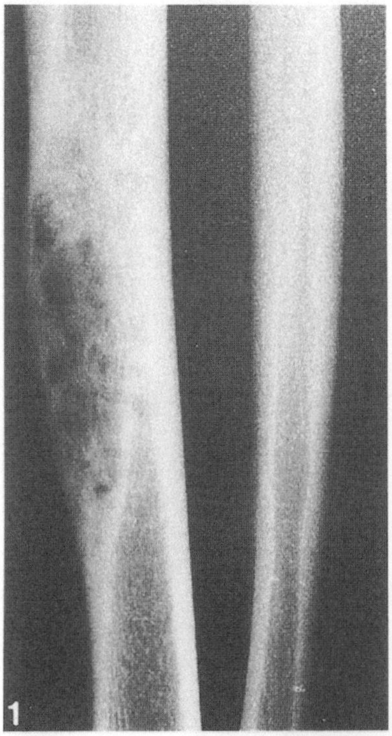

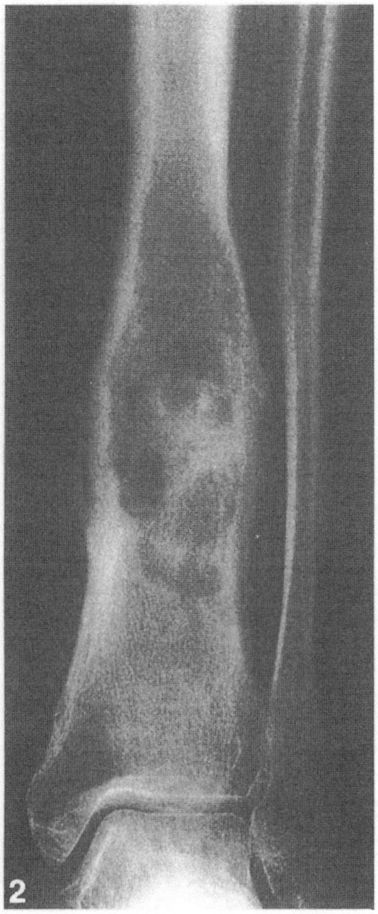

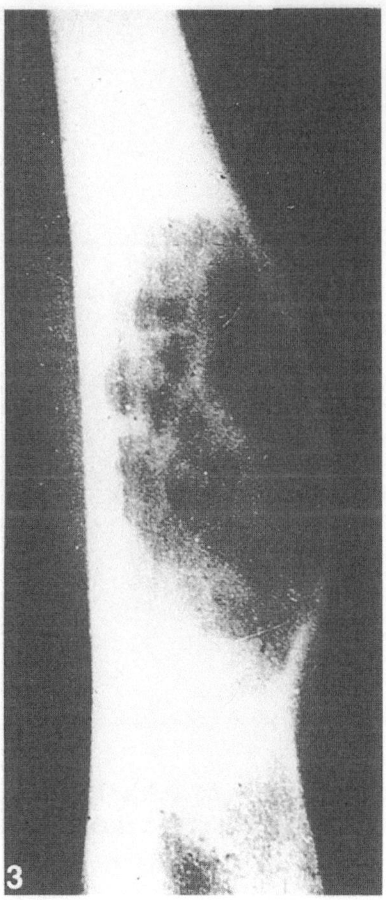

Fig. 1. Adamantinoma, middle third of tibia, excentric, multilocular, minor osteosclerotitc reaction. Woman of 21

Fig. 2. A different case: the tumour is ill-defined in its proximal part. The cortex persists, but is ballooned by periosteal bony apposition

Fig. 3. A compartmented aspect of tumour and very definite boundaries are classical but not pathognomonic features. In this boy of 12, cure of the femoral adamantinoma was obtained at the cost of amputation, after local recurrence

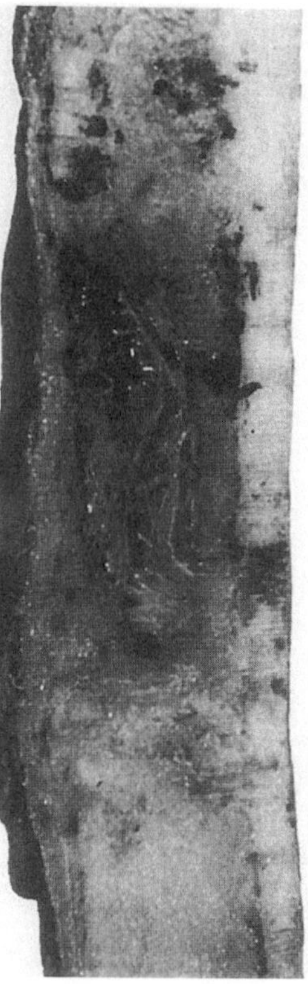
4

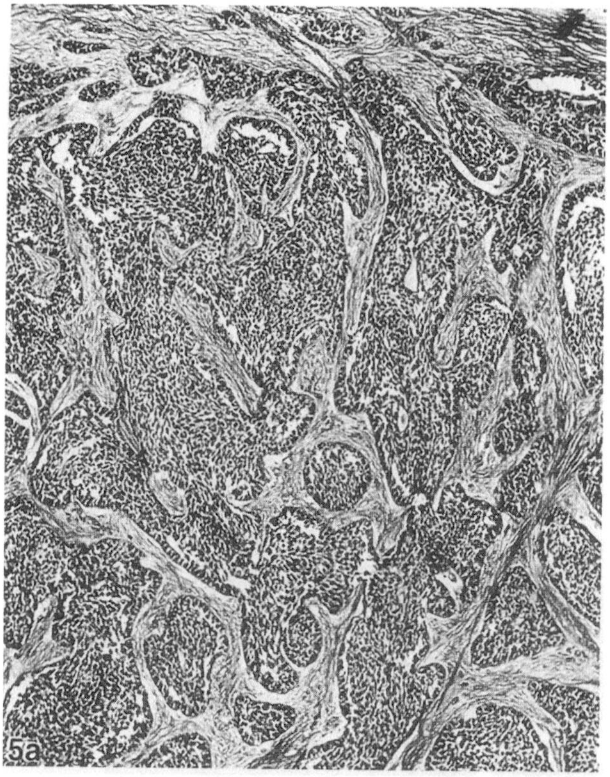

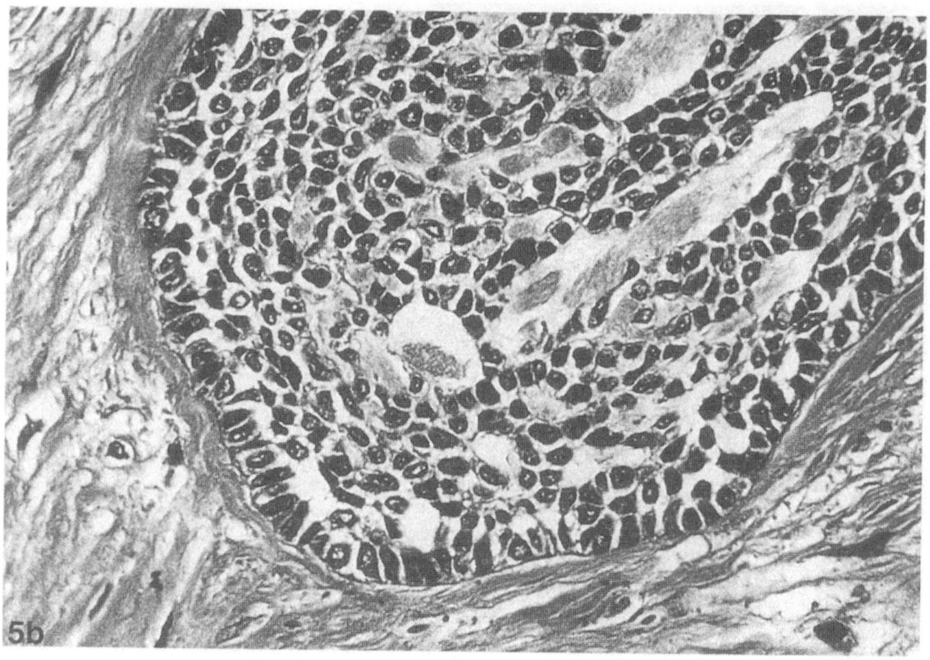

Fig. 4. Longitudinal section, bone resection for adamantinoma of tibia, woman aged 35. Multiple cavities filled with mucoid material are bounded by fibrous bands. At both ends of the tumour, reactive osteogenesis obstructs the medullary canal almost entirely

Fig. 5 a, b. Another adamantinoma of the tibia. **a** Low magnification: the zones of dark epithelial cells are bordered by cells of the same type but cubo-cylindrical in shape. **b** Higher magnification shows acellular spaces occupied by mucoid material. The epithelial zones are surrounded by fibrous tissue. The general appearance suggests adamantinomatous tissue

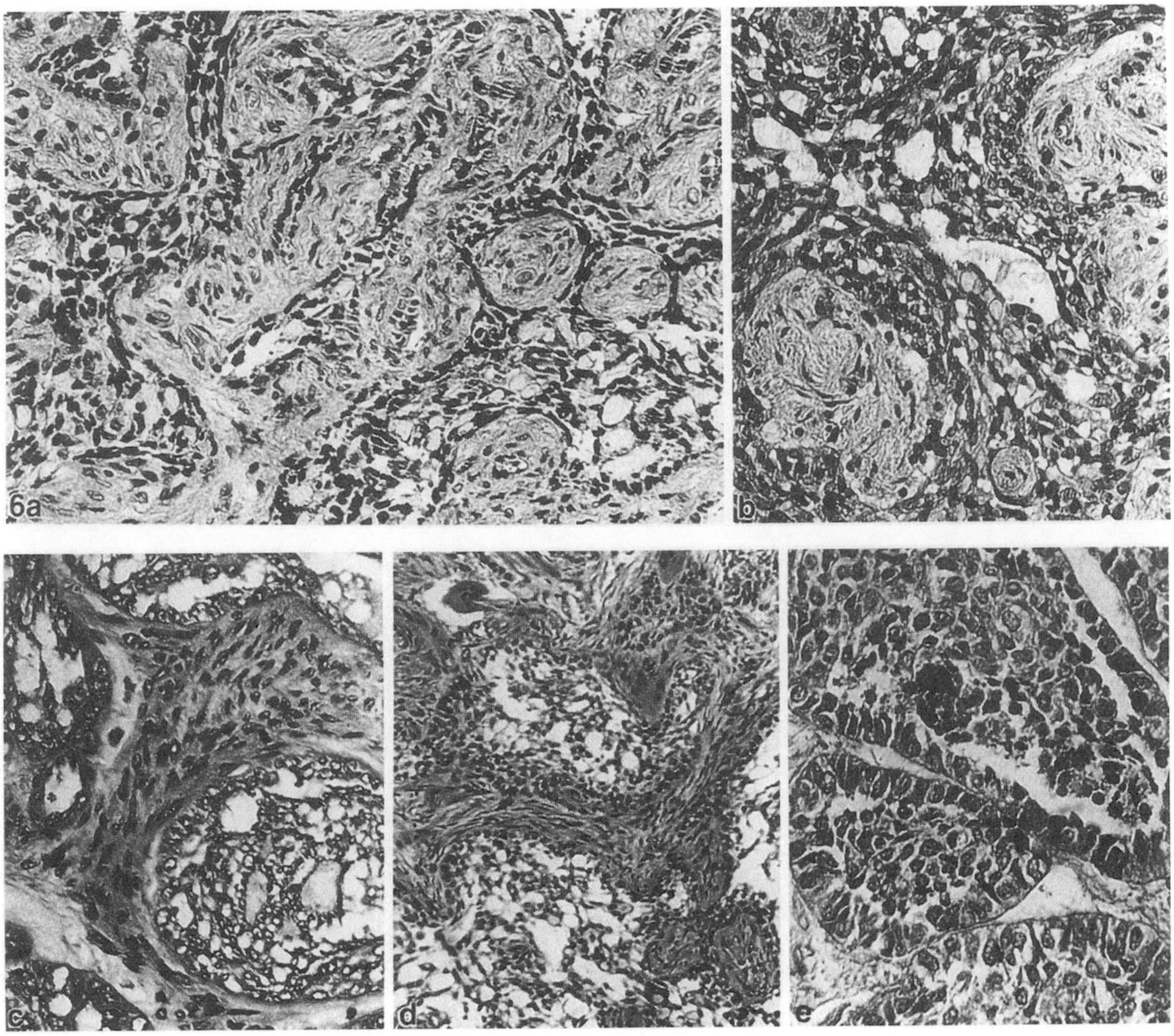

Fig. 6. a Strands of dark epithelial cells seem to be stretched out between wide bands of fibrous tissue. **b, c, d** The epithelial zones hollow out small compartments filled with mucus, some bordered by cubical cells, others by cells flattened as if displaced by secretion. **e** The cell islands bordered by cubical cells may suggest metastasis from a glandular epithelioma

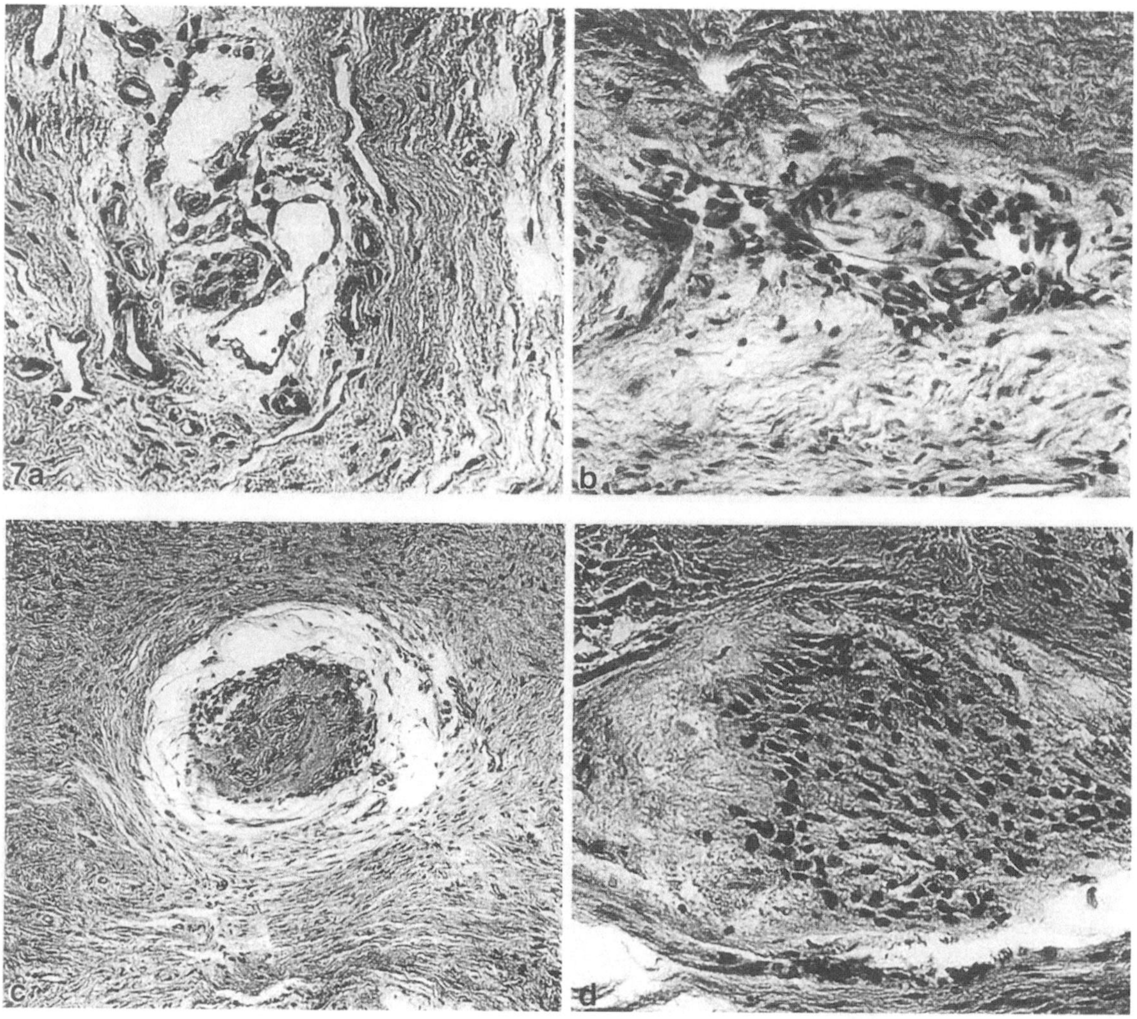

Fig. 7 a-d. This tibial adamantinoma is of fibrous type. The four microphotographs are intended to stress the fact that minuscule cellular islands, often near the vessels and scattered in an abundant fibrous tissue, should arouse attention and instigate the production of numerous sections in a search for characteristic features

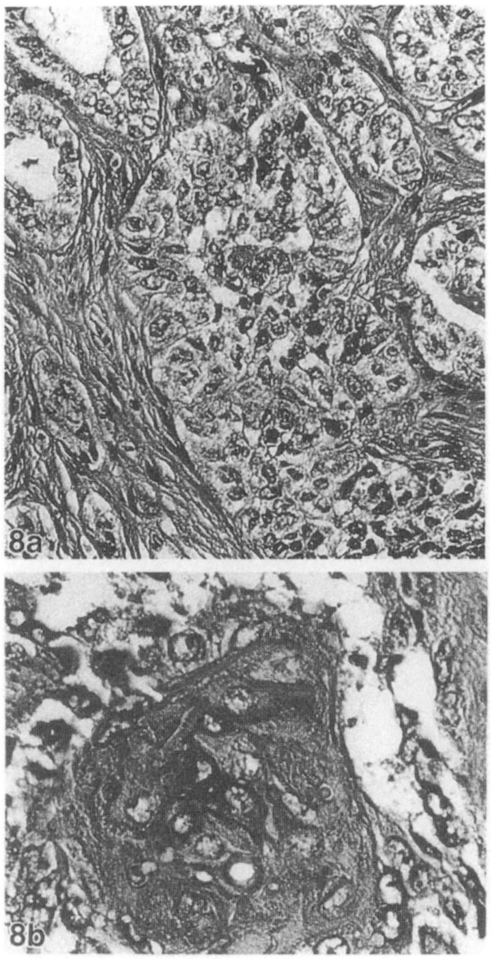

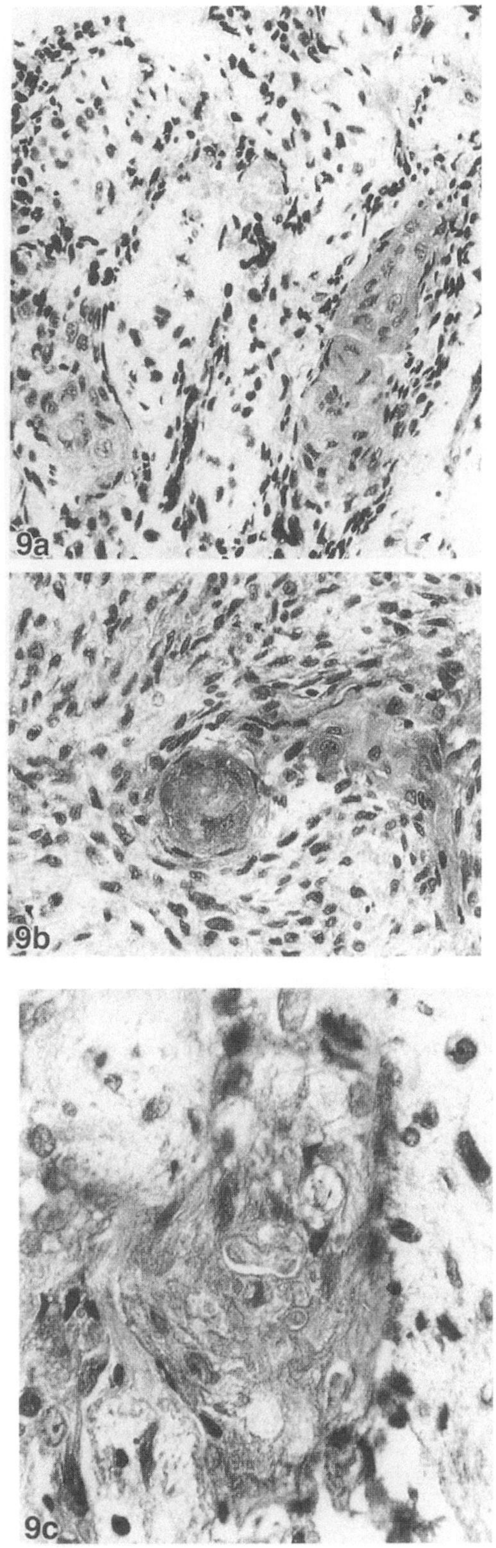

Fig. 8. Dense cellular zones, glând-like appearances (**a**) and a partly keratinised malpighian island coexist in this adamantinoma (**b**)

Fig. 9 a-c. These epithelial appearances with whorled zones and keratinisation are those of a periosteal adamantinoma

20. Chordoma

Chordoma is a tumour which develops along the median longitudinal axis of the body from the base of the skull to the coccyx, originating from vestiges of the notochord. The concept of notochordal development and its role in morphogenesis has extended and is intra- or juxtavertebral. It is the only bone tumour of dysembryoplastic origin. Because of its slow and insidious growth, diagnosis is often delayed, making complete ablation of the tumour difficult or even impossible.

Case histories

Case 1. Monsieur B., aged 53, was admitted to the department of gastroenterology for disturbances of bowel transit which had become progressively worse over some ten months, but with practically no pain. There was nothing of note in the history and no change in his dietary regime could be blamed for the delay in transit. Examination revealed the presence of a firm tumour in the pelvis extending to the sacrum. Imaging confirmed the presence of this tumour, which attacked the rectum, displacing it forward and laterally; it was attached to the anterior aspect of the sacrum, effacing the first sacral foramina. Biopsy allowed an easy diagnosis of chordoma from the typical histological appearances.

Case 2. A biopsy, accompanied by these simple words arrived in the laboratory. "Biopsy of sacrum, woman of 60". The cells, grouped in small islands or scattered in pools of mucus, contained PAS-positive droplets. At low magnification, this appearance might suggest a chordoma but closer examination of the cells on the one hand, and of numerous sections on the other, revealed numerous cellular anomalies, mitoses, and in places arrangements of cubo-cylindrical cells which suggested glandular layering. A glance at the case-notes revealed that the patient had been operated for carcinoma of the colon four years previously.

General considerations

This is a rare tumour, 3-4% among primary tumours of bone, but which constitutes 20-30% of primary malignant spinal tumours [Fuentes et al 1990]. Chordoma is approximately twice as common in men as in women. It can develop at any age but its maximum incidence is in the 4th to 7th decades. Most chordomas are detected at around the age of 45, but sacro-coccygeal tumours occur slightly later (50 years).

The commonest site (80% of cases) is in the fixed parts of the spine. Of these cases 50% are in the sacrum and 30% at the base of the skull in the vicinity of the spheno-occipital synostosis and the clivus of Blumenbach: 38% of 155 cases at the Mayo Clinic [Heffelfinger et al 1983]; 12-20% of cases affect the movable parts of the spinal column [Chevalier et al 1990].

Clinical features and course

The tumour is often asymptomatic for years before the first clinical signs appear. These are signs of compression, either of nerve roots or of the rectum or bladder, that betray a sacral chordoma developing anteriorly, but posterior development of a sacral chordoma may only be recognised by the presence of a tumour which displaces the skin in the sacro-gluteal region [Konrad et al 1981]. In tumours of the sacral region the average duration of symptoms before the first consultation is 12 months. Increased pain in the seated position has been reported in coccygeal chordomas.

Table 1.

	PS100	EMA	KL1	ACE	Vimentin
Chordoma	+ (90%)	+	+	+ (50%)	+
Chondroid chordoma	+	–	–	–	+
Chondro-sarcoma	+	–	–	–	+

Chordomas of the skull base have a more polymorphous symptomatology. Sometimes they extend towards the cranial cavity, destroying the pituitary and compressing the optic nerves; sometimes they develop towards the retropharyngeal space and nasal fossae, and manifest with otorhinolaryngological features [Eisemann 1980, Campbell et al 1980]. Even in this site, their latency is sometimes surprising and I have had the occasion to make this diagnosis from a biopsy made by a dentist in a child of 12 at a routine dental inspection. In contrast to this anterior development, spheno-occipital growth has been described. Chavany and Hagenmuller (1956) reported one case in a woman of 50 which gave rise to a complex neurological syndrome.

The prognostic factors in these spheno-occipital tumours is apparently varied. In the statistics of Mitchell et al (1993), based on 41 cases, survival at 15 years was markedly greater in patients under 40 years of age. But O'Connell et al (1994) found the 10-year survival assessed in 62 patients to be 20% for women and 63% for men. The comments of Briand Jeffrey et al (1995) attempt to provide an explanation for these apparent diversities.

Lesions which are multiple from the outset, and do not metastasise, are certainly exceptional such as the case reported by Anderson and Meyers (1968) in a man of 59 who had a double lesion, at the skull-base and the sacral region. Chordomas of the flexible spine, whether cervical, thoracic or lumbar, manifest with pain of late onset.

If complete excision is not done, progress occurs inexorably to invasion of the adjacent organs leading to death from compression phenomena and local infection, a course only briefly retarded by radiotherapy. Chordoma is usually regarded as not much given to metastasis; however, in the study of Kaiser et al (1984) of 63 patients followed up for 2-24 years, there were 25% of metastatic cases. Usually the metastases involve the lymph nodes and lungs. Local tumour recurrences are relatively common but patients who have had a satisfactory operation aimed at cure have a 5-year survival of over 50%. Three of the 6 patients reported by Laurent et al (1981) survived for more than 7 years. If we consider only chordomas of the cervical spine, the incidence of early and rapidly fatal recurrences reduces the mean survival to less then 2 years [Griffet et al 1988]. This is to acknowledge that the most daring surgical resections, palliative radiotherapy, cryotherapy - techniques all with serious local risks - obtain only a relatively mediocre result in the treatment of this tumour, whose stealthy and insidious behaviour does not allow of diagnosis until it is too advanced for cure.

Imaging

The radiological aspects of chordoma have been carefully studied in the thesis of Laredo (1981). In sacrococcygeal chordomas, the osteolysis, which is often paramedian at the outset, obliterates a sacral foramen and then extends towards the lower part of the sacrum and coccyx. This osteolysis is well-defined but without marginal sclerosis; in 25% of cases there is calcification in the tumour. Opacification of the hollow organs reveals their displacement by the tumour. In lateral views, presacral tumour opacity is usually evident.

In the thoracolumbar spine (fig. 5), the lesion is often limited to a single vertebra for a long time and is of mixed type, both lytic and sclerosing. Its site is usually midline, at the back of the vertebral body. It provokes a posterior collapse of the body and extends posteriorly to the internal cortex of the pedicles. In addition, there is often a reactive prevertebral osteogenesis and, in half the cases, a spindle-shaped image.

At the cervical level, two types of lesions may be distinguished: osteolysis of a vertebral body which may or may not extend to the posterior arch, with a visible image in the adjacent retropharyngeal or anterolateral soft parts; a widening of the intervertebral foramen and a tumour that is mainly lateral.

At the base of the skull (figs. 2, 3), the osteolysis of the chordoma in its posterior progress displaces the sella turcica. In its forward spread the tumour is visible as a rounded opaque mass which displaces the pharyngeal wall. CT and MRI studies (fig. 4) are essential in preoperative assessment for precise identification of the extent of the lesions; however explicit the imaging, diagnostic certainty is provided by the anatomical and pathological examination.

Pathological anatomy and histopathology

The tumour is smooth, knobbly, and elastic in consistency, features which recall those of cartilaginous tumours. Sacrococcygeal chordomas are apparently encapsulated except at their bony attachment. On section, the tumour is semi-elastic in consistency or softer and gelatinous. Some calcified zones may be seen. Spheno-occipital chordomas have the same characteristics; they displace the soft tissues but infiltrate the bony tissue in which they arise.

In perusing large surfaces of a section at low magnification some polymorphism is seen, both architectural and cellular [Volpe et al 1983]. The cells are grouped in islands or in strands of epithelial appearance (fig. 5) in an amorphous mucoid and amphophil or slightly fibrillary matrix. Some collagen septa lobulate the tumour. Several authors have described different types of tumour cells which actually correspond to different developmental stages of the same cellular element [Cesarini et al 1971, Lagacé et al 1975, Thiery et al 1977]. The cells most commonly observed have an eosinophil cytoplasm laden with fine droplets which fix stains for fats and glycogen (fig. 8). The cells form small groupings or strands in the midst of the mucoid matrix (fig. 13); more rarely, they exhibit pseudoglandular layering. Sometimes the concentric arrangement of flattened cells assumes a variably keratinised bulbiform aspects (fig. 9). Overall, the appearance is frankly one of epithelial proliferation. There are also dense compact chordomas made up of massive epithelial islands separated from one another by some connective tissue flows, traversed by vessels and likely to be infiltrated by mononuclear inflammatory cells. The epithelial nature of the tumour is a feature which should suggest a diagnosis of chordoma.

In an ultrastructural study, J.-P. Thiery et al (1977) distinguished five evolutional stages of these tumour cells, whose main features are also to be found in the cells of the embryonal notochord. Staining with PAS permits ready characterisation of the different types. The small cells of type I contain no glycogen. In type III, the glycogen is very concentrated and in type V (vacuolated cells) the glycogen is reduced. Cell types II and IV are intermediate. In these different cell types the nuclei vary greatly in size, are often irregular and sometimes multiple. Mitoses are very rare. The physaliphorous cells are regarded by many authors as characteristic. They are bulky structures of 10 to 100 microns whose cytoplasm is hollowed out by numerous vacuoles, which displace the nucleus. Between the vacuoles the weakly staining cytoplasm forms a radiate network (fig. 6 b). Physaliphorous cells may be absent from a biopsy specimen and consequently in a fine-needle aspiration [Thompson & Callery 1988].

In some cases, spontaneously or after irradiation, a fusiform-cell sarcomatous appearance may be substituted for the characteristic histological aspects [Miettinen et al 1987, Hruban 1990]. Development towards a malignant fibrous histiocytoma has also been reported after irradiation [Halpern et al 1984]. These malignant transformations are discussed under the title of "dedifferentiated chordoma" [Meis et al 1987, Smith et al 1989]. Zones of dedifferentiation coexist with areas of quiescent chordoma; the transition between the two appearances is sometimes sharp, sometimes gradual. Most often the tumour appearance resembles a fibroblastic sarcoma.

The histochemical and immunohistological reactions are a valuable aid to diagnosis. We have seen variations of PAS staining of the cell cytoplasm with cell type (I-V). PAS stains the intercellular substance weakly and this staining is virtually unchanged after hyaluronidase. This same intercellular substance is not stained by the reaction of Gordon and Sweet, nor by phosphotungstic acid haematoxylin, unlike classic chordoma. Staining with alcian blue is positive, as it is for the chondroid substance of chondrosarcoma.

Strong positivity of the reaction to 5'-nucleotidase localised to the cell membrane is important for the differential diagnosis between chondrosarcoma and ependymoma [Bottles et al 1984]. The anti-cytokeratin (44-54 kDa) antibodies and the epithelial membrane antigen give a positive reaction [Salisbury et al 1985, Abenoza et al 1986, Coindre et al 1986] in nearly 95 to 100% of cases. The same reactions are negative in chondrosarcomas. The antivimentin and anti-protein S100 antibodies give a positive reaction in virtually all chordomas and chondrosarcomas, at least for a considerable number of cells. The reaction against neurofilaments (gliofibrillary acid protein) is negative. In the fusiform cells of dedifferentiated chordomas the reaction with antikeratin is positive in frozen sections; it is negative with anti-protein S100 antibody.

The smears from fine-needle aspiration allow valuable cytological studies [Lefer et al 1978, O'Dowd et al 1983, Plaza et al 1989], but their diagnostic value has been assessed cautiously [Benoît et al 1990]. Cytogenetic analysis of two sacral chordomas [Gibas et al 1992] showed remodelling of chromosome 21. The authors suggest, while awaiting other observations to confirm their findings, that involvement of chromosome 21q22 is directly related to chordoma.

Chondroid chordoma

A particular histological problem is raised by certain spheno-occipital chordomas categorised as chondroid chordomas. They combine chordal and cartilaginous tissue in very varying proportions. From the clinical aspect they do not differ from other chordomas of the base of the skull and manifest with a rhinopharyngeal symptomatology and/or pareses or paralyses of the cranial nerves and violent headaches. Unlike the chordomas they seem commoner in women than in men. They affect younger patients and the average age of detection is around 35 years. Several cases have been reported in children. One case of a double basicervical and sacral location has been reported; this patient showed no nodal or other spread at post-mortem examination.

The macroscopic appearance of chondroid chordoma does not greatly differ from that of pure chordomas but histologically it combines areas of chordal and cartilaginous appearance. The cartilaginous areas are represented by immature stellate cells dispersed in a mucoid material. These zones coexist with appearances of chordoma characterised by cell alignments of epithelial appearance and vacuolated cells at different stages of evolution towards the physaliforous cell.

In an immunohistological study of 14 cases of typical chordomas and 5 cases of chondroid chordomas, Walker et al (1991) reported major differences between these two tumours. Whereas the antigenic expression of vimentin, protein S100 and NSE was close to 100% for both tumours, that for the epithelial membrane antigen and antikeratin was positive in up to 100% of typical chordomas but negative in the 5 cases of chondroid chordoma, as it is in chondrosarcoma. Further, HMB-45, whose reaction is positive in half of typical chordomas, is negative in chondroid chordomas. The authors suggest that it would be more appropriate to classify this latter tumour in the group of chondrosarcomas of low grade malignancy.

By ultrastructural examination, some authors have demonstrated the presence of both desmosomes and microtubular inclusions; these latter are also reported in extraskeletal myxoid chondrosarcomas. Others assert that ultrastructural examination shows that the zones of cartilaginous appearance are of an epithelial nature, like those in typical chordomas. Based on ultrastructural and immunohistochemical studies, Mierau et al (1987) consider chondroid chordoma to be a variant of chordoma and not a tumour derived from chondrocytes. This is the position of Brian Jeffrey et al (1995) who, in a major review of the literature, considered that at least three entities have been reported under the term of chondroid chordoma, viz: chondrosarcomas of a low grade of malignancy, hyalinised chondromas, and more rarely what the authors term "dedifferentiated chordoma". The 64 cases of tumours of the base of the skull studied (5 chondroid chordomas, 46 chordomas and 13 chondrosarcomas) led to the conclusion that chondroid chordoma exhibits some zones of chordal appearance and others of cartilaginous appearance, but that this is not a biphasic tumour. The immunological reactions for cytokeratin, EMA and PS100 are positive in both the chordoid and chondroid zones. Moreover, ultrastructural study of the chondroid zones demonstrates tonofibrils and desmosomes, confirming their epithelial nature. The authors suggest the term "hyalinised chordoma" for this tumour, whose prognosis seems identical to that of pure chordoma.

In practice, when the problem of distinguishing chondrosarcoma and chordoma arises because some zones appear cartilaginous, the positive immunological reactions for epithelial cells permit easy classification.

Diagnosis

The diagnosis of chordoma is easy to make in most cases; the appearance of the cells and their grouping, which suggest an epithelial formation, guide the diagnosis. However, sacral osteolysis may be the consequence of a metastasis from a colonic carcinoma; the size of the pseudoglandular cell groups and the frequency of mitoses, and often of atypical mitoses, should permit this diagnosis to be made. In a small sample, the clear cells may also suggest a metastasis from a renal epithelioma. But the cells of the renal tumour have a less chromophil nucleus, surrounded by a clearer cytoplasm. The vascularisation is usually different with an endocrinoid appearance. Lastly, but not invariably, in chordomas mucoid areas may be seen in which the chordal cells, dissociated or dispersed in small strands, resemble the histology of the nucleus pulposus. Finally, it has been established that tumours located outside the median axis of the body and described by the name of chordoid sarcomas are extraskeletal chondrosarcomas.

References

Abdelwahab IF, O'Leary PF, Steiner GC, Zwass A (1986) Chordoma of the fourth lumbar vertebra metastasizing to the thoracic spine and ribs. Skeletal Radiol 15: 242-246

Abenoza P, Sibley RK (1986) Chordoma: an immunohistologic study. Hum Pathol 17: 744-747

Alezais, Peyron A (1920) Sur l'évolution cellulaire du tissu notochordal dans les tumeurs. C R Soc Biol 83: 368-370

Anderson WB, Meyers Hl (1968) Multicentric chordoma. Report of a case. Cancer 21: 126-128

Benoit J, Videcoq PH, Hardy PH, Durigon M (1990) Les chordomes rachidiens. A propos d'un cas de chordome de L3. Rev Rhum Mal Osteoartic 57: 557-561

Bottles K, Beckstead JH (1984) Enzyme histochemical characterization of chordomas. Am J Surg Pathol 8: 443-447

Briand Jeffrey P, Biava CG, Davis RL (1995) Chondroid chordoma. A hyalinized chordoma without cartilaginous differentiation. Am J Clin Pathol 103: 271-279

Campbell WM, McDonald TJ, Unni KK, Laws ER (1980) Nasal and paranasal presentations of chordomas. The Laryngoscope 90: 612-618

Cesarini JP, Bonneau H (1971) A propos de l'étude ultrastructurale d'un chordome sacré. Arch Anat Path. 12: 95-102

Chavany JA, Hagenmuller D (1956) Sur une variété gravissime, heureusement rare, de tumeur intracrânienne, la forme postérieure des chordomes sphéno-occipitaux. Sem Hop (Paris) 77: 4154-4157

Chevalier X, Voisin MC, Brugières P, Ducou P, Lepointe H, Avouac B, Marty M, Martigoy J, Hernigou PH, Goutellier D, Villiaumey J, Larget-piet B (1990) Chordomes du rachis mobile. A propos de 9 cas. Revue de la littérature. Rev Rhum Mal Osteoartic 57: 767-778

Coindre JM, Rivel J, Trojani M, De Mascarel I, De Mascarel A (1986) Immunohistological study in chordomas. J Pathol 150: 61-63

De Vries J, Oldhoff J, Hadders HN (1986) Cryosurgical treatment of sacrococcygeal chordoma. Report of four cases. Cancer 58: 2348-2354

Eisemann ML (1980) Sphencocipital chordoma presenting as a nasopharyngeal mass. A case report. Ann Otol (St Louis) 89: 271-275

Fuentes JM, Benezech J, Iborra F, Marty M, Monthieu JY (1990) Les tumeurs rachidiennes primitives, résultats d'une enquête nationale. Rachis 2: 301-310

Gibas Z, Miettinen M, Sandberg AA (1992) Chromosomal abnormalities in two chordomas. Cancer Genet Cytogenet 58: 169-173

Griffet J, Perraud L, Lacour C, Paquis P, Grellier P (1987) Chordome du rachis cervical. Rev Chir Orthop 74: 299-301

Halpern J, Kopolovic J, Catane R (1984) Malignant fibrous histiocytoma developping in irradiated sacral chordoma. Cancer 53: 2661-2662

Heffelfinger MJ, Dahlin DC, McCarty CS, Beabout JW (1973) Chordomas and cartilaginous tumors at the skull base. Cancer 32: 410-420

Horwitz T (1941) Chordal ectopia and its possible relations to chordoma. Arch Pathol Lab Med 31: 354-362

Hruban RH, May M, Marcove RC, Huvos AH (1990) Lumbosacral chordoma with high-grade malignant cartilaginous and spindle cell components. Am J Surg Pathol 14, 4: 384-389

Hruban RH, Traganos F, Reuter VE, Huvos AG (1990) Chordomas with malignant spindle cell components. A DNA flow cytometric and immunohistochemical study with histogenetic implications. Am J Surg Pathol 137: 435-447

Kaiser TE, Pritchard DJ, Unni KK (1984) Clinicopathologic study of sacrococcygeal chordoma. Cancer 54: 2574-2578

Kay S, Schatzki PF (1972) Ultrastructural observations of a chordoma arising in the clivus. Hum Pathol 3: 403-413

Konrad AE, Meister P, Lob G, Lessler M (1981) Chordoma with a predominant retrosacral tumor mass. J Cancer Res Clin Oncol 101: 213-217

Lagacé R, Delage C (1975) Ultrastructure d'un chordome sacré. Ann Anat Pathol 20: 479-488

Laredo JD (1981) Les chordomes rachidiens et sacro-coccygiens. Description des différents aspects radiologiques. A propos de 27 cas. Thèse Doct Méd Paris

Laurent P, Linarte R, Noblia B, Senegas J, Le Rebeller A, Houton JL (1981) Chordomes vertébraux. Problèmes diagnostiques et thérapeutiques (Suppl II). Rev Chir Orthop 67: 1937-1940

Lefer LG, Rosier RP (1978) The cytology of chordoma. Acta Cytologica 22: 51-53

Mastuno T, Kaneda K, Nojima T (1987) Myxopapillary ependymoma of filum terminale with massive bone destruction of sacrum. Skeletal Radiol 16: 485-488

Meis JM, Raymond AK, Evans HL, Charles ER, Giraldo AA (1987) "Dedifferentiated" chordoma. A clinicopathologic and immunohistochemical study of three cases. Am J Surg Pathol 11: 516-525

Mierau GW, Weeks DA (1987) Chondroid chordoma. Ultrastructural Pathology 11: 731-737

Miettinen M, Karaharju E, Jarvinen H (1987) Chordoma with a massive spindle-cell sarcomatous transformation. A light and electron microscopic and immunohistological study. Am J Surg Pathol 11, 7: 563-570

Miettinen M, Lehto VP, Dahl D, Virtanen I (1983) Differential diagnosis tumors as aided by anti-intermediate filament antibodies. Am J Pathol 112: 160-169

Mitchell A, Scheithauer BW, Unni KK, Forsyth PJ, Wold LE, McGirney DJ (1993) Chordoma and chondroid neoplasms of the spheno-occiput. An immunohistochemical study of 41 cases with prognostic and nosologic implications. Cancer 72: 2943-2949

O'Connell J, Renard LG, Liebsch NJ, Efird JT, Muzenrider JE, Rosenberg AE (1994) Base of skull chordoma. A correlative study of histologic and clinical features of 62 cases. Cancer 74: 2261-2267

O'Dowd GJ, Schumann GB (1983) Aspiration cytology and cytochemistry of coccygeal chordoma. A case report and review of the literature. Acta Cytol 27: 178-183

Persons DL, Bridge JA, NeffJR (1991) Cytogenetic analysis of two sacral chordomas. Cancer Genet Cytogenet 56: 197-201

Plaza JA, Ballestin C, Perez-Barrios A, Martinez MA, De Augustin P (1989) Cytologic, cytochemical, immunocytochemical and ultrastructural diagnosis of a sacrococcygeal chordoma in a fine needle aspiration biopsy specimen. Case report. Acta Cytol 33, 1: 89-92

Ribbert H (1894) Über die Ecchondrosis Physalifora Sphenooccipitalis. Zentralbl Allg Path 5: 457-461

Rich TA, Schiller A, Suit D, Mankin HJ (1985) Clinical and pathologic review of 48 cases of chordoma. Cancer 56: 182-187

Roddie M, Adam A, Lambert H, Pickering D, Barker F (1989) Lumbar vertebral chordoma causing sclerosis of affected vertebra (3rd lumbar vertebra). Skeletal Radiol 17: 611-613

Salisbury JR, Isaacson PG (1985) Demonstration of cytokeratins and an epithelial membrane antigen in chordomas and human fetal notochord. Am J Surg Pathol 9: 791-797

Smith J, Reuter V, Demas B (1989) Anaplastic sacrococcygeal chordoma (dedifferentiatod chordoma). Skeletal Radiol 18: 561-564

Spoden JE, Bumsted RM, Warner ED (1980) Chondroid chordoma. Case report and literature review. Ann Otol (St Louis) 89: 279-285

Thiery JP, Mazabraud A, Mignot J, Durigon M (1977) Etude au microscope électronique d'un chordome sacré. Caractérisation de diverses étapes évolutives des cellules tumorales. Ann Anat Path (Paris) 22: 193-204

Thompson SK, Callery RT (1988) Cytologic diagnosis of a chordoma without physaliforous cells. Diagn Cytopathol 4: 144-147

Volpe R, Mazabraud A (1983) A clinicopathologic review of 25 cases of chordoma (a pleomorphic and metastasizing neoplasm). Am J Surg Pathol 7: 161-170

Walker WP, Landas SK, Browley MC, Sturm MTM (1991) Immunohistochemical distinction of classic and chondroid chordomas. Modern Pathol 4, 5: 661-666

Wyatt RB, Schochet SS, McCormick WF (1971) Ecchordosis physaliphora. An electron microscopy study. J Neurosurg 34: 672-677

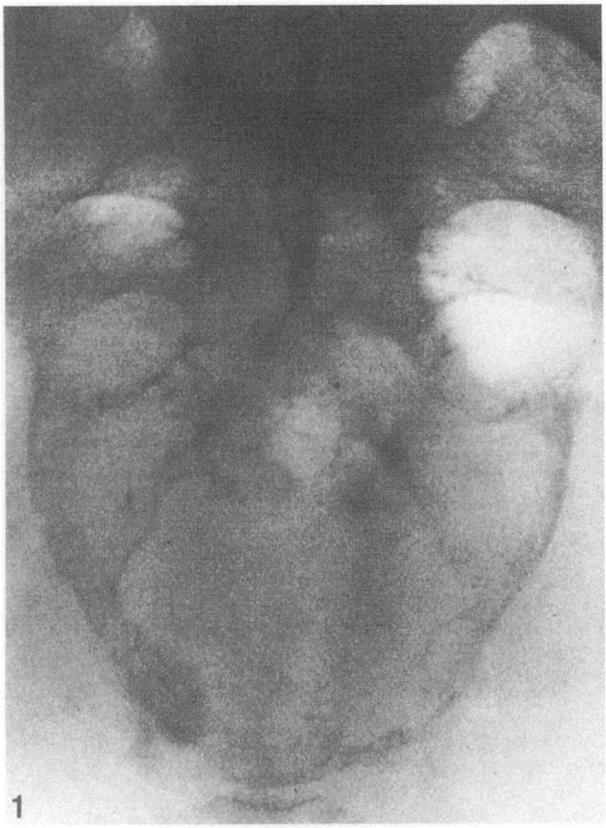

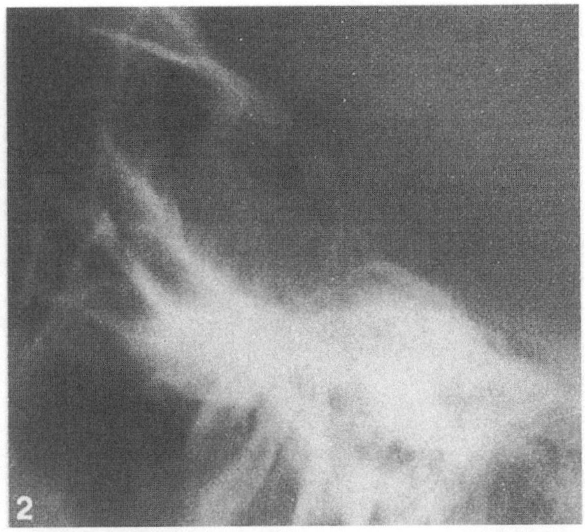

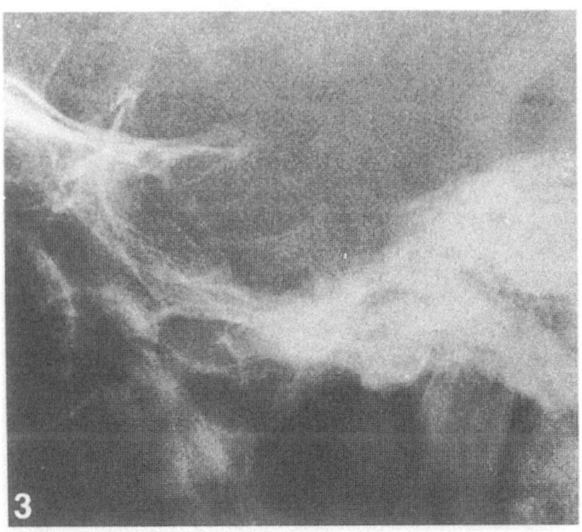

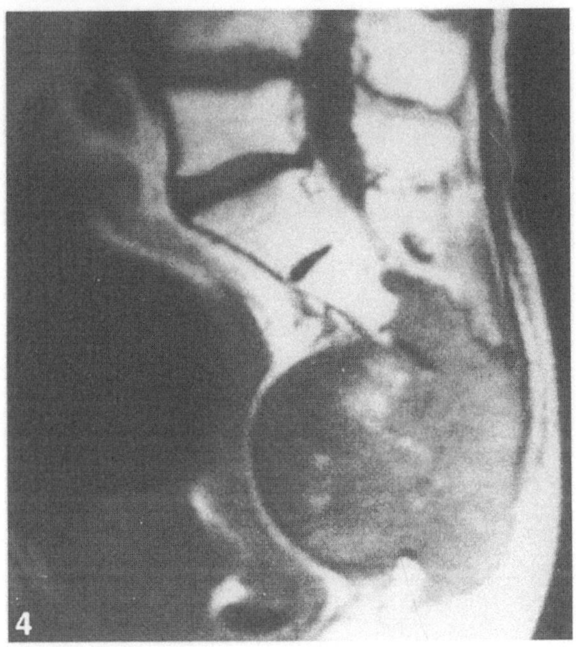

Fig. 1. A lytic tumour obliterates the lower sacral segments; only the first three sacral foramina are visible. Man of 48

Fig. 2. Sphenoidal chordoma filling the posterior part of the sphenoidal sinus, prebasilar shadow and decreased size of sella turcica. Woman of 53

Fig. 3. Major destruction of sella turcica by tumour

Fig. 4. Sacral chordoma, recurrence after radiotherapy. In this sagittal MRI section (T1 weighted, TR600, TE20), the tumour mass is heterogeneous and separated from the rectum by a clear line of fatty tissue. Posteriorly, the tumour reaches the spinal canal. The first two sacral vertebrae are intact; like L5, they have a more marked fatty content than the vertebrae above and are "whiter" because of the radiotherapy

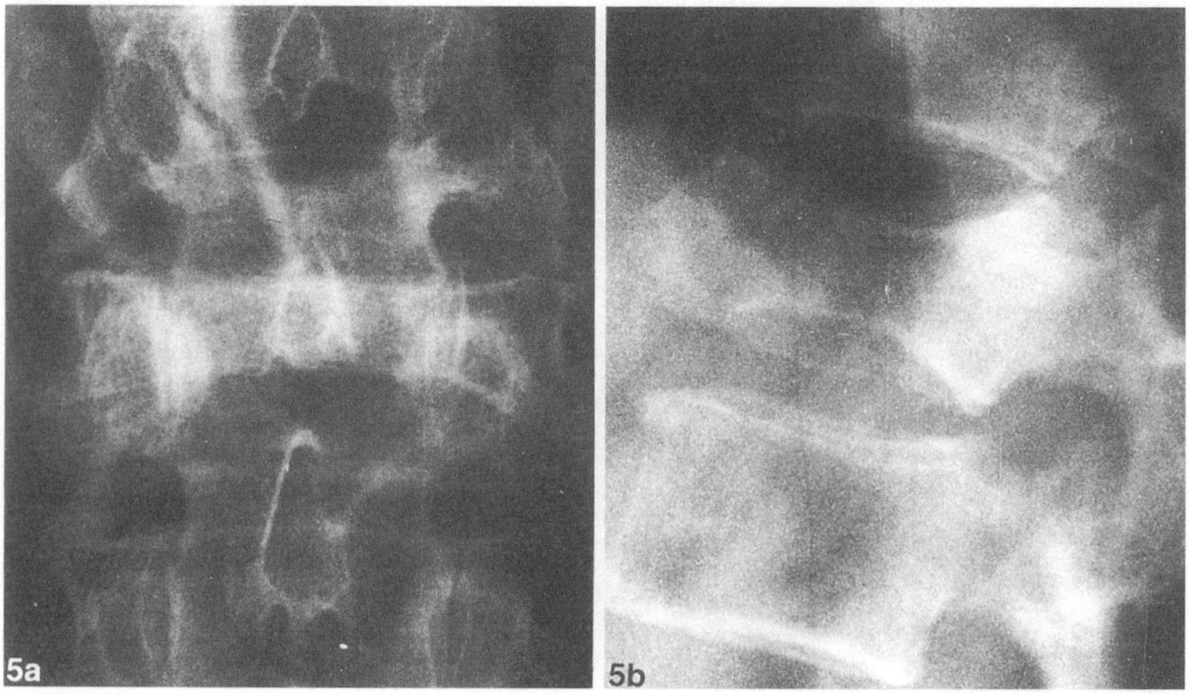

Fig. 5 a, b. Collapse of the body of L1, whose anteroposterior diameter seems increased in the lateral view

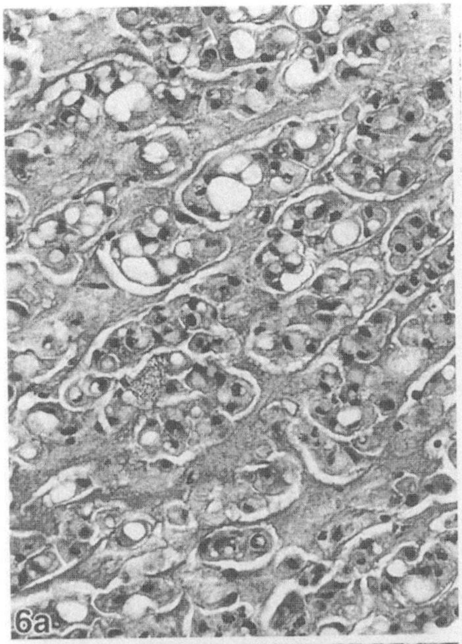

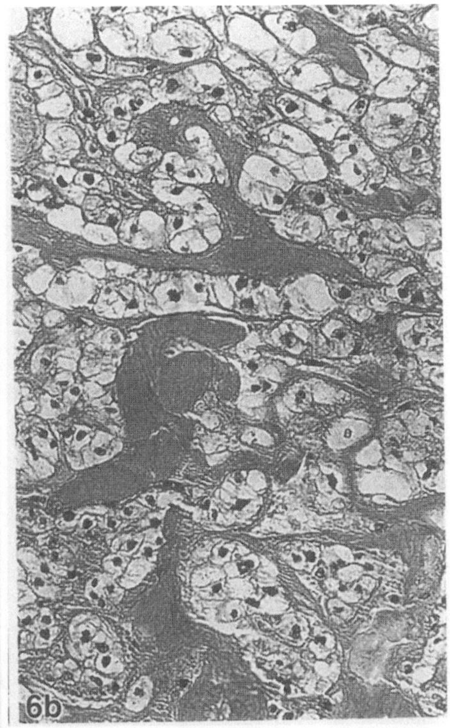

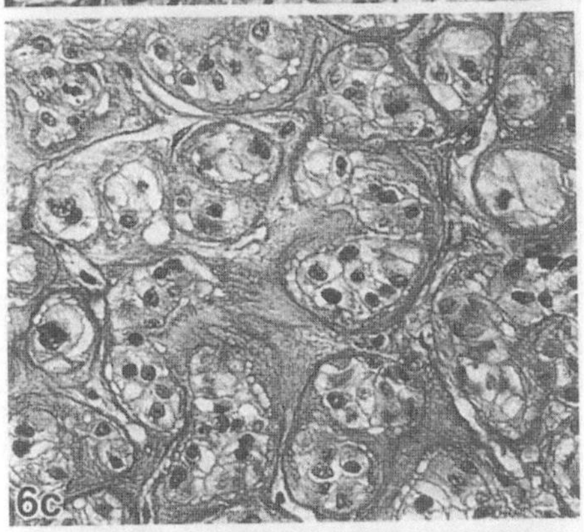

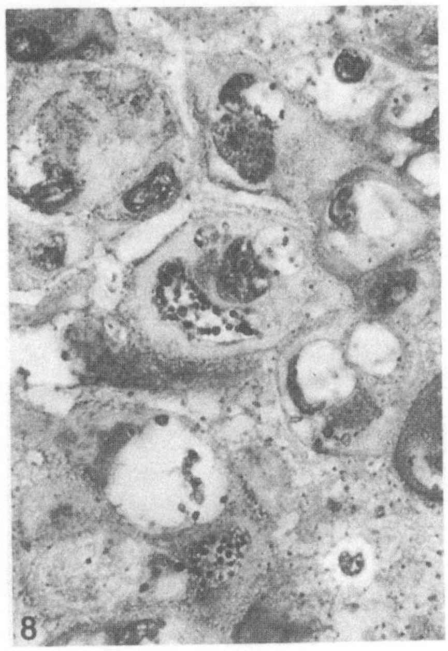

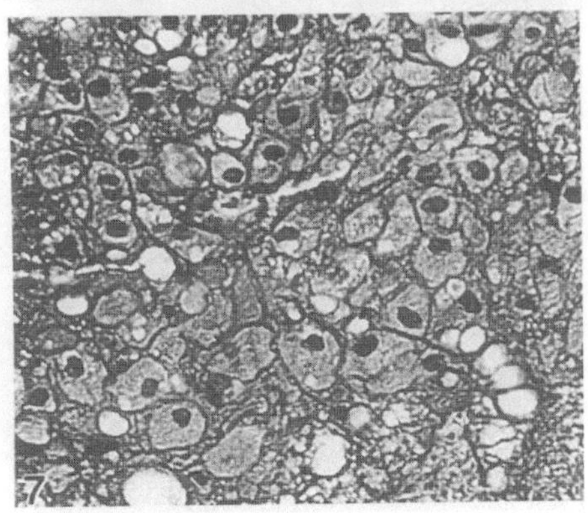

Fig. 6 a-c. The tumour cells are grouped in small islands and strands. At this magnification, the cell inequality is obvious; the very chromophil nuclei are central in the cell or displaced to the periphery by one or two vacuoles. A weakly chromophil ground substance surrounds the cell groups

Fig. 7. Here the cytoplasm is finely granular (grayish aspect in photograph) and clear vacuoles are rarer than in fig. 1. The epithelial appearance cannot be missed on examination of these different cellular preparations

Fig. 8. Multiple small fine granules, stained by Best's carmine (seen here as deep black) are scattered in the cytoplasm

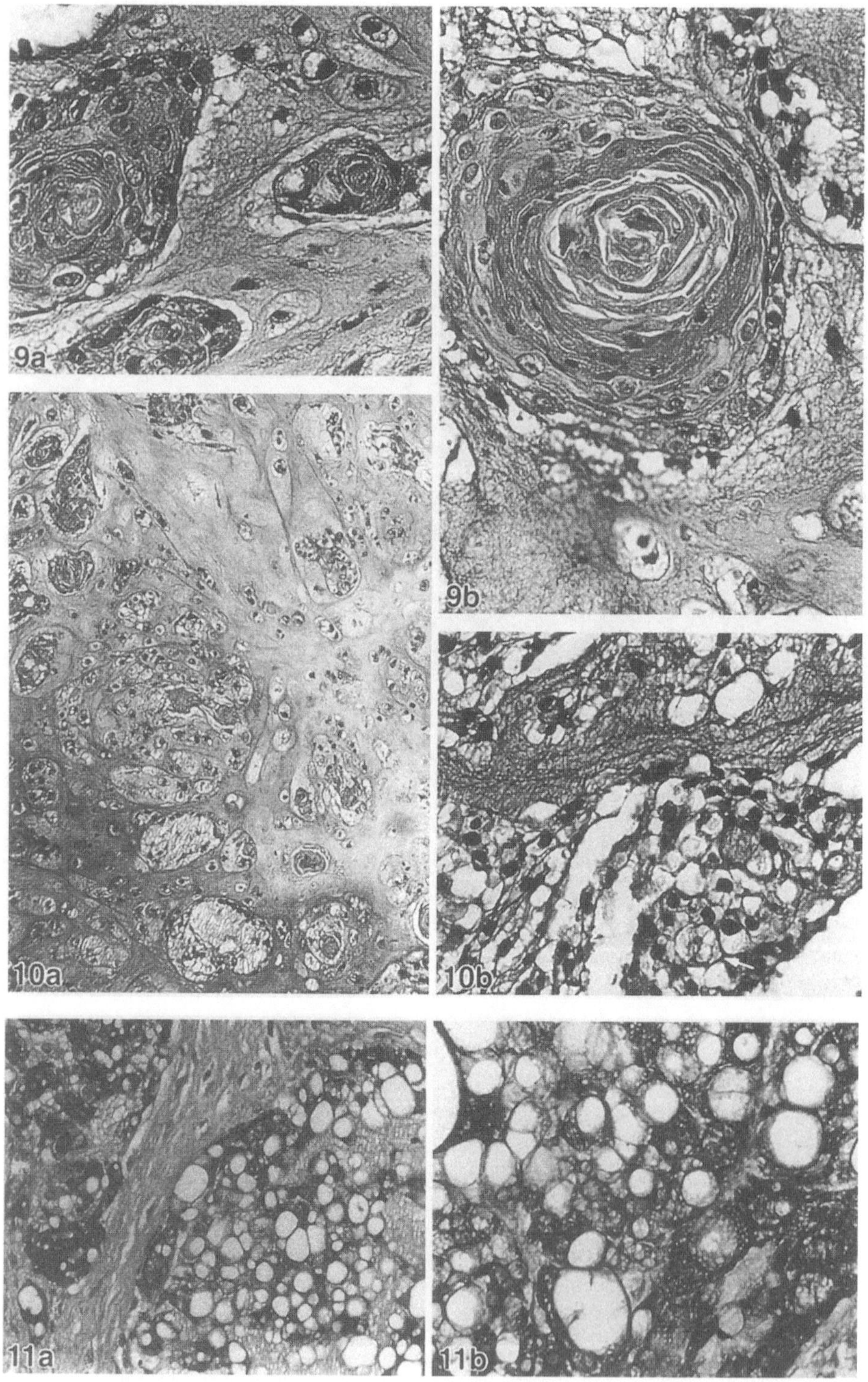

Fig. 9 a, b. Markedly keratinised bulbiform epithelial whorls

Fig. 10. a "Chondrocytic" appearance of isolated cells in the ground substance. **b** Vacuolated cells, one of which is larger with a central nucleus, giving the appearance of a physaliphorous cell (*arrow*)

Fig. 11. a Strongly positive reaction with antikeratin (KL1); the cytoplasm is deep black in these microphotographs. **b** Higher magnification, a physaliphorous cell in the upper left corner

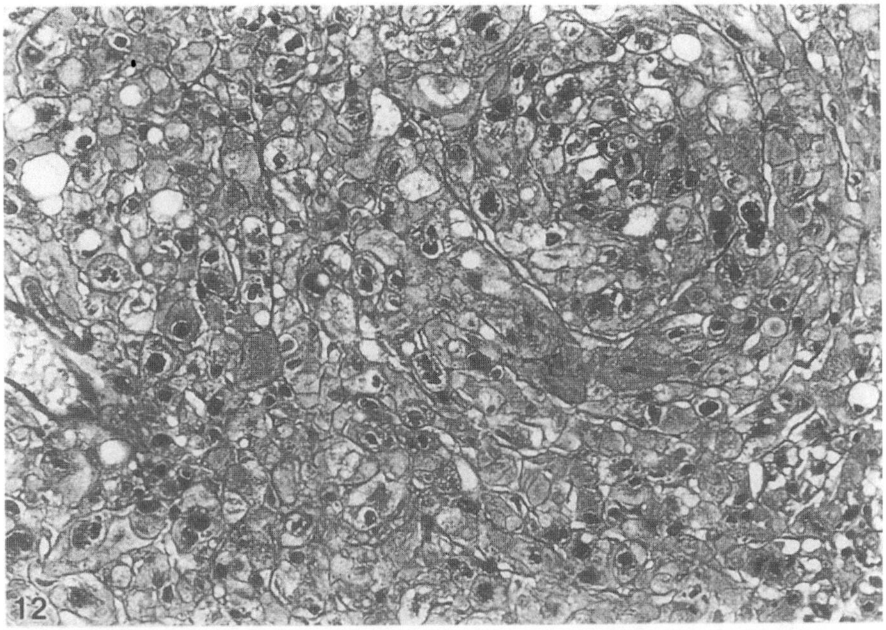

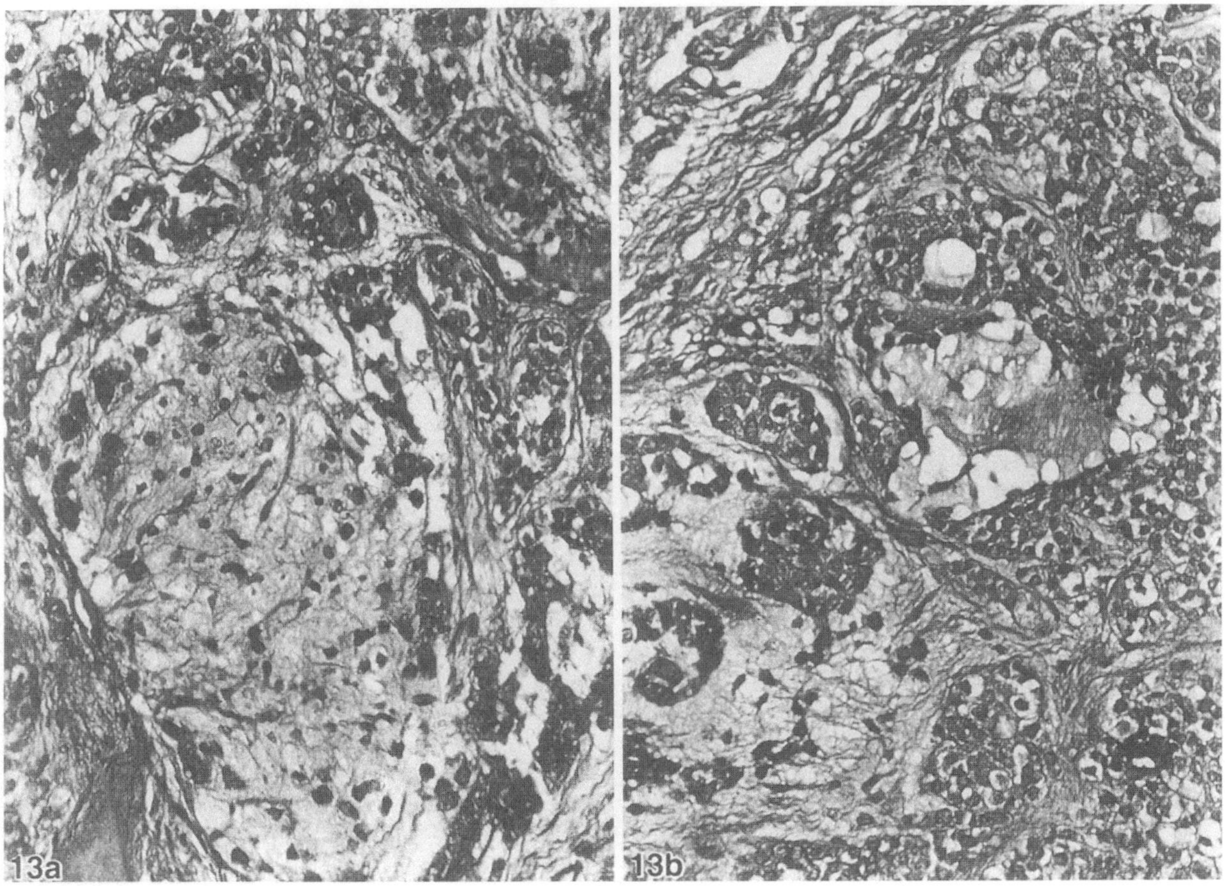

Fig. 12. Densely whorled appearance of epithelial cells with sharp borders, considerable anisonucleosis

Fig. 13 a, b. The cells are isolated or grouped in small islands scattered in pools of mucus

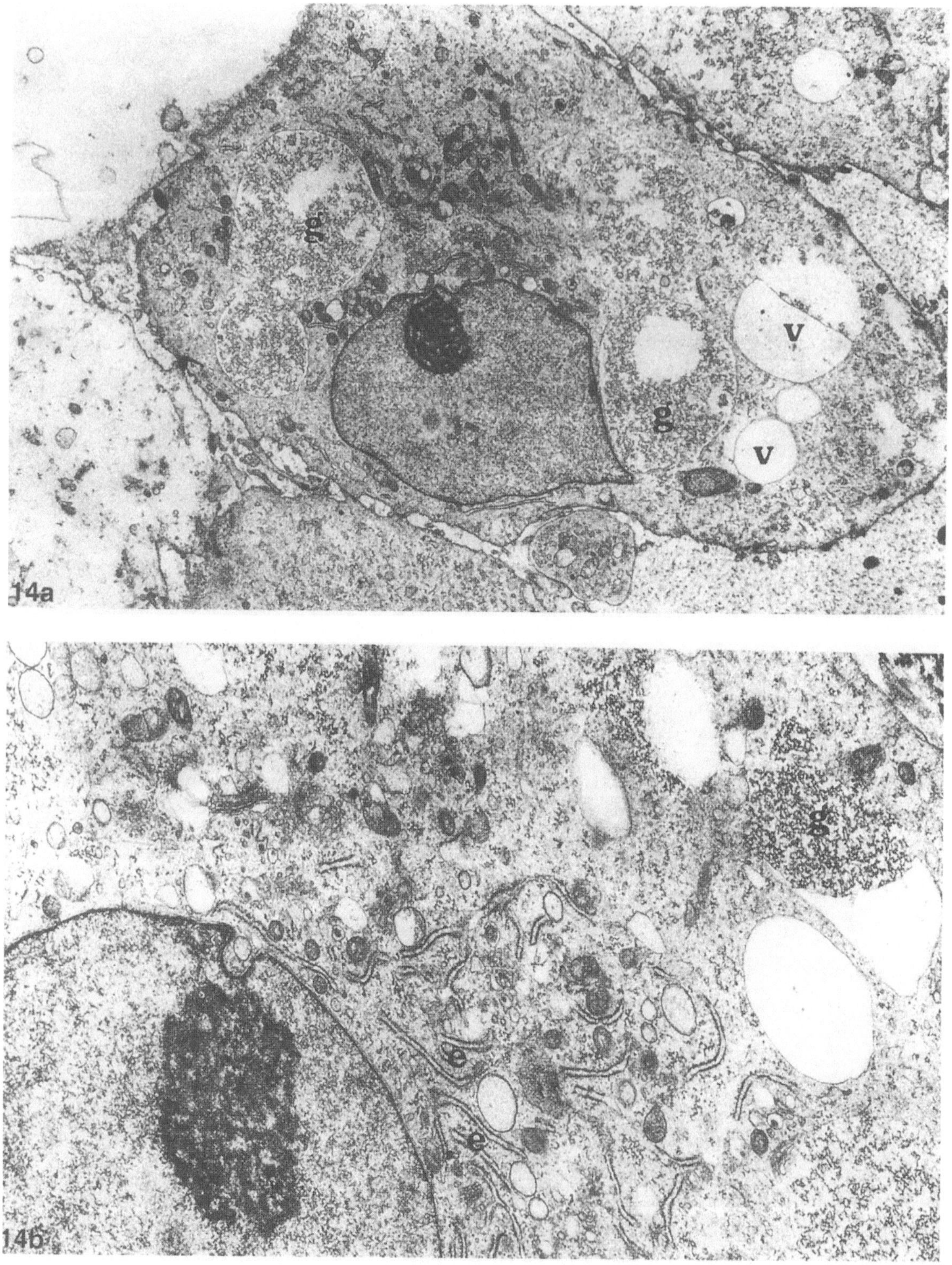

Fig. 14 a, b. Electron microscopy: x 5700 and x 22,000. The chromatin in the nucleus is dispersed in fine clumps, the nucleoli are dense, some small accumulations of glycogen (*g*) in the vicinity of vacuoles of reduced size. The cytoplasmic organelles are collected near the nucleus. (*e*) ergastoplasm (J.-P. Thiery)

21. Giant-cell tumour

Benign giant-cell tumour

Historically, this lesion was first a sarcoma "à myéloplaxes", became then known as a benign tumour with giant cells [Nélaton 1860]. It is a disturbing lesion because its course cannot be predicted histologically (this is not the pathologist's favourite tumour!). Confusion and debate have been fostered by the established dogma that the giant cell was the specific histological element. This attitude led to the classification in the same general category of aneurysmal cysts, chondroblastomas, telangiectatic sarcomas, and probably what we now recognise as malignant fibrous histiocytoma with giant cells. A vestige of this attitude persists in recent textbooks, which still use the term "stromal cells" to designate those tumour cells which are mononuclear.

Case histories

Case 1. Mrs R., aged 40, a farmer actively engaged in work of a diversified nature, decided to attend an orthopaedic clinic in extremis. For 5-6 months she had suffered with her right knee, first mainly when tired and then more constantly; at the same time the joint underwent a change in shape. On examination, the lower end of the femur was enlarged and slightly warmer than the opposite knee. Imaging demonstrated metaphyseo-epiphyseal lysis, well circumscribed on the shaft side, but destroying the internal cortex. The diagnosis of giant-cell tumour was plausible, but so was that of anaplastic sarcoma. Histological examination of the biopsy confirmed the diagnosis of giant-cell tumour without signs of malignancy.

Case 2. A woman of 30 attended a rheumatology department. As far as the history could determine the onset of symptoms, she had suffered pain in the right shoulder for 3-4 months. On examination, the shoulder was slightly deformed, but imaging showed virtually complete destruction of the head of the humerus. These very disturbing clinical and radiological features contrasted with the histological findings in the biopsy - a typical giant-cell tumour without cellular anomalies. It is understandable that such a discrepancy is sometimes difficult to accept by our colleagues responsible for treatment. So it was with a friendly insistence that the pathologist confronted with this problem, firm in his conviction, was compelled to answer for the histologically benign nature of the tumour... in the fragment examined. In the case mentioned here, excision of the humeral head was followed by definitive cure, a fortunate outcome for both patient and pathologist!

Preliminary remarks

True giant-cell tumour develops in a mature skeleton in the metaphyseo-epiphyseal region of the long bones of the limbs. The normal course of an untreated tumour leads to ulceration of the skin and suppuration, without either histological or other modification of the benign nature of the lesion. "Benign" histology at biopsy is not predictive of recurrences metastases, or sarcomatous transformation.

Some authors have stressed the existence of episodes of progression, unrelated to any hormonal factor for some instances but, interdependent with the stages of reproductive life in women for others. It is important to note that any "giant-cell tumour" (but not any tumour with giant cells) which develops on a long bone outside the metaphyseo-epiphyseal regions, or in any other bone of the skeleton, or in the metaphyseo-epiphyseal zone in a patient outside the usual age group, requires that calcium/phosphorus metabolism be examined. This should include at minimum the estimation of blood levels of calcium and phosphorus and possibly an esti-

Table 1. Diagnosis of giant-cell tumour

Site: metaphyseo-epiphyseal, long bones of limbs
Age: 3rd and 4th decades mainly
Histology: amphophil cells, interconnected by fine prolongations, possible small osteoid areas. Numerous mitoses (in exacerbation period) suggest resection rather than curettage.
If the age and/or site are atypical (immature skeleton, diaphyseal location), caution is necessary: think of brown tumour of von Recklinghausen; chondroblastoma; aneurysmal cyst; reparative granuloma, giant-cell tumour in Paget's disease, fibrous defect, anaplastic sarcoma.
Vertebral location is very special. Exclude: aneurysmal cyst, osteoblastoma; multifocal forms have been reported
Multiple non-progressive metastases: around 3% of cases
If there are signs of malignancy, consider: anaplastic sarcoma, malignant fibrous histiocytoma
1-2% of giant-cell tumours diagnosed as benign progress towards malignancy

mation of parathyroid hormone, unless Paget's disease is known to affect the incriminated bone. Before making a diagnosis of giant-cell tumour in a patient under 20 years of age, and still more under 15, one must formally exclude an aneurysmal cyst and especially a telangiectatic anaplastic sarcoma, whether or not with giant cells. Finally a reparative granuloma with giant cells must be excluded.

General considerations

Giant-cell tumour represents around 5-7% of all bone tumours, and around 20% of benign tumours. The statistics show a slight female predominance (55-60%). It is rare before the age of 20 and exceptional before 15 and is seen mainly in the 3rd and 4th decades [Dahlin et al 1970, Dahlin & Unni 1986]. About 75% are localised near the end of a long bone at a metaphyseo-epiphyseal site.

Half the cases develop around the knee, followed by the lower end of the radius, sacrum and lower end of ulna and fibula. The phalanges, carpal and metacarpal bones, vertebrae and some skull bones (frontal, sphenoid) may also be affected. Rib lesions are very rare, of the order of 0.6% of the total [Hanna et al 1992]. Giant-cell tumour is very rare in the patella, around 1-4 per thousand bone tumours; but in 210 patellar tumours collected from the literature [Mercuri et al 1991] giant-cell tumour was nevertheless the commonest (28% of cases).

Clinical features and course

The patient attends either for disabling pain or for a tumour. In half the cases the symptoms go back up to 6 months before the first consultation. In the long bones, presentation is with fracture in 5-8% of cases.

Properly treated, cure is obtained in the great majority of cases, even if it is necessary to reoperate for local recurrences and solitary pulmonary metastases [Vanel et al 1983, Wray et al 1990]. The percentage of local recurrence is in great part dependent on the operation, but in general should not exceed 10-15%. As for pulmonary metastases of benign tumours, these occur in 2-6% in different series; a figure of 3% is probably closer to reality [Vanel et al 1983, Rock 1984, Bertoni et al 1985, 1988, Wray et al 1990]. A malignant course, histologically unpredictable, occurs in 1-2% of cases [Hutter et al 1962, Nascimento et al 1979, Sanerkin 1980].

The various published series differ considerably from one another and allow only some general remarks; sites where surgical intervention is likely to lead to incomplete removal of the tumour have a less favourable prognosis, and apart from death attributed to "malignant transformation", death may occur from sudden massive haemorrhage from ulceration of great vessels.

Imaging

The relatively characteristic radiological appearance will suggest the diagnosis in the majority of cases. It is a clear, round or oval, lytic lesion with its long axis parallel to that of the limb, in a metaphyseal or metaphyseo-epiphyseal site (figs. 1, 2). Radiologically, there may be distinguished tumours whose osteolysis is well circumscribed, particularly towards the medullary canal, by a fine line of ossification concave towards the articulation (fig. 3). The cortex is preserved, though possibly ballooned (figs. 5, 6). The joint surface is intact. "Septa" are often described which do not partition the tumour, as may be seen in the resection specimens. These are actually bony ridges elongated along the long axis of the bone which correspond to cortical zones, probably still dense and not destroyed by the tumour proliferation. An alveolar appearance is rare and does not suggest a diagnosis of giant-cell tumour specifically (fig. 8). Tumours that have destroyed the cortex and whose boundaries are punched (figs. 2, 4) are also seen. These two appearances are very difficult or even impossible to reconcile with the histological lesion and clinical course. In any case, though this osteolysis is relatively characteristic for the long bones, it is less suggestive in the sacrum and the mobile spine (fig. 7).

Pathological anatomy and histopathology

Macroscopically (figs. 9-11), the tumour is reddish and soft, with denser zones corresponding to fibrous areas or to small osteoid masses. It is enclosed in a bony cavity unrelated to the soft tissues and articular cartilage, from which it is separated by a bony band of varying width. If the tumour is more advanced it may destroy the cortex, separated from the soft tissues only by a fine fibrous septum. In the most advanced cases it invades the periarticular tissues, ulcerates the skin and penetrates into the adjacent joint. In the knee it follows the cruciate ligaments, less often a collateral ligament, and infiltrates into the articulation via a perforation of very small diameter hollowed out against the attachment of a ligament. Rarely two adjacent bones are affected: radius and ulna, tibia and fibula.

Histological examination demonstrates a monomorphous proliferation of round or slightly oval cells which constitute a uniform background against which the multinucleate giant cells stand out (figs. 13, 14). The nucleus of the mononucleate cells is rounded, its chromatin is fine, the clearly visible nucleolus is small, and mitoses are rare. The nuclei of the giant cells are of the same type as those of the mononucleate cells. The giant cells are often irregularly distributed. They are bulky, and have 40-100 nuclei (figs. 14, 15). The nuclei are often grouped in the central part of the cytoplasm, which also contains inclusions and vacuoles of varying size (fig. 25). There are some zones of foamy histiocytes (fig. 21), siderophages and possibly some inflammatory cells often associated with these two cell types (fig. 18). Collagen formation, usually absent in the central part, may appear more or less discretely at the periphery; in these zones the mononuclear cells assume a fusiform appearance.

Silver staining reveals a reticulin network and in frozen sections histochemical reactions demonstrate the presence of acid phosphatases in the cytoplasm of the giant cells and of some mononuclear cells (fig. 20).

The following three points are of value to the pathologist:

- Staining with haematoxylin-eosin gives the section an overall slightly mauve colour, due to the amphophil nature of the cytoplasm of most of the tumour cells.
- Often, fine cytoplasmic prolongations may connect adjacent cells.
- In virtually every case where it is possible to examine the connective tissue adjoining the tumour in numerous sections, small tumour fragments are found in dilated vessels. More rarely a lesion of the vessel wall is seen. These observations seem to have no prognostic significance (fig. 19).

Variants in the typical appearance

Examination of numerous sections often shows the presence of small osteoid or bony areas, sometimes in the very midst of the tumour. This finding is without diagnostic or prognostic implications (fig. 21). If numerous mitoses are found, possibly associated with some atypical cells and especially present fusiform cells outside the peripheral zones of collagen formation, they must be scrupulously mentioned in the report. The finding indicates that the surgical procedure should be a wide resection rather than curettage. The statistics then show a better outcome in these cases than in forms that are apparently "tranquil" in a simple biopsy, but in which curettage does not give a 100% guarantee against local recurrence. Very exceptionally, the presence of small cartilaginous islands has been reported in these tumours; I have not seen this myself, but it is not always easy to differentiate between osteoid and chondroid tissue.

During examination of the biopsy, it is important to remember that the histological appearance varies from one zone to another and that progression in discrete exacerbations is necessary. Correlations between the course of the tumour, the radiological appearances and the histological appearance is not close enough to attach real value to grading, and DNA study has not been shown to have any prognostic value [Ladanyi 1989, Sara et al 1990]. The most reliable prognostic factor is the nature of the surgical procedure, effective surgery alone provides a good result.

Differential diagnosis

We have noted the elements of a positive diagnosis and here stress the fact that the diagnosis of giant-cell tumour is no exception to the general rule; it is based on concordance of the clinical, radiological and histological findings. Unfortunately, despite their precision, immunohistological studies [Doussis et al 1992] are not of much help in the diagnosis of giant-cell tumour.

Brown tumour

The brown tumour of parathyroid osteosis (von Recklinghausen's disease of bone) may be histologically impossible to distinguish from a giant-cell tumour. Collagen fibers and osteoid strands are inconstant and inadequate to identify it; its considerable vascularisation may be suspicious unless it suggests an angioma or an aneurysmal cyst. It is wise and simple to request the estimation of phosphorus and calcium almost routinely when the diagnosis of giant-cell tumour is in question, and this becomes imperative if the lesion is not metaphyseo-epiphyseal, if radiological examination reveals other bone lesions, or if the patient's age is outside the normal range. In such cases, a study of calcium/phosphorus metabolism and/or the level of parathormone are the more necessary.

Giant-cell tumour in Paget's disease

Cases of "giant-cell tumour" have also been reported in Paget's disease. The quite special context and often cranial localisation usually permit diagnosis [Schajowicz & Slullitel 1966].

Chondroblastoma

Chondroblastoma is relatively easy to identify. The cells are rounded and strongly eosinophil, unlike those of giant-cell tumour which are amphophil. Commonly, a fine clear margin is seen around these cells, separating them from one another or isolating them in a rudimentary deposit of chondroid substance. This intercellular material forms typical cartilaginous islands in places. Lastly, and especially, the epiphyseal site and the often early age of the patient are incompatible with the diagnosis of giant-cell tumour.

Cortico-metaphyseal fibrous defect

Cortico-metaphyseal fibrous defects pose no special problem. Bundles of fusiform cells with fine elongated nuclei, between which are collagen fibers and areas of foamy histiocytes, and irregularly distributed giant cells which are rarely numerous complete the histological picture of a biopsy made in a child, and so enable clinicians to reassure the parents who may have been worried by the radiological examination, despite its characteristic appearance.

Aneurysmal cyst

Aneurysmal cyst may be much more difficult to diagnose. One must seek biopsy tissue fragments for long osteoid bands bordering the blood-filled spaces. Here again, the frequent youthfulness of the patient, the epiphyseal site and the radiological appearances are valid arguments against the diagnosis of giant-cell tumour.

Giant-cell sarcoma

A giant-cell sarcoma, completely devoid of tumour zones with non-sarcomatous giant cells, must be distinguished from an exceptional giant-cell tumour in process of sarcomatous transformation in which both aspects coexist (the grade 3 giant-cell tumour of some authors).

Osteogenic sarcoma

Anaplastic telangiectatic osteogenic sarcoma is a very vascularised tumour in which small osteoid strands can be seen, often bordering on the wall of a vascular cavity. The atypical aspect of the osteogenesis and above all the cytonuclear anomalies shape the diagnosis, which is based equally on both clinical and radiological findings.

Malignant fibrous histiocytoma and fibroblastic sarcoma

Malignant fibrous histiocytoma and fibroblastic sarcoma are histologically different from a giant-cell tumour. They should not be regarded as the malignant evolution of giant-cell tumour: authentic areas of giant-cell tumour can be found in biopsy or resection specimens.

Reparative granuloma with giant cells

Reparative granuloma with giant cells was described by Jaffe in 1953 in the maxilla and then in other bones of the craniofacial skeleton, a diagnosis made by Ackerman and Spjut in 1962 in the bones of the phalanges. In 52 lytic lesions of the hands and feet with giant cells, Picci et al (1986) diagnosed 11 reparative granulomas as against 9 giant-cell tumours. The label "giant cell reaction", proposed by Helpap et al (1981) for a lytic and expanding lesion of the diaphysis of a 2nd metatarsal is more realistic. It is possible, at least in some cases, that this granuloma is related to a local haemorrhage.

General considerations

This is a rare lesion, less than 10% of maxillary tumours, and an even smaller percentage when compared with tumours of the bones of the hands and feet. It may seem surprising to assess the frequency of a granuloma against tumours of the same sites. However, the problem raised by the clinical picture and imaging is precisely the need to eliminate a true tumour. There is a slight female predominance and, although the granuloma may be seen at any age, it is commoner before 25. The lesions are mainly localised in the craniofacial skeleton, particularly the maxillae, but more often in the ethmoid, temporal and sphenoid bones. It also affects the phalanges of the hands and feet and the tarsal and carpal bones. Lorenzo and Dorman (1980) reported 8 cases in the small bones of the hands and feet, 1 vertebral and 2 costal lesions. Picci et al (1986) reported 11 cases in the bones of the hands and feet.

Clinical features and course

The clinical picture is one of pain and swelling; sometimes a pathological fracture calls for radiological examination. In 25% of cases the history is one of local injury. The period between the first symptoms and consultation extends from a few weeks to several years. The blood-levels of calcium and phosphorus are normal. The course is favourable, even after several recurrences.

Imaging

Imaging displays a clear rounded or oval osteolytic zone, accompanied by bony expansion. Usually this area of osteolysis measures between 1.5 and 2.5 cm in diameter and is sometimes veined by some trabeculae appearing as persistent ridges in a thinned cortex. There is no sclerosis but CT examination may demonstrate an opacity corresponding to peripheral osteoid formation.

The granuloma, if in the tubular bones of the hands and feet, is sited in the diaphysis or metaphysis; in one case, however, reported by Lorenzo and Dorman (1980), the metatarsal epiphysis was involved. It may appear superficial and subperiosteal (fig. 26).

Pathological anatomy and histopathology

At operation the lesion is reddish-brown and friable; sometimes there is a collection of blood. The reports generally refer to the well defined edges of the granuloma.

The giant cells in the histological sections are scattered in a background of fusiform or more or less polyhedral cells. These giant cells phagocytose some red corpuscles and haemosiderin pigment. Mitoses are rare. Generally the granuloma is very vascular and contains little collagen. Silver impregnation shows a rich reticulin network.

Some appearances depart from this general description: the giant cells are grouped in clumps, often around the vessels, and not dispersed throughout the granuloma; cystic aspects filled with red corpuscles may resemble an aneurysmal cyst. In some granulomas, osteoid or osseous metaplasia appears amidst the fibrous proliferation.

Differential diagnosis

The clinical features, age, site and histological examination usually point to the diagnosis. But from the histological viewpoint alone, it may be impossible to distinguish a granuloma from the brown tumour of von Recklinghausen's disease. Estimation of plasma calcium and phosphorus levels and perhaps of parathormone will then be required.

Difficulties and controversies

Localisation

Adding together the cases reported in the publications of Verbiest (1965), Larson et al(1975) and Dahlin (1977), involving the vertebrae of the mobile spine and one case in the sacrum, we note that 29.7% of patients are under the age of 20. Based on 31 cases affecting only the mobile spine, Dahlin has suggested, given the age of the patients (7 in the second decade, 2 in the first), that these vertebral tumours are fundamentally different from other giant-cell tumours. However this may be, the prognosis was frankly good in patients who were followed up, most for many years, despite the treatment employed at that time. This generally involved curettage followed by radiotherapy, often after one or two local recurrences. With current procedures one may therefore expect an excellent prognosis.

The clinical picture of these tumours is of the presence of local pain, and of variable neurological manifestations depending on the site and size of the tumour; hypoesthesia, muscular atrophy, motor impairment and signs of cord compression may all be found.

In radiographs, the tumour develops mainly in the vertebral body but can invade the posterior arch and extend beyond the vertebral body, either into the paravertebral connective and muscular soft tissues, or towards the spinal canal. If the cells are smaller or exhibit a fusiform tendency, the most important duty is to ensure absence of signs of malignancy.

Two possible benign lesions must be considered: aneurysmal cyst and osteoblastoma. The latter is markedly commoner in the vertebrae than giant-cell tumour.

Currently, complete excision of a vertebra is practicable, but a sacral tumour, often diagnosed late, still poses serious problems. It is in the context of this tumour that some authors have suggested cryotherapy as a supplementary treatment.

Forms with multiple (bony) lesions have been reported, without a hyperparathyroid syndrome [Deburge & De Grandmaison 1980, Peimer et al 1980,

Tornberg et al 1975, Sim et al 1977, Kaiser et al 1993, Ogihara et al 1994, Bacchini et al 1995].

Fain et al (1993) have reported two cases of a tibial shaft lesion in patients aged 21 and 27. Beyond the restrictions I have already stressed, this poses a diagnostic problem, especially from an anaplastic sarcoma.

Giant-cell tumour in the immature skeleton

Giant-cell tumour may develop in the growing skeleton, or when growth is, exceptionally, completed before the age of 15 [Reckling et al 1979]. Although the percentage quoted is quite variable in different sources, giant-cell tumour before 15 years is rare. If we exclude some rare and abnormally high figures, the percentage varies between 1.1 and 2%. Picci et al (1983), in a paper dealing with experience at the Rizzoli Institute (326 cases) found 6 cases occurring in the growing skeleton. The skeleton was so defined when there complete obliteration of the growth-plate had not yet occurred. The series of Schütte and Taconis (1993) is quite typical. Of 402 patients, 49 were under 19; 10.6% of the giant-cell tumours thus developed in children and adolescents. Lipszyc (1990), in his thesis, describes a giant-cell tumour of the lower end of the femur in a girl aged 10 1/2 years (fig. 25).

The delay between the first symptoms and diagnosis is of the order of some months. The radiological image is identical to that of giant-cell tumour in adults: an eccentric metaphyseal osteolytic zone adjacent to the epiphysis, which may be invaded. The cortex is not invaded. The elective sites are the metaphyses at the knee.

The histological features are no different from those in adults. One cannot overstress the caution with which this diagnosis must be made in every case where the tumour develops outside the usual range of age and site. Before the age of 15 it is proper to seek signs of precocious maturity, as expressed by the secondary sexual characteristics, and to scrupulously monitor the image of the state of the growth-plate.

Histological grading of malignancy

The problem of the histological grade of malignancy is a disturbing one. The attribution of a designation of grade 1 to a tumour which may show about 2% of sarcomatous evolution is unhelpful. In support of this position, which some may consider to represent disillusion, I quote the work of Fukanaga et al (1992). These authors studied 26 cases of giant-cell tumour and their conclusions show little predictive value for DNA analysis by flow cytometry; there is no significant correlation between DNA ploidy, histological grading of malignancy and the presence or absence of pulmonary metastases.

Grade III histological malignancy merits the name of giant-cell sarcoma, which does not necessarily correspond to the term of malignant giant-cell tumour as the lesion may be a malignant fibrous histiocytoma or a fibroblastic sarcoma with giant cells.

Viral inclusions

Viral inclusions have been reported in the osteoclasts of Paget's disease and in the giant cells of giant-cell tumour [Mills & Singer 1976, Le Charpentier et al 1977, Mirra et al 1981]. Their nature and role are uncertain.

Acid phosphatase

This has been demonstrated in the osteoclasts and giant cells of the tumours. This phosphatase is contained in abundance in the collected lysosomes in defined cytoplasmic territories. As a result of these findings, J.-P. Thiery et al (1975) proposed the hypothesis that this acid phosphatase, excreted locally in abundance, could enter the general circulation and increase the level of plasma phosphatase. This was confirmed by study of the plasma of patients taken before and after resection of the tumour [Motais de Narbonne et al 1977]. The presence of this osteoclastic acid phosphatase in the blood is revealed by electrophoresis on polyacrylamide gel, where it is characterised by the appearance of a minimum of two close bands in the zone of slow migration (figs. 31, 32). The reappearance of these bands in a plasma which had returned to normal after excision of the tumour allows the firm diagnosis of the development of recurrence when the radiological images are unclear between postoperative remodelling or recurrence.

Histogenesis

Observations taken from immunological studies, cultures and certain clinical facts led Athanasou and Quinn (1990) to the conclusion that the osteoclastic line on the one hand and the macrophagic monocyte line on the other have a monoblast or a promonocyte in common. They suppose that the cell which is at the origin of the osteoclast separates at a very early stage from that which gives rise to the (monocyte) macrophage. This would explain the presence of common cytoplasmic and surface antigens (CD45, CD54, CD68) but also of numerous different antigens. Given that no specific osteoclastic antigen has been identified, the distinction between osteoclast and multinuclear macrophage must be based on the inability to demonstrate antigens which are expressed only by the multinuclear macrophages (CD11 a, b, c, CD18, CD14).

Various opinions have been given regarding the formation of giant cells. It is virtually impossible to observe a mitosis in a giant cell; even when searching for them routinely, I have seen a mitotic nucleus only three times in a giant cell. In culture mitoses may be seen. Like J.-P. Thiery we believe that the most likely process is multiplication by mitosis without division of the cytoplasm.

Treatment

Treatment is by complete surgical excision. Recurrences are commoner after curettage than after resection. Dreinhöfer et al (1995) state that pathological fracture does not contraindicate classical treatments, but of 15 patients treated 4 (26%) recurred. In cases which could not be completely excised and were treated by supplementary irradiation, the statistics record malignant transformation of the order of 20-25%. Adjuvant cryotherapy has been suggested, but is not without local risks [Marcove et al 1973, 1994]. In every case prolonged surveillance is necessary, both clinical and radiological. Solitary pulmonary metastases should be excised and the prognosis remains favourable.

Kaiser et al (1993) report a case where interferon treatment had a spectacular effect on bilateral pleural and pulmonary metastases in a woman of 37 who presented with bone and skin lesions; but the follow-up period was relatively short (less than two years).

Malignant giant-cell tumour (figs. 12, 22, 23)

A giant-cell tumour is diagnosed as benign. Following several local recurrences - without irradiation - the histological image is transformed to become that of a sarcoma with fusiform cells, atypical mitoses, necrosis, giant cells of irregular shape and size. It is not possible, in principle, to exclude the possibility of malignant transformation of a benign tumour, but such malignant transformation is rare, perhaps of the order of 1-2%. This figure provides the first question: does not a 1-2% rate of malignant transformation fall within the limits of error of histological examination, limits below which it is impossible to go in the conditions imposed by optical microscopy? We are too familiar with the alleged "chondroblastomas" and "osteoblastomas" which are merely very differentiated chondrosarcomas and ostesarcomas of slow evolution. From this angle, does the persistence of histologically benign areas permit one to consider that there has been a malignant transformation?

It would be wiser to acknowledge that giant-cell tumour is a benign tumour, variably aggressive locally, capable in certain cases of giving rise to discrete metastases, easily cured by surgery; in 1-2% of cases, sarcomatous evolution, unpredictable by optical microscopy, corresponds in great part to a fundamental inadequacy of the morphological examination and, to a much lesser degree, to a true malignant transformation. Awareness of the limitations and inadequacies of a technique does not traduce those who use it.

But other questions lie in wait for the pathologist. Let us suppose that a benign giant-cell tumour is irradiated and 4-10 years later an obviously malignant tumour develops. Is this a giant-cell sarcoma, a malignant fibrous histiocytoma, an anaplastic telangiectatic osteosarcoma or a fibroblastic sarcoma? If a malignant giant-cell tumour is diagnosed at the first biopsy, is this a giant-cell tumour or a malignant fibrous histiocytoma? If a giant-cell tumour develops in Paget's disease, it is important to remember that not every giant-cell tumour in a pagetic bone is necessarily a sarcoma and the very extent of the pagetic remodelling may render this diagnosis very difficult. Lastly, the appearance of a pulmonary metastasis in the months following excision of a benign giant-cell tumour is worrying for the patient and the pathologist, but it is very possible that both metastasis and tumour exhibit the same benign histology.

References

Benign giant-cell tumour

Allen JM, Gockerman J (1964) Electrophoretic separation of multiple forms of particle associated acid phosphatases. Ann N Y Acad 121: 616-633

Aoki J, Moser RP, Vinh TN (1989) Giant-cell tumor of the scapula. A review of 13 cases. Skeletal Radiol 18: 427-434

Aparisis T, Arborgh B, Ericsson JLE (1978) Giant-cell tumor of bone. Fine structural localization of alkaline phosphatase. Virchows Arch (Pathol Anat) 378: 287-295

Aqel NM, Springle JAS, Horton MA (1988) Cellular heterogeneity in giant-cell tumor of bone (osteoclastoma): an immunohistological study of 16 cases. Histopathology 13: 675-685

Athanasou NA, Quinn J (1990) Immunaphenotypic differences between osteoclasts and macrophage polykaryons: immunohistochemical distinction and implications for osteoclast ontogeny and function. J Clin Pathol 43: 997-1003

Bacchini P, Bertoni F, Ruggieri P, Campanacci M (1995) Multicentric giant-cell tumor of skeleton. Skeletal Radiol 24: 371-374

Bertoni F, Present D, Enneking WF (1985) Giant-cell tumor of bone with pulmonary metastases. J Bone Joint Surg (Am) 67A: 890-900

Bertoni F, Sudanese A, Baldini N, Baldini P, Present D, Campanacci M (1988) Giant-cell tumor of bone with pulmonary metastases. Six cases reports and a review of the literature. Clin Orthop 237: 265-285

Bloodgood JC (1924) The giant-cell tumor of bone and the specter of the metastasizing giant-cell tumor. Surg Gynec Obstet 38: 784-789

Brecher ME, Wilbur AF, Simon MA (1986) Immunohistochemical study of mononuclear phagocyte antigens in giant-cell tumor of bone. J Pathol 125: 252-257

Butler MG, Dabir GA, Schwartz HS (1993) Molecular analysis of transforming growth factor beta in giant cell tumor of bone. Cancer Genet Cytogenet 66: 108-112

Caballes RL (1981) The mechanism of metastasis in the so-called benign giant-cell tumor of bone. Hum Pathol 12: 762-767

Campanacci M, Baldini N, Boriani S, Sudanese A (1987) Giant-cell tumor of bone. J Bone Joint Surg (Am) 69A: 106-114

Chambers TJ (1980) The cellular basis of bone resorption. Clin Orthop 151: 283-293

Codman EA (1931) Epiphyseal chondromatous giant-cell tumors of upper end of humerus. Surg Gynecol Obstet 52: 543-548

Dahlin DC (1977) Giant-cell tumor of vertebrae above the sacrum. A review of 31 cases. Cancer 39: 1350-1356

Dahlin DC, Cupps RE, Johnson EW (1970) Giant-cell tumor: a study of 195 cases. Cancer 25: 1061-1070

Dahlin DC, Unni KK (1986) Bone tumors general aspects and data on 8,542 cas. 4th edn. Charles C Thomas, Springfield

Daroca PJ, Reed RJ, Martin PC (1990) Metastatic amelanotic melanoma simulating giant-cell tumor of bone. Hum Pathol 21: 9

Deburge A, De Grandmaison P (1980) Tumeur à cellules géantes bifocale. Un cas. Rev Chir Orthop 66: 323-326

Doussis IA, Puddle B, Athanasou NA (1992) Immunophenotype of multinucleated and mononuclear cells in giant-cell lesions of bone and soft tissue. J Clin Pathol 45: 398-404

Dreinhöfer KE, Rydhol MA, Baver HCF, Kricbergs (1995) Giant-cell tumors with fracture at diagnosis. Curettage andacrylic cementing in ten cases. J Bone Joint Surg 77B: 189-193

Fain JS, Unni KK, Beabout JW, Rock MG (1993) Non epiphyseal giant-cell tumor of long bones. Cancer 71: 3514-3519

Fukunaga M, Nikaido T, Shimoda T, Ushigome S, Nadamori K (1992) A flow cytometric DNA analysis of giant-cell tumors of bone including two cases with malignant transformation. Cancer 70: 1886-1894

Geschickter CF, Copeland MM (1930) Tumors of giant-cell group, a pathologic entity. Arch Surg 21: 145-156

Guilleminet M, Faysse R (1954) Résultats du traitement des tumeurs à myéloplaxes du squelette (à propos de 18 cas). Rev Chir Orthop 40: 3-14

Hanna RM, Kyriakos M, Quinn SF (1992) Giant-cell tumor of rib. Skeletal Radiol 21: 482-488

Herman SD, Mesgarzadeh M, Bonakdarpour A, Dalinka MK (1987) The role of magnetic resonance imaging in giant-cell tumor of bone. Skeletal Radiol 16: 635-643

Hindman BW, Seefer LL, Stanley P, Forrester DM, Schwinn CP, Tan SZ (1994) Multicentric giant-cell tumor: report of five new cases. Skeletal Radiol 23: 187-190

Hunter RL, Markert CL (1957) Histochemical demonstration of enzymes separated by zone electrophoresis in starch gels. Science 125: 1294-1295

Hutter VP, Worcester JN, Francis KC, Foote FW, Stewart FW (1962) Benign and malignant giant-cell tumors of bone: a clinicopathological analysis of the natural history of the disease. Cancer 15: 653-690

Jacobs TP, Michelsen J, Polay JS, D'Adamo AC, Canfiels RE (1979) Giant-cell tumor in Paget's disease of bone: familial and geographic clustering. Cancer 44: 742-747

Jaffe HL, Lichtenstein L, Portis RB (1940) Giant-cell tumor of bone: its pathologic appearance, grading, supposed variants and treatment. Arch Pathol 30: 993-1031

Kaiser U, Newmann K, Havemann K (1993) Generalised giant-cell tumour of bone: successful treatment of pulmonary metastases with interferon, a case report. J Cancer Res Clin Oncol 119: 301-303

Kirby EJ, Buchalter JS, Kastenbaum DM, Kenan S, Kummer FJ, Lewis MM (1990) CO2 laser cauterization of giant-cell tumor margins. Clin Orthop 253: 231-239

Larsson SE, Lorentzon R (1975) Giant-cell tumors of the spine and sacrum causing neurological symptoms. Clin Orthop 111: 201-211

Le Charpentier Y, Le Charpentier M, Forest M, Daudet Monsac M, Lavenu-Vacher MC, Louvel A, Sedel L, Abelanet R (1977) Inclusions intranucléaires dans une tumeur osseuse à cellules géantes. Mise en évidence au microscope électronique. Nouv Presse Med 6: 259-262

Lichtenstein L (1951) Giant-cell tumor of bone. Current status of problems in diagnosis and treatment. J Bone Joint Surg 33A: 143-150

Lipszyc H (1990) Tumeur à cellules géantes chez l'enfant, à propros d'un cas. Thèse de doctorat Université de Reims

Marcove RC, Lyden JP, Huvos AH, Bullough PB (1973) Giant-cell tumors treated by cryosurgery. A report of twenty-five cases. J Bone Joint Surg 55A: 1633-1644

Marcove RC, Weis LD, Vaghaiwalla MR, Pearson R, Huvos AG (1978) Cryosurgery in the treatment of giant-cell tumors of bone: a report of 52 cases. Cancer 41: 957-969

Marcove RC, Sheth DS, Brien EW, Huvos AG, Healey JH (1994) Conservative surgery for giant cell tumors or the sacrum. The role of cryosurgery as a supplement to curettage and partial excision. Cancer 74: 1253-1260

Mechlin MB, Kricum ME, Schwamm HA (1984) Giant-cell tumor of tarsal bones. Skeletal Radiol 11: 266-270

Mercuri M, Casadei R, Ferraro A, Cristofaro (de) A, Balladelli A, Picci P (1991) Tumours of the patella. Int Orthop 15: 115-120

Merle d'Aubigné R, Mazabraud A (1962) A propos de 22 observations de "vraies" tumeurs à cellules géantes. Lyon Chir 58: 389-403

Merle d'Aubigné RM, Thomine JM, Mazabraud A, Hannouche D (1968) Evolution spontanée et post-opératoire des tumeurs à cellules géantes: indications thérapeutiques à propos de 39 cas dont 20 suivis 5 ans et plus. Rev Chir Orthop 54: 689-714

Mills BG, Singer FR (1976) Nuclear inclusions in Paget's disease of bone. Science 194: 201-202

Mirra JM, Bauer FC, Grant TT (1981) Giant-cell tumor with viral-like intranuclear inclusions associated with Paget's disease. Clin Orthop 158: 243-251

Motais de Narbonne J, Thiery JP, Magdelenat H, Mazabraud A (1977) Mise en évidence de la phosphatase acide ostéoclastique dans le sérum de malades atteints de tumeurs à cellules géantes. Bull Cancer 64: 31-36

Moulonguet P, Ronsin R (1954) Le sarcome ostéolytique à cellules géantes. J Chir 70: 669-690

Nascimento A, Huvos AG, Marcove RC (1979) Primary malignant giant-cell tumor of bone: study of eight cases and review of the literature. Cancer 44: 1393-1402

Nelaton E (1860) "Mémoire sur une nouvelle espéce de tumeur bénigne des os ou tumeur à myéloplaxe". Thèse, Paris

Oberling F, Rousselot P (1967) Les tumeurs à myéloplaxes malignes. Ann Anat Path 12: 71-78

Ogihara Y, Sudo A, Shiokawa Y, Takeda K, Kusano I (1994) Multiple giant-cell tumor of bone (symmetrical lesions in both humeral heads). Skeletal Radiol 23: 487-489

Onimus M, Belot V, Vauzelle JL (1984) A propos d'un cas de kyste anévrismal du rachis. Rev Chir Orthop. 70: 335-341

Ores R, Rosen P, Ortiz J (1969) Localization of acid phophatases activity in a giant-cell tumor of bone. Arch Pathol 88: 54

Peimer CA, Schille AL, Mankin HJ, Smith RJ (1980) Multicentric giant-cell tumor of bone. J Bone Joint Surg 62A: 652-656

Peirce CB (1932) Giant-cell bone tumor; a consideration of the morphology of this neoplasm, the response to surgical and radiation therapy, and report in detail of two apparently malignant cases. Am J Roentgenol 28: 167-188

Picci P, Manfrini M, Zucchi V, Gherlinzoni F, Rock M, Bertoni F, Neff JR (1983) Giant-cell tumor of bone in skeletally immature patients. J Bone Joint Surg 65A: 486-490

Present D, Bertoni F, Hudson T, Enneking WF (1986) The correlation between the radiologic staging studies and histopathologic findings in aggressive stage 3 giant-cell tumor of bone. Cancer 57: 237-244

Rebel A, Bregeon CH, Basle M, Malkani K (1975) Les inclusions des ostéoclastes de la maladie osseuse de Paget. Rev Rhum 42: 637-664

Rebel A, Malkani K, Basle M (1974) Anomalies nucléaires des ostéoclastes de la maladie osseuse de Paget. Nouv Presse Med 3: 1299-1301

Rebel A, Malkani K, Basle M, Bregeon CH (1974) Particularités ultrastructurales des ostéoclastes de la maladie de Paget. Rev Rhum 41: 767-771

Reckling FW, Gurtler RA, Mantz FA (1979) Recurrent giant-cell tumor of bone in a thirteen-year-old girl. J Bone Joint Surg 61A: 281-285

Roche I, Courtois J (1972) Les phosphatases. Exposés annuels de biochimie médicale. Edn Masson, Paris 30: 219

Rock MG, Pritchard DJ, Unni KK (1984) Metastases from histologically benign giant-cell tumor of bone. J Bone Joint Surg 66A: 269-274

Rozenszajn L, Eplein Y, Shoham D, Arber J (1968) The acid phosphatase isoenzymes in normal and pathological sera and in tissue homogenates. J Lab Clin Med 72: 786-793

Sanerkin NG (1980) Malignancy, aggressiveness, and recurrence in giant-cell tumor of bone. Cancer 46: 1641-1649

Sara AS, Ayala AG, El-Naggar A, Raymond AK, Muray JA (1990) Giant-cell tumor of bone. A clinicopathologic and DNA flow cytometric analysis. Biologic Behavior Cancer 66: 2186-2190

Schajowicz F (1961) Giant-cell tumors of bone (osteoclastome): a pathological and histochemical study. J Bone Joint Surg 43A: 1-29

Schajowicz L, Slullitel I (1966) Giant-cell tumor associated with Paget's disease of bone. A case report. J Bone Joint Surg 48A: 1340-1349

Schütte HE, Taconis WK (1993) Giant-cell tumor in children and adolescents. Skeletal Radiol 22: 173-176

Shankman S, Greenspan A, Klein MJ, Lewis MM (1988) Giant-cell tumor of the ischium. A report of two cases and review of the literature. Skeletal Radiol 17: 46-51

Shuffstall RM, Gregory JE (1953) Osteoid formation in giant-cell tumors of bone. Am J Pathol 29: 1123-1131

Sim FH, Dahlin DC, Beabout JW (1977) Multicentric giant-cell tumor of bone. J Bone Joint Surg 59A: 1052-1060

Thiery JP, Mazabraud A, Voisin MC, Baviera E, Lacroix G (1975) Etude cytologique de la tumeur à cellules géantes. Microscopie électronique et cytoenzymologie. Rev Chir Orthop 61: 377-386

Trifaud A (1955) Les tumeurs osseuses à myéloplaxes. Marseille Chir 7: 5-33

Tornberg DN, Dick HM, Johnson AD (1975) Multicentric giant-cell tumors in the long bones: a case report. J Bone Joint Surg 57A: 420-422

Vacher-Lavenu MC, Louvel A, Daudet-Monsac M, Le Charpentier Y, Abelanet R (1981) Inclusions tubulo-filamenteuses intranucléaires dans les cellules multinucléées des tumeurs à cellules géantes des os. Etude ultrastructurale d'une série de 31 tumeurs. Présentée par Merle d'Aubigné R. CR Acad Sci, Paris, 293

Vanel D, Contesso G, Rebibo G, Zafrani B, Masselot J (1983) Benign giant-cell tumours of bone with pulmonary metastases and favourable prognosis. Report on two cases and review of the literature. Skeletal Radiol 10: 221-226

Verbiest H (1965) Giant-cell tumours and aneurysmal bone cysts of the spine. With special reference to the problems related to the removal of a vertebral body. J Bone Joint Surg 47B: 699-713

Wray CC, MacDonald AW, Richardson RA(1990) Benign giant-cell tumour with metastases to bone and lung one case studies over 20 years. J Bone Joint Surg 72B: 486-489

Malignant giant-cell tumour

Ackerman LV, Spjut HL (1962) Giant-cell reaction. Tumors of bone and cartilage. In Atlas of tumor pathology, sect II, fasc 4 1st series. Armed Forces Institute of Pathology, Washington DC: 282

Helpap B, Totovic V, Bechtelsheimer H (1981) Giant-cell reaction in the small tubular bones. J Cancer Res Clin Oncol 101: 219-226

Hermann G, Abdelwahab IF, Klein MJ, Berson BD, Lewis MM (1990) Giant-cell reparative granuloma of the distal end of right femur. Skeletal Radiol 19: 367-369

Jaffe HL (1953) Giant-cell reparative granuloma, traumatic bone cyst and fibrous (fibro-osseous) dysplasia of the jaw bones. Oral Surg 6: 159-175

Jernstrom P, Stark HH (1971) Giant-cell reaction of a metacarpal. Am J Clin Pathol 55: 77-81

Lorenzo JC, Dorman HD (1980) Giant-cell reparative granuloma of short tabular bones of hand and feet. Am J Surg Pathol 4: 551-563

Picci P, Baldini N, Sudanese A, Boriani S, Campanacci M (1986) Giant-cell reparative granuloma and other giant-cell lesions of the bones of the hands and feet. Skeletal Radiol 15: 415-421

Smet (de) AA, Travers H, Neff JR (1982) Giant-cell reparative granuloma of left femur arising in polyostotic dysplasia. Skeletal Radiol 8: 314-318

Wold LE, Dobyns JH, Swee RG, Dablin DC (1986) Giant-cell reaction (giant-cell reparative granuloma) of the small bones of the hands and feet. Am J Surg Pathol 10: 491-496

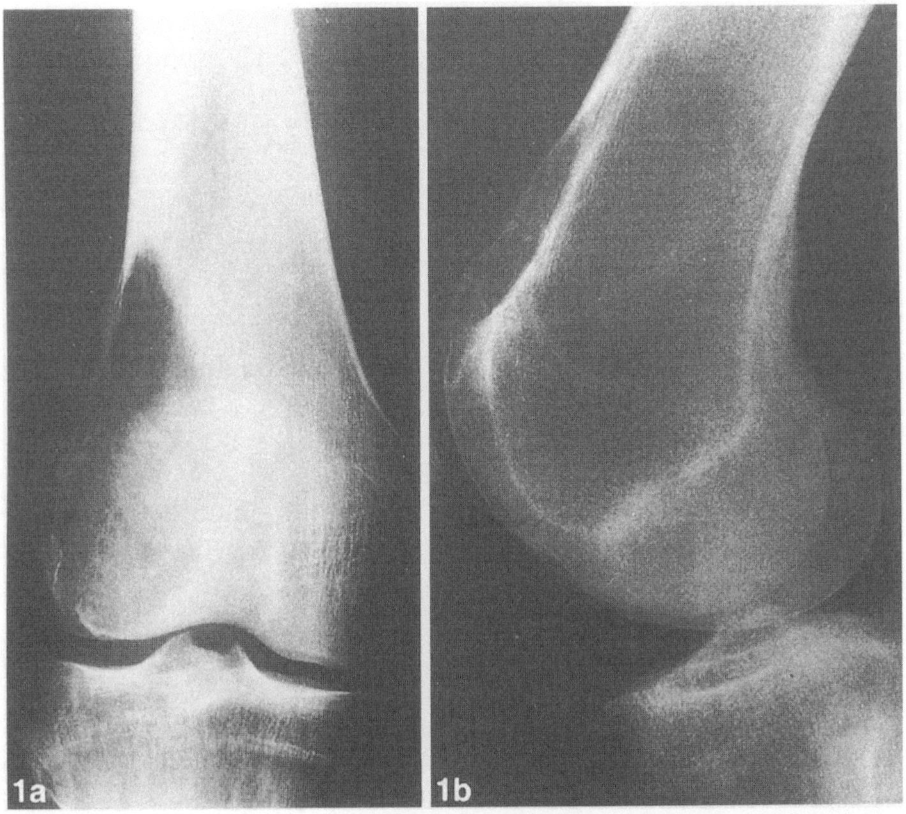

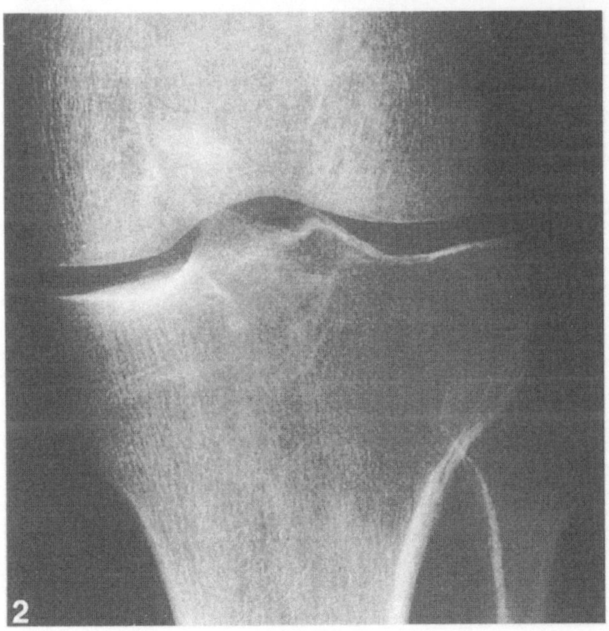

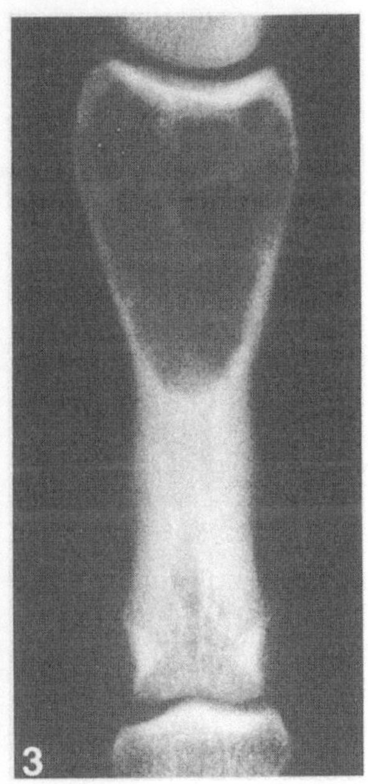

Fig. 1 a, b. This enormous tumour osteolysis of the metaphyseo-epiphyseal region spares the cortex and articular cartilage

Fig. 2. Osteolysis of outer half of upper end of tibia, poorly circumscribed, particularly at its internal border; however, the histological appearances were those of a quiescent tumour

Fig. 3. Alveolar pattern in midst of tumour osteolysis of base of first phalanx of middle finger

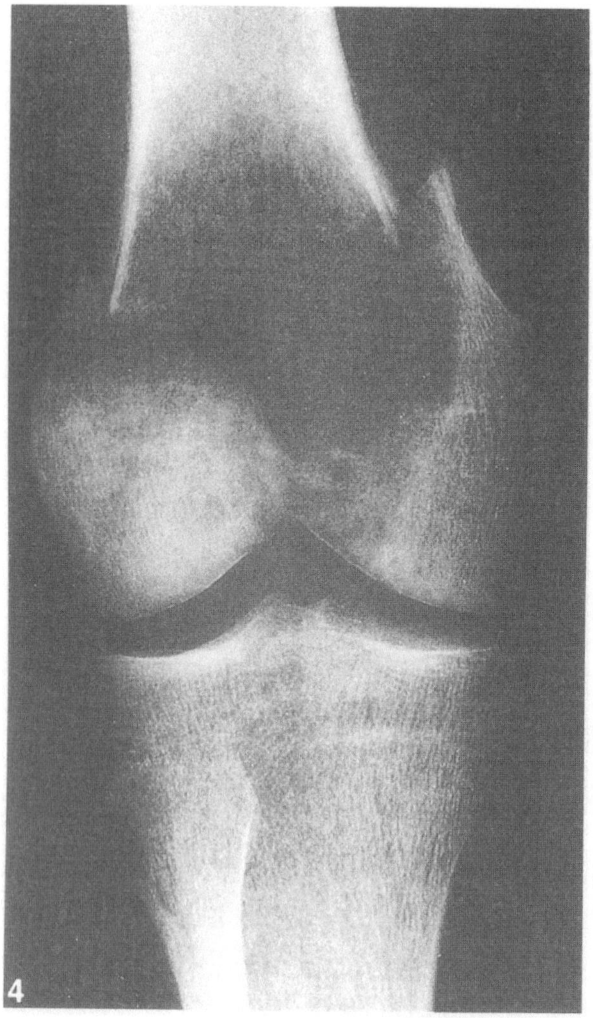

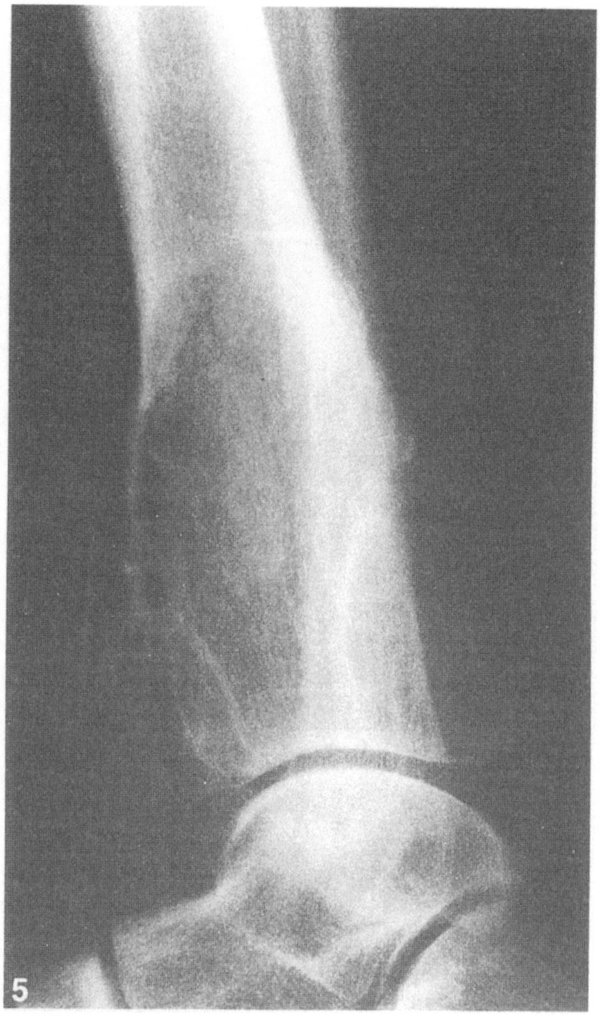

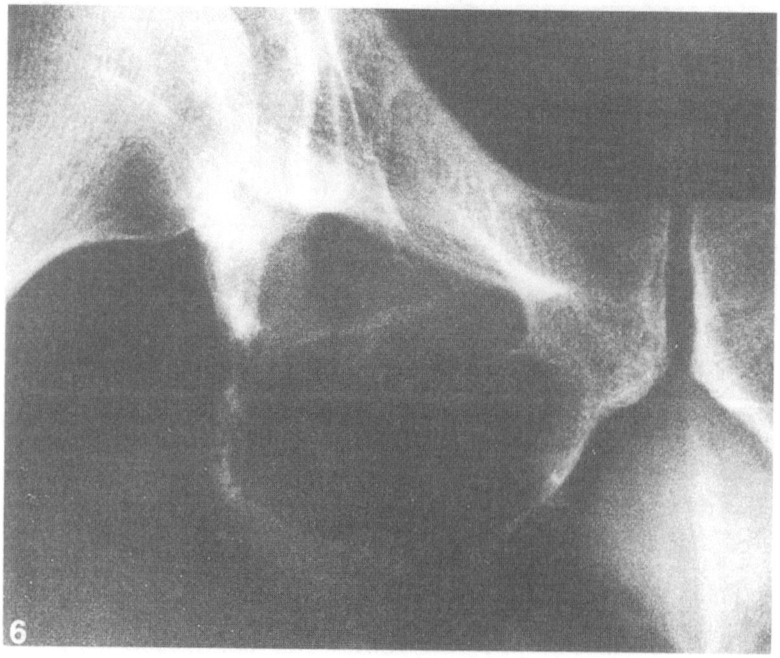

Fig 4. This indolent tumour of the lower end of the femur was revealed by fracture

Fig. 5. The persistence of bony ridges on the deep aspect of the cortex gives the impression of partitioning of this tumour of the lower end of the tibia

Fig. 6. This rapidly growing giant-cell tumour balloons the ischiopubic ramus

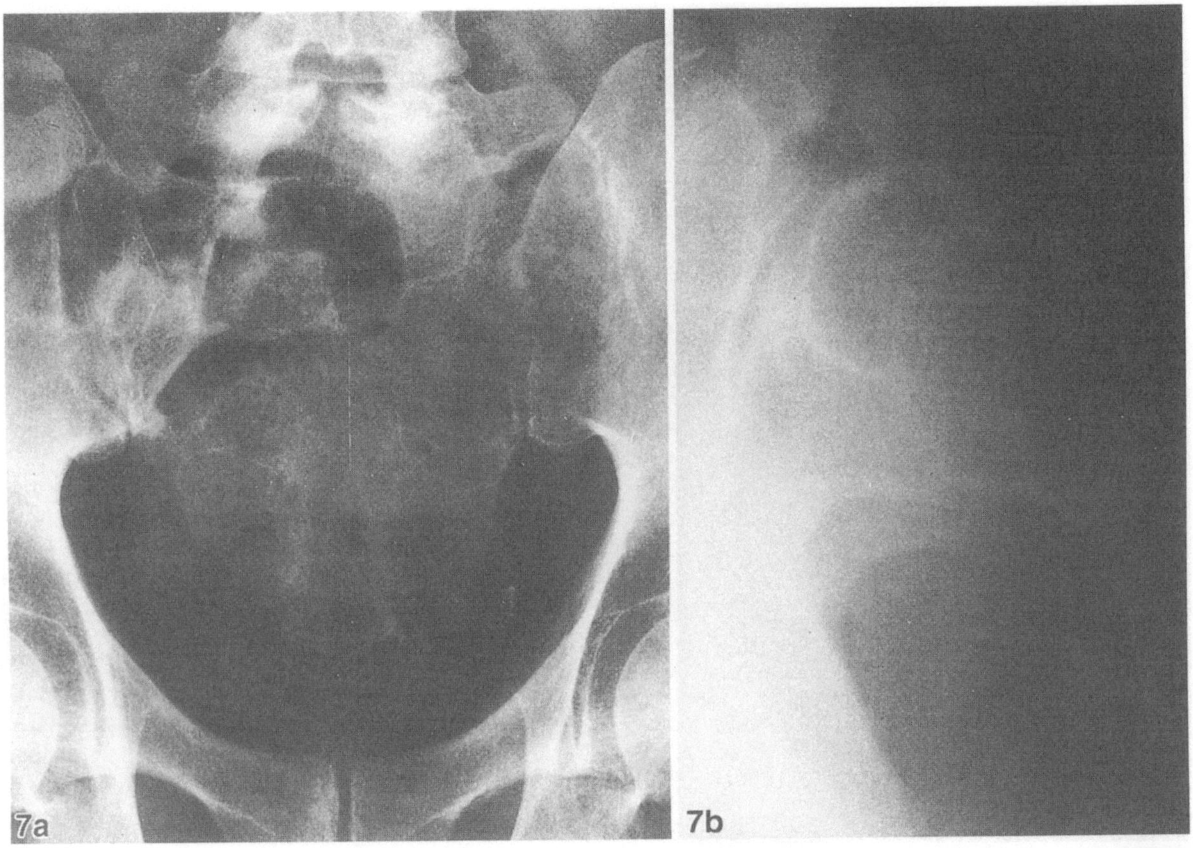

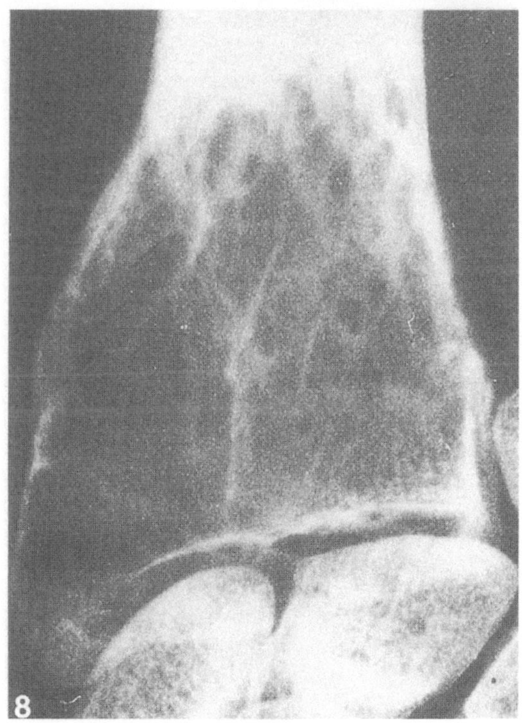

Fig. 7 a, b. The tumour obliterates the outlines of the first sacral foramina and the bony structure of the left sacral wing

Fig. 8. The particular architecture of the bony ridges of the deep aspect of the cortex outlines this alveolar appearance sometimes observed in giant-cell tumour

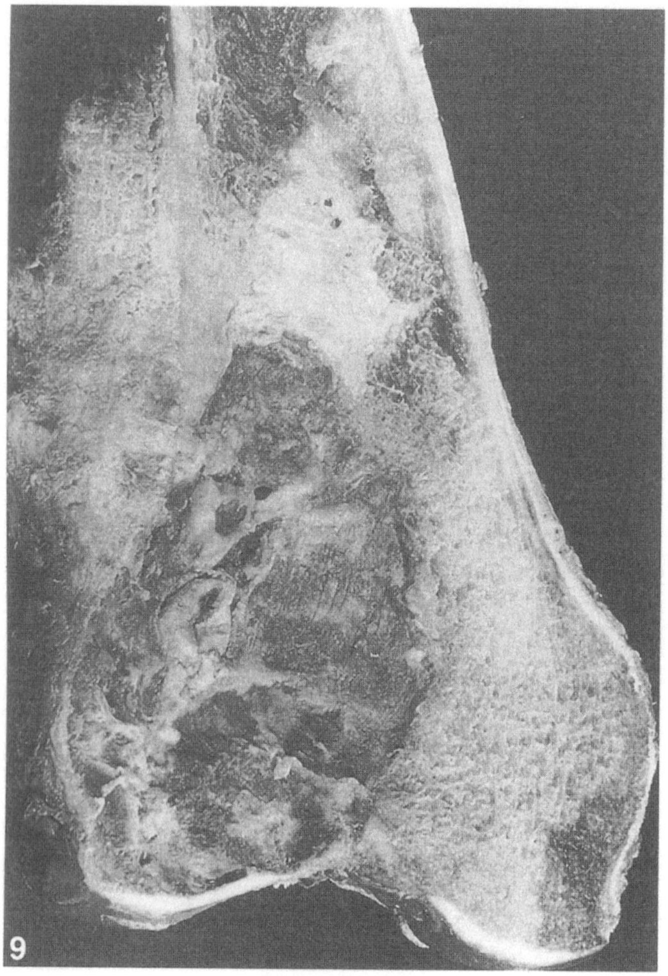

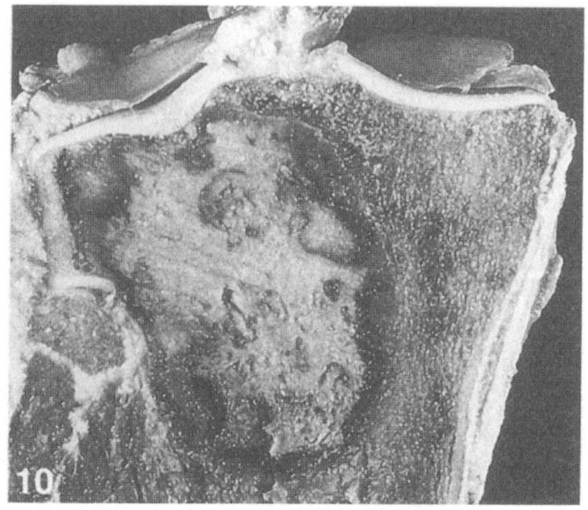

Figs. 9, 10. These two metaphyseo-epiphyseal tumours have partly destroyed the cortex but have spared the articular cartilage

Fig. 11. This large tumour of the lower end of the femur has widely invaded the soft tissues. At the center, there are cystic and haemorrhagic zones. Laterally and in the central part of the joint, the tumour follows the lateral and cruciate ligaments from their femoral attachments

Fig. 12. Lytic invasive tumour, histologically sarcomatous and rich in giant cells, better qualified as anaplastic sarcoma rather than malignant giant-cell tumour

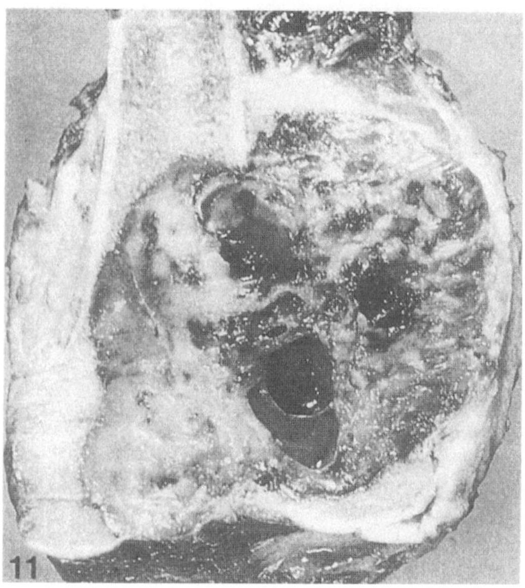

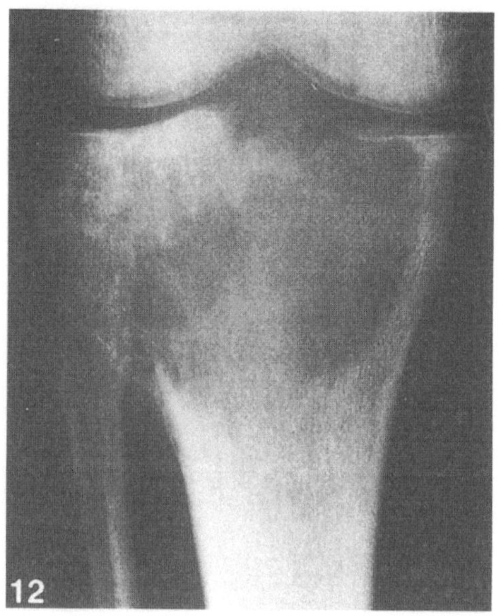

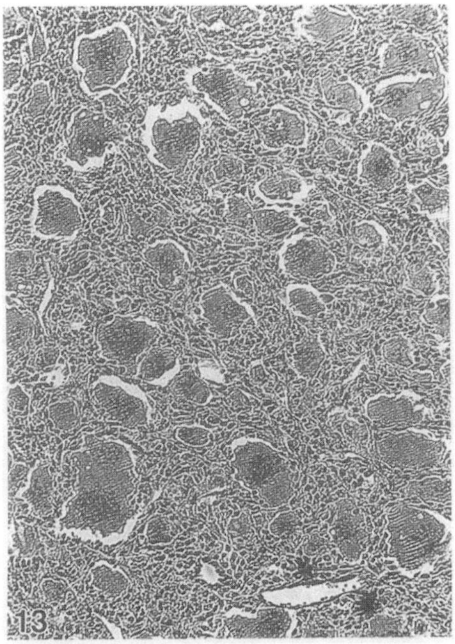

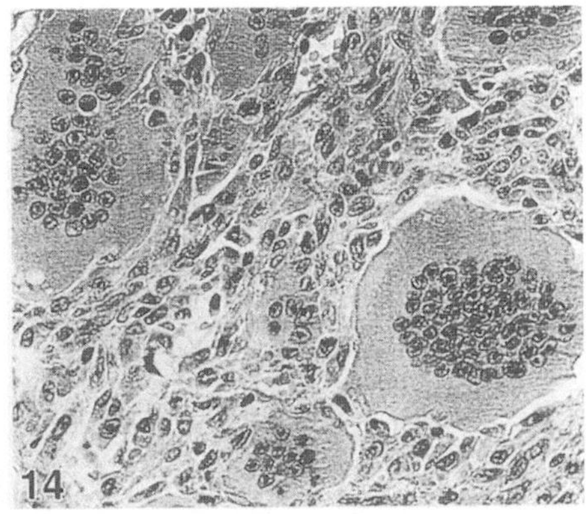

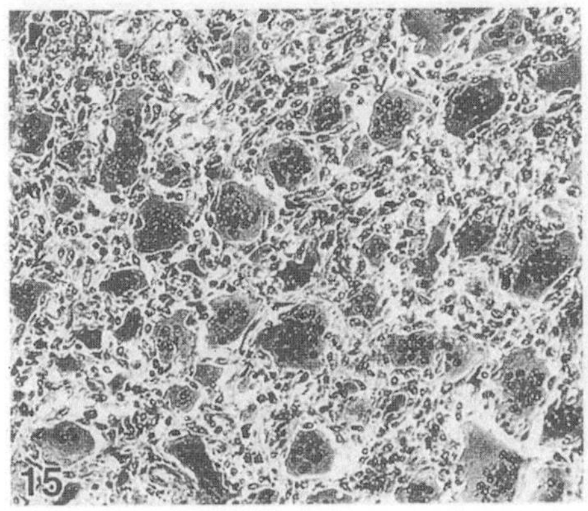

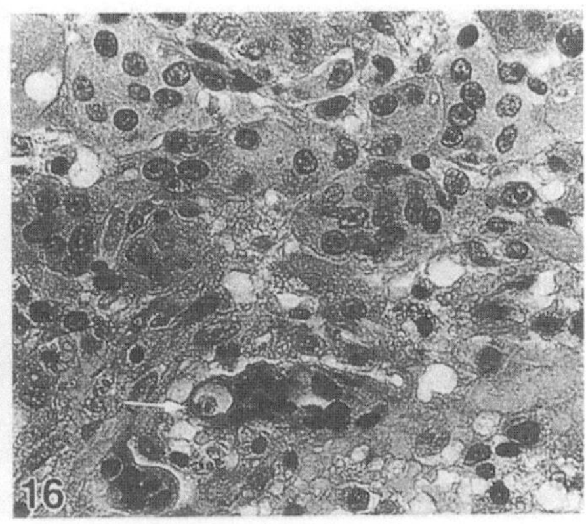

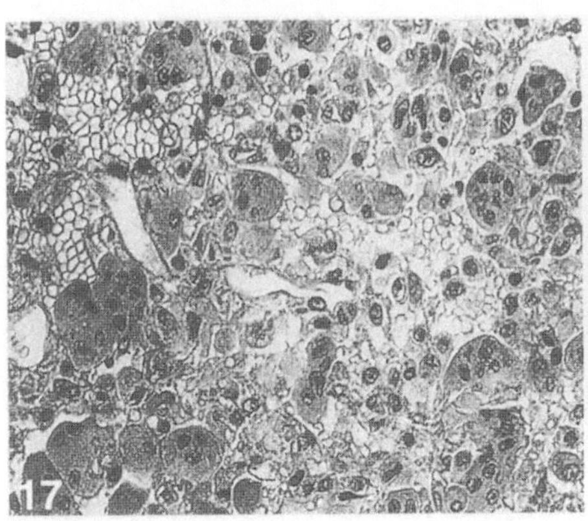

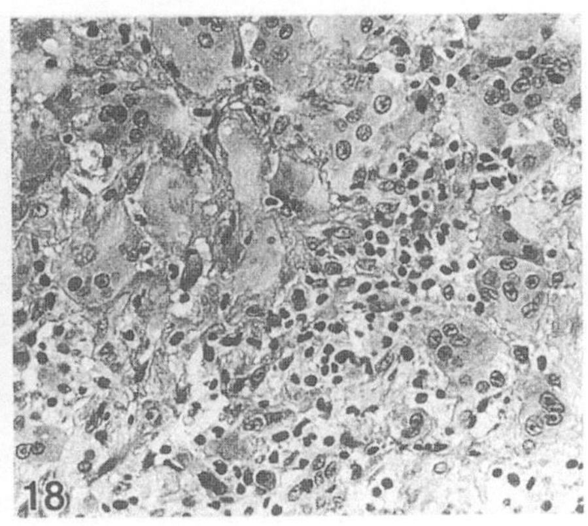

Fig. 13. General view: quite regularly distributed giant cells against background of mononuclear tumour cells

Fig. 14. The nuclei are grouped in the central part of the cytoplasm of the giant cells

Fig. 15. Giant cells of irregular shape and unequal size, an indication to confirm that the mononuclear cells retain their normal characteristics

Fig. 16. The cytoplasm of the giant cells is vacuolated. In the cytoplasm of one giant cell a phagocytosed cell is in course of degeneration *(arrow)*

Fig. 17. The tumour tissue is often dispersed by a haemorrhagic effusion

Fig. 18. Inflammatory infiltrations without haemorrhagic or suppurative phenomena

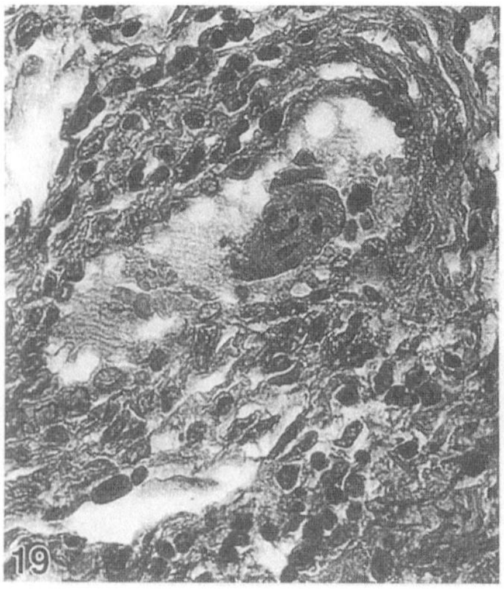

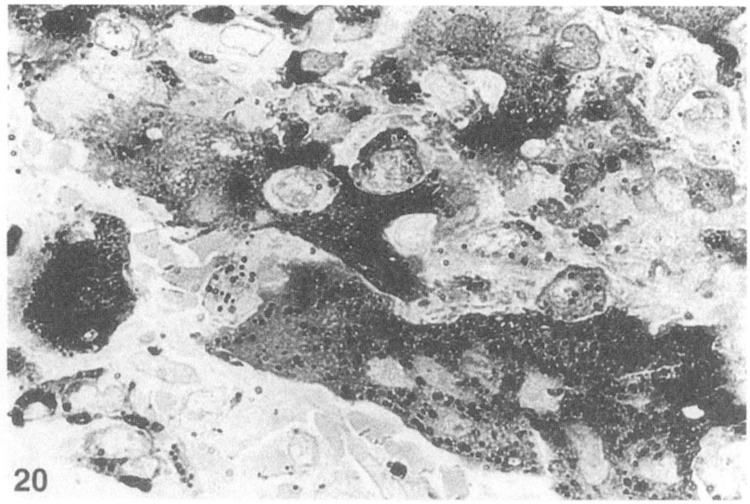

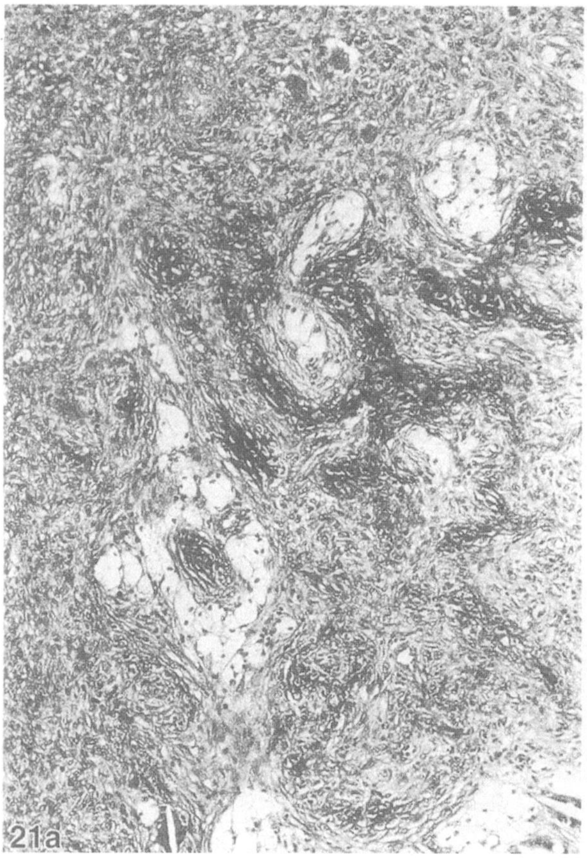

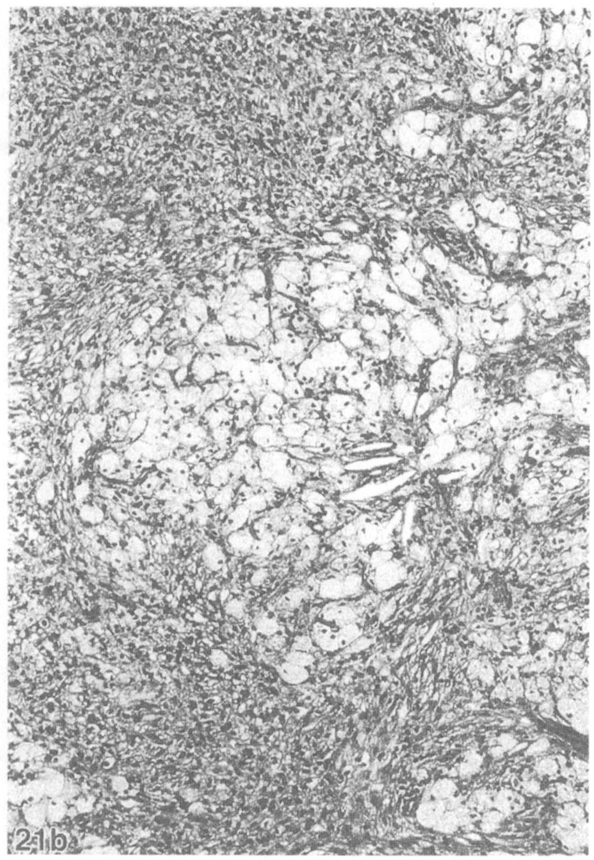

Fig. 19. The presence of giant cells and/or tumour fragments in the vessels of the peritumour tissue is commonplace and of no prognostic significance

Fig. 20. Optical microscopy: a black intracytoplasmic precipitate reveals acid phosphatases in the giant cells and some mononuclear cells

Fig. 21 a, b. These two microphotographs show (**a**) zones of osteogenesis and (**b**) an area of histiocytes in the midst of a giant-cell tumour

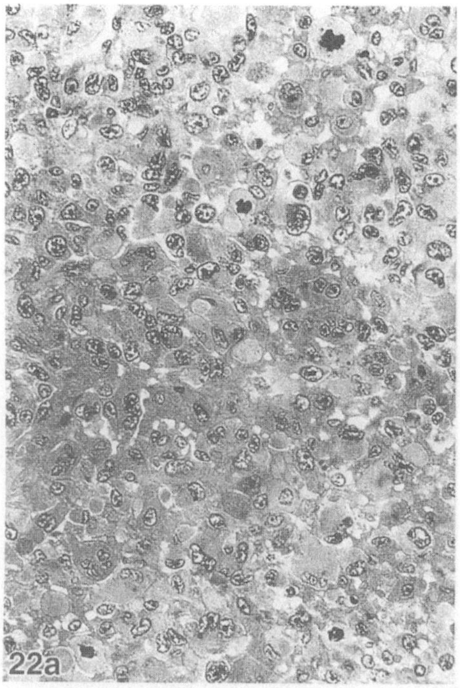

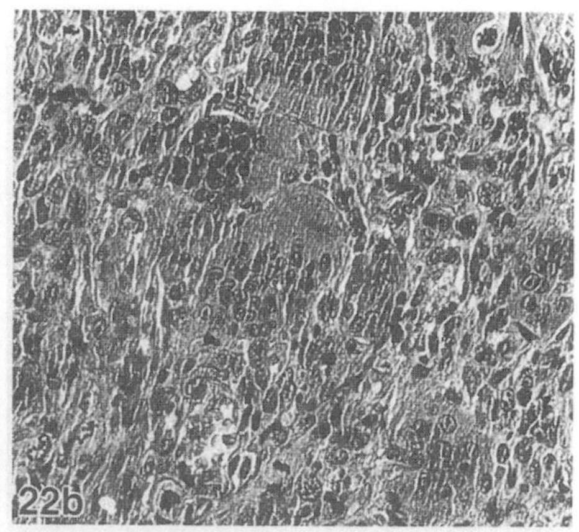

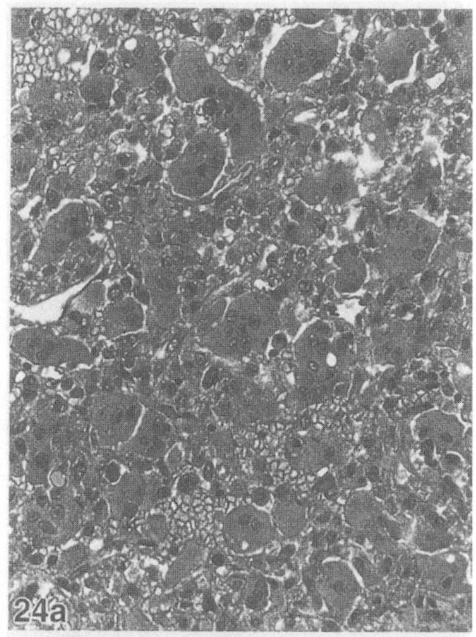

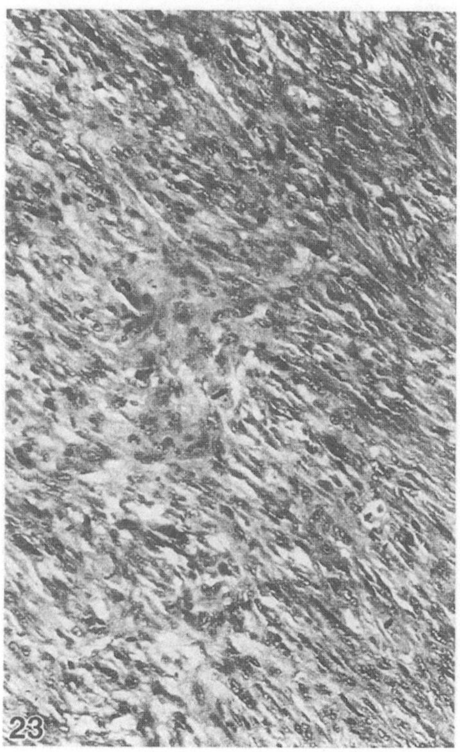

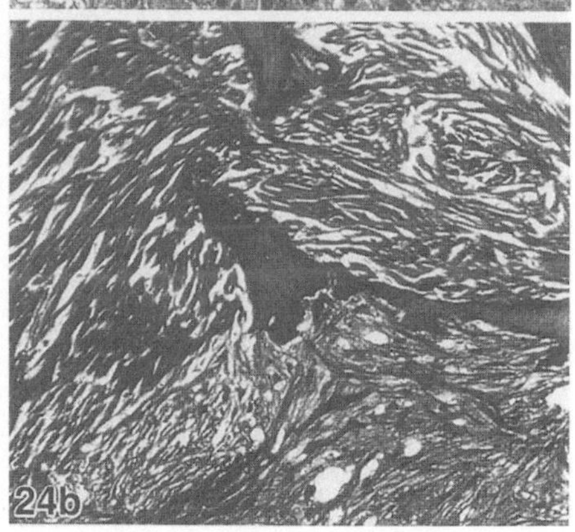

Fig. 22 a, b. The radiographic appearance and clinical course of this giant-cell sarcoma are related to active cellular proliferation. This unambiguous label seems preferable to that of giant-cell tumour grade III or IV (depending on the scale of malignancy chosen)

Fig. 23. This sarcoma with fusiform and giant cells may be secondary to a giant-cell tumour. The fact is doubtless a possibility, but it is better to call things by their proper names

Fig. 24. a Giant-cell tumour of sacrum showing paucinuclear giant cells and increased nuclear-cytoplasmic ratio of some mononuclear cells. **b** This tumour, at that time judged inoperable, was treated by irradiation. Radiotherapy achieved stabilisation at the cost of histological changes rendering the interpretation of subsequent biopsies equivocal

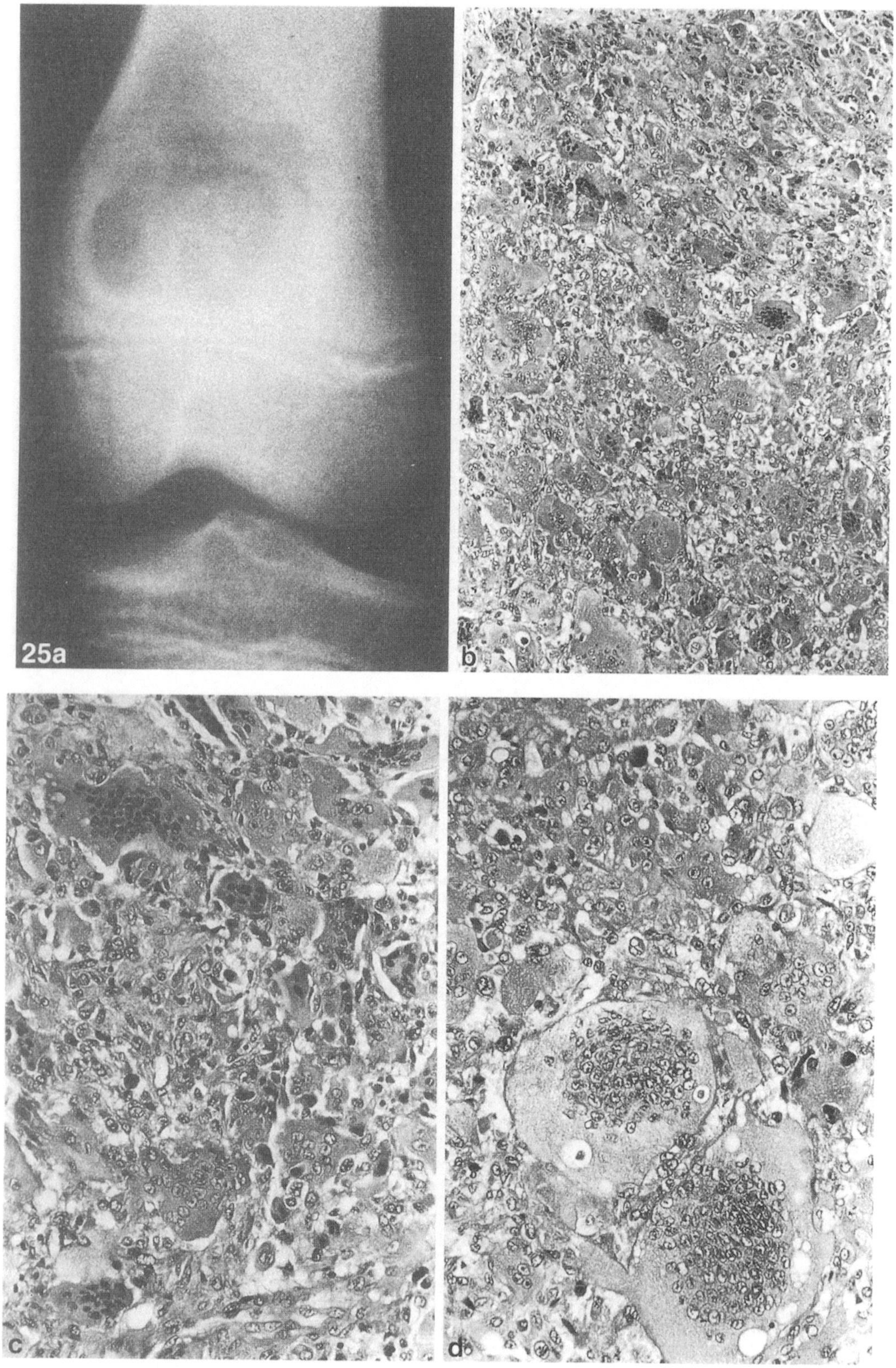

Fig. 25 a-d. In this growing skeleton (girl of 10 1/2 years) the metaphyseal tumour (**a**) does not cross the growth plate. At different enlargements (**b, c, d**) the histology of this tumour is benign (Courtesy of Dr Lipszyc from his thesis, Reims 1990)

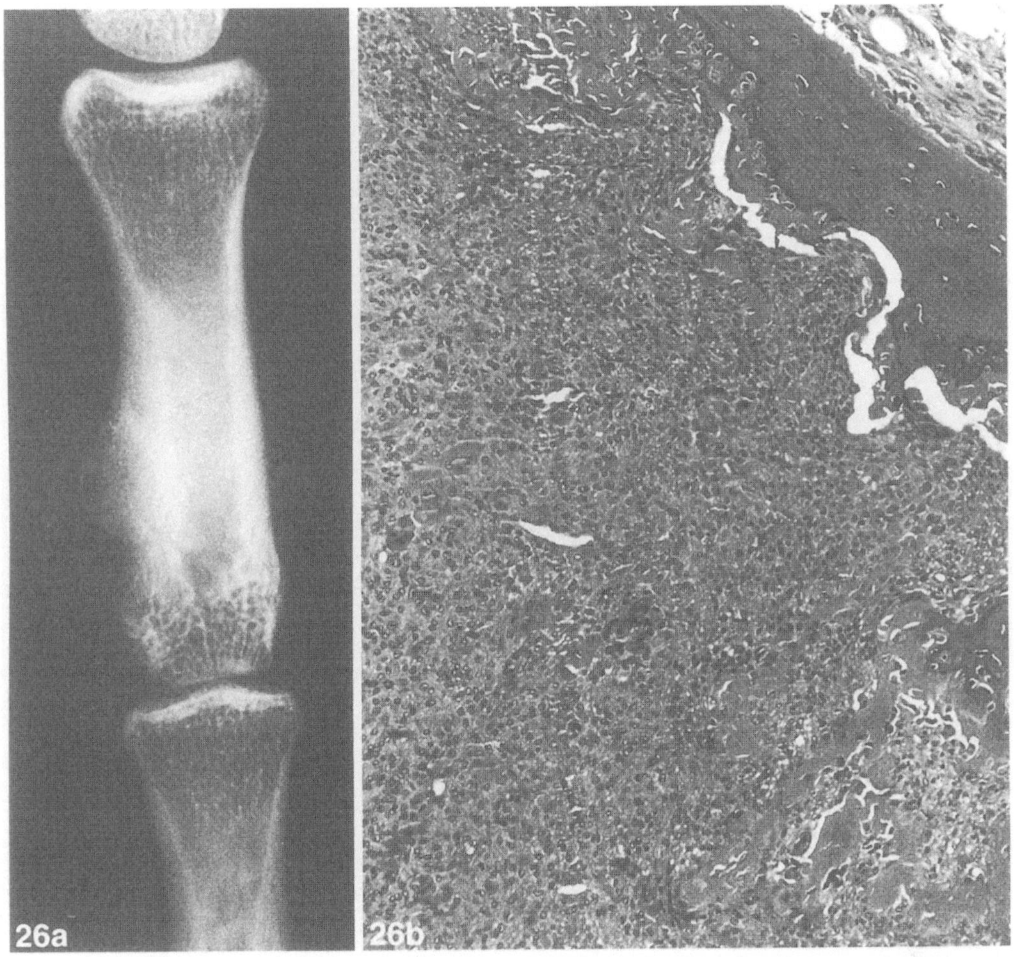

Fig. 26 a, b. Superficial location of a giant-cell granuloma on the first phalanx of the middle finger. The presence of inflammatory cells and of rudimentary peripheral osteoid formation is evident

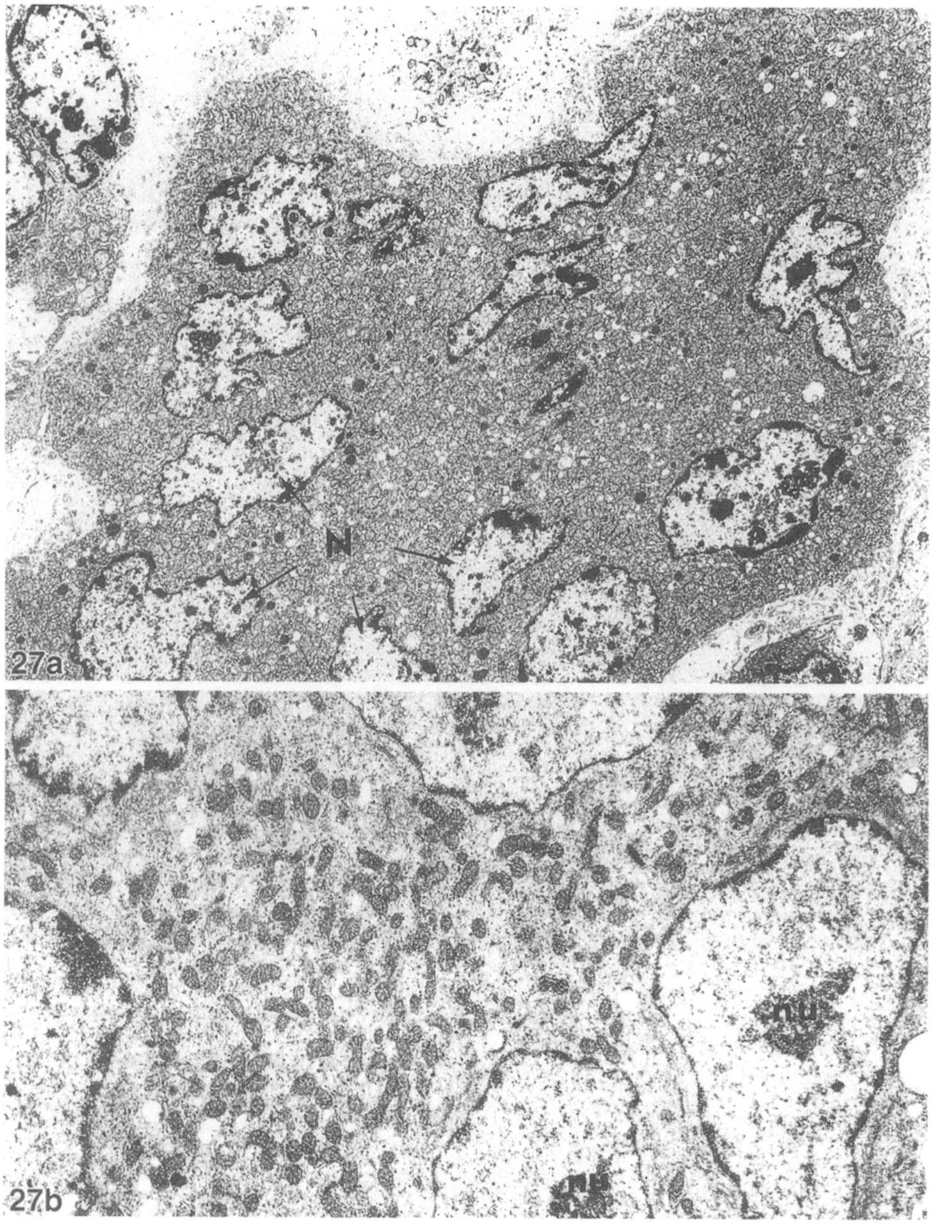

Fig. 27. a At this enlargement (x 2000) the nuclei (*N*) of a giant cell are clear; the dense chromatin is situated at the margin. **b** At higher magnification (x 5200) numerous mitochondria are seen. *nu*: nucleolus

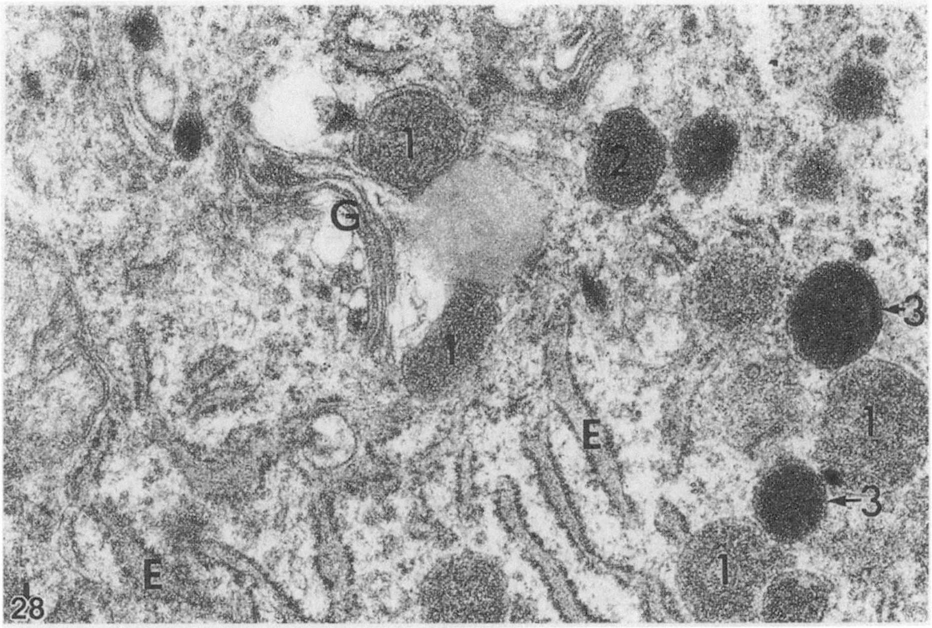

Fig. 28. Lysosomes in a giant cell (x 36,000). Lysosomes at different stages of formation 1, 2, 3, in the Golgi apparatus (G). (E) Ergastoplasm

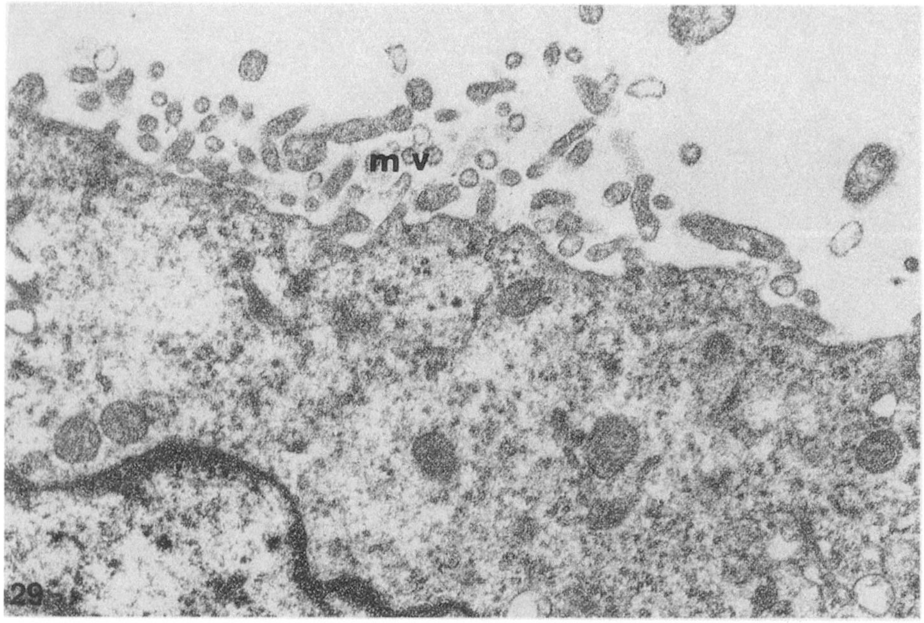

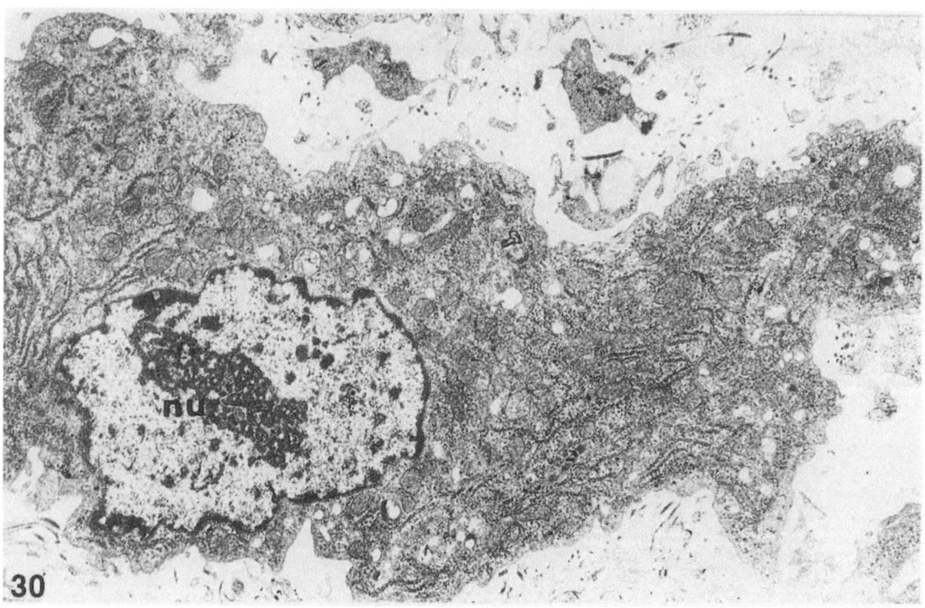

Fig. 29. Numerous microvillosities (*mv*) at margin of a giant cell (x 19,000)

Fig. 30. Mononuclear cell exhibiting cytoplasmic features of a giant cell. Nucleolus (*nu*) (x 6600) (These ultrastructural views have also been published in Étude cytologique de la tumeur à cellules géantes. J.-P. Thiery et al, Rev Chir Orthop 61: 377-386)

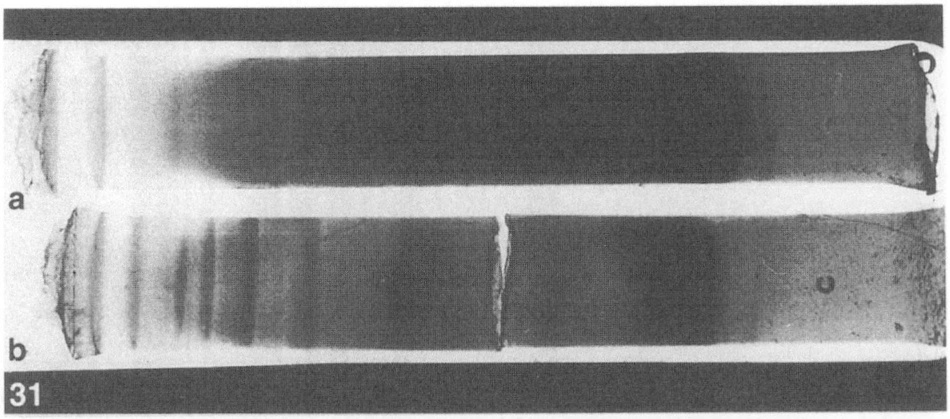

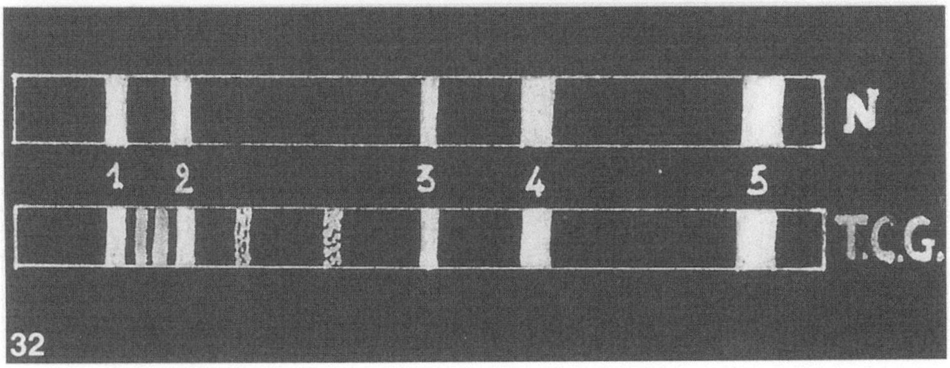

Fig. 31 a, b. Demonstration of osteoclastic phosphatases by serum electrophoresis. **a** Photograph of zymogram on acrylamide gel (acid phosphatases) of plasma of a normal subject. **b** Same technique performed on plasma of a patient in whom biopsy gave a diagnosis of giant-cell tumour

Fig. 32. Schema of 2 zymograms. Bands 1 to 3: osteoclastic phosphatases; band 4: prostatic and platelet phosphatases; band 5: hepatosplenic phosphatases. In the plasma of the patient, several close bands appear in the slow migration zone between bands 1 and 2 (cf Motais de Narbonne, [J.-P. Thiery et al 1977])

22. Haemangioendothelioma

The pathological and clinical variants of this tumour have given rise to debates of a nosologic, pathogenic and therapeutic nature; a debate which will doubtless lead to a better understanding of these lesions and more adequate treatment programs. There seems to be every degree of aggression in this type of lesion. At the two extremes, there are the slowly-growing and possibly curable forms (histiocytoid or epithelioid haemangioendothelioma, myxoid haemangioendothelioma); at the other extreme are the forms which are rapidly fatal despite mutilating surgical procedures and chemotherapy (anaplastic, sarcomatous form). Between these two forms there are types whose lethal course extends over 1 to 5 years. Although classification into histological grades of malignancy does not provide a precise prediction of the course of the lesion its application to haemangioendotheliomas is generally perfectly legitimate.

Case histories

Case 1. A woman of 31 attended for rather vague pain in the right thigh. The radiograph of the femur demonstrated some small cavities. The rest of the examination supplied no further information; in particular, the radiographs of the entire skeleton showed no other lesion. For family reasons the patient refused operation and surveillance consisted essentially of annually repeated radiography. The lesions extended in the femur and new cavities developed. A fracture of the upper end of the femur united with simple plaster immobilisation. Ten years after the first symptoms the lesions, still exclusively femoral, had progressed materially. The patient finally accepted disarticulation, followed by cure as noted at 10-year follow-up.

The histological appearance of the lesions and the evolution followed over 10 years allow us to class this angioendothelioma as grade 1 of histological malignancy (figs. 1-3, 10-17).

Case 2. A man of 50 attended an orthopaedic clinic for pain in the lower end of the right femur. There was no remarkable history and clinical examination gave no guidance. The standard radiograph showed irregular lysis, poorly circumscribed, of the lower third of the femur. Skeletal survey revealed no other lesion. Biopsy supplied the diagnosis of angiosarcoma, but without predicting the fulminating course, which was to kill the patient in a few months after virtual generalisation of the lesions (fig. 26).

Epithelioid haemangioendothelioma

The histiocytoid (or epithelioid) haemangioendotheliomas represent less than 0.5% of malignant tumours of bone. The term "haemangioendothewoma" was suggested by Weiss and Enzinger in 1982; in some publications this tumour is reported under the name of benign histiocytoid haemangioendothelioma. While recognising the absence of bizarre nuclei and of necrosis, the clinical course, which often requires mutilating procedures, has led most authors to classify this tumour with haemangoendotheliomas of grade 1 malignancy.

General considerations

The rarity of this tumour excludes statistical considerations; of the 14 cases described by Tsuneyoshi et al (1986), 11 were male. In the same report the ages varied between 10 and 73 years, with a mean age of 32 years. Any bone may be affected, but there is possibly a predilection for the long bones of the limbs. In a fourth of cases, the tumour is multifocal [Jaffe et al 1989], but with unilateral distribution.

Clinical features and course

The clinical features often amount to vague pain, so vague that sometimes it is only a spontaneous fracture or signs of nerve compression that alert the patient. At superficial sites, near certain joints for instance, the tumour may be palpable and slightly tender. For years the lesion may remain localised to a single bone.

Surgical intervention is usually by resection with reconstruction if the case allows, though this does not always act as a guarantee against recurrence. Amputation is necessary in very advanced cases.

Metastasis is certainly very rare. In some cases it has been preceded by irradiation, and the short interval between this treatment and the development of the metastases leaves some doubt as to the correctness of the diagnosis.

Imaging

Imaging is of major importance and will suggest the diagnosis; however, other possible diagnoses include malignant lymphoma, Ewing's sarcoma or metastases, because of the variety of the images and their non-specific appearance.

There is sometimes a rounded and well-circumscribed zone of osteolysis and sometimes irregular osteolysis, an appearance of moth-eaten bone that directs the diagnosis elsewhere. Multiple lesions, especially localised to a single bone, are a diagnostic feature. In every case, CT, MRI, scintigraphy and angiography provide precise information as to the nature and extent of the lesions.

Pathological anatomy and histopathology

In this lesion, the macroscopic appearance may be very suggestive at the time of operation. At macroscopic examination the femur (illustrated here) exhibits scattered multiple dark-red nodules, isolated in places, confluent in others, within well-circumscribed cavities bordered by a periosteal or endosteal osteogenic reaction. In other zones, invasion of the bony tissue is poorly limited and irregular.

On section, the histological lesions seen in the same case are very variable and may correspond to the heterogeneous radiographic appearance of the images observed in a single patient. The soft reddish tumours are striated by several grayish fibrous septa. In histological section, the tumour consists of compact tissue zones of large eosinophil cells with definite margins, whose nuclei are dotted with a clearly visible nucleolus. Sometimes the cells are arranged in stout strands, sometimes they surround a lumen filled with red corpuscles. In the peripheral zones, the cells are more dispersed in a myxoid matrix. At some sites there is a fine lumen between several cells, at others a hollowed-out intracytoplasmic vacuole displaces the nucleus, demonstrating all the rudiments of an embryonic vessel. In the peripheral zones there is a polymorphous inflammatory infiltrate. Also to be seen at the periphery are large vascular clumps which it would be difficult to distinguish as tumour vessels or simple vascular hyperplasia.

Deceptive appearances are portrayed by tumour cell columns, separated from one another by clear gaps, which may be taken for an angiopericytoma (fig. 14). In practice, there are many areas in which the reticulin pattern removes any doubt (fig. 16). In spite of the epithelioid appearance, which may suggest a metastatic lesion, the ultrastructure and the immunohistology with antibodies anti-factor VIII and Ulex europeus I supply proof that these are endothelial cells.

The appearance may be even more atypical with cells separated from one another in an abundant matrix or grouped in fine columns. Some cells are hollowed out by a clear vacuole, or two or three cells surround a small vascular cavity (figs. 23, 24). Ultrastructural studies [Tsuneyoshi et al 1986, Martinez-Tello et al 1989] allow study of the different stages of angiogenesis based on these signet-ring cells.

Myxoid haemangioendotheliomatosis (a possible variant of histiocytoid haemangioendothelioma)

General considerations

Reed described this disorder in 1982. Mirra and Kameda reported a case in 1985 under the term of myxoid angioblastomatosis of the bones, in order to indicate the angioblastic nature of the cells and the multiplicity of sites. This was in a woman aged 24 whose first lesions had occurred at the age of 12. Radiological examination showed lesions of the right elbow (humerus and radius) and lateral malleolus of the right ankle, with a multilocular cystic appearance. Though the course was particularly insidious and slow, comparable to that described in the first case history, the histological appearance was entirely different.

However, localisation may be monostotic, as in the case we present (fig. 9) and the literature provides accounts of very varied radiological aspects.

Clinical features and course

The clinical picture is identical to that described above for histiocytoid haemangioendothelioma. This tumour more often affects the vertebrae and skull; but multiple lesions may develop in the bones of the skull, trunk and limbs.

The course in such cases is sometimes fatal because of the multiplicity of bony and visceral lesions, but the precise classification of this lesion remains in dispute between a low-grade malignant tumour or a hamartomatous lesion of possibly fatal import.

Pathological anatomy and histopathology

The macroscopic appearance is deceptive, more suggestive of a metastasis or a primary fibrous tumour than a vascular tumour, hence the need for excellent imaging.

In histological sections the cells are isolated, or grouped in fine columns or small islands scattered in a fibromucoid matrix. Some islands are hollowed by a central lumen but numerous cells show a clear vacuole displacing the nucleus, and some have a signet-ring appearance. All these clear intracellular lacunae represent so many embryonal vessels. Alcian blue staining of the abundant intercellular substance is positive; the cell proliferation is strongly positive for the antibody anti-factor VIII and Ulex europeus I.

Ultrastructural study confirms the endothelial nature of the cells by showing the presence of Webel-Palade bodies and numerous perinuclear intermediary filaments and intercellular junctions. The intercellular substance, which contains dense bodies, consists of a fibrillary network.

Differential diagnosis

The differential diagnoses to be considered from standard staining in optical microscopy are numerous and include adenocarcinomatous metastases, liposarcoma, myxoid chondrosarcoma and angiosarcoma. These diagnoses are easily excluded by immunohistological reactions. Both forms, histiocytoid and myxoid, may be classified as of grade 1 malignancy, considering that the myxoid form is a possible anatomo-clinical variant of epithelioid haemangioendothelioma. Further studies based on a larger number of cases may allow a more exact classification.

I have no personal knowledge of the bony lesion of fusiform-cell haemangioendothelioma of a low grade of malignancy, as described by Weiss and Enzinger in 1986.

Haemangioendothelioma of grade 3 malignancy (haemangioendotheliosarcoma, angiosarcoma)

This tumour corresponds to histological malignancy grade 3. In his report of an angiosarcoma of the sternum in a man of 51, Pollak (1949) ascribed the origin of the term malignant endothelioma to Golgi, in 1869. The aetiology is unknown, but some malignant haemangioendotheliomas develop on preexisting lesions (infarcts, osteitis) or in contact with metallic material (bullet-wounds, rarely prostheses). Jennings et al (1988) report 3 cases of angiosarcoma associated with the presence of foreign bodies, and Himmer et al (1991) one after a knee prosthesis.

Clinical features and course

There is a male predominance. All the bones of the skeleton may be affected. The course is rapid; in weeks or 2-4 months following biopsy of an apparently solitary tumour, diffuse metastatic spread appears affecting the long bones of the limbs, vertebrae, and pelvis, while pulmonary lesions develop simultaneously. Death usually occurs during the two years following appearance of the first symptoms.

Imaging

At the onset, the radiological image is of blurred osteolysis with ill-defined boundaries, recalling that observed in anaplastic telangiectatic osteogenic sarcoma. After resection or amputation, other lesions appear and the osteolytic zones progress rapidly.

Pathological anatomy and histopathology

The biopsy removes disintegrated bony tissue whose splinters are bathed in a haemorrhagic layer, but this appearance is not sufficiently characteristic to supply a precise diagnosis. Although the surgical procedure of biopsy in this friable tissue can only add to the architectural disruption, two main appearances can nevertheless be distinguished in most cases.

In one, the anaplastic tumour cells are grouped in columns and small compact areas; mitoses, bizarre cells, large hyperchromatic nuclei and necrosis make it easy to recognise a grade 3 malignant tumour. The whole is bathed in an haemorrhagic lake, in which fragments of necrotic bony trabeculae are scattered.

In the other, at first sight, there is only haemorrhage in spongy bone, while tumour cells are rare. Here and there they are dispersed along a fine connective tissue layer, are endosteal or are seen on a rudimentary vessel-wall, or to adhere to a bone splinter. They are frankly atypical (fig. 26).

Differential diagnosis

The anaplastic nature of the tumour may suggest various diagnostic hypotheses, but the haemorrhagic appearance and the rapid development of other lesions of the same type leave little doubt as to the diagnosis and its high malignancy. In such very undifferentiated cases it is best not to expect confirmation from the immunohistological reactions. It is obvious that, between the extreme types we have just described, some haemangioendotheliomas are histologically malignant since they have bizarre cells and increased number of mitoses, but do not possess the alarming character of the previous form. Malignancy may be confirmed, but such tumours are classed in grade 2 of histological malignancy, and if necessary their endothelial origin can be demonstrated by the immunohistological reactions. Lastly, the diagnosis is purely histopathological.

It is fundamental to recognise the histiocytoid haemangioendothelioma, whose prognosis is relatively favourable. It may be regarded as of grade 1 malignancy and responds to conservative treatment [Campanacci et al 1980]. It is interesting to consider the case reported by Morgenstern et al (1969) of an angiosarcoma of the clavicle (diagnosis confirmed by Stout), in which cure was obtained by irradiation, with a follow-up of 14 years. The excellent but unfortunately sole microphotograph strongly invites one to think that this tumour falls in the context of epithelioid haemangioendothelioma. At the opposite end of the scale, grade 3 histological malignancy carries a high mortality. In 12 cases of grade 3 reported by Campanacci, the incidence of metastasis was 92% despite complex treatment regimes combining the various modalities currently available. He notes in particular that the tumour is moderately radiosensitive.

Tumours of intermediate malignancy (grade 2) react more favourably to treatments supplementary to surgery, but their prognosis remains very poor.

References

Abrahams TG, Bula W, Jones M (1992) Epithelioid hemangioendothelioma of bone. A report of two cases and review of the literature. Skeletal Radiol 21: 509-513

Angervall L, Kindblom LG, Karlsson K, Stener B (1985) Atypical hemangioendothelioma of venous origin. A clinicopathologic, angiographic, immunohistochemical and ultrastructural study of two endothelial tumors within the concept of histiocytoid hemangioma. Am J Surg Pathol 9: 504-516

Boccara M, Foucault D, Dumesnil de Maricourt, Gerbal JL, Mazabraud A, Quillard J, Manigand G, Deparis M (1978) L'hémangioendothéliome des os. A propos d'une observation anatomoclinique. Sem Hop Paris 54: 1278-1282

Boyle WJ (1972) Cystic angiomatosis of bone. A report of three cases and review of the literature. J Bone Joint Surg 54B: 626-636

Bundens WD, Brighton CT (1965) Malignant hemangioendothelioma of bone. Report of two cases and review of the literature. J Bone Joint Surg 47A: 762-772

Campanacci M, Boriani S, Ginnti A (1980) Hemangio endothelioma of bone: a study of 29 cases. Cancer 46: 804-814

Cayla J, Roger M, Rondier J, Guiraudon C, Malherbe M, Grellet J (1977) Les hémangioendothéliomes malins osseux. A propos d'un cas. Rev Rhum 44: 354-358

Chow RW, Wilson CF, Olsen ER (1970) Angiosarcoma of the skull. Report of a case and review of the literature. Cancer 25: 902-906

Cone RO, Hudkins P, Nguyen V, Merriwether WA (1983) Histiocytoid hemangioma of bone: a benign lesion which may mimic angiosarcoma. Skeletal Radiol 10: 165-169

Corrin B, Manners B, Millard M, Weaver L (1979) Histogenesis of the so-called "intravascular bronchioloalveolar tumor". J Pathol 128: 163-167

Costello SA, Sdeywright M (1990) Postirradiation malignant transformation in benign hemangioma. European J Surg Oncol 16: 517-519

Craver WL, Brown BS (1979) Hemangioendothelioma of bone with pulmonary metastases: a 25 year course. Report of a case. Cancer 43: 1917-1923

Dail DH, Liebow AA (1975) Intravascular bronchioloalveolar tumor. Am J Pathol 78: 6a

Desproges-Gotteron R, Dunoyer J, Loubet R, Rousseau J, Claude M, Leroy V (1972) A propos d'un cas d'angiomatose diffuse et extensive du squelette. Rev Rhum 39: 306-311

Dube VE, Fischer DE (1972) Hemangioendothelioma of the leg following metallic fixation of the tibia. Cancer 30: 1260-1266

Garcia-Moral CA (1972) Malignant hemangioendothelioma of bone. Review of world literature and report of two cases. Clin Orthop 82: 70-79

Gilbert EF, Jones B, Majzoub HS (1971) Malignant hemangioendothelioma of bone in childhood. A report of a case and review of the literature. Am J Dis Child 121: 410-414

Gutierrez RM, Spjut HL (1972) Skeletal angiomatosis: report of three cases and review of the literature. Clin Orthop 85: 82-97

Hartmann WH, Stewart FW (1962) Hemangioendothelioma of bone. Cancer 15: 846-854

Himmer O, Lootvoet L, Deprez P, Monfor L, Ghosez JP (1991) Angiosarcome après prothèse totale du genou. Rev Chir Orthop 77: 125-129

Jaffe JW, Mesgarzadeh M, Bonakdarpour A, Edmonds PR (1989) Histiocytoid hemangioendothelioma of right 10th rib. Skeletal Radiol 18: 50-54

Jennings TA, Peterson L, Axiotis CA, Friedlaender GE, Cooke RA, Rosai J (1988) Angiosarcoma associated with foreign body material. A report of three cases. Cancer 62: 24362444

Kaufmann S, Stout AP (1961) Malignant hemangioendothelioma in infants and children. Cancer 14: 1186-1196

Larson SV, Lorentzon B, Boquist L (1975) Malignant hemangioendothelioma of bone. J Bone Joint Surg 57A: 84-89

Leader M, Collins M, Patel J, Henry K (1986) Staining for factor VIII related antigen and ulex europaeus agglutinin I (UEA-I) in 230 tumours. An assessment of their specificity for angiosarcoma and Kaposi's sarcoma. Histopathology 10: 1153-1162

Martinez-Tello FJ, Marco-Robles J, Blanco-Lorenzo F (1989) Primary epithelioid hemangioendothelioma of bone (polyostotic). Skeletal Radiol 18: 55-59

Maruyama N, Kumagai Y, Ishida Y (1985) Epithelioid hemangioendothelioma of the bone tissue. Virchows Arch (A) 407: 159-165

Miettinen M, Holthofer H, Lehto VP, Miettinen A, Virtanen I (1983) Ulex europaeus I lectin as a marker for tumors derived from endothelial cells. Am J Clin Pathol 79: 32-36

Mirra JM, Arnold WD (1973) Skeletal hemangiomatosis in association with hereditary hemorrhagic telangiectasia. J Bone Joint Surg 55A: 850-854

Mirra JM, Kameda N (1985) Myxoid angioblastomatosis of bones. A case report of a rare, multifocal entity with light, ultramicroscopic, and immunopathologic correlation. Am J Surg Pathol 9: 450-458

Morgenstern P, Westing SW (1969) Malignant hemangioendothelioma of bone. Fourteen-year follow-up in a case treated with radiation alone. Cancer 23: 221-224

Mukai K, Rosai J, Burgdorf WC (1980) Localization of factor VIII-related antigen in vascular endothelial cells using an immunoperoxidase method. Am J Surg Pathol 4: 273-276

Ose D, Vollmer R, Shelburne J, McComb R, Harrelson J (1983) Histiocytoid hemangioma of the skin and scapula. A case report with electron microscopy and immunohistochemistry. Cancer 51: 1656-1662

Otis J, Hutter RWP, Foote FW, Marcove RC, Stewart FW (1968) Hemangioendothelioma of bone. Surg Gynecol Obstet 127: 295-305

Pollak A (1949) Angiosarcoma of the sternum. Am J Surg 77: 522-527

Reed R (1982) Consultation case: malignant angioblastoma of bone. Am J Surg Pathol 6: 159-163

Rosai J, Gold J, Landy R (1979) The histiocytoid hemangiomas. A unifying concept embracing several previously described entities of skin, soft tissue, large vessels, bone and heart. Hum Pathol 10: 707-730

Schajowicz F, Rebecchini AC, Bosch-Mayol G (1979) Intracortical hemangioma simulating osteoid osteoma. J Bone Joint Surg 61B: 94-95

Smet (de) AA, Debra I, Neff JR (1989) Histiocytoid hemangioma of the distal end of the right humerus. Skeletal Radiol 18: 60-65

Steiner GC, Dorfman HD (1972) Ultrastructure of hemangioendothelial sarcoma of bone. Cancer 29: 122-135

Stout AP (1943) Hemangioendothelioma: a tumor of blood vessels featuring vascular endothelial cells. Ann Surg 118: 445-464

Sweterlitsch PR, Torg JS, Watts H (1970) Malignant hemangioendothelioma of the cervical spine a case report. J Bone Joint Surg 52A: 805-808

Tsuneyoshi M, Dorfman HD, Bauer TW (1986) Epithelioid hemangioendothelioma of bone. A clinicopathologic, ultrastructural and immunohistochemical study. Am J Surg Pathol 10: 754-764

Volpe R, Mazabraud A (1982) Hemangioendothelioma (angiosarcoma) of bone: a distinct pathologic entity with an unpredictable course? Cancer 49: 727-736

Weiss SW, Enzinger FM (1982) Epithelioid hemangioendothelioma. A vascular tumor often mistaken for a carcinoma. Cancer 50: 970-981

Wold LE, Unni KK, Beabout JW, Ivins JC, Bruckman JE, Dahlin DC (1982) Hemangioendothelial sarcoma of bone. Am J Surg Pathol 6: 59-70

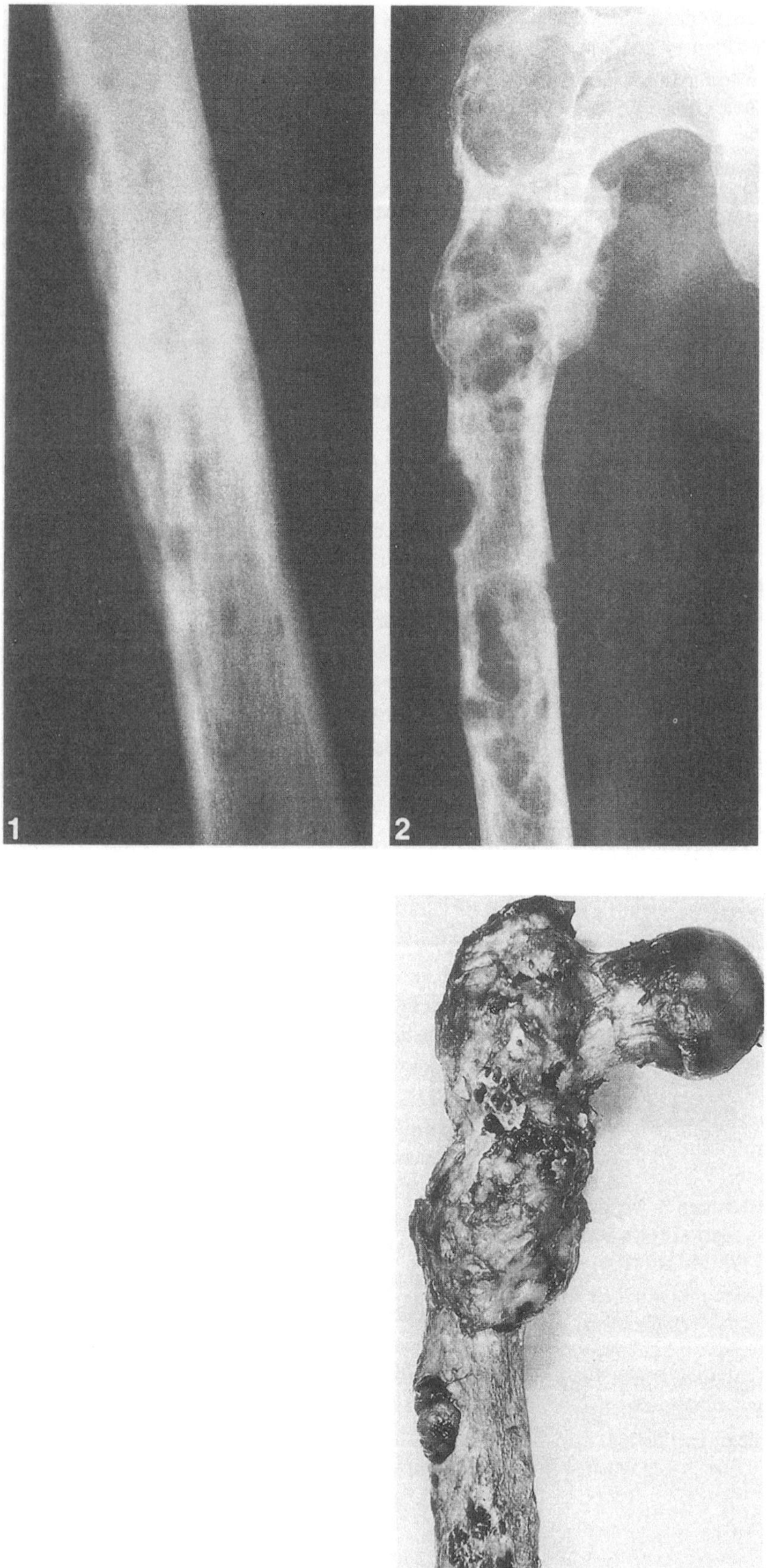

Figs. 1-3. The history of this 31-year-old woman serves to introduce the section on histiocytoid haemangioendothelioma. **1** After 2-3 years' progress, the femur is riddled with numerous cavities and there is endosteal and periosteal reaction. **2** After 10 years, the lesions have invaded the entire femur. **3** In the amputation specimen, the cavities hollowed out in the cortex are quite limited. There was no other tumour

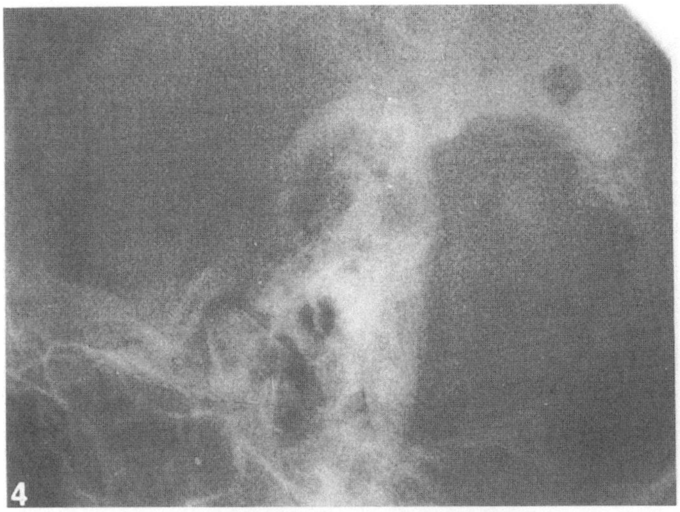

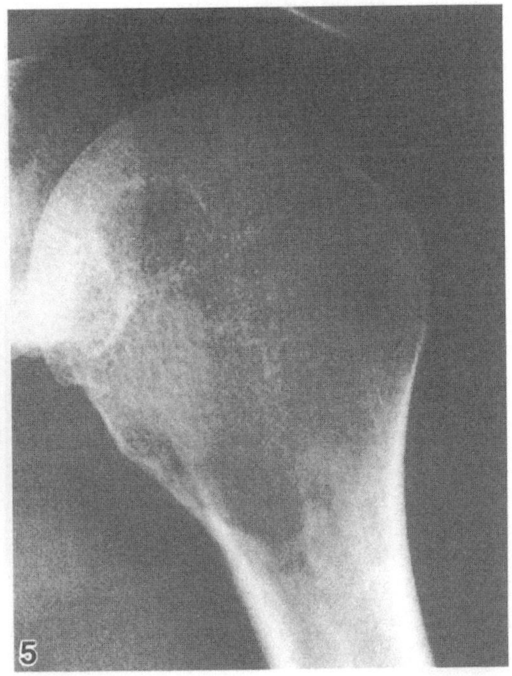

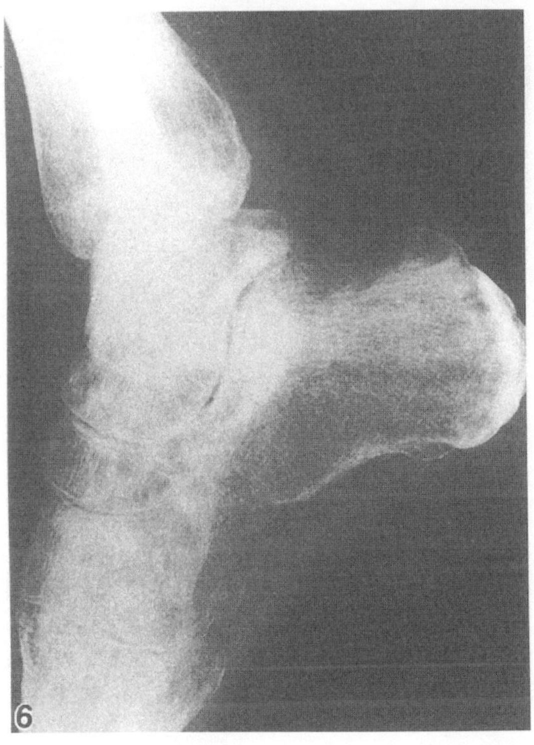

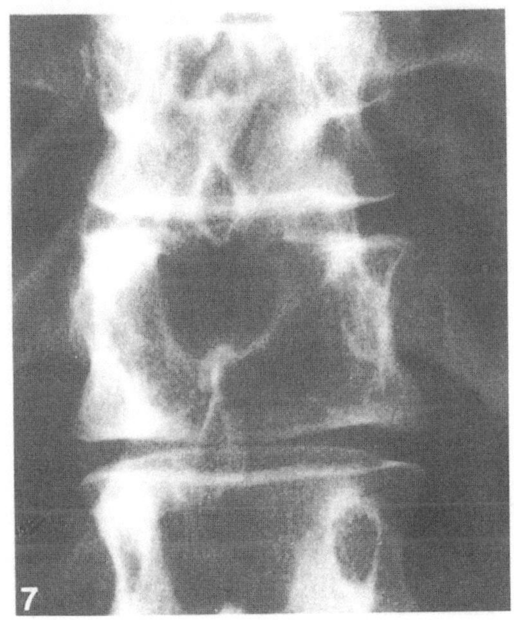

Figs. 4-8. Woman of 28. The onset of the disorder was marked by vertigo and tinnitus. In the following years, mastoid, clavicular and iliac lesions developed. After a course of 6 years, the disease became generalised: long bones of limbs, vertebrae, bones of feet. Death occurred 7 years after the onset of clinical features

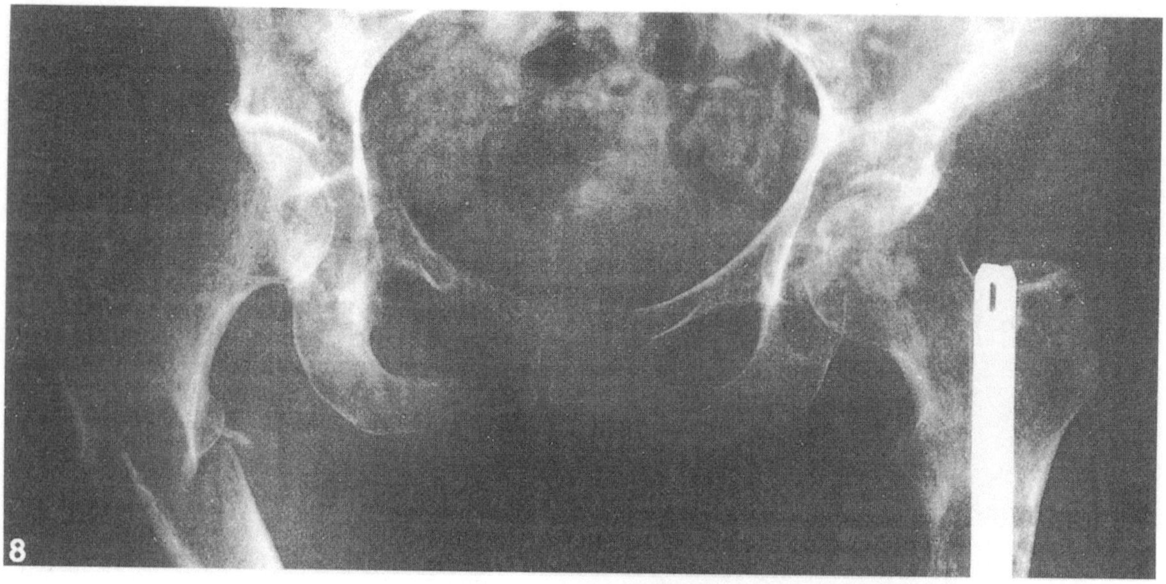

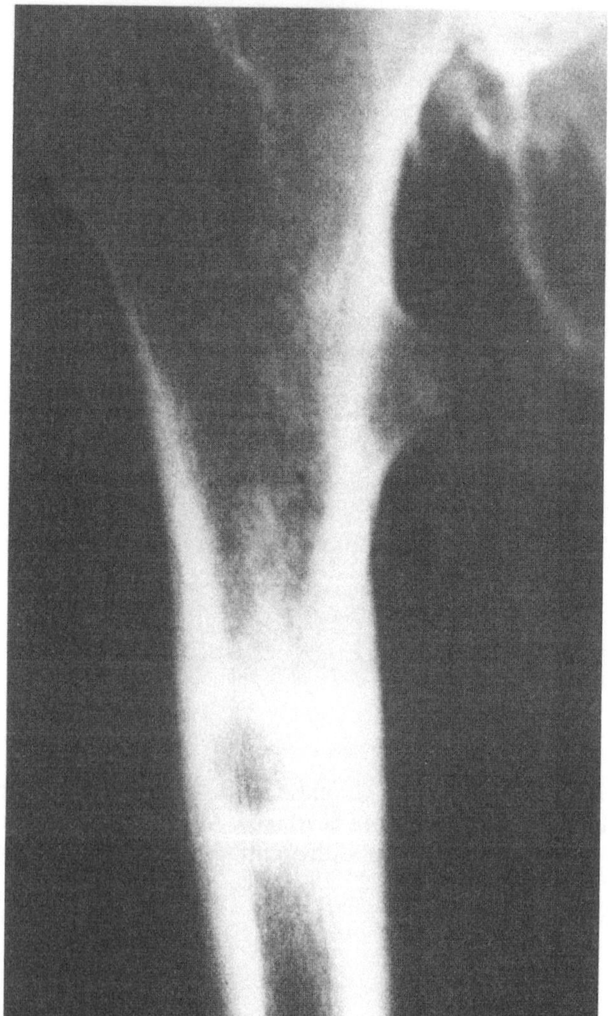

Fig. 9. Solitary femoral lesion of haemangioendothelioma. The round well-circumscribed lacuna is surrounded by bony condensation represented mainly by apposition of periosteal bony lamellae

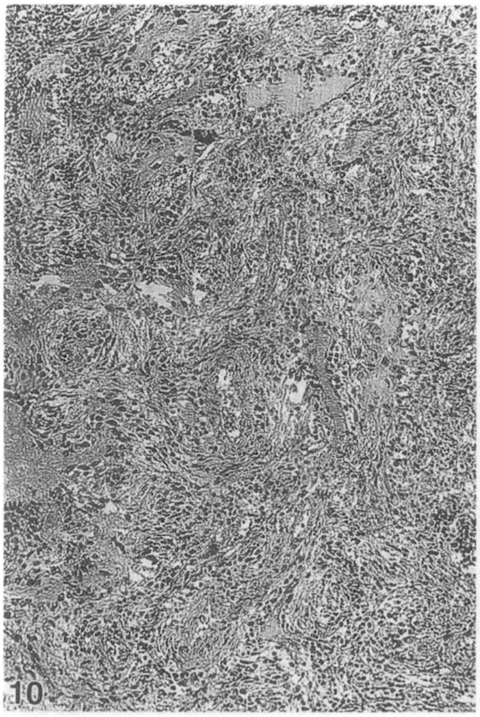

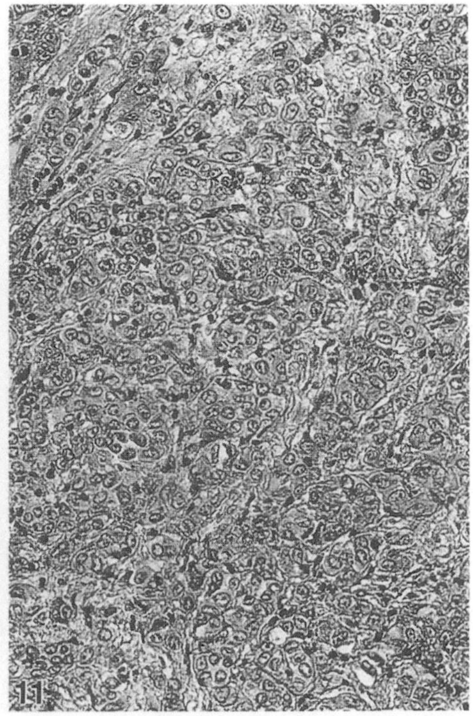

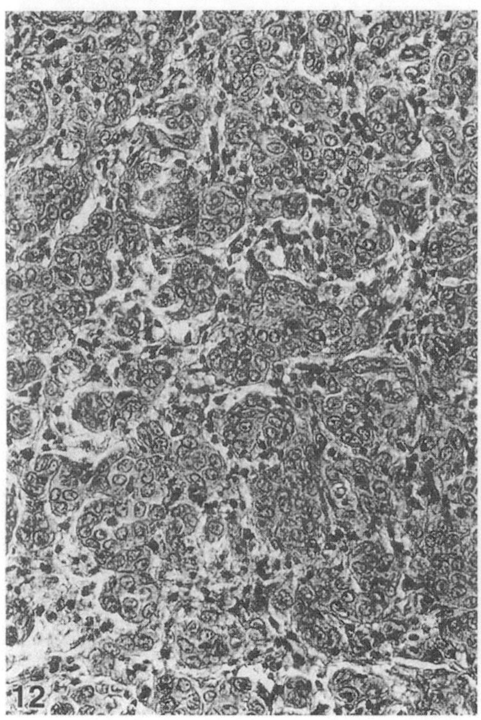

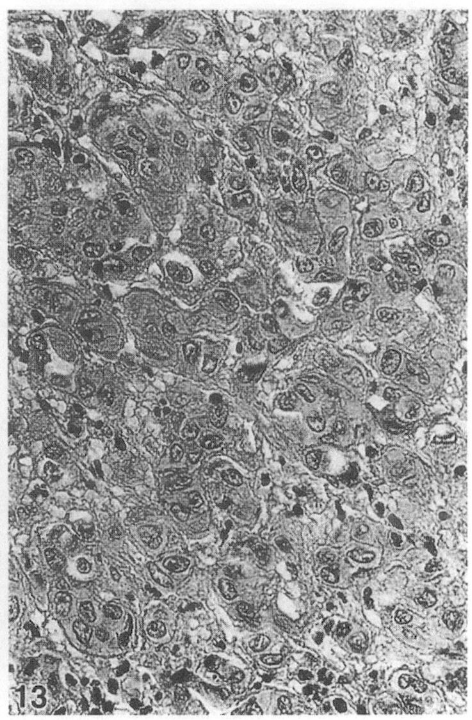

The microphotographs 10-17 are of an histiocytoid haemangioendothelioma whose clinical history has been reported (figs. 1-3)

Figs. 10, 11. The overall appearance is that of a compact tumour, hollowed out by rare vascular cavities

Fig. 12. The tumour cells are grouped in small dense islands

Fig. 13. The compact islands are bounded by a thick membrane. The nuclear-cytoplasmic ratio is not disturbed. This appearance may suggest a metastatic tumour

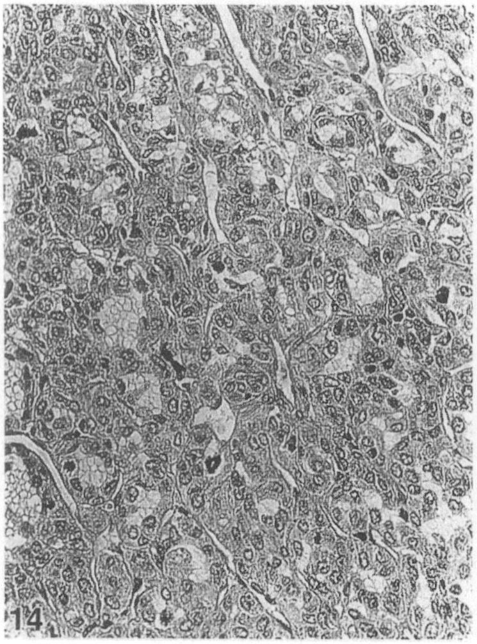

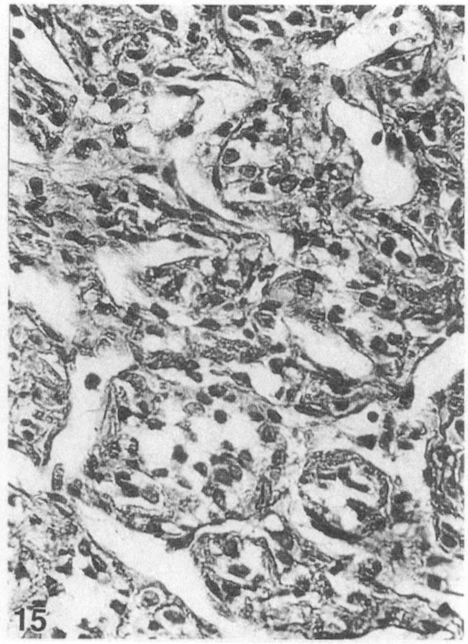

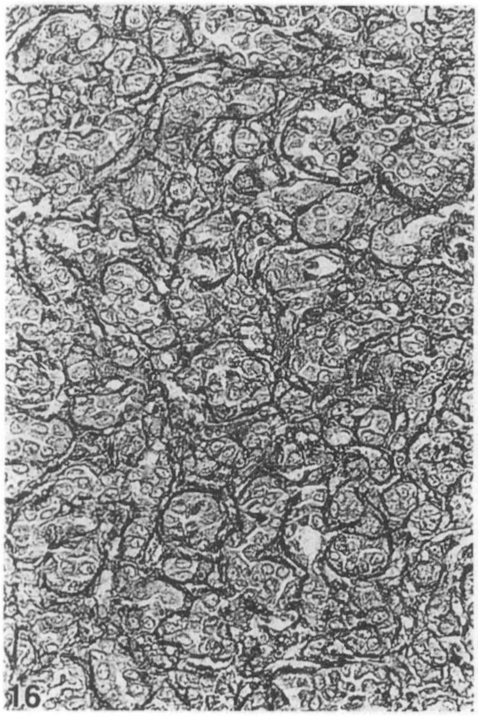

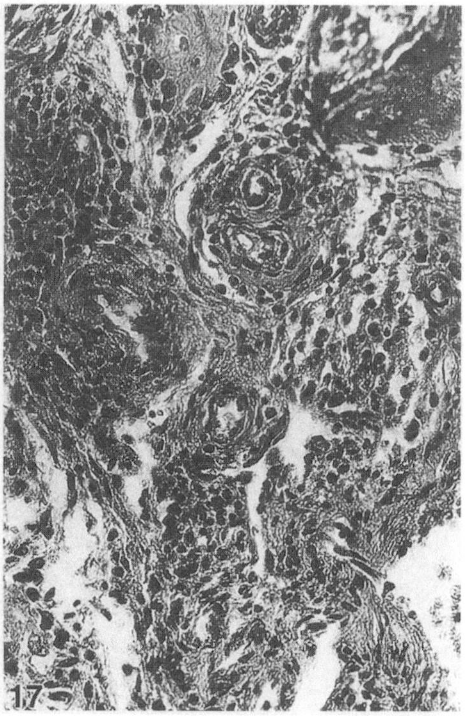

Fig. 14. In this zone, the cells bound cavities filled with erythrocytes

Fig. 15. The endothelial strands are separated from one another by a loose oedematous tissue; this appearance may suggest a haemangiopericytoma (some reports mention associations of angiopericytoma and haemangioendothelioma, but these extraordinary cases should be strictly monitored before publication)

Fig. 16. The very significant reticulin network surrounds endothelial tumour cells

Fig. 17. At the periphery, some vascular clumps formed of vessels with well-defined walls, possibly the pedicles of tumour nodules, are surrounded by inflammatory cells. These peripheral inflammatory infiltrates are reported in most publications

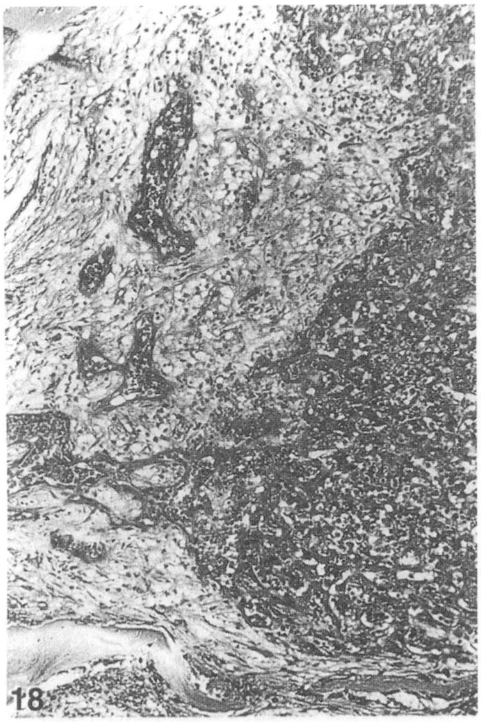

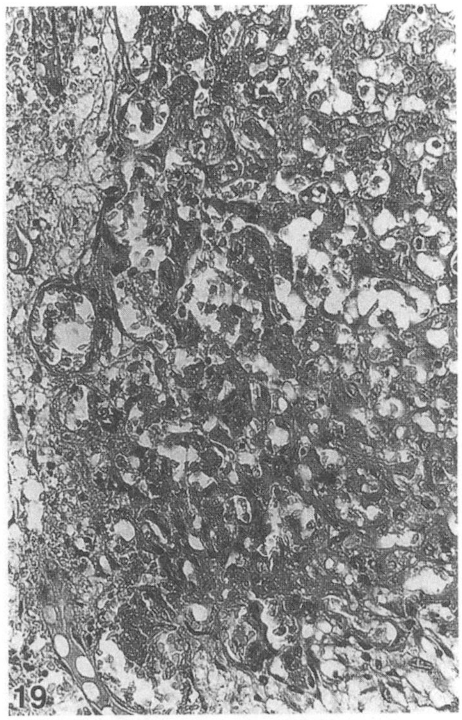

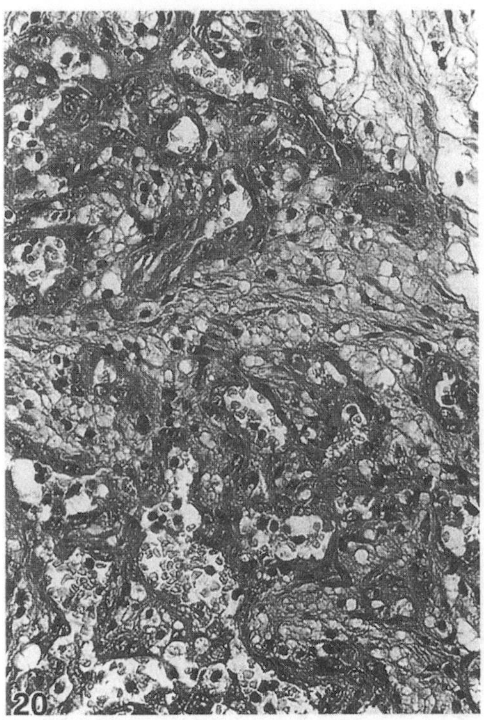

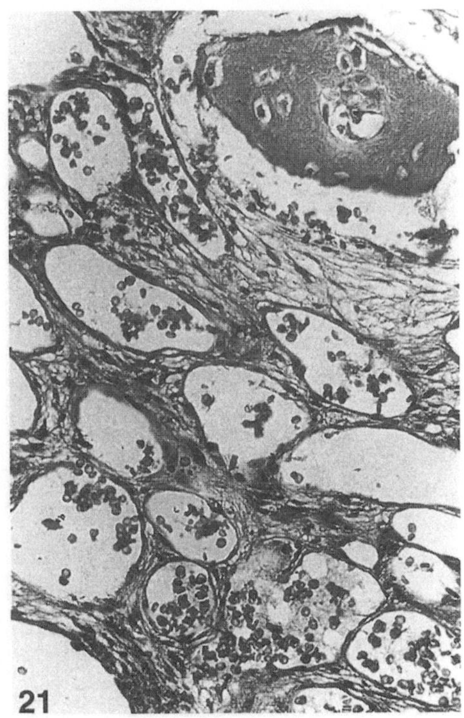

Fig. 18. In this costal haemangoendothelioma the angioblastic islands have developed in a loose fibrous marrow. Swarms of angiomatous formations are characterised by disorderly proliferation in anastomotic cell strands

Figs. 19, 20. The meshes of this network are filled with erythrocytes. The vessels (fig. 20) seem better individualised; here and there an endothelial cell with a large nucleus projects into a vascular lumen

Fig. 21. Peripherally, wide vascular dilatations are bordered by rare flat endothelial cells. A biopsy carried out only in this peripheral zone would probably lead to erroneous interpretation, at least as to the histological grade of malignancy (in which case a "spontaneous exacerbation" of the developing lesion could always be blamed for the bad prognosis)

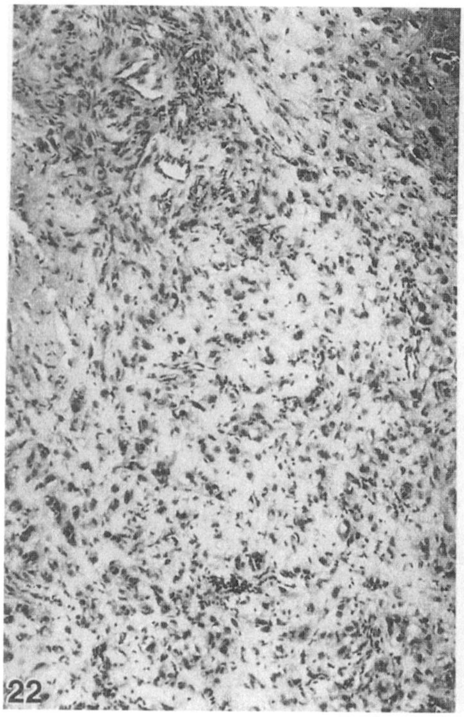

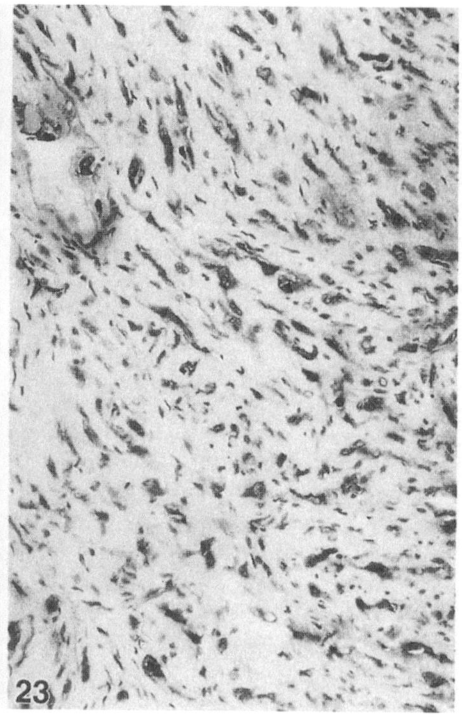

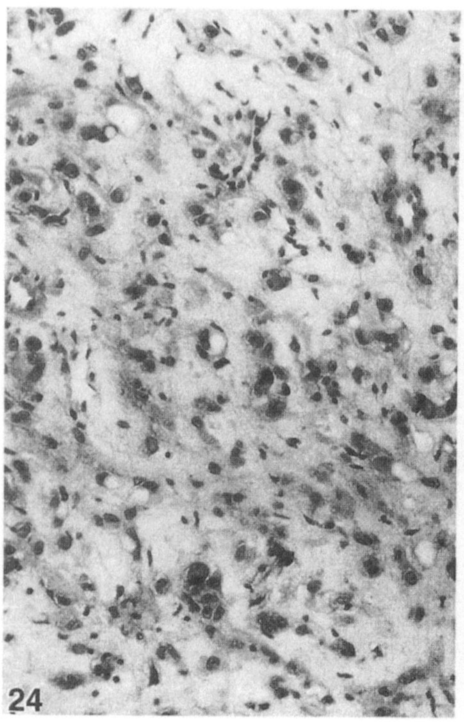

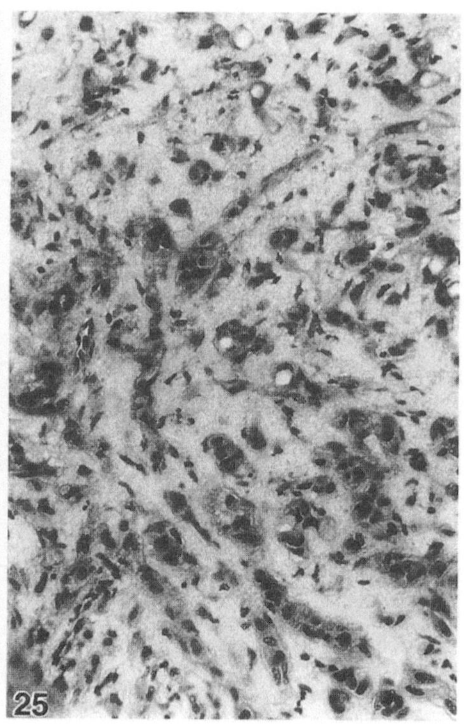

Fig. 22. Histiocytoid haemangioendothelioma. Proliferation of independent cells scattered in a fibromucoid matrix (alcian blue-positive) or grouped in small chains of a few components

Fig. 23. Small fusiform, sometimes rounded cells, the rudiments of vascular cavities. Immunohistological reaction with antibody anti-factor VII is strongly positive

Figs. 24, 25. Rudimentary vascular cavities are more visible here than in the previous microphotograph: cells grouped around a lumen or a simple small intracellular cavity displacing the nucleus (signet-ring image)

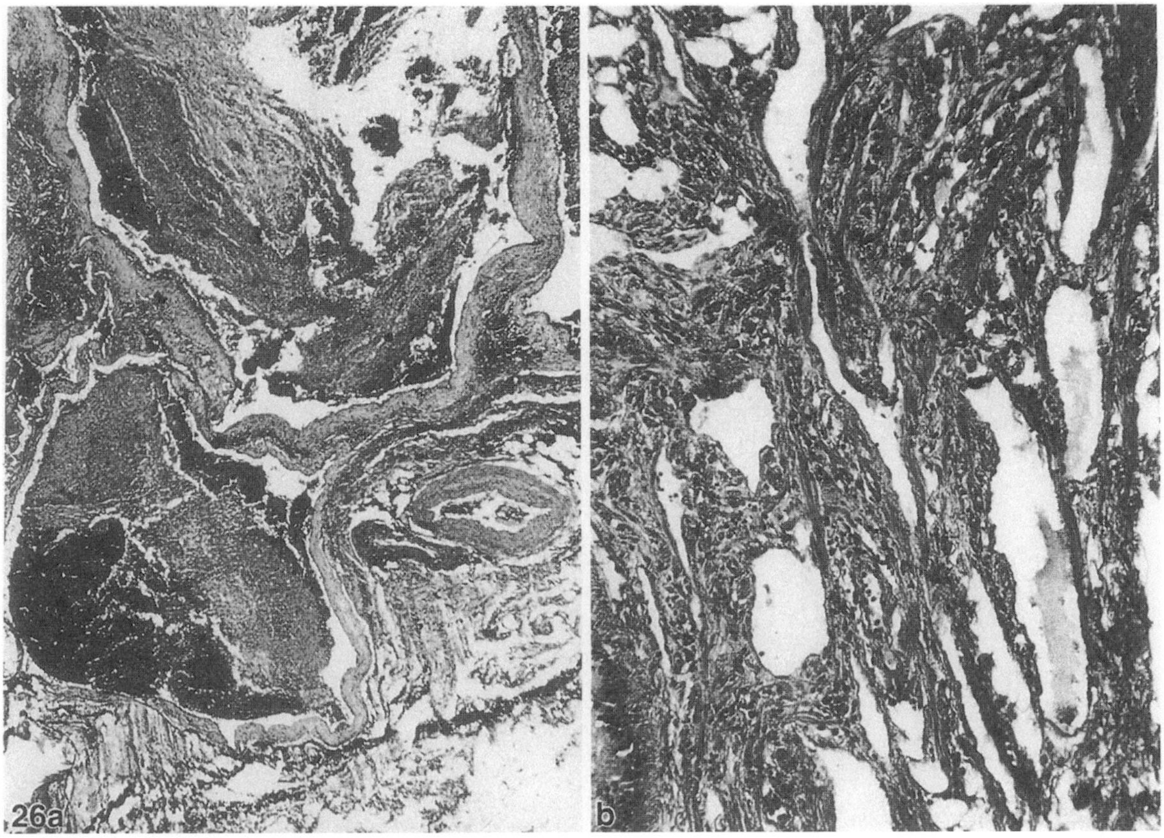

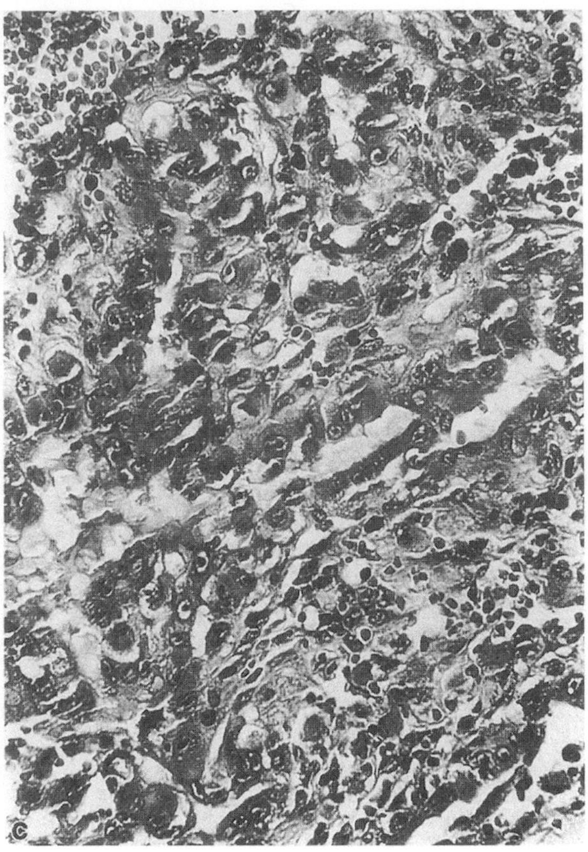

Fig. 26 a-c. Depending on the zones examined, the biopsy of this tibial lesion in a man of 65 shows very different appearances, but progress towards spread of the lesions to numerous parts of the skeleton was fulminating. Such samples illustrate the hazards of bone biopsy in these heterogeneous tumours

23. Haemangiopericytoma

In their 1942 publication, Stout and Murray reported nine cases of a tumour of organoid nature which they distinguished clearly from glomus tumour, and which they had previously proved, by tissue culture, to consist of cells derived from the pericytes of Zimmermann. It also differed from haemangioma by the presence of perivascular cells which they identified as pericytic in nature. The authors suggested the descriptive term of haemangiopericytoma for this tumour.

Case history

The patient, a man of 32, attended for a large tumour deforming the retro- and submandibular region. The skin was of normal colour; the tumour was knobbly, firm in consistency, not tender. The history revealed that this was the second recurrence of an angiopericytoma of the mandible operated on four years previously. Local invasion prevented a surgically satisfactory procedure. This third operation was followed by local irradiation, which may possibly have further delayed progress of the lesion.

General considerations

This is a rare tumour, and Dahlin (1986) could find only seven cases in the statistics of the Mayo Clinic. Haemangiopericytoma is twice as common in males. The maximum incidence is around the 4th and 5h - decades but cases have been reported at all ages, from infancy to the 9th decade. The commonest sites are the pelvis and long bones of the lower limbs [Tang et al 1988] but cranial, vertebral and multifocal lesions have been reported [Puech et al 1965].

Clinical features and course

The tumour is painless for a long time and may slowly destroy the bony cortex and project under the skin by the time the patient first attends. Numerous cases have been reported of local recurrences and malignant forms, either from the outset or after recurrences, with metastatic pulmonary lesions, more rarely bony or nodal. In the female patient of Marcial-Rojas (1960), local recurrence and pulmonary dissemination were discovered 11 months after resection of the clavicle and adjacent tissues.

Conversely, some reports refer to cure at follow-up for over 10 years after local treatment [Dube & Paulson 1974]. But this tumour is capable of metastatic dissemination delayed until 15 and even 20 years after the first treatment. The case reported by May et al (1970) is difficult to interpret. Multiple bony lesions revealed the tumour in a man of 26. Six months later, a lesion of the scalp appeared which the authors regarded as the probable origin of the diffuse bony metastases.

Imaging

The radiographic image is that of osteolysis, often with cortical destruction and invasion of the soft tissues. A discrete periosteal reaction is sometimes evident. The boundaries between bone and tumour are sharp or ill-defined in different cases. Intratumour calcification may be seen. CT examination, and angiography if the diagnosis of a vascular tumour is suggested, supply information on the extent of the tumour and the modifications of the adjacent circulation.

Pathological anatomy and histopathology

At macroscopic examination the tumour is firm, grayish-white and located within or both within and outside the bone.

Histologically, the appearance is quite uniform, due to the proliferation of large areas of ovoid or fusiform cells with round nuclei and abundant eosinophil cytoplasm. These cells are arranged around a vascular lattice with multiple branches of very variable diameter. Wide lumens coexist with numerous elongated vascular slits associated with cell proliferation, often leading to the so-called "staghorn" appearance. However, some biopsies are more evocative at first sight of a compact "epithelioid" proliferation (fig. 1). In these cases silver impregnation of the reticulin fibers reveals the existence of numerous associated vessels and shows up a network of fine reticulin fibers originating from the vascular lumena with surrounding layers of pericytes (fig. 4).

When their lumens are visible, the vessels may contain some red corpuscles, but are mainly reduced to a flat non-proliferative endothelium (figs. 2, 3). They are sometimes lined with a hyaline cuff, which may orient the diagnosis towards a neural tumour, the more so since in this type of cell proliferation a palisaded arrangement of the pericytic nuclei may be observed as in some other tumours.

Ultrastructural studies [Battifora 1973, Chomette 1978, Nunnery 1981] have clearly demonstrated the pericytic nature of the tumour cells. Each is surrounded by a basement membrane which separates it completely from the vascular endothelium. The many fine cell ramifications are closely lined with this basement membrane. Small bundles of filaments are detectable in the cytoplasm. In some cells differentiation of smooth muscle type is also noted.

Despite these ultrastructural findings, there are no immunohistological tests capable of identifying these tumour. Whereas normal pericytes express the smooth muscle type of actin (recognised by the antibody alpha-SM1), the reaction is negative in tumour cells.

Diagnosis

Depending on the way they develop, the bony lesions may suggest different diagnoses. The bulky cells with their eosinophil cytoplasm suggest a carcinoma and more especially a metastasis from an endocrine carcinoma. But the cellular monotony, the absence of atypical mitoses and the negativity to epithelial markers and protein S100 are arguments in favor of the diagnosis of haemangiopericytoma.

Leiomyoma or intraosseous schwannoma are very rare tumours but should be considered; haemangioma or glomus tumour may also be discussed as may an haemangioendothelioma; in the latter case, the reticulin and the immunohistology are valuable factors in differentiation.

In mesenchymal chondrosarcomas, one can see identical appearances reproduced by reticulin around some vessels, but there is no cartilaginous tissue in a haemangiopericytoma. Another problem is the assessment of the histological gradient of malignancy. The principle adopted by most French cancer centers (based on differentiation, necrosis, mitoses) satisfies this requirement. The histological grade of malignancy may increase with recurrences, but interpretation of biopsies made on tumours irradiated because they are inoperable is very difficult. However, there seem to exist variants which are malignant from the outset and are recognised as such at the first biopsy. Partly preserved overall architecture suggests the diagnosis, but the cytonuclear anomalies are obvious. In the radiographs of some cases sent to this laboratory, the osteolysis clearly suggested a malignant tumour (figs. 5-8). Treatment, essentially surgical, does not prevent a recurrence rate of over 50%, often followed by generalised metastatic spread.

References

Battifora H (1973) Hemangiopericytoma: ultrastructural study of five cases. Cancer 31: 1418-1432

Biraben J, Lagarde C, Hugues A (1961) Hémangiopéricytome malin. Ann Anat Pathol 6: 515-519

Chomette G, Auriol M, Tereau Y (1978) Hémangiopéricytome malin: à propos de l'analyse ultrastructurale et histoenzymologique d'une observation. Ann Anat Pathol 23: 41-51

Dahlin DC, Unni KK (1986) Bone tumors general aspects and data on 8,542 cases. 4th edn. Charles C Thomas, Springfield, p. 394

Dube V, Paulson DF (1974) Metastatic hemangiopericytoma cured by radiotherapy: a case report. J Bone Joint Surg 56A: 833-835

Dunlop I (1973) Primary hemangiopericytome of bone. Report of two cases. J Bone Joint Surg 55B: 854-857

Enzinger FM, Weiss S (1988) Soft tissue tumors 2nd edn Mosby, pp 596-613

Faure C, Verspyck R, Parienty R (1964) Le syndrome angiographique de l'hémangiopéricytome. Ann Radiol 7: 181-187

Kennedy JC, Fischer JH (1960) Hemangiopericytoma: its orthopedic manifestations. J Bone Joint Surg 42B: 80-85

Legre G, Payan H, Aubert M (1966) Hémangiopéricytome osseux. Rev Chir Orthop 52: 551-559

Marcial-Rojas RA (1960) Primary hemangiopericytoma of bone. Review of literature and report of the first case with metastases. Cancer 13: 308-311

May VC, Lièvre JA, Attali P, Lièvre JA (1970) Hémangiopéricytome avec localisations osseuses. Rev Rhum 37: 809-815

Mittal KR, Gérald W, True LD (1986) Hemangiopericytoma of breast: report of a case with ultrastructural and immunohistochemical findings. Hum Pathol 17: 1181-1183

Murad TM, Von Haam E, Murthy MSN (1968) Ultrastructure of a hemangiopericytoma and a glomus tumor. Cancer 22: 1239-1249

Nemes Z (1992) Differentiation markers in hemangiopericytoma. Cancer 69: 133-140

Nunnery EW, Kahn LB, Reddick RL, Lipper S (1981) Hemangiopericytoma: a light microscopic and ultrastructural study. Cancer 47: 906-914

Puech A, Pujol H, Mlle Dermenghen, Chavanne F (1965) Hémangiopéricytome à localisation cutanée, abdominale, pulmonaire et osseuse. Montpellier Med 68: 179-192

Saunders TS, Fitzpatrick TB (1957) Multiple hemangiopericytomas; their distinction from glomangiomas (glomus tumors). Arch Dermatol 76: 731-734

Sehested M, Hou-Jensen K (1981) Factor VIII-related antigen as an endothelial cell marker in benign and malignant diseases. Virchows Arch (A) 391: 217-225

Stout AP (1949) Hemangiopericytoma: a study of twenty-five new cases. Cancer 2: 1027-1035

Stout AP (1956) Tumors featuring pericytes: glomus tumor and hemangiopericytoma. Lab Invest 5: 217-223

Stout AP, Murray MR (1942) Hemangiopericytoma: a vascular tumor featuring Zimmermann's pericytes. Ann Surg 116: 26-33

Tang JSH, Gold RH, Mirra JM, Eckardt J (1988) Hemangiopericytoma of bone. Cancer 62: 848-859

Tewifk TL, Finlayson M, Attia EL (1981) Hemangiopericytoma of the temporal bone. J Otolaryngol 10: 72-77

Unni KK, Ivins JC, Beabout JW Dahlin DC (1971) Hemangioma, hemangiopericytoma, and hemangioendothelioma (angiosarcoma) of bone. Cancer 27: 1403-1414

Vang PS, Falk E (1980) Hemangiopericytoma of bone. Acta Orthop Scand 51: 903-907

Vathana P (1984) Primary hemangiopericytoma of bone in the hand: a case report. J Hand Surg (Am) 9A: 761-764

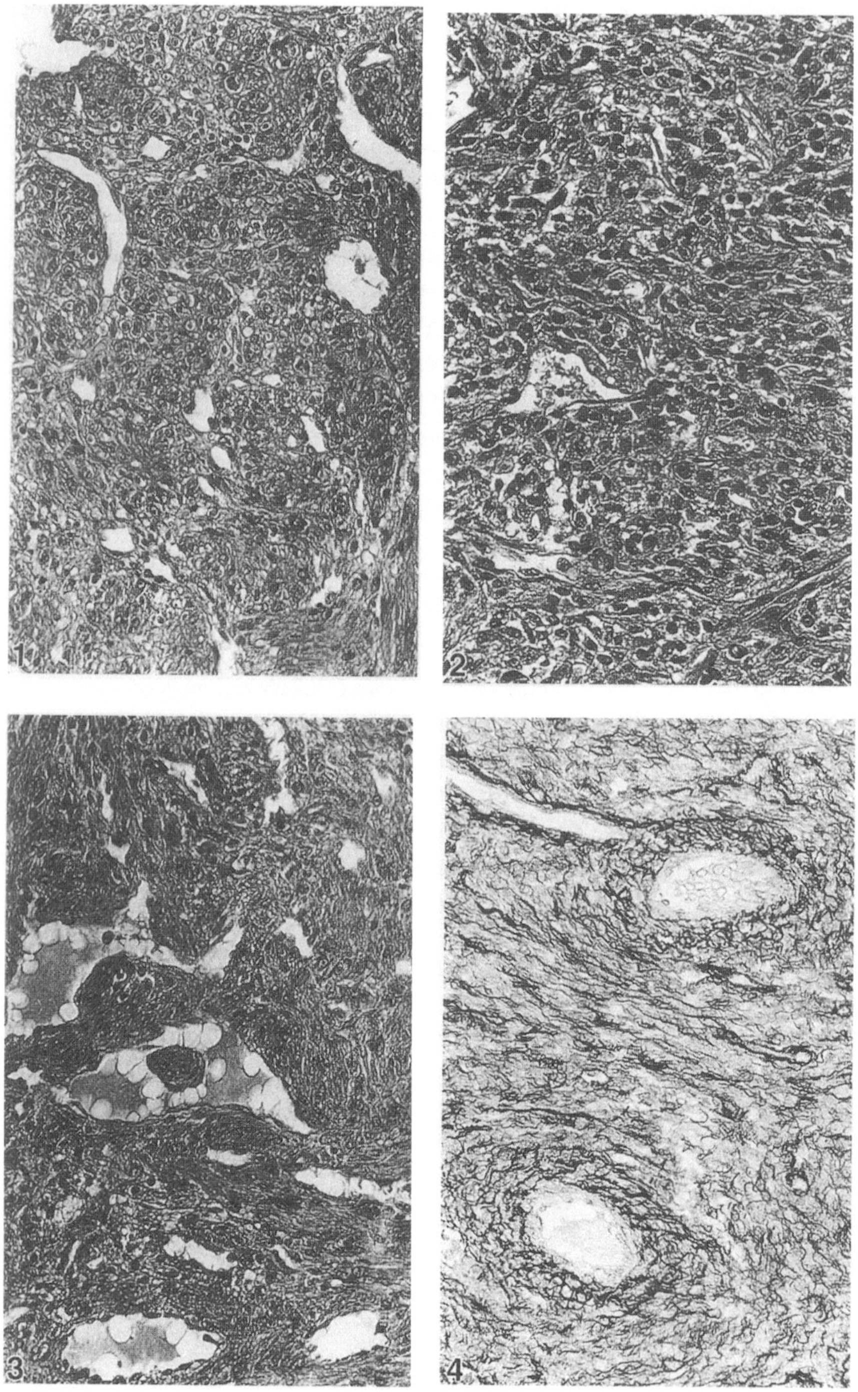

Figs. 1, 2. In this haemangiopericytoma of the frontal bone, the cells, whose boundaries are clearly visible, form compact areas around vessels stretched into crescentic shape; their cytoplasm is markedly eosinophil and the rounded nuclei are very chromophil

Fig. 3. The endothelium of the vessels is flat and though some cells project slightly into the lumen there is no intravascular cell proliferation

Fig. 4. The reticulin fibers which surround each cell make very characteristic layers around the vessels

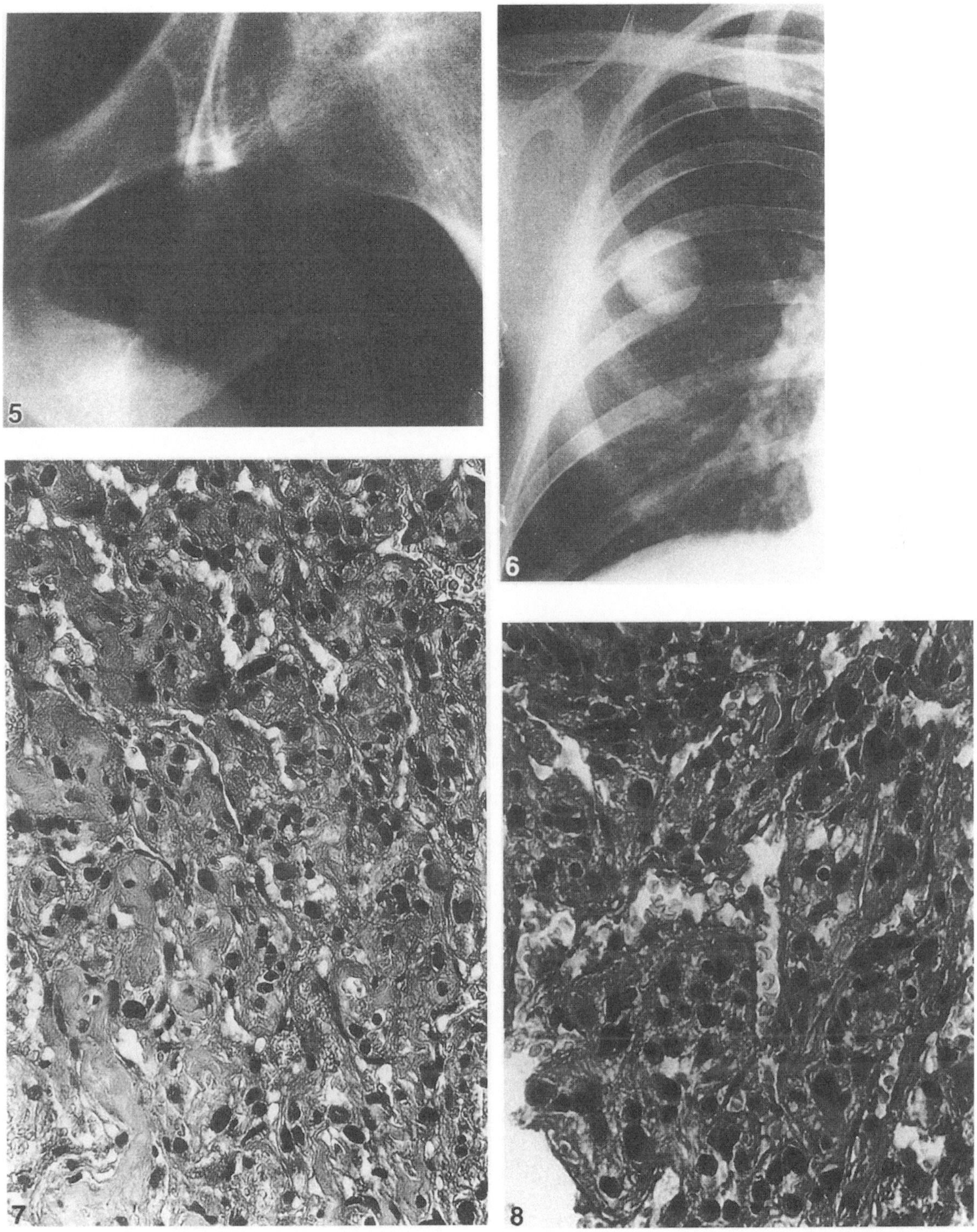

Figs. 5-8. The poorly defined osteolysis of the ischiopubic ramus extends to the iliac wing. A year later this man of 32, despite local irradiation, has a pulmonary metastasis and locally the acetabular region was totally destroyed. In the histological sections, the cells are of unequal size and have large nuclei. The vessels are reduced to vascular slits in this malignant haemangiopericytoma

24. Glomus tumour

Rare cases of intraosseous glomus tumours have been reported. It was Masson, in 1924, who described the "neuro-arterial glomus of the tactile regions and its tumours" in the soft tissues.

Case history

An upholsterer of 55 attended for increasingly severe pain in the terminal phalanx of the left middle finger. The history revealed nothing specific except that the fingers of this man were necessarily exposed to various injuries. In the radiographs, a rounded and well-circumscribed osteolysis occupied much of the phalanx. The cortex was uninvolved. There was no central calcification. The severity of the pain might have suggested an osteoid osteoma, but also a glomus tumour.

General considerations, clinical features and course

The tumour is usually located in the phalanges. However, cases have been reported in the femur, fibula, and pubis, whether or not preceded by trauma [Simmons et al 1992]. Some have affected children, others adults [Leger et al 1960, Bjorkengren 1986]. The presenting feature is usually pain, which is sometimes intolerable. Surgical removal, usually by simple curettage, is followed by permanent cure.

Imaging

The radiographic image is that of rounded osteolysis with sharp borders, suggestive in a phalanx of chondroma, epidermoid cyst, or metastasis. This intraosseous lesion must be distinguished from the impression that may be made by a juxtaosseous tumour of the soft tissues, such as an angioma.

Pathological anatomy and histopathology

Surgical intervention removes a small firm rounded structure, sometimes reddish, sometimes whitish.

From the histological viewpoint, there is nothing to contradict the supposition that the varieties described by Masson (1924-1937) in glomus tumours of the soft tissues may be expressed in bone. It is possible to see a predominantly cellular epithelioid tumour of angiomatous or neuromatous nature, and even the appearance reported by Enzinger and Weiss (1988), characterised by a progressive transformation of the glomus cells into fusiform cells of smooth muscle type representing 10% of glomus tumours of the soft tissues.

The intraosseous glomus tumour illustrated here (figs. 1-4) was located in an ungual phalanx and had developed for several years after a major injury. The globoid cells of epithelioid appearance were grouped in small compact islands and inter-anastomosing strands and the tumour was partly hyalinised. The vascular lumina, surrounded by a hyaline wall, were clearly evident with standard stains. Some nerve bundles were also observed, probably correlated with the painful symptoms which had revealed the tumour.

Differential diagnosis

The pain, well-circumscribed osteolysis and location in an ungual phalanx are features which will indicate the diagnosis. It is essential not to confuse this lesion with an endothelioma, whose prognosis is doubtful, to avoid the useless amputation of a digit. At other sites - the long bones of the limbs, pelvis - it is unlikely that the diagnosis will be suggested by the radiographs initially.

This tumour has given rise to much histogenetic debate. According to Masson (1924), it is an abnormal development of a neurovascular glomus and is to be classified as an arterial angioneuromyoma. The existence of glomus tumours outside the zones in which histologists have described neurovascular glomuses is explained by the presence of the glomus in a heterotopic site which happens here to be intramedullary.

Murray and Stout (1942), from their tissue culture studies, believed that the cells of glomus tumours were no different from pericytes. But ultrastructural studies [Venkatachalam & Greally 1969] demonstrated the presence of actin filaments in the cytoplasm of these cells, which resemble smooth muscle cells more than pericytes; the more so since, in addition to myofibrils, there are zones of densification of these filaments, condensations quite characteristic of smooth muscle cells. These agglomerated filaments terminate at the inner aspect of the membrane, an appearance often noted in smooth muscle cells, but only rarely in pericytes. In optical microscopy, our predecessors had already identified the presence of muscle cells and neural structures by means of Masson's trichrome staining and that of Bodian.

For Enzinger and Weiss (1988), pericytes, glomus cells and muscle cells are closely related; and the probable passage from one type to another would explain both the presence of glomus tumours in regions where there are normally no glomuses and certain cases of tumours whose equivocal histiological appearance combines zones of haemangiopericytic type with zones characteristic of glomus tumour.

Nuovo et al (1990) studied the immunohistological reactions with various antibodies in 40 glomus tumours. They noted that, while all the tumours were marked by antivimentin and anti-actin antibodies, the antidesmin antibody marked only 73% of cases and the number of positive cells as well as the intensity of the reaction varied greatly from one tumour to another; no tumour was marked by the anticytokeratin antibody.

References

Bjorkengren AG, Resnick D, Haghighi P, Sartoris DJ (1986) Intraosseous glomus tumor: report of a case and review of the literature. AJR 147: 739-741

Enzinger FM, Weiss SW (1988) Soft tissue tumors, 2nd edn. Mosby, St Louis, pp 581-595

Leger L, Bitry-Boely C, Gritton PH, Lapeyre J (1960) Tumeurs glomiques multiples ou glomangiomatoses. Présentation d'un cas et revue de la littérature. Presse Med 68: 2261-2264

Masson P (1924) Le glomus neuro-artériel des régions tactiles et ses tumeurs. Lyon Chir 11: 915

Masson P, Géry L (1927) Les tumeurs glomiques sous-cutanées en dehors des doigts (angio-neuromyomes artériels). Ann Anat Pathol 4: 153-165

Murad TM, Von Haam E, Murray MSN (1968) Ultrastructure of a hemangiopericytoma and a glomus tumor. Cancer 22: 1239-1249

Nuovo MA, Grimes MM, Knowles DM (1990) Glomus tumors: a clinicopathologic and immunohistochemical analysis of forty cases. Surg Pathol 3: 31-45

Simmons TJ, Bassler TJ, Schwinn CP, Forester DM (1992) Primary glomus tumor of bone. Skeletal Radiol 21: 407-409

Sunderraj S, Al-Khalifa AA, Pal AK, Pim HP, Sabri SH (1989) Primary intra-osseous glomus tumor. Histopathol 14: 532-536

Tarnowski WM, Hashimoto K (1969) Multiple glomus tumors. An ultrastructural study. J Invest Dermatol 52: 474-478

Tocker C (1969) Glomangioma: an ultrastructural study. Cancer 23: 487-492

Venkatachalam MA, Greally JC (1969) Fine structure of glomus tumor: similarity of glomus cells to smooth muscle. Cancer 23: 1176-1184

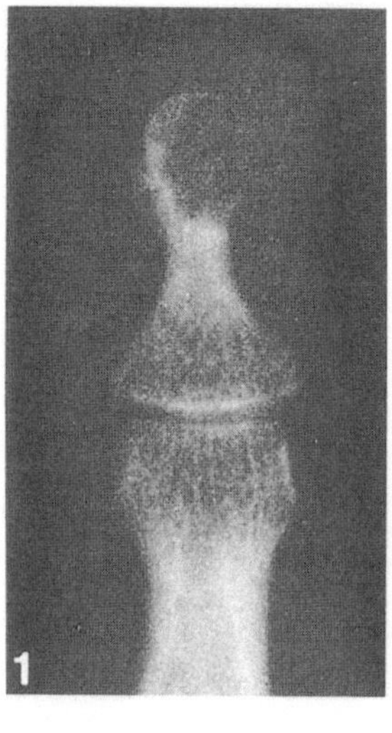

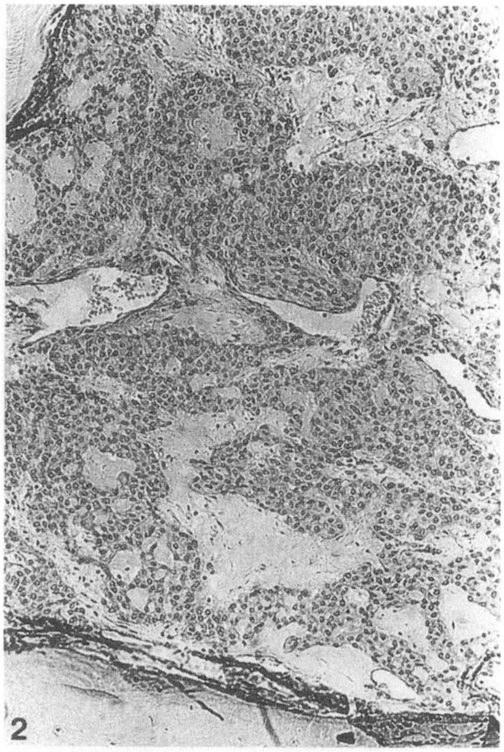

Fig. 1. In this young woman of 21, the tumour occupies the distal part of the ungual phalanx of the right ring finger. At the age of 4, she had suffered a severe injury to this phalanx

Fig. 2. At low magnification, the appearance of this intraosseous glomangioma is characteristic and quite similar to that of the soft tissue tumour

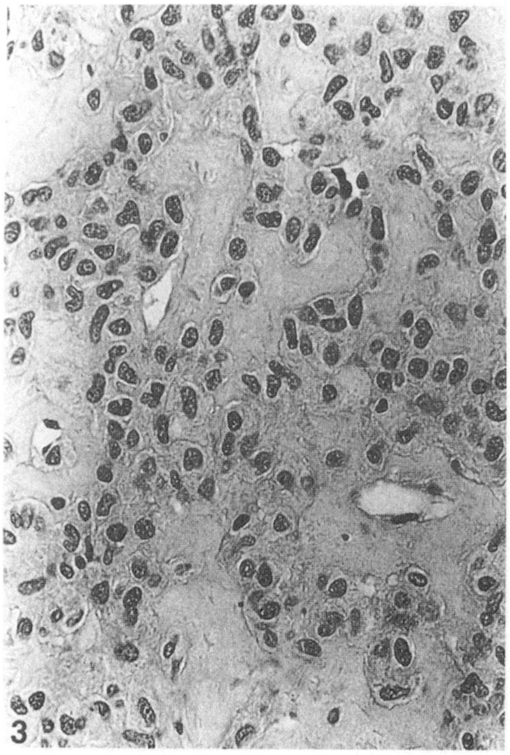

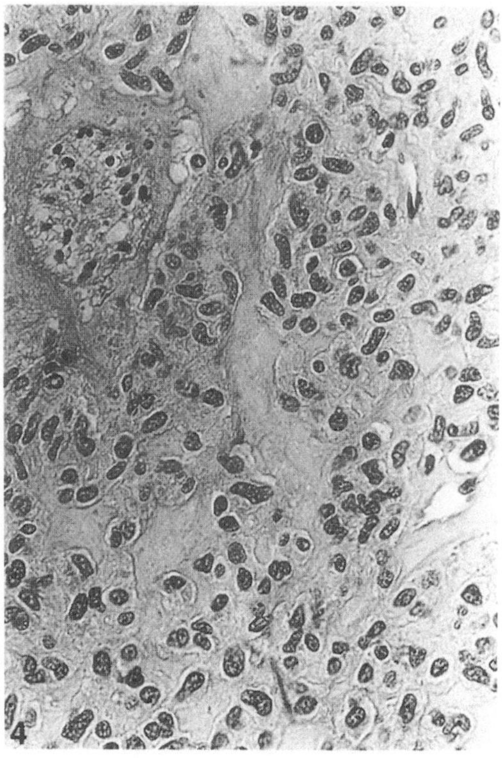

Fig. 3. The perivascular hyalinisation is more obvious in this microphotograph

Fig. 4. Top left: a relatively large nerve in the midst of the tumour

25. Haemangioma

Benign in itself, whether hamartoma or tumour, the prognosis of a haemangioma depends on its site and extent, which determine the treatment possibilities.

Angioma

Case history

A biopsy sample labelled "cutaneous angioma, outer aspect of lower end of leg, young girl of 18" was sent to the laboratory. The biopsy involved the skin and subcutaneous zones. The histological appearance was that of a typical angioma formed of well-differentiated vessels with lumina of unequal size. There was no endothelial cell proliferation. The regularly arranged endothelial cells projected slightly into the vascular channels. As this was a "soft issue" lesion, no radiograph accompanied the sample, and the histological report was followed by the remark: "What is the state of the underlying tibia? These cutaneous angiomas are sometimes the visible manifestation of a much deeper tumour involving the subjacent bone. It is wise to ensure by a skeletal survey that here is no other bony lesion". The angioma of our young patient was confirmed as solitary, but it involved the lower end of the tibia widely and raised the problem of preservation or arthrodesis of the tibio-tarsal joint, the most dysfunctional of articular ankyloses of the lower limb.

General considerations

Angioma of bone is a rare tumour. Women are affected 2-3 times as often as men and it is seen at all ages, but mainly between 30 and 60 years of age. The vertebrae and craniofacial skeleton account for about 70% of cases, followed by the femur, ribs and pelvis; virtually any bone may be affected.

Clinical features and course

Symptoms consist only of some pain. In the case cited above, it was the superficial cutaneous development that attracted attention but angioma may be asymptomatic and discovered during a radiological examination performed for some other reason.

The clinical implications of an angioma relate essentially to its site and extent and lastly to treatment possibilities. Vertebral angiomas may give rise to cord compression. Serious consequences are related to the level of the compression (paraplegia, rarely quadriplegia). Paraplegia usually has a rapid onset, which may or may not be preceded by pain; but sometimes there is a regional angiomatosis which extends far beyond the vertebral body. Baker et al (1996) reported 4 cases of vertebral angiomas presenting with neurologic of features including hyperesthaesia and decreased muscle power or simply thoracic or thoracolumbar pain preceding vertebral collapse.

In some cases, the clinical features arise during pregnancy with girdle pain and paresthesiae. The pain is exacerbated by coughing and straining, but many vertebral angiomas are asymptomatic. On the whole, asymptomatic vertebral angiomas remain relatively stable.

There is a diffuse form of familial cystic angiomatosis of benign course; Reid et al (1989) reported 12 cases in the same family involving the ends of the long bones. This asymptomatic cystic angiomatosis involved each of four generations. In the radiographs, the cysts were surrounded by a fine border of sclerosis and the course was towards sclerosis with obliteration of the cyst. These authors link this form of hereditary angiomatosis to the hamartomas.

Spontaneous malignant transformation of an angioma is rare but after irradiation there is some risk of malignant transformation.

Imaging

The radiological image of vertebral angioma is quite characteristic, at least in its typical form. The vertebra is more radiolucent than the vertebrae above and below. The vertebral body appears "meshed" or "combed out" due to the persistence of the supporting vertebral bony columns only. The osteolysis may extend to the posterior arch in varying degree. The vertebral body may have a barrel-shaped deformity; more rarely, there is vertebral collapse, due to fracture of the vertebral body. In the long bones of the limbs, the zone of osteolysis is quite well circumscribed and sometimes even surrounded by a sclerotic border.

Some appearances are more suggestive of a cyst or polycystic lesion than of an angioma (fig. 1). Angiomas of the craniofacial skeleton, which are often osteoangiomas, produce an opaque prominence in the outer table of the skull bones. In the face, they sometimes cause considerable hypertrophy of the bone affected (figs. 4, 5).

The various imaging techniques - CT, MRI, angiography and possibly isotope scanning - define the precise boundaries of the lesion, the state of the bony cortex and any extension into the soft tissues. It is useful to exclude the association of an angioma with chondromatosis (Maffucci's syndrome).

Pathological anatomy and histopathology

The macroscopic appearance at operation varies with the stage of development of the angioma and its structure. Sometimes the appearance is that of a haemorrhagic cyst (fig. 2), sometimes that of a compact tumour, the vascular proliferation being masked by the cell proliferation surrounding the vessels, whose lumen is often collapsed. In other zones a stratum of barely projecting endothelial cells surrounds wide lumens containing red corpuscles, which appear as if scooped out in dense connective tissue with numerous folds (figs. 9-12). In vertebral haemangiomas, the tumour occupies the vertebral body and possibly part of the posterior arch. The fine-walled vessels are elongated in a fatty marrow or bounded by dense connective tissue. Their narrow or dilated lumen is filled with erythrocytes (figs. 13-16). Such appearances may be noted in the biopsy of a chondroblastoma if this has been taken too peripherally, but an appearance of hypervascularisation may also suggest a metastasis, and in cases where presentation is with fracture it may be considered to be a reactive state.

When discovered at autopsy the angioma may be reduced to a small reddish-brown area in the spongy bone of the vertebral body. Cranial angiomas may be lytic or productive and these osteoangiomas are quite characteristic (cf Chapters 10 & 38).

Differential diagnosis

Histological diagnosis is easy in most cases but one cannot conclude that the tumour is an angioma, and only an angioma, without an acquaintance with the clinical history and imaging. The pathologist must assure himself that the tumour is a solitary lesion, that there are no associated chondromas, and that it is not a lymphangioma in which the vessels are filled with erythrocytes because of surgical haemorrhage.

The angiomatous appearance observed in a biopsy may be a manifestation of an osteoblastoma but also of hyperparathyroidism, a disorder which must be excluded routinely (search for a parathyroid tumour, study of calcium-phosphorus metabolism, estimation of parathormone). An angiomatous condition may be seen in some cases of multiple metastases, particularly from renal carcinomas.

Once the diagnosis of an angioma has been established, one must exclude a haemangioendothelioma with proliferation of endothelial cells in its "histiocytoid" form and angiosarcoma in its very malignant forms. A histiocytoid haemangioma with atypical vascular proliferation with "histiocytoid" cells in an inflammatory setting may also cause confusion.

The prognosis is favourable when a surgical procedure is possible under good conditions. Irradiation of cases judged inoperable should not be undertaken routinely in view of the risk of malignant transformation.

Cystic angiomatosis

Following the description of the entity "cystic angiomatosis of the skeletal system" by Jacobs and Kimmelstiel in 1953, a relatively small number of cases have been reported under this heading, either with localised skeletal lesions (in the skull), or diffuse and often associated with cystic angiomatosis of the viscera and/or soft tissues. The disorder is seen mainly in the 20s or 30s and affects the long bones of the limbs, but in many cases also involves the limb-girdles, ribs and skull. The zones of osteolysis are surrounded by a discrete sclerosis but there is no periosteal reaction. The visceral angiomatosis often found in association may be manifest or discovered during examination. The term "angiomatosis", though lacking in precision, has been retained simply because the authors recognise that it is difficult to distinguish between cystic haemangioma and lymphangioma. Further, some reports seem to confirm skeletal haemangiomatosis accompanied by a visceral lymphangiomatosis in the same patient. The possible differential diagnoses include Langerhans histiocytosis, fibrous dysplasia, hyperparathyroidism and, more rarely, metastases or lymphoma [Zenny et al 1981, Lateur et al 1996, Levey et al 1996].

Histiocytoid haemangioma

General considerations

In 1979, Rosai, Gold and Landy described a variety of angioma characterised essentially by a particular appearance of the endothelial cells which they called, for lack of a better term, "histiocytoid endothelial cells". In addition to this histiocytoid aspect of the endothelial cells there were inflammatory infiltrations varying in extent in different cases but rich in eosinophils. In their study, they reported seven cases, two at a bony site: the upper end of the tibia and the lower end of the femur, both at the epiphysis. In both cases, one in a man of 21 and the other in a girl of 10, the course was slow and curettage was followed by cure. The other five cases were lesions of the soft tissues, one at a periosteal site. According to various reports it seems that in the soft tissues the preferential sites are cranial (scalp) and sometimes cervical. Ose et al (1983) reported a case of histiocytoid haemangioma of the scalp in a man of 50, accompanied by three lesions in the form of skin papules, of the same histological appearance as the bony lesion. In the same year, Cone et al (1983) described a case with multiple bony lesion in a man of 52 who developed two verrucous lesions of the sole of the foot. The case reported by Desproges-Gotteron et al in 1972 under the name of angiomatosis and characterised by multiple bony lesions and lesions of the scalp involving the cranial bones probably forms part of this group.

No valid statistical conclusions can be drawn from the published cases as to frequency, site or gender predominance.

Imaging

Imaging reveals a zone of osteolysis with an irregular outline but the lesion is often well-circumscribed and usually without periosteal reaction. In the case reported by De Smet et al (1989) at a humeral epiphyseal site there were two small areas of posterior cortical rupture. Isotope scan with ^{99m}Tc demonstrates major fixation of the isotope, but often reveals other lesions. These lesions are either present at the first examination or become evident in the months following the first lesion. However, in every case the bony lesion may be associated with cutaneous or visceral involvement.

Clinical features and course

The bony lesion is usually revealed by pain, relatively acute when it is situated at an epiphysis, exacerbated by movement and partly relieved by immobilisation. In some cases laboratory tests have shown mild eosinophilia. The course is benign but the risk of articular complications is considerable.

Curettage, if need be repeated after recurrence, is followed by definitive cure. The patients of De Smet and Cone remained cured after 7 and 10 years' surveillance respectively, in the latter patient after treatment of multiple bony lesions (femoral, vertebral, metatarsal). In one of the cases reported by Rosai, a woman of 34 was admitted for multiple scalp nodules. The diagnosis made was that of Kaposi's sarcoma. After excision, the nodules recurred at 2 and 7 years after the first operation, with lysis of the outer table of the frontal bone. At operation the lesion, which extended to the dura mater, was treated by diathermy; cure seems definitive 10 years after the onset of the disease.

Pathological anatomy and histopathology

Macroscopically, this is a reddish spongy haemorrhagic structure which contains some bony fragments.

At microscopic examination there is a vascular proliferation composed of vessels of very variable size. The lumen of the larger vessels is filled with erythrocytes. Some reports mention mucinous degeneration of the vascular walls which appears as a subendothelial basophil material. The endothelial cells are large and proliferative, of cuboid shape and with eosinophilic cytoplasm. The nucleus, oval and often plicated, is dotted with one or two very evident nucleoli, an appearance resembling that of histiocytes. In some cases the abundance of these endothelial cells in the vessel lumen suggests metastasis from an adenocarcinoma.

Other cells of the same type proliferate in the loose intervascular connective tissue, either solitary or in small compact groups. Some vacuolated cells resemble signet-ring cells, the rudiments of new vessels. Every intermediate form exists between the cavernous types and the rudimentary new vessels. However histiocytoid or epithelioid the cells may be, ultrastructural studies demonstrate their endothelial nature.

A fundamental feature of histiocytoid haemangioma is the presence of an inflammatory infiltrate accompanying the vascular proliferation. This may be dispersed in the connective tissue or grouped in dense nodules. It consists of lymphocytes, plasmocytes, macrophages, neutrophils and eosinophils, the last sometimes predominating. Some haemorrhagic zones and fibrin deposits may also be seen. However, there is no tumour necrosis and no cytological evidence of malignancy.

A number of endothelial cells do not express factor VII; the bulkier the cell, the less likely is a positive reaction [Ose et al 1983].

Diagnosis

The relative frequency of epiphyseal location in the radiographs has suggested the diagnoses of chondroblastoma, osteomyelitis and eosinophil granuloma.

From the histological aspect, the diagnostic reservations of pathologists confronted with histiocytoid haemangiomas of the soft tissues are important; they are entirely determined by the possible predominance of one or other of the components of the polymorphous picture. The diagnoses proposed initially are of varying proximity to the truth: Kaposi's sarcoma, malignant angiomatosis, atypical endothelial vascular proliferation, angiomatoid hyperplasia with eosinophilia, angiomatosis and, for bony lesions, eosinophil granuloma, chronic osteomyelitis and haemangioendothelioma. This list of diagnoses demonstrates the four main areas of confusion. The first is the vascular and haemorrhagic nature, which directs the diagnosis towards Kaposi's sarcoma and the second the predominance of inflammatory phenomena, which, in bone, raise the possibility of osteomyelitis. Thirdly, the "histiocytoid" dominance and eosinophil infiltration may suggest the diagnosis of histiocytosis, and finally the "histiocytoid" cell proliferation, virtually devoid of inflammatory infiltration, which evokes a haemangioendothelioma of low-grade malignancy.

To conclude that there is a sort of spectrum ranging from angioma to angiosarcoma may be intellectually satisfactory but does not resolve the fundamental problem of the pathologist. Whatever its presentation and whatever the predominance of any one component, the essential fact is the absence of cytological anomalies, which forbids the pathologist to classify the vascular lesion he has to diagnose as a malignant tumour.

References

Acquaviva R, Tamic PM, Kerdoudi H, Thevenot CH, Bru P, Lévy-Lebar JP, Varga LA (1968) Les compressions médullaires par hémangiomes vertébraux. A propos de neuf observations personelles. J Med Maroc IV: 271-311

Baker ND, Greenspan A, Neuwirth M (1986) Symptomatic vertebral angiomas: a report of four cases. Skeletal Radiol 15 :458-463

Carpentier EB, Strawn LM (1963) Hémangiomatose du cubitus et des muscles fléchisseurs de l'avant-bras avec rétraction secondaire en flexion du poignet et de la main. J Bone Joint Surg 45A: 1472-1478

Cone RO, Hudkins P, Nguyen V, Merriwether WA (1983) Histiocytoid hemangioma of bone. A benign lesion which may mimic angiosarcoma. Report of a case and review of literature. Skeletal Radiol 10: 165-169

D'Eshougues JR, Ferrand J, Smadja A, Bensaid J (1961) Hémangiome capillaire de l'apophyse coracoïde. Presse Med (Paris) 69: 2264-2265

De Smet AA, Inscore D, Neff JR (1989) Histiocytoid hemangioma of the distal end of the right femur (case report). Skeletal Radiol 18: 60-65

Desproges-Gotteron, Dunoyer J, Loubet R, Rousseau J, Claude M, Leroy V (1972) A propos d'un cas d'angiomatose diffuse et extensive du squelette. Rev Rhum (Paris) 39: 306-311

Enzinger FM, Weiss S (1988) Soft tissue tumors. CV Mosby, pp. 491-508

Jacobs JE, Kimmelstiel P (1953) Cystic angiomatosis of the skeletal system. J Bone Joint Surg 35A: 409-420

Lateur L, Simoens CJ, Gryspeerdt S, Samson I, Mertens V, Van Damme B (1996) Skeletal cystic angiomatosis. Skeletal Radiol 25: 92-95

Levey DS, MacCormack LM, Sartoris DJ, Haghighi P, Resnick D, Thorne R (1996) Cystic angiomatosis: case report and review of the literature. Skeletal Radiol 25: 287-293

Moseley JE, Starubin MD (1964) Cystic angiomatosis of bone: manifestation of a hamartomatous disease entity. Am J Roentgen 94: 1114-1120

Ose D, Vollmer R, Shelburne J, McComb R, Harrelson J (1983) Histiocytoid hemangioma of the skin and scapula. A case report with electron microscopy and immunohistochemistry. Cancer 51: 1656-1662

Pope TL, Fecher RE, Keats TE (1986) Hemangiome of the nasal bone. Skeletal Radiol 15: 327-329

Reid AB, Reid IL, Johnson G, Hamonic M, Major P (1989) Familial diffuse cystic angiomatosis of bone. Clin Onhop 238: 211-218

Rosai J, Gold J, Landy R (1979) The histiocytoid hemangiomas. A unifying concept embracing several previously described entities of skin, soft tissue, large vessels, bone and hean. Hum Pathol 10: 707-730

Wallis LA, Ash T, Maisel BW (1964) Diffuse skeletal hemangiomatosis. Report of two cases and review of literature. Am J Med 37: 545-563

Weible ER, Palade GE (1964) New cytoplasmic components in arterial endothelia. J Cell Biol 23: 101-112

Zenny JC, Leclère J, Boccon-Gibod L, Fauré C (1981) L'angiomatose kystique diffuse des os ou ectasies capillaires intra-osseuses. A propos d'un cas suivi sur cinq ans. J Radiol 62: 43-46

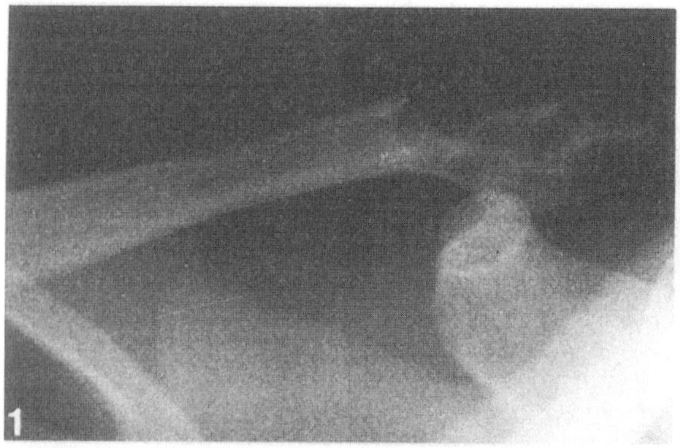

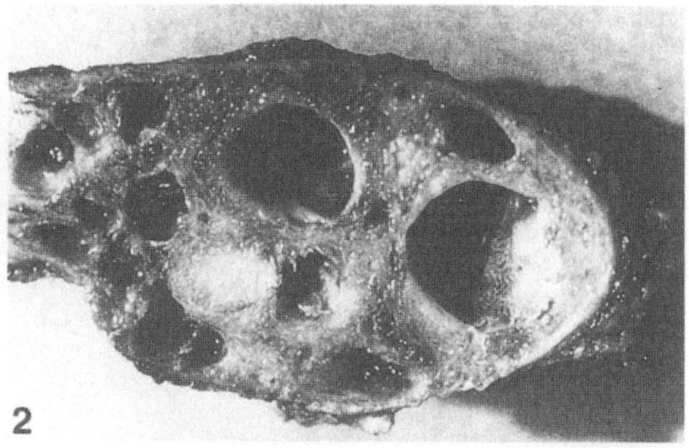

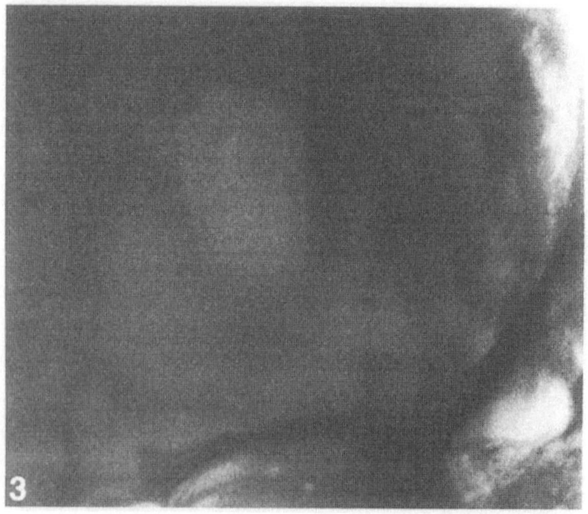

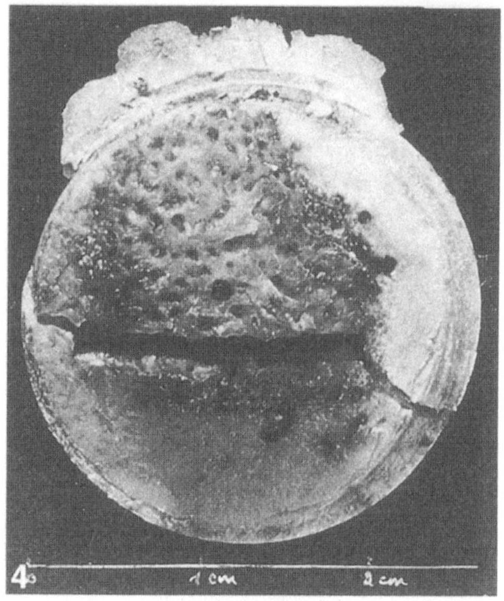

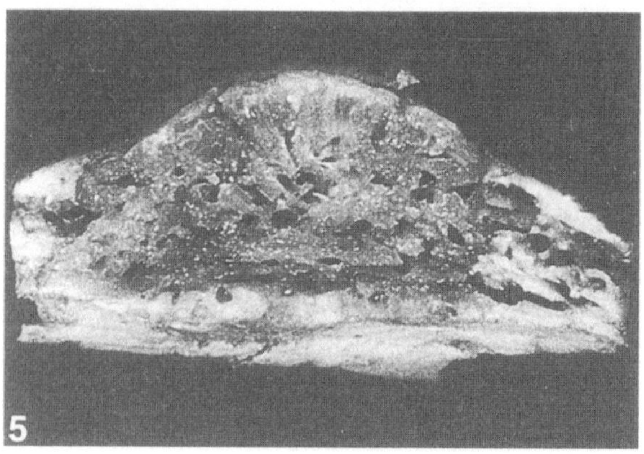

Figs. 1, 2. Angioma of clavicle of polycystic appearance: in the macroscopic section the fine-walled vessels form large cavities lined with endothelium

Figs. 3-5. Angioma of frontal bone, developing one year after injury. The osteoangioma made a firm tender prominence and gave rise to frontal headache

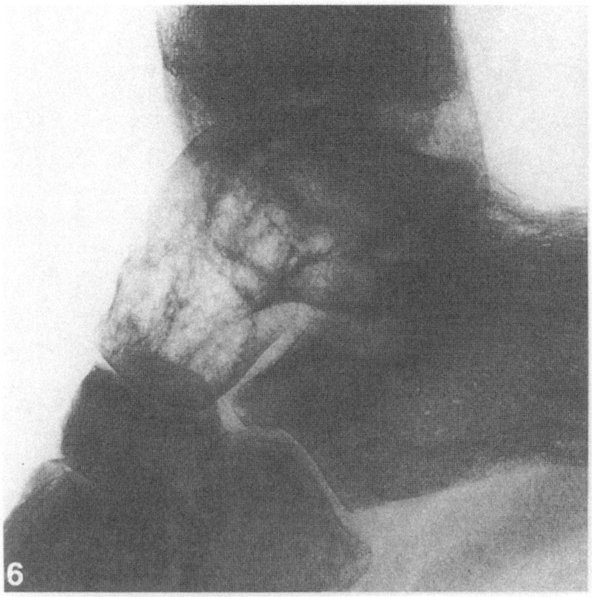

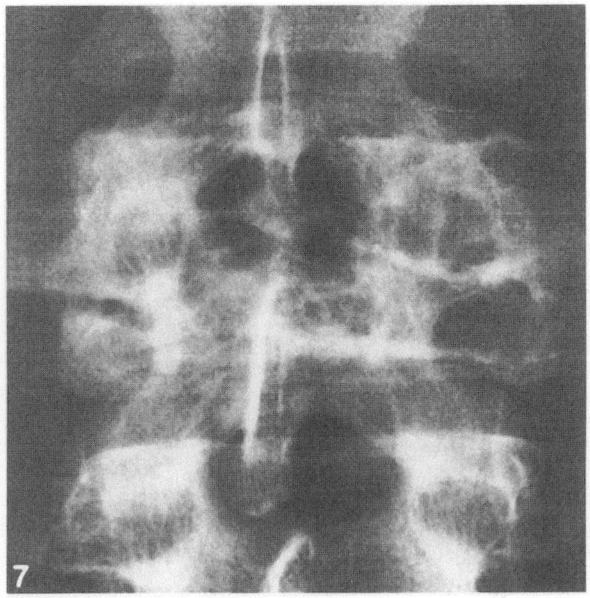

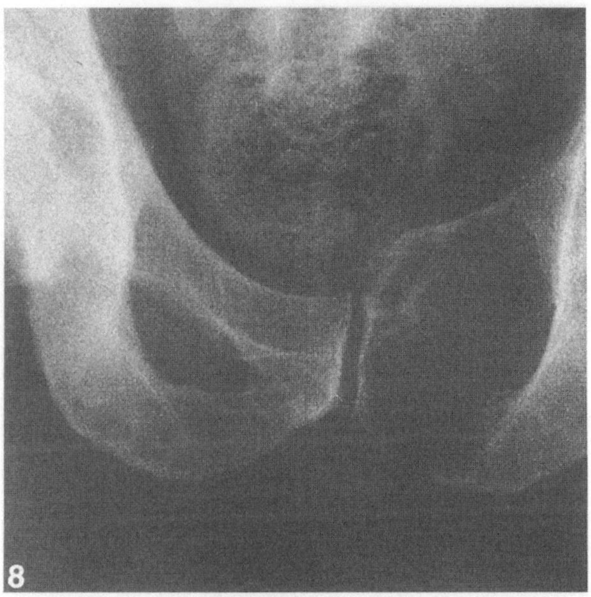

Fig. 6. This angioma of the talus is one of the lesions of widespread angiomatosis

Fig. 7. This man of 22 suffered from a vertebral angioma of L3. After an initial biopsy the angioma was irradiated and then treated surgically a year later

Fig. 8. The slow and painless course of this angioma did not lead to consultation until it had destroyed the greater part of the ischio- and ilio-pubic rami

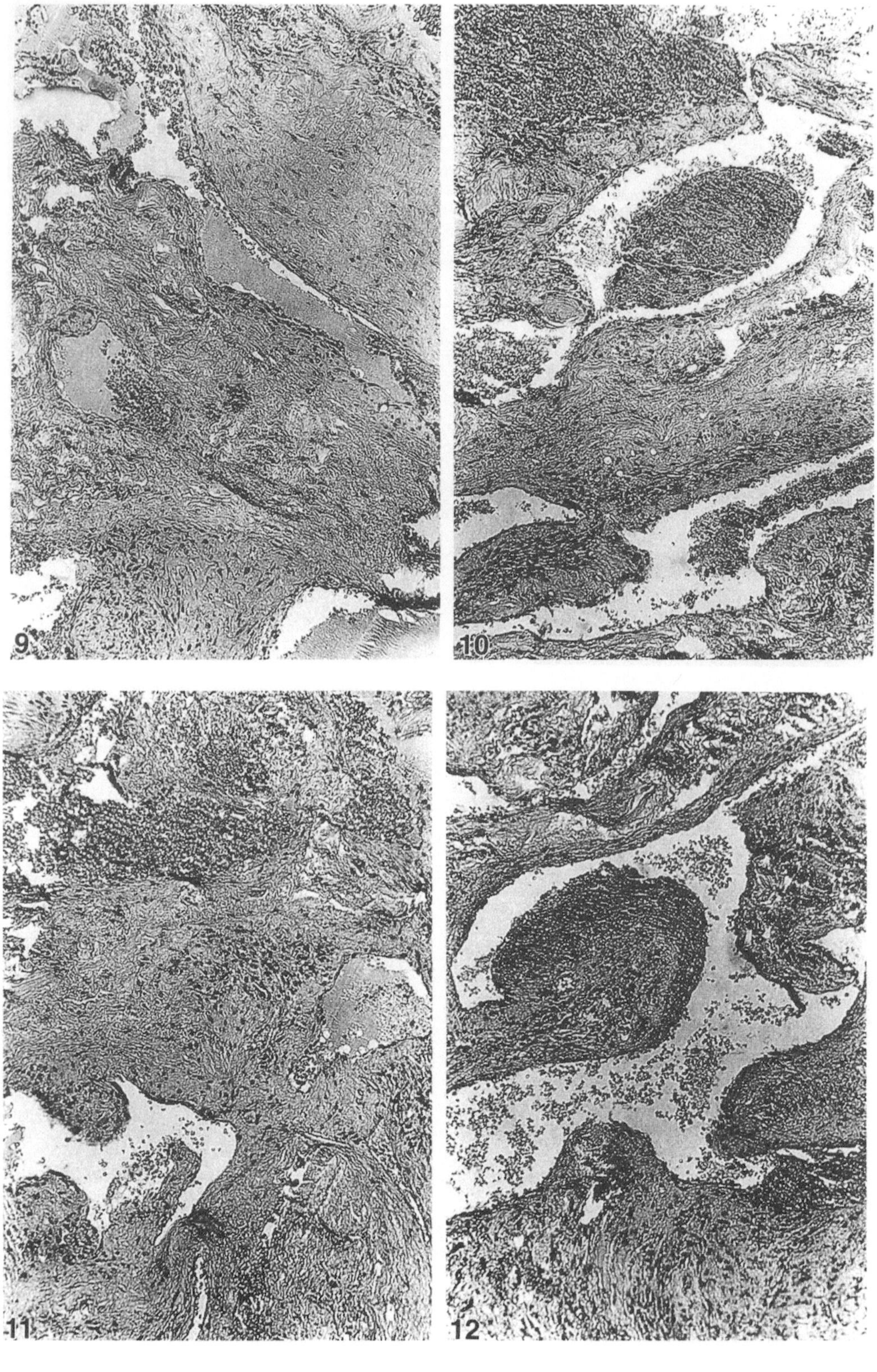

Figs. 9-12. Vertebral haemangioma: vessels with wide lumen developing in dense fibrous connective tissue. They are lined by an endothelium clearly visible in figs. 10 and 11. In fig. 12 a parietal fibrous fold is covered by a fibrinous deposit, the possible start of a thrombosis

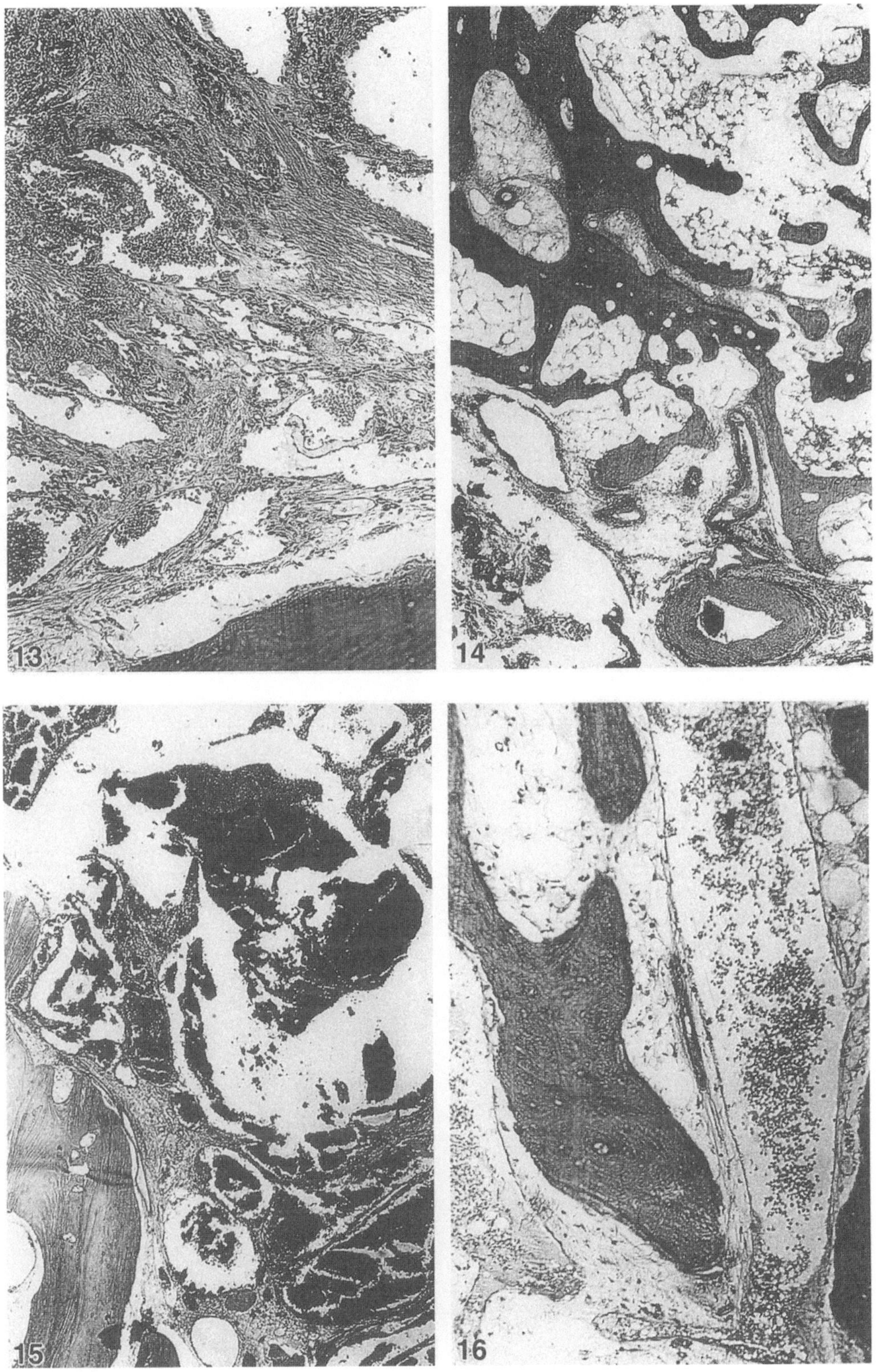

Figs. 13-16. Haemangiomatosis. The vessels, mostly fine-walled, develop in a fibro-adipose marrow. More rarely, some thick-walled vessels (**14**, lower part) probably represent a pedicle. Vast lacunae filled with erythrocytes (**15**). No endothelial proliferation was found in sections of the biopsies made at various sites of this angiomatosis

26. Lymphangioma

Bone is normally devoid of lymphatic vessels and yet certain types of bony lesions seem to be related to lymphatic proliferations. These lesions range from a small solitary cavity, clinically silent, to a generalised and fatal lymphangiomatosis. These same lymphatics are also held responsible for the so-called "idiopathic" osteolyses, either massive or localised to the extremities.

These conflicts between lymphatic vessels and bone are not always elucidated by biopsy. It is essential to identify an angioma and perhaps even a lymphangioma, but this does not go far to clarify the mechanism of the bone resorption and the prognosis of the disorder. In the majority of cases only a synthesis of the pathological, clinical and radiological concepts can embrace the developmental possibilities by classifying the disorder more precisely within one of the existing schemas.

Review of the principal syndromes

Diffuse lymphangiomatosis

Case history

A boy of 13 was brought to the rheumatology department for pain in the right forearm. In the radiographs made at this first attendance there were confluent cavitary lesions of the lower third of the radius. There was also a suspect image in the left humerus. At operation the bone was friable, the cortex of the radius seemed thinned and the surgical opening was immediately invaded by a bloody effusion. In the sections the architecture was relatively well preserved; the cortex, of irregular thickness, covered spongy bone whose fine parallel strands bounded cavities occupied by vessels. These vessels had fine walls, barely separated from strands of porotic bone by some collagen fibers. Here and there some flattened cells were scattered on the endothelium. Erythrocytes filled the specimen due to the operative trauma. In sum, in this porotic bone there was an angioma, either a haemangioma of capillary type or a lymphangioma. The lesion rapidly became generalised, causing weakness and spontaneous fractures; the child became bedridden and died about four months after the first manifestations. Nothing in the small sample from the radius could have allowed the prediction of such a course (figs. 1-9).

General considerations

Diffuse lymphangiomatosis is usually discovered in adolescence, though actually the bony modifications develop in childhood including unequal limb length and joint deformities. There is often cutaneous hyperpigmentation and one of the zones of election for skin lesions is the scrotum. When the diagnosis of lymphangiomatosis is suggested in a small boy, biopsy of the scrotum may show the characteristic appearances of lymphangioma. In these grave cases with diffuse bone lesions, spontaneous or repeated fracture may be the presenting feature.

Regional lymphangiomatosis

Case history

A young man of 16 was referred by his physician to the rheumatology center for cavitary lesions of the upper end of the femur, bony anomalies associated with thickening of the adjacent soft tissues and a particular appearance of the skin of the femoral triangle. The skin discharged a clear, somewhat syrupy fluid through minute slightly prominent orifices. The radiographs showed images in the acetabular region identical to the femoral lesions.

In the sections of the skin biopsy, the dermis and hypodermis were transformed into a quite dense fibrous tissue in which the lymphatics were totally collapsed; not only to narrow slit, but with actual adhesion of the thin endothelial walls which must be identified as evidence of this angiomatosis. In such circumstances the immunohistological reactions are very important, if positive. Matters might have stayed as they were, but generalisation of the lesions could not be formally excluded and the histology did not offer any prognostic guidance.

General considerations

Regional lymphangiomatosis affects one or more bones and the adjacent soft tissues. When skin involvement is demonstrated by the oozing of clear free-flowing fluid, the diagnosis of the underlying bony lesion is obvious, but histological examination is unable to specify whether this is the first stage of a generalised lymphomatosis or not.

Some observations are difficult to categorise with certainty (cf Chapter 25). In children and adolescents the bony lesions are sometimes associated with chylous ascites, with or without pleural effusions. The bone biopsy reveals vascular ectasia with spaces usually filled by a haemorrhagic effusion. Given the context, it seems logical to classify the disorder among the lymphangiomatoses rather than to envisage a haemolymphangiomatosis. Fessard et al (1974) reported two cases and collected 17 more from the literature. Formally - but without contrasting them - the authors distinguish cases where the bony lesions are diffuse and multiple (mean age 6 years) and those where the bony involvement is localised but evolves towards massive osteolysis (mean age 16 years).

Cystic lymphangioma

Case history

"Cavity in lower third of tibia in a man of 39, discovered because of vague pain. The rest of the skeleton is normal. Biopsy of the wall of the cavity, which contained only a few drops of clear fluid which was immediately stained by minor parietal haemorrhage. Radiograph accompanies specimen".

In the standard radiograph, the cavity was clearly defined. In the sections, the bony wall of the cavity was covered by a flat thin endothelium, completely resembling that of a lymphatic vessel, whose nature was confirmed by the immunohistological reactions. In this case, what other diagnosis could be made than that of a solitary cystic lymphatic structure?

Jumbelic et al (1984) reported a case of polycystic lymphangioma of the humerus developing in a girl aged 2 years and 11 months. Some of the cystic cavities, devoid of erythrocytes, contained small endothelial tufts, contrasting with the flat endothelium covering the cavities as a whole.

General considerations

The solitary cystic form described by the German authors seems very rare and its diagnosis quite difficult. This diagnosis is based on the identification of a lymphatic endothelium lining the wall of an apparently ordinary cyst [Hayes & Brody 1961, Moseley & Starubin 1964]. The necessary decalcification does not facilitate immunohistological reactions. I have ventured to make this diagnosis three or four times, without knowing whether this is too many or too few.

Massive osteolysis, Gorham's syndrome, phantom bone, idiopathic osteolysis

Case history

A woman was referred to the Institut Curie for osteolysis of the outer third of the clavicle and part of the acromion. Then there was progressive disappearance of part of the rib-cage and proximal part of the humerus.

At biopsy, the bony tissue was replaced by dense fibrosis. Endothelial adhesion of the walls of collapsed lymphatics was seen between the collagen bundles. Another biopsy was taken from a bony region adjacent to the osteolysis. Apart from the presence of wide vessels without endothelial proliferation and without peripheral muscle, rare osteoclasts were seen and in places there was a discrete osteoid osteoblastic layering.

General considerations

Gorham's syndrome (1954) is a rare and insidiously developing disorder evidenced by progressive absorption of contiguous bony structures which is rarely fatal. The thoracic forms are the most to be feared. Gorham's disease is also related to a lymphangiomatosis but the precipitating cause remains unknown. This massive osteolysis is seen in children and adults, and is twice as common in females. The maxillofacial region is particularly affected but the pelvic girdle and femur, shoulder-girdle and humerus, ribs and adjacent vertebrae may all be involved [Tuker 1967, de Sèze et al 1968, Imbert & Picaut 1974, Damron et al 1993, Takeda 1987].

The disorder passes through an initial stage of active bone destruction which is slightly painful. This gives way to a quiescent phase in which the bony tissue is replaced by fibrous tissue traversed by lymphatic vessels. Laboratory tests do little to clarify the situation. The hydroxyproline-creatinine ratio, related to bone destruction, may have some value but modern imaging is more instructive.

Spontaneous arrest of the course of the disease is possible, hence the difficulties in assessing the possible value of radiotherapy. The insertion of bone grafts is usually followed by their dissolution.

The precipitating cause remains unknown. Infection and injury have been suggested, even the minimal trauma which may suggest the syndrome of osteoporosis described by Destot-Sudeck-Leriche, but which involves the blood-vessels [Lagier & Van Linthoudt 1978, Arlet et al 1978].

Acro-osteolysis

Numerous cases have been reported. It seems that the lesions are comparable to those observed in massive osteolysis. Among these osteolyses, various syndromes have been defined: Hajdu-Cheney, carpo-tarsal osteolysis, and idiopathic acro-osteolysis of all three phalanges. These syndromes are accompanied by anomalies of maxillofacial structure. Another recently described syndrome develops after an infective episode and combines the bony lesions with major skin lesions (see also Maroteaux: Les maladies osseuses de l'enfant, p. 385).

References

Arlet J, Duroux R, Theallier JP, Mazières B, Bouteiller G (1978) Histopathologie des lésions osseuses dans 9 cas d'algodystrophie de la hanche. Rev Rhum (Paris) 45: 691-698

Beals RK, Bird CB (1975) Carpal and tarsal osteolysis. A case report and review of the literature. J Bone Joint Surg 57A: 681-686

Behram P, Horvath K, Lack EE (1987) Seventeen year follow-up and autopsy findings in a case of massive osteolysis. Skeletal Radiol 16: 291-297

Bickel WH, Broders AC (1947) Primary lymphangioma of the ilium. Report of a case. J Bone Joint Surg 29: 517-522

Bullough PG, Goodfellow JW (1976) Solitary lymphangioma of bone. J Bone Joint Surg 54A: 418-419

Damron TA, Brodke DS, Heiner JP, Swan JS, De Souky S (1993) Gorham's disease (Gorham-Stout syndrome) of scapula. Case report. Skeletal Radiol 22: 464-467

Fessard CI, Boulesteix C, Boudil Ch, Grynblat N, Fondimare A, Dumas R, Jean R, Daily R (1974) Ascite chyleuse, chylothorax et ectasies capillaires intra-osseuses. A propos de deux observations. Arch Fr Pediatr 31: 489-506

Goldstein MR, Benchimol A, Cornell W, Long DR (1969) Chylopericardium with multiple lymphangioma of bone. New Engl J Med 19: 1034-1037

Gorham LW, Stout AP (1955) Massive osteolysis (acute spontaneous of bone, phantom bone, disappearing bone). Its relation to hemangiomatosis. J Bone Joint Surg 37A: 985-1004

Gorham LW, Wright AW, Shultz HH, Mxon FC (1954) Disappearing bones: a rare form of massive osteolysis. Report of two cases, one with autopsy findings. Am J Med 17: 674-682

Hayes JT, Brody GL (1961) Cystic lymphangiectasis of bone. A case report. J Bone Joint Surg 43A: 107-117

Heffeez L, Doku HC, Carter BL, Feeney JE (1983) Perspectives on massive osteolysis: report of a case and review of the literature. Oral Med Oral Pathol 55: 331-343

Imbert JC, Picaut C (1974) Ostéolyse massive idiopathique ou maladie de Jackson-Gorham. A propos d'une nouvelle observation. Rev Chir Orthop 60: 73-80

Jackson JBS (1838) A singular case of absorption of bone (a boneless arm). Boston Med Surg J 18: 368-369

Joseph R, Nezelof CH, Guéraud l, Job JC (1959) Acro-ostéolyse idiopathique familiale. Ann Pediatr 35: 622-629

Jumbelic M, Feverstein IM, Dorfman HD (1984) Solitary intraosseous lymphangioma. J Bone Joint Surg 66A: 1479-1481

Lagier R, Rutishauser E (1965) Osteoarticular changes in a case of essential osteolysis an anatomical and radiological study. J Bone Joint Surg 47B: 339-353

Lagier R, Van Linthoudt D (1978) Dystrophie de Sudeck de l'arrière-pied. Confrontation anatomo-radiologique. Ann Radiol 21: 539-544

Lamy M, Maroteaux P (1961) Acro-ostéolyse dominante. Arch Pediatr 18: 693-702

Maraoteaux P (1985) Les maladies osseuses de l'enfant. 3ème edn. Flammarion, p. 385

Mialaret J (1953) Résorption spontanée de la paroi thoracique. Mem Acad Chir (Paris) 79: 212-213

Moseley JE, Starubin MD (1964) Cystic angiomatosis of bone: manifestation of a hamanomatous disease entity. Am J Roentgenol 91: 1114-1120

Petit P, Fryns JP (1986) Distal osteolysis, short stature, mental retardation, and characteristic facial appearance: delineation of an autosomal recessive subtype of essential osteolysis. Am J Med Genet 25: 537-541

Rosenquist CJ, Wolfe DC (1968) Lymphangioma of bone. J Bone Joint Surg 50A: 158-162

Sacrez R, Klein F, Levy JM (1969) Lymphangiectasies osseuses disséminées. Arch Fr Pediatr 26: 537-546

Santos (dos) Carneiro R, Steglich V (1987) Disappearing bone disease in the hand. J Hand Surg 12A: 629-634

Sèze (de) S, Debeyre J, Schweisguth O, Mazabraud A, Langumier Solnica J, Bussière JL (1968) A propos de deux cas de lymphangiome osseux. J Belge Rhumatol Med Physique 23: 281-288

Sèze (de) S, Hubault A (1956) Ostéolyse essentielle scapulothoraco-brachiale. Rev Rhum (Paris) 23: 517-522

Takeda Y, Kuroda M, Suzuki A, Fujioka F, Takayama K (1987) Massive osteolysis of the mandibule. Acta Pathol Jpn 37: 677-684

Tucker AS (1964) Lymphangiectasis benign and malignant. Am J Roentgenol 91: 1104-1113

Tucker SM (1967) Bilateral chylothorax with multiple osteolytic lesions? Generalized abnormality of lymphatic system. Proc R Soc Med (pediatrics) 60: 17-20

Van Den Houten BR, Kate T, Gerding JC (1985) The Hajdu-Cheney syndrome. A review of the literature and report of three cases. Int J Oral Surg 14: 113-125

White AA (1971) Disappearing bone disease with arthropathy and severe scarring of the skin. A report of four cases seen in South Vietnam. J Bone Joint Surg 53B: 303-309

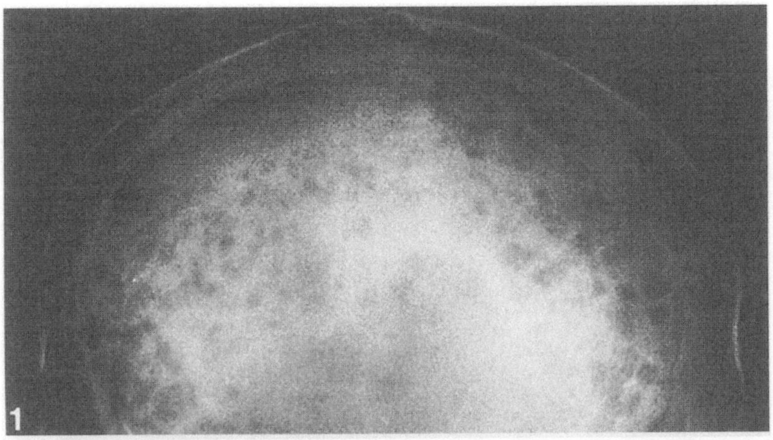

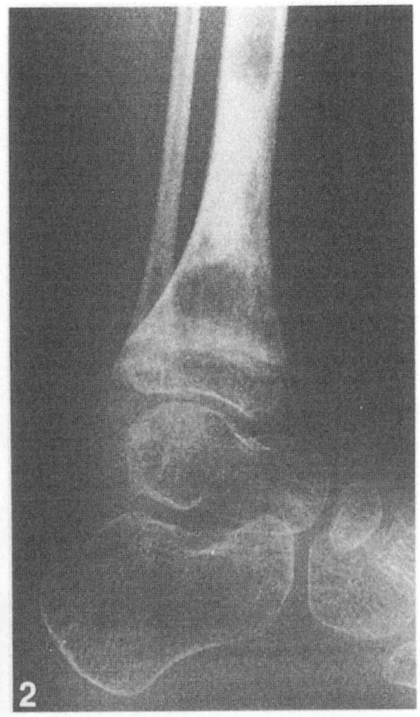

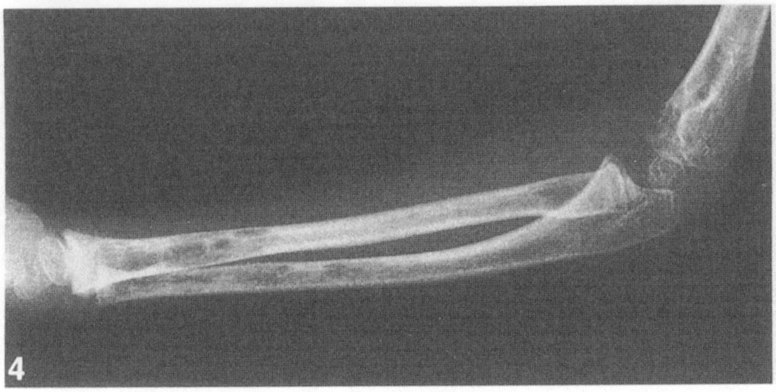

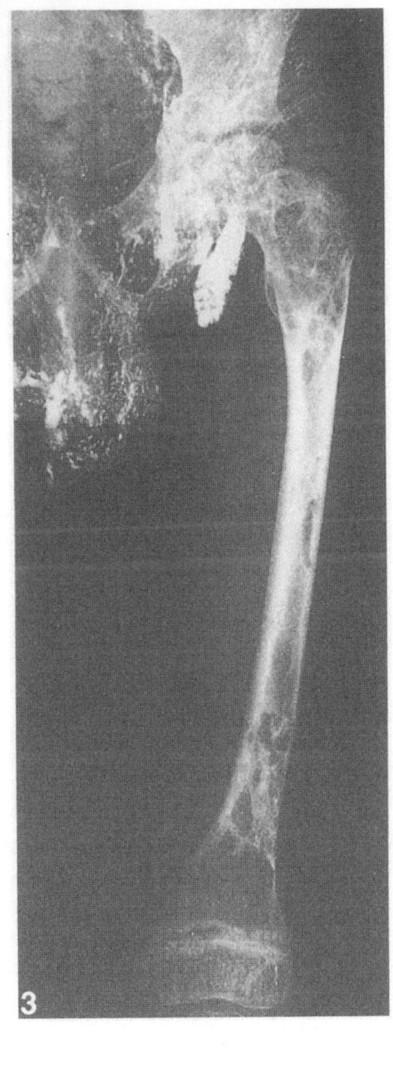

Figs. 1-4. These illustrations are from the case history of the boy of 13 referred to in this chapter. The radiographs show the dissemination of the lesions in the skull, pelvis and long bones. The lymphangiogram (3) shows the anomalies of the deep lymphatic system and the extension to the soft tissues and skin

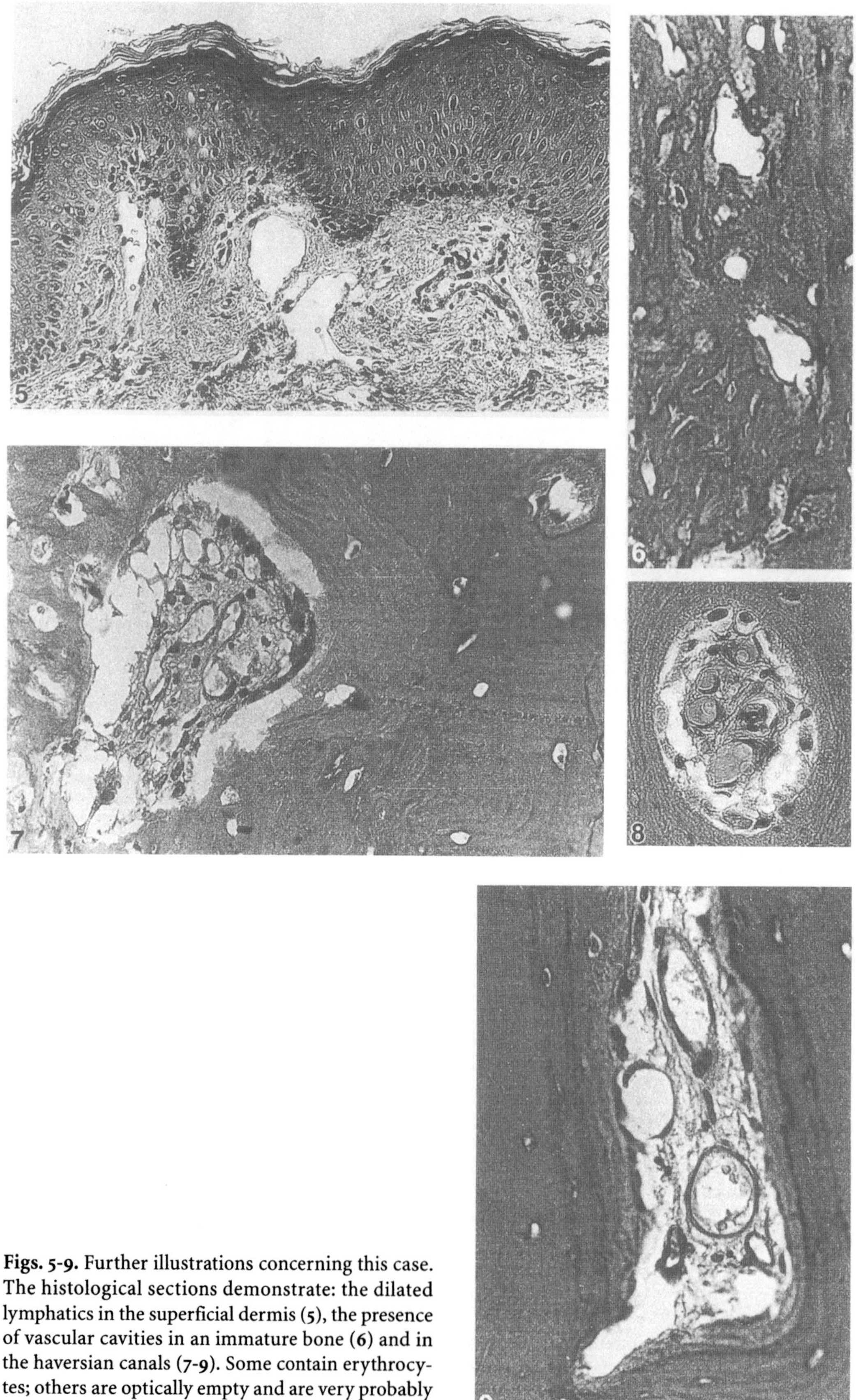

Figs. 5-9. Further illustrations concerning this case. The histological sections demonstrate: the dilated lymphatics in the superficial dermis (5), the presence of vascular cavities in an immature bone (6) and in the haversian canals (7-9). Some contain erythrocytes; others are optically empty and are very probably lymphatics

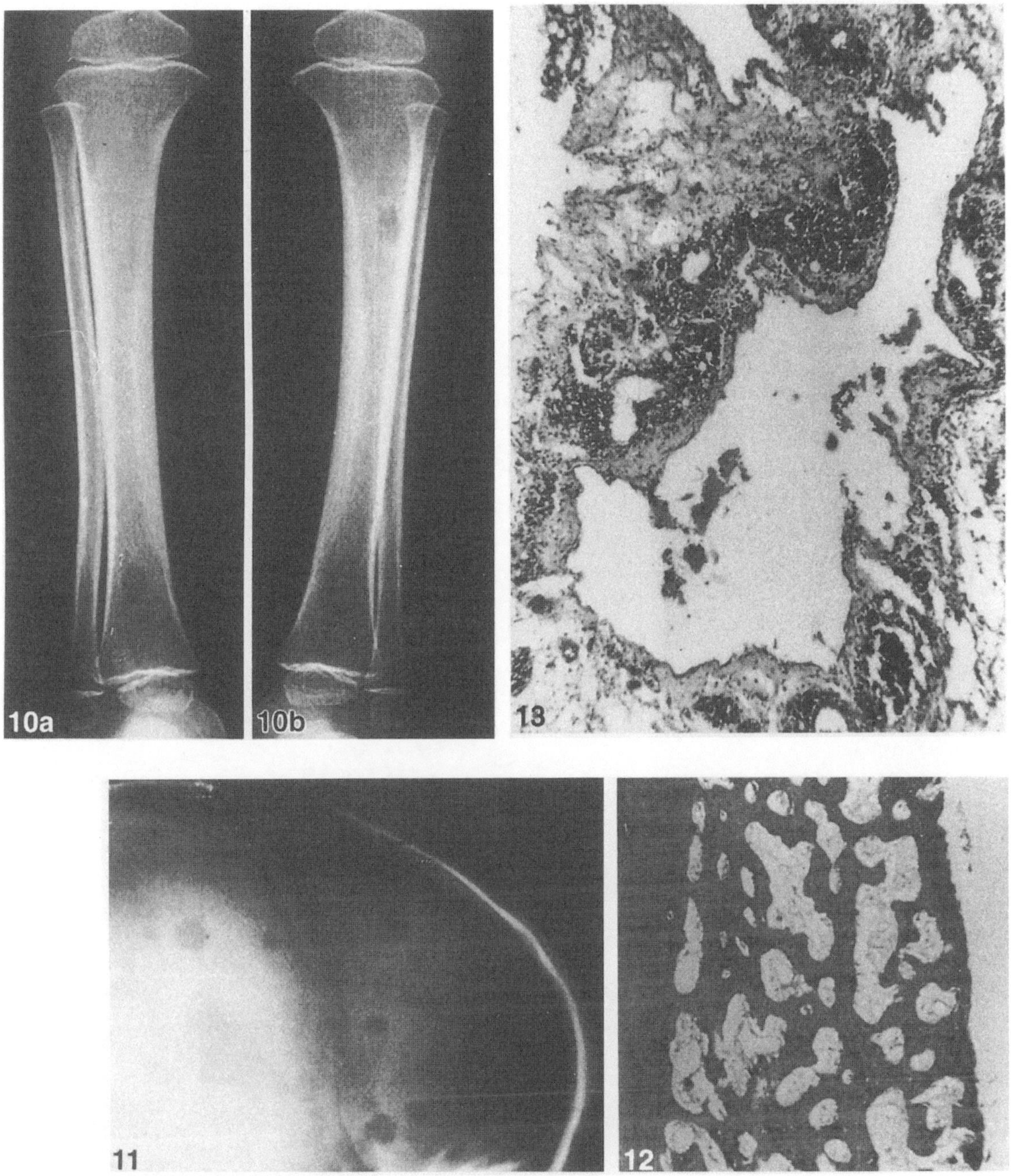

Figs. 10-13. Another case of lymphangiomatosis in a girl of 2. Small rounded islands of osteolysis, bounded by a discrete osteosclerosis, are disseminated throughout the skeleton (10, 11). In a partially destroyed rib periosteal, osteogenesis has occurred in which the intertrabecular spaces are filled by a network of numerous large vessels devoid of erythrocytes and lined by a simple endothelium (12). Lymphangiomatous dilatations in the soft tissues in the vicinity of the bony lesion (13)

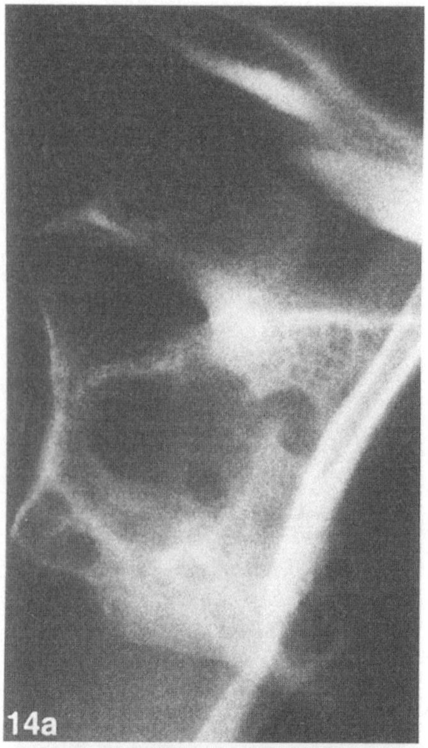

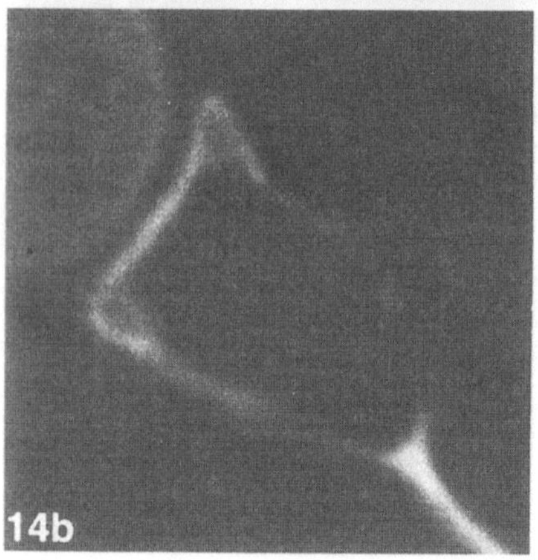

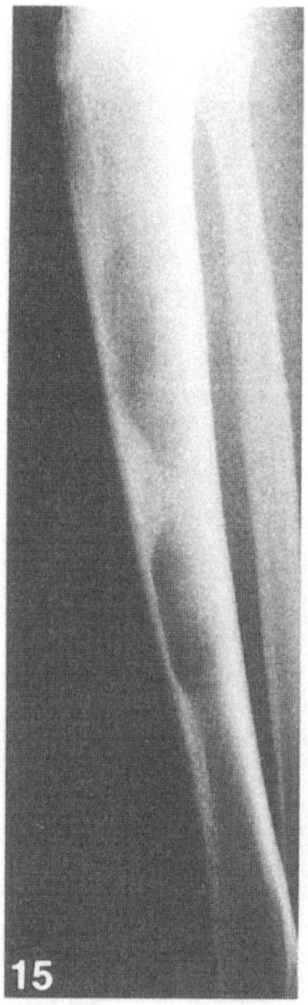

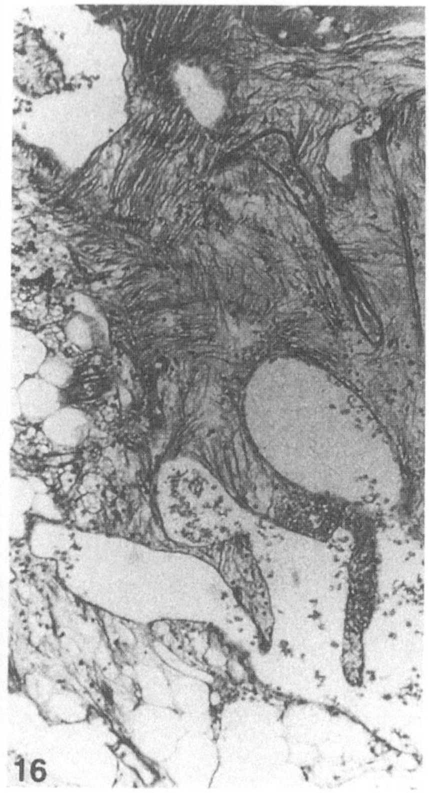

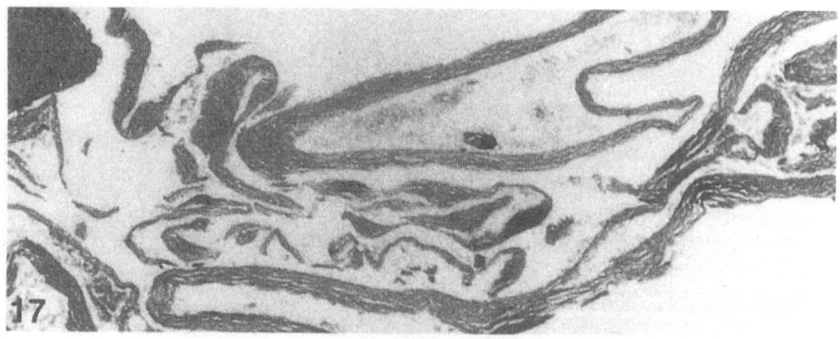

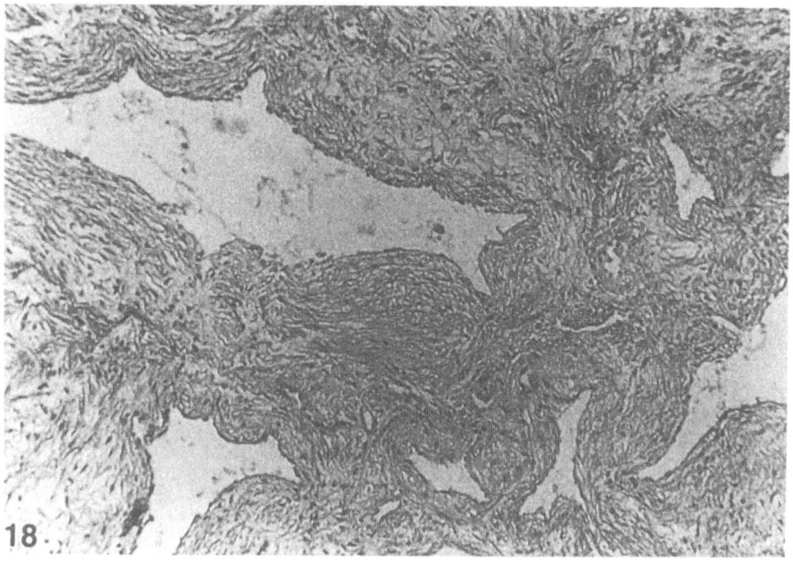

Fig. 14. a Cystic lesion of multilocular appearance in the neck of the scapula in a standard film. **b** The CT sections suggest that this is a solitary cavity with persistence of parietal bony ridges

Fig. 15. Cystic appearance in tibial shaft in an adolescent boy in which the histological sections were interpreted as being those of a cystic lymphangioma

Figs. 16, 17. These isolated cystic formations are difficult to interpret. Their fine connective tissue walls are lined by an endothelium. Presence or absence of erythocytes is not a helpful finding, unlike when such lesions are accompanied by lymphangioma of the soft tissues

Fig. 18. The very different appearance of a typical lymphangioma developing in the upper end of the ulna of a woman of 40

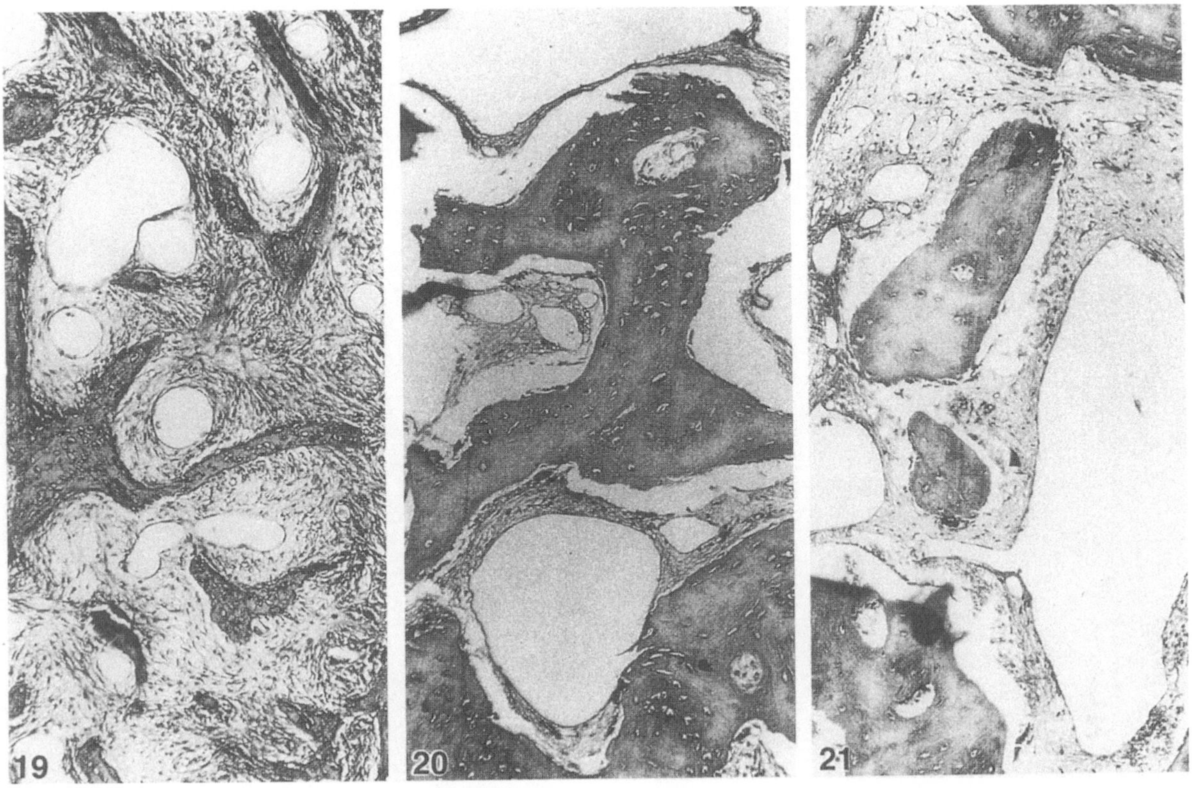

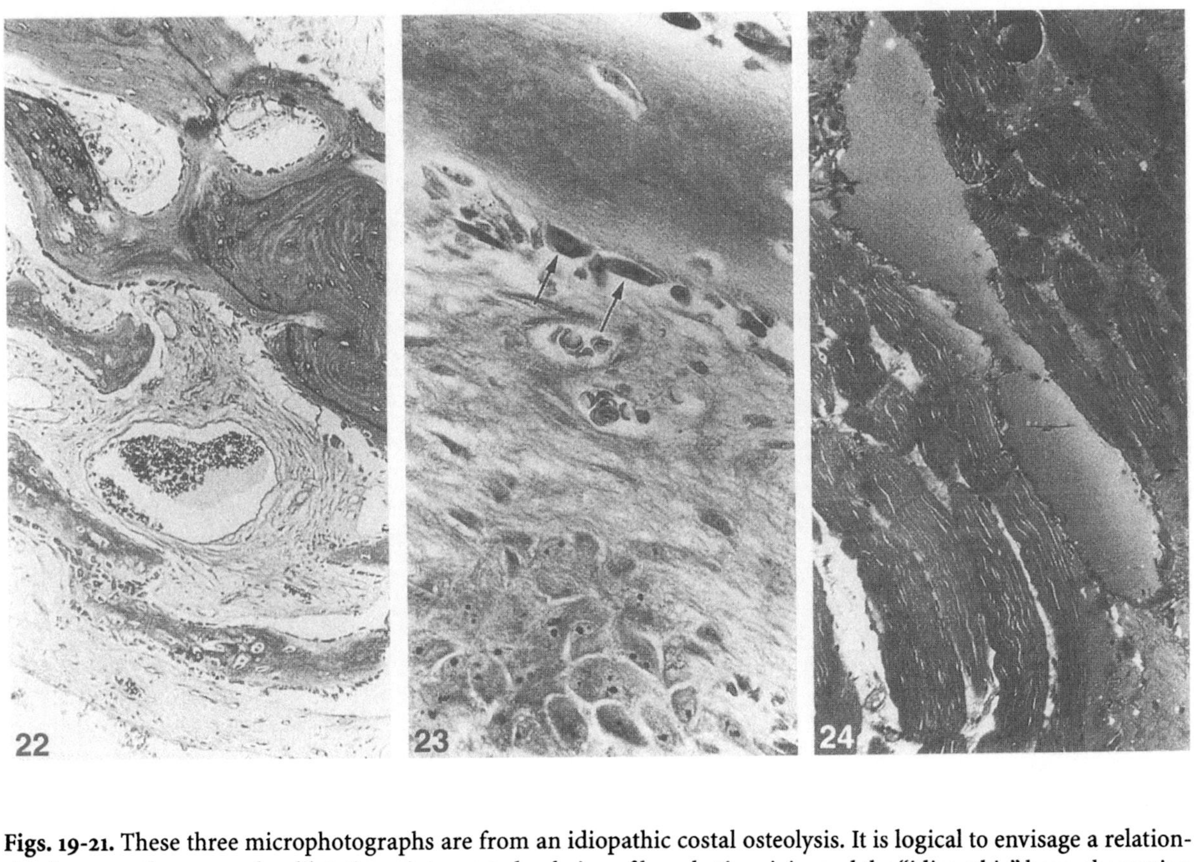

Figs. 19-21. These three microphotographs are from an idiopathic costal osteolysis. It is logical to envisage a relationship between these vascular dilatations, interpreted as being of lymphatic origin, and the "idiopathic" bony absorption

Figs. 22-24. Gorham's disease in a woman of 34 whose case history is given in this chapter. **22** Bulky osteoid apposition on strands of old bone, partly necrosed. **23** On this poorly calcified osteoid strand the function of the two cells adherent to its lower border (*arrows*) is not obvious. In this region of major osteolysis, the osteoclasts are few and localised to few zones, but mononuclear cells can behave like osteoclasts. At the lower part of the photograph is an island of very quiescent osteoblasts. **24** The lymphangiomatosis extends into the adjacent soft tissues: connective-adipose and muscular

27. Lipoma, liposarcoma

Despite the constant presence of adipocytes in major quantities in the bone marrow, intraosseous lipomas are rare; the first case was reported by Brault in 1901 in Cornil and Ranvier's textbook of histology.

Intraosseous and juxtacortical lipomas

Case histories

Case 1. A young woman of 23 attended for intermittent pain, not severe, in the lower end of the right lower limb. There was no remarkable previous history and the biochemical variables were normal. But in the standard radiograph there was a clear, finely bounded image occupying part of the metaphyseo-diaphyseal region of the tibia. Such an image suggested the diagnoses of non-ossifying fibroma, a cyst of unknown aetiology, or a large cortico-metaphyseal fibrous defect. The only certainty was that the development of this lesion had been insidious and slow to attain such a size with a minimum of clinical features.

Operative approach revealed a surprise by exposing a monomorphous lipomatous structure occupying the whole of the osteolytic zone, without any haematopoiesis; there were no cellular anomalies or angiomatous vascularisation. The only possible diagnosis was that of intraosseous lipoma, despite some small myxoid zones.

Case 2. A woman of 33 attended for a "tumour" developing in the middle of the thigh. The tumour was difficult to palpate since it was covered by muscle masses. In the radiograph there was a periosteal reaction of moderate extent but the image of a lipoma was barely visible.

At operation, a lipoma was removed which displaced the soft tissues and adhered to the periosteum by its calcified base of implantation. Here again, the various biochemical variables were normal and the previous history was unremarkable. Histological examination could only confirm the diagnosis of juxtacortical lipoma.

General considerations

Although rare, cases of intraosseous or juxtacortical lipoma have been reported affecting the tibia, radius, calcaneum, fibula, frontal bone, sacrum, jaws and ribs. They are seen mainly in the third to sixth decades.

Clinical features and course

The symptoms are vague: mild intermittent pain, increased by fatigue. In the case of juxtacortical lipomas, it is often the palpable tumour that attracts the patient's attention, unless compression of a vein or nerve produces signs of stasis or sharp pain [Bombart et al 1970]. Given surgical removal, the prognosis is entirely favourable. Sarcomatous transformation is certainly very rare [Milgram 1990].

Imaging

Imaging demonstrates a clear image, either intraosseous and finely bordered, possibly with some vaulting of the cortex, or an ovoid structure displacing the soft tissues (figs. 1-4) in which the periosteal base of implantation is more or less calcified or ossified [Bombart et al 1970, McLean et al 1985, Goldman et al 1993].

Pathological anatomy and histopathology

Macroscopically, this is a mass which is entirely adipose or contains zones of more mucoid consistency or is still traversed by some relics of the bony trabeculae (figs. 5, 6).

From the histological aspect, the lipocyte proliferation lacks noticeable anomalies. Sometimes there are some calcifications in amorphous material resembling that seen in bone infarcts [Lagier 1980, Gero & Kahn 1988, Jones et al 1984]; however, the expansive nature of the lipoma, which balloons the bone, differentiates it from infarction. No focus of haematopoiesis is found.

Three particular features should be mentioned the presence of myxoid areas (fig. 6), which do not justify the diagnosis of myxoma, the abundant vascularisation, as may be seen in lipomas of the soft tissues, consonant with the term of angiolipoma and a reactive osteosclerosis which may or may not go hand in hand with trabecular osteogenesis in the mass of fatty tissue.

Differential diagnosis

The histological diagnosis of lipoma is easy, though lipomyxomas have been reported; however, this term is acceptable only when as the myxoid component amounts to at least 80% of the sectional surface. An angiomatous component or association has been reported. The diagnosis may be too easy to make. I am not certain that a small clear zone in which MRI confirms the presence of adipose tissue should be included in the category of lipomas. It seems justified only if the lesion shows well-defined boundaries and/or balloons the bone in which it develops.

The diagnosis of the osteoporotic lesion of Destot-Sudeck-Leriche in its final stage has to be considered. The cause may pass unnoticed among so many possible factors. The bone is reduced to a fine cortex enclosing fatty tissue in which the spongy bone has virtually disappeared. Haematopoiesis is absent. At a less advanced stage, an abundant plasmostasis indicates the severity of the local circulatory disturbance. The bone retains its normal shape and the lesion is not expansive.

Lastly, one must ensure that the lipoma is solitary and that it does not form part of the syndrome of hyperlipoproteinemia type IV associated with multiple intraosseous lipomas and often complicated by fractures [Freiberg et al 1974].

The major differential diagnosis is from liposarcoma, but here the imaging shows an ill-defined tumour whose course is more rapid and painful, while the cytological anomalies should confirm the diagnosis. As for the diagnoses of fibroma or cyst, suggested in the standard radiographs, current (MRI) imaging should virtually exclude these even before pathological examination [Levin et al 1996].

Liposarcoma

General considerations

Primary intraosseous liposarcoma is a very rare tumour. It has no gender preference and is seen mainly between the 2nd and 5th decades. The lower end of the femur, the tibia, fibula and humerus are the sites most often reported.

Clinical features

The presenting feature is pain, usually moderate. Exceptionally, presentation is with fracture or by discovery of an entirely silent liposarcoma during a radiological examination.

Imaging

The radiological image is of an ill-defined clear zone of osteolysis with slight bulging due to periosteal apposition. In advanced cases there is a breach of the cortex and invasion of the soft tissues. In the tumours described as osteoliposarcoma or malignant mesenchymoma, osteogenesis is found together with the osteolytic image [Schajowicz et al 1966], but this may also indicate relics of incompletely destroyed bony trabeculae. Current imaging techniques allow identification of the lipomatous nature of the tumour.

Pathological anatomy and histopathology

At operation the tumour is firm, grayish-white and lobulated. It may contain small haemorrhagic zones, bony strands and patches of calcification.

At histological examination, though the cellular anomalies and polymorphism suggest a diagnosis of malignancy, the histological characteristic remains the presence of intracytoplasmic lipid droplets. As well as the lipoblasts, which are sometimes frankly monstrous, there are often zones of fusiform cells and myxoid appearances which may suggest a diagnosis of malignant fibrous histiocytoma. In fact, this polymorphism is not at all abnormal, bearing in mind the histological variants of liposarcoma and lipoma of the soft tissues [Enzinger & Harvey 1975].

The zones of marked calcification, sometimes in contact with newly-formed bony tissue of pagetoid appearance, may suggest the presence of a primary bone infarct, but there may be malignant transformation of a preexisting lipoma, as in the cases reported by Milgram (1981); in such conditions the appearances of benign lipoma and of liposarcoma coexist.

Differential diagnosis

From the histological viewpoint, a metastasis from a clear cell renal carcinoma is easily excluded. A very rare intraosseous lipoma may pose the same problems as those of atypical lipomas of the soft tissues and fusiform-cell lipomas.

Though one may make a diagnosis of liposarcoma, it remains to be proved that it is primarily of intraosseous origin; and this is impossible from a single biopsy. Such a diagnosis of localisation must necessarily be based on the imaging, the macroscopic findings and even more on the clinical report. McLean et al (1985) reported a case of liposarcoma in a man of 47 in which the diagnosis of malignancy was made only on the appearance of bony metastases from a tumour of the soft tissues, diagnosed as a benign lipoma on two occasions.

However, the possibility of fusiform-cell or pleomorphic lipomas [Azzopardi et al 1983] at a bony site risks making a wrong diagnosis of malignancy.

The existence of liposarcoma is denied by some authors; others [Schajowicz et al 1966, Ross et al 1968, Cremer et al 1981] have described a "malignant mesenchymoma", characterised by a liposarcomatous predominance associated with an osteosarcomatous component.

References

Intraosseous and juxtacortical lipomas

Azzopardi JG, Ioceo J, Salm R (1983) Pleomorphic lipoma: a tumor simulating liposarcoma. Histopathology 7: 511-523

Barcelo M, Pathria MN, Abdul-Karim FW (1992) Intraosseous lipoma. A clinicopathologic study of four cases. Arch Pathol Lab Med 116: 947-950

Bombart M, Thomine JM, Mazabraud A, Liorzou G (1970) Lipome para-osseux. Rev Chir Orthop 56: 563-570

Brault A (1901) Des tumeurs. In: Cornil V, Ranvier L. Manuel d'histologie pathologique. 3ème edn, vol 1. Baillière et Cie Paris, pp. 393-395

Downey EF, Brower AC, Holt RB (1983) Cortical ossifying lipoma of femur. Skeletal Radiol 10: 189191

Enzinger FM, Harvey DA (1975) Spindle cell lipoma. Cancer 36: 1852-1859

Freiberg RA, Air GW, Glueck CJ, Ishikawa T, Abrams NR (1974) Multiple intraosseous lipomas with type-lV hyperlipoproteinemia. A case report. J Bone Joint Surg 56A: 1729-1732

Gero MJ, Kahn LB (1988) Intraosseous lipoma of the distal end of the fibula with focal infarction. Skeletal Radiol 17: 443-446

Goldman AB, Dicarlo EF, Marcove RC (1993) Coincidental parosteal lipoma with osseous excrescence and intramuscular lipoma. Skeletal Radiol 22: 138-145

Hall FM, Cohen RB, Grumbach K (1986) Intraosseous lipoma (angiolipoma) of right third rib. Skeletal Radiol 15: 401-403

Hart JAL (1973) Intraosseous lipoma. J Bone Joint Surg 55B: 624-631

Jones JG, Habemmann ET, Dorfman HD (1981) Parosteal ossifying lipoma of femur. Skeletal Radiol 18: 537-540

Lagier R (1980) Lipoma of the calcaneus with bone infarct. Skeletal Radiol 5: 267-269

Lagier R (1985) Fibular lipema with areas of bone infarct calcification. Eur J Radiol 5: 226-227

Levin MF, Vellet AD, Munk PL, McLean CA (1996) Intraosseous lipoma of the distal femur: MRI appearance. Skeletal Radiol 25: 82-84

Longuet YJ, Saks P (1947) Lipome profond de l'avant bras. Mem Acad Chir (Paris) 73: 199-200

McLean RG, Caligeros D, Nayanar V, Murray PC (1985) Metastatic liposarcoma. Case report. Skeletal Radiol 13: 84-88

Milgraum JW (1981) Intraosseous lipomas with reactive ossification in the proximal femur. Report of eight cases. Skeletal Radiol 7: 1-13

Moon N, Marmor L (1964) Parosteal lipoma. J Bone Joint Surg 46A: 608-614

Moulonguet P (1946) Lipomes profonds des membres. Lipomes périostés. Mem Acad Chir 72: 301-303

Moulonguet P, Bachy F, Dobkevith S (1939) Lipomes périostés. Rev Chir 58: 1-9

Trillat A, Mounier-Kuhn A, Dejour J (1965) Lipome paraosseux de l'extrémité supérieure du radius. Lyon Chir 61: 92-94

Zorn DT, Cordray DR, Randels PH (1971) Intraosseous lipoma of bone involving the sacrum. J Bone Joint Surg 53A: 1201-1204

Liposarcoma

Bolen JW, Thorning D (1984) Liposarcomas. A histogenic approach to the classification of adipose tissue neoplasms. Am J Surg Pathol 8: 3-17

Catto M, Stevens J (1963) Liposarcoma of bone. J Pathol Bacteriol 86: 248-253

Coste F, Lapresle J, Basset F (1959) Un cas de liposarcome à point de départ vraisemblablement osseux et ayant intéressé secondairement la moelle épinière. Presse Med 67: 834-837

Cremer H, Koischwitz D, Tismer R (1981) Primary osteoliposarcoma of bone. J Cancer Res Clin Oncol 101: 203-211

Enzinger FM, Harvey DA (1975) Spindle cell lipoma. Cancer 36: 1852-1859

Kenan S, Klein, Lewis M (1989) Juxtacortical liposarcoma. A case report and review of the literature. Clin Orthop 243: 225-229

Mandard JC, Mandard AM, Le Gal Y (1973) Les liposarcomes primitifs de l'os. A propos de 5 cas. Revue de la littérature. Ann Anat Pathol 18: 329-346

Milgram JW (1990) Malignant transformation in bone lipomas. Skeletal Radiol 19: 347-352

Milosevic D (1971) Liposarcome du péroné. Contribution à la discussion sur l'origine des liposarcomes osseux. Rev Chir Orthop. 57: 225-228

Retz LD (1961) Primary liposarcoma of bone. Report of a case and review of the literature. J Bone Joint Surg 43A: 123-129

Ross CF, Hadfield G (1968) Primary osteo-liposarcoma of bone (malignant mesenchymoma). J Bone Joint Surg 50B: 639-643

Schajowizc F, Cuevillas AR, Slberman FS (1966) Primary malignant mesenchymoma of bone. A new tumor entity. Cancer 19: 1423-1428

Schwartz A, Shuster M, Becker SM (1970) Liposarcoma of bone. Report of a case and review of the literature. J Bone Joint Surg 52A: 171-177

Stewart FW (1931) Primary liposarcoma of bone. Am J Pathol 7: 87-94

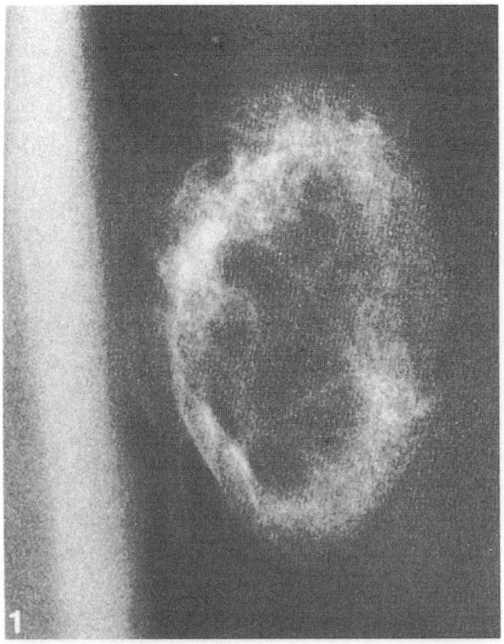
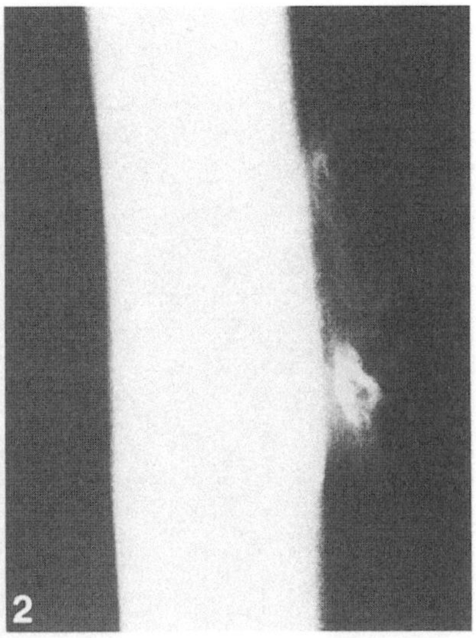
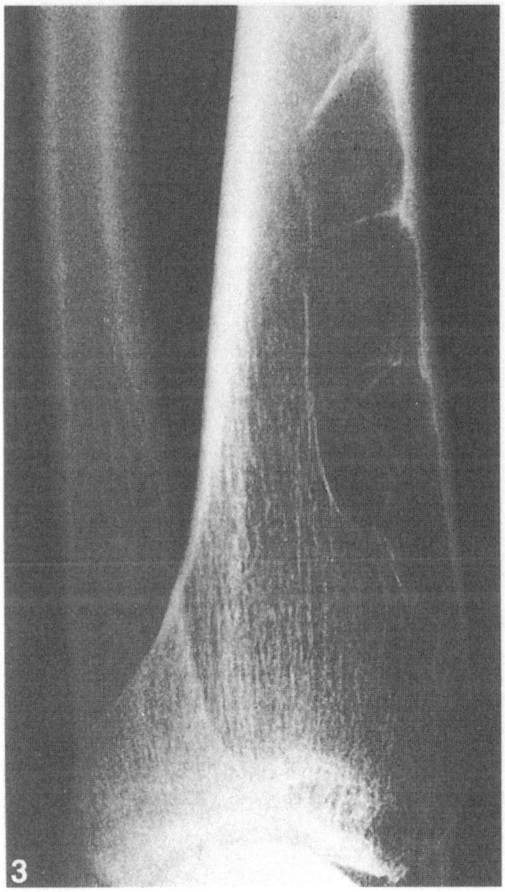
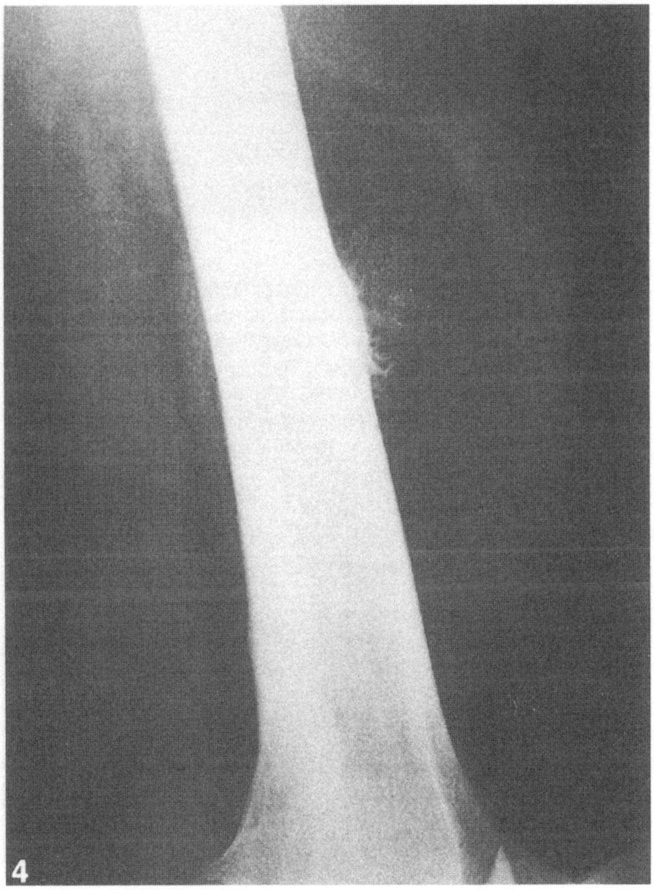

Figs. 1, 2. Two juxtaosseous lipomas. One is partly calcified (1), the other shows only ossification at the contact zone with the bony cortex (2)

Fig. 3. Intraosseous lipoma of lower third of tibia: clear image bounded by a fine border of sclerosed bone

Fig. 4. Juxtaosseous lipoma whose implantation site is ossified. The voluminous clear image of the lipoma pushes the soft tissues into a regular ring which neatly delimits the tumour (courtesy of Prof. Fauré)

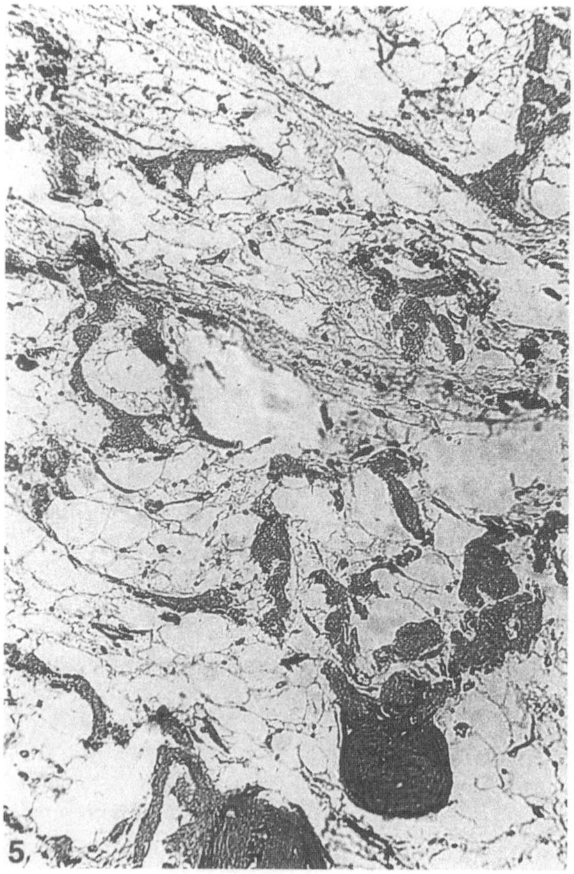

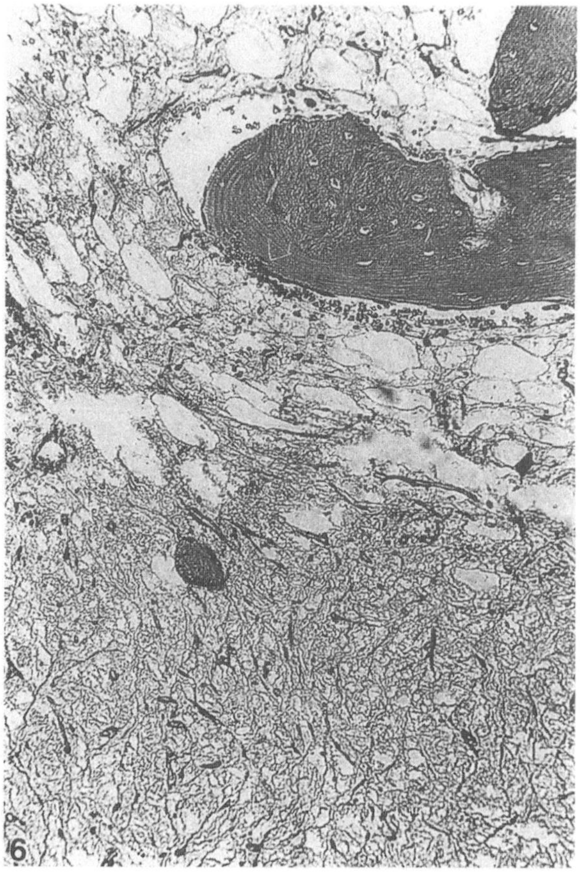

Fig. 5. This lipoma contains numerous small areas of osteogenesis

Fig. 6. A lipomyxoid zone in the same tumour

28. Myxoma, fibromyxoma

Whether intra- or juxtaosseous, myxomas and fibromyxomas are considered to be true tumours. Their rarity in the long bones contrasts with their relative frequency in the mandible and maxilla.

General considerations

The presenting symptom is usually pain, varying in intensity with the case; sometimes the lesion is a radiographic discovery.

Imaging

The radiographs show a lytic image, possibly expansive and with a border of from 1 to 5 cm in diameter. In some cases the tumour is dotted with several calcifications.

Pathological anatomy and histopathology

At operation, the lesion is well circumscribed, of gelatinous consistency and grayish in colour.

In sections, fine fusiform or stellate cells are seen scattered in a mucoid matrix and adherent to the fibers of a loose reticulin network demonstrable by silver impregnation. The nuclei are hyperchromatic and the cytoplasm scanty, but some cells may contain vacuoles, usually of lipids. In the case of Hill et al (1978), some cells had a signet-ring appearance. Mitoses are rare, there are no cytonuclear monstrosities and vessels are very rare. There is a positive reaction to alcian blue, mucicarmine, and colloidal iron. After hyaluronidase has acted on the mucopolysaccharides, the reaction to alcian blue is negative, but these reactions are quite difficult to obtain after decalcification. If denser areas of collagen are observed here and there the term fibromyxoma applies. There may be small cystic formations but there is no lobular appearance and no cartilaginous islands.

Differential diagnosis

The diagnostic difficulties relate to the radiological image, which may suggest a chondroma, a chondromyxoid fibroma or cyst, but also to the fact that a myxoid appearance is seen in numerous tumours and is therefore not specific. It may be found in the peripheral zone of a chondroma, chondrosarcoma, fibroma, lipoma or certain metastases. It may also be a component of a chondromyxoid fibroma, an adamantinoma or the myxoid form of a fibrous dysplasia.

The pathologist is therefore automatically obliged to seek elsewhere in the sections, and to be completely informed as to the clinical features, imaging and history of the patient. The presence of cartilaginous, fibroblastic or lipocytic areas may guide the diagnosis into other paths.

The vacuolated cells and the abnormal presence of vascularisation may suggest a liposarcoma. In fact, the virtual non-vascularisation of a myxoma contrasts with the plexiform capillary network of a liposarcoma.

A chondromyxoid fibroma, which may be suggested by the metaphyseal location of a myxoma, normally appears in the first two decades of life and its histological picture must comprise the three characteristic components.

It may be concluded that the diagnosis of myxoma is made by elimination, after having excluded any other possibility in the light of the clinical picture, the imaging and study of the histological sections.

References

Adler CP (1981) Fibromyxoma of the femoral neck. J Cancer Res Clin Oncol 101: 183-189

Bauer WH, Harell A (1954) Myxoma of bone. J Bone Joint Surg 36A: 263-266

Bloodgood JC (1924) Bone tumors, myxoma. Second paper with report of three cases. Ann Surg 80: 817-833

Chacha PB, Tan KK (1972) Periosteal myxoma of the femur. J Bone Joint Surg 54A: 109-1094

Enzinger FM (1965) Intramuscular myxoma. A review and follow-up study of 34 cases. Am J Clin Pathol 43: 104-113

Goldman AB, Vigorita VJ (1983) Fibromyxoma of the femur. Skeletal Radiol 10: 197-200

Milgram JW, Preininger RE (1973) Calcifying myxoma. J Bone Joint Surg 55A: 401-405

Stout AP (1948) Myxoma. The tumor of primitive mesenchyme. Ann Surg 127: 706-719

29. Idiopathic cyst, juxta-articular and related cysts, epidermoid cyst, hydatid cyst

Cysts (from Greek *kustis*: bladder) are not tumours, but in pathology the term covers a number of disparate entities; in bone pathology they share a very similar radiological image. The relative specificity of the radiological image and the particular circumstances of their development are the justification for surgical biopsy.

Superficial "necrobiotic cysts" in the weight-bearing zones of arthrotic joints are excluded from this chapter since they pose no diagnostic problems. It is convenient, though no doubt rather too schematic, to distinguish several apparently clear-cut categories: juxta-articular cysts, idiopathic cysts, post-traumatic cysts; but a cyst of the patella may be both post-traumatic and juxta-articular; and a cyst of the calcaneum may be post-traumatic, idiopathic or the delayed manifestation of a vascular disorder. Hydatid and epidermal cysts have a well defined aetiology but here the term "cyst" refers only to a radiological image of limited osteolysis, the multiple causes of which may have many surprises for the pathologist.

Idiopathic cyst (figs. 1-22)

General considerations

This is a relatively common lesion which is seen twice as often in boys as in girls, chiefly in the first two decades. The cyst is usually situated in the long bones, initially at the metaphysis, near the growth plate. It moves away from the latter as it grows older. This "migration" towards the shaft is the result of growth in length of the bone (fig. 1). The commonest site is at the upper end of the humerus; then come the upper ends of the femur and tibia, the short bones, and calcaneum, while the pelvic bones (fig. 2) are not immune.

There are numerous hypotheses about its aetiology: dystrophy, ischaemic necrosis [Lefranc & Nezelof 1957], the latter seemingly founded on firm anatomical bases. An infectious origin (osteomyelitis) or tumour related cause, a cyst following the "liquefaction" of a fibroma have both been abandoned as putative causative factors.

Clinical features and course

The lesion may be revealed by a spontaneous fracture, pain or, more rarely, by a radiological examination performed for some other reason. The capricious course of these cysts has given rise to many forms of treatment, more or less based on the pathogenic hypotheses. Whether curetted, grafted, bridged or injected with cortico-steroids, they heal or recur (fig. 3). If they fracture, they heal at the same time as the fracture unites (fig. 4). Spontaneous cure is possible and the cyst which has migrated towards the diaphysis is regarded by definition as "cured", or at least not progressing, unlike that which remains in contact with the growth plate.

Lastly, the indication for operation may be based on the damaged caused by the progressive nature of a cyst which remains in contact with the epiphyseal cartilage, or fear of a fracture, or when a fracture has actually occurred. Though the lesion is benign, it may restrict the activities of young patients for long months or even years. Sometimes cure occurs only after multiple fractures, leaving relatively severe deformities and often shortening of the limb.

Imaging

In the radiographs the cyst is usually unilocular (fig. 10a), but sometimes the persistence of bony ridges gives it a multilocular appearance (fig. 10b). It is ovoid and central and slightly balloons the thinned cortex.

Table 1. Cysts: some aspects and particular problems

Idiopathic cyst:
- moves away from the epiphyseal plate during growth and normally separates from it
- spontaneous cure possible after fracture
- histological specimen from a fractured cyst: haemorrhage, osteoclasts, cartilage and vascular proliferation may suggest an aneurysmal cyst or skeletogenic sarcoma
- the fact that it is benign does not necessarily save adolescents from the severe handicap of recurrences
- the multiplicity of proposed treatments is evidence of their qualified efficacy
- it is very unlikely that the histological evidence alone will allow distinction from cystic fibrous dysplasia from an idiopathic cyst; the clinical and imaging findings are essential

Juxta-articular cyst:
- a major pitfall, eg: some cavities beneath the clearly arthrotic cartilage of the tibial plateau; actual diagnosis: metastasis betraying an epithelioma

Epidermoid cyst:
- rare, often post-traumatic, terminal phalanx, no problems in histological diagnosis
- maxillary lesions: think of basal-cell nevomatosis

Its boundaries are sharp, separated from the medullary canal by a fine bony concave shell, the so-called "egg-cup" (fig. 5).

Pathological anatomy and histopathology

Surgical approach to the cyst by disruption of its bony shell, often thin in the humerus, sometimes quite thick in the femur, leads, without much bleeding, into a cavity which usually contains some millilitres of yellowish or serohaemorrhagic fluid. The bony wall is sometimes lined by a fine fibrous membrane, sometimes with thick fibrous tissue (fig. 6b). In some operative reports it is stated that the cyst was empty and that its walls were devoid of any lining, on at least one that was macroscopically identifiable.

Histological examination of the outermost wall of the cyst shows a fine layer of atrophic cortical bone in which the osteoplasts are partly uninhabited (fig. 11). The periosteum covering this cortex is rather inactive, considering the age of the patient. In the connective tissue which clothes the inner aspect of this cortex, osteogenesis is observed which becomes more bizarre, dystrophic and protean the closer it is to the cavity. There are osteoid strands covered with a row of osteoblasts (figs. 12, 14), fine atrophic bony trabeculae, partly necrotic (fig. 12) and osteoid strands which are irregularly calcified, sometimes in their peripheral and sometimes in their central part (figs. 11, 13, 14). Bands of collagen with wavy outlines, bordered here and there by some flattened cells may be seen and their central part is almost devoid of cell inclusions (figs. 16, 19). It may be supposed that they represent an abortive attempt at osteogenesis, especially since some of them are continuous with markedly osteoid trabeculae (fig. 14); but this is merely a hypothesis. The osteoid strands and collagen bands are strongly safranophil with metaplastic ossification with large fibers which resembles what may be seen in the majority of heterotopic ossifications (fig. 15). Coin-shaped patches of ossification very similar to those observed in fibrous dysplasia.

The hypothesis of a lesion of fibrous dysplasia becoming cystic has been advanced. We should remember that there is a rare form of cystic fibrous dysplasia which causes much chagrin among pathologists, since the course of the disorder usually provides them with proof of their inadequacy.

The fibrous tissue in which these different types of osteogenesis take place is itself also quite special; a paucicellular and possibly myxoid connective tissue which in places may be partitioned by some interanastomosing collagen bands (figs. 17, 18). The vascularisation is ensured by fine-walled vessels. In some cases, angiomatous and perhaps lymphangiomatous appearances (figs. 19, 20) may give rise to certain aetiopathogenic theories; but at the periphery the absorption is of the osteoclastic type (fig. 21).

Curiously, at its poles the cyst is separated from the medullary canal by a fine bony membrane which completely corresponds to the radiological description of this axial "egg-cup" boundary.

Differential diagnosis

The lesion is usually surgically accessed after the diagnosis of a cyst based on standard radiography. It is removal by operation and the pathological examination that make it possible to state whether it is a compact tumour (cartilaginous or giant-cell) or whether this cavitary lesion has some special aetiology. Solitary cystic lymphangioma seems very rare and is metaphyseal in location; it does not balloon the cortex and is bounded by a dense bony layer (cf Chapter 26). A sometimes serious difficulty is created by a fractured idiopathic cyst. The inner wall, covered with tissue rich in macrophages, the cavity filled with erythrocytes and a rudimentary cartilaginous callus with its inevitable cellular anomalies, may be suggestive of an aneurysmal cyst or a telangiectatic sarcoma.

Every pathologist knows, or should know, that the differential diagnosis between aneurysmal cyst and telangiectatic sarcoma based on the small biopsy fragments supplied to us is one of the most difficult diagnoses in the field of bone pathology.

Another rare and very difficult diagnosis is posed by examination of the wall of a cyst arising in a child of some ten years, the solitary manifestation of a fibrous dysplasia in its cystic form (fig. 8). In the radiographs, the somewhat disquieting extension of this cavity fully justifies operation to remove a parietal fragment of a macroscopically empty cavity. A histological study which does not distinguish between this fibrous wall and that of an idiopathic cyst and confirms the macroscopic findings may be reassuring, but the course is less so (cf Chapter 32).

Juxta-articular and related cysts

(figs. 23-34)

Some of these are directly related to an arthrosis; they are superficial and actually necrobiotic lesions. Others are remote from the articular surfaces, which are relatively well preserved. The lesions are sometimes voluminous as in the femoral neck (which may be bilateral). Various mechanisms have been suggested for the origin of these cysts; necrobiosis and cartilaginous perforation (due to increased synovial fluid pressure), are two explanations that have not been formally confirmed.

Juxta-articular cysts

General considerations

In view of their latency, the true incidence of these formations is difficult to estimate; many are discovered fortuitously in radiographs made for some other reason.

A routine radiographic study of the wrist at the Institute of Pathology in Geneva has shown the presence of cysts in 47% of cases [Bugnion 1951]; the capitate and lunate bones accounted for 31% of the lesions. There is a slight female predominance. These cysts are usually detected in adults of between 25 and 55 years of age. After the wrist, come the ankle, elbow, upper end of femur, acetabulum and upper end of tibia; indeed, they have been found in every bone of the skeleton.

Clinical features and course

Many are latent; others are mildly painful and lead to radiographic examination. Some are stable; others, particularly those adjacent to the larger joints - femoral head and neck, upper end of tibia - progress from year to year. This expansion of the cyst weakens the affected bone and may give rise to a fracture or collapse of a joint surface, for example, justifying preventive operation.

Imaging

In the radiographs there is a round or oval clear image, sometimes with a polycyclic outline, situated in the epiphysis close to the articular cartilage. It is usually bounded by a fine band of osteosclerosis.

Pathological anatomy and histopathology

The macroscopic appearance is variable and may be related to the stage of the lesion. The cavity, bordered by a relatively thick membrane, is often occupied by a myxoid material identical to that seen in degenerative cysts of the soft tissues. In these cases the cavity is filled with a straw-coloured fluid. Sometimes it is empty and its wall devoid of fibrous covering. It is rare to demonstrate any communication between the cyst and the joint cavity; in some cases, the cyst is situated 1-1.5 cm from the articular cartilage. When there is a communication between the cavities of the cyst and the joint the cyst may open into the joint or vice versa.

Histologically, the cyst wall is formed by fibrous tissue with few cells, covered by a fibrinous deposit. More rarely this wall is covered with eosinophil cells forming a sort of discontinuous layer, an extension of the synovium with which the cyst communicates. This layer covers only part of the surface, which suggests that the perforation connecting the cyst and the joint cavity is secondary and that the cyst has been "sown" by cells of synovial origin.

The difficulty is to identify the synovial origin of the intracystic tissue, but the reaction to the antikeratin antibody is positive only in that tumour labelled, perhaps somewhat facilely, synovial sarcoma. When the fibrous wall bounds a cavity occupied by a mucoid material, the appearance may be identical to that of the tendino-aponeurotic cysts so common at the wrist.

Diagnosis

The pathologist must identify the cyst, study its wall scrupulously and possibly suggest its aetiology. The possibilities include necrobiosis (in a cyst remote from a weight-bearing zone and probably related to a vascular disturbance), increased pressure of synovial fluid and, most commonly, an idiopathic origin.

The following may have a cystic presentation: chondroblastoma, a pseudo-aneurysmal cyst-like appearance associated with an other lesion, an infective or parasitic lesion. In particular, it is important to exclude a genuine aneurysmal cyst, a cavity hollowed out by an aggressive villonodular synovitis, a pseudo-cavity, abnormally hollowed out at a tendinous attachment, a metastasis masked as a rounded lytic image in a standard film and a cavity of gouty origin.

Cystic or related pseudo-cystic structures

Various lytic lesions of more or less definite aetiology often designated as cysts, sometimes only on the imaging evidence: cystic formations related to arthrosis, fracture or simple trauma and superficial cortical cysts probably of periosteal origin [Byers & Wadsworth 1970, Grange 1978, McCarthy et al 1983] are included in this. Some cysts are hollowed out in the subjacent cortex and for some of these a traumatic origin is fairly obvious. When opened, they contain mucoid material reminiscent of tendino-aponeurotic cysts. In arthroses, the cystic structures usually contain a mucoid material and fine fibrous strands with few cells. These necrobiotic cysts often communicate with the joint, but some "cystic images" in arthrotic femoral heads actually correspond to small newly-formed cartilaginous islands situated in the superficial spongiosa. Absorption of a haematoma and inclusion of adipose tissue are pathogenic hypotheses advanced for cavities developing after a fracture or other injury.

Epidermoid cyst (figs. 35-38)

This is a relatively rare lesion of bone. The epithelial tissue is introduced by a traumatic or surgical infraction, or it may be a persistent inclusion from the first stages of fetal development. However this may be, epidermoid cysts mainly develop in bones close to the skin cover (phalanges, skull, mandible).

General considerations

Most are found in the phalanges of the hands; cysts of the ungual phalanges are mostly post-traumatic. They are commoner in men, particularly in manual workers aged between 25 and 55.

Clinical features and course

Their clinical expression is limited to a painful swelling, whether in the phalanges, skull or mandible. Cure is obtained by curettage.

Imaging

The radiological image is that of a clear cavity, often surrounded by a sclerotic layer. In the phalanges the lesion suggests a chondroma, possibly a glomangioma, or a gouty lesion.

Pathological anatomy and histopathology

The macroscopic appearance is quite characteristic: the curette extracts a whitish or colourless magma from a spherical cavity.

Microscopic examination identifies a malpighian epithelium whose superficial strata desquamate into necrotic cells composing this whitish curdled substance, which occupies the central cavity of the cyst. At the periphery, the relations between bone and epithelium are quiescent. The bone is protected from aggression by a fine sclerotic shell in such a way that no cortical reaction is seen. More rarely, the bony-epithelial relations are the site of some osteoclastic activity, but here too the first contacts between the two tissues are not available to us; it is likely that they are more eventful to lead to this complete osteolysis which easily measures 7-8 mm across in a phalanx.

Three special features should be mentioned. Firstly, the relative frequency of epidermoid cysts of the mandible and skull, where the well-circumscribed osteolysis may nevertheless destroy both outer and inner tables. The radiographs may suggest a diagnosis of meningioma or, in children, that of histiocytosis X. Secondly, the presence of multiple cysts of the jaws, which should instigate a search for other cutaneous and bony manifestations of basal-cell nevomatosis. Finally, the development of cholesteatoma, usually consequent on an otitis. Curettage removes a malpighian epithelial wall and numerous cholesterol crystals accompanied by a macrophagic foreign body reaction and inflammatory cells. The epithelial inclusion may be primary or secondary (epithelialisation of the cavity).

Hydatid cyst (figs. 39-42)

Echinococcosis of bone is rare, exceptionally so in the long bones. In all the records examined from 1962 to

1992 at the Hôpital Parnet in Algiers, the bony lesion was rarely primary [Prof. Zidane, personal communication]. This is also the opinion of Ilidi et al (1992) who give bony involvement as 0.8 to 2% of hydatid lesions, a disease predominantly of the liver and lungs. However, some cases of vertebral and iliac lesions considered as primary have been reported [Von Sinner & Aktar 1994].

General considerations

There is a slight female predominance. The age distribution is very extensive, with a mean at about 35. The preferential sites are the vertebral column (40-50% of cases), pelvis (20%), the long bones of the limbs and then the skull.

Clinical features and course

The lesion presents with moderate pain or a swelling. A fracture with lesions in the long bones or a secondary infection may also be the first signs of a cyst, which develops insidiously and sometimes reaches a considerable size before discovery. In 12 cases with bony lesions, of which 9 appeared solitary and revealed the disorder [Ilidi et al 1992], 3 had a sinus of which one suppurated. It is cardinal, when a bony lesion is the presenting feature, to seek evidence of visceral lesions. The prognosis depends on the surgical possibilities.

Imaging

The standard films demonstrate a lysis of cavitary appearance; in the vertebrae involvement of the vertebral body is often associated with affection of the posterior arch. The lesion is usually multilocular in the iliac wing and scapula. More effective imaging (CT, MRI) will suggest the diagnosis by demonstrating images of the density of water.

Pathological anatomy and histopathology

Operation exposes a voluminous cyst or an agglomeration of small structures of cystic appearance. In the long bones, the lesion invades the medullary canal progressively. In the spongiosa this infiltrative character, possibly accompanied by an inflammatory reaction, is quite peculiar to this lesion. The bony cortex may be breached. Some accounts mention a discrete periosteal reaction.

Study of the sections demonstrates, apart from necrotic debris and granulation tissue, some fragments of hyaline membrane, with or without macrophage reaction on contact, easily identifiable by positive PAS staining. Hexacanth scolices of *Taenia echinococcus* and the strongly fuschinophil and birefringent hooks (like rose thorn) are seen on examination under polarised light.

Diagnosis

The diagnosis may be suggested by the imaging, but this may also suggest a hyperparathyroid lesion or some other type of cyst. It is the immunological reactions and the histological examination that will confirm the diagnosis.

References

Idiopathic and related cysts

Abdelwahab IF, Lewis MM, Klein MJ, Barbera C (1989) Simple (solitary) bone cyst of the calcaneus. Case report. Skeletal Radiol 17: 607-610

Bensahel (1969) Kyste solitaire des os. Etude diagnostique et thérapeutique. Rev Prat XIX: 2121-2130

Broder HM (1968) Possible precursor of unicameral bone cysts. J Bone Joint Surg 50A: 503-507

Bugnion JP (1951) Lésions nouvelles du poignet. Thèse n°2026 Genève

Byers PD, Wadsworth TG (1970) Periosteal ganglion. J Bone Joint Surg 52B: 290-295

Capanna R, Van Horn J, Ruggieri P, Biagini R (1986) Epiphyseal involvent in unicameral bone cysts. Skeletal Radiol 15: 428-432

Cope R, Marsan R, Castelli MJ (1992) Gout presenting as a large pseudotumor (tophus) in the proximal end of the tibia. Skeletal Radiol 21: 269-270

Ehara S, Kattapuram SV, Khurana JS (1989) Intraosscous ganglion of olecranon with vacuum phenomenon. Skeletal Radiol 18: 329-330

Ehara S, Rosenberg AE, EL-Khoury GY (1990) Sacral cysts with exophytic components. Skeletal Radiol 19: 117-119

Foucar E, Buckwalter J, El-Khoury GY (1984) Gout presenting as a femoral cyst. J Bone Joint Surg 66A: 294-297

Grange WJ (1978) Subperiosteal ganglion. J Bone Joint Surg 60B: 124-125

Janecki CJ, Nelson CL, Dohn DF (1972) Intrasacral cyst. J Bone Joint Surg 54A: 423-428

Journées orthopédiques franco-vénitiennes (1979) Les kystes essentiels osseux. Rev Chir Orthop 65: 3-10

Kambolis C, Bullough PC, Jaffe HL (1973) Ganglionic cystic defects of bone. J Bone Joint Surg 55A: 496-505

Lefranc J, Nezelof C (1957) Les kystes essentiels des os longs étude anatomopathologique et traitement chirurgical. Rev Chir Orthop 43: 385-406

Malghem J, Maldague B (1987) Post-traumatic cyst-like lesions. Skeletal Radiol 16: 403-406

McCarthy EF, Matz, Steiner GC, Dorfman HD (1983) Periosteal ganglion: a cause of cortical bone erosion. Skeletal Radiol 10: 243-246

Moore TE, King AR, Travis RC, Allen BC (1989) Post-traumatic cysts and cyst-like lesions of bone. Skeletal Radiol 18: 93-97

Nezelof C, Laurent M (1966) Inclusions capsulo-synoviales intra-osseuses. Rev Chir Orthop 52: 225-240

Rutishauser E, Jacqueline FR (1953) Lésions de nécrose et hernies capsulaires dans les os du poignet de l'adulte (confrontation anatomo-radiologique). Rhumatologie 4: 179-194

Sanerkin NG (1979) Old fibrin coagula and their ossification in simple bone cysts. J Bone Joint Surg 61B: 194-199

Schajowicz F, Clavel Sainz M, Slullitel JA (1979) Juxta-articular bone cysts (intra-osseaus ganglia). A clinicopathological study of eighty-eight cases. J Bone Joint Surg 61B: 107-116

Scholder P (1952) Vascularisation osseuse et pseudokystes du poignet. Thèse no.-2100, Genève

Scholder P (1953) Vascularisation osseuse et pseudokystes du poignet. Rev Chir Orthop 39 (suppl 1 bis): 1-56

Schultz E, Gretuspan A (1986) Simple bone cyst (traumatized). Skeletal Radiol 15: 405-407

Sim FH, Dahlin DC (1971) Ganglion cysts of bone. Mayo Clin Proc 46: 484-488

Södergard J, Karaharju EO (1990) Kystes du calcanéum; diagnostic, traitement. Rev Chir Orthop 76: 502-506

Struhl S, Edelson C, Pritzker H, Seimon LP, Dorfman HD (1989) Solitary (unicameral) bone cyst. Skeletal Radiol 18: 261-265

Ucla E, Tomeno B (1990) Kystes sous-chondraux (inclusions capsulo-synoviales). A propos de 25 cas. Rev Chir Orthop 76: 533-537

Woods CG (1961) Subchondral bone cysts. J Bone Joint Surg 43B: 758-766

Epidermoid cyst

Jean C, Hould J (1964) Kyste épidermoïde des os. Laval Med 45: 894-900

Lerner MR, Southwick WD (1968) Keratin cysts in phalangeal bones. Report of an unusual case. J Bone Joint Surg 50A: 365-372

Oda Y, Hashimoto H, Tsuneyoshi M, Ono N (1992) Intraosseous epidermoid cyst arising in the fifth metacarpal bone. Skeletal Radiol 21: 343-345

Hydatid cyst

Abelanet R, Forest M, Palangié A, Meary R,Tomeno B, Languepin A (1975) L'échinococcose osseuse, à propos de 6 observations anatomocliniques. Ann Anat Pathol 20: 133-140

Acquaviva R, Tamic A, Kerdoudi H, Bru P, Levy-Lebar JP, Ouradou J, Thevenot CH, Bouflet-Lahlou S, François-Bensimon SS (1967) L'hydatidose de la moelle et du rachis. J Med Maroc 3: 289-330

Acquaviva R, Tamic, Kerdoudi H, Levy-Lebar JP, Lebascle J, Bru P (1968) L'échinococcose des os du crâne. J Med Maroc 4: 245-264

Argenson C, Griffet J, Lacour C, Arcamone H, Lovet J, Peretti (de) F (1989) L'hydatidose vertébrale. A propos de deux cas. Rev Chir Orthop 75: 267-270

Ilidi R, Yaakoubi MT, Ladel MF, Ben Ayeche ML, Ghannouchi G, Moula T (1992) L'hydatidose osseuse. 12 cas. Ann Pathol 12: 98-101

Von Sinner WN, Aktar M (1994) Primary spinal echinococcosis of lumbosacral spine case report. Skeletal Radiol 23: 220-223

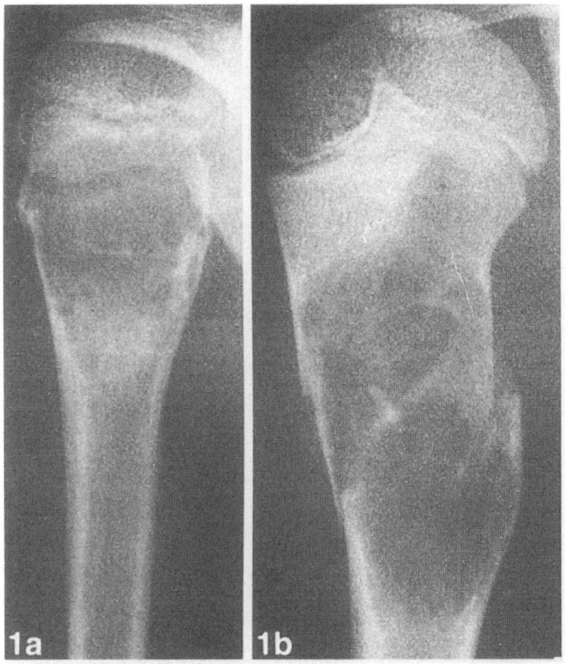

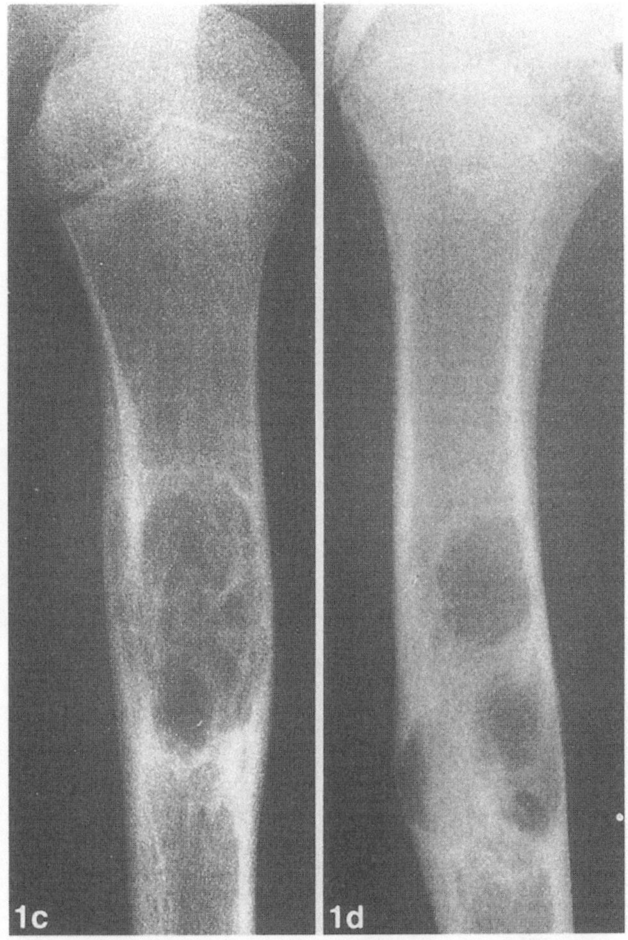

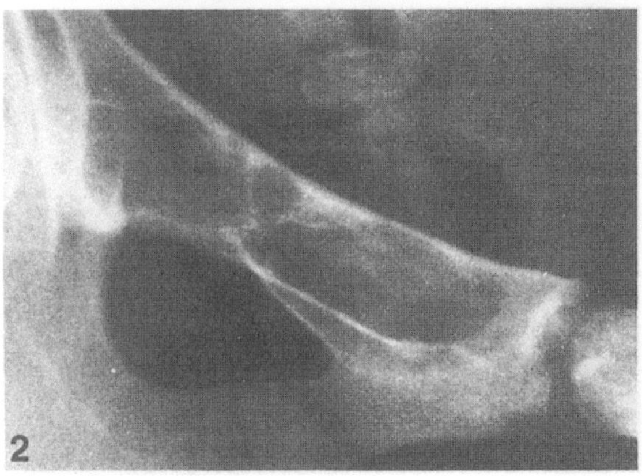

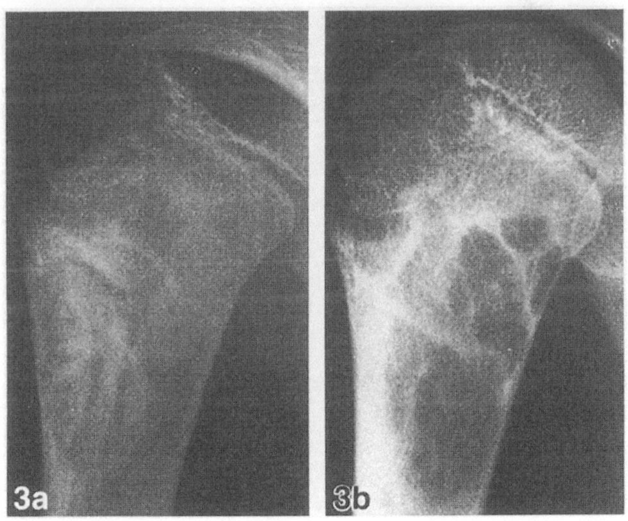

Fig. 1 a-d. In 1962, a fracture revealed the presence of a cyst of the upper humeral metaphysis in a boy of 7 (**a**). In 1964, the cyst fractured for the second time; there is slight ballooning of the bone (**b**). In 1967, the cyst is now diaphyseal, oval, well defined by a margin of dense bone and seemingly in process of cure (**c**). In 1970, it appears multicavitary (**d**); it has not healed spontaneously even after two fractures in its 8-year course. This sequence of radiographs well demonstrates the "migration" of the cyst from the metaphysis towards the diaphysis

Fig. 2. Multilocular cyst of iliopubic ramus in a woman of 20

Fig. 3. a This cyst of the upper end of the humerus in a boy of 8 has been curetted and packed with spongy bone-grafts. **b** Six months later the grafts have been absorbed and the cyst has recurred

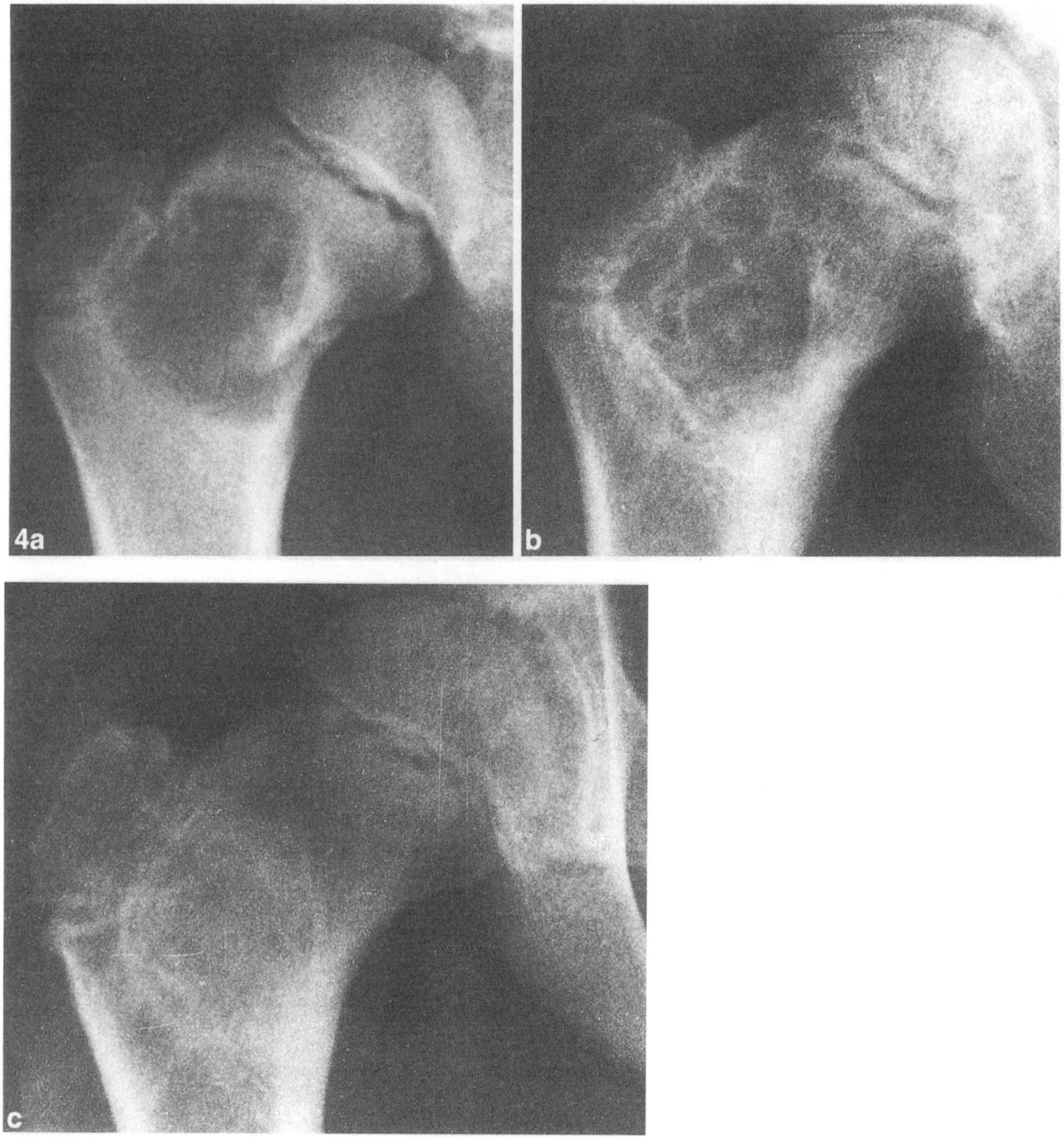

Fig. 4. a Cyst of upper end of femur with fracture at medial border of neck cure two years later (**b, c**), possibly due to the fracture

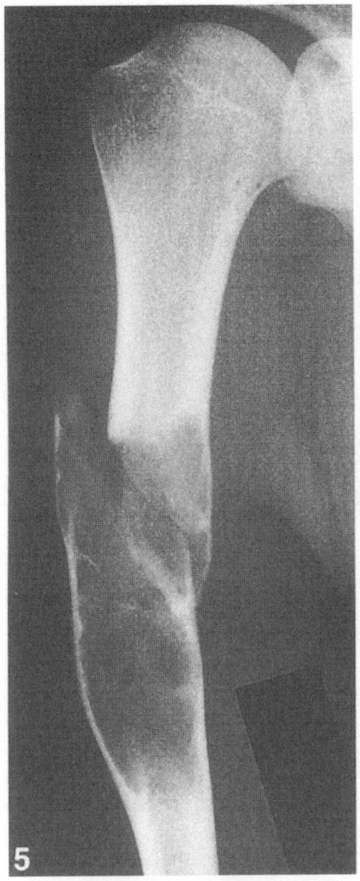

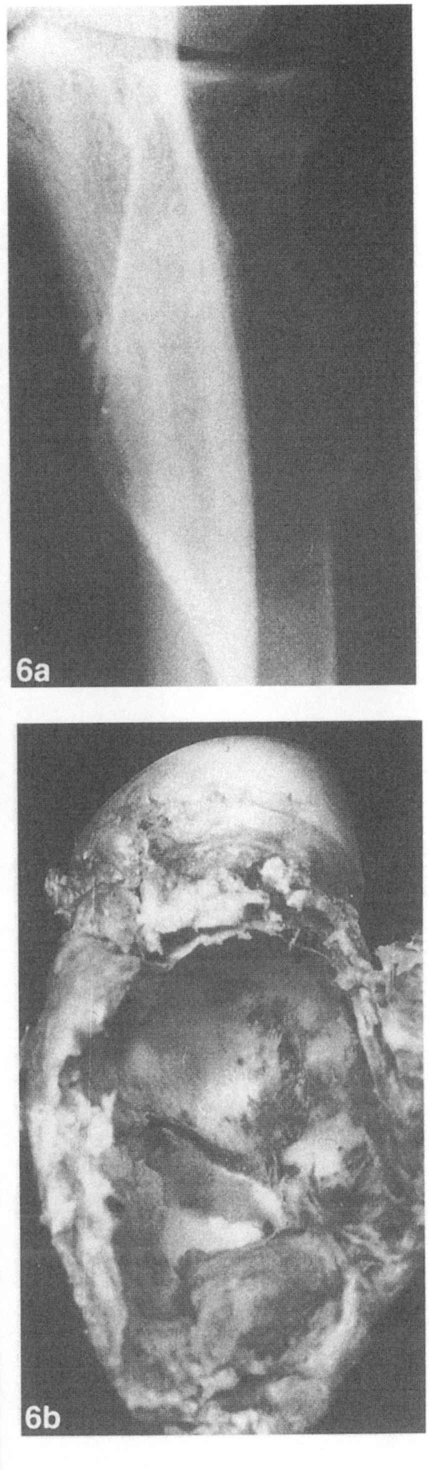

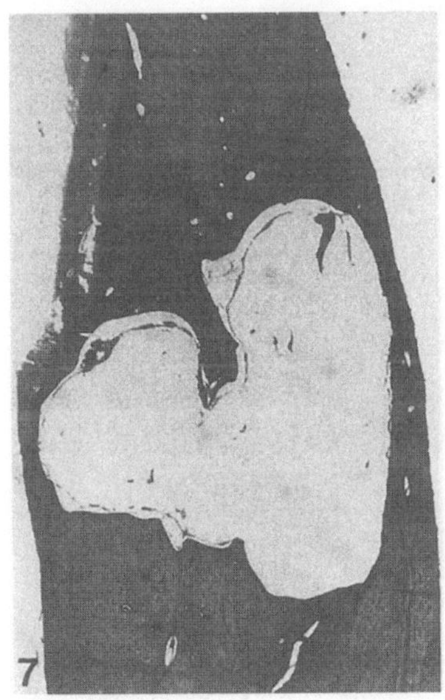

Fig. 5. Cyst in diaphyseal position in man of 24, slight ballooning of humerus, fracture of very thinned cortex

Fig. 6. a This ill-defined cyst balloons the upper metaphysis of the radius in a woman of 44. **b** In the specimen the bony wall of the cyst is covered with a smooth fibrous membrane; no specific aetiology was detected

Fig. 7. Three years after a fracture of the lower end of the radius this cystic lesion developed in a girl of 15. The cavity is bordered by a fine membrane and involves the entire thickness of the cortex

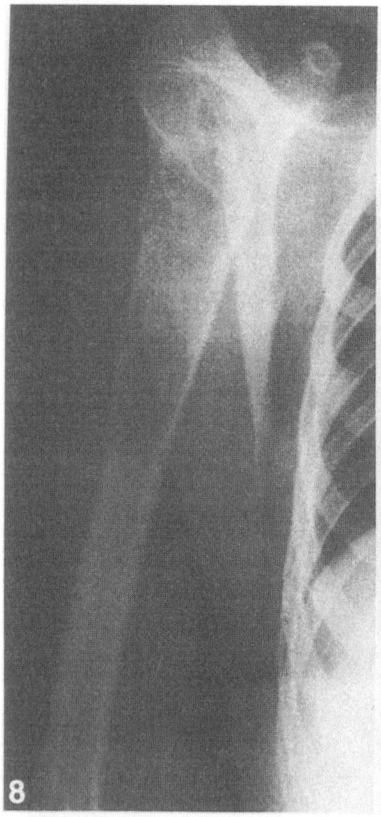

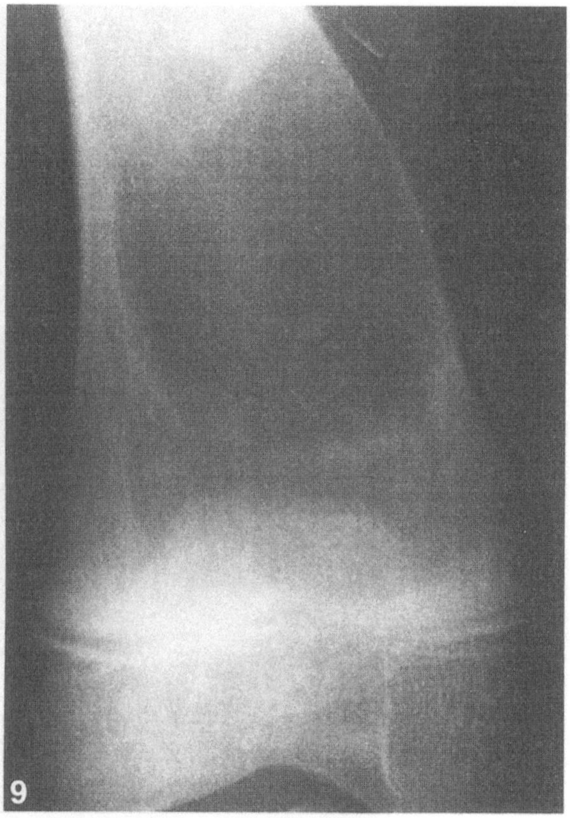

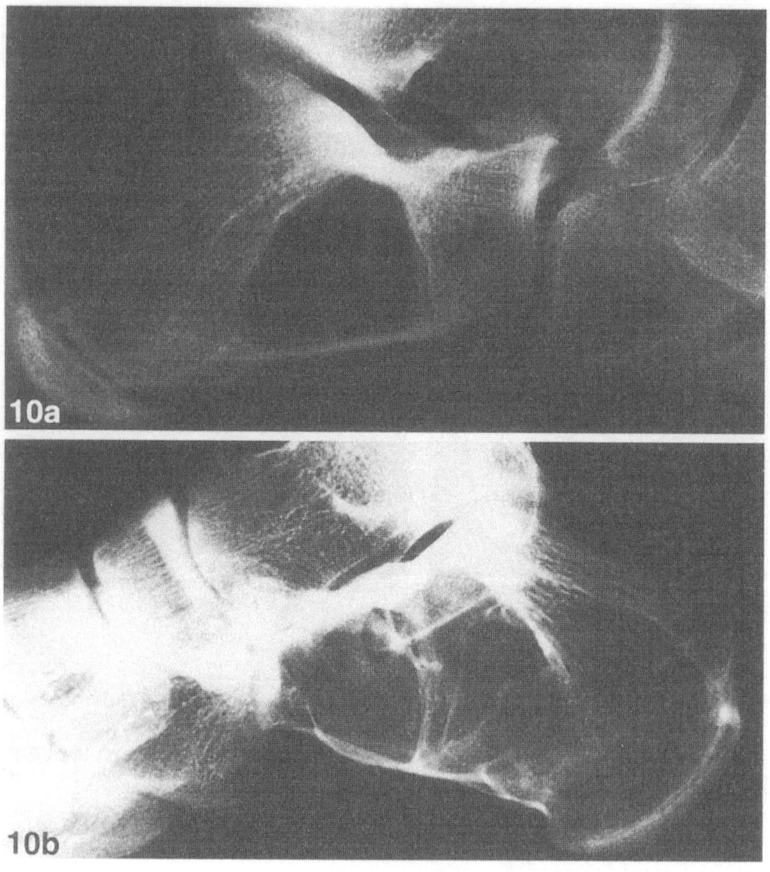

Fig. 8. In a young woman a fracture revealed extensive lesions of the upper third of the humerus. There is a cystic image, well-circumscribed at its lower end, and the cortices are thinned; in fact this is not an idiopathic cyst but a cystic form of fibrous dysplasia. The course of the radiological changes over 23 years is described in Chapter 32, fig. 8

Fig. 9. Large metaphyseal cystic formation in boy of 12. Biopsy provided no clue as to aetiology

Fig. 10. Cysts of calcaneum in an immature bone (**a**), and in adult bone (**b**). Calcaneal cysts are relatively common but cystic tumours of the calcaneum also occur (chondroblastoma)

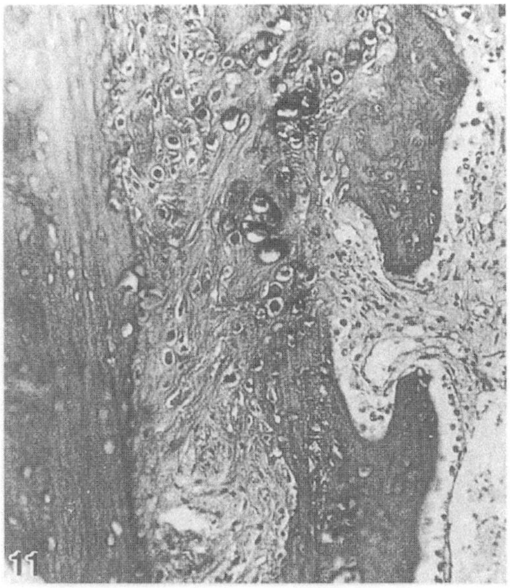

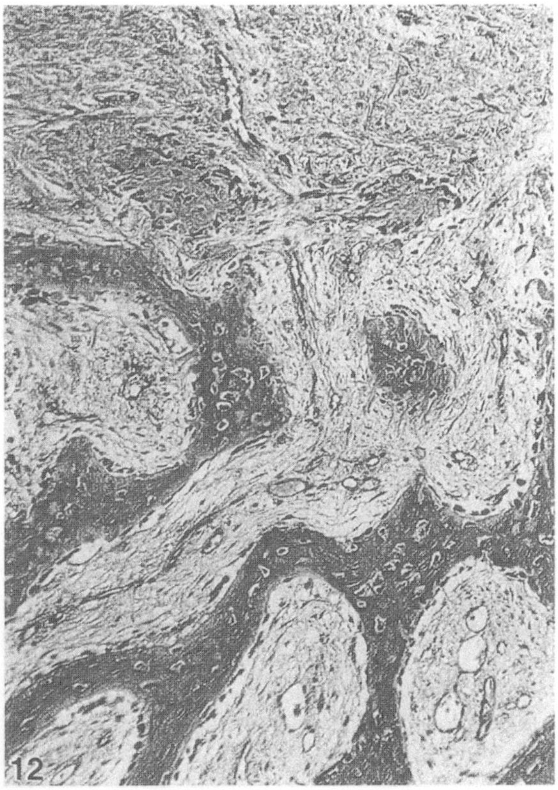

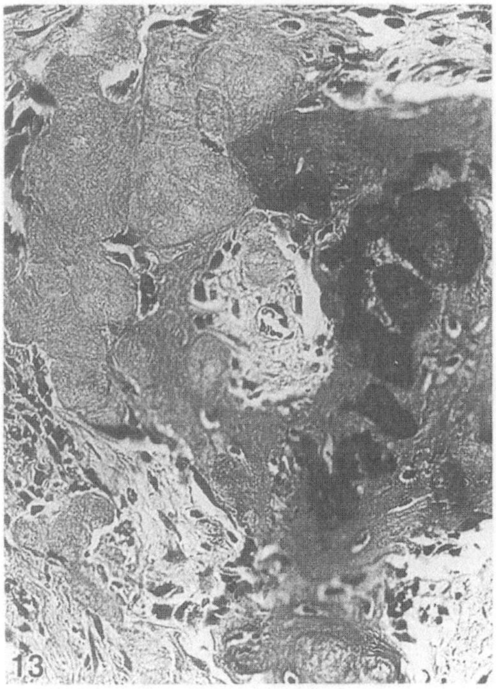

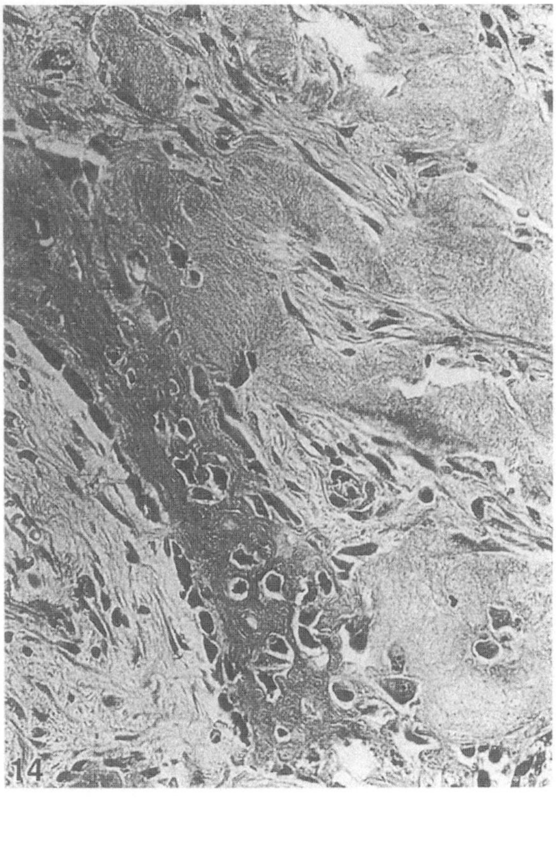

Fig. 11. In the cyst wall a dystrophic osteogenesis is adherent to an atrophic cortical residue (left side of microphotograph). Cyst developed in a boy of 14

Fig. 12. Relatively regular osteogenesis forming inter-anastomosing strands of immature bone, bordered by a row of osteoblasts, in this fibrous wall of an idiopathic cyst. Boy of 12

Fig. 13. Formation of collagen, osteoid and partly calcified osteoid. Boy of 9

Fig. 14. Wide band of collagen, possibly an abortive attempt at osteogenesis, in continuity with an immature bony trabecula. Boy of 10

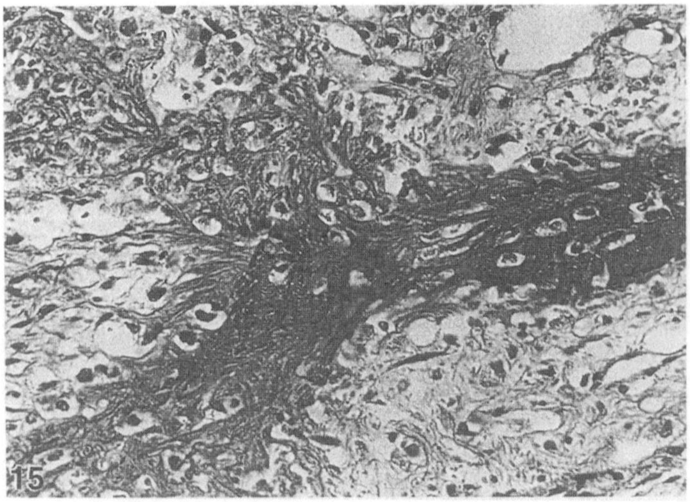

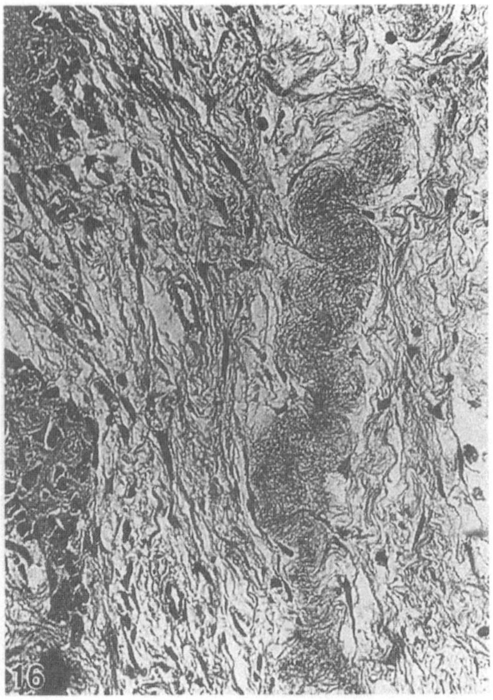

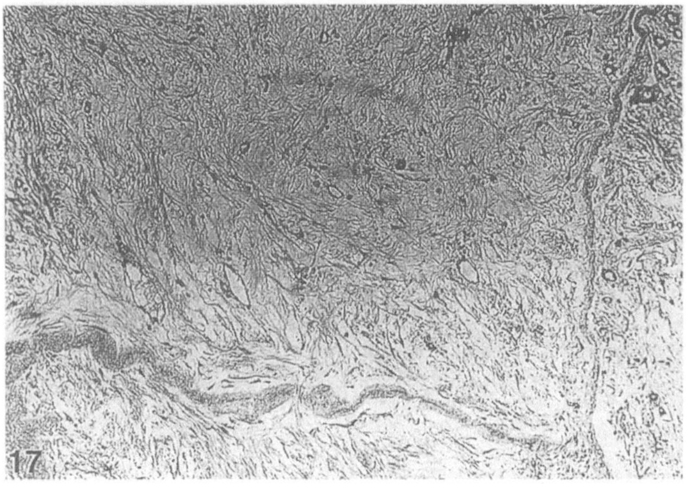

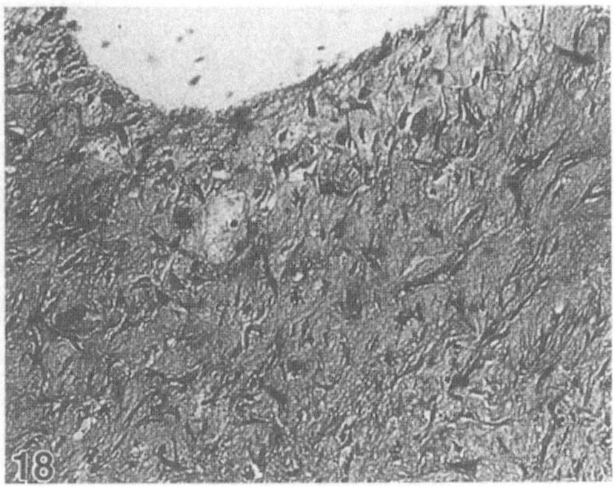

Fig. 15. Metaplastic ossification with wide collagen fibers

Fig. 16. Large and virtually acellular collagen band

Fig. 17. These fine inter-anastomosed collagen strands in the fibrous wall of a cyst in a child of 12 are possibly only aborted formation of dystrophic bony trabeculae

Figs. 18, 19. The paucicellular connective tissue contains elements which are sometimes fusiform and sometimes stellate. It forms the wall of the cavity

Fig. 20. The ectasias of the capillaries give this cyst wall an angiomatous appearance. In the loose fibrous tissue, the newly-formed bony trabeculae are surrounded by osteoblasts

Fig. 21. Stripping of the endosteum, to which the osteoclasts remain adherent, clearly reveals the jagged pattern of the subjacent bony tissue

Figs. 22 a, b. Areas of irregular calcification (**a**), with rudimentary osteogenesis (**b**) in the wall of an idiopathic cyst strongly suggest foci of infarction

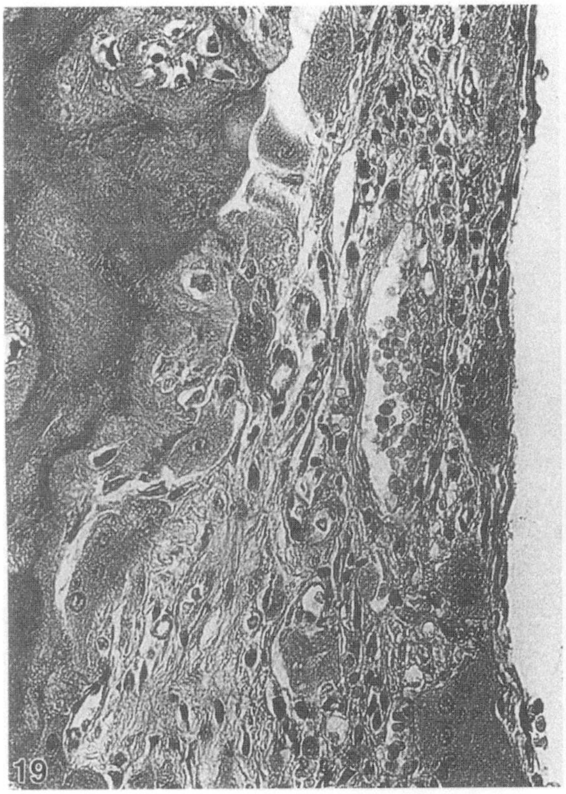
19

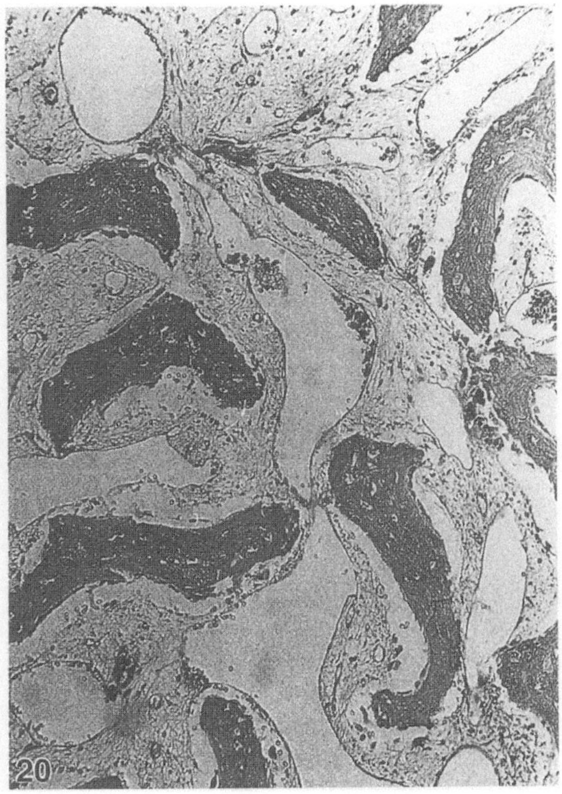
20

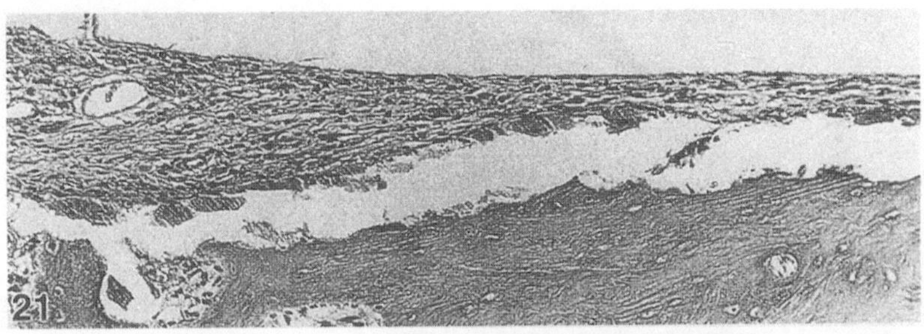
21

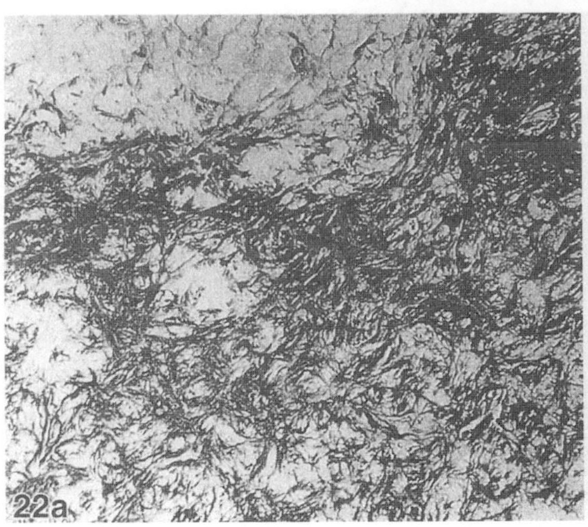
22a

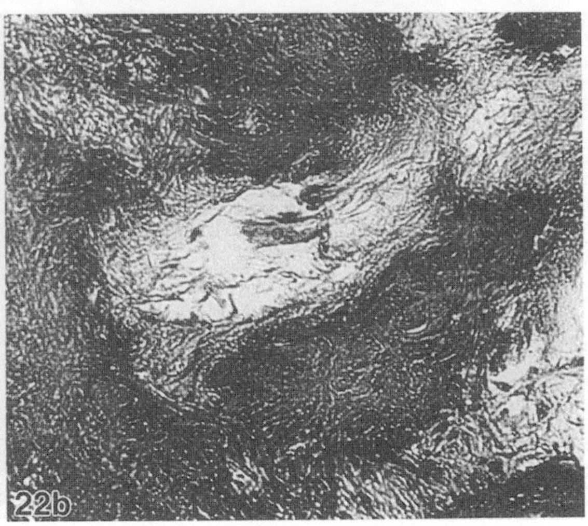
22b

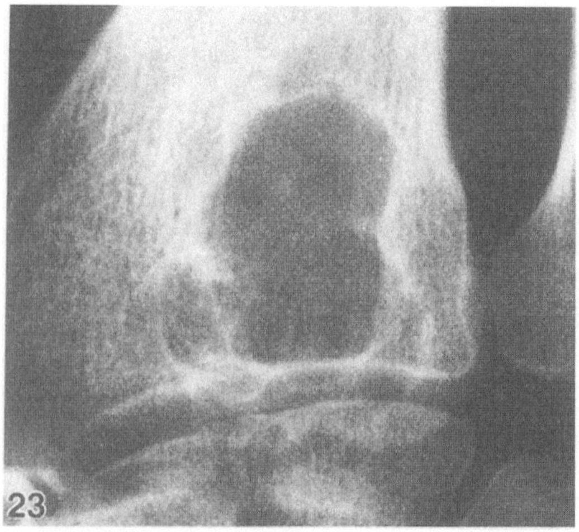

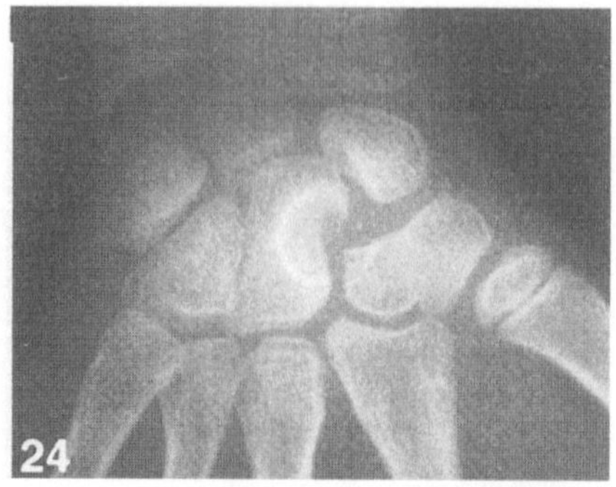

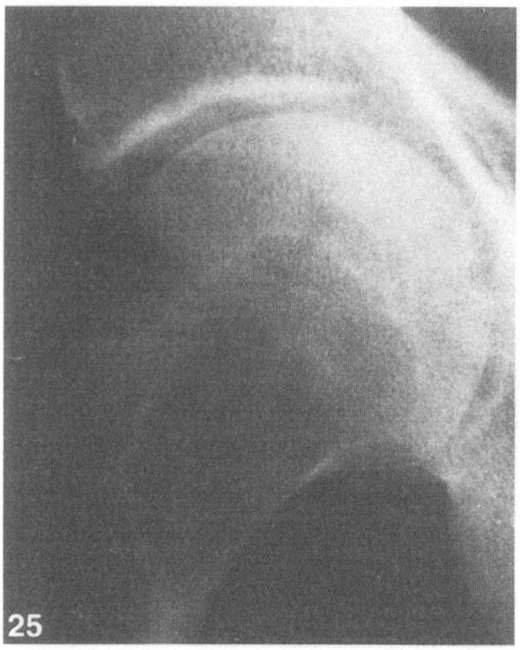

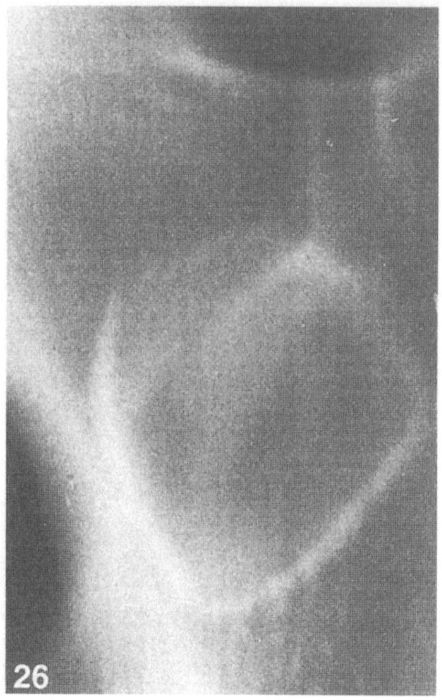

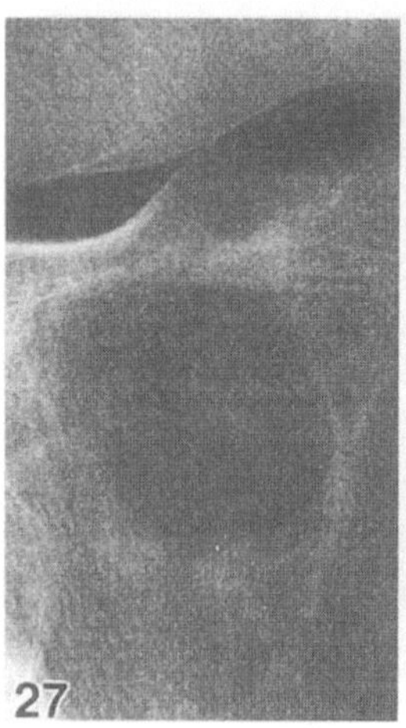

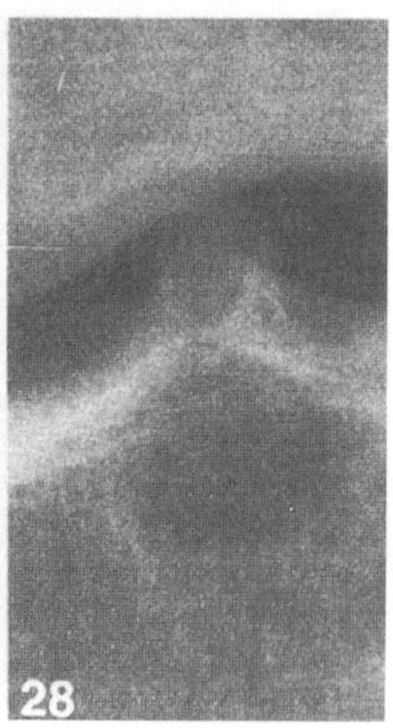

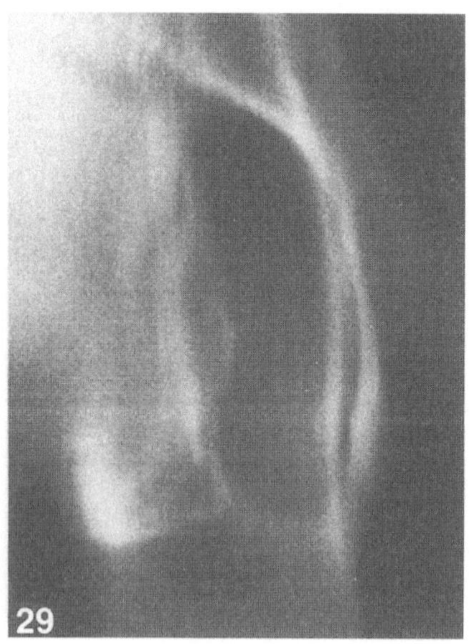

Fig. 23. Large cyst of lower end of radius with polycyclic outline in a man of 50. It is bounded by a fine shell of sclerosed bone. Histologically, it is lined by a thick fibrous membrane

Fig. 24. This cyst of the capitate is filled with a mucoid material completely identical with that of tendo-aponeurotic cysts. It is possible that this is simply the impression of a degenerative aponeurotic "cyst" on the bony tissue

Fig. 25. Cystic lesion of femoral head and neck; such lesions are sometimes bilateral and extend from year to year

Fig. 26. Cyst with well-marked borders at level of intertrochanteric line; its wall is clothed with a thick fibrous membrane

Figs. 27, 28. These two cysts have developed in the median zone of the upper tibial epiphyseal region

Fig. 29. Tomograph of cyst in posterior column of acetabulum, communicating with hip joint

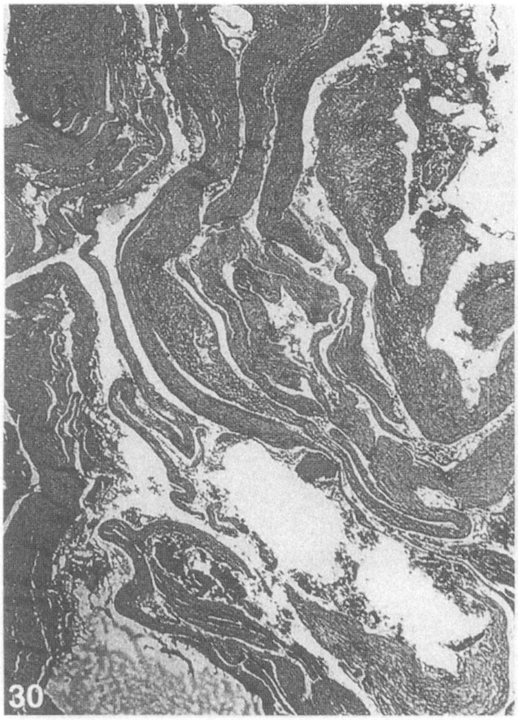

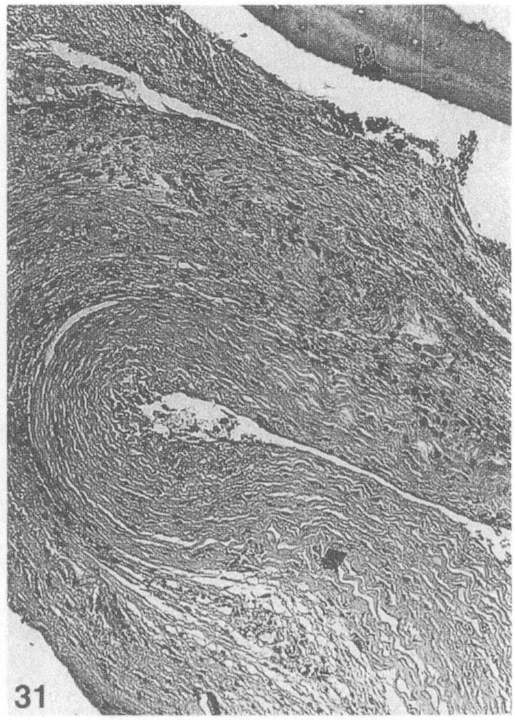

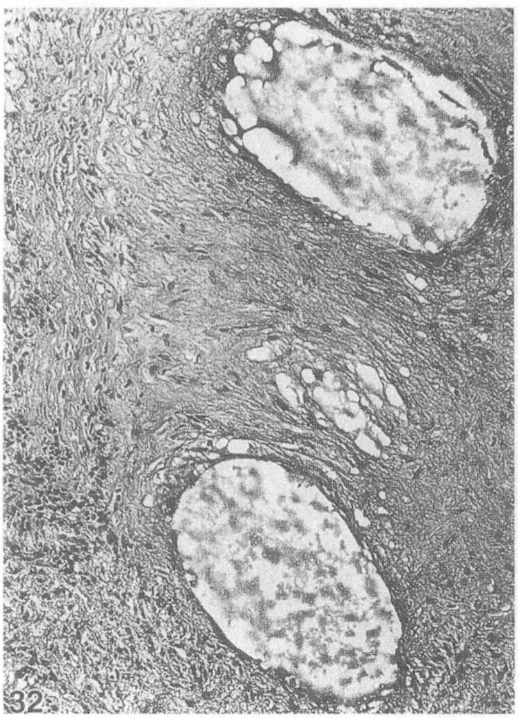

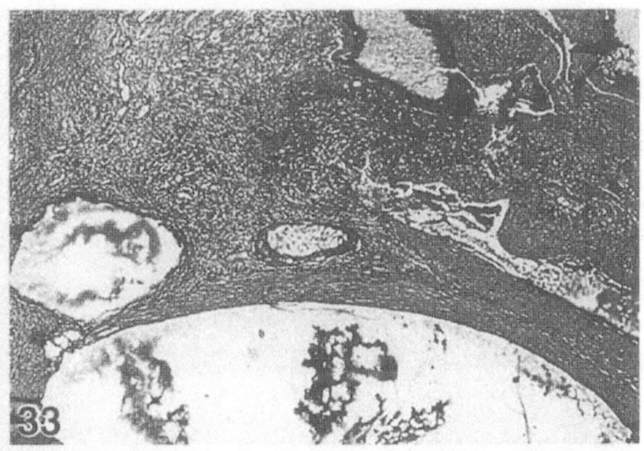

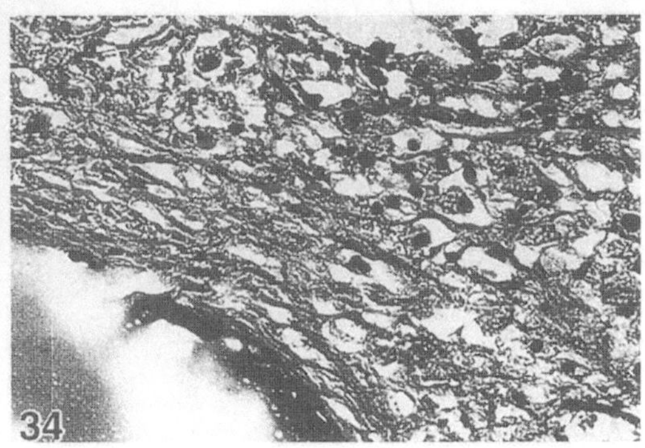

Figs. 30, 31. Cyst of acetabular lip in woman of 42. The thick fibrous wall of this cyst consists of parallel collagen fibers with few cells; there is a discrete inflammatory reaction

Fig. 32. In the fibrous tissue of a cyst wall, zones of mucoid degeneration outline two secondary cavities; between them is a third zone of degeneration. Discrete inflammatory infiltration in the left half of the microphotograph

Fig. 33. The mucoid material may be in direct contact with the bony tissue

Fig. 34. Histiocytic reaction in the parietal connective tissue at the margin of the zone of cavitary degeneration

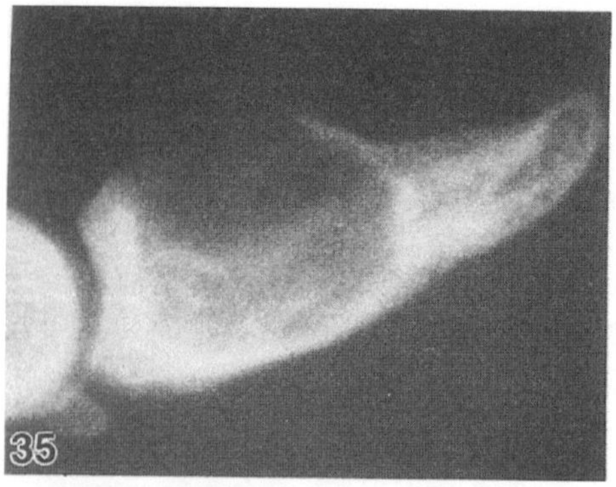

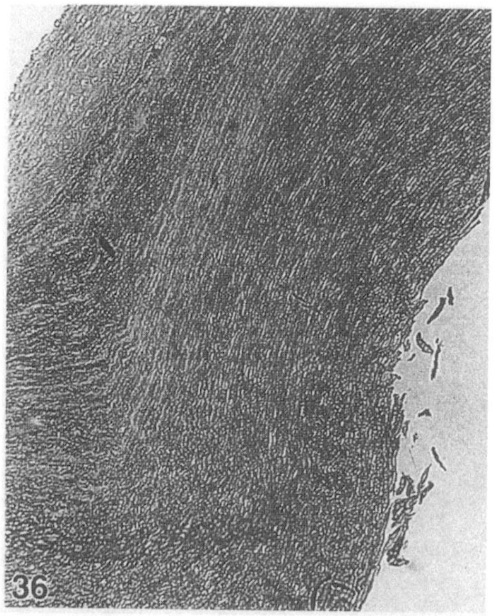

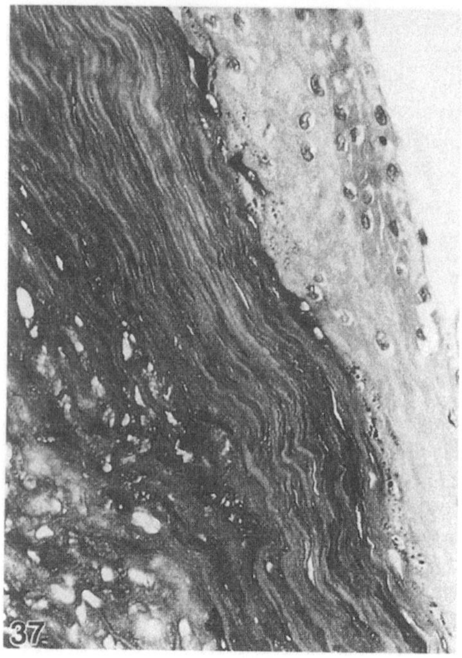

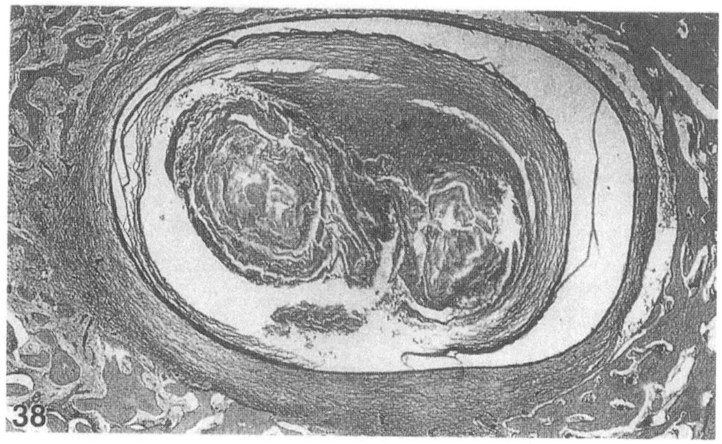

Fig. 35. The radiological appearance of this epidermoid cyst is of a vast cavity at the base of the ungual phalanx of thumb, sharply bounded by sclerosed bone

Figs. 36, 37. Low magnification (36): note the major thickness of the epithelium clothing this cyst of an ungual phalanx. Higher magnification (37): cellular maturation is obvious and there is a layer of cells containing granules (stratum granulosum)

Fig. 38. Overall view of cyst of mandible

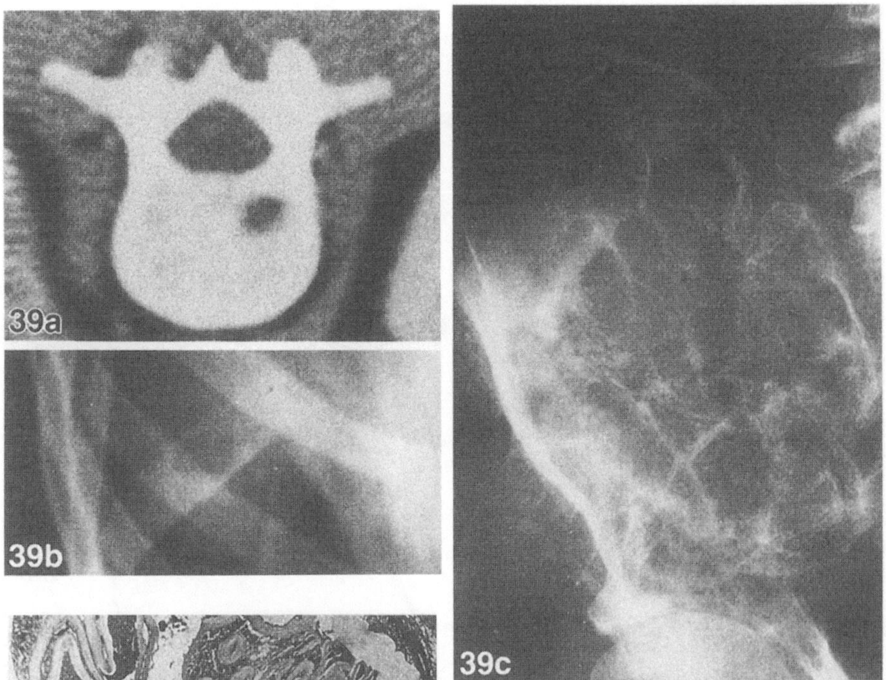

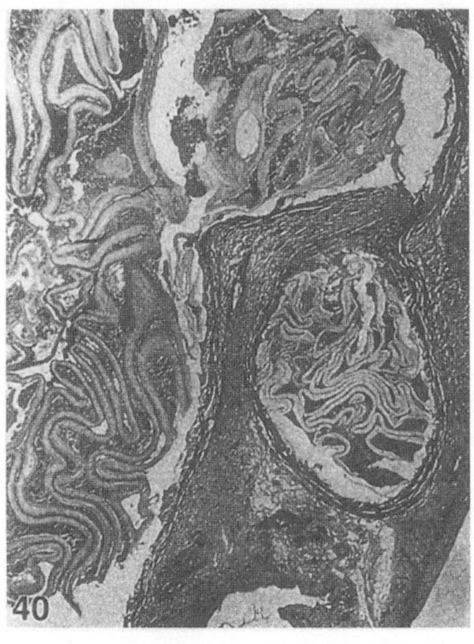

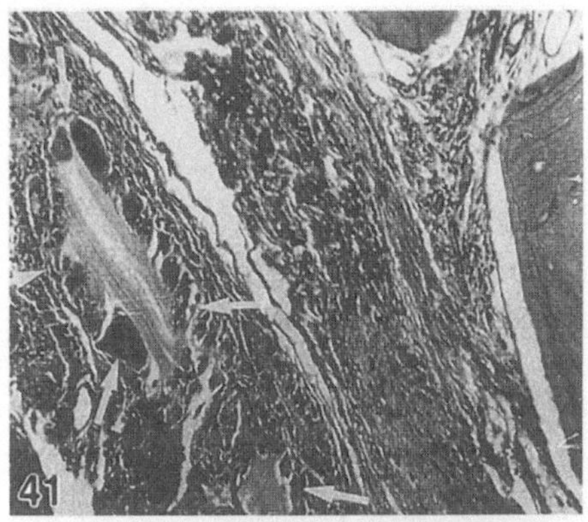

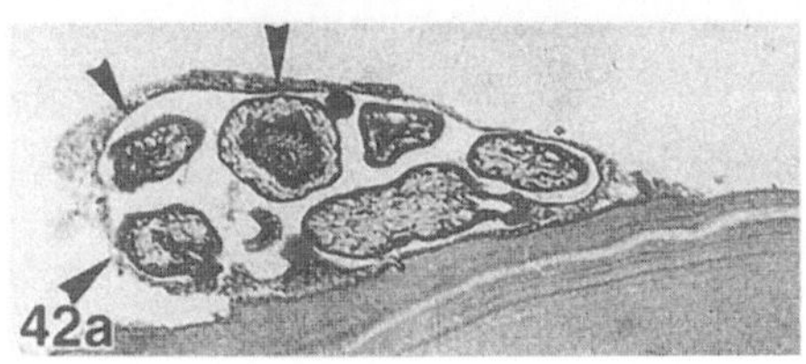

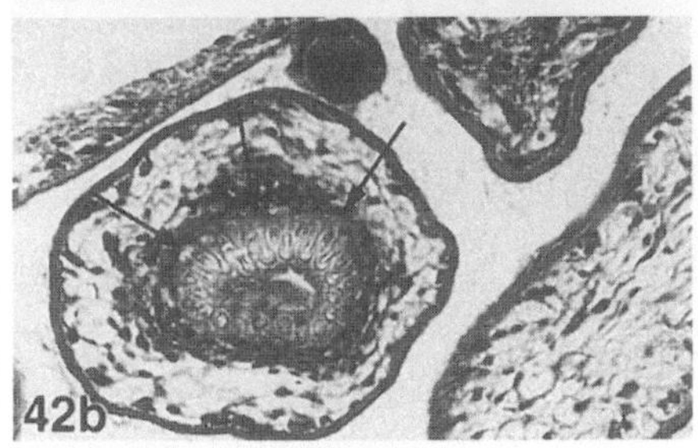

Fig. 39 a-c. Hypodense MRI image (**a**) in a vertebra in a patient with several vertebral lesions (*Echinococcus granulosus*) (courtesy Hôpital Pasteur, Nice). (**b**) Hydatid cyst of rib and (**c**) multicavitary iliac lesion (courtesy Prof. Zidane and Dr. Bouhadef, Hôpital Parnet, Alger)

Fig. 40. Sections involving cavitary formations partly filled with membranes. The hyaline appearance of these membranes is very suggestive but requires the demonstration of scolices, or of their hooks (fuschinophil, Ziehl -Nielsen + and birefringent)

Fig. 41. In the fibrous tissue adjacent to a bony trabecula there is a macrophage reaction with giant cells (*arrows*) around membrane debris

Fig. 42 a, b. In a daughter vesicle (**a**) the scolices (*arrows*) are attached to the proligerous membrane. At higher magnification (**b**), birefringent hooks can be seen arranged in a circlet (*arrows*) (courtesy Dr Ravisse, Institut Pasteur, Paris)

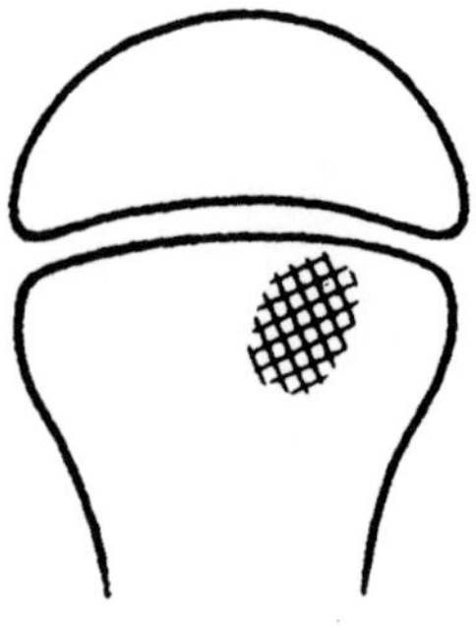

1a

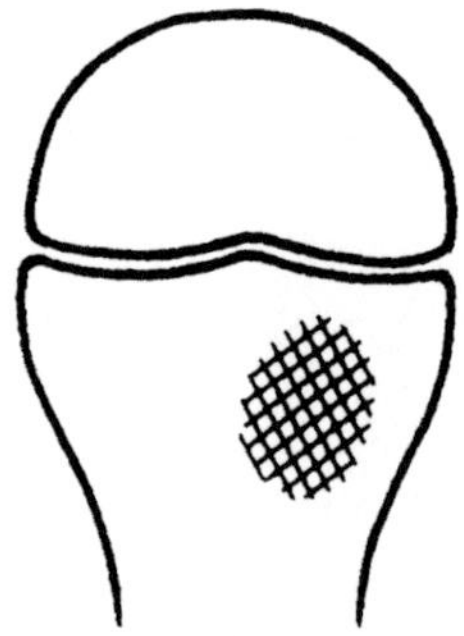

b

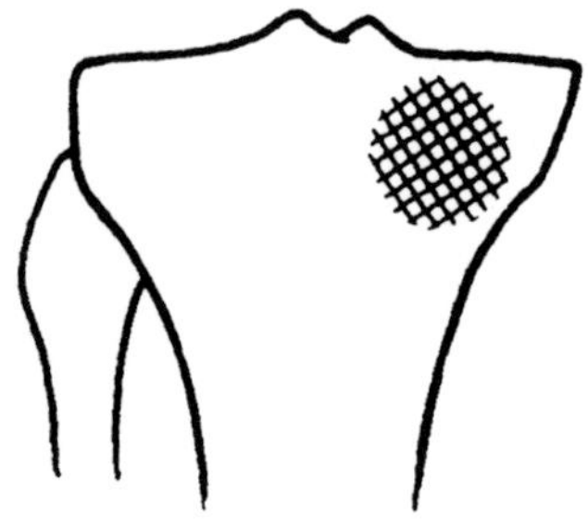

2

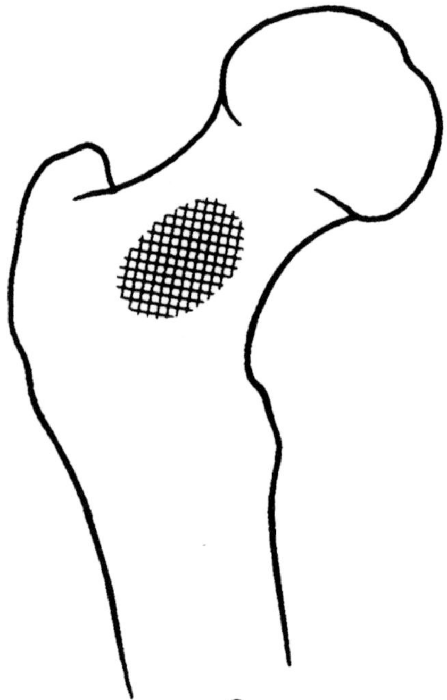

3

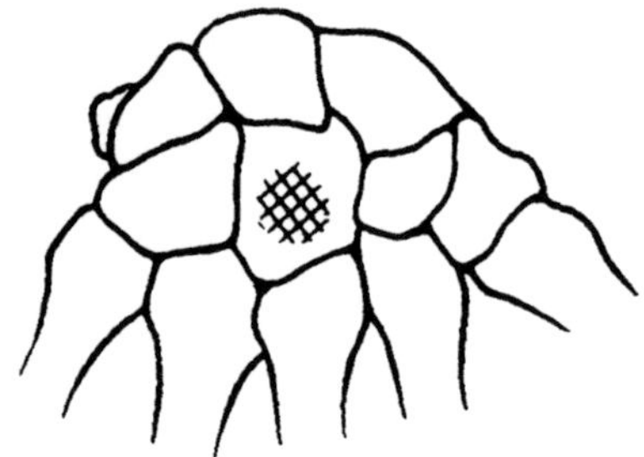

4

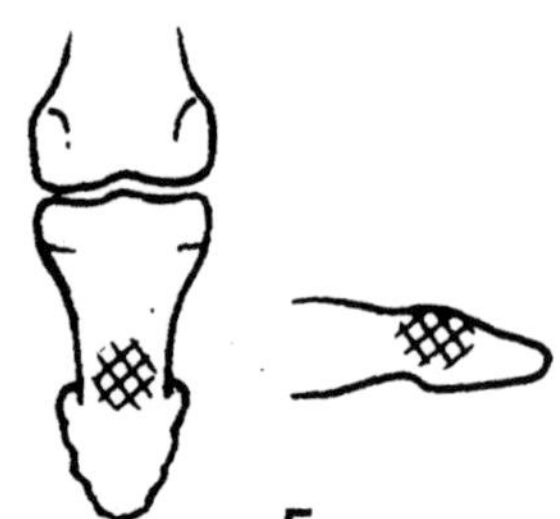

5

Diagrammatic representation of sites of some cysts and tumours:

Diagram 1. a Idiopathic cyst in very young child, still in contact with growth plate. **b** As ossification continues, the cyst has lost contact with the cartilage

Diagram 2. Relatively common site of juxta-articular cyst (the joint is often arthrotic)

Diagram 3. Cyst of femoral neck, possibly "associated" with coxofemoral arthrosis; the cause is probably ischaemic necrosis

Diagram 4. Cyst of carpal bone, common

Diagram 5. Epidermoid cyst

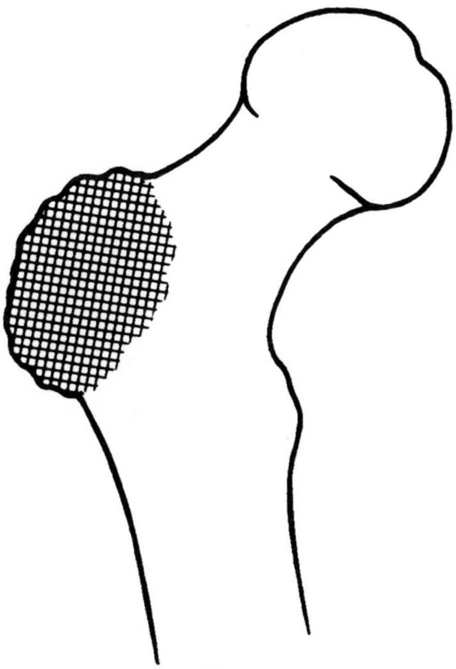

6

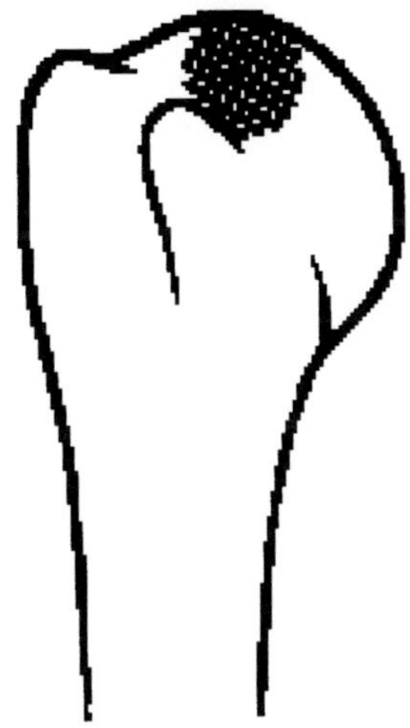

7

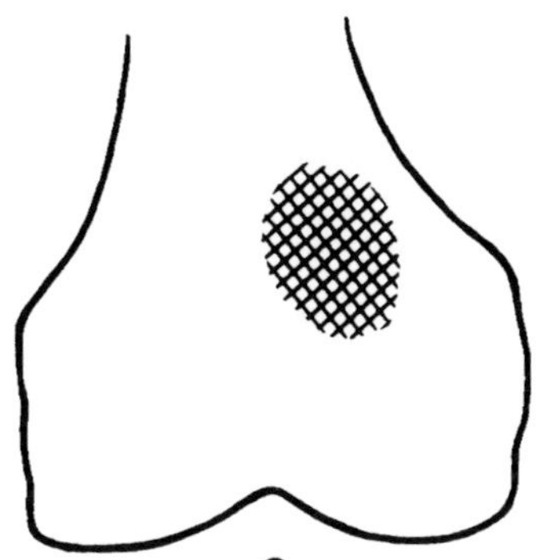

8

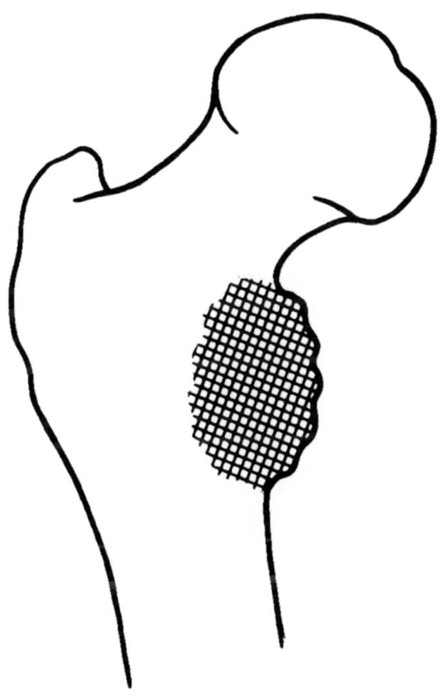

10

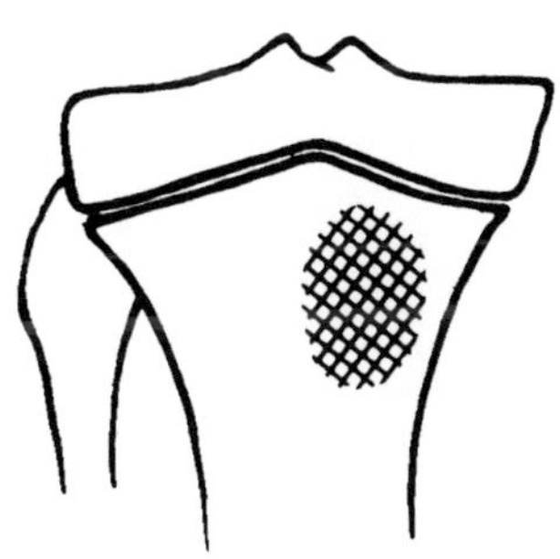

9

Diagram 6. Possible site of aneurysmal cyst

Diagram 7. Chondroblastoma: epiphyseal, possibly cystic

Diagram 8. Giant-cell tumour: metaphyseal or metaphyseo-epiphyseal, plate fused

Diagram 9. Chondromyxoid fibroma: metaphyseal, growth-plate patent

Diagram 10. Possible site of aneurysmal cyst but also of telangiectatic osteosarcoma, clear-cell chondrosarcoma and other lesions

30. Aneurysmal cyst

This rare lesion was described by Jaffe and Lichtenstein in 1942. Though histologically benign, it nevertheless carries a serious prognosis because of the frequency of local recurrences and, especially in children, because of its important sequelae. From the pathological standpoint, aneurysmal cyst may be confused with certain benign and malignant cystic angiomatous neoplasms, and in particular with anaplastic sarcoma of telangiectatic type.

Case history

Pierre X., aged 15, had complained for about two months of persistent pain in the right shoulder. Examination revealed a slight outward vaulting of the upper end of the humerus. The radiographs showed a clear, ballooned but limited image. The outer cortex was replaced by a fine periosteal bony layer as if distended by increased underlying pressure, giving the tuberosity a swollen appearance. The patient's age and the site of this cystic image, which was ballooning the bone, suggested the diagnosis of aneurysmal cyst, which was confirmed by both macroscopic and microscopic examination. But this benign lesion, followed by two recurrences after curettage, was to prevent this adolescent from normal school attendance and any sporting activity, and finally led to near-total destruction of the upper end of the humerus and its growth cartilage.

General considerations

The incidence of aneurysmal cyst is difficult to define. Dahlin estimates it at around half that of giant-cell tumour. In France and other countries where the orthopaedic surgery of children and adults is carried out in independent departments, the data are collected in a way which makes estimates difficult. From various series, there appears to be a slight female predominance, of the order of 55:45. The lesion is usually discovered in the adolescent or young adult; about 75% of patients are under the age of 20.

The site of election is the metaphysis of the long bones, where it occupies an eccentric position (fig. 12). In the adolescent it is limited by the growth-plate, but in adults it may extend towards the epiphysis (fig. 8); more rarely, the cyst is diaphyseal in position (figs. 6, 9). It may also affect the vertebrae (figs. 4, 11, 12), more often the posterior arch than the body, but also the ribs, pelvis and craniofacial region, mainly the temporal bone and mandible.

In the long bones, 50% of the lesions are distributed equally between the proximal and distal extremities. In the study of Vergel de Dios et al (1992) dealing with 238 cases, the lower epiphysis of the femur and upper epiphysis of the tibia accounted for 22% of cases, the short bones for 15%, the vertebrae for 15% and the flat bones for 20%.

Clinical features and course

The clinical picture varies in terms of the site and spontaneous course. There is moderate pain in some 50% of cases, a hard palpable swelling in about 35% and sometimes both pain and swelling. More rarely there is a limp, protective spinal rigidity or sciatica due to compression. The cyst may also rupture but only exceptionally does it cause a fracture.

The course is quite unpredictable. Surgical curettage may be followed by definitive cure, but recurrence or even exacerbation are not uncommon. However, in view of the expansile nature of the lesion a surgical procedure may be necessary to avoid destruction of an adjacent joint, to decompress nerve structures, or eliminate the risk of fracture.

There may well be a spontaneous course towards cure [Macqueen et al 1985]. It is quite likely that some stable large ossifications, the ballooning of a spinal apophysis or the upper end of a fibula, may represent the appearances of resolution of an aneurysmal cyst. Nature does (with less risk of malignant transformation) what radiotherapy does in those cases judged to be inoperable.

Therapy has passed through different phases. In view of the frequency of recurrences after surgery alone, some have advocated low-dose irradiation, but this indication is considerably restricted by the risks of possible sarcomatous transformation, the irradiation of adjacent organs or the arrest of growth. Cristofaro et al (1992) regard selective arterial embolisation as the treatment of choice for aneurysmal cysts and angiomas of the vertebrae, sacrum and pelvis, locations where surgery is likely to cause haemorrhage. Marcove et al (1995) propose a combination of surgery and cryosurgery. Recurrences tend to occur within 3-4 months after curettage, but their frequency varies greatly with the series; the mean rate of 20-25% after curettage is higher in very young patients.

Inequality of limb length is due to destruction of the epiphyseal growth plate. Neurological complications from compression due to expansion of a cyst of the posterior vertebral arch usually regress after operation. It is certain that, apart from the aggressivity of the lesion, the treatment employed may also carry the risk of damaging the growth plate in the long bones, or the neural structures in vertebral and sacral lesions in particular.

Imaging

In most cases the radiological appearance is very suggestive. The cyst is manifest by a clear eccentric image, predominantly metaphyseal. The lesion forms a sort of bubble which effaces the cortex and displaces the soft tissues, from which it is separated only by a thin bony shell secreted by the periosteum displaced by expansion of the cyst (figs. 1, 3, 5, 8b).

In the long bones this image may trespass on the diaphysis and epiphysis. In a rib or the ischiopubic ramus (fig. 5), the cyst is seen as a more or less globular swelling bounded by a thin shell of newly-formed periosteal bone, but within these bounds the bony structure is virtually completely obliterated. However, some lesions may suggest a chondroma; the superficial lesions may resemble a fibroma (figs. 6, 7); a lower femoral metaphyseal lesion a sarcoma, and so on.

Pathological anatomy and histopathology

Surgical approach leads to a fine layer of periosteal bone bounding a cavity of variable size. Usually, this cavity is subdivided into or surrounded by cavities of unequal size forming a multilocular structure (fig. 13). These cavities are filled with a blood-stained brownish-red fluid which does not coagulate. The cavities are bordered by variably thick walls, which may be ossified or calcified in places. Cysts can also be formed of a reddish-brown friable tissue which very much resembles a giant-cell tumour; the haemorrhagic cavitary central zone being of reduced size. In such cases, treated by curettage, the fragmentation of the tissue and its disruption by haemorrhage leaves no chance of reconstructing its general topography. Only the examination of numerous sections will reveal all of the characteristic elements. Sometimes it is a relatively dense fibrous tissue which lines the bony wall and bounds a large haemorrhagic cavity. It may be that these are virtually stabilised cysts. In very progressive forms, aggressive either from the outset or during an accelerated growth phases closely following the first operation, the cyst invades the soft tissues (fig. 14) and only rare fragments of periosteal bone remain.

On examining large sections at low magnification, the presence of multiple rounded lacunae separated from one another by septa which may be thick or thin is very suggestive (fig. 15). These cavities are occupied by abundant erythrocytes held in an eosinophil coagulum. Their walls may or may not be bordered by endothelial cells but are devoid of complete arterial or venous blood vessels (figs. 18-20). The septa separating these vascular spaces are formed of connective tissue which may be oedematous or more or less fibrous, in which bands of osteoid tissue stand out, often very close to the endothelium (or to the free border devoid of endothelium), but sometimes in the midst of the fibrous septa (figs. 20, 21). These vascular spaces may represent virtually all the "tumour" or may, on the contrary, be accompanied by an abundant very cellular tissue resembling a giant-cell tumour (fig. 24). Whatever the nature of the cyst wall, deposits of haemosiderin, extracellular or contained in the histiocytes, are frequent.

As the cyst grows, the periosteum lays down bone with wide collagen fibers whose deeper part is doomed to destruction by the progress of the cyst (fig. 25). More rarely, there are small tissue zones here and there whose morphology may suggest fibrous dysplasia [Levy et al 1975, Forest et al 1977, Diereks et al 1986].

The mitotic index is very variable from one case to another. Though a raised index evidences a locally progressive character, cases of spontaneous malignant transformation, if they exist, are certainly extremely rare.

In their very well-documented report from the Mayo Clinic, Vergel de Dios et al (1992) single out 5% of "solid forms", in which, apart from the absence of obvious vascular spaces, the histology is identical to that of more typical aneurysmal cysts. This non-cystic variant has been described by Sanerkin et al (1983) in 3 vertebral cases and one ethmoidal case. It combines proliferation of fibrohistiocytes, osteoblasts and osteoclasts with osteoid production; but there are still some dilated vessels and some foci of calcified fibromyxoid tissue. It should be noted that these 4 cases were situated in vertebrae or bones of similar origin, whose reactions to aggression are known to differ from those of the long bones. But is this a variant or a precystic evolutional stage?

For their part, Dahlin and Unni (1986) dealing with 31 cases of vertebral giant-cell tumours, have stressed the particular cellular characteristics (smaller cells of fusiform tendency) and the good prognosis of these vertebral lesions. For these authors, none of their 31 cases had the characteristics of variants of an aneurysmal cyst or of osteoblastoma.

Diagnosis

In many cases the diagnosis is easy. The radiological appearances, site and youth of the patient are often very suggestive and the macroscopic findings at operation will evoke the diagnosis. Ignoring the extremes of age reported in some publications, this diagnosis may logically be considered between the ages of 5 and 30, without forgetting that this age-group is not predisposed to an aneurysmal cyst. However, the radiological appearances of superficially developing forms, especially at the early stages of their development, entail consideration of other lesions arising juxtacortically. It is then examination of the biopsy specimen that must be relied on for the diagnosis.

In practice, the pathologist is essentially faced with three diagnoses, each of which calls for a specific treatment: anaplastic telangiectatic sarcoma, giant-cell tumour and a fractured idiopathic cyst. Other differential diagnoses, though less common, are no less difficult to exclude and it would be unreasonable to attempt to make a diagnosis on material obtained by aspiration.

Anaplastic telangiectatic sarcoma. While it is true that certain pathological diagnoses are made from examination at low magnification, there are others for which examination of the cells at high magnification is essential and aneurysmal cyst is one of these. With this lesion, frozen section is the main source of confusion with telangiectatic sarcoma. If this error is made, the sarcoma will be treated by curettage and recurrence will follow with-in 6-8 weeks. The risks that the erroneous diagnosis is not corrected by the second biopsy are far from negligible.

The bloodstained and fibrinous effusion filling the cavity after curettage is surrounded by newly-formed tissue in which histiocytofibroblastic proliferation participates as widely as tumour cell proliferation. It is essential to re-examine the sections of the first biopsy. Anaplastic telangiectatic sarcoma may simulate an aneurysmal cyst at low magnification. What happens in these cases is that the tumour allows the proliferation of narrow tissue bands only, forming septa between the bloodlakes. These anaplastic cells rarely secrete osteoid lamellae in the intervascular septa.

Only scrupulous examination of the cells will demonstrate the characteristic anomalies of sarcoma; in a biopsy sample mitoses may be very rare. Some reports, doubtless related to aggressive forms of aneurysmal cyst, stress the abundance of (normal) mitoses but it is wise to regard a diagnosis of aneurysmal cyst sceptically if there are cell anomalies [Vergel de Dios et al 1992].

Giant-cell tumour. The problem may remain unsolved by biopsy. We may recall the findings of Martinez and Sissons (1988) in 96 giant-cell tumours, in 14 of which they listed an "association" with an aneurysmal cyst. Rightly or wrongly, I have several times reported "a giant-cell tumour in process of cyst formation" on the finding of cavitation occupying a fifth or sixth part of the tumour. There is no doubt that some would have reported "aneurysmal cyst associated with giant-cell tumour". Is this an evolution of giant-cell tumour, in young patients? In these circumstances the age of the patient and the imaging provide real guidance. It is to be recalled that in the vertebrae giant-cell tumour is commoner in the body, and cysts in the posterior arch.

Fractured idiopathic cyst. Here again, the haemorrhagic fluid, the dystrophic osteogenic reaction and the cellular proliferation accompanied by numerous osteoclasts sometimes may simulate an aneurysmal cyst. Study of the results of imaging is an essential factor in diagnosis.

Other differential diagnoses must be considered. Angioma is a relatively easy diagnosis. While one may hesitate between the diagnoses of angioma and aneurysmal cyst, other possibilities must be considered such as certain types of cystic and haemorrhagic fibrous dysplasia and osteoblastoma. Certain osteoblastomas, whether of the long bones or the posterior vertebral arch, may simulate an angioma or cyst. Search must be made for foci of ossification rich in osteoblasts and true nests of osteoblasts; these appearances are not always observable in a small biopsy. The osteoblasts are usually large, even bizarre, but without monstrosities. Chondroblastoma, cystic or not, is located in an epiphysis or apophysis. The particular appearance of the cells (cf Chapter 5), which secrete a chondroid material, should give the diagnosis. The newly-formed cartilage is quite different from a fragment of growth cartilage removed "accidentally" during the curettage of an epiphyseal or metaphyseal lesion adjoining the growth plate. Non-ossifying fibroma and cystic fibrous dysplasia are rich enough in fusiform cells for the diagnosis of aneurysmal cyst to be excluded even if associated with some giant cells and haemosiderin-laden macrophages. The idiopathic cyst of the very young child has a degree of cellularity in its wall and the presence of giant cells has led some colleagues to speak readily of aneurysmal cyst. This is not my opinion and I do not know who is right. But when the soft tissue wall of a cyst, if large, is reduced at this stage, the course following curettage in unfavourable cases is not that of development of an expansile lesion but the reproduction of a "cystic" cavity.

Pseudo-aneurysmal cyst or "related aneurysmal cyst"

Eight years after having distinguished the aneurysmal cyst, Jaffe recognised the possibility that an identical histological picture might coexist with preexisting bony lesions.

In 1988, reviewing 639 bony tumours, Martinez and Sissons listed 15% with the appearance of aneurysmal cyst in giant-cell tumours and chondroblastomas, and a markedly lower percentage in chondromyxoid fibromas, non-ossifying fibromas, osteoblastomas, fibrous histiocytomas, fibrous dysplasias and osteosarcomas. In the preceding pages we have stressed the possibility of a very similar appearance in different tumours, in particular in anaplastic telangiectatic sarcoma. The first and fundamental importance of the work of Martinez and Sissons is to alert the pathologist against too ready a diagnosis of a cyst based on the findings at the margin of a haemorrhagic cyst lined with an osteoid layer and reproducing what is observed in a pure aneurysmal cyst, but which may coexist with a true tumour. The second point is to raise the question: What is an aneurymsal cyst? Is it an entity, or a stage in the evolution of certain tumours, or a mode of reaction to a cause of which we are ignorant?

The hypothesis of an arteriovenous aneurysm has been proposed, but it is a strange aneurysm which is accompanied by such a cellular proliferation that it sometimes represents virtually the entire lesion. In adult pathology, it is rather the exceptional diagnosis of aneurysmal cyst which is difficult to confirm, but it is certain that between 20 and 30 years of age the diagnosis may be confused with that of giant-cell tumour of telangiectatic appearance. In paediatric pathology, it is the diagnosis of a rare giant-cell tumour which may be difficult to make. In cystic chondroblastoma, the tissue surrounding the haemorrhagic cavity is usually quite characteristic, even without mentioning the detection of the presence of cartilaginous islands, which sometimes require numerous sections. This association in chondroblastoma is not without prognostic significance since in such cases recurrence after curettage is 4-5 times as common as in chondroblastomas lacking these appearances.

Although the radiological and histological appearances are not absolutely specific, they are generally sufficiently characteristic to identify an aneurysmal cyst despite our ignorance of its aetiology and physiopathology.

When similar appearances coexist with those of a benign or malignant tumour, it is the terminology appropriate to the tumour which must be retained since this usually determines the treatment and course. It is the tumour that recurs rather than the cyst. Why cloud the issue? It is simpler to speak of a cystic zone, or report that the tumour is of a cystic nature, or even that there is a cavity resembling an aneurysmal cyst than to speak of "a lesional association". This attitude seems to be confirmed by a study of 238 cases of aneurysmal cysts by our colleagues at the Mayo Clinic [Vergel de Dios et al 1992], from which it emerges that this cyst is a distinct pathological entity.

Aneurysmal cyst of the soft tissues

Rodriguez-Peralto et al (1994) describe an aneurysmal cyst of the soft tissues. Previously, Salm and Sissons (1972) had described "giant-cell tumours of the soft tissues", some of which were cystic, without going so far as to consider them as being aneurysmal cysts.

References

Arlet V, Rigault P, Padovani JP, Mallet JF, Finidori G, Thouzet PH (1987) Le kyste anévrismal des os chez l'enfant. Etude de 28 cas. Rev Chir Orthop 73: 337-348

Berson B, Abdelwahab IF, Hermann G, Klein MJ (1989) Aneurysmal bone cyst of the acetabulum (case report). Skeletal Radiol 18: 547-549

Biesecker JL, Marcove RC, Huvos AG, Miké V (1970) Aneurysmal bone cysts. A clinicopathological study of 66 cases. Cancer 26: 615-625

Billey T, Dromer C, Massri A, Ginesty E, Gigaud M, Foumic B, Lassoued S (1993) Kyste anévrismal osseux cervical. A propos de deux observations. Rachis 5: 133-136

Buraczewski J, Dabska M (1971) Pathogenesis of aneurysmal bone cyst. Relationship between the aneurysmal bone cyst and fibrous dysplasia of bone. Cancer 28: 597-604

Bumstein MI, De Smet AA, Hafez GR, Heiner JP (1990) Subperiosteal aneurysmal bone cyst of tibia (case report). Skeletal Radiol 19: 294-297

Campanacci M (1986) Unicameral and aneurysmal bone cysts. Clin Orthop 204: 25-26

Capanna R, Abbisinni U, Calderoni P, Campanacci M, Springfield S (1975) Aneurysmal bone cyst of the spine. J Bone Joint Surg 67A: 527-531

Capanna R, Van Horm JR, Biagini R, Ruggieri P (1989) Aneurysmal bone cyst of the sacrum. Skeletal Radiol 18: 109-113

Coltalorda J, Bollini G, Panvel M, Scheiner C, Jouve JL, Labriet C, Bouyala JM (1993) Le kyste anévrismal des os chez l'enfant. Rev Chir Orthop 79: 272-280

Copin G, Heckel T, Dosch JC (1990) Kyste anévrismal de l'os: à propos de deux cas au niveau de la cheville. Med Chir Pied 63: 139-141

Cristofaro (de) R, Biagini R, Ricci S, Ruggieri P, Rossi G, Fabbri N, Roversi R (1992) Selective arterial embolization in the treatment of aneurysmal bone cyst and angioma of bone. Skelatal Radiol 21: 523-527

Dabska M, Buraczwski J (1969) Aneurysmal bone cyst: pathology, clinical course and radiological appearance. Cancer 23: 371-389

Daffner RH, Linetsky L, Zabklar JH (1987) Aneurysmal bone cyst of T8. Skeletal Radiol 16: 428-432

Dahlin D, Unni KK (1986) Bone tumors: general aspects and data on 8,542 cases. 4th edn. Charles C Thomas, Springfield, pp 420-430

Dahlin DC, Mcleod RA (1982) Aneurysmal bone cyst and other non neoplastic conditions. Skeletal Radiol 8: 243-250

Daudet M, Faysse MJ, Vauzelle JL, Baulieu J, Rebouillat J, Lapras C (1971) Le kyste anévrismal osseux chez l'enfant. Ann Chir Inf 12: 7-33

Diereks RL, Sauter AJM, Mallens WMC (1986) Aneurysmal bone cyst in association with fibrous dysplasia. J Bone Joint Surg 48B: 144-146

Forest M, Le Charpentier Y, Carlioz A, Abelanet R, Tomeno B, Postel M, Maurer P, Kerboul M (1977) Le kyste anévrismal des os: maladie ou symptôme. Nouv Presse Med 6: 2889-2890

Hay MC, Paterson D, Taylor TKF (1978) Aneurysmal bone cysts of the spine. J Bone Joint Surg 60: 406-411

Jaffe HL (1950) Aneurysmal bone cysts. Bull Hosp Joint Dis 11: 3-13

Kein GM, Spector HL, Nernoff J (1982) Aneurysmal bone cyst of stemum (case report). Skeletal Radiol 8: 299-302

Kyriakos M, Hardy D (1991) Malignant transfommation of aneurysmal bone cyst, with an analysis of the literature. Cancer 68: 1770-1780

Levy WM, Miller AS, Bonakdarpour A, Aegerter E (1975) Aneurysmal bone cyst secondary to other osseaus lesions. Report of 57 cases. Am J Clin Path 63: 1-8

Lichtenstein L (1950) Aneurysmal bone cyst, a pathological entity commonly mistaken for giant-cell tumor and occasionnaly for hemangioma and osteogenic sarcoma. Cancer 3: 279-289

Lichtenstein L (1953) Aneurysmal bone cysts. Further observations. Cancer 6: 1228-1237

Macqueen M, Chalmers J, Smith GD (1985) Spontaneous healing of aneurysmal bone cysts, a report of two cases. J Bone Joint Surg (br vol) 67: 310-312

Marcove RC, Sheth DS, Takemoto S, Healey JH (1995) The treatment of aneurysmal bone cyst. Clin Orthop and Relat Res 311: 157-163

Martinez V, Sissons HA (1988) Aneurysmal bone cyst. A review of 123 cases including primary lesions and those secondary to other bone pathology. Cancer 61: 2291-2304

Misasi N, Gigala F, Iaccarino V, Cozzolino F, Sadlle F, Marasco E (1982) Selective arterial embolisation in aneurysmal bone cysts. Int Orthop (SICOT) 6: 123-128

Moreau CA (1981) Kystes anévrismaux. Ann Orthop Ouest 13: 47-53

Nezelof C, Michel J, D'Amato J (1960) Le kyste anévrismal de l'os. Ses principaux caractères anatomo-radiologiques. Rev Chir Orthop 46: 369-383

Nobler MP, Higinbatham NL, Phillips RF (1968) The cure of aneurysmal bone cyst. Irradiation superior to surgery in an analysis of 33 cases. Radiology 90: 1185-1192

Onimus M, Belot, Vauzelle JL (1984) A propos de kyste anévrismal du radius. Problèmes pathogéniques et thérapeutiques. Rev Chir Orthop 70: 335-341

Rodriguez-Peralto JL, Lopez-Borea F, Sanchez-Herrera S, Atienza M (1994) Primary aneurysmal bone cyst of soft tissue (extraosseous aneurysmal bone cyst). Am J Surg Pathol 18: 632-636

Ruiter DJ, Lindeman J, Haverkate F, Noordhoek Hegt V (1975) Fibrinolytic activity in aneurysmal bone cysts. Am J Clin Pathol 64: 810-816

Ruiter DJ, Van Rijssel THG, Van Der Velde EA (1977) Aneurysmal bone cysts: a clinicopathologic study of 105 cases. Cancer 39: 2231-2239

Salm R, Sissons HA (1972) Giant-cell tumours of soft tissues. J Pathol 107: 27-39

Sanerkin NG, Mott MG, Roylance J (1983) An unusual intra-osseous lesion with fibroblastic, osteoclastic, osteoblastic, aneurysmal and fibromyxoid elements. "Solid" variant of aneurysmal bone cyst. Cancer 51: 2278-2286

Tillman BP, Dahlin DC, Lipscomb RR, Stewan JR (1968) Aneurysmal bone cyst: an analysis of ninety-five cases. Mayo Clin Proc 43: 478-495

Vade A, Wilbur A, Puollowski R, Ghosh L (1989) Osteoblastoma of sacrum with secondary aneurysmal bone cyst (case report). Skeletal Radiol 18: 475-480

Verbiest H (1965) Giant-cell tumours and aneurysmal bone cysts of the spine with special reference to the problems related to the removal of a venebral body. J Bone Joint Surg 47A: 699-713

Vergel De Dios A, Bond JR, Shives TC, McLeod RA, Unni KK (1992) Aneurysmal bone cyst. A clinicopathologic study of 238 cases. Cancer 69: 2921-2931

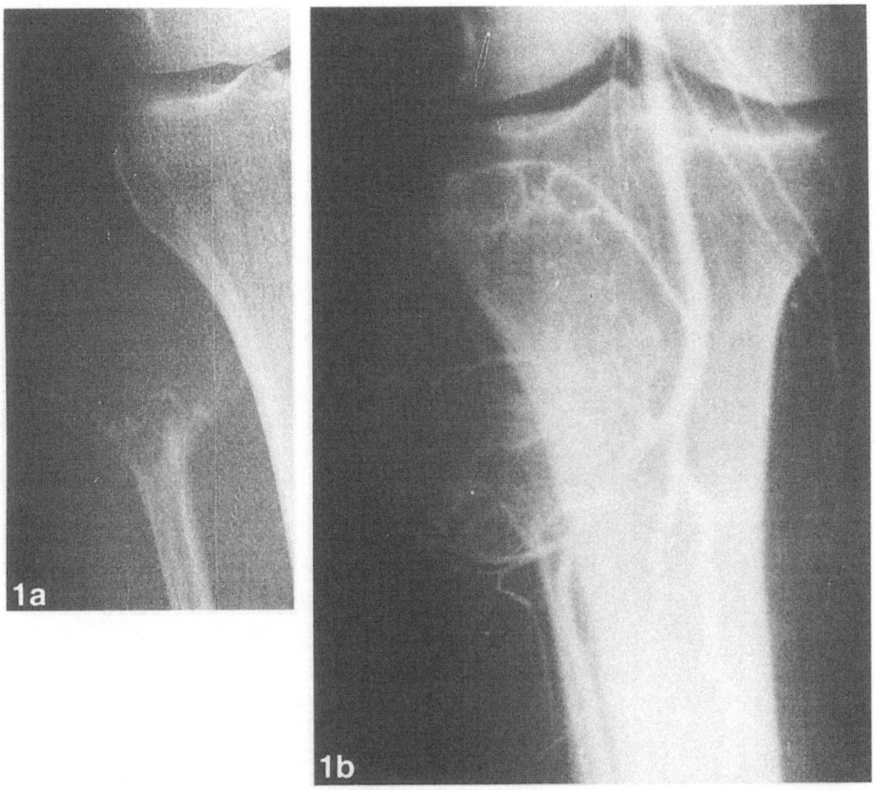

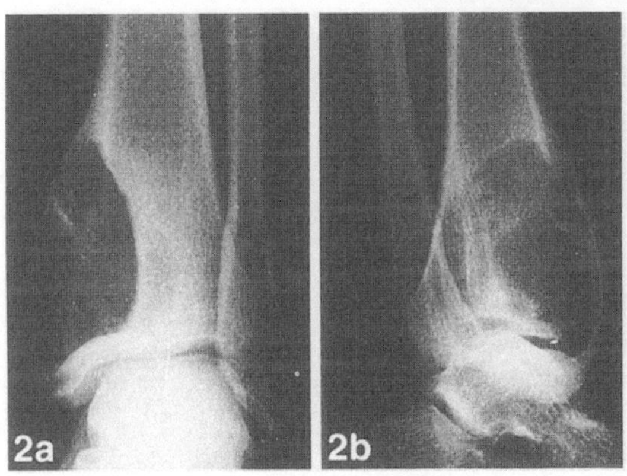

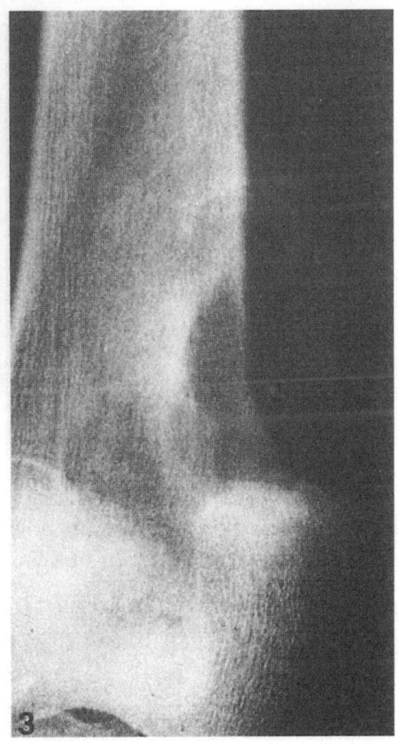

Fig. 1. a Aneurysmal cyst of upper end of fibula, metaphyseal and epiphyseal. **b** Angiography shows the peripheral arterial plexus but does not inject the cystic cavities

Fig. 2. a Cyst of medial malleolus of girl of 16, well circumscribed. **b** It occupies the anteroposterior thickness of the malleolus

Fig. 3. Cyst developing in lower femoral metaphysis, mainly superficial

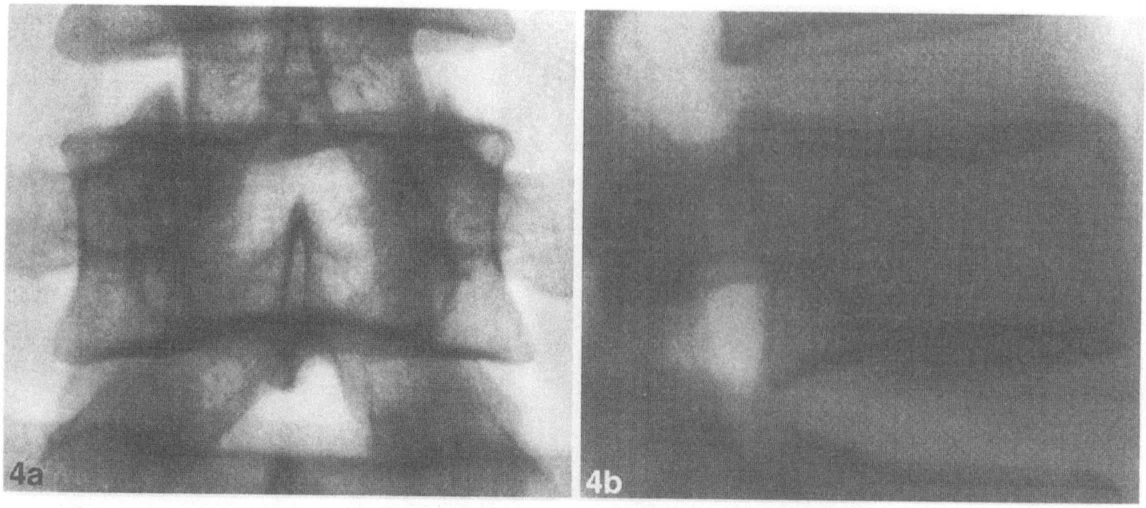

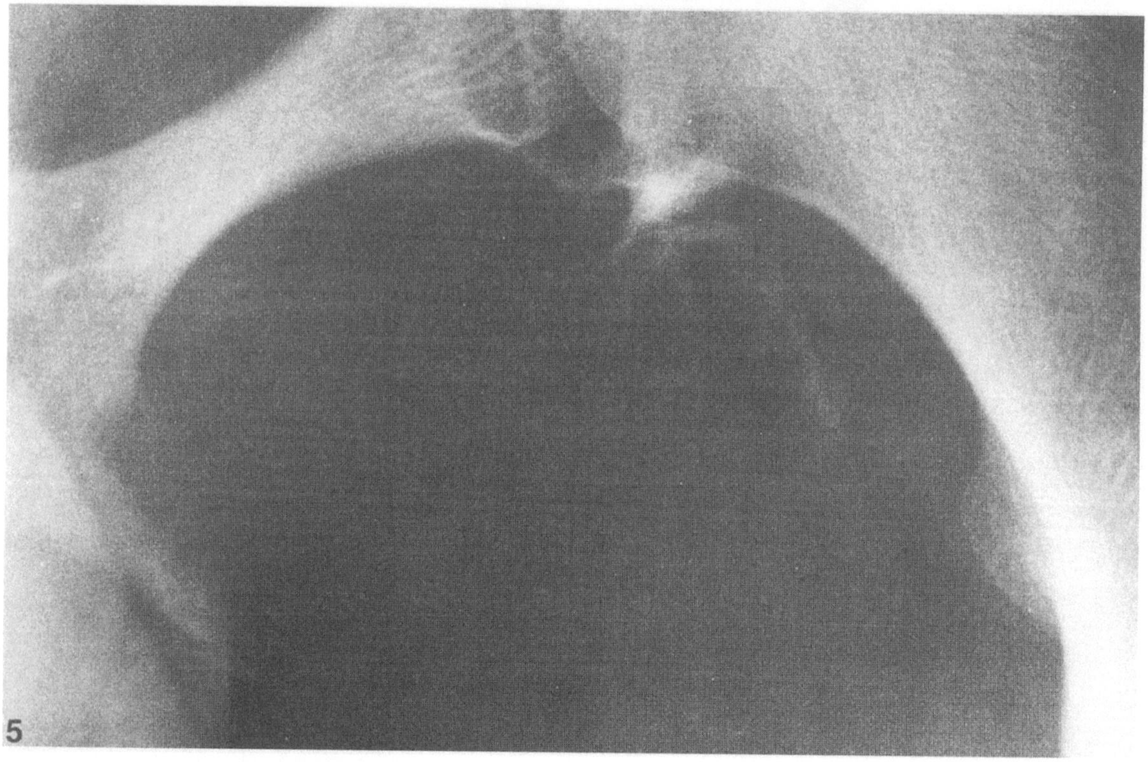

Fig. 4 a, b. Though aneurysmal cysts usually arise in the posterior vertebral arch, this one occupies the vertebral body of L4 in a man of 27 suffering from Ehlers-Danlos disease

Fig. 5. The ischiopubic ramus is completely destroyed by a large aneurysmal cyst whose boundaries are visible only in the vicinity of the ilium on the one hand and the pubis on the other

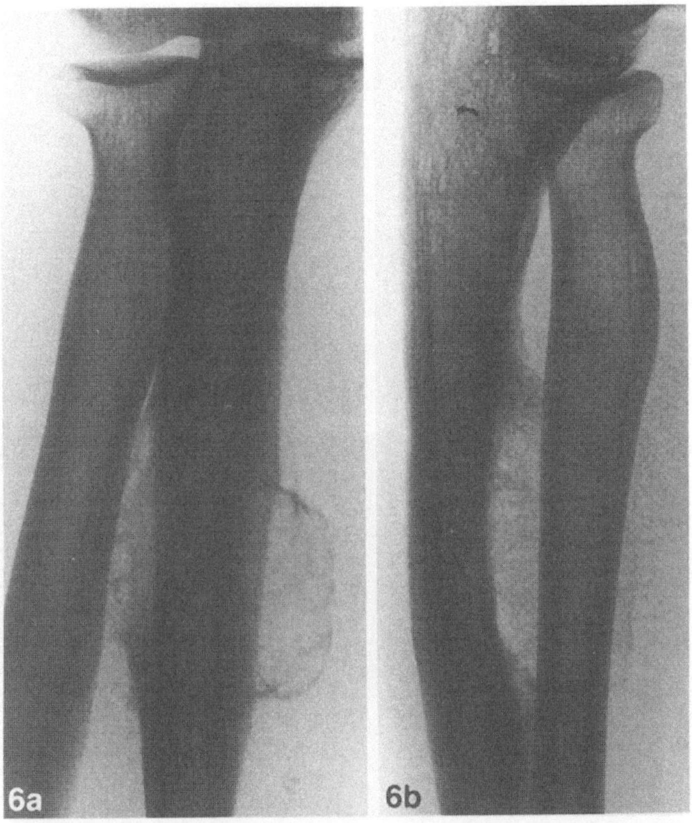

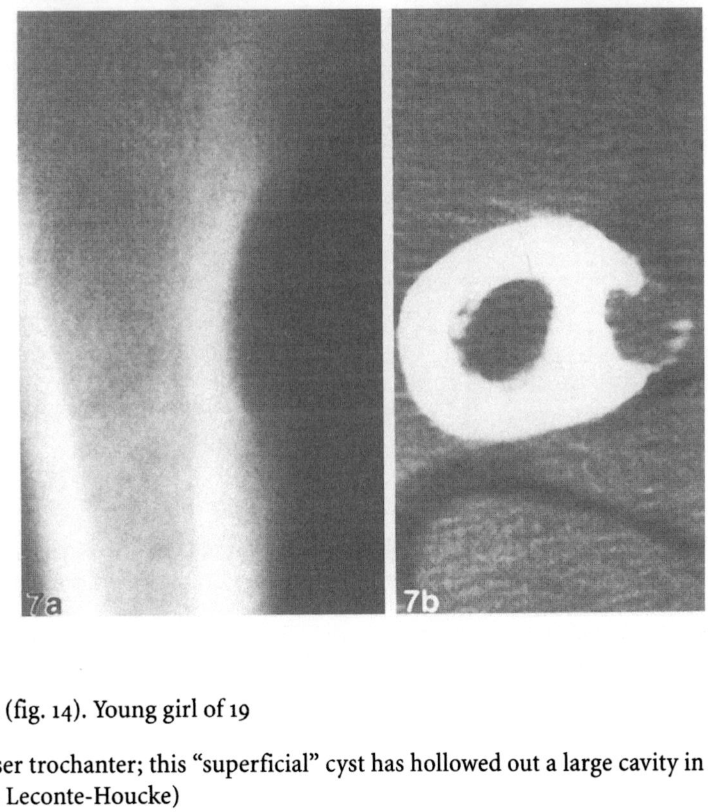

Fig. 6 a, b. Diaphyseal cyst ensheathing the ulna (fig. 14). Young girl of 19

Fig. 7 a, b. Medial aspect of femur below the lesser trochanter; this "superficial" cyst has hollowed out a large cavity in the cortex (young man of 19). (Courtesy of Prof. Leconte-Houcke)

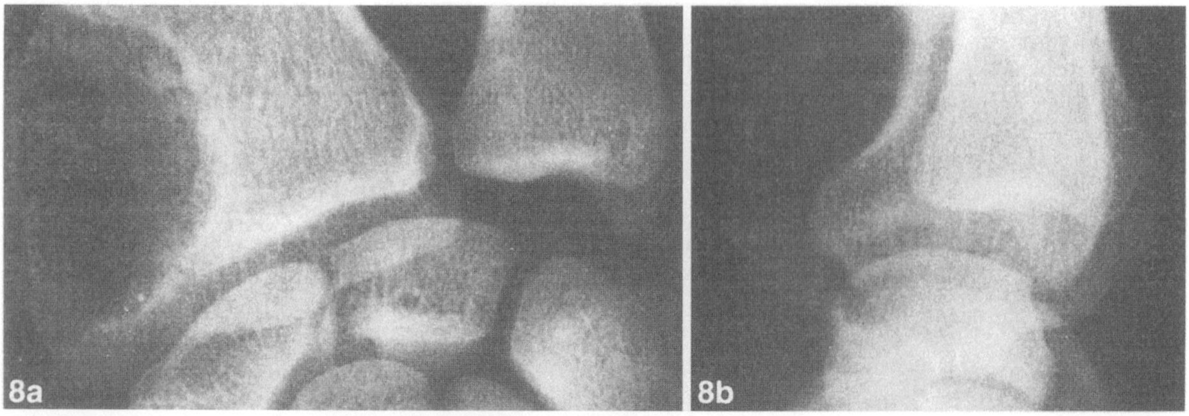

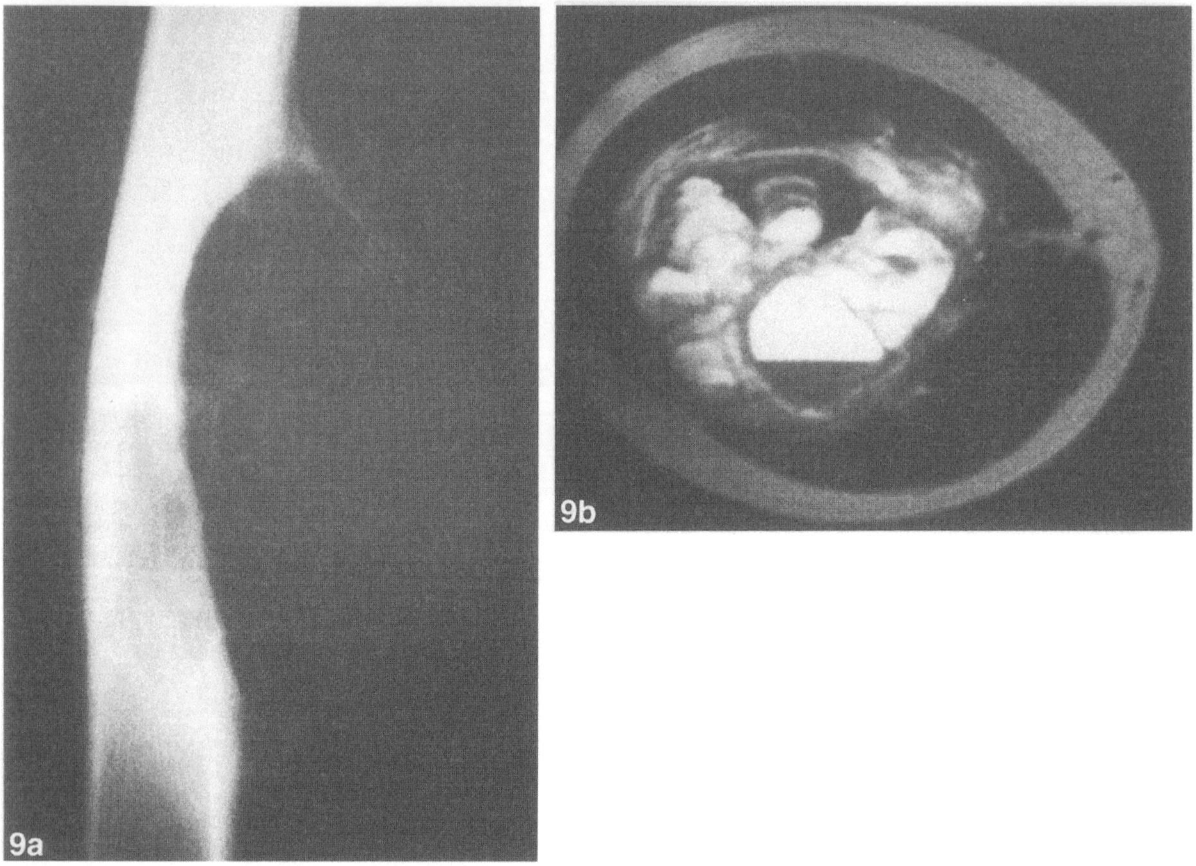

Fig. 8 a, b. In the frontal view (**a**), the cyst seems to have developed entirely within the lower end of the radius. The lateral view (**b**) demonstrates the expansile nature of this lesion, with an "egg-cup" image due to periosteal apposition

Fig. 9 a, b. Aneurysmal cyst, mass in right femur. **a** Standard lateral view: very well circumscribed lytic diaphyseal lesion with periosteal spurs. Girl of 16. **b** MRI [axial section, T2 weighting (TR2000, TR100)]: the lesion consists of multiple cavities containing a horizontal level; the upper part is white, the lower black. Visualisation of deposit of cells and haemoglobin degradation products in cavities containing blood with slow circulation

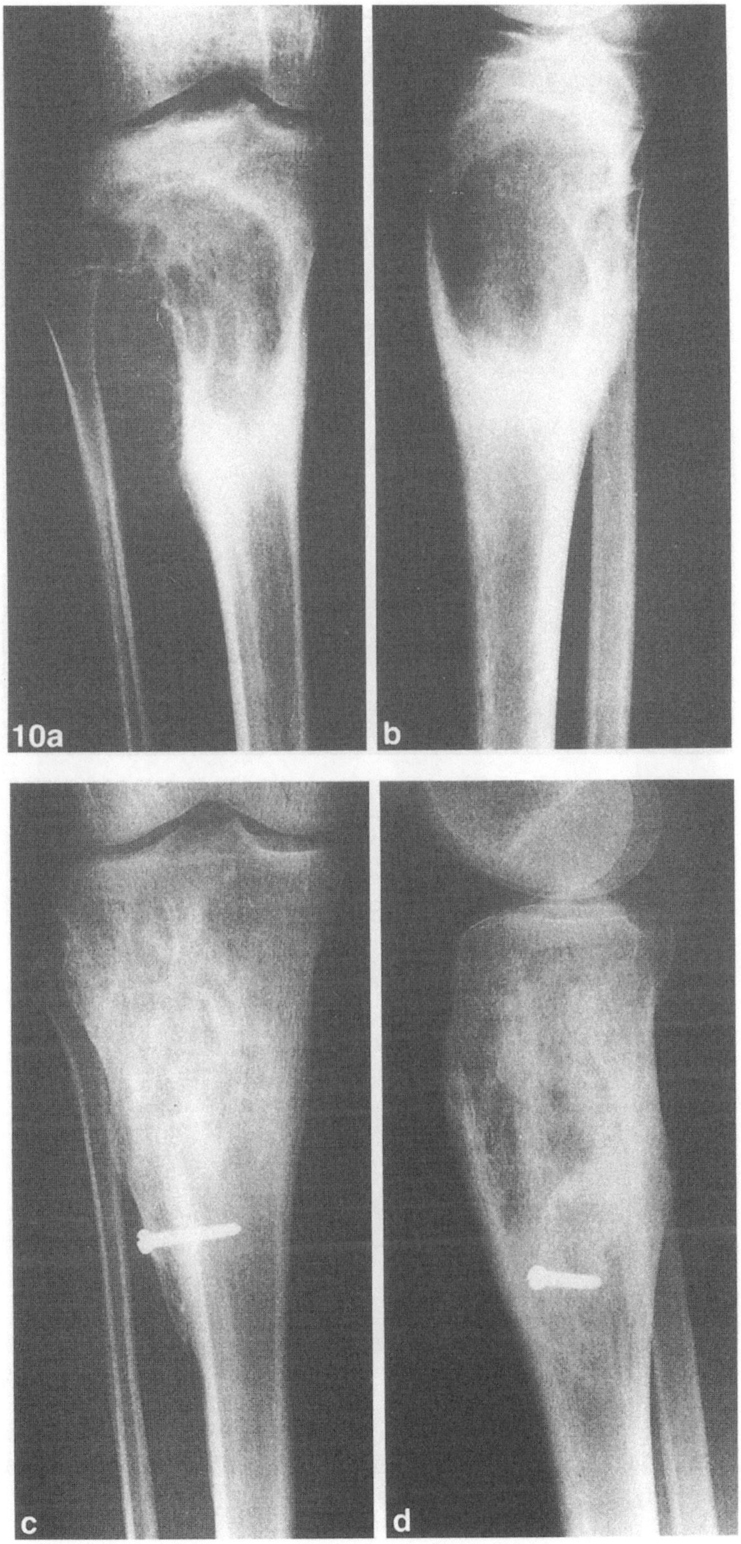

Fig. 10 a-d. Cyst of upper end of tibia in which the lateral view shows limitation of the lesion by the growth plate (**a, b**). Three years after surgical intervention (curettage and packing) the tibia is slowly regaining its normal structure (**c, d**)

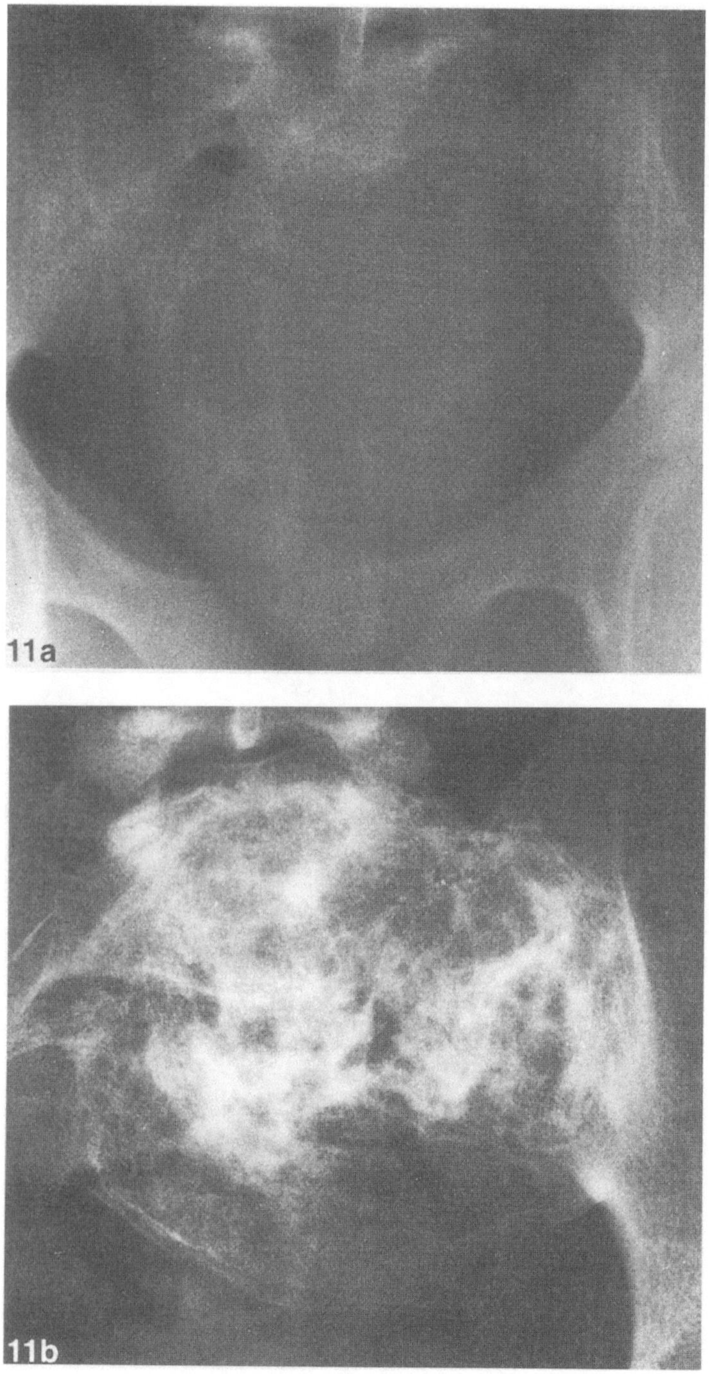

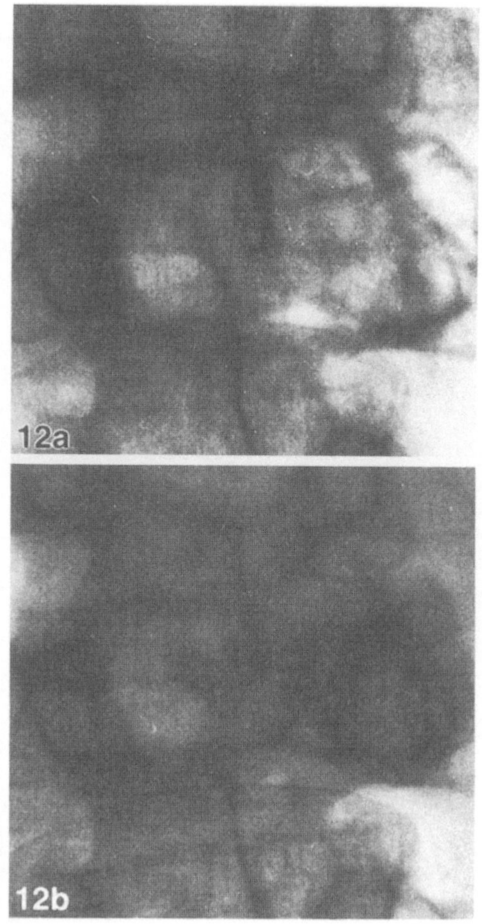

Fig. 11 a, b. At the age of 13, this girl suffered from sciatica. Radiography showed major lysis of the sacrum (**a**). Histological examination led to a diagnosis of aneurysmal cyst. The lesion was irradiated and 10 years later (**b**) it is calcified and apparently stabilised (archive records)

Fig. 12 a, b. This aneurysmal cyst of the posterior hemi-arch of L2 with invasion of part of the vertebral body has been irradiated (**a**). This treatment was followed by virtually total recalcification (archive records) (**b**)

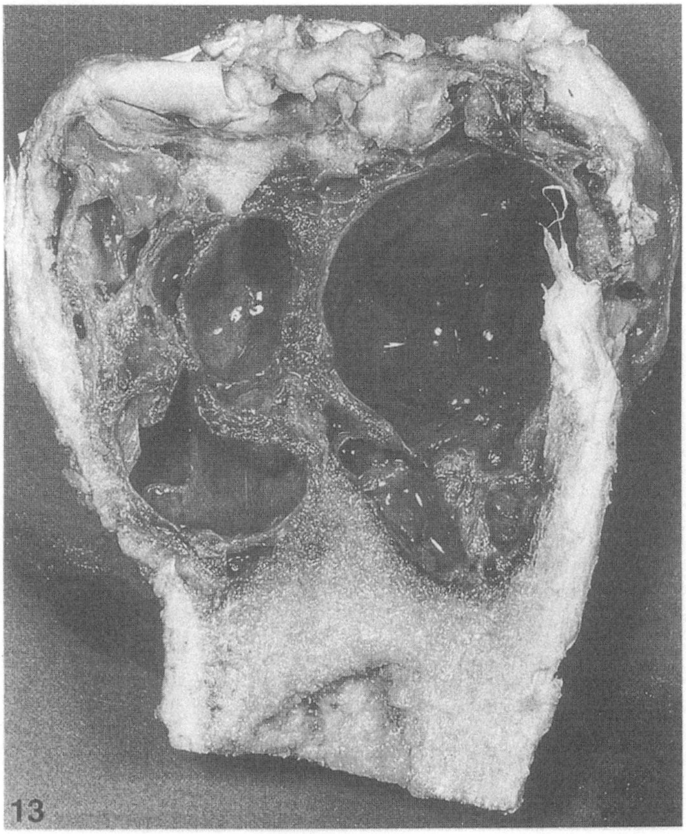

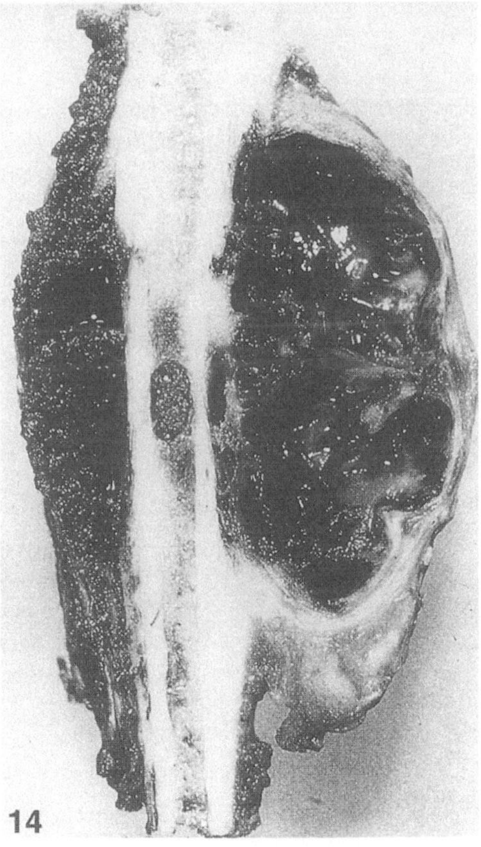

Fig. 13. Resection of upper end of tibia after recurrence following curettage (lad of 17). The main cavity, sited anteriorly, communicates with several smaller cavities situated in the posterior part of the metaphysis. These smooth-walled cavities were occupied by a blood-stained effusion. The whole of this structure is well demarcated

Fig. 14. The cyst ensheaths the ulna (fig. 6), destroys the outer part of the cortex and penetrates the medullary canal. At the upper and lower limits of the cyst the cortex is thickened by the periosteal reaction

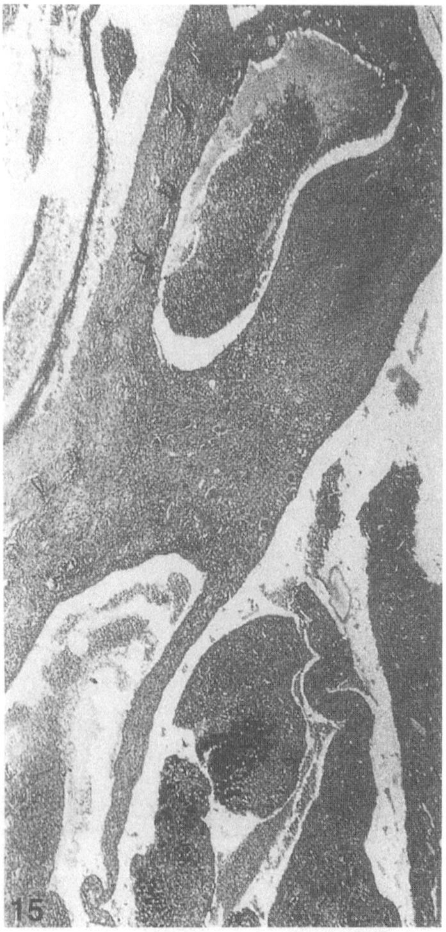

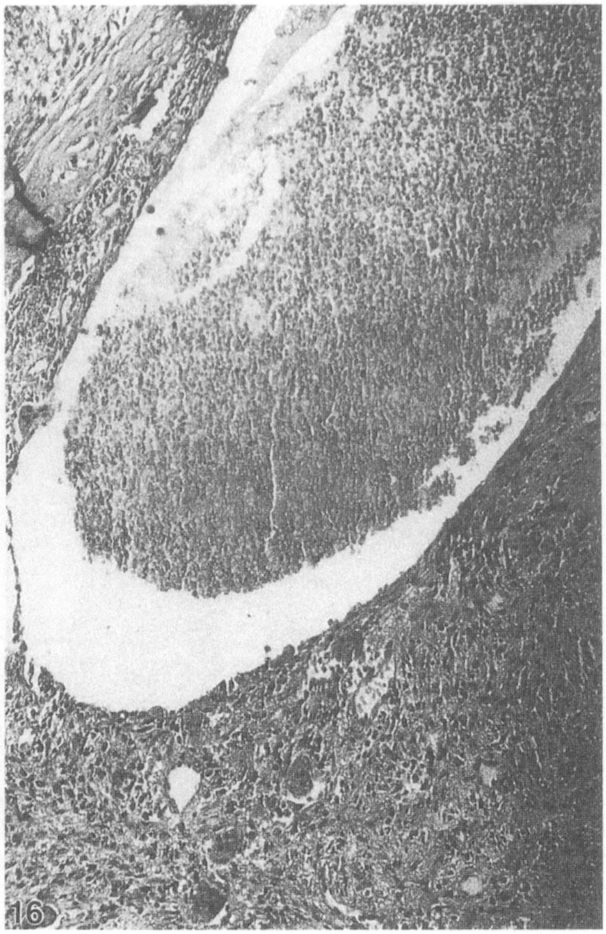

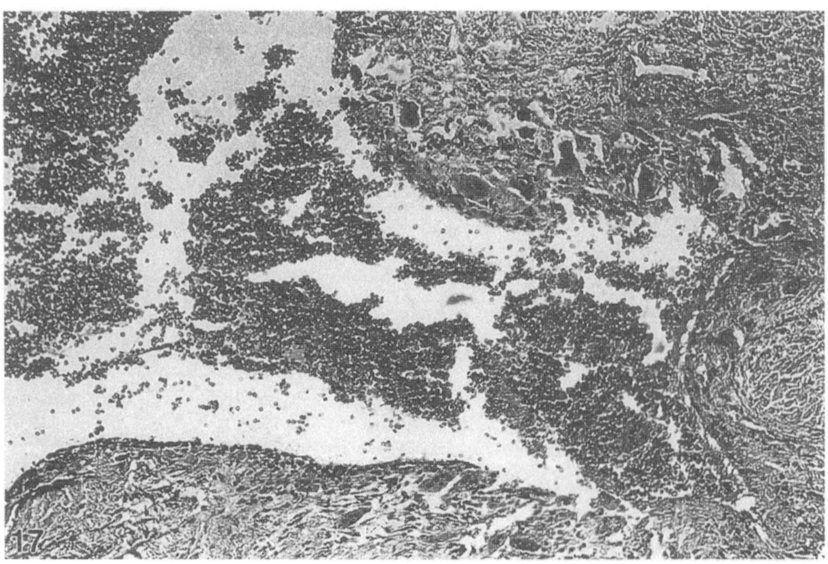

Fig. 15. In this sectional plane, the microphotograph demonstrates cavities separated from one another by septa of varying thickness

Figs. 16, 17. At this magnification erythrocytes are seen, in the walls of the multinuclear cells and the lumen, sometimes in clumps and sometimes separate from one another. In fig. 17 the cavity is bounded on the right by a fine hyaline osteoid band based on fibrous tissue

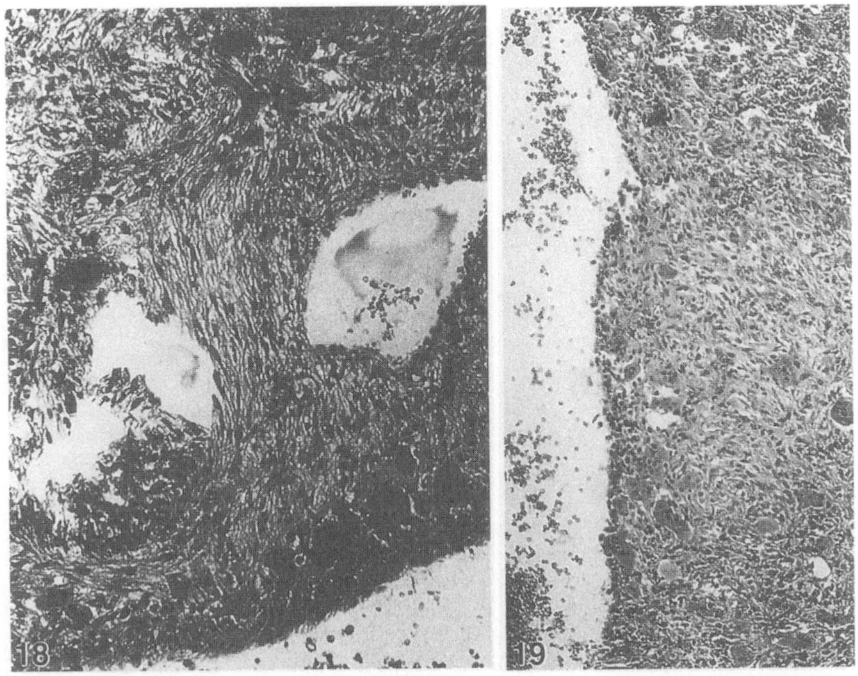

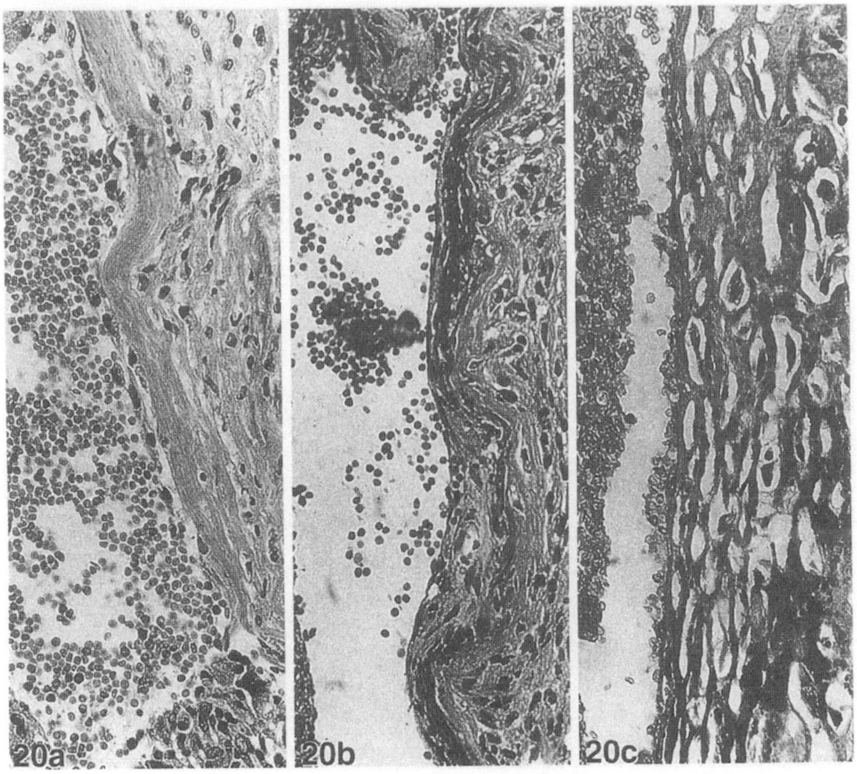

Figs. 18, 19. In fig. 18 band of fibrous tissue separates two cavities. In fig. 19 the cavity is bordered by a moderately cellular tissue without discernable endothelium. Presence of some multinuclear giant cells

Fig. 20. a, b, c show different aspects of an osteoid band, partly calcified in **b** and **c**. The osteoid is separated from the blood cavity only by a fine cellular layer in **a** and **b** which may represent an endothelium

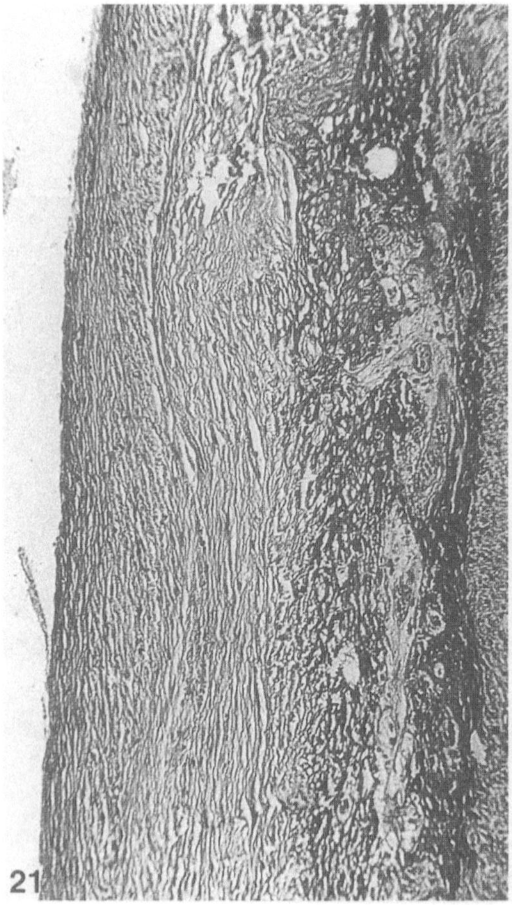

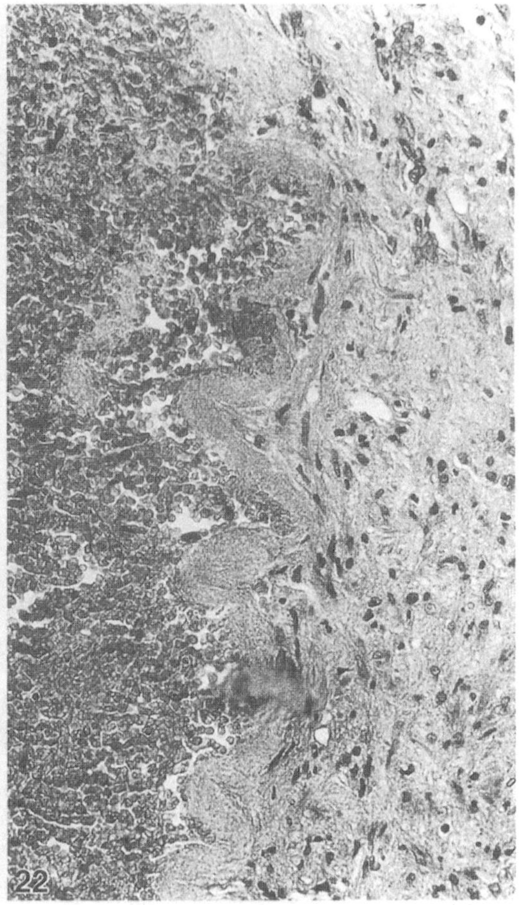

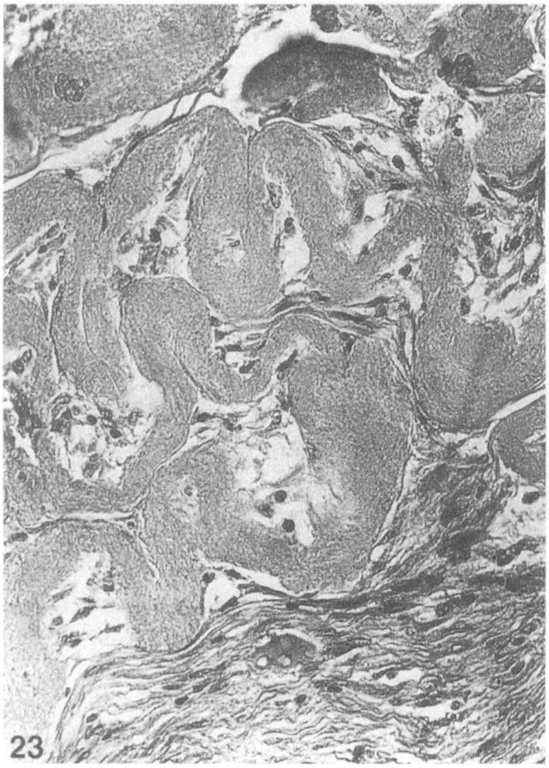

Fig. 21. The zone of calcified osteoid tissue is separated from the cavity by dense fibrous tissue

Fig. 22. It is commonplace to observe a band of hyaline tissue bordering a blood cavity; its wavy aspect is probably related to the technique

Fig. 23. This hyaline tissue may be the beginning of osteoid tissue (purely hypothetical)

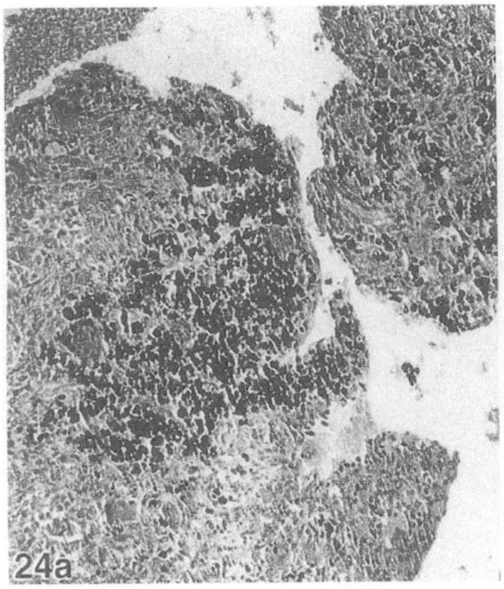

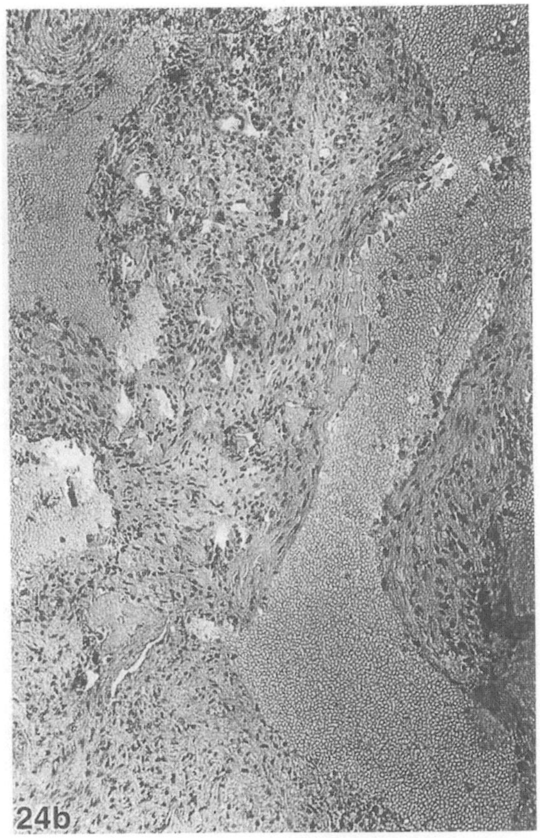

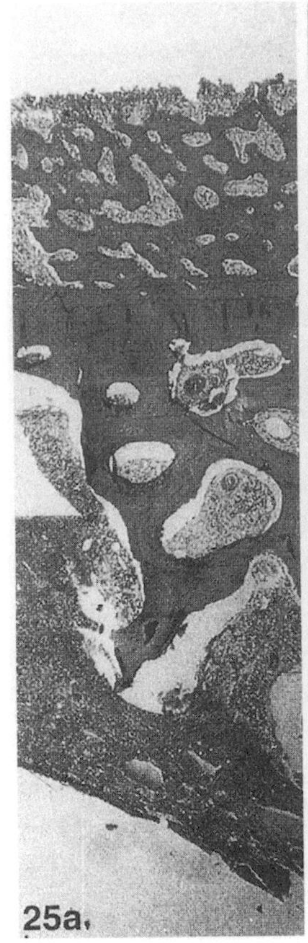

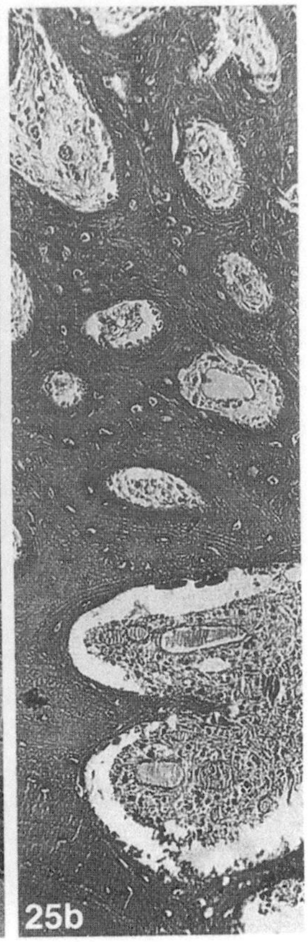

Fig. 24 a, b. Cyst of a cervical vertebra. The cavities are filled with red cells. There is no osteoid border but some calcified zones here and there (**a**)

Fig. 25. a From below upwards, the cyst lumen, its histiocyto-fibroblastic wall, the spongy cortical bone and the reactive periosteal osteogenesis. **b** From below upwards, cortical haversian bone of lamellar type, then immature periosteal bone with stout fibers

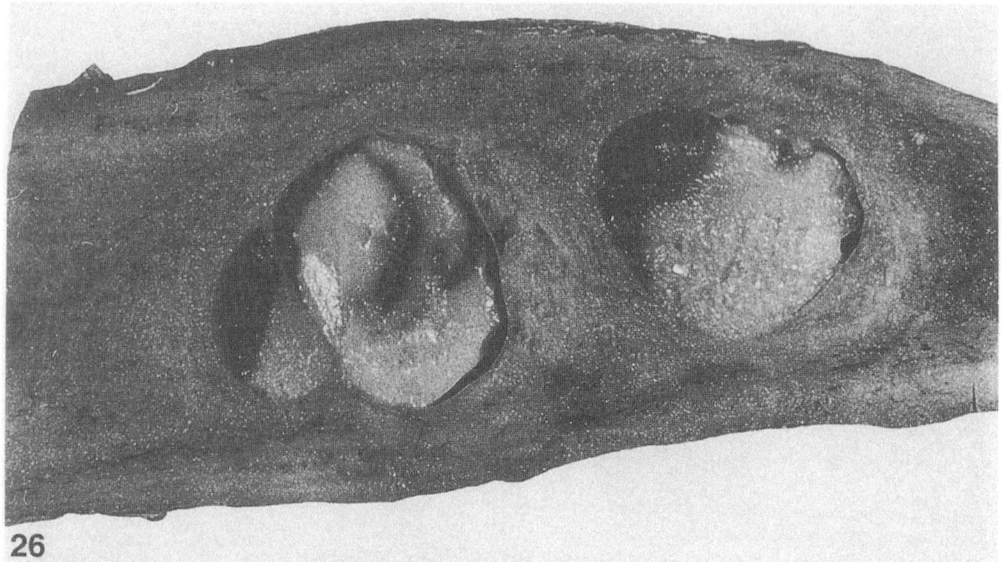

26

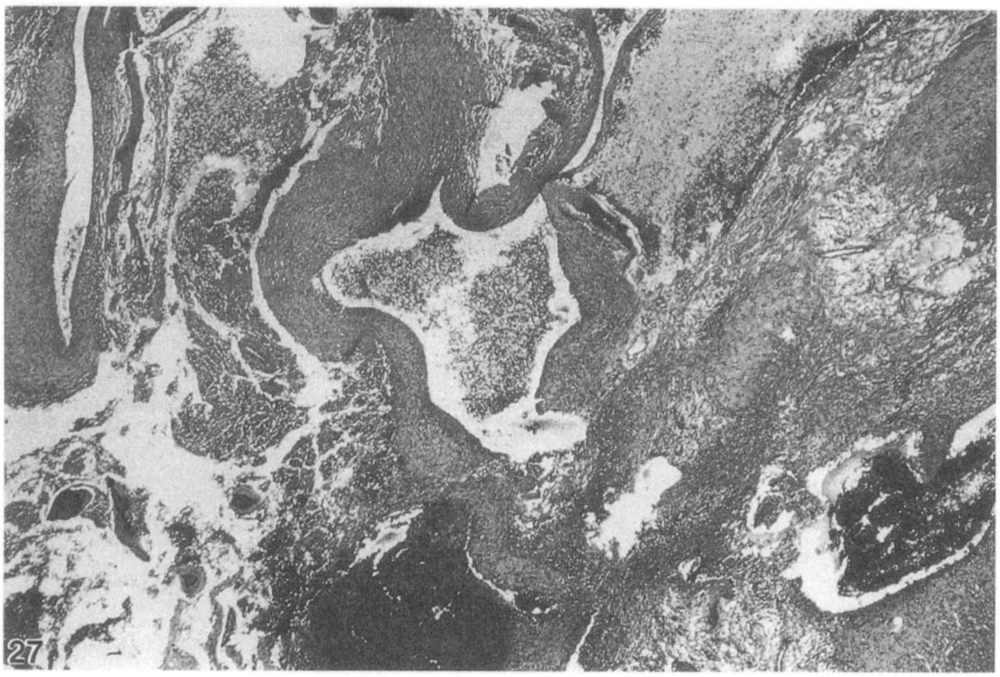

27

Fig. 26. Resection of a rib "blow-out". The blood cavities are surrounded by fibrous tissue and the rib is enlarged by periosteal apposition. This is not an angioma, nor an aneurysmal cyst, but fibrous dysplasia which has undergone cyst formation. After resection it was not the pseudo-aneurysmal cyst that recurred but the fibrous dysplasia, in a compact form without cavity formation

Fig. 27. A case of cavitation which could be confused with an aneurysmal cyst. This too is fibrous dysplasia

31. Langerhans'cell histiocytosis: histiocytosis X, eosinophil granuloma

The almost uniform affection of the bone in this disorder explains the frequency of biopsies sent by orthopaedists.

Clinical review

The finding by clinicians of intermediate stages between eosinophil granuloma and Hand-Schüller-Christian disease on the one hand, and between the latter and Letterer-Siwe disease on the other, led Jaffe in 1953 to suggest the grouping of these entities under the title of histiocytosis X.

In 1956, ultrastructural studies [Basset, Turiaf & Basset, Nezelof] demonstrated a particular structure in the cytoplasm of the histiocytes of bony and visceral lesions providing a new argument in favor of a unitary concept. Lastly, since 1973 [Nezelof et al 1973] the Langerhans cell origin of histiocytosis X has been widely accepted on the basis of both the clinical and morphological findings, the marker of the histiocytic cells of histiocytosis X being identical to the Langerhans cell granules. These proliferative disorders of the Langerhans cell system and its physiological role have been remarkably well discussed in the work of Barbey and Nezelof (1986).

Histiocytosis is now classified as:

- localised (bony: eosinophil granuloma, unifocal and pulmonary);
- disseminated, acute and subacute (Letter-Siwe disease);
- disseminated, chronic (multifocal eosinophil granuloma, Hand-Schüller-Christian disease).

The cure of eosinophil granuloma may lead to a restitution ad integrum; a collapsed vertebra may become a virtually normal vertebra again (fig. 3). No information from the examination of sections can foretell if the bony lesion examined will remain solitary or if other lesions will appear.

Letterer-Siwe disease is an acute disseminated form which affects children under the age of two years. The osteolytic lesions are often accompanied by an inflammatory syndrome with hepatosplenomegaly, erythemato-squamous rash, pulmonary involvement, anaemia and thrombocytopaenia. This thrombocytopaenia is regarded as indicating a poor prognosis; until recently, the mortality was of the order of 40%.

Hand-Schüller-Christian disease is seen essentially in later childhood and adolescence. The bony lacunae may be associated with diabetes insipidus and exophthalmos, and though the prognosis is better than that of the previous form its cure may leave complications.

While in children a histiocytosis X that remains silent for 3 years may be considered to be cured, we have seen the appearance of new lesions in adults after intervals of 4-6 years. It should be noted that a multiplicity of lesions is regarded as a bad prognostic factor.

Eosinophil granuloma

General considerations

Localised eosinophil granuloma is seen mainly in older children and young adults. There is a male predominance. Lesions of the bones of the skull (35-40%) and of the pelvis are commoner before the age of 20; then come the scapulae, ribs, vertebrae and proximal ends of the long bones [Sessa et al 1992]. Lesions in the bones distal to the elbow and knee are much more rare, and the observation of Strousse et al (1992) of symmetric lesions of eosinophil granuloma in both tibiae is unusual. In the study of Lieberman et al (1996) dealing with 238 patients, the disorder was manifested in most cases during the first 15 months of life and males were affected predominantly.

Imaging

The radiographic image is of a lacunar osteolysis with often very clear-cut outlines. In the flat bones (including the skull) destruction of both tables is complete. In the ilium (fig. 4) the lesions sometimes assume the appearance of multilocular cysts. Involvement of the temporal bone may be associated with an otitic syndrome. The vertebral lesions affect either the body (vertebral compression) or the posterior arch. In the long bones the lesion is metaphyseal (figs. 6, 7) or diaphyseal in different series. The bony lacuna may be accompanied by a lamellar periosteal reaction. In the case reported by Thyn et al (1990) in a girl of 2, the entire fibular shaft was ballooned by an expansile lesion.

In the disseminated forms some lacunae may regress and disappear during the course of the disease, while others appear de novo.

Pathological anatomy and histopathology

Some essential concepts must be familiar to pathologists faced with a bone biopsy. It is important to emphasise that the pathological nuances described between Letterer-Siwe disease, Hand-Schüller-Christian syndrome and eosinophil granuloma are more presumptive than factual and that the essential common feature is the histiocytoid Langerhans cell. The pathological appearances may vary from case to case and from one lesion to another in the same patient and the duration of the course and the age of the lesion are factors in this diversity. Finally the identification of a bony lesion in no way permits prediction of the course of the disorder, but indicates the need for a complete examination in the search for other bony and visceral lesions.

In its typical forms, the granuloma is remarkable for its polymorphism, its richness in histiocytes, the presence of numerous eosinophil granulocytes and of some small areas of necrosis (figs. 11-14). The histiocytes are variable in size; their cytoplasm is weakly eosinophil, often laden with granules and vacuoles (fig. 16). Depending on the case, the boundaries of the cytoplasm are well-defined or indistinct. The nucleus of the histiocytic cell is quite characteristic: ovoid, kidney-shaped, notched, sometimes with twisted outlines (fig. 15). Some nuclei have a sort of fine ridge parallel to the main axis of the nucleus, a kind of longitudinal median plication. Mitoses are usually few. The granulocytes are sometimes abundant, sometimes rare or even absent. They are grouped in clumps or may be scattered. Nezelof (1963) stressed the fact that these eosinophil granulocytes are likely to be situated in the vicinity of foci of necrosis. Often clearly visible in standard staining, they are best shown by the Giemsa and Mann-Dominici stains. There are also multinuclear histiocytes, polynuclears, lymphocytes, plasmocytes and mononuclear macrophages. Intermediate forms exist between bi- or trinuclear histiocytes and giant cells with 8-10 nuclei. Necrosis often affects numerous small areas but may also be completely absent in a small biopsy.

Differential diagnosis

The sometimes considerable morphological variation does not always permit certainty in diagnosis. The cellular proliferation may be predominantly histiocytic, but the histiocytes may assume a foamy appearance. Fibrosis is sometimes very marked, leaving only a few persistent granulomatous foci.

The pathological appearance may also depart from the typical form by rarity or absence of eosinophil granulocytes, absence of necrosis, an abundant proliferation of polynuclear cells and a very modest histiocytic proliferation. Such appearances may lead to the consideration and subsequent exclusion of infective lesions (bacterial or mycotic osteitis) or of tumours (sarcomatous histiocytic proliferation, Hodgkin's disease).

In some cases the diagnostic difficulties are resolved by immunohistological techniques. A positive reaction to antibodies CD68, CD1 and often CD4 will support a diagnosis of histiocytosis X or Langerhans'cell histiocytosis. Mayo-Smith et al (1989) stressed the positivity of Langerhans cells to the antigenic markers PS100 and CD1. Feng Ye et al (1990) studying 27 cases of histiocytosis X, noted a strongly positive reaction of the histiocytes to the S100 protein in 23 cases; but such a positive reaction does not confirm the diagnosis, given the ubiquitous nature of this protein. More important is the possible demonstration of an epitope of antigen CD1a present on the surface of the mononuclear cells of a Langerhansian histiocytosis [Krenacs et al 1993, Emile et al 1995]. This technique, using antibody 010, works in paraffin-embedded sections of tumours fixed in bouin or formalin.

Lastly, ultrastructural study will reveal the typical pentolamminar granules of Langerhans (or of Birbeck) in the cytoplasm of the histiocytic cells (figs. 18-21). The ultrastructural appearances minutely described by Basset and Nezelof (1969) in an attempt to identify criteria of malignancy have led to the conclusion that an atypical morphological appearance of the Langerhans cells observed in a biopsy does not allow prediction of the clinical outcome of the disorder.

References

Barbey S, Nezelof C (1986) Le système Langerhansien. Définition, modification physiologiques et pathologiques. Patn Biol 34: 259-273

Basset F, Nezelof C (1969) L'histiocytose X. Microscopie électronique. Culture "in vitro" et histo-enzymologie. Discussion à propos de 21 cas. Rev Fr Et Clin Biol 14: 31-45

Basset-Lacronique FR (1966) L'histiocytose X. Presse Med 74: 2459-2460

Ben-Ezra J, Bailey A, Azumi N, Delsol G (1991) Malignant histiocytosis X. A distinct clinicopathologic entity. Cancer 68: 1050-1060

Calzada LD, Chaussain JL, Job JC (1978) Le retard de croissance au cours de l'histiocytose X. Exploration antéhypophysaire. Sem Hop Paris 54: 41-42

Cheyne C (1971) Histiocytosis X. J Bone Joint Surg 53B: 366-382

Christian MA (1920) Defects in membranous bone, exophthalmos and diabetes insipidus. An unusual syndrome of dyspituitarism. Med Clin North Am 3: 849-871

Compere EL, Johnson WE, Coventry MB (1954) Vertebra plana (Calvé's disease) due to eosinophilic granuloma. J Bone Joint Surg 36A: 969-978

Elema JD, Atmosoerodjo-Briggs JE (1984) Langerhans'cells and macrophages in eosinophilic granuloma: an enzyme-histochemical, erizyme-cytochemical, and ultrastructural study. Cancer 54: 2174-2181

Emile JF, Wechsler J, Brousse N, Boulland ML, Cologon R, Fraitag S, Voisin MC, Gaulard P, Boumsell L, Zafrani E-S (1995) Langerhans' cells histiocytosis. Definitive diagnosis with the use of monoclonal antibody 010 on routinely paraffin-embedded samples. Am J Surg 19: 636-641

Emile JF, Donadieu J, Thomas C, Brousse N (1995) L'histiocytose langerhansienne. Données récentes sur le diagnostic et la physiopathologie. Ann Pathol 15: 252-259

Enriquez P, Dahlin DC, Hayles AB, Henderson ED (1967) Histiocytosis X: a clinical study. Mayo Clin Proc 42: 88-99

Farber S (1941) The nature of "solitary or eosinophilic granuloma" of bone. Am J Pathol 17: 625-629

Feng Ye, Shu-Wei Huang, Hang-Ji Dong (1990) S-100 protein, peanut agglutinin, and transmission electroscopy study. Am J Clin Pathol 94: 627-631

Fowles JV, Bobechko WP (1970) Solitary eosinophilic granuloma in bone. J Bone Joint Surg 52B: 238-243

Fox JL, Berman B (1983) T6-antigen cells in eosinophilic granuloma of bone. JAMA 249: 3071

Hand A (1921) Defects of membranous bones. Exophthalmos and polyuria in childhood in dyspituitarism. Am J Med Sci 16: 509

Imamura M, Muroya K (1971) Lymph node ultrastructure in Hand-Schaller-Christian disease. Cancer 27: 956-964

Krenacs L, Tissalvicz L, Krenacs T, Boumsell L (1993) Immunohistochemical detection of CD1 a antigen in formalin-fixed and paraffin-embedded tissue sections with monoclonal antibody 010. J Pathol 171: 99-104

Letterer E (1924) Aleukamische reticulose. Frankf Ztschc F Pathol 30: 377-394

Lichtenstein L (1953) Histiocytosis X. Integration of eosinophilic granuloma of bone, "Lettrer-Siwe disease" and "Schaller-Christain disease" as related manifestations of a single nosologic entity. AMA Arch Pathol 56: 84-102

Lichtenstein L (1964) Histiocytosis X (eosinophilic granuloma of bone, Letterer-Siwe disease, and Schaller-Christian disease). Further observations of pathological and clinical importance. J Bone Joint Surg 46A: 76-90

Lieberman PH, Jones CR, Fillipa DA (1980) Langerhans cell (eosinophilic) granulomatosis. J Invest Dermatol 75: 71-72

Makley T, Earter JR (1986) Eosinophilic granuloma of bone. Clin Orthop 204: 37-44

Lieberman PH, Ray Jones C, Steinman RM, Erlandson RA, Smith J, Gee T, Huros A, Garin-Chesa P, Filippa DA, Urmacher C, Gangi MD, Sperber M (1996) Langerhans cell (eosinophilic) granulomatosis. A clinicopathologic study encompassing 50 years. Am J Surg Pathol 20: 519-522

Marie J, Hennequet A, Levêque B, Debauchez CL, Desbois CL, Watchi JM (1968) La réticulose histiocytaire du nourrisson ou maladie de Letterer-Siwe. Etude clinique et thérapeutique. Ann Pediatr 45: 2717-2732

Mayo-Smith W, Rosenthal DI, Kattapuram SV, Rosenberg AE (1989) Eosinophilic granuloma of femur case report. Skeletal Radiol 18: 245-247

Navert C, Zornora J, Ayala A, Harle TS (1983) Eosinophilic granuloma of bone: diagnosis and management. Skeletal Radiol 10: 227-235

Nezelof C (1980) Histiocytosis X: a histological and histogenetic study. Perspect Pediatr Pathol 6: 153-178

Nezelof C, Basset F, Rousseau MF (1973) Histiocytose X: histogenic arguments for a Langerhans cell origin. Biomedecine 18: 365-371

Nezelof C, Guibert C (1963) L'histiocytose X. Nosologie et pronostic. Etude fondée sur l'évolution contrôlée de 52 observations personnelles. Arch Fr Pediatr 20: 1063-1103

Poirier J, Dadavne JP (1968) La cellule de Langerhans de l'épiderme. Presse Med 76: 1729-1731

Rigault P, Finidori G (1977) Les localisations vertébrales de l'histiocytose X. Aspect orthopédique. Rev Chir Orthop 63: 190-194

Schajowicz F, Slullitel J (1973) Eosinophilic granuloma of bone and its relationship to Hand-Schaller-Christian and Letterer-Siwe syndromes. J Bone Joint Surg 55B: 545-565

Schüller A (1915) Über eigenartige Schardeldelakte in Ugendalter. Forstchr A D Geb D Rontgen 23: 12-18

Schüller A (1921) Über eine einartige Syndrom von Dyspituitarismus. Wien Med Wschr 71: 510

Sessa S, Sommelet D, Gabet F, Cavave S, Lascombes P, Prevot J (1992) Les localisations osseuses de l'histiocytose X. Rev Chir Orthop 78: 112-123

Shenouda NF, Azouz EM (1991) Langerhansts cell histiocytosis (LCH) of the skin, skull, and mandible with calcifications in associated soft-tissue masses. Case report. Skeletal Radiol 20: 620-623

Siegal GP, Dehner LP, Rosai J (1985) Histiocytosis X (Langerhan's cell granulomatosis) of the thymus. A clinicopathologic study of four childhood cases. Am J Surg Pathol 9: 117-124

Siguier F, Godeau P, Camus JP, Lévy R, Ben Hamida (1963) L'association diabète insipide granulome éosinophile des os. Sem Hop Paris 39: 615-620

Siwe S (1949) The reticulo-endotheliosis in children. Adv Pediatr 4: 117-143

Strouse PJ, Ellis BI, Shifrin LZ, Shah AR (1992) Symmetrical eosinaphilic granuloma of the lower extremities (proven) and Erdbeim-Chester disease (probable). Skeletal Radiol 21: 64-67

Thijn CJP, Martijn A, Postma A, Molenaar WM (1990) Histiocytosis X (eosinophilic granuloma of the fibula) case report. Skeletal Radiol 19: 309-311

Turpin R, Véron P, Bocquet L, Gorin R, Caille B, Lafourcade J, Roustan B, Cruveiller J (1965) Maladie granulomateuse histiocytaire (histiocytose X). A propos de deux observations. Ann Pediatr 41: 6-23

Tusques J, Pradal G (1969) Analyse tridimensionnelle des inclusions rencontrées dans les histiocytes de l'histiocytose X en microscopie électronique. Comparaison avec les inclusions des cellules de Langerhans. J Microscopie 8: 113-122

Wolfson WL, Gossett T, Pagani J (1976) Systemic giant-cell histiocytosis. Report of a case and review of the the adult form of Letterer-Siwe disease. Cancer 38: 2529-2537

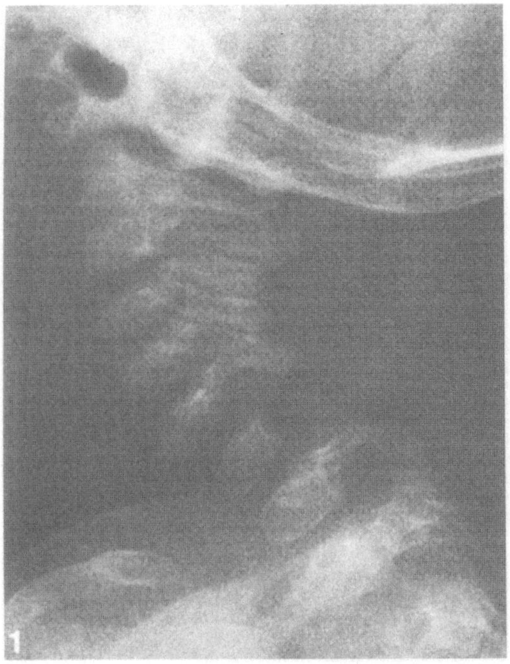

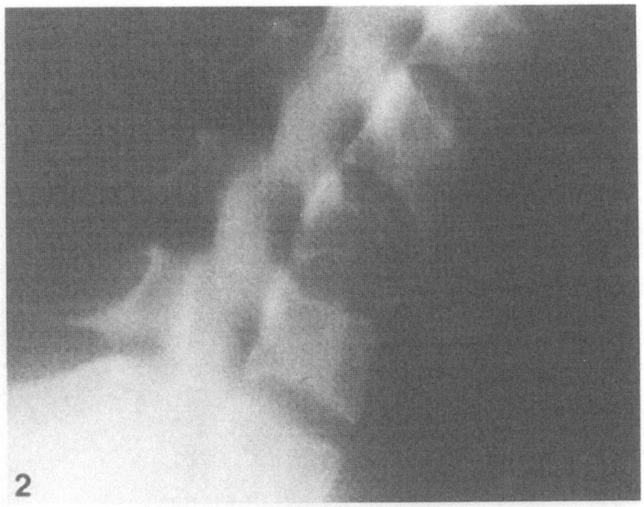

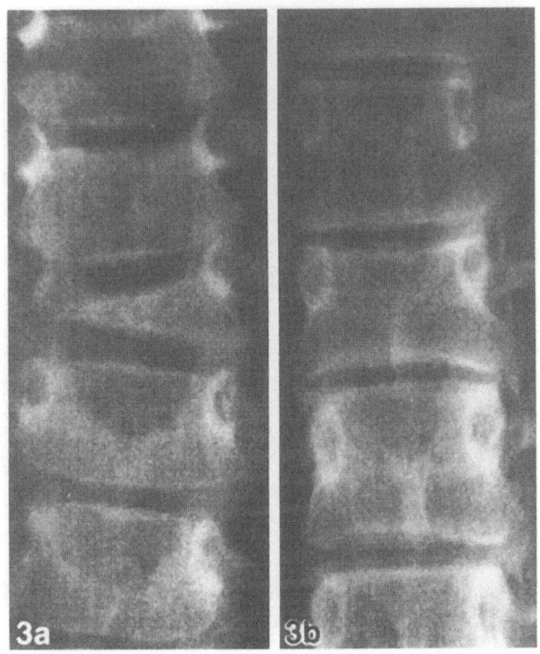

Figs. 1, 2. These radiographs of the cervical spine illustrate destruction of the posterior arch (1) and that of the vertebral body (2)

Fig. 3 a, b. The affected vertebra D7 is collapsed in this child of 3 (**a**). At 14 years of age, vertebral reconstruction is almost perfect, leaving only slight decrease of height of the body compared with the vertebrae above and below (**b**) (courtesy of Dr Dubousset)

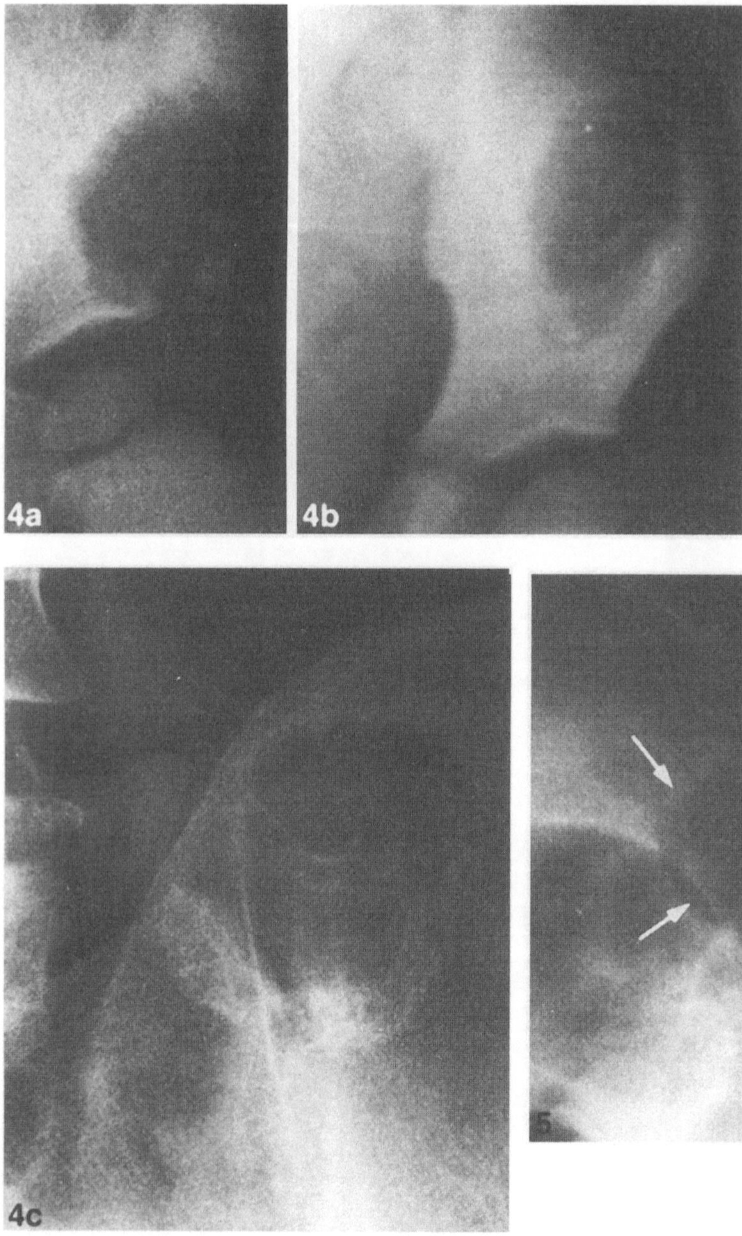

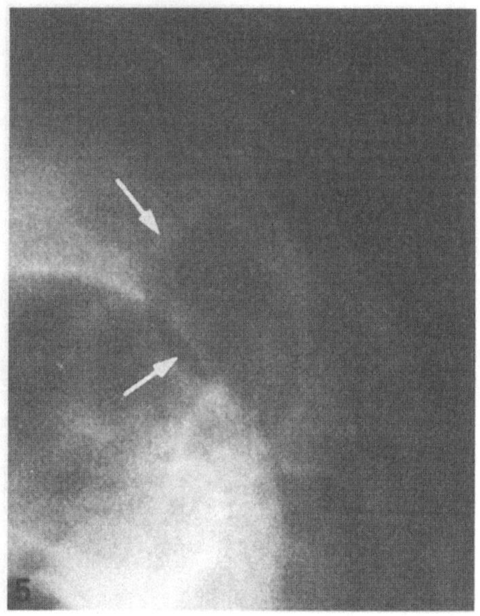

Fig. 4 a-c. Cavitary appearances in the ilium in patients aged 2 years (**a**), 4 years (**b**), and 41 years (**c**)

Fig. 5. Left fronto-orbital lesion in a child of 8. The rounded, sharply-bordered zone of osteolysis breaches the contour of the orbital cavity in its supero-lateral part (*arrows*)

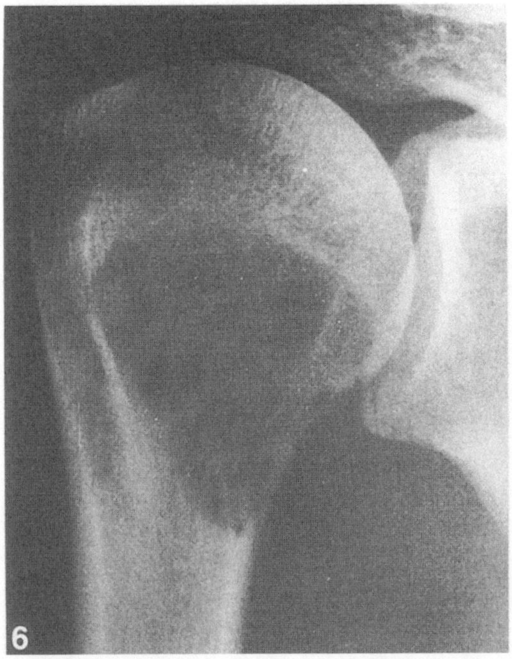

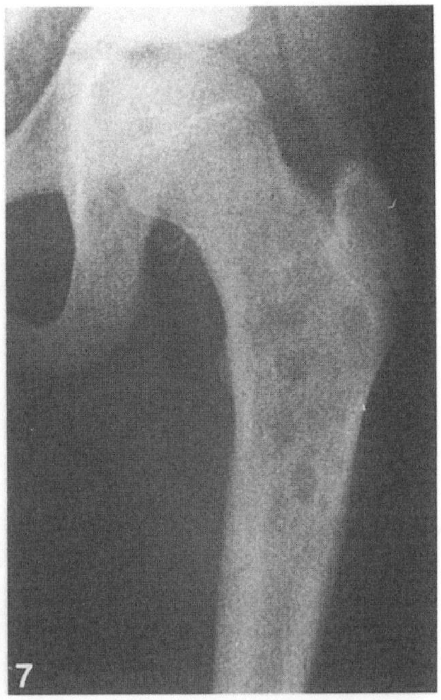

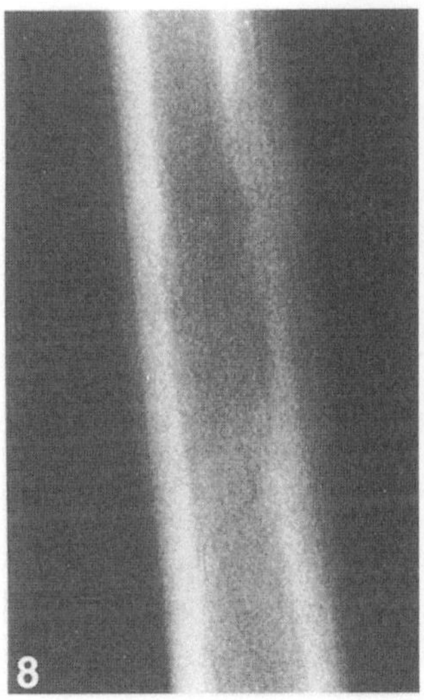

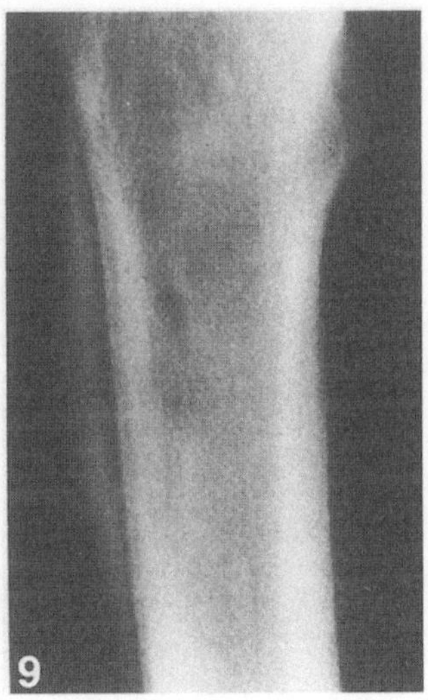

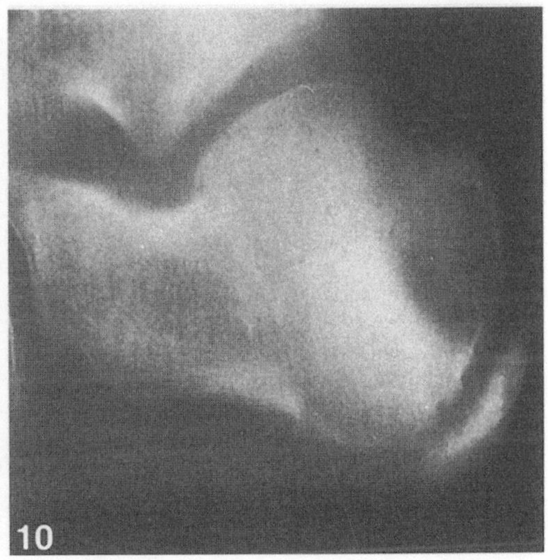

Figs. 6, 7. Osteolysis of the upper humeral metaphysis, less clearly defined than in the flat bones (**6**). This feature is still more obvious in the upper femoral metaphysis, where the irregularly absorbed cortex gives an ill-defined multicavitary image (7)

Fig. 8. Cortical osteolysis: the periosteal apposition on the femur of a girl of 5 had suggested a sarcomatous lesion

Fig. 9. Major periosteal apposition: girl of 4

Fig. 10. Lesion in posterior tuberosity of calcaneum (boy of 9): some bony sclerosis bounds the osteolysis anteriorly

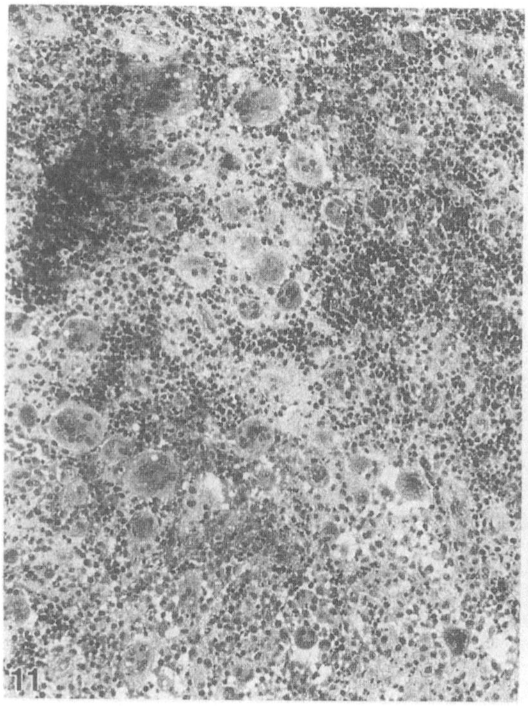

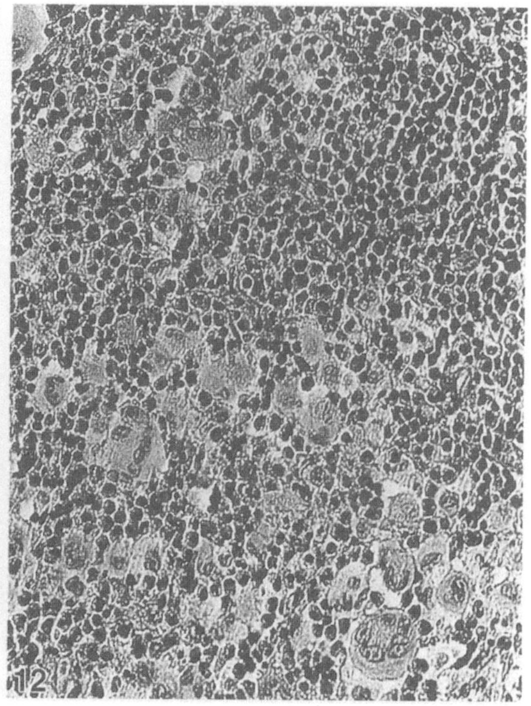

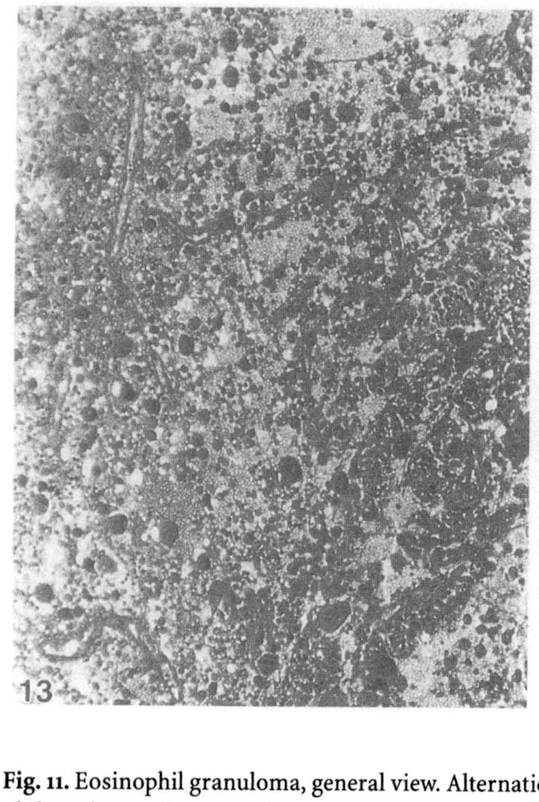

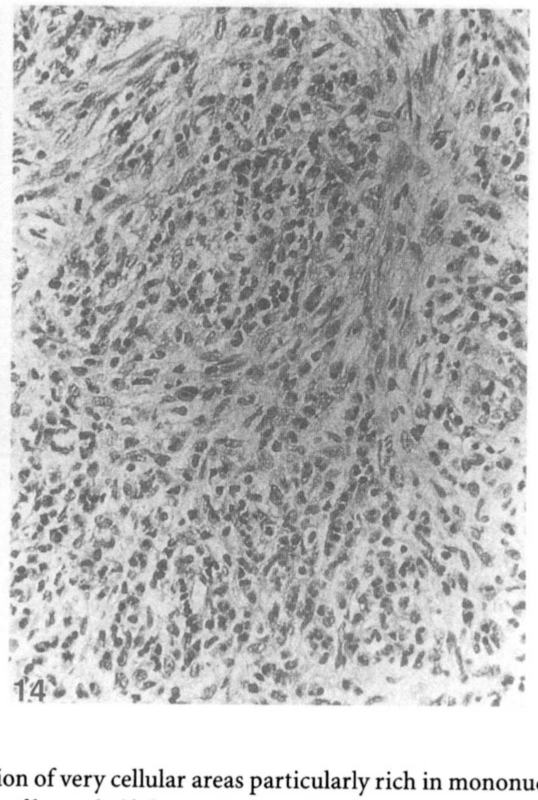

Fig. 11. Eosinophil granuloma, general view. Alternation of very cellular areas particularly rich in mononuclear eosinophils and areas dominated by giant cells. Middle part of lower half shows absence of nuclear staining corresponding to a necrotic zone

Fig. 12. Mononuclear proliferation interrupted by larger mono- or multinuclear cells with clear cytoplasm and a nucleus very characteristic of histiocytic cells

Fig. 13. Necrosis is common in histiocytosis X. The residues of giant cells and less distinct mononuclear cells are seen, but there are no disintegrated polynuclears

Fig. 14. Islands of mononuclear cells separated from one another by some fibroblastic bundles

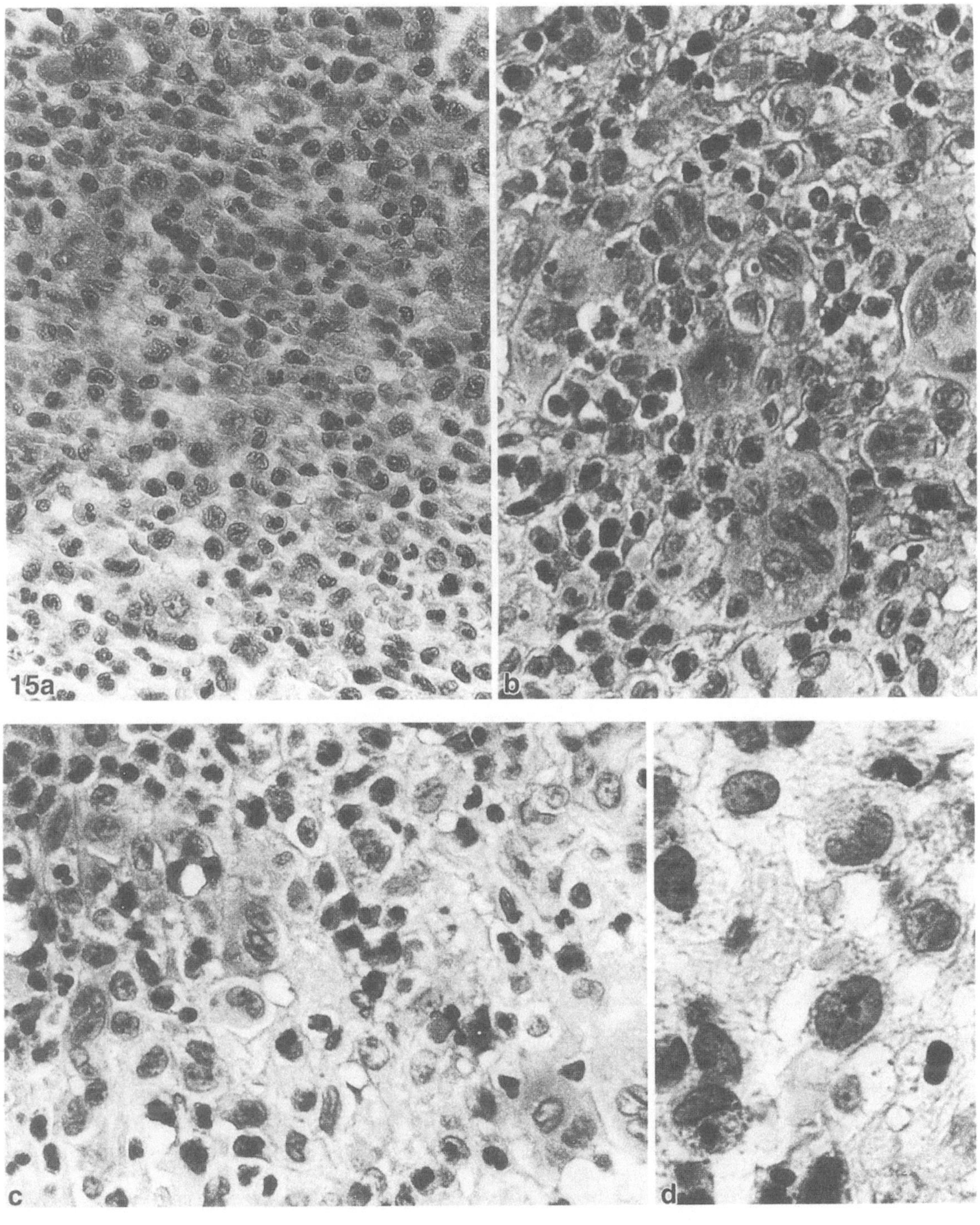

Fig. 15 a-d. These four microphotographs at different enlargements show the cellular polymorphism and cytological features of the histiocytes. **a** At the lower magnification there are mononuclear cells, polynuclears, lymphocytes and giant cells. **b** The giant cells have a relatively reduced number of nuclei, which exhibit the same morphology as those of the mononuclear histiocytes. **c** The kidney-shaped, bilobed, twisted appearance of the histiocytic nuclei appears in this microphotograph as well as the fold, a sort of median ridge parallel to the long axis of the nucleus, better visualised under immersion in **d**

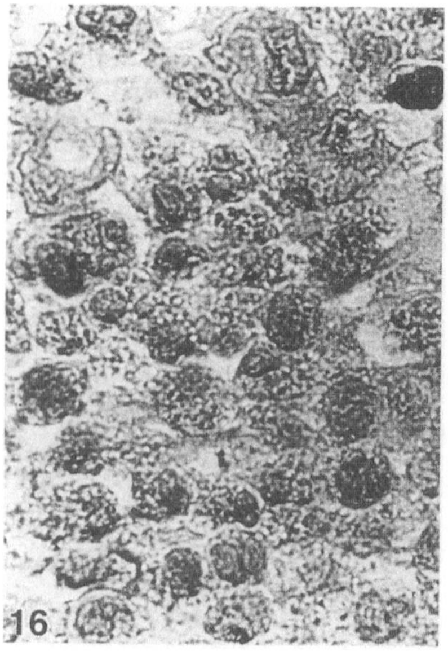
16

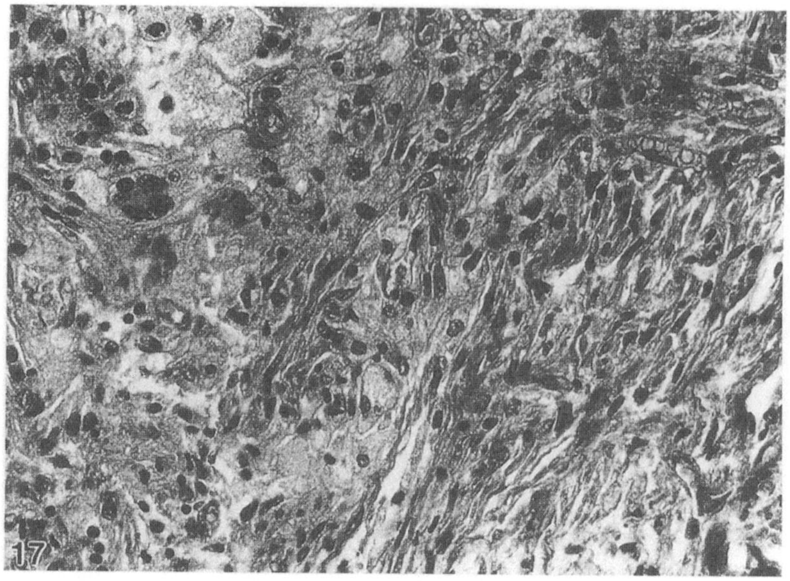
17

Fig. 16. The eosinophil granules are difficult to demonstrate in a black and white film, except by "cheating" a little with the lighting

Fig. 17. This biopsy was made after irradiation for histiocytosis X. There is a degree of sclerosis but the histiocytic proliferation persists, evidence of incomplete cure

→

Fig. 18. Overall view of a pathological histiocyte. The characteristic granules are numerous in the lower half of the cell and frequently in continuity with the cell membrane (x 4250, reduced to 80%)

Fig. 19. Detail of lower border of preceding image (x 15,750, reduction to 80%)

Fig. 20. Fragment of a pathological histiocyte showing numerous characteristic granules in an anastomomic network and frequently continuous with the cell membrane. On the right, an identical image in contact with another contiguous cytoplasmic expansion (x 15,000, reduced to 80%)

Fig. 21. Cells in process of necrosis. Above: the nucleus is relatively well preserved whereas the cytoplasmic organelles are very disintegrated as well as the cell membrane, which is interrupted. The characteristic "granules" appear multiplied. Below and right: clumps of fibrin very opaque to electrons (x 20,000, reduced to 80%)

Thanks are due to Mme Dr. Basset for furnishing these ultrastructural illustrations.

See illustrations pages 365-366

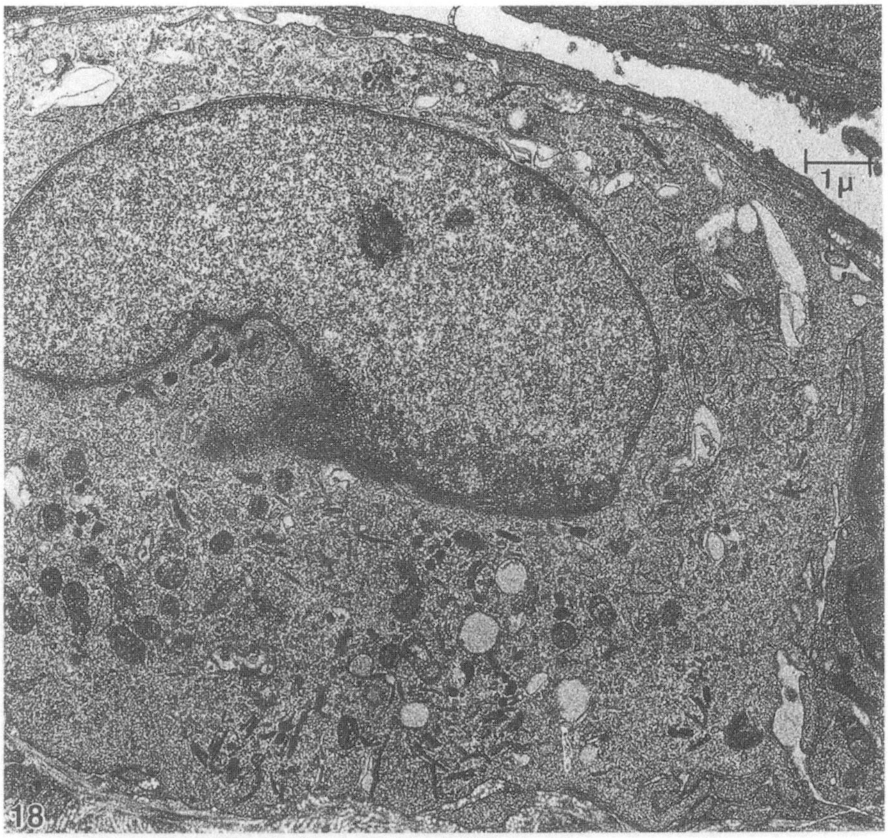
1 μ
18

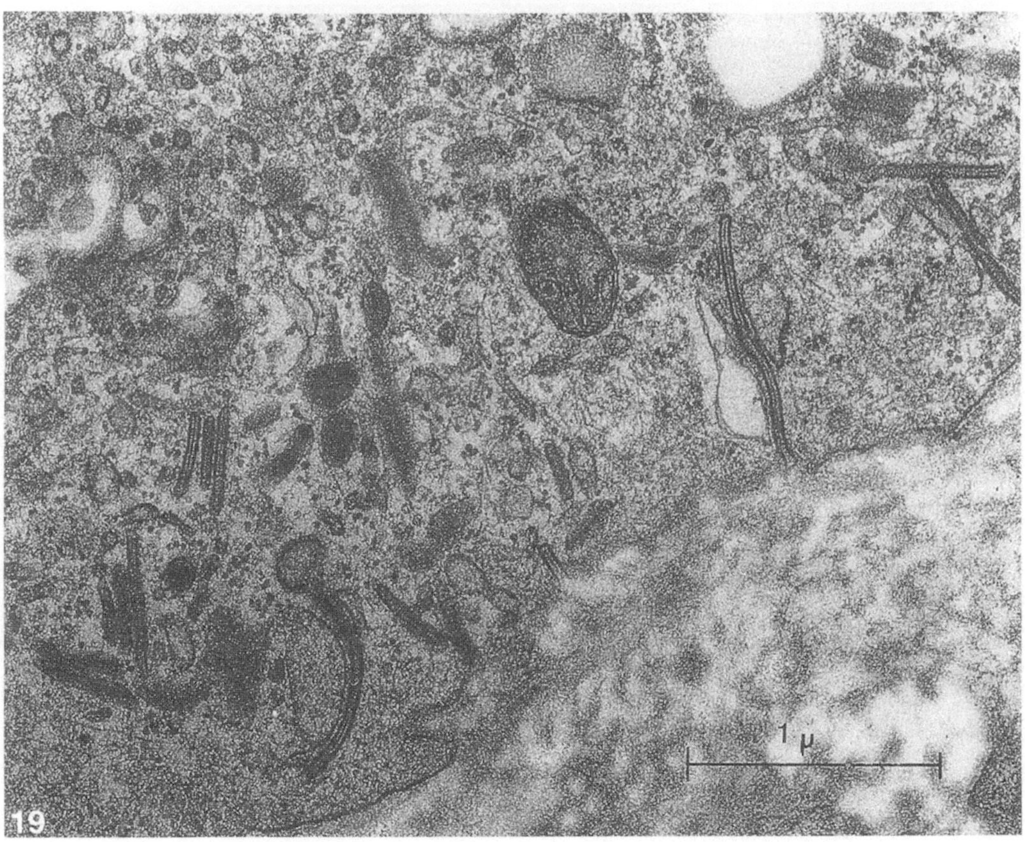
1 μ
19

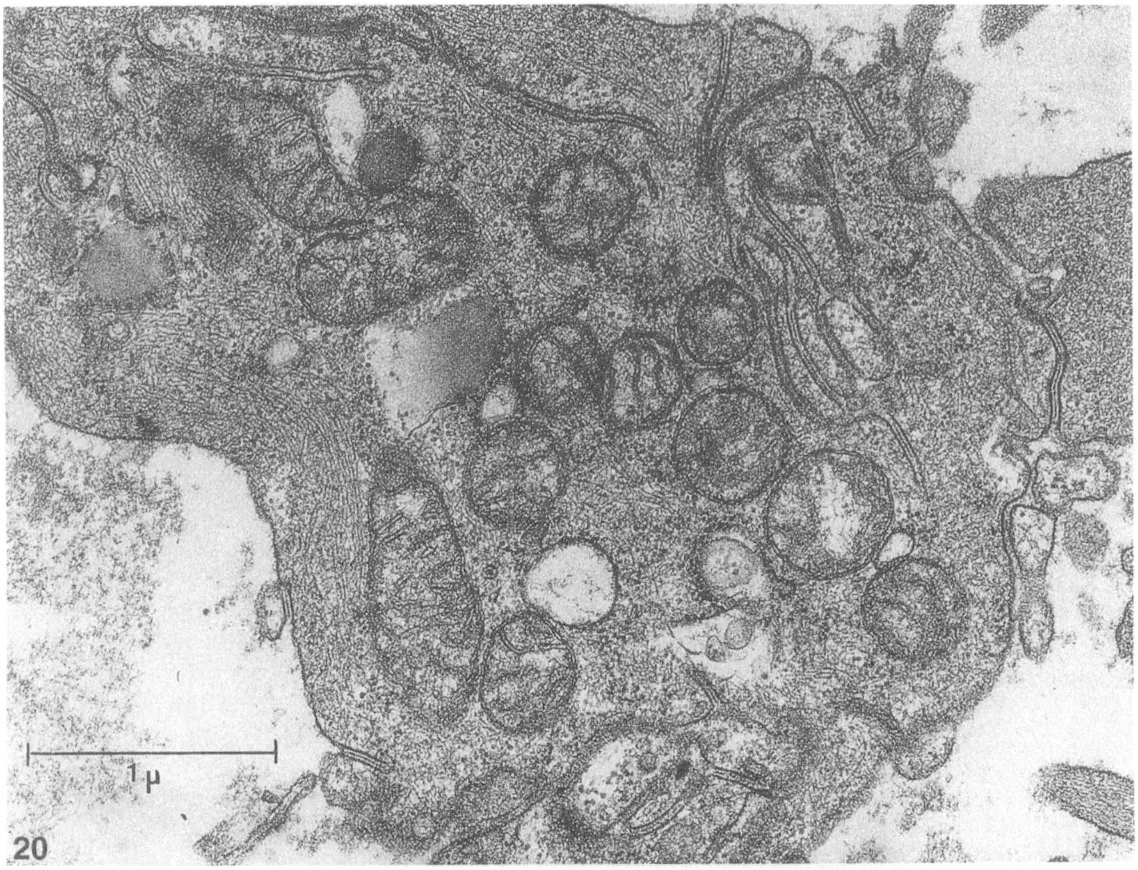
1 μ
20

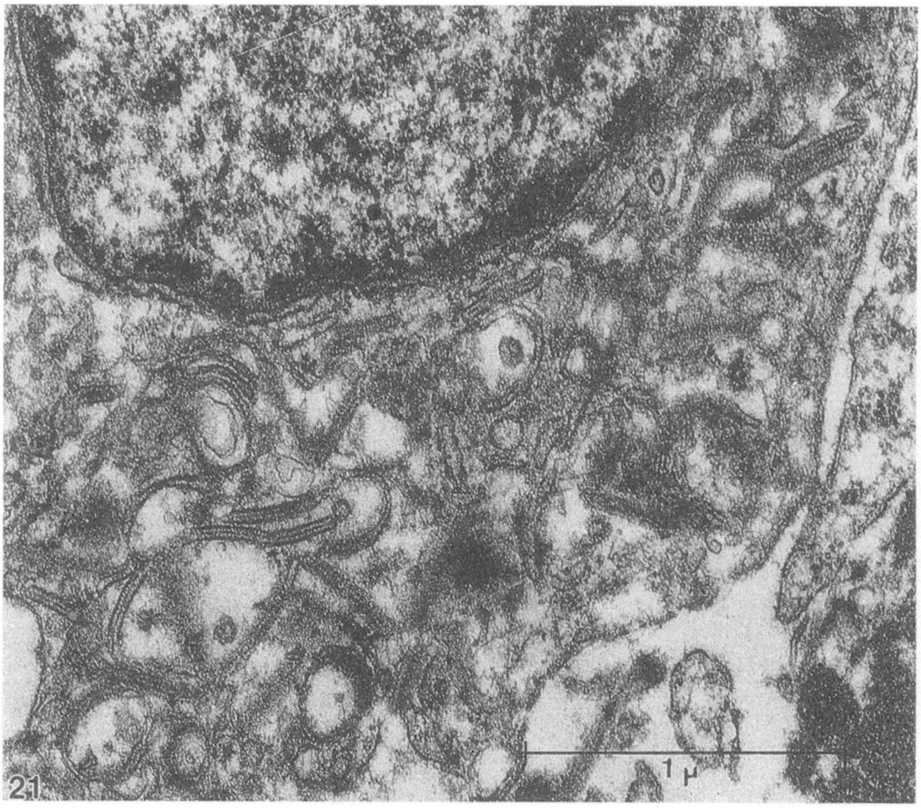
1 μ
21

32. Fibrous dysplasia

The multiple clinical presentations of this non-hereditary disorder, whose aetiology remains unknown, justifies the taking of biopsies, particularly in monostotic "occult" forms. This chapter, devoted to fibrous dysplasia, is only a simple anatomical and clinical review of the disorder.

Case histories

Case 1. A radiograph made in a man of 40 complaining of pain localised to the right hemithorax revealed a lytic costal lesion slightly ballooning the bone. At operation there was a firm whitish tumour which breached the cortex and infiltrated the musculo-aponeurotic soft tissues.

Case 2. The surgical approach to the lower end of the humerus in a woman of 35 exposed tissue of a soft consistency resembling that of a myxoma.

Case 3. A man of 50 was referred to the rheumatology department exhibiting firm nodular structures situated in the gluteal muscles and immobilised by muscular contraction. These nodules were painless; on examination they were found to be situated at the musculotendinous junctions.

Case 4. A woman of 30 attended for slight vaulting of the inner aspect of the right tibia. The radiographic appearances suggested an adamantinoma. The macroscopic findings at operation were compatible with this diagnosis.

Case 5. In a girl of 11 a cyst of the upper metaphysis of the humerus did not cease growing and, unlike every evolving idiopathic cyst, persisted in retaining contact with the cartilaginous growth plate. It was the radio-clinical context rather than the biopsy, devoid of really specific features, that made the diagnosis of fibrous dysplasia in its cystic form (fig. 8).

Case 6. A woman of 70 was admitted to a cancer unit for a malignant tumour of the tibia. The biopsy allowed a ready diagnosis of skeletogenic sarcoma, both osteogenic and chondrogenic, arising in fibrous dysplasia with scattered cartilaginous islands.

General considerations

In 1937, Albright et al described a syndrome characterised by disseminated fibrous osteitis associated with areas of skin pigmentation and with precocious puberty in girls. In the same year, Jaffe and Lichtenstein gave an anatomic account of fibrous dysplasia of bone and regarded Albright's syndrome as one of its variants. A rare disorder of unknown aetiology, fibrous dysplasia may affect a single bone (monostotic form) but more often affects multiple parts of the skeleton. The mean age when the disorder is detected is between 5 and 10 years, but there is a very wide range from the first months of life to the 6th and 7th decades. There does not seem to be any gender predominance.

All the bones may be affected: the long bones of the limbs, ribs, craniofacial bones (cf Chapter 38), metacarpals, often the 4th, and the metatarsals.

Fibrous dysplasia represents 7% of all benign lesions of bone and is the commonest of all benign lesions affecting the ribs [Lucas et al 1995]. In the long bones its preferentially metaphyseal site excludes any effects on the joint for a long period. The commonest femoral lesion is at the upper metaphysis (fig. 7).

Clinical features and course

Whether the disease is monostotic or polyostotic, it may be revealed by pain, disturbance of gait, bony deformity or pathological fractures and should lead to a complete examination of the skeleton.

In Albright's syndrome the precocious puberty or the presence of flat yellowish-brown skin patches are often the first manifestations. There can be little doubt that quite a number of monostotic forms are asymptomatic and escape diagnosis. In any case, diagnosed polyostotic forms are commoner than monostotic forms. Although the disorder has no characteristic tumour related finding, about 20% of cases have been reported with a slight increase in the alkaline phosphatases which seems to be unconnected with the extent of the lesions.

The effect of the disorder on the skeleton is characterised by an acceleration of bony maturation, but this premature growth ceases precociously and usually leads to slight decrease in the patient's height. Other factors are involved in this loss of height including scoliotic or kyphotic deformity in cases of vertebral lesions and bowing of the upper end of the femur (coxa vara).

It is classically accepted that the progress of the disorder ceases with growth of the skeleton, but this is only partly true. The periodic exacerbations are marked by fractures and bony curvature, and some authors have noted a coincidence between these exacerbations and normal or pathological stages of female reproductive life.

In addition to Albright's syndrome, which combines pigmented skin patches and hormonal disturbances with the bony lesions, other associated lesions have been reported; there are vascular, renal and ocular malformations and fibromyxomas of the musculo-aponeurotic junctions. These fibromyxomas are often multiple and appear successively during the course of the disorder. They are usually situated in the same segment of the limb as the bony lesions. The term "fibromyxoid nodule" would be more appropriate than that of fibromyxoma since all the cases so far reported in the literature have an excellent prognosis, without recurrence or malignant transformation. The prognosis of the disorder seen as a whole is good, though severe forms exist. In children an extensive form has an adverse functional outcome due to deformities and repeated fractures. In adults, a monostotic lesion in a weight-bearing bone may pose serious orthopaedic problems.

Certain craniofacial forms are particularly severe (cf Chapter 38) because of the severity of nerve compressions. Sarcomatous transformation is very rare, and is usually skeletogenic in nature; it is particularly seen in forms where chondrogenesis is more marked, as in the case reported by Roze et al (1967).

Imaging

The radiological appearances in fibrous dysplasia are relatively typical. Sometimes there is a clear oval lacuna, or several adjacent lacunae, in the tibia or femur, the lesion being slightly expansile. Sometimes the image is more characteristic, a ground-glass opacity which invades the medullary canal and cortex and has an oblique boundary (fig. 3). Lesions in a weight-bearing bone are often associated with deformity. Many cases present with unilateral predominance of the lesions. Bilaterally symmetrical forms are very rare.

Pathological anatomy and histopathology

Macroscopically, the fibrous tissue proliferation totally destroys the spongy bone, fills the medullary canal of long bones, and leaves only a shell of periosteal bone after having destroyed the cortical haversian systems. In lesions of the ribs the bony cortex is usually destroyed. The diseased tissue is white or slightly grayish and firm. It contains small rounded or oblong more or less calcified structures, but sometimes also cartilaginous areas. Some rusty-brown zones may be seen, indicative of the presence of haemosiderin deposits. In some cases this tissue is hollowed out into cavities, which may or not be surrounded by softened zones of mucoid appearance. These pseudocysts contain either a clear fluid or a haemorrhagic effusion (cf Chapter 30, figs. 26, 27).

At microscopic examination, under low magnification, the lesion appears monomorphous, with some formations of osteoid and sometimes chondroid appearance standing out against a fibrous background. The lesion consists of collagen fibers between which there develops a proliferation of fusiform or polyhedral cells with an often notched nucleus. These fibroblasts are often abnormally short; collagen formation varies in different cases and the collagen is usually densely safranophil (figs. 9, 12). Vascularisation is via unequally sized vessels, sometimes surrounded by a clear zone of loose connective tissue resembling that observed in the fibromatoses. In some cases the fibrous tissue is traversed by numerous capillaries. Here and there the monotony of this fibrous background is interrupted by metaplastic chondroid or osteoid formation (figs. 11, 12). The chondroid metaplasia may lead to the formation of very differentiated cartilage (fig. 17). The osteoid metaplasia arises in irregularly woven collagen fibers and leads to the formation of trabecular primary bone. There is no osteoblastic margin but an osteoblastic metamorphosis of the cells which will participate in the elaboration of these bony strands. These strands, which do not inter-anastomose, are mineralised in their central part. In places, this bony tissue forms long strands outlining images of broken rings, circles or letters. Without being pathognomonic, this architecture is nevertheless very specific (figs. 12, 13, 16, 25).

Small, strongly basophil, coin-shaped formations resembling calco-spheroids are quite characteristic. Some seem to be related to the vessels, others are continuous with the bony tissue, still others are scattered in the fibrous production (figs. 18, 19). One can only support the view of Sissons et al (1993) and of Voytek et al (1995) that these calcified spherules are in no way specific. Their presence in an osteofibrous lesion of bone, apart from the jaw bones, in no way allows a diagnosis of cementoma or fibrocementoma.

In some fibrous dysplasias, a considerable number of mastocytes is seen (fig. 14) laden with granules metachromatic to toluidine blue. Bertrand et al (1978), in an ultrastructural study, stress the rosette pattern of these granules and recall that this type of granulation is predominant in fetal mastocytes. At the periphery the fibrous proliferation is poorly circumscribed, and invades the medullary spaces between the bony strands, which are in large part persistent.

Pathological variants

Ishida and Dorfman (1993) report 8 cases of fibrous dysplasia with abundant cartilaginous differentiation. They stress the risk of making a diagnosis of chondrosarcoma due to ignorance of the benign nature of the cartilaginous areas. These authors suggest the term of fibrocartilaginous dysplasia, which it might be more proper to regard as a variant of fibrous dysplasia.

The fibrous tissue may be loose and myxoid, perhaps more especially after repeated biopsies, but sometimes from the outset. This appearance is sometimes described as a particular form of fibrous dysplasia but a simple biopsy does not provide a complete picture of the lesion and it may be a matter of local remoulding or a stage in the development. Some fibrous dysplasias are excavated, and the cavities are sometimes occupied by a bloodstained effusion; in addition, some giant cells are often present in the margins of these pseudocysts, so that the pathologist has the impression of witnessing the birth of an aneurysmal cyst.

Associated lesions

The commonest associated lesions are fibromyxomas of the musculo-aponeurotic and musculo-tendinous junctions. These junctional nodules are rounded and slightly elongated in the direction of muscle pull. They are surgically removable but their extraction tears the tendino-aponeurotic and muscle fibers which adhere to their surface and from which they are indissociable. Slightly bluish in colour, they measure 4-8 cm in diameter but may reach considerable size in very rare cases. On section they are translucent, formed of a sort of jelly partitioned by some septa arising from their musculo-aponeurotic wall (figs. 21, 22).

Microscopically, these nodules are formed of a loose network of fine reticulin fibers, and some collagenous septa retain in their meshes a weakly amphophil amorphous substance, slightly positive to mucicarmine staining and PAS-positive. In this substance there are scattered some fusiform or stellar mesenchymal cells, often with large nuclei. This myxoid-like tissue infiltrates and separates the tendino-aponeurotic and muscular fibers (figs. 23, 24).

Ultrastructural study confirms the fibroblastic nature of the stellate and fusiform cells but also shows cells of a foamy appearance, possibly endowed with macrophagic activity. Special staining supports the hypothesis of the mucopolysaccharide nature of the content of the vacuoles and of the granular material which covers the cells.

Vessels are extremely rare or absent. To regard these lesion as true "myxomas", a term which suggests a benign tumour lesion, is probably incorrect. To regard them as degenerative lesions is possibly nearer the truth. These degenerative lesions should be distinguished from true myxomas (if they exist). In a recent publication, Meis and Enzinger (1992) report 65 cases of juxta-articular myxomas but cautiously conclude that they cannot clearly distinguish between a neoplastic or a reactive process.

Differential diagnosis

The diagnosis of fibrous dysplasia in its typical appearances in the long bones is easy in the light of the clinical and radiological findings and provided that the biopsy is of adequate size. It is certain that a needle aspiration which demonstrates a proliferation of short and slender cells allows only compatibility with the suggested clinical diagnosis. A solitary lesion of the ilium or rib, with firm whitish tissue invading the soft tissues is sometimes sent to the laboratory with a diagnosis of a possibly malignant tumour.

The pathological variants, mainly in solitary lesions, raise some problems. A myxoid appearance may suggest the diagnosis of intraosseous myxoma, but this diagnosis is very rare and cannot be considered before thinking of commoner disorders capable of assuming, at least locally, a myxoid character, including fibrous dysplasia. The cystic forms may simulate an idiopathic cyst and their diagnosis is quite difficult in the radiological and clinical context. Haemorrhagic cavities should not lead to too rapid a diagnosis of angioma or aneurysmal cyst.

Some fibrous dysplasias are particularly rich in cartilage [Ishida et al 1993] and suggest a diagnosis of chondroma, chondrosarcoma, or the very rare fibrocartilaginous mesenchymoma [Dahlin et al 1984, Bulichova et al 1993]. In mesenchymoma the fusiform cells which surround the cartilaginous zones are quite different from the fine short cells of fibrous dysplasia. Moreover, in fibrocartilaginous mesenchymoma (Dahlin's tumour) two very characteristic features are seen: cartilaginous plaques which reproduce the metaphyseo-epiphyseal cartilaginous growth plate and others which resemble the cartilage cap which overlies exostoses.

Lastly, in some rare cases, where the fibrous nature of the dysplasia is abnormally marked, fibroma must be excluded as a possible cause, including desmoid fibroma, but here again the appearance of the fibroblastic cells with nuclei that are often hyperchromatic is quite different.

References

Bertrand G, Minard MF, Simard C, Rebel A (1978) Etude ultrastructurale d'un cas de dysplasie fibreuse monostotique. Ann Anat Pathol 23: 81-90

Biagini R, Ruggieri P, Borani S, Picci P (1987) The Mazabraud's syndrome: case report and review of the literature. Ital J Orthop Traumatol 13: 105-111

Bulychova IV, Unni KK, Bertoni F, Beabout JW (1993) Fibrocartilaginous mesenchymoma of bone. Am J Surg Pathol 17: 830-836

Cozzutto C, Cornaglio-Ferraris (1991) Fibrocartilaginous mesenchymoma of bone. Pathol Res Pract 187: 279-283

Dahlin DC, Bertoni F, Beabout JW, Campanacci M (1984) Fibrocartilaginous mesenchymoma with low-grade malignancy. Skeletal Radiol 12: 263-269

Enzinger FM (1965) Intramuscular myxome. Am J Clin Pathol 43: 104-113

Feintuch T (1973) Chondrosarcoma arising in a cartilaginous area of previously irradiated fibrous dysplasia. Cancer 31: 877-881

Ford KB, Palmer PES, Tesluk H (1985) Fibrous dysplasia of calvaria (multiple sclerotic lesions). Skeletal Radiol 13: 68-71

Gober GA, Nicolas RW (1993) Skeletal fibrous dysplasia associated with intramuscular myxoma. Case report. Skeletal Radiol 22: 452-455

Huvos AG, Higinbotham NL, Millert R (1972) Bone sarcomas arising in fibrous dysplasia. Am J Clin Pathol 57: 266 (Abst)

Ishida T, Dorfman HD (1993) Massive chondroid differentiation in fibrous dysplasia of bone (fibrocartilaginous dysplasia). Am J Surg Pathol 17: 924-930

Lejeune E, Bouvier M, Vauzelle JL, Queneau P, Thomas JD, Chaudy J, Leung TK, Deplanet JP (1972) Dysplasie fibreuse et myxomes des tissus mous. Rev Rhum 39: 281-288

Le Merrer M, Maroteaux P (à paraître) Mazabraud's syndrome: fibrous dysplasia of bone and intramuscular myxoma. Pediatr Radiol

Lichtenstein L, Jaffe (1942) Fibrous dysplasia of bone. A condition affecting one, several or many bones, the graver cases of which may present abnormal pigmentation of skin, premature sexual development, hyperthyroidism or still other extra-skeletal abnormalities. Arch Pathol 33: 777-816

Lièvre JA, Mme Lièvre JA, Ract A (1966) La dysplasie fibreuse des os. Une série de 34 observations. Nosologie et pathogénie. Sem Hop Paris 53: 3252-3263

Louyot P, Gaucher A, Jeanblanc J, Fresse B (1965) Neuf cas de dysplasie fibreuse des os de Jaffe-Lichtenstein. Rev Rhum 12: 745-750

Lucas E, Sudaram M, Boccini T (1995) Polyostotic fibrous dysplasia. Orthop Int 3: 279-280

Mazabraud A, Girard J (1957) Un cas particulier de dysplasie fibreuse à localisation osseuses et tendineuses. Rev Rhum 9/10: 1-8

Mazabraud A, Semat P, Roze R (1967) A propos de l'association de fibromyxomes des tissus mous à la dysplasie fibreuse des os. Presse Med 75: 2223-2228

Mazabraud's syndrome: intramuseular myxoma associated with fibrous dysplasia of bone. Aust NZ J Surg 60: 825-828

Meis JM, Enzinger FM (1992) Juxta-articular myxoma: a clinical and pathologic study of 65 casses. Hum Pathol 23: 639-646

Perkinson NG, Higinbatham NL (1955) Osteogenic sarcoma arising in polyostotic fibrous dysplasia. Cancer 8: 396-402

Pons A, Arlet J, Alibelli MJ, Fabre J, Carton M, Combes PF (1974) Deux cas de dégénérescence maligne osseuse sur dysplasie fibreuse des os. J Radiol Electrol 55: 268

Roze R, Mazabraud A, Semat P (1967) Dysplasie fibreuse de os et myxomes des tissus mous. Dégénérescence sarcomateuse localisée. J Radiol Electrol 48: 527-536

Shapeero LG, Vanel D, Ackerman LV, Terrier-Lacombe MJ, Housin D, Schwaab G, Sigal R, Masselot J (1993) Aggressive fibrous dysplasia of the maxillary sinus. Skeletal Radiol 22: 563-568

Sissons A, Steiner C, Dorfman D (1993) Calcified spherules in fibro-osseous lesions of bone. Arch Pathol Lab Med 117: 284-290

Taconis WK (1988) Osteosarcoma in fibrous dysplasia. Skeletal Radiol 17: 163-170

Van Horn PA, Dahlin DC (1963) Fibrous dysplasia: a clinical pathologie study of orthopedic surgical cases. Proc Mayo Clin Rochester 38: 175-196

Virenque J, Gaubert J, Bouissou H (1965) Aspects radiographiques de la maladie de Jaffe-Lichtenstein. Presse Med 73: 1-4

Voytek TM, Ro JY, Edeiken J, Ayala AG (1995) Fibrous dysplasia and cemento-ossifying fibroma: a histologic spectrum. Am J Surg Pathol 19: 775-781

Wirth WA, Leavitt D, Enzinger FM (1971) Multiple intramuscular myxomas. Another extraskeletal manifestation of fibrous dysplasia. Cancer 27: 1167-1173

Zimmer JF, Dahlin DC, Pugh DG, Clagett OT (1956) Fibrous dysplasia of bone analysis of bone: analysis of 15 cases of surgically verified costal fibrous dysplasia. J Thoracic Surg 31: 488-496

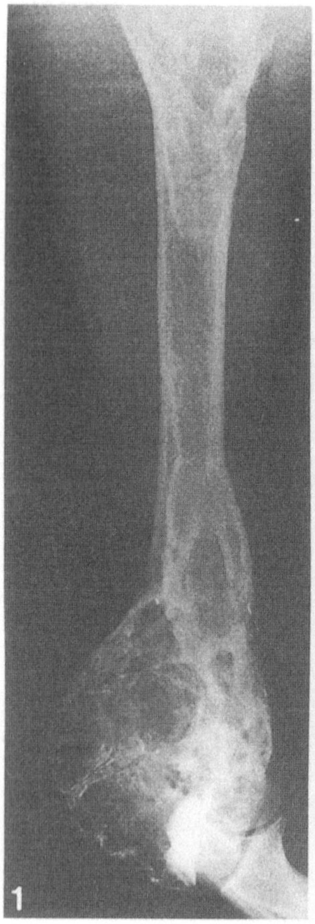

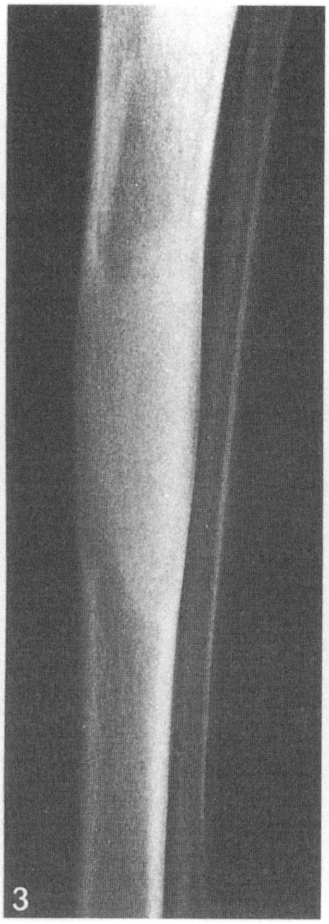

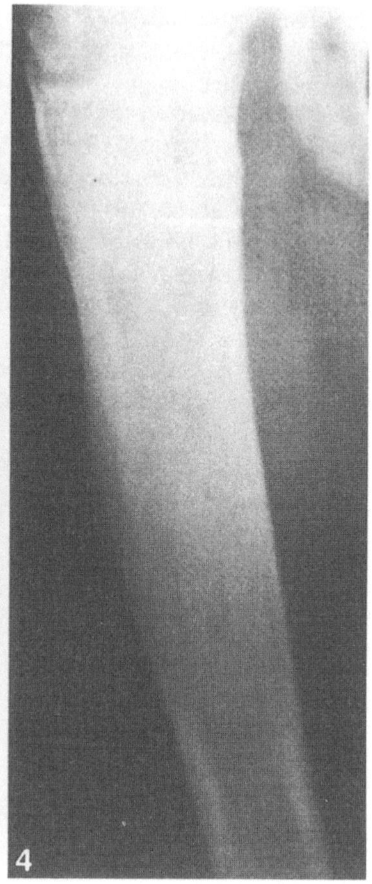

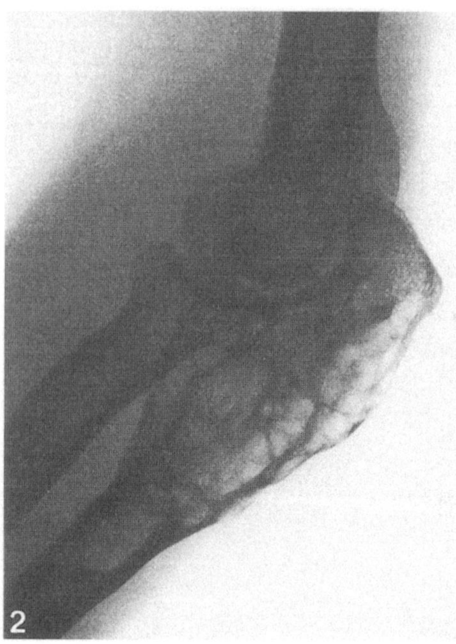

Fig. 1. Man of 72, referred for the presence of several nodules situated at the musculo-tendinous junctions of the pectoral and gluteal muscles. This was a currently multifocal fibrous dysplasia. The bony lesions were stabilised, but at the age of 20 the lesion at the lower end of the humerus, probably solitary, was considered to be a giant-cell tumour and irradiated following a fracture

Fig. 2. Large lesion of alveolar "soap-bubble" appearance at the upper end of the ulna

Fig. 3. Tibial lesion in a boy of 14. The diaphysis is very slightly ballooned at the level of this homogeneous "ground glass" area with an oblique lower limit

Fig. 4. Dysplasia of upper third of femur, slight thickening, cortex and medulla confused in a homogeneous area

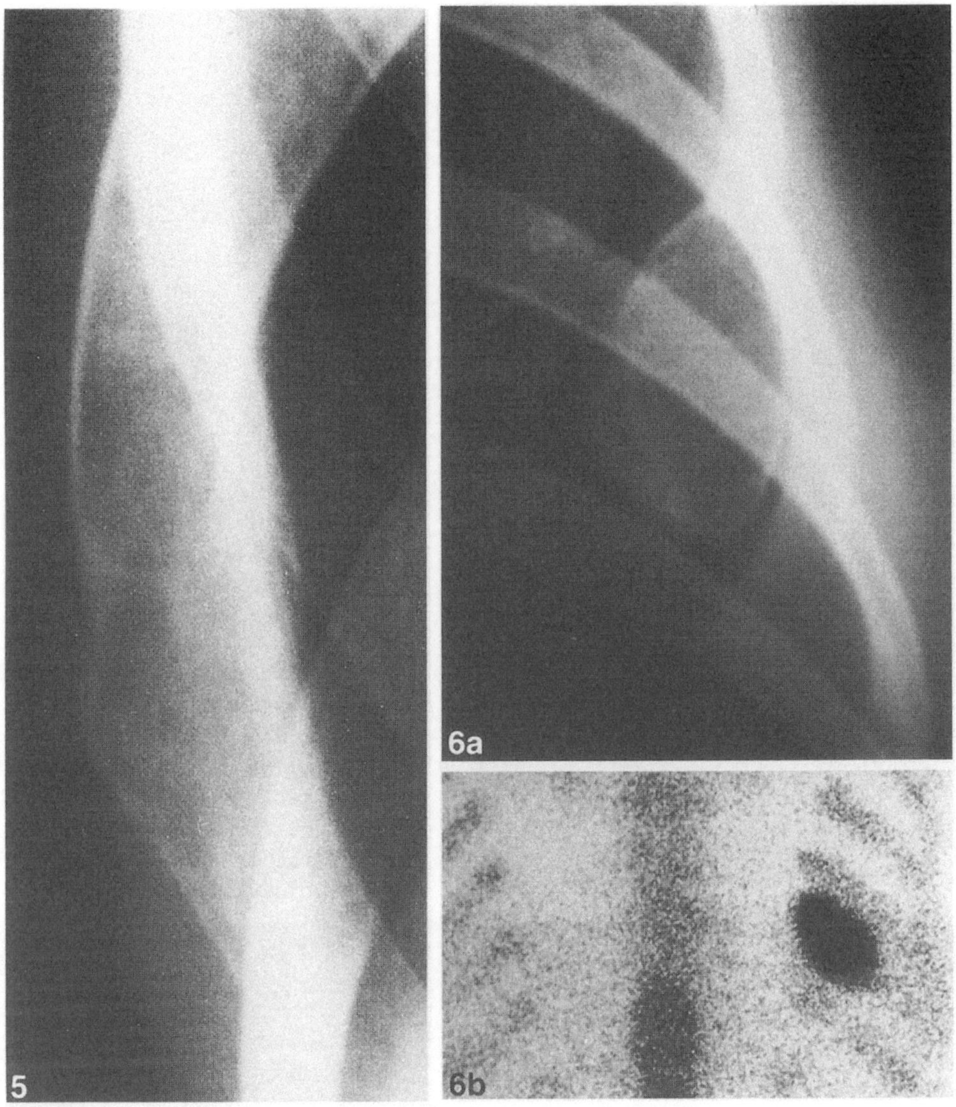

Fig. 5. In the ribs, fibrous dysplasia often assumes a tumour-like appearance with breaching of the cortex and invasion of the soft tissues. It is also often cystic and these cysts are haemorrhagic cavities

Fig. 6 a, b. Radiological appearance (**a**) and bone scan (**b**) of a lesion of tumour-like appearance developing in the anterior arch of the 5th rib in a woman of 31

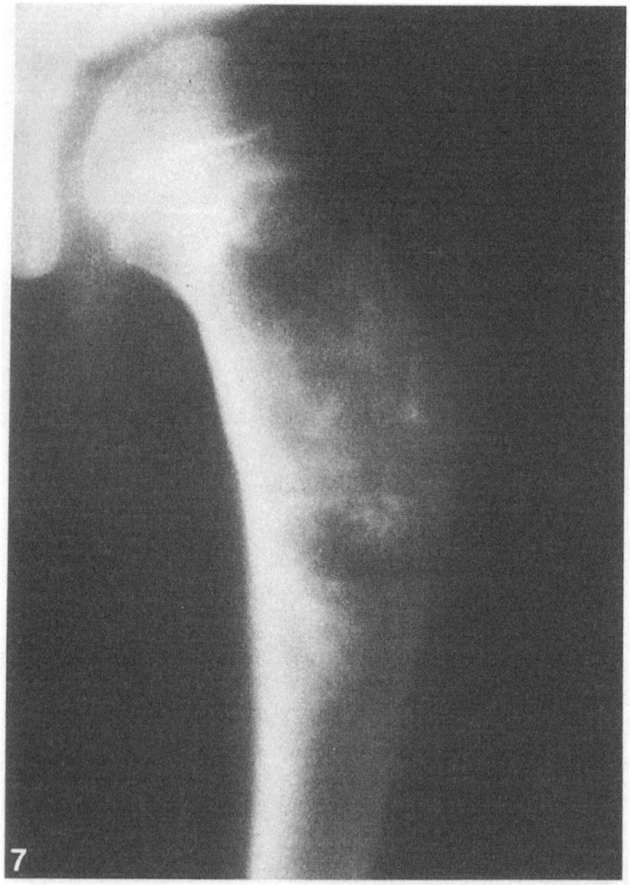

Fig. 7. The fuzzy, patchy, slightly ballooned appearance of the upper third of the femur suggests the possibility of partly calcified osteoid plaques in this fibrous dysplasia

Fig. 8. Cystic fibrous dysplasia. **a** This relatively rare form of fibrous dysplasia first affected the upper end of the right humerus in 1963 and then extended progressively to virtually the entire humerus by 1964 (**b**) and 1971 (**c**), ending in 1990 (**d**) with global involvement of the bone with angular deformity due to repeated fractures (courtesy of Prof. Dunoyer, CHU, Limoges)

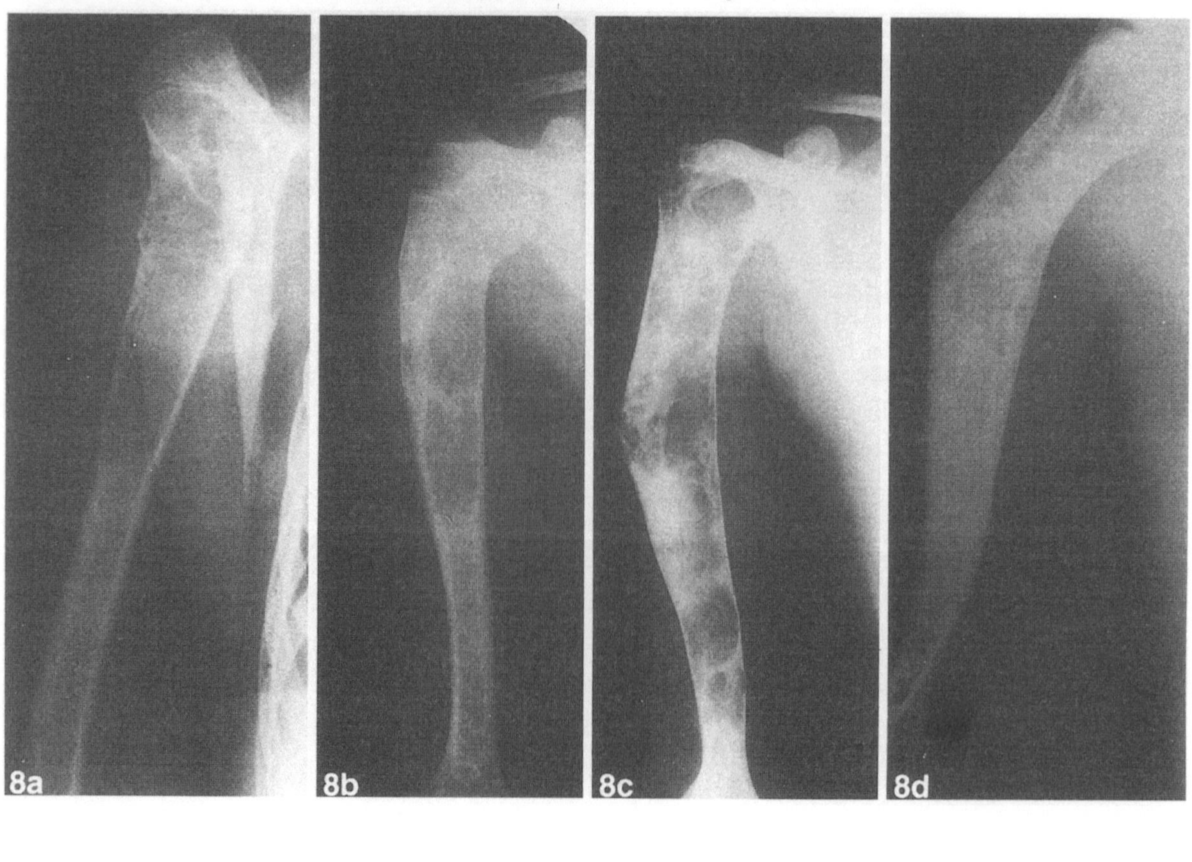

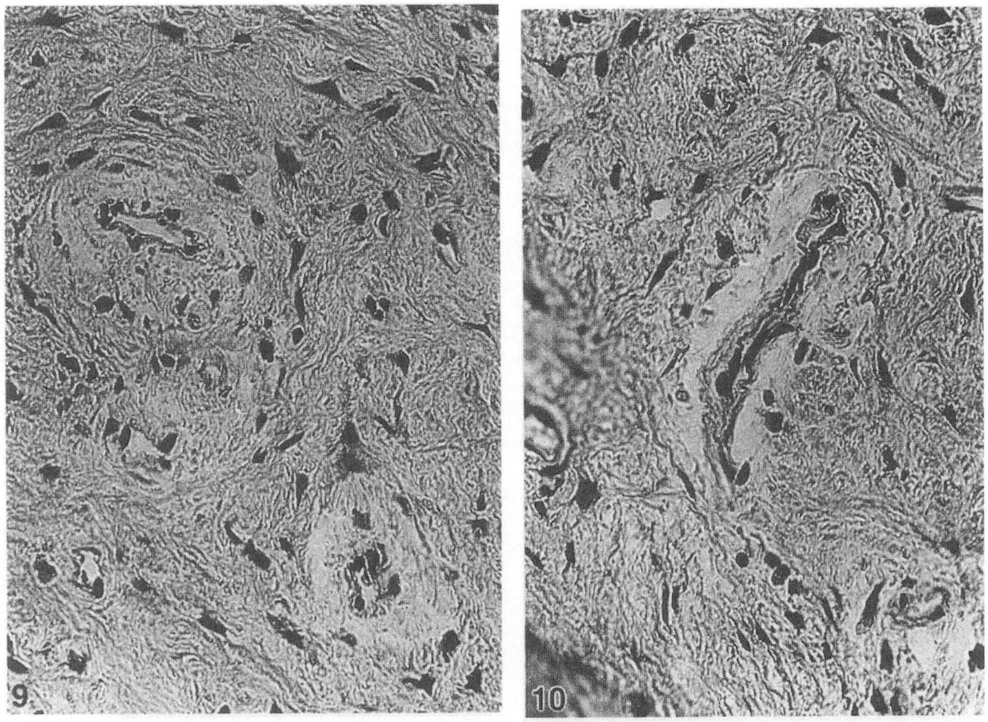

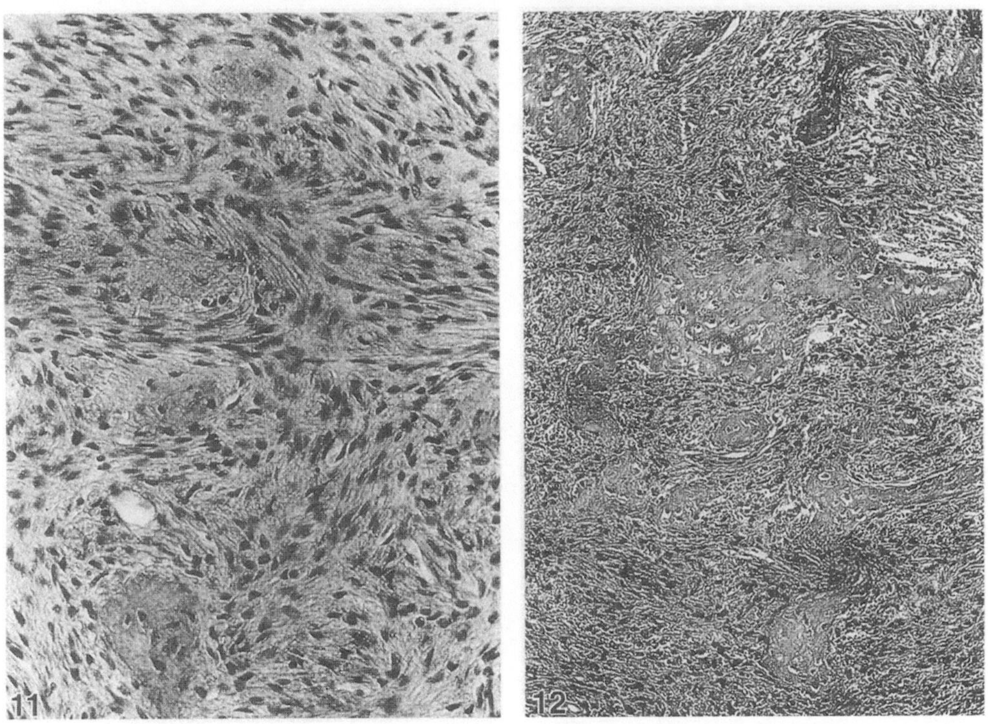

Figs. 9, 10. The fusiform or slightly polyhedral cells are regularly distributed along the thick collagen fibers. The vessels are surrounded by a loose tissue resembling that of fibromatoses of the soft tissues

Figs. 11, 12. Chondroid or osteoid metaplasia by metamorphosis of the ground substance, which becomes hyaline and uniform, while the cellular metamorphosis assumes a chondrocytic or osteocytic appearance

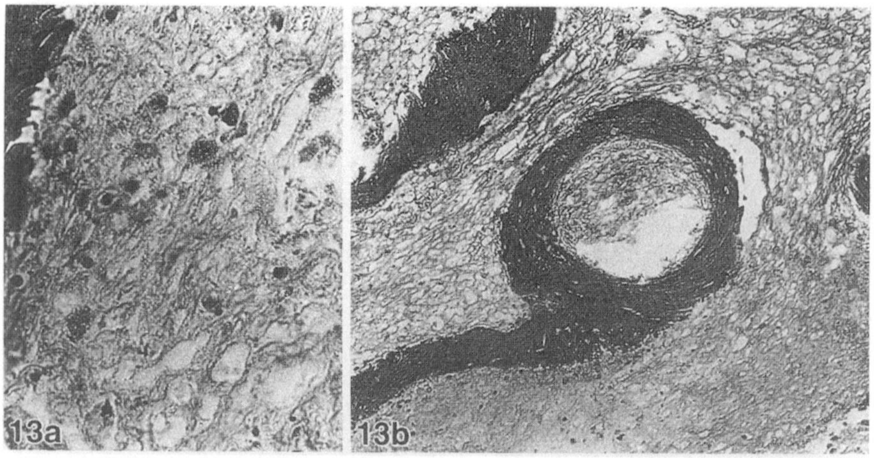

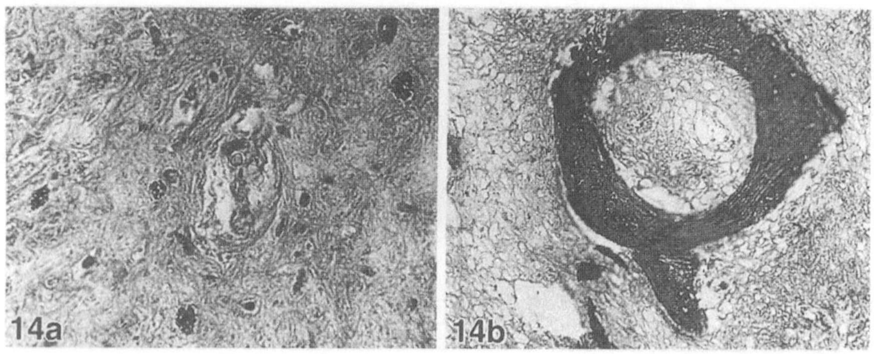

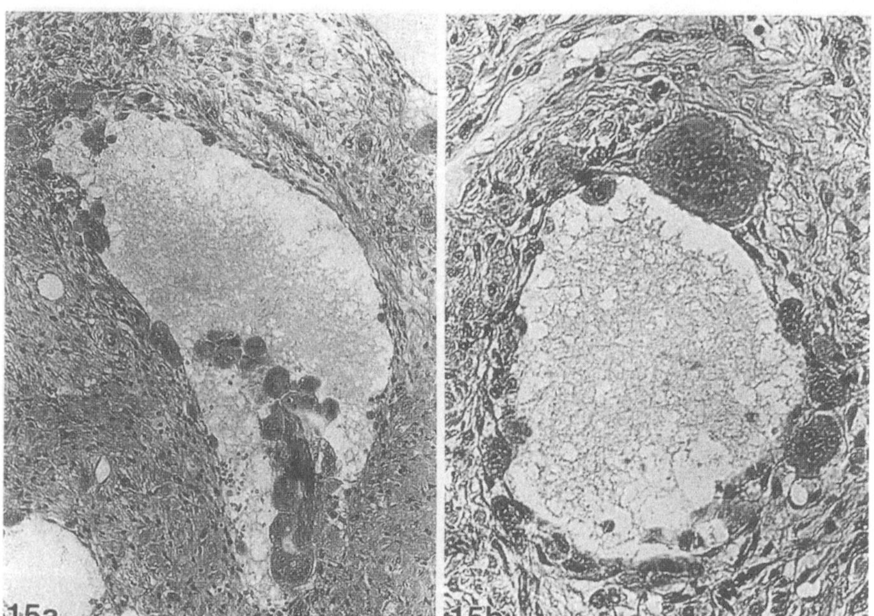

Fig. 13 a, b. Particular appearances of osteogenesis as "letters" or "Chinese characters"

Fig. 14 a, b. Mastocytes in fibrous dysplasia

Fig. 15 a, b. These large lacunae surrounded by some multinucleated giant cells may be the beginning of the cystic formations seen in some cases of dysplasia

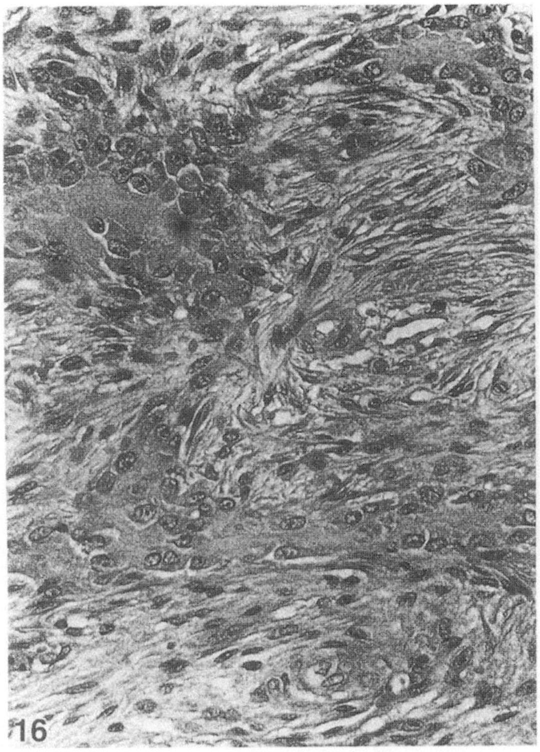

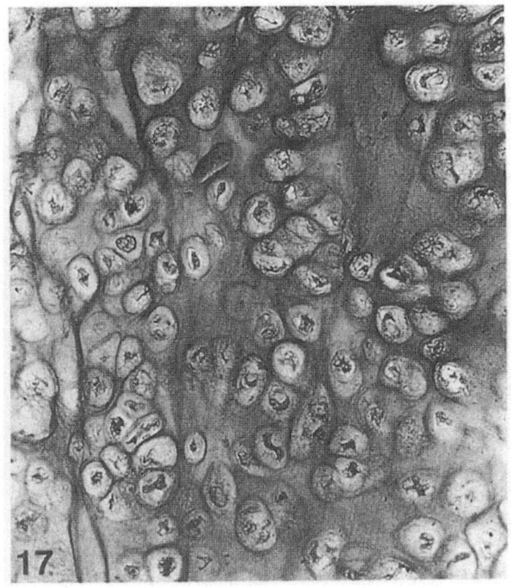

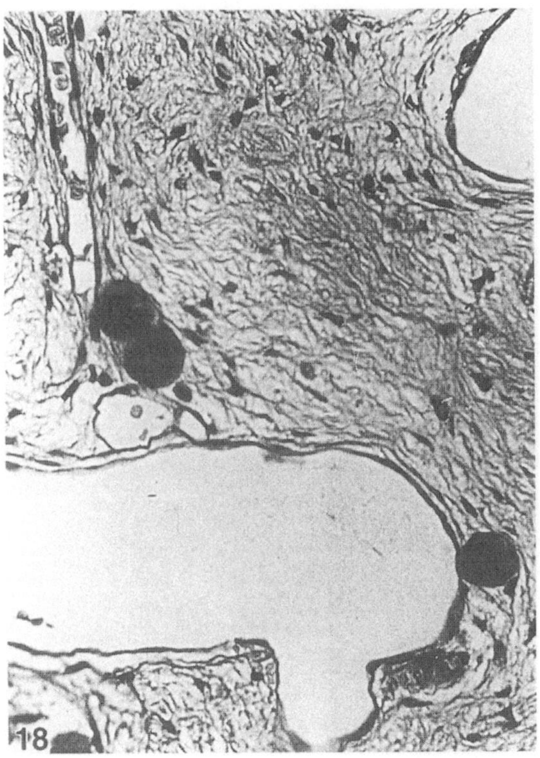

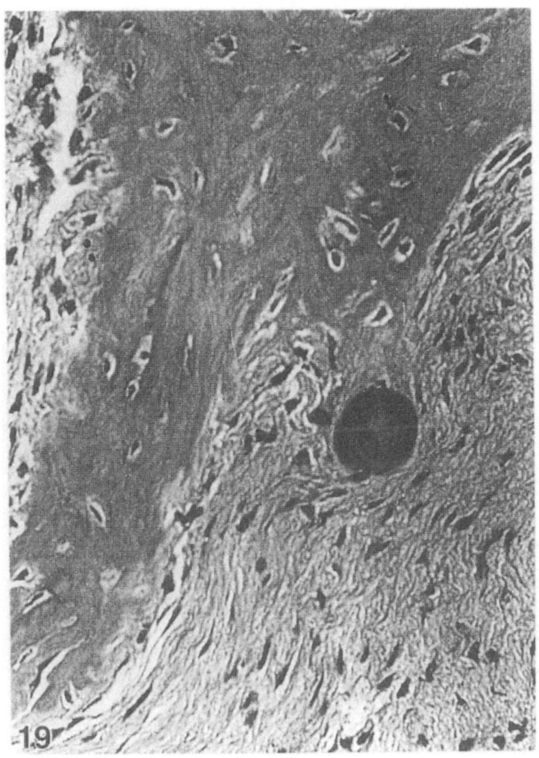

Fig. 16. Osteoid metamorphosis may be accompanied by cell proliferation resembling osteoblastic metamorphosis

Fig. 17. Area of well-differentiated metaplastic cartilage

Figs. 18, 19. Small rounded calcified formations with strongly haematinophil concentric annular reinforcement

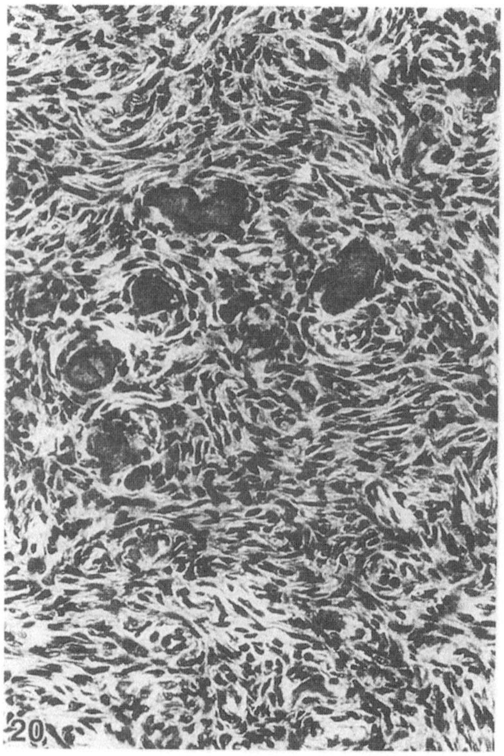

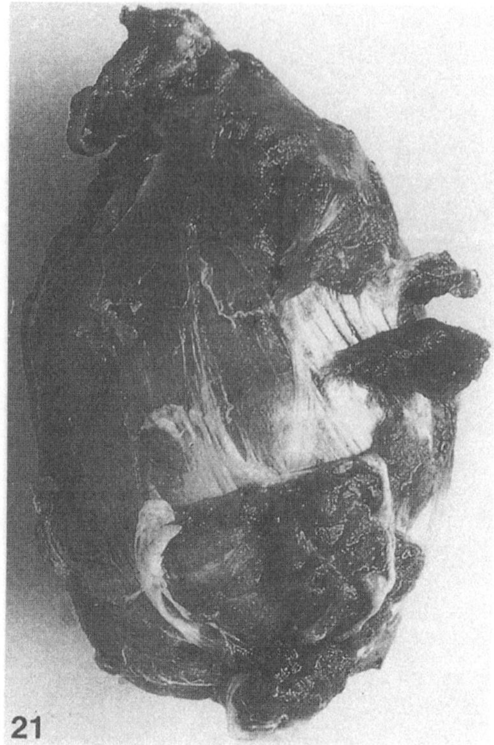

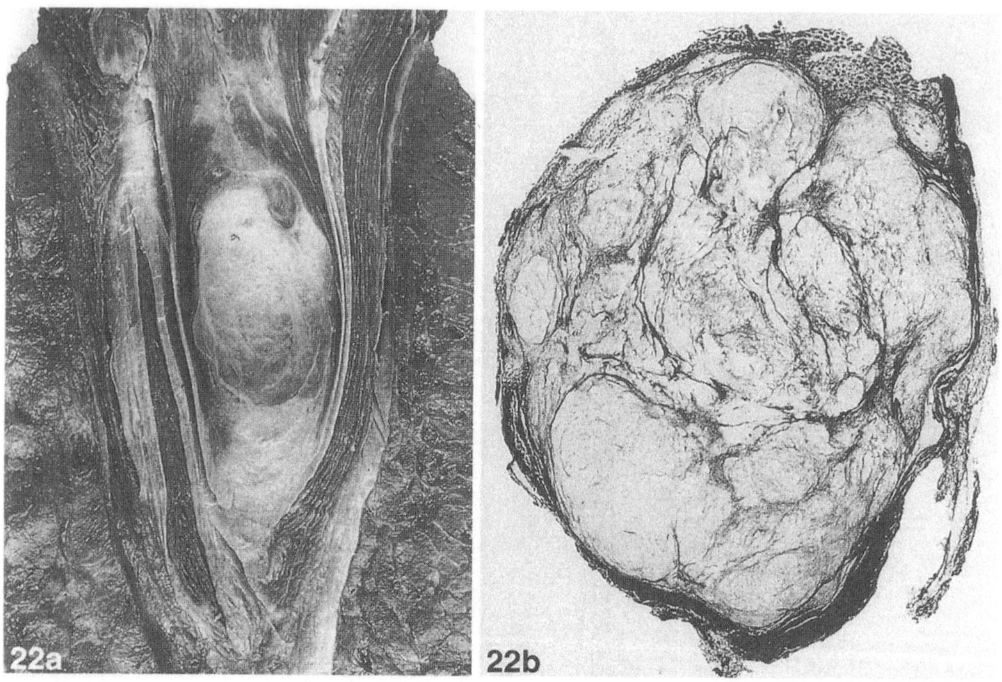

Fig. 20. Appearance of fibrous dysplasia in a case of Albright's syndrome. In this orbital lesion the appearance is identical to that of dysplasia in the long bones

Fig. 21. "Myxoma" of a musculo-tendinous junction (quadriceps). Autopsy specimen

Fig. 22. a "Myxoma" with adherent muscle and aponeurotic fibers. **b** In the section some fibrous septa lobulate a mucoid substance

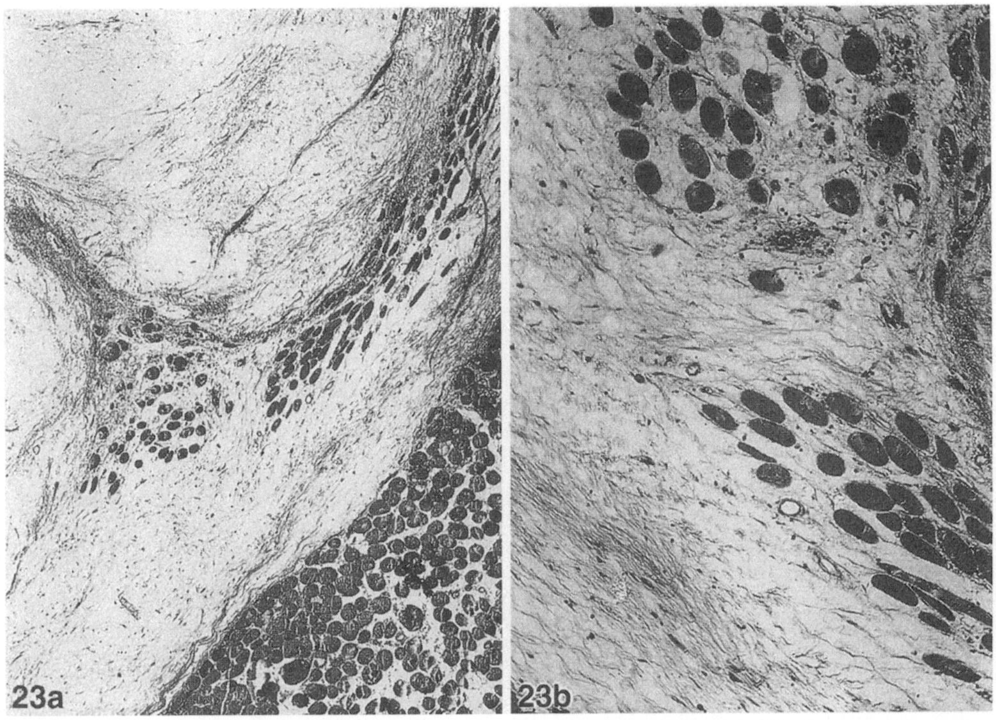

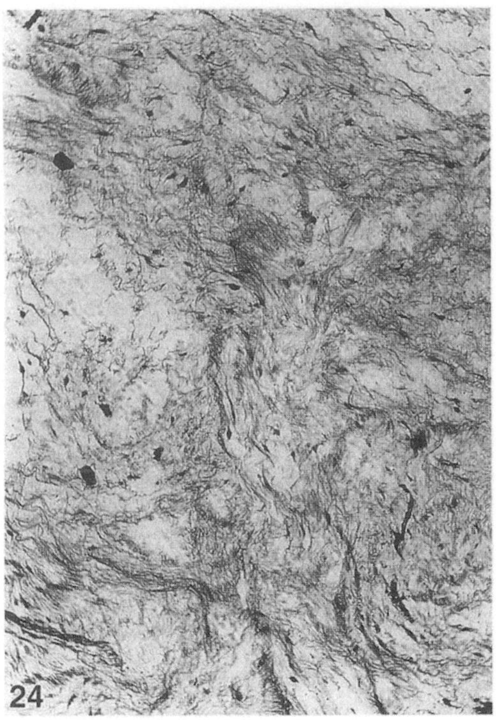

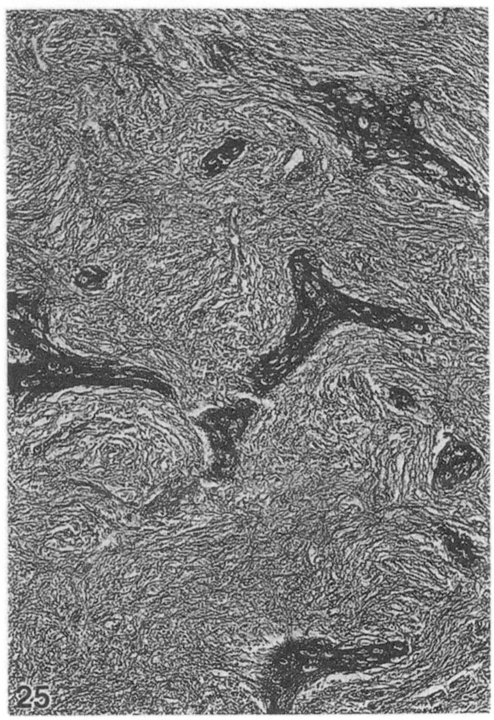

Fig. 23 a, b. There are no definite boundaries in the section; this myxoid appearance infiltrates the muscle bundles

Fig. 24. The lesion has few cells and is poorly vascularised, but is rich in fine reticulin fibers

Fig. 25. Same patient: zone of fibrous dysplasia; silver impregnation reveals the abundant reticulin network surrounding the metaplastic bony trabeculae

33. Metastases (secondary cancers of bone)

In a book about bone tumours this chapter can only hope to deal with matters of differential diagnosis. The metastatic process itself is not considered in this chapter, but simply, after a brief general review, some of the problems metastases create for pathologists.

General considerations

In adults, metastases to bone are about four times as common as primary malignant tumours. According to different sets of data, they are the presenting feature in about 10 to 30% of cases. In another 50% of cases they develop in the five years following detection of the primary tumour; but they can appear 15 years and more after that tumour has been treated.

Some carcinomas have the reputation of preferring bony sites, including prostatic, mammary, renal, thyroid and bronchopulmonary tumours; their relative incidence varies considerably from one hospital department to another. In a series of 380 patients affected by metastases from carcinoma of the breast (Finsen Institute, Copenhagen) 40% had only bony metastases and no other localisation. The statistics of the Alexis-Vautrin Center of Nancy [Conroy et al 1988], relating to 429 cases of bony metastases, mention 32.6% breast carcinomas, 22.1% lung carcinomas, 7.7% prostatic carcinomas and 7.4% carcinomas of the upper respiratory and alimentary tracts. At this same center bony metastases were the presenting feature of a bronchial tumour in 13.7% of cases, whereas they were the original manifestation in 30.3% of cases of prostatic cancer.

Depending on the hospital department concerned and its environment, the highest percentage is sometimes that of breast cancer, sometimes that of prostatic or bronchopulmonary cancer. Without denying a degree of bone preference in these tumours, it can be shown in a specialist department that the percentage of bony metastases in osteosarcomas is of the order of 15%, not allowing for the osteosarcomatoses (about 4%) or for skip metastases. Eighty per cent of metastases affect the spine and pelvis, followed by the ribs, femur, skull, scapulae and more rarely the distal bones [Bouvier et al 1982, Kernin 1983, Libson et al 1987]. Despite the rarity of distal metastases, 167 cases of metastases in the bones of the hand and 94 in those of the feet have been reported. About half the metastases in the foot bones affect the tarsus, a fourth being localised to the calcaneum. Opinions and statistics diverge as to the relative frequency of involvement of the carpus and the long bones. Carcinomas situated above the diaphragm metastasise more readily to the dorsal spine; conversely, carcinomas of the colon, rectum and prostate metastasise more readily to the lumbar spine.

The incidence of femoral involvement in carcinoma of the breast was 51.9% in the statistics of the Alexis-Vautrin center. In the same series, for cancers as a whole, bony metastases were the presenting feature in 22.6%; in 10.9% of cases investigations did not succeed in revealing the primary tumour, but here again there are wide variations from one publication to another.

Presenting features

The presenting features are pain, neurological signs and more rarely spontaneous fracture. Signs of inflammation are seen particularly in metastases of the extremities.

Table 1. Diagnosis of metastases

Adults

Essential: knowledge of the history and the radiological and clinical findings
The choice of immunohistological reactions must be guided by the morphology
The detection of one antigen in the tumour cells does not allow identification of the nature of the original tissue in every case
Epithelial appearance dominant (confirmed by antibodies). Investigate: prostate, thyroid, breast
- Traps: chordoma, adamantinoma, mesothelioma, schwannoma, meningioma

Fusiform-cell appearance dominant (confirmed by +ve vimentin reaction)
- Primary or secondary sarcoma? Previous history, clinical study
- Cellular polymorphism may suggest the origin: schwannian, muscular, histiocytofibroblastic
- Vimentin -ve, keratin +ve: consider fusiform-cell epithelioma (especially upper respiratory/alimentary tracts)

Clear cell appearance dominant
- Any epithelioma may be clear-celled: consider kidney, epithelioid sarcoma, clear-cell sarcoma, neuroendocrine tumour
- Traps: primary bone tumour of cartilaginous, adipose or vascular nature, some Ewing's tumours

Anaplastic appearance
- The immunology may suggest an epithelial tumour. If not, consider anaplastic osteosarcoma, melanoma, etc.

Children

Common: neuroblastoma, haemopathies (Langerhans histiocytosis has been discussed in Chapter 31)
Uncommon: metastases from osteosarcomas (the special case of osteosarcomatosis is discussed in Chapter 11). Metastases from embryonal rhabdomyosarcoma, mesenchymal nephroblastoma, clear-cell sarcoma of the kidney

Epithelial markers +	Epithelial markers – (vimentin +)
- Metastatic carcinoma • NSE, chromogranin +: neuroendocrine differentiation • PSA, PhAP +: prostatic origin • thyroglobulin +: thyroid origin • GCDFP, hormonal receptors: mammary origin - certain connective tissue tumours: adamantinoma, chordoma, epithelioid sarcoma, synovial sarcoma, mesothelioma	- PS100 +: schwannoma, malignant melanoma, clear-cell sarcoma - desmin, muscular actin +: muscle tumour, malignant fibrous histiocytoma

Imaging

The radiological appearances are many and various. Imaging may reveal bony metastasis, single or multiple, in patients regularly monitored after treatment of a carcinoma but it is bony metastases as a presenting feature that pose a real problem.

The osteolysis may have sharp boundaries more suggestive of a plasmocytic lesion or benign chondroma, but is more often ill-defined with fuzzy borders, suggesting a malignant structure. Less common are sclerosing forms which are often vertebral (breast, prostate) and which may suggest myelofibrosis, sclerosing myeloma, mastocytosis or sarcoidosis [Pederson et al 1976, Galasko 1982, Silverman 1991]. In some cases a sclerosing (osteoblastic) metastasis may be a response to chemotherapy [De Martini et al 1983], especially those where the sclerosis seems to correspond to a stabilisation of the metastatic lesion.

Usually the appearance is not so characteristic and there is a mixed appearance: a pagetoid, cloudy or woolly appearance, unaccompanied by thickening of the invaded bone, is a phenomenon characteristic of Paget's disease; a pseudosarcomatous type with a periosteal reaction may be suggestive of a primary tumour [Bloom et al 1987].

Pathological anatomy and histopathology

Macroscopically, every intermediate stage is possible between a firm, whitish tumour and a necrotic, haemorrhagic, encephaloid tumour. A haemorrhagic appearance is often mentioned in the operative report, especially with metastases from renal carcinoma. But there is at least one metastasis where the diagnosis is sometimes obvious: that of malignant melanoma, when the bony tissue is frankly pigmented and blackish.

In sections, osteolytic metastases occupy a zone devoid of bony trabeculae. At the periphery, the osteoclastic reaction is often obvious, but in certain cases the osteoclasts are only fusiform eosinophil cells with one or two nuclei and adherent to the bony tissue. In some sections there is major bony necrosis, probably related to vascular injury. The epithelial cells form small irregular islands; sometimes small groups of cells (often several small groups) are situated in the lumen of a dilated capillary (fig. 7). In other cases there is a largely dominant fibrous reaction occupying the greater part of the section surface and numerous parts must be searched to identify small foci of metastatic cells. The same applies to sclerosing forms or to a fragment of eburnated bone where some cell groups, usually prostatic or mammary, are detected in minute medullary areas.

Prognostic implications

In the course of carcinomas the presence of metastatic bony lesions is usually regarded as an unfavourable prognostic factor; however, survival of patients affected by bony metastases also depends on the organ affected, the efficacy of treatment, the duration of the latent period and the existence of other, non-bony, metastases [Conroy et al 1988]. A major statistical study has shown that 5-year and 10-year survival of patients with soft tissue sarcomas of a high grade of malignancy where the tumour invades nerves, vessels or bones, was significantly better than that of patients with lymph node lesions [Ruka et al 1988]. Toma et al (1993) followed 60 patients affected with vertebral metastases; the mean survival after discovery of the metastases was 40.4 months. Korkala and Karaharju (1991) treated 42 patients with metastatic fractures of the long bones from 1976 to 1980; only 5 survived for 6 years or more. Progress in chemotherapy may give some hope of an improvement of these results.

Diagnostic groups (mainly in adults)

The site of the primary cancer is known

The lesion, usually osteolytic, has appeared 3-5 years after the end of treatment and the biopsy is intended only to confirm a strong clinical suspicion.

Comparison of tumour and metastatic morphology

The metastasis may be identical to the primary tumour but may also be more or less differentiated, or structurally altered by treatment. Again, tumour cells find a singular support in the bony tissue and cylindrical cells may be seen arranged along the bony trabeculae as if on a basement membrane. It is not unusual to see cases where the morphology of the metastatic lesion is so different from that of the primary tumour that it is impossible to assert that it is the same tumour. Immunohistological reactions may help.

Abnormally long latent period

There is a risk that the primary tumour, even if not forgotten, is not mentioned on the request for examination. This may involve a genuine metastasis, but it may also be true for another tumour, either primary or a metastasis from a second, undiagnosed, tumour of which the metastasis is the presenting feature.

Tumours that rarely metastasise

These include the chemodectomas and certain skin tumours. In the light of the patient's history the report must be very cautious if the metastasis is not typical.

Bone lesions after irradiation

There is a common problem in maxillofacial surgery after irradiation of a carcinoma: is the zone of mandibular osteolysis observed a metastatic lesion, a post-irradiation osteolysis, or, if some years have passed, a radiation-induced sarcoma?

The first two problems are of limited difficulty but in putative radiation-induced sarcoma we may find no reason to incriminate the irradiation from the pathological findings. But if the lesion has developed in an irradiated zone the probability is very high. Further, in recent decades we have seen a decrease in the interval between the irradiation and the development of sarcoma.

Is this a metastasis, a second tumour, or a multifocal syndrome?

This question, often posed to the pathologist, will not find an answer solely on the microscope stage. The types of difficulty presented are say a giant-cell tumour with 2 or 3 lesions, but the problem may be more complex. A child of 14 had an amputation for a sarcoma of the left leg. Two years later, I received a biopsy from a sarcoma of the right tibia, radiologically an apparent primary. It is not clear what is represented by the multiple bony lesions in this patient femur, scapula and ribs. Is this a mesenchymal chondrosarcoma? What is represented by multiple lesions of a malignant angioendothelioma developing over time? It is likely that these are metastases but certainty is difficult.

The site of the primary cancer is not known

The radiological appearance suggests a primary tumour

A lateralised osteolytic image in a long bone with periosteal reaction typical of a primary sarcoma (fig. 1) and a request for histological examination may arrive with this provisional diagnosis; but this radiographic appearance will not present histological difficulties.

Pagetic or pagetoid radiological appearances

The characteristic thickening of pagetic bone is quite different from the pagetoid appearance without thickening of the bone so characteristic of a vertebra or iliac bone. But there may be considerable difficulty for the pathologist, especially if the lesion is a sclerotic one; the greater part of the sectional surface is occupied by bone and the medullary spaces which control ossification are reduced, so that it is necessary to study more sections and to know how to distinguish a small grouping of 5 or 6 cubo-cylindrical cells from an osteoblastic proliferation.

A solitary lesion and its histological appearance suggest a primary non-bony tumour

A sacral or vertebral metastasis from a colonic carcinoma may simulate a chordoma. If the morphology is not evident in a small sample, histochemical and immunohistological reactions may provide the diagnosis. Some adamantinomas resemble epitheliomatous metastases, others an angiosarcoma.

Undifferentiated fusiform-cell tumour

Is this a primary tumour or a metastasis from an undiagnosed sarcoma or epithelioma? Some metastases from carcinoma of the kidney and upper respiratory-alimentary tracts may consist solely of fusiform cells. In renal metastases the operative report often mentions the signally haemorrhagic nature of the lesion. But it may also be a fibroblastic sarcoma - despite its effacement by malignant fibrous histiocytoma - or a primary leiomyosarcoma, even after the pathologist has been assured that the patient has not undergone a hysterectomy for "fibroma" in previous years (fig. 13).

Immunology may render great service and suggest other investigations but it may also leave the problem unresolved.

Primary tumour, local invasion by an adjacent tumour, or a metastasis?

This problem often arises in connection with a biopsy made on a flat bone (ilium, sternum, mandible), where epithelial inclusions or fusiform-cell sarcomas have very rapidly destroyed the cortical bone. It may be imprudent to affirm a metastatic origin.

Presentation with pathological fracture

Spontaneous fracture is ten times as often the presenting feature in an orthopaedic department as in a rheumatology clinic. Though it occurs in patients having generally reached the age where osteoporosis is common, this is not always the case.

When a biopsy is made some days after the fracture, new formation of cartilage and bone is already visible in addition to the haemorrhage and fibrinous coagulum. Only an adequate surgical sample will allow the diagnosis of a focus of small-cell proliferation (osteosarcoma, epithelioma, neuroepithelial tumour, lymphosarcoma); the age and history (smoking) may be suggestive but the histochemical and immunohistological reactions are very important.

Metastases in children and adolescents

The commonest metastases are those from Ewing's sarcoma, osteosarcoma and neuroblastoma (fig. 4); then come metastases from Wilms tumour, rhabdomyosarcoma and medulloblastoma. If there is any uncertainty, the report should make use of the supplementary studies (imaging, biochemical assays) which allow identification of the primary tumour.

Metastases from medulloblastomas have several times been reported as a cause of osteosclerosis.

In children treated for retinoblastoma, it should be remembered that the risks of developing an osteosarcoma are three times as great as those in a healthy subject.

Metastasis to a diseased bone

No normal bone, including a sesamoid and the patella in particular, is immune from harboring a metastatic proliferation; but diseased bones may also be affected, including irradiated or pagetic bone [Crouzet and Beraneck 1990] as I have twice observed.

Routine search by needle aspiration

This involves aspiration of the iliac crests and guided aspiration [Troussier et al 1980]. These techniques allow confirmation of malignancy in nearly half the cases explored, according to Vinceneux et al (1983).

The detection of antigens, initially wide-spectrum and then more specific, permits and will increasingly permit the recognition of metastatic cells and definition of their origin.

Uses and limitations of current techniques

Current techniques in molecular biology allow the location and amplification in a tumour sample of any DNA sequence whose nucleotide sequence is known. Sequences can thus be detected which correspond to the chromosomal translocations characteristic of chronic lymphoid leukaemia and nodular lymphoma as examples. This methodology makes it possible to detect one tumour cell among 10^5 or 10^6 normal cells. In principle, it may be employed whenever a tumour is associated with a characteristic DNA modification; but does the detection of tumour cells in a sample of circulating blood, for instance, necessarily imply the existence of bony metastases?

This investigation may be complemented by scintigraphic investigation using organo-phosphates labelled with ^{99m}Tc, which allows a complete skeletal survey with an irradiation dose less than that of standard radiography of the entire skeleton (figs. 5, 6). Schematically, the two appearances observed are a zone of hyperfixation or, on the contrary, a clear zone of nonfixation; prostatic metastases belong to the first category and those from the kidney and thyroid to the second. Metastases from breast carcinoma may belong to either of these two types.

An attempt to distinguish between primary tumours and metastases, based on study of the patient's serum, was made by Shinozaki et al (1992). The radioimmunological technique applied to several markers left them with the tissue polypeptide antigen (TPA) as being the most discriminant. The other antigens studied, including alpha-fetoprotein and carcino-embryonal antigen, were of no value. Specific antibodies may specify the origin of a metastasis, a practice virtually limited to thyroid and prostatic carcinomas.

References

Aoki J, Yamamoto I, Hino M, Shigeno C, Kitamura N, Sone T, Shiomi K, Konishi J (1988) Osteoclast-mediated osteolysis in bone metastasis from renal cell carcinoma. Cancer 62: 98-104

Berrettoni BA, Carter JR (1986) Mechanism of cancer metastasis to bone. J Bone Joint Surg 68A: 308-312

Bloom RA, Libson E, Husband JE, Stoker DJ (1987) The periosteal sunburst reaction to bone metastases. A literature review and report of 20 additional cases. Skeletal Radiol 16: 629-634

Blythe JG, Ptacek JJ, Buchsbaum HJ, Latourette HB (1975) Bony metastases from carcinoma of cervix. Occurrence, diagnosis, and treatment. Cancer 36: 475-484

Bouvier M, Lejeune E, Bonvoisin B, Brion P (1982) Les métastases osseuses distales du membre supérieur. Sem Hop Paris 58: 2736-2739

Chomette G, Auriol M, Pinaudeau Y, Brocheriou C (1964) Les métastases osseuses des tumeurs malignes. Dénombrement, répartition topographique, réaction du mésenchyme ostéomédullaire (à propos de 119 cas). Bull Cancer 51: 181-202

Coerkamp EG, Kroon HM (1988) Cortical bone metastases. Radiol 169: 525-528

Conroy T, Malissard L, Dartois D, Luporsi E, Stines J, Chardot C (1988) Histoire naturelle et évolution des métastases osseuses. A propos de 429 observations. Bull Cancer 75: 845-857

Contreras E, Ellis LD, Lee RE (1972) Value of the bone marrow biopsy in the diagnosis of metastatic carcinoma. Cancer 29: 778-783

Crouzet J, Beraneck L (1990) Maladie de Paget et métastases d'épithélioma sur le même os. 11 nouvelles observations et revue de la littérature. Rev Rhum 57: 517-520

De Martini AL, Buzdar AU, Blumenschein GR (1983) Osteoblastic metastatic disease as a therapeutic response to adjuvant chemotherapy in breast cancer. J Surg Oncol 22: 32-34

Dubost JJ, Galtier B, Ristori JM, Sauvezie B, Bussière JL, Rampon S (1987) Maladie de Paget et cancer prostatique. Un difficile problème diagnostique illustré par 3 observations. Rev Rhum 54: 771-114

Fornasier VL, Horne JG (1975) Metastases to the vertebral column. Cancer 36: 590-594

Galasko CSB (1982) Mechanism of lytic and blastic metastatic disease of bone. Clin Orthop 109: 20-27

Gellad FE, Sadato N, Numaguchi Y, Levine AM (1990) Vascular metastatic lesions of the spine: preoperative embolization. Radiology 176: 683-686

Goorin AM, Shuster JJ, Baker A, Horowitz ME, Meyer WH, Link MP (1991) Changing pattern of pulmonary metastases with adjuvant chemotherapy in patients with osteosarcoma: results from the multi-institutional osteosarcoma study. J Clin Oncol 9: 600-605

Greenspan A, Norman A (1988) Oteolytic cortical destruction: an unusual pattern of skeletal metastases. Skeletal Radiol 17: 402-406

Gricouroff G (1947) Sur la pathogénie des métastases tardives dans le cancer. J Belge Radiol 30: 1-7

Hosenpud JD, Thoming D, Greenberg G (1980) Liposarcoma metastatic to bone marrow presenting as myelophthisic anemia. A case report. Cancer 45: 345-348

Ishimura E, Iwamoto H, Kobashi Y, Yamabe H, Ichijima K (1983) Malignant chondroid syringoma. Report of a case of pertinent literature. Cancer 52: 1966-1973

Jacobs SG (1983) Spread of prostatic cancer to bone. Urol 21: 337-344

Johnston WW, Szpak CA, Schlom J, Lortich SC, Thor A (1986) Use of a monoclonal antibody (B72.3) as a novel immunohistochemical adjunct for the diagnosis of carcinomas in fine needle aspiration biopsy specimens. Hum Pathol 17: 501-513

Kamby C, Vejborg 1, Dugaard S, Guldhammer B, Dirksen H, Rossing N, Mouridsen HT (1987) Clinical and radiologic characteristics of bone metastases in breast cancer. Cancer 60: 2524-2531

Kattapuram SV, Shurana JS, Scott JA, El-Koury GY (1990) Negative scintigraphy with positive magnetic resonance imaging in bone metastases. Skeletal Radiol 19: 113-116

Kerin R (1983) Metastatic tumors of the hand: a review of the literature. J Bone Joint Surg 65A: 1331-1334

Khurana JS, Kattapuram SV, Ehara S, Rosenberg AE, Yaw K (1989) Metastatic paranganglioma. Skeletal Radiol 18: 565-567

Kim ED, Deland FH, Maruyama Y (1978) Decreased uptake in bone scans (cold lesions) in metestatic carcinoma. Two case reports. J Bone Joint Surg 60A: 844-846

Korkala OL, Karaharju EO (1991) Metastatic fractures of long bones. Int Orthop 15: 105-109

Le Charpentier Y, Tomeno B, Carlioz A, Chevrot A, Abelanet R (1979) Métastases osseuses simulant un chondrosarcome. A propos de 3 cas. Rev Chir Orthop 65: 351-352

Libson E, Bloom RA, Husband JE, Stoker DJ (1987) Metastatic tumours of bones of the hand and foot. A comparative review and report of 43 additional cases. Skeletal Radiol 16: 387-392

Litton GJ, Ward JH, Abbatt RM, Williams HJ (1991) Isolated calcaneal metastastis in a patient with endometrial adenocarcinoma. Cancer 67: 1979-1983

Maillefert JF, Tebib J, Huguenin MC, Chauffert B, Pascaud F, Peere T, Chatard C, Tavernier C, Strauss J (1993) Les métastases osseuses révélatrices: recherche du cancer primitif. Etude d'une série de 15 cas. Sem Hop Paris 69: 372-378

Marsot-Dupuch K, Cauquil P, Muntalak H, Mazabraud A, Jaqueux Y (1984) Métastases osseuses d'un hémangiopéricytome. J Radiol 65: 41-45

McLean RG, Caligeros D, Vimala N, Murray IPC (1985) Metastatic liposarcoma. Skeletal Radiol 13: 84-88

McLennan MK (1991) Malignant epithelial thymoma with osteoblastic metastases. Skeletal Radiol 20: 141-144

Miller F, Whitehill R (1984) Carcinoma of the breast metastatic to the skeleton. Clin Orthop 184: 121-127

Mir R, Philips SL, Schwartz G, Mathur R, Khan A, Kahn LB (1987) Metastatic neuroblastoma after 52 years of dormancy. Cancer 60: 2510-2514

Muggia FM, Hansen HH (1972) Osteoblastic metastases in small-cell (oat-cell) carcinoma of the lung. Cancer 30: 801-805

Nielsen OS, Munro AJ, Tannock IF (1991) Bone metastases: pathophysiology and management policy. J Clin Oncol 9: 509-524

Nottebaert M, Exner GU, Von Hochstetter AR, Schreiber A (1989) Metastatic bone disease from occult carcinoma: a profile. Int Orthop 13: 119-123

Okazaki N, Yoshimo M, Yoshida T, Hikohasshi S, Kishi K, Simosato Y (1985) Bone metastasis in hepatocellular carcinoma. Cancer 55: 1991-1994

Pederson RT, Haldak DJ, Ferris RA, Macdonald JS, Schein PS (1976) Osteoblastic bone metastasis in Zollinger-Ellison syndrome. Radiology 118: 63-64

Pedro TV, Azouz EM, Hoeffel JC (1989) Metastases to bone in medulloblastoma. A report of 5 cases. Skeletal Radiol 18: 445-449

Piedbois P, Breau JL, Morere JF, Israel L (1987) Sweat gland carcinoma with bone and visceral metastases prolonged complete remission lasting 16 months as a result of chemotherapy. Cancer 60: 170-172

Rochet N, Pages M, Lassoued S, Poey C, Fournié B, Fournié A (1991) Métastase phalangienne de la main. A propos d'une observation. Rev Rhum 58: 73-78

Ruka W, Emrich LJ, Driscoll DL, Karakousis CP (1988) Prognostic significative of lymph node metastasis and bone, malor vessel, or nerve involvement in adults with high-grade soft tissue sarcomas. Cancer 62: 999-1006

Schlumberger M, Tubiana M, De Valthaire F, Hill C, Gardet P, Travagli JP, Fragu P, Lombrosso J, Caillou B, Parmentier C (1986) Long-term results of treatment of 283 patients with lung and bone metastases from differentiated thyroid carcinoma. J Clin Endoc Metab 63: 960-967

Serre H, Simon L, Lamboley C (1970) Les métastases osseuses des cancers cutanés. Cahiers Méd 11: 1231-1243

Shapeero LG, Couanet D, Vanel D, Ackerman LV, Terrier-Lacombe MJ, Flamant F, Contesso G, Lumbroso J (1993) Bone metastases as the presenting manifestation of rhabdomyosarcoma in childhood. Skeletal Radiol 22: 433-438

Shinozaki T, Chigira M, Kato K (1992) Multivariate analysis of serum tumor markers for diagnosis of skeletal metastases. Cancer 69: 108-112

Silverman JM (1991) Metastatic osteoblastic carcinoid tumor (primary in pancreas or gallbladder). Skeletal Radiol 20: 149-151

Simon MA, Bartucci EJ (1986) The search for the primary tumor in patients with skeletal metastases of unknown origin. Cancer 58: 1088-1095

Thompson J, Zimmermann W (1988) The carcinoembryonic antigen structure expression and evolution. Tumor Biol 9: 63-83

Toma S, Valenturino A, Sogno G, Formica C, Bignotti B, Bonassi S, Palumbo R (1993) Metastatic bone tumors. Non surgical treatment. Outcome and survival. Clin Orthop 295: 246-251

Tomita T, Das L, Radkowski MA (1990) Bone metastases of medulloblastoma in childhood; correlation with flow cytometric DNA analysis. J Neuro Oncol 8: 113-120

Troussier B, Pillon P, Masri B, Grauer JL, Boiszel R, Jacquot F, Phelip X (1988) Métastases osseuses révélatrices d'une tumeur carcinoïde du pancréas. Presse Med 17: 1411

Troussier B, Zagala A, Tarel V, Couderc P, Juvin R, Phelip X (1986) La ponction-biopsie osseuse systématique de crête iliaque dans les cancers secondaires des os. A propos de 67 observations. Sem Hop Paris 62: 3407-3412

Valette F, Dryll A, Sèze (de) S (1969) Le cancer secondaire des os d'origine pulmonaire en rhumatologie. A propos de 41 observations. Rev Rhum 36: 1-18

Vieco PT, Azouz EM, Hocffel JC (1989) Metastases to bone in medulloblastoma a report of five cases. Skeletal Radiol 18: 445-449

Vinceneux P, Cramer E, Grossin M, Kahn MF (1983) Diagnostic des métastases osseuses. Intérêt de la ponction dirigée et la ponction-biopsie systématique en crête iliaque postérieure. Presse Med 12: 873-876

Wassef M, Cywiner-Golenzer CH (1979) Les métastases osseuses des cancers: retentissement sur le tissu osseux et médullaire. Arch Anat Cytol Pathol 27: 337-342

Yazawa Y, Frassica FJ, Chao EYS, Pritchard DJ, Sim FH, Shives TC (1990) Metastatic bone disease. A study of the surgical treatment of 166 pathologic humeral and femoral fractures. Clin Orthop 251: 213-219

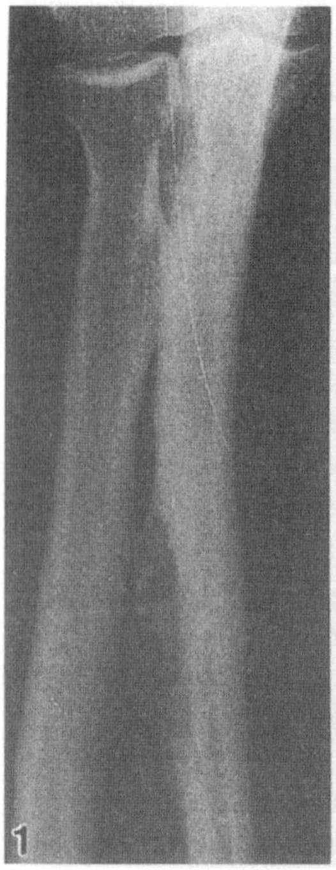
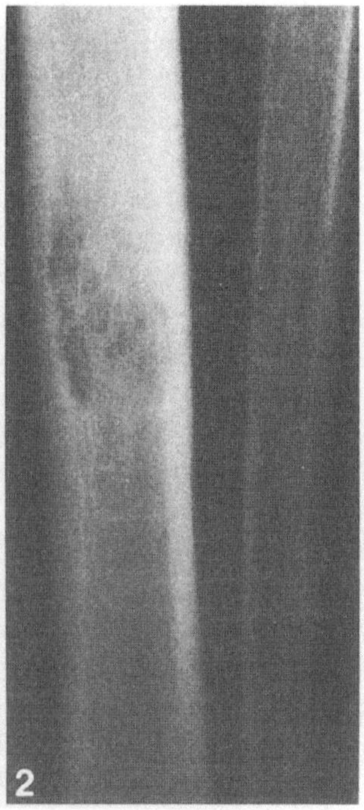
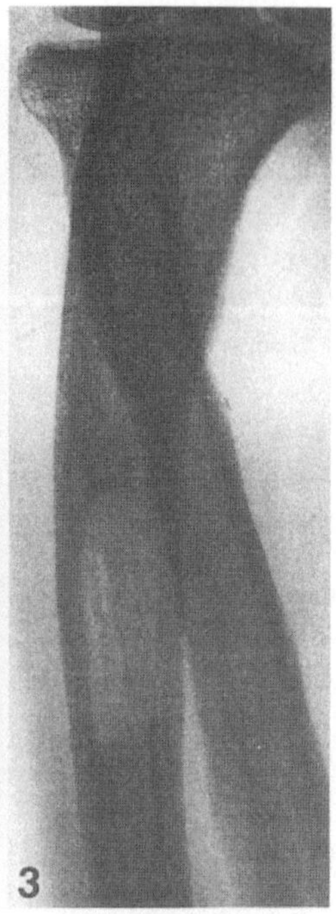
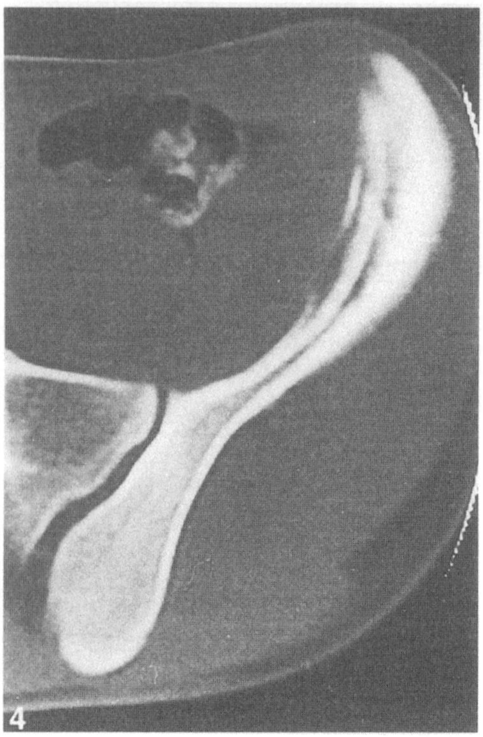
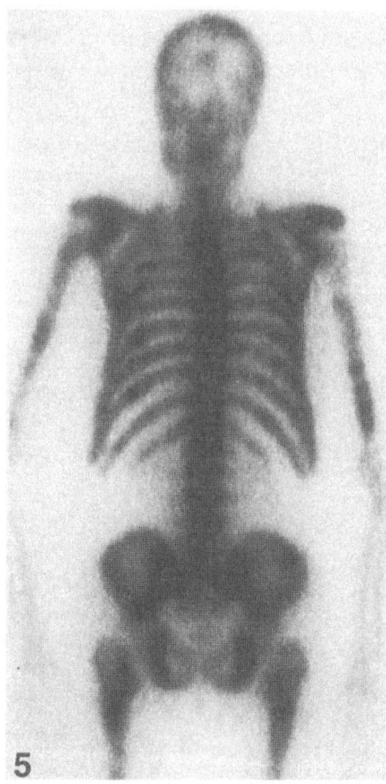
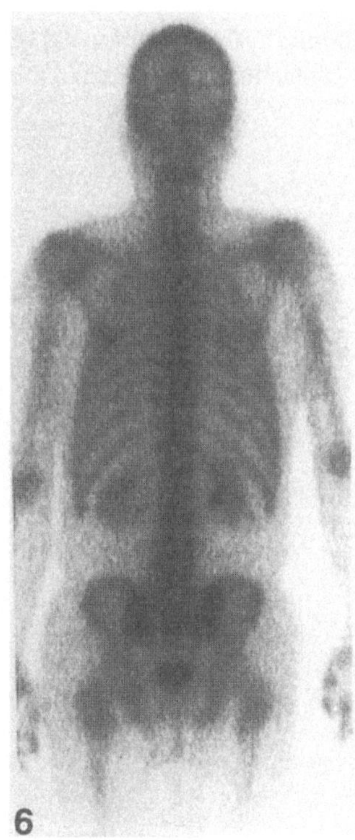

Fig. 1. This cortico-periosteal metastasis may suggest a chondroma or a chondrosarcoma, but it is a metastasis from a malignant melanoma

Fig. 2. This tibial diaphyseal metastasis may suggest a diagnosis of adamantinoma, but it is a carcinoma

Fig. 3. In a porotic forearm this well-defined lytic area does not correspond to a metastasis or a plasmocytoma; it is a lesion of parathyroid osteoporosis

Fig. 4. CT image of a metastasis in the iliac crest from a neuroblastoma

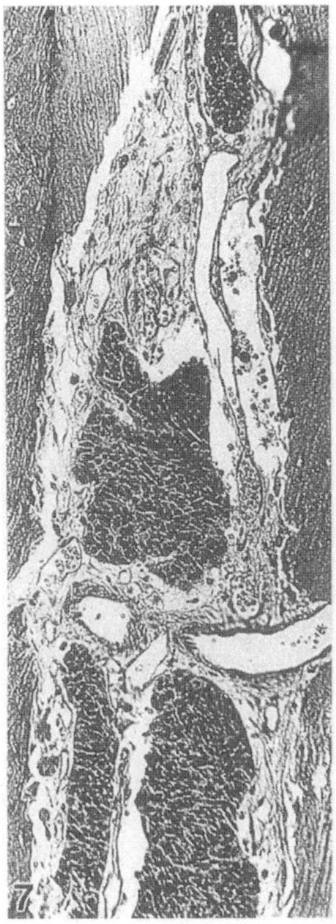

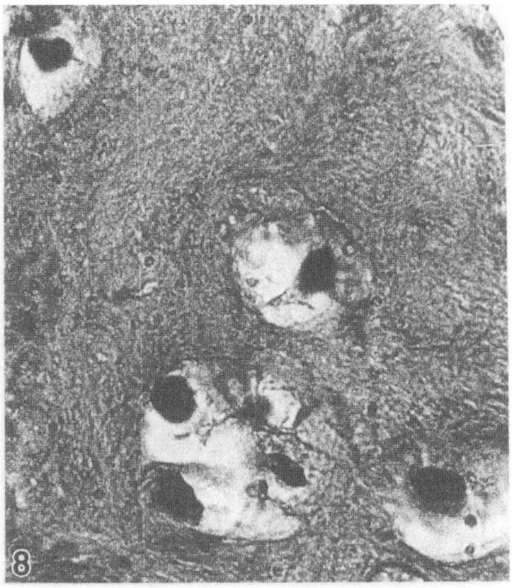

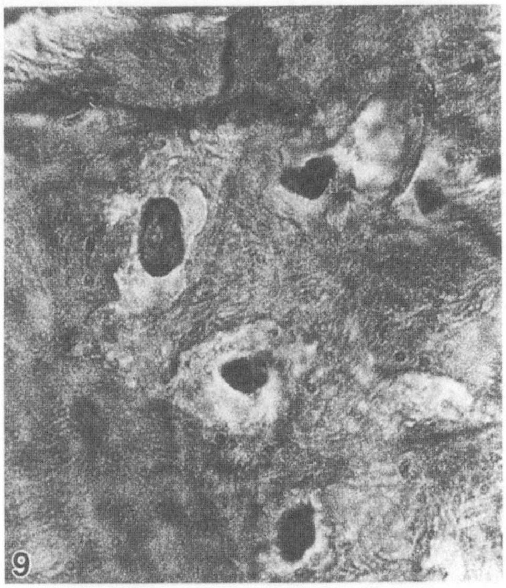

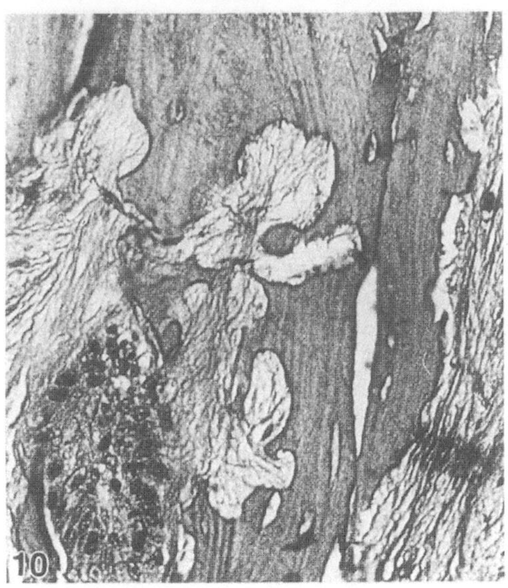

Fig. 7. Intravascular location of a bronchial carcinoma. The osteoclasis develops in the fibrous marrow away from the tumour islands, perhaps to reabsorb bone that is already necrotic due to circulatory disorders created by tumour embolism

Figs. 8, 9. Tumour cells of mammary origin trapped in osteoid tissue or possibly participating in its formation

Fig. 10. Metastasis from a bronchial carcinoma. This fragment of cortical bone, partly absorbed by multiple osteoclastic engulfment, is sequestrated in a paucicellular fibrous marrow

←

Fig. 5. Scintigraphic image (^{99m}Tc-MDP). Search for bony lesions from cancer of the prostate in a man aged 81. The lesions are multiple and very contrasted; there is a major concentration of the isotope by the prostatic metastases. The great sensitivity of the numerous rib and humeral lesions allowed their detection 4 and 6 months before their appearance in a standard radiograph

Fig. 6. Depending on the nature of the tumour, there are great differences of affinity for the radioactive tracer. In this woman of 65, although the bony lesions from a thyroid carcinoma are numerous, scintigraphy (^{99m}Tc-MDP) only shows the iliac lesions and one costal lesion (8th rib), whereas iodine scintigraphy demonstrated multiple costal, spinal and cranial lesions

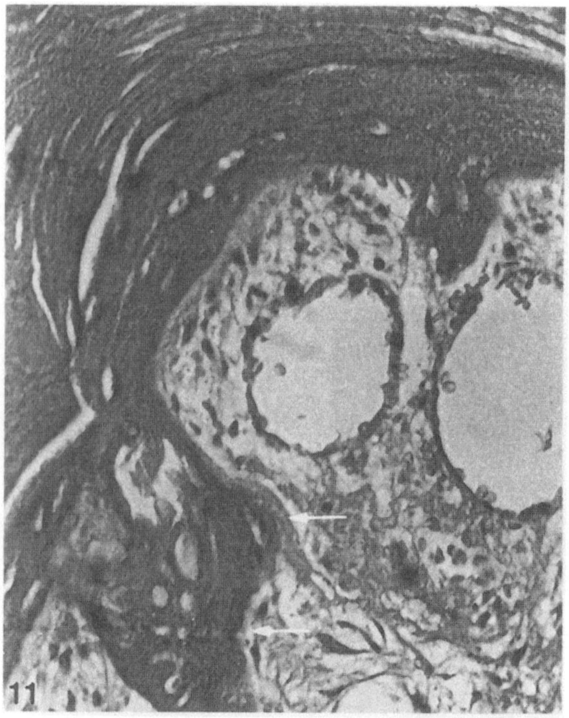

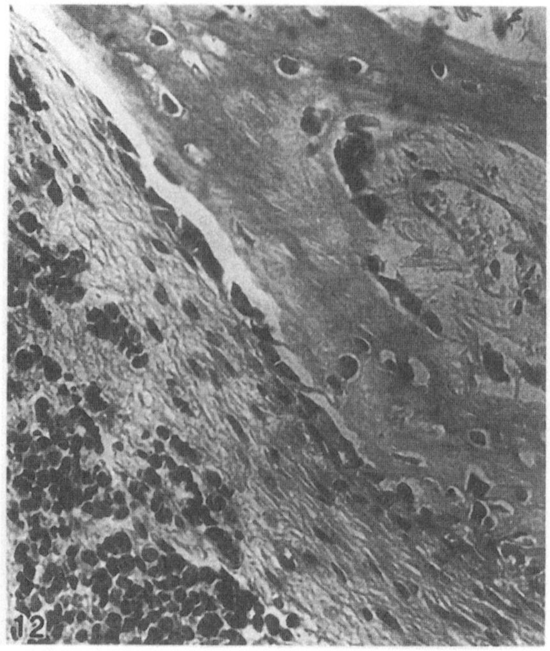

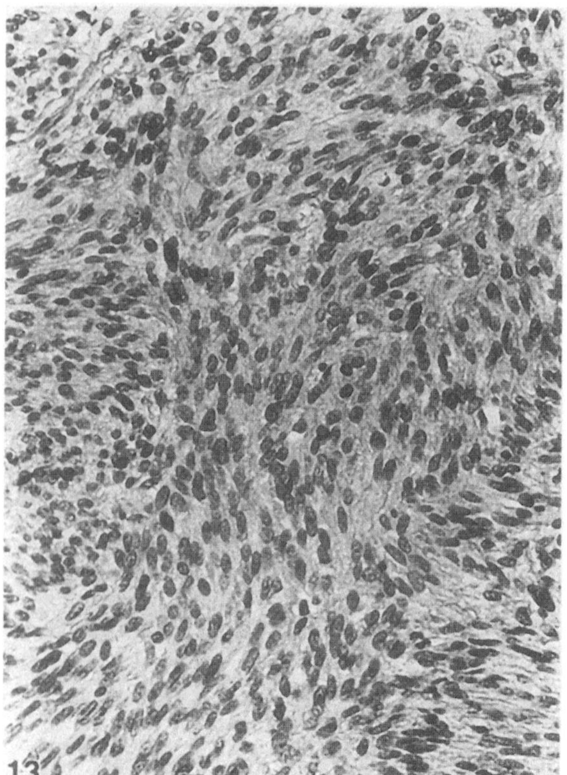

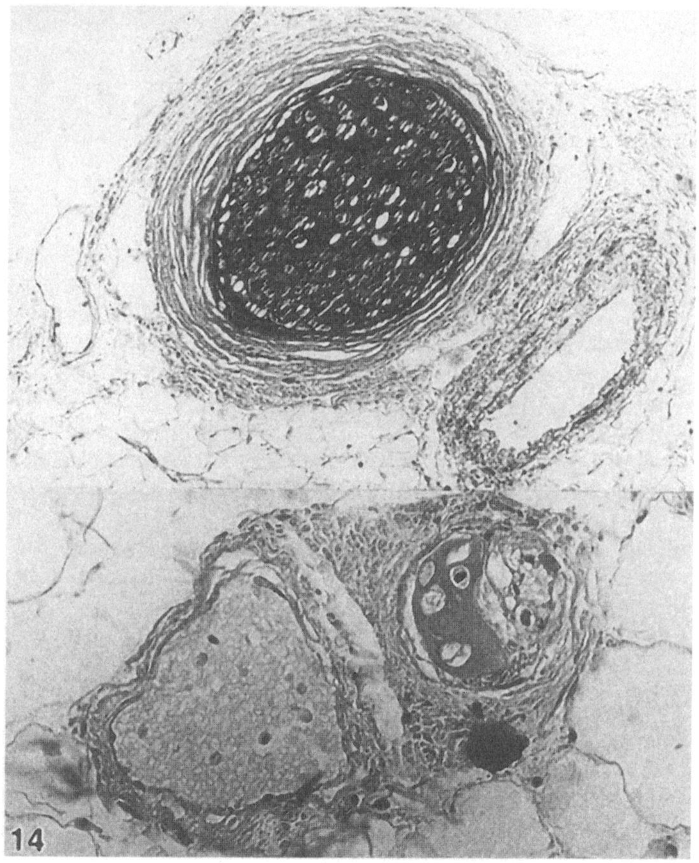

Fig. 11. Apposition of metaplastic bone (*arrows*) on preexisting bony lamellae

Fig. 12. Bone formation of osteoblastic type in the immediate vicinity of a metastasis from a retinoblastoma

Fig. 13. Trochanteric metastasis from a uterine sarcoma

Fig. 14. The "rapid arterial route" has allowed this chondrosarcoma of the shoulder to metastasise to all the distal tissues of the upper limb, including the distal phalanges and soft tissues

34. Malignant lymphoma

Our understanding of the malignant lymphomas has advanced considerably in recent years helped by the development of immunohistological methods. Everything that has been discovered about nodal lymphosarcomas is by definition applicable to the extranodal lymphosarcomas and the reader may consult specialist works on this subject. The following section concerns only those lymphomas with primarily bony manifestations which usually lead to biopsy (Hodgkin's or non-Hodgkin's lymphomas).

Malignant non-Hodgkin's lymphomas with primary localisation in bone

(figs. 1-17 and Diagram 1)

The primary malignant lymphomas of bone occupy a special place in the generality of non-Hodgkin's lymphomas. First identified in 1939 by Parker and Jackson under the name of "reticulosarcoma", their incidence among the extranodal forms of non-Hodgkin's lymphomas is quite rare (about 1%) and their symptomatology is often that of a localised tumour whose spread is very slow, though it may come to involve other bony or nodal structures, when the initial picture is identical with that of all non-Hodgkin's lymphomas. The term "reticulosarcoma" has been abandoned in the modern classifications of non-Hodgkin's lymphoma; it nearly always refers to the "large-celled" lymphomas, which are the commonest histological forms of primary malignant lymphomas of bone.

Case histories

Case 1. A young man of 17 attended for pain in the left shoulder of some weeks' duration. The radiographs of the humerus showed a very peculiar appearance with small confluent zones of osteolysis, but no breach of the cortex, suggesting a lymphosarcomatous tumour. Biopsy confirmed the diagnosis and indicated that it was a large-celled lymphoma, while further investigation revealed no other bony, visceral or nodal lesion. The prognosis was excellent, after a short course of chemotherapy followed by radiotherapy to the affected bone. The complications were minimal.

Case 2. A secretary of 55 had had pain in the elbow for over a year; a radiograph had shown nothing suggesting a diagnosis. After a year she fractured the lower end of the humerus during housework. The arm was then immobilised in plaster in the hope of securing union of the fracture but the pain increased and a new radiograph showed virtually total lysis of the lower third of the humerus. The biopsy then made allowed a diagnosis of malignant non-Hodgkin's lymphoma. It is interesting to note that despite the long delay there was no other evidence of spread than a slightly suspect homolateral axillary node. Chemotherapy appropriate to the type of lymphoma (immunoblastic) was at once instituted. The results were spectacular; not only did the lesion cease to progress but in a few months the humerus was virtually reconstituted. Recovery without functional complications allowed the patient to resume her work; all treatment has been discontinued for 5 years.

Case 3. The orthopaedic department sent a biopsy of a partly destroyed vertebral body in a man of 50. As in the two previous cases the search for spread revealed no other lesion.

General considerations

The lymphomas represent not more than 3 to 5% of all tumours of bone. Male predominance is of the order

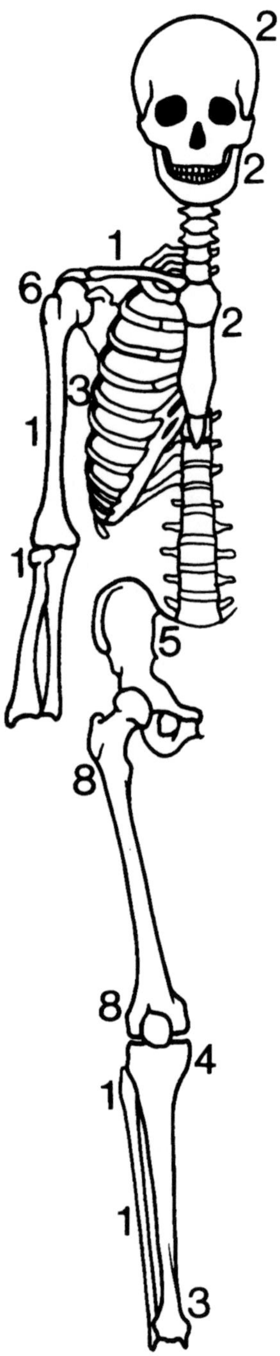

Diagram 1. Localisation of 45 lymphosarcomas of bone [Dumont et al 1983]

of 3:2. These tumours are very rare before the age of 15, though Howat et al (1987) reported 7 cases of malignant lymphoma in children, of whom the eldest was under 15 and the youngest only 18 months. The rarity of this tumour in children is demonstrated by the fact that during the same period these authors had treated 88 patients with Ewing's sarcoma. The age range is however very broad, with a peak in the 5th and 6th decades.

The bones most often affected are the femur and ilium followed by the humerus, tibia and radius, skull and face, vertebrae and scapulae. Diagram 1 represents the localisations of 45 cases studied with Dr Dumont at the Institut Curie in 1979.

Clinical features

The presenting feature is usually bone pain, which may precede discovery of the lesion by many months and is attributed only subsequently to the tumour. More rarely, there may be an initial pathological fracture or a palpable swelling. In one of our patients there was a frankly rounded structure, radiologically well-circumscribed, of the lower end of the thigh; it was situated partly within the metaphysis and partly in the soft tissues, which were displaced. Maroteaux (1995) stresses bone involvement in children during acute leukaemias, where bone pain reveals the disease in nearly 25% of cases. Any fracture which is suspected of being "spontaneous" calls for biopsy (case history, fig. 3).

Imaging

The radiological images are either solely lytic and relatively well-defined, or more fuzzy with appearances of infiltration; sometimes a major lamellar periosteal bony reaction develops. In some patients there is a large tumour mass (ilium, scapula) which may suggest other diagnoses than lymphoma. In others, several bony lesions may be discovered.

Pathological anatomy and histopathology

The classification of non-Hodgkin's lymphomas (NHL) has become complex and whatever is formulated may change as international standards are regularly brought up to date. The most recent [Blood 1994] is the fruit of a European-American collaboration; it describes the lesions together with the most current immunohistological results. However, it risks being superseded in turn, if only by the WHO classification currently in process of being edited. What is most important is to make the diagnosis of NHL and to assess the degree of its potential aggressivity. If necessary, we can always call in aid one of our specialist haematologist colleagues.

Macroscopically, the tumour destroys the cortex and displaces and infiltrates the musculo-aponeurotic tissues. On section it is grayish-white with small scattered zones of necrosis or haemorrhage. When the tumour is still intraosseous the periosteal bony lamellae are easily undermined, the subjacent cortex infiltrated by the tumour is partly destroyed and curettage removes a pink tissue containing small fragments of bony debris. Attendance of the pathologist in the operating-room allows him to ensure macroscopically (and if need be histologically) that the samples are of sufficient size and contain non-necrotic tissue fragments. The slide smears which should be made routinely in the operating-room for all bone tumours are particularly necessary in these cases of lymphosarcoma.

Histologically, the proliferation is often very polymorphous and structures of the lymphoid series are easily recognised. The appearances are in general very similar to those of nodal lesions of large-celled lymphosarcoma, with frequent predominance of large round or notched cells, sometimes with a varying proportion of immunoblasts and "multilobular" cells. The "polymorphous" nature of the lesion and its very frequent association with fibrosis of varying extent, is quite peculiar to the bony lesions of malignant non-Hodgkin's lymphomas. However, though the large-celled type is predominant, other histological varieties of lymphoma may be seen, and in practice all the varieties as described in the international classification may be encountered. Lymphomas of low malignancy very rarely give rise to striking primary bony lesions, and very malignant lymphomas also usually have a very different clinical picture. The result is that it is especially the so-called intermediate histological varieties which are most often represented. This may account for their rarity during childhood, since it is known that the non-Hodgkin's lymphomas of children are histologically highly malignant; this was the case in 395 children treated for NHL [Fitch et al 1989], of whom only 3.8% presented with primary bony lesions.

B lymphomas are commoner than T lymphomas, but there are some T lymphomas with a primary bony location.

The immunohistological reactions are useful in two circumstances: when there is hesitation between a primary lymphomatous lesion and a metastasis or some other kind or round-celled tumour, or if the exact cell type of the NHL is of therapeutic importance.

In the first case, classical reactions distinguish the lymphoid line (pan-leukocytic antibodies) from epitheliomatous lines (antikeratin antibodies or epithelial markers) so that the distinction is easy. In the second case, the different pan-B or pan-T markers will attribute the lymphoma to one of these two lines, even though we know that, either for technical reasons or in a small number of lymphoma cases, none of these different markers may be positive, including the pan-leukocytic antibody. When there are small round monomorphous immature cells, it may be difficult to distinguish between a lymphoblastic form of lymphosarcoma and a possible Ewing's tumour.

In each of these tumours, the usual immunohistological markers may prove totally negative, and methods capable of making the distinction, such as cellular apposition or cytogenetic study, may not always be available. Other factors exist which may help in differential diagnosis including the age of the patient. Ewing's tumour is essentially a tumour of young children unlike primary lymphoma of bone; the radiological images, the architectural pattern of the tumour and the frequency of intracytoplasmic PAS-positive deposits may all help (cf Chapter 18).

In adults, distinction may be difficult from certain lesions of Hodgkin's disease, myeloma, or even from benign lesions such as chronic osteomyelitis, which may be associated with a mononuclear cell reaction and much fibrosis.

Differential diagnosis

When diagnosing primary lymphoma of bone, it is necessary to search for involvement of other parts of the skeleton or lymphoid organs. In addition to the usual assessment for lymphoma, it is recommended to look for other localisations by bone scintigraphy. Bipolar localisation is possible and does not necessarily have a bad prognosis.

Prognosis

Treatment depends on the stage and histological type. As primary lymphomas of bone are very often localised and nearly always large-celled, treatment may consist of initial chemotherapy followed by local irradiation. The chemotherapy produces a rapid relief of pain, and while the bony image is rarely restored to normal, cure is nevertheless obtained in over 90% of cases.

Orthopaedic complications may require surgical procedures; the fixation of a fracture in a weakened bone, sometimes even the insertion of a prosthesis as a preventive measure when a weight-bearing bone has been weakened by the tumour. There is no indication for amputation. Complications associated with radiotherapy are very rare.

References

Blood (1994) 84: 1358-1391

Chan JKC, Ng CS, Hui PK, Leung WT, Sin VC, Lam TK, Chick KW, Lam WY (1991) Anaplastic large cell Ki-1 lymphoma of bone. Cancer 68: 2186-2191

Chassard JL, Chassard E (1971) Le sarcome de Parker et Jackson. Cahiers Med Lyon 47: 4385-4391

Clayton FC, Butler JJ, Ayala AG, Ro JY, Zornoza J (1987) Non-Hodgkin's lymphoma of bone. Pathologic and radiologic features with clinical correlates. Cancer 60: 2494-2501

Coley BL, Higinbotham NL, Groesbeck HP (1950) Primary reticulum-cell sarcoma of bone: summary of 37 cases. Radiology 55: 641-658

Dosoretz DE, Raymond AK, Murphy GF, Doppke KP, Schiller AL, Wang CC, Suit HD (1982) Primary lymphoma of bone. The relationship of morphology diversity to clinical behavior. Cancer 50: 1009-1014

Dumont J, Mazabraud A (1979) Primary lymphomas of bone (so-called "Parker and Jackson's reticulum cell sarcoma"): histological review of 75 cases according to the new classifications of non Hodgkin's lymphomas. Biomedicine 31: 271-275

Dumont J, Mazabraud A (1983) Les tumeurs de Parker et Jackson. Concours Med 105: 2845-2855

Furman WC, Fitch S, Hustu HO, Callihan T, Murphy SB (1989) Primary lymphoma of bone in children. J Clin Oncol 7: 1275-1280

Howat AJ, Thomas H, Waters KD, Campbel PE (1987) Malignant lymphoma of bone in children. Cancer 59: 335-339

Huvos AG (1979) Bone tumors. Diagnosis treatment and prognosis. Saunders Compagny 1: 392-402

Klimo P, Connors JM (1985) MACOP-B chemotherapy for the treatment of diffuse large cell lymphoma. Ann Int Med 102: 596-602

Lennert K, Feller AC (1992) Histopathology of non-hodgkin's lymphomas. 3rd edn. Springer-Verlag, Heidelberg

Maroteaux P (1995) Les maladies osseuses de l'enfant. 3ème edn. Médecine-Sciences Flammarion

Oberling CH (1928) Les réticulosarcomes et les réticulo-endothéliosarcomes de la moelle osseuse (sarcome d'Ewing). Bull Cancer (Paris) 17: 259-296

Oberling CH, Raileanu C (1932) Nouvelles recherches sur les réticulosarcomes de la moelle osseuse (sarcome d'Ewing). Bull Cancer 21: 333-347

Ostrowski ML, Unni KK, Banks PM, Shives TC, Evans RG, O'connell MJ, Taylor WF (1986) Malignant lymphoma of bone. Cancer 58: 2646-2655

Paker F, Jackson H Jr (1939) Primary reticulum cell sarcoma of bone. Surg Gynecol Obst 68: 45-53

Pettit CK, Zukerberg LR, Gray MH, Ferry JA, Rosenberg AE, Harmon DC, Harris NL (1990) Primary lymphoma of bone. AB-cell neoplasm with a high frequence of multilobated cells. Am J Surg Pathol 14: 329-334

Reimer RR, Chabner BA, Young RC, Reddick R, Johnson RE (1877) Lymphoma presenting in bone. Results of histopathology, staging, and therapy. Ann Int Med 87: 50-55

Valls J, Musculo D, Schajowicz F (1952) Reticulum-cell sarcoma of bone. J Bone Joint Surg 34B: 588-598

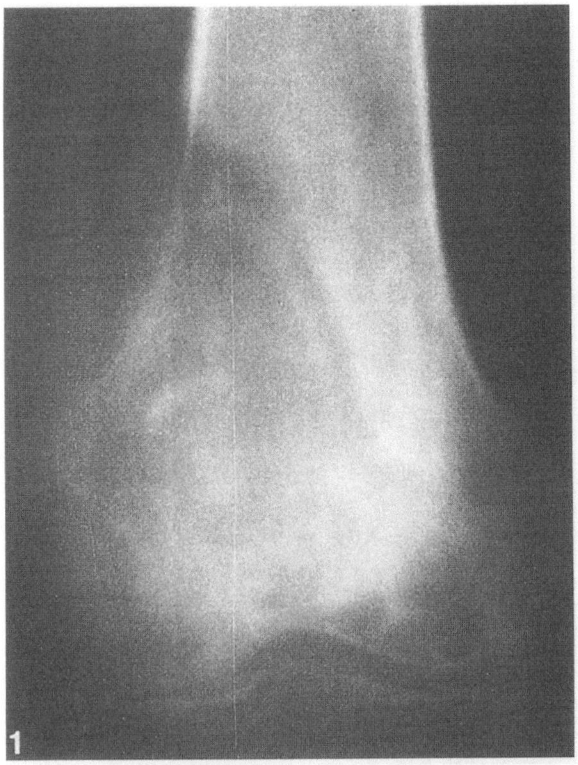

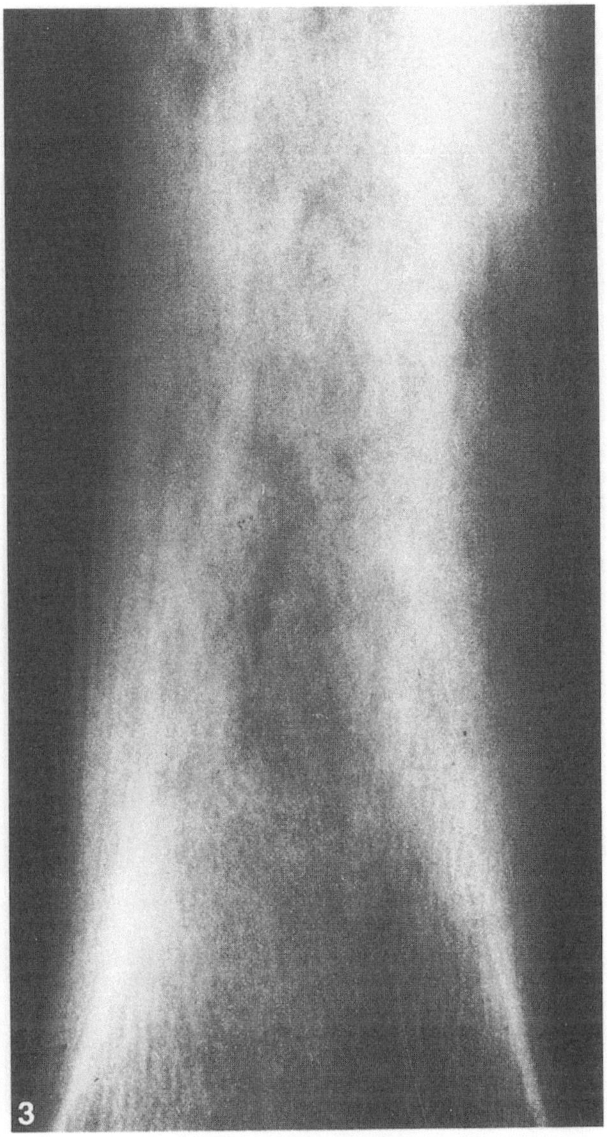

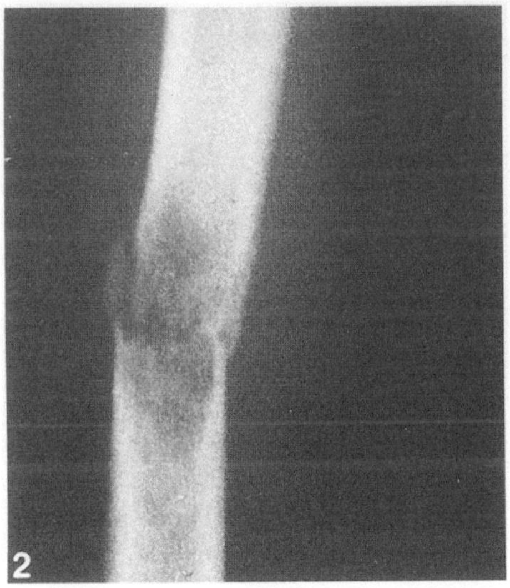

Fig. 1. Large solitary tumour, slightly painful, deforming the lower end of the thigh, first manifestation of lymphosarcoma

Fig. 2. The fracture of the shaft of the humerus was the presenting feature and sole lesion in this woman of 60

Fig. 3. Remodelling of the lower end of the femur has punched out the inner and outer borders of the cortex; there is also periosteal lamellar apposition. Man of 19

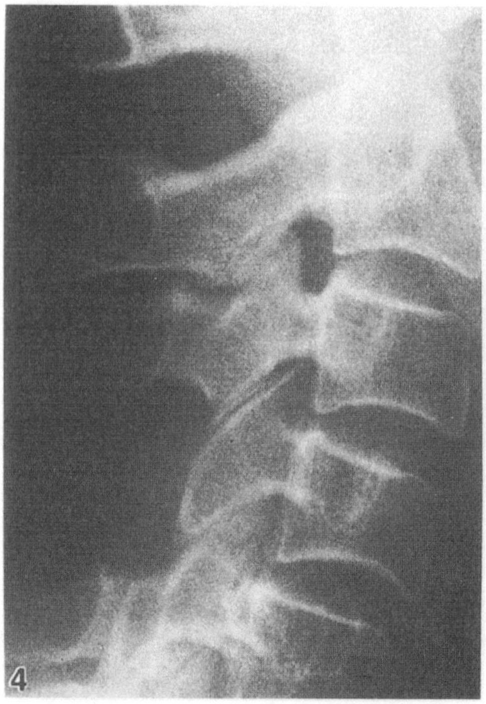

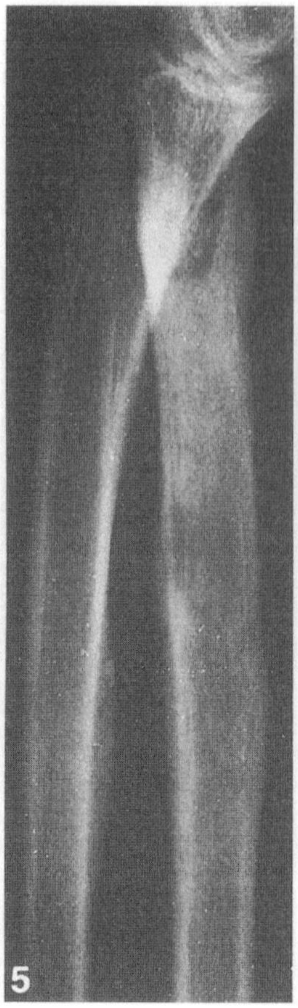

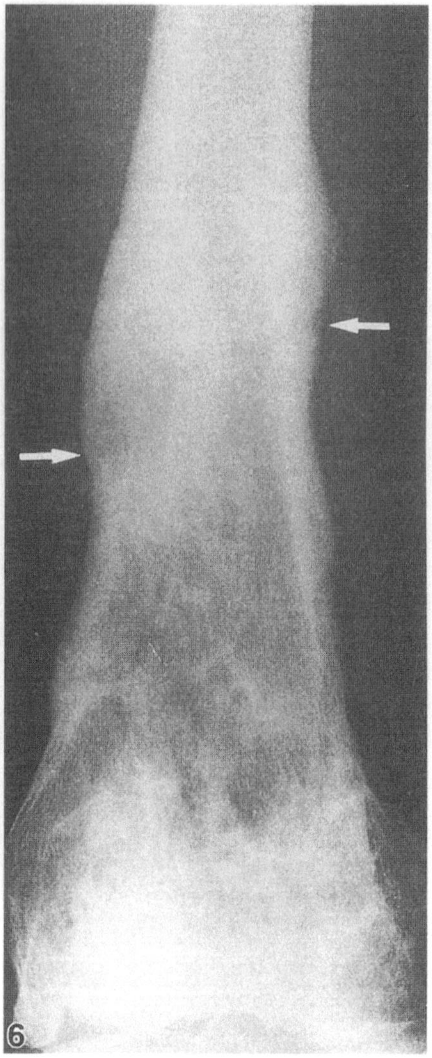

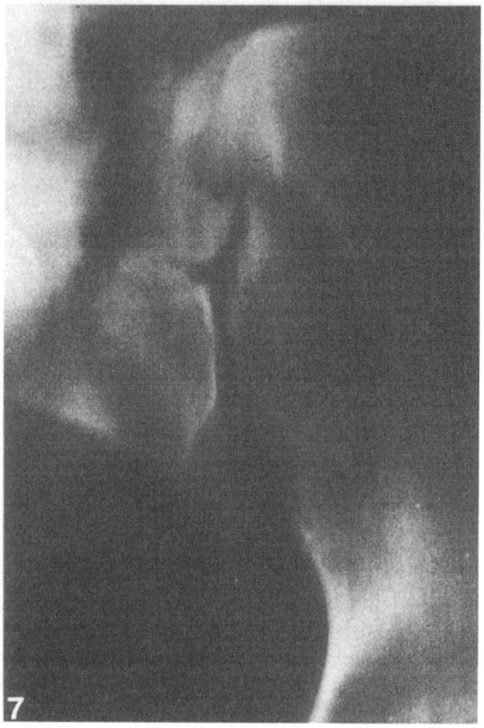

Fig. 4. Neck pain and disappearance of the spinous process are the features of a second localisation of a lymphosarcoma which began in an iliac crest

Fig. 5. The bony remodelling of the radius demonstrates an architecture arranged parallel to the long axis of the bone, somewhat similar to that in the femur (weight-bearing bone) in fig. 3. Man of 38

Fig. 6. Lymphosarcoma treated by radiotherapy: 7 years later the bone is transversely thickened, very dense and has fractured (*arrows*). Biopsy confirmed the absence of any tumour. Woman of 24

Fig. 7. Pain and sacroiliac osteolysis are the manifestations of a lymphosarcomatous lesion. Woman of 48

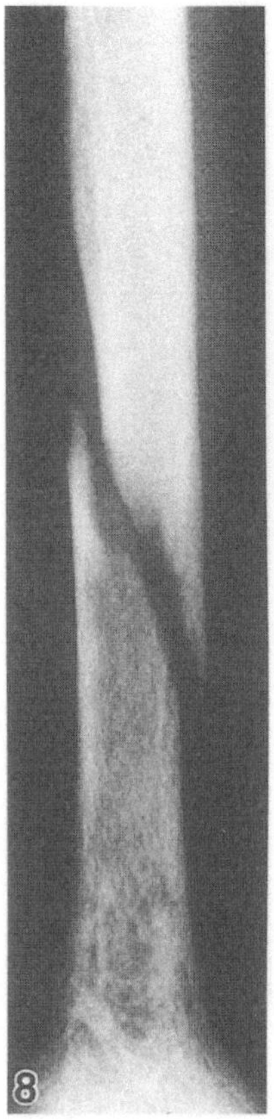

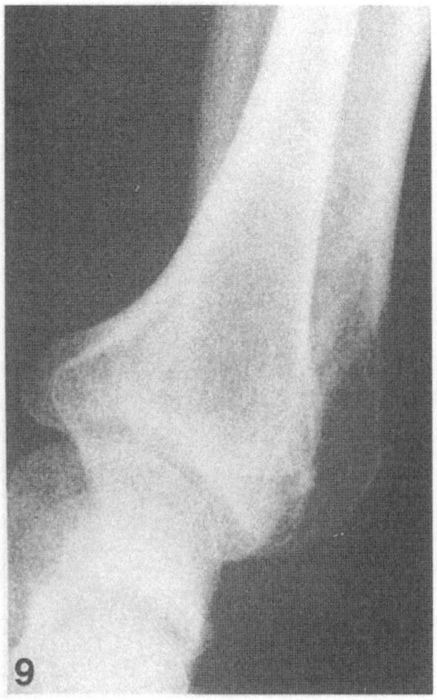

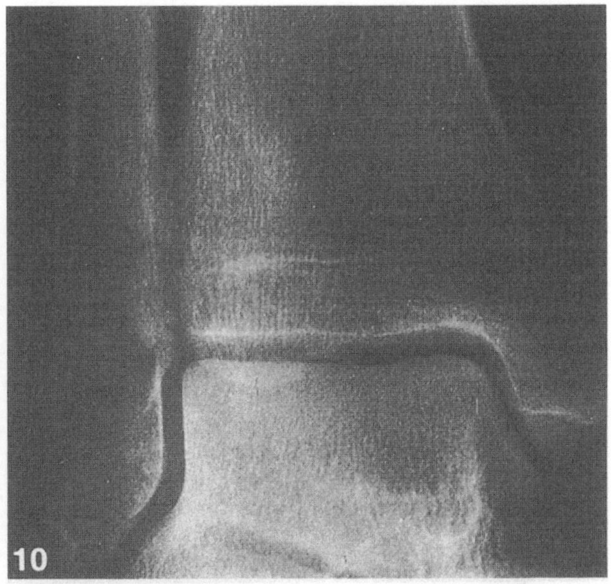

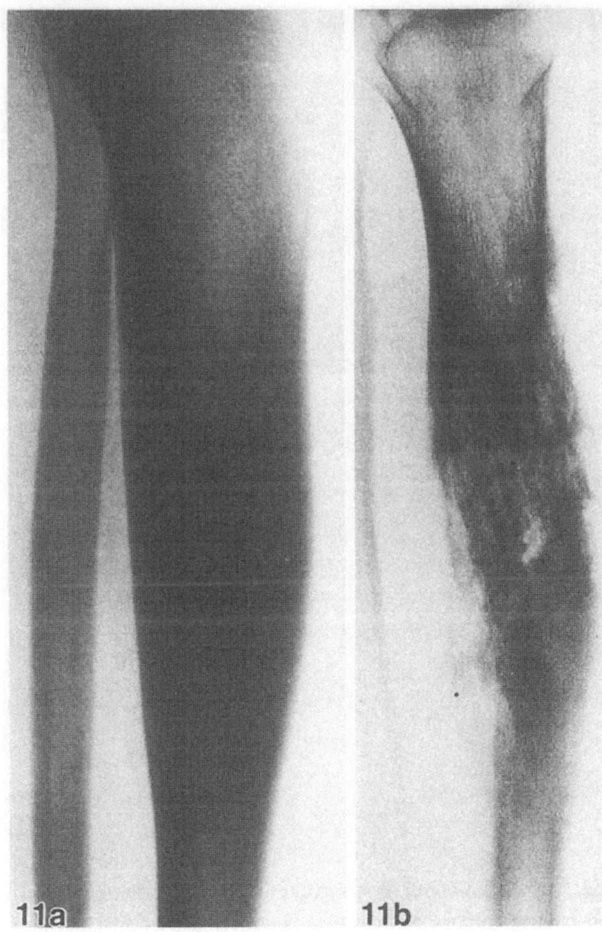

Fig. 8. Pathological fracture of humerus, solitary lesion, manifestation of lymphosarcoma (see case history)

Fig. 9. Quite unusual appearance of lymphosarcomatous osteolysis, which strangely spares a fine cortex at the lower end of the radius

Fig. 10. Unlike the previous case, the osteolysis of the lower end of the fibula has completely destroyed the cortex

Fig. 11. a Biopsy of a diaphyseal tibial sclerosis gave a diagnosis of osteomyelitis. The young girl, aged 12, was treated intensively with antibiotics for 6 years until a new biopsy allowed the diagnosis of lymphosarcoma. **b** The tumour was eventually treated by irradiation. Thirty-two years later the patient is in perfect health. Note that the tumour extended progressively for 6 years but remained strictly localised to the tibia. The fallibility of pathological examination is evident

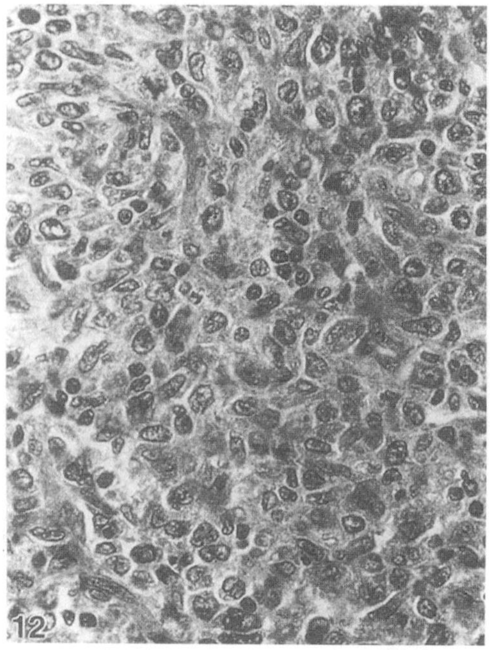

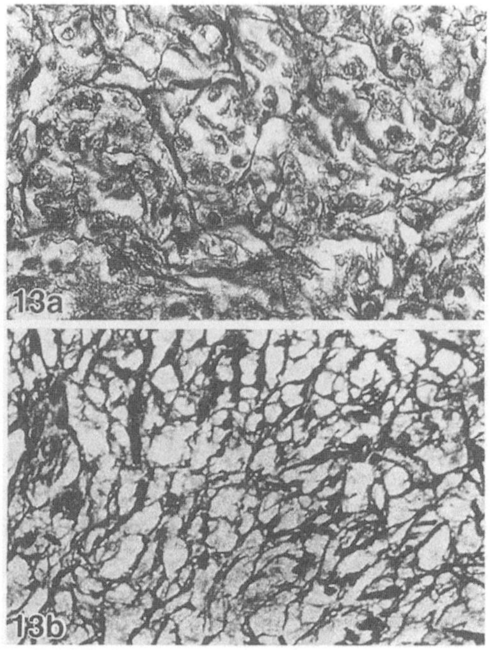

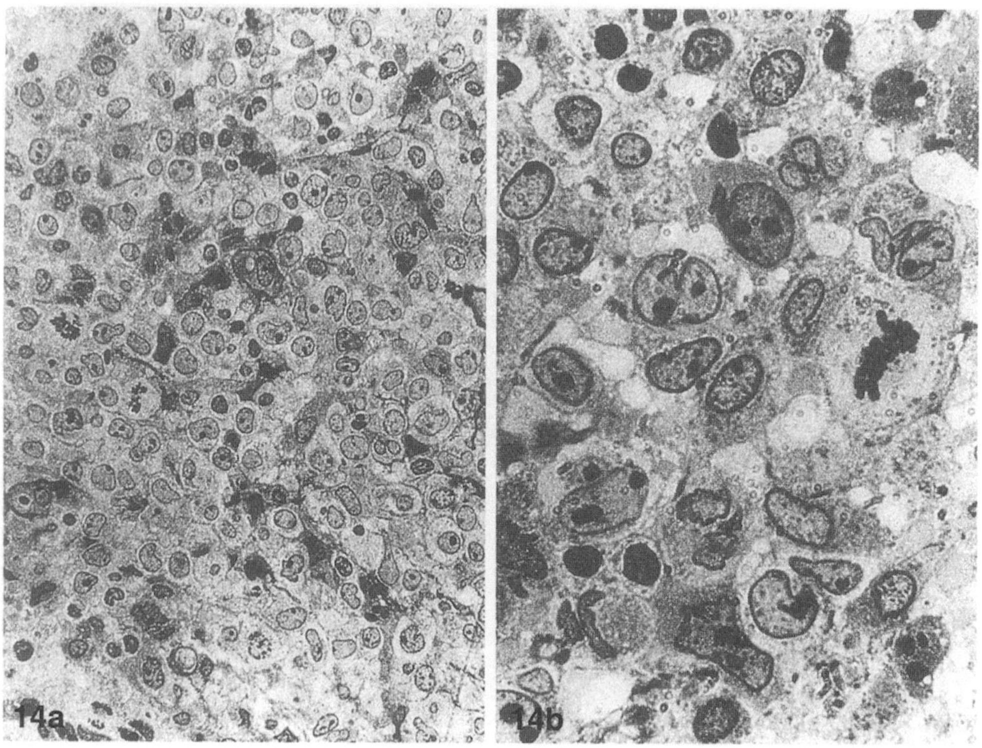

Fig. 12. Typical appearance: polymorphous lymphoid cells of predominantly immature form, with rounded or notched nuclei, presence of some mature forms. Note a degree of fibrosis, practically always present except in very highly malignant forms

Fig. 13 a, b. Increase of the reticulin network, which ensheaths the cell islands or solitary cells

Fig. 14. a Lymphoma with predominance of large round cells (semifine sections, J.-P. Thiery). This is the commonest form in bony lesions. **b** Higher magnification: a mixture of large round cells and notched cells; sometimes the latter predominate

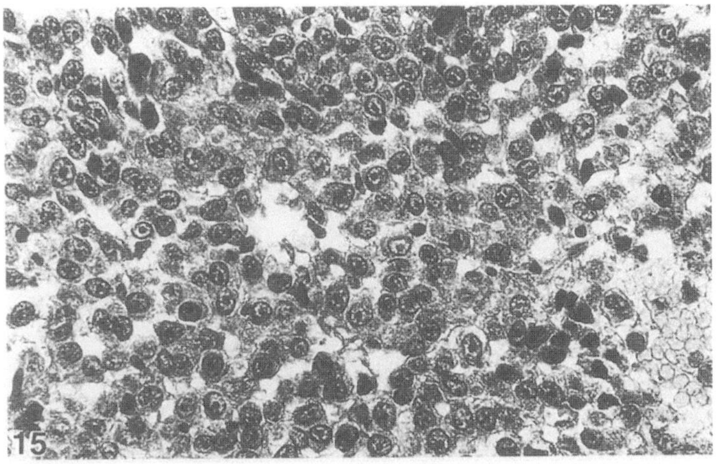

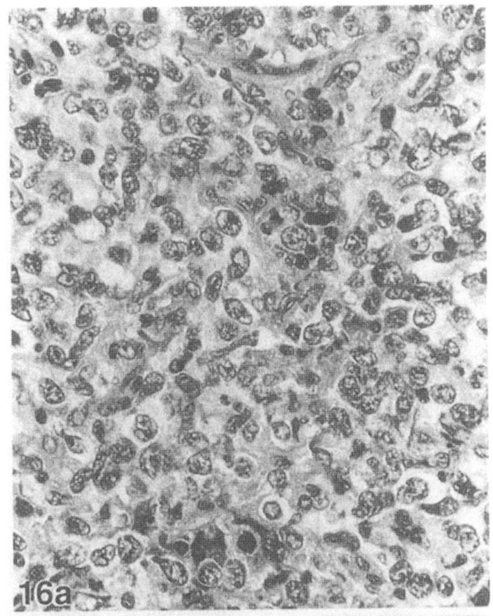

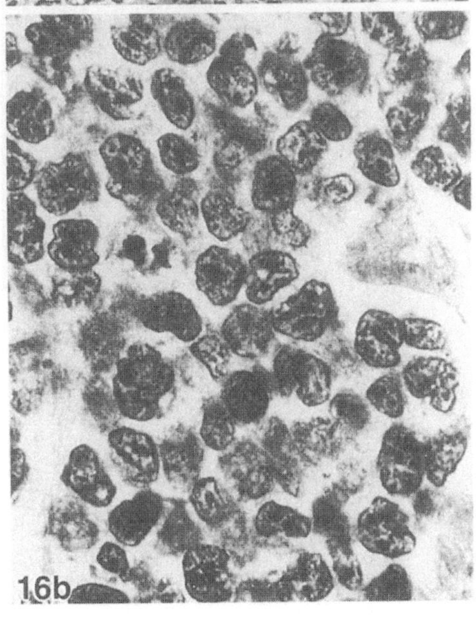

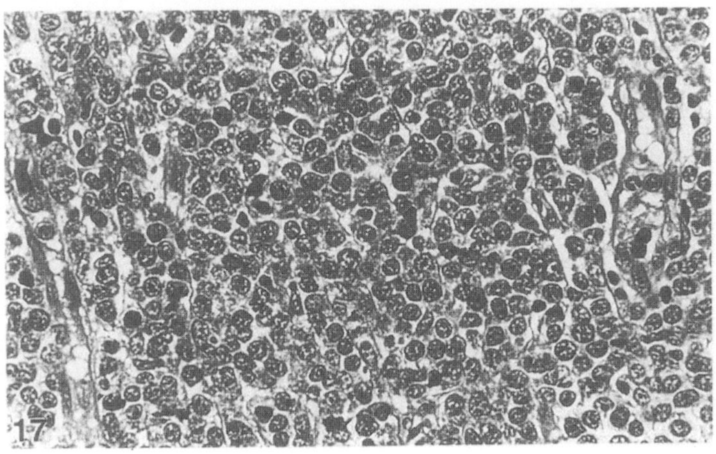

Fig. 15. Immunoblastic form with rounded and slightly eccentric nuclei and central nucleoli

Fig. 16. a Form with irregular bossed nuclei with multiple nucleoli (T lymphoma). **b** At higher magnification the very immature nuclei with bossed outlines are clearly visualised

Fig. 17. Forms of low malignancy (with small mature lymphocytes) are rarely responsible for bony tumours; the bony lesions are usually asymptomatic. The appearance of bony features proper (pain, radiological lysis) during a known lymphocytic haemopathy suggests transition to a more aggressive histological form

35. Hodgkin's disease

Unlike the non-Hodgkin's lymphomas, it is exceptional for an apparently solitary bone lesion to reveal Hodgkin's disease. It does happen, and I have seen it several times. This finding does not necessarily imply that a primary bony form of Hodgkin's disease exists. The diagnosis rests on examination of the biopsy of a (generally osteolytic) zone discovered in the radiographs made for a locally painful syndrome.

Case histories

Case 1. For some weeks an adolescent boy had complained of pain near an iliac crest, more marked after sporting exertion. A radiograph of the pelvis made because of the persistence and worsening of this pain revealed a zone of osteolysis extending over 2-3 cm along the iliac crest and about 1 cm broad. A large biopsy provided the diagnosis (fig. 6).

Case 2. An adult complained of persistent deep bone pain for several weeks, which he localised to the upper third of the femur, without radiological image in standard films. Biopsy performed on the painful area provided the diagnosis.

General considerations

The relatively restricted number of reported cases does not permit a valid calculation of the incidence of this disorder, which however seems of little importance as a presenting feature of the disease. The published cases indicate much the same number of patients of either sex. Usually the patients are adolescents and young adults. Virtually all the bones of the skeleton may be affected including the vertebrae, flat bones of the pelvis and shoulder and long bones of the limbs.

Clinical features

The symptoms are often no more than insidious but persistent pain. In some cases the ingestion of alcohol provokes pain at the site of the bony lesions

Imaging

The standard films show an irregular zone of osteolysis, possibly with a periosteal reaction. The overall appearance is non-specific and not suggestive of the diagnosis of a Hodgkin's lesion, but may promote a clinical and radiological search for adenopathies.

Pathological anatomy and histopathology

Although few studies have been devoted to this subject, it seems that the size of the bony lesion is, in some degree, correlated with its histological aggressiveness. Types I and II of Hodgkin's disease are rarely associated with bone destruction. However, it must be recognised that it is very difficult to attribute a reliable histological type to a solitary bony lesion of Hodgkin's disease (as for any non-nodal organ). The original diagnoses reported in the literature, made from a first biopsy, were Paget's disease, osteomyelitis, eosinophil granuloma, metastasis, primary sarcoma (and doubtless, in a number of cases, no diagnosis at all). However this may be, these honestly reported diagnostic errors should urge us to insist on the need for a large initial sample. Despite its rarity, one should beware of this diagnosis and examine numerous sections in the search for characteristic lesions. The bony lesions are often associated with an abundant fibrosis which markedly exceeds the lymphoid proliferation which itself contains more or less typical Sternberg cells. The same problem arises in those cases where fibrosis is considerable, when it is necessary to study marrow biopsies to assess the extent of an already diagnosed Hodgkin's disease. When large cells with a big nucleolus and a multilobed nucleus are present, the differential diagnosis is simplified, except perhaps in certain so-called anaplastic forms of non-Hodgkin's lymphomas which include cells rather like the Sternberg cells but in much greater abundance.

In some cases the immunohistological reactions may be useful. The anti-Ber H2 antibody, which is localised on the large cells, marks both the Sternberg cells and those of anaplastic lymphoma. The latter also stain equally well with the anti-EMA antibody, which is very rarely positive in Hodgkin's disease except in some type I forms. The anti-BNH9 antibody, positive in over half of anaplastic lymphomas, makes a useful distinction since it hardly ever marks the Sternberg cells. Conversely, these are marked by the anti-Leu M1 antibody. Pan-B or T antibodies are less useful in resolving the problems of differential diagnosis. Many anaplastic lymphomas are marked by pan-T.

In practice, morphology remains very important, since in cases of Hodgkin's disease originating in bone there is nearly always dense fibrosis and a plasmocytic accompaniment usually absent in anaplastic lymphomas. Moreover, immunohistological reactions are not always possible after decalcification of the bone specimens.

The plasmocytic infiltration and fibrosis may suggest osteomyelitis; we repeat that for every bone lesion in which the diagnosis depends entirely on the biopsy it is imperative to make slide smears in the operating-room and to send a tissue fragment to the bacteriology laboratory. The diagnosis can be confirmed only if the presence of Sternberg cells is certain. Discovery of the bony lesion is necessarily followed by an assessment of extent identical to that made in other lymphomas.

Prognosis

Treatment, if rapidly instituted, is curative in over 80% of cases. It must be stressed that a bony lesion is not in itself a bad prognostic factor and that it responds to treatment as rapidly as lesions elsewhere; the chemosensitivity of the lesions is currently the best criterion of their course.

References

Bourgeois M (1972) Les formes osseuses révélatrices de la maladie d'Hodgkin. Thèse, Lille

Bouvier M, Lejeune E, Deplante JP, Le Provost C (1975) Les manifestations osseuses révélatrices de la maladie de Hodgkin. Rhumatologie: 177-193

Brannstein EM (1980) Hodgkin disease of bone: radiographic correlation with the histological classification. Radiology 137: 643-646

Chan KW, Rosen G, Miller DR, Tan CTC (1982) Hodgkin's disease in adolescents presenting as a primary bone lesion. A report of four cases and review of literature. Am J Pediatr Hematol Oncol 4: 11-17

Ferrant A, Rodhain J, Michaux JL, Sokal G (1977) L'atteinte osseuse et médullaire dans la maladie de Hodgkin. Nouv Rev Fr Hematol 18: 545-554

Gross SB, Roberton WN, Lange BJ, Bunin NG, Drummond DS (1992) Primary Hodgkin's disease of bone a report of two cases in adolescents and review of the literature. Clin Orthop 283: 276-280

Huvos AG (1979) Bone tumors. Diagnosis, treatment and prognosis. Saunders Compagny, Philadelphia, pp 406-412

Lacombe MJ, Le Charpentier Y, Carlioz A, Mathiot C, Tomeno B, Dumont J, Abelanet R (1979) Localisations osseuses d'allure tumorale de la maladie de Hodgkin. A propos de 2 cas simulant une tumeur primitive. Rev Chir Orthop 65: 409-412

Mills SE, Sloop FB, Thiele AL, Miller CW, Zazakos CP (1983) Hodgkin disease, nodular sclerosing variant, primary form. Skeletal Radiol 10: 287-289

Papillon J, Croizat P, Revol L, Chassard JL, Brothier F, Coste J (1964) Les localisations osseuses de la lympho-granulomatose maligne. J Radiol Electrol 45: 109-116

Weiss RB, Brunning RD, Kennedy BJ (1975) Hodgkin's disease in the bone marrow. Cancer 36: 2077-2083

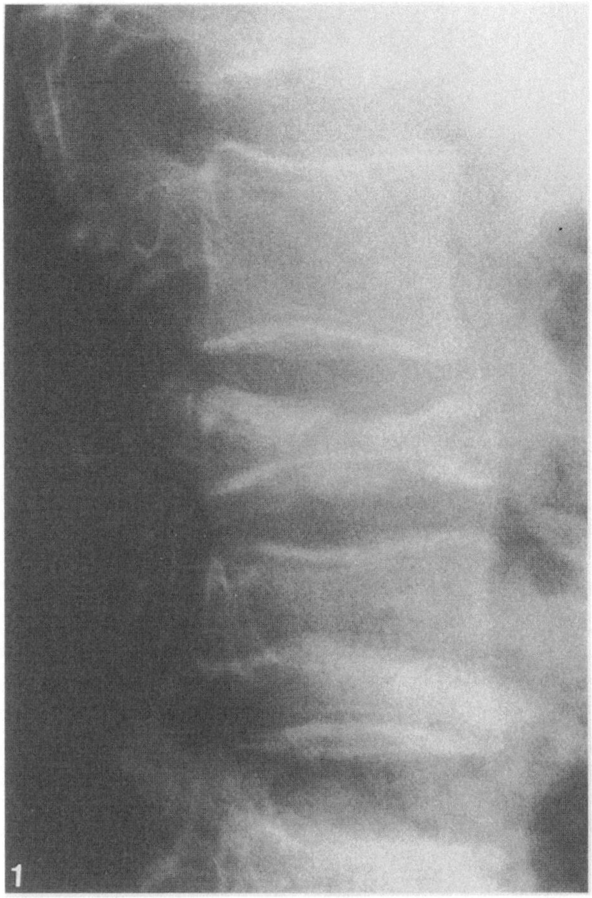

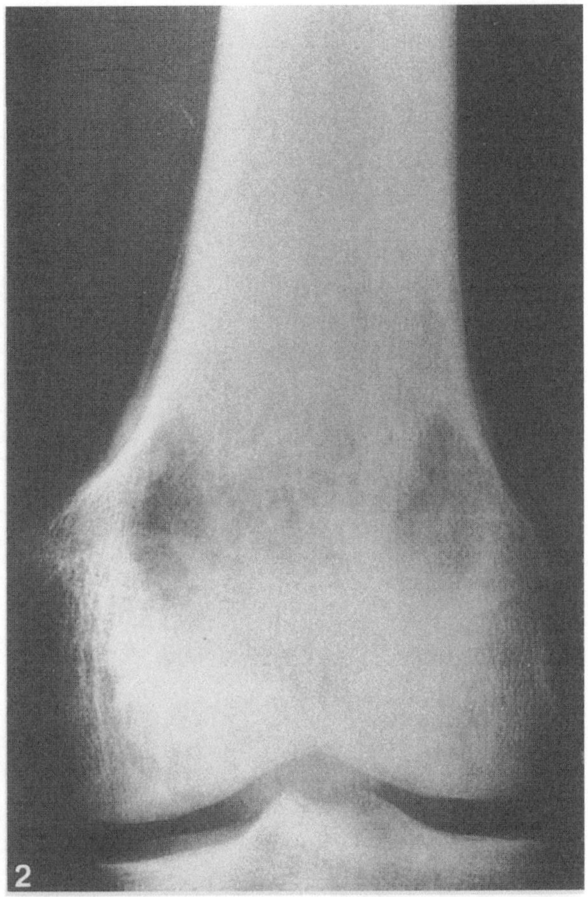

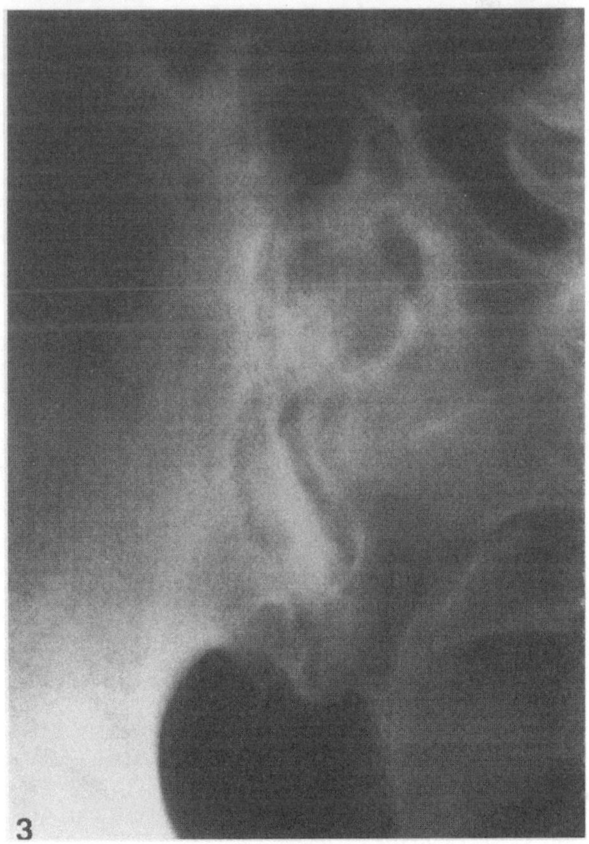

Fig. 1. The L3 vertebra is flattened between two well-preserved disks; this is a crush fracture, due to collapse of multiple bone trabeculae thinned and rarefied by the development of the tumour

Fig. 2. The bony rarefaction of the lower end of the femur is associated with an ossified periosteal reaction, well shown in this film

Fig. 3. Sacroiliac involvement marks the clinical onset of the disorder in this woman of 51. There is also an osteogenic reaction, apparently endosteal, which circumscribes the osteolytic foci

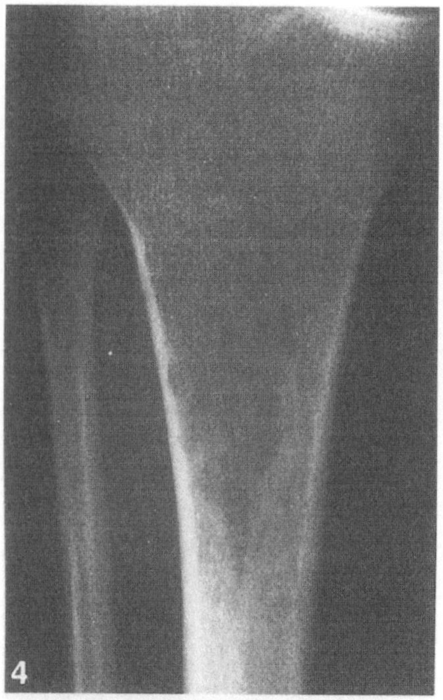

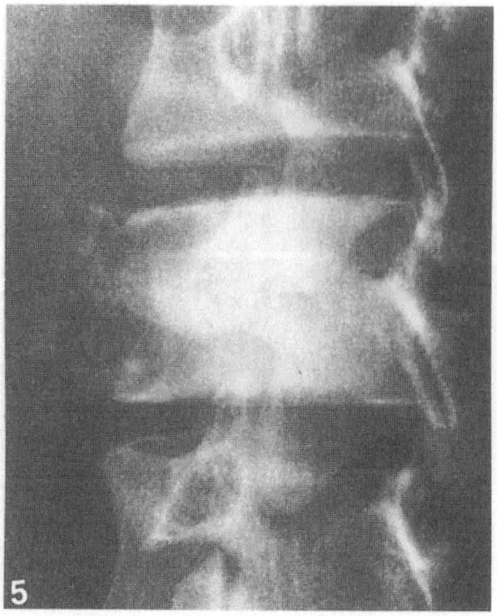

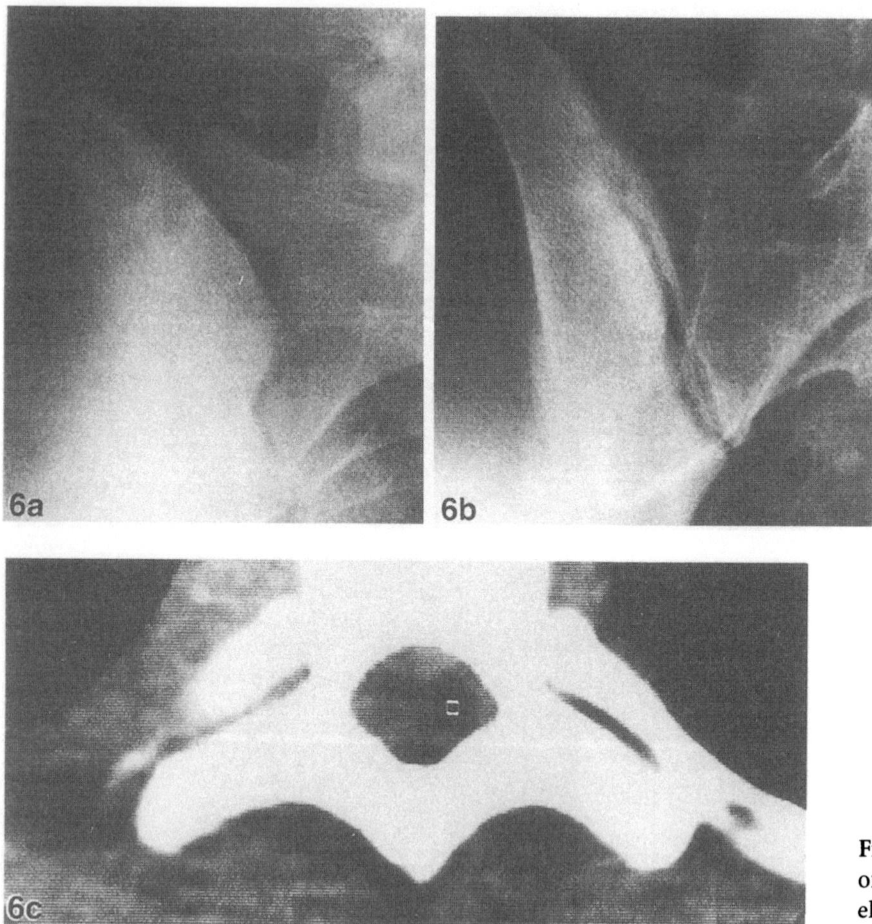

Fig. 4. Osteolysis of the upper end of the tibial diaphysis with crenellated borders due to osteoclastic absorption (fig. 7)

Fig. 5. Involvement of the vertebral body by tumour with proliferation in the soft tissues

Fig. 6. a, b Lesion in the vicinity of the posterior part of the iliac crest, standard radiographs. **c** The lysis appears much more extensive in the CT image

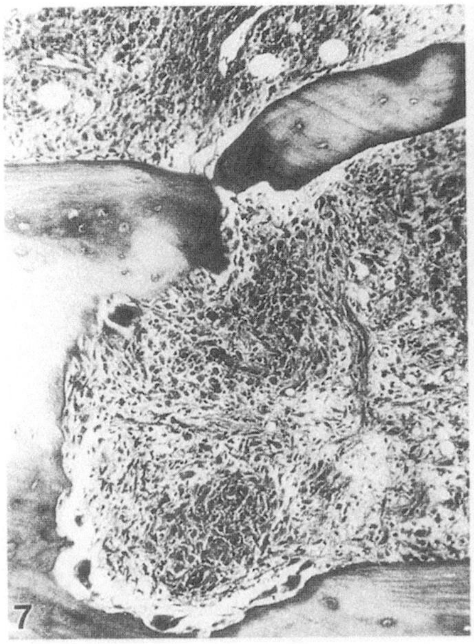

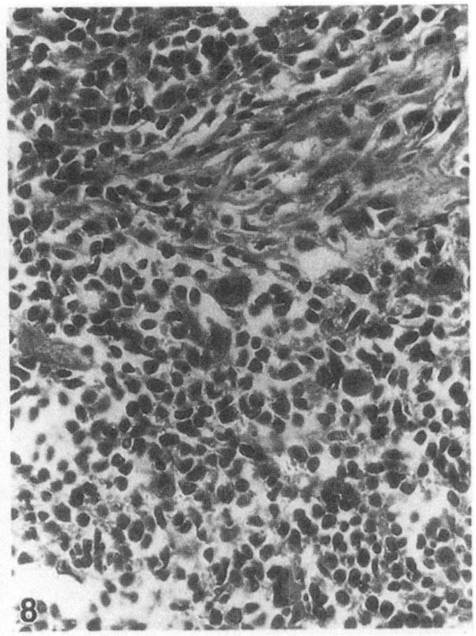

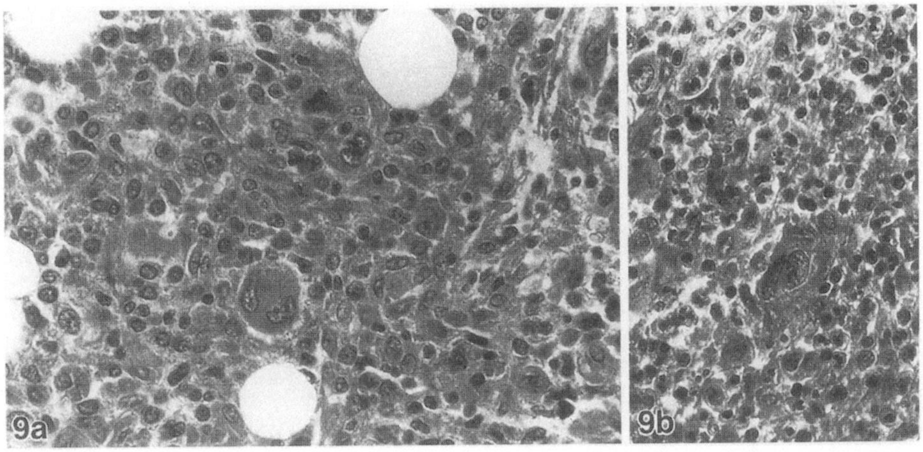

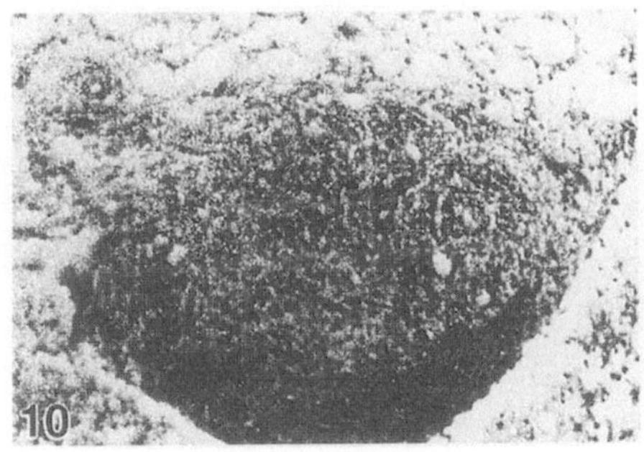

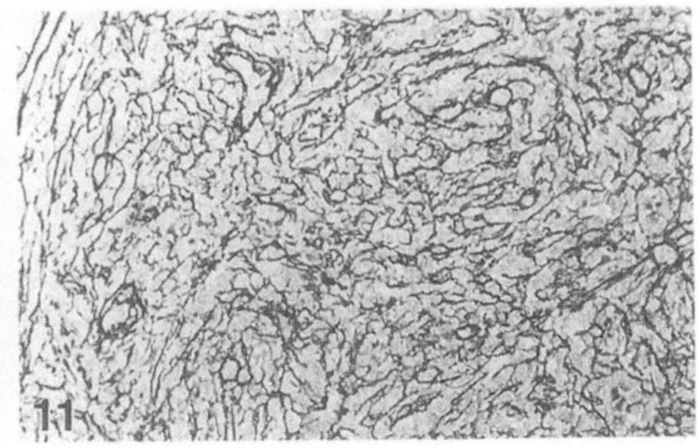

Fig. 7. Hodgkin's nodule (femur). The lesion is well individualised amidst a partly preserved myeloid tissue, structured by fibrosis that is always present and even very abundant, deforming the cells

Fig. 8. At higher magnification it is possible to identify small lymphoid cells and a few large cells with deformed and multiple nuclei, some plasmocytes and immunoblasts

Fig. 9. a Typical granuloma with cells suggestive of Hodgkin's disease. **b** Another appearance in the same patient: only a few solitary cells suggest the diagnosis, striking in their size and nuclei

Fig. 10. Reticulin network in the midst of the same lesion

Fig. 11. Hodgkin's nodule in a marrow biopsy made during a routine assessment of the extent of Hodgkin's disease diagnosed by examination of cervical adenopathy; note a degree of fibrosis and aplasia of the myeloid tissue around the nodule

36. Plasma-cell proliferations

Although they have been known throughout the world (and for a very long time, since myelomatous lesions have been found in the skulls of prehistoric skeletons), plasma-cell proliferations are common in Western countries, rare in the East and very common in Blacks where the age of onset seems lower.

Case histories

Various clinical presentations initiate the diagnostic process but pain often directs the patient to a rheumatology clinic.

Case 1. A man of 60 attended for diffuse pain, mainly over the spine. Bony and biochemical anomalies very quickly led to the diagnosis.

Case 2. A woman of 70, affected by severe osteoporosis, hardly noted any increase in pain, but anaemia and a very high sedimentation rate served to guide the investigations.

Case 3. A man of 45 had a painful hip; the pelvic radiographs showed a solitary lytic image. All the biochemical manifestations were negative, but a bone biopsy was decisive.

Clinical features

The incidence of myeloma is difficult to assess but is of the order of 0.03% of all cancers. Male predominance is of the order of 2:1. The mean age is 55, the maximum incidence being between 45 and 70 years.

Imaging

The multiple clinical presentations have different radiological appearances. In the majority of cases of plasma-cell myeloma the radiological studies demonstrate an abnormal transparency of the skeleton, indicative of osteoporosis or osteomalacia, often with a combination of both lesions. This decalcification may embody the bony anomaly; it predominates at the sites richest in bone marrow (the axial skeleton and the proximal ends of the humerus and femur). This appearance may be the sole radiological sign of the disease, but more often, as the disorder advances, small foci of osteolysis are added; a major involvement may lead to fractures of the long bones or vertebrae (vertebral crush fractures). This "demineralisation", whether osteoporosis or osteomalacia, has no very specific appearance but it is relatively suggestive in middle-aged patients. Several radiological appearances correspond to localised lesions. Rounded lacunae, usually multiple and with sharp borders, are particularly suggestive.

Images with osteolysis, sometimes of "soap-bubble" appearance, may suggest an aneurysmal cyst or a hyperparathyroid lesion in the iliac bones or sacrum. A solitary tumour in the metaphysis of a long bone, destroying the cortex and invading the soft tissues, initially suggests a primary tumour rather than a plasmacytoma.

Presentation may be with fracture, as in 6% of the 364 cases of myeloma in the study of Schneider et al (1959). In the vertebral bodies and ribs such a fracture raises the possible diagnosis of a metastatic lesion; the vertebral pedicles are more often respected than is the case with metastases and tumour extension into the soft tissues is common.

An osteosclerotic reaction is seen in about 3% of cases; it may be diffuse or focal. A combination of lytic and sclerosing images is possible. There is also a purely sclerosing form which represents a special type of myeloma. Lastly, we should recall that the first manifestation may be arthropathy or bone infarct; appearances which correspond to a deposit of amyloid material but where radiological diagnosis remains very uncertain.

Pathological anatomy and histopathology

Diagnosis is based on the coexistence of bony lesions, the demonstration of secretion of immunoglobulin in the plasma (usually of a light chain) and the discovery of plasma-cell proliferation.

Obviously, the pathologist is often more involved in cases of non-secretory plasmacytoma or solitary plasmacytoma. From a practical viewpoint it has to be remembered that the polymorphism of the radiological lesions is correlated with very varied diagnostic ideas accompanying the biopsy sample (chondrosarcoma, giant-cell tumour, metastases, may all be mentioned). The sample is obtained by surgical biopsy or needle aspiration; in the latter case the decreased bone mass confirms the diagnosis of osteoporosis or osteomalacia. This is a formidable trap, since osteoporosis or osteomalacia (or both) do exist in myeloma and are often more obvious than a small plasmocytic island. However, it is the demonstration of plasma-cell proliferation that suggests the diagnosis and the proof of its monoclonal nature can be made with the sample removed.

The morphological diagnosis of plasmocytic proliferation is easily made from the biopsy and in many cases marrow aspiration from the iliac crest will provide the diagnosis. In the histological sections the plasma-cells may appear mature, with an eccentric nucleus and the chromatin arranged like the spokes of a wheel, but often they are more immature with asynchrony of nuclear-cytoplasmic maturation and clearly visible nucleoli. They may contain Russell's bodies in their cytoplasm or crystals. Multinuclear forms are commonplace during malignant plasmocytic proliferations.

Even if the diagnosis of myeloma is already made, a biopsy of the bone marrow may be sent to the pathologist to assess the degree of plasmocytic infiltration as an aid to prognosis. This means analysis of the distribution and size of the plasmocyte islands, the morphology of the plasmocytes (especially their maturity), the extent of the subjacent fibrosis and that of the residual haematopoiesis. Certain pathologists have attempted to correlate these different data with the prognosis [Bartl 1988]. Once the plasma-cell line has been identified (or even suspected in anaplastic forms) the pathologist can prove that this is indeed a lymphoid cell carrying monoclonal cytoplasmic immunoglobulins: IgG, IgD, IgM, IgA... K and for the light chains, only one of these is present in the malignant monoclonal proliferations. Immunological or molecular biological methods will confirm the monoclonal character of the proliferation in the section, which is important to demonstrate when the monoclonal protein is not secreted in the plasma in sufficient amounts to be demonstrable by immunoelectrophoresis.

The so-called «benign» monoclonal gammapathies

A marrow biopsy may be sent to the pathologist following the discovery of a monoclonal protein in the plasma of a patient without any other skeletal or clinical disorder suggestive of a malignant pathology. These monoclonal proteins are often monitored for years and can give rise to repeated marrow biopsies. The problem posed to the pathologist is that of the presence in this biopsy of lesions suggestive of the onset of a malignant proliferation, particularly if there is a plasmocyte population of some magnitude.

The demonstration of the monoclonal nature of the plasmocyte proliferation by modern methods is important, although it does not constitute formal proof of an underlying malignant pathology. One must therefore be extremely cautious in such reports, and especially endeavour to see if the extent of the plasmocyte proliferation increases during successive biopsies or if its monoclonal nature becomes accentuated.

References

Bartl R (1988) Histological classification and staging. Hematol Oncol 6: 107-113

Bataille R, Sany J, Serre H (1981) Plasmocytomes apparemment solitaires des os. Aspects cliniques et pronostiques (à propos de 114 cas). Nouv Presse Med 10: 407-411

Bataille R, Sany J, Serre H (1978) Le plasmocytome solitaire des os: à propos de 25 cas. Rev Rhum Mal Osteoartic 45: 229-239

Brandon C, Martel W, Weatherbee L, Cape KP (1989) Osteosclerotic myeloma. Skeletal Radiol 18: 542-546

Brown TS, Paterson CR (1973) Osteosclerosis in myeloma. J Bone Joint Surg 55B: 621-623

Calle R, Graic Y, Mazabraud A, Schlienger P (1972) Plasmocytome osseux solitaire: à propos de quatre cas. Bull Cancer (Paris) 59: 395-404

Canioni D, Kermarec J (1982) Interprétation des plasmocytoses médullaires minimes dans les dysglobulinémies monoclonales. Ann Pathol 4: 279-292

Corwin J, Lindberg RD (1979) Solitary plasmocytoma of bone vs. extramedullary plasmacytoma and their relationship to multiple myeloma. Cancer 43: 1007-1013

Delauche-Cavallier MC, Laredo JD, Wibier M, Bard M, Mazabraud A, Le Bail Darne JL, Kuntz D, Ryckewaert A (1988) Solitary plasmacytoma of the spine. Cancer 61: 1707-1714

Engels EP, Smith RC, Krantz S (1960) Bone sclerosis in multiple myeloma. Radiol 75: 242-247

Ennuyer A, Bataini P (1972) Plasmocytes et tumeurs plasmocytaires. Séance du 18-12-72 de l'Association Française pour l'étude du cancer. Bull Cancer 59: 353-417

Feldann JL, Guedri M, Ohana N, Menkes CJ, Amor B (1984) Le plasmocytome solitaire vertébral. Ann Med Interne 135: 259-264

Hall FM, Gore SM (1988) Osteosclerotic myeloma variants. Skeletal Radiol 17: 101-105

Laredo JP, Chiche Portiche V, Bondeville JM, Bard M (1990) In: De Sèze et coll. L'actualité rhumatologique. L'expansion Scientifique, Paris, pp 219-230

Mazabraud A, De Sèze S (1962) Aspects anatomopathologiques des lésions osseuses du myélome. Sem Hop Paris 15: 951-957

Meis JM, Butler JJ, Osborne BM, Nelson C, Ordonez NG (1987) Solitary plasmacytomas of bone and extramedullary plasmacytomas. A clinicopathologic and immunohistochemical study. Cancer 59: 1475-1485

Menkes CJ, Herreman JL, Prud'homme JL, Godeau P, Delbarre F (1972) Myélome à plasmocyles non excrétants (à propos de deux nouvelles observations). Nouv Presse Med 1: 309-312

Meyer JE, Schulz MD (1974) Solitary myeloma of bone. A review of 12 cases. Cancer 34: 438-440

Peterson LC, Brown BA, Crosson JT (1986) Application of the immunoperoxydase technic to bone marrow biopsies in the classification of patients with monoclonal gammapathies. Ann J Clin Pathol 85: 688-693

Porter EC (1961) Osteogenesis in multiple myeloma. Report of a case. Radiol 76: 457-458

Schneider M, Mazabraud A (1959) Les signes révélatrices du myélome et leur fréquence relative. Rev Rhum 11: 660-675

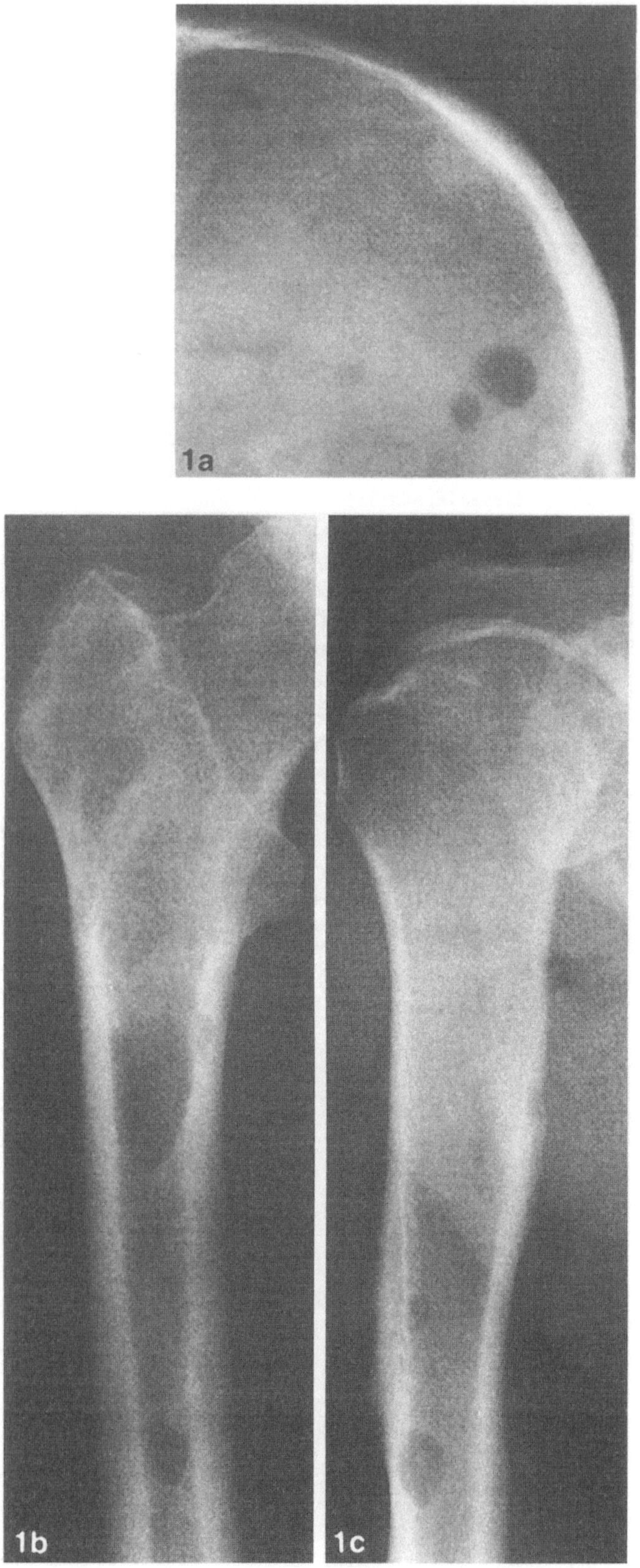

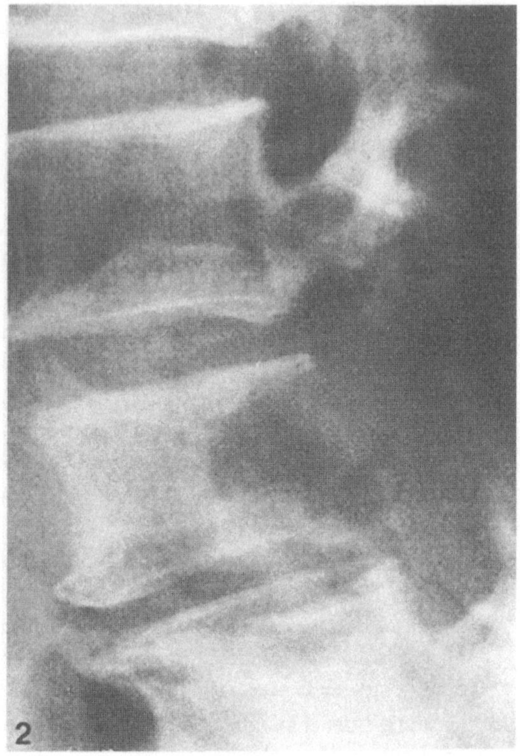

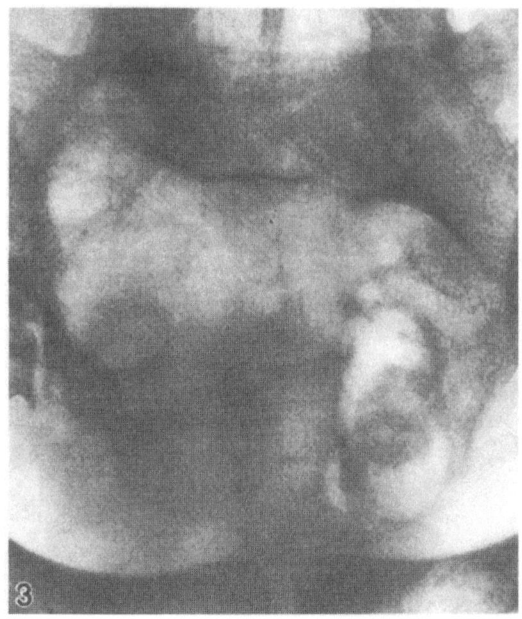

Fig. 1 a-c. The pathologist sometimes receives a biopsy from a bony lacuna, thought to be solitary. The plasmocyte proliferation he discovers, atypical and polymorphous, suggests supplementary investigations. These three radiographs are only intended to show the punched-out appearance of these lacunae

Fig. 2. Plasmacytoma of L1: destruction of posterior vertebral arch and posterior half of vertebral body

Fig. 3. Solitary plasmacytoma of sacrum, presenting with right sciatica. Irradiation led to recalcification and stabilisation over a 9-year period (archive record)

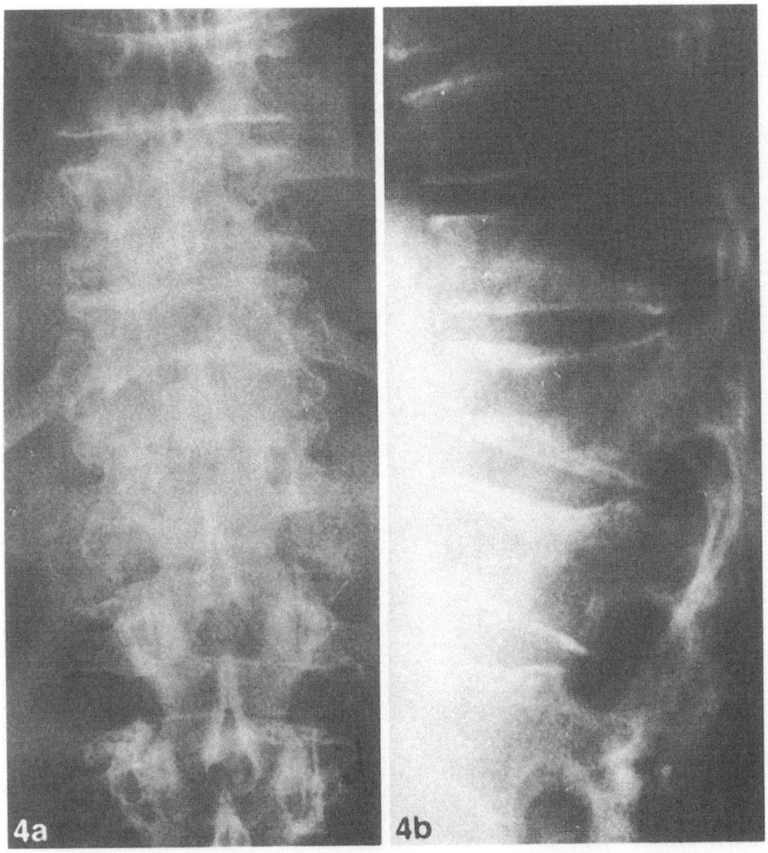

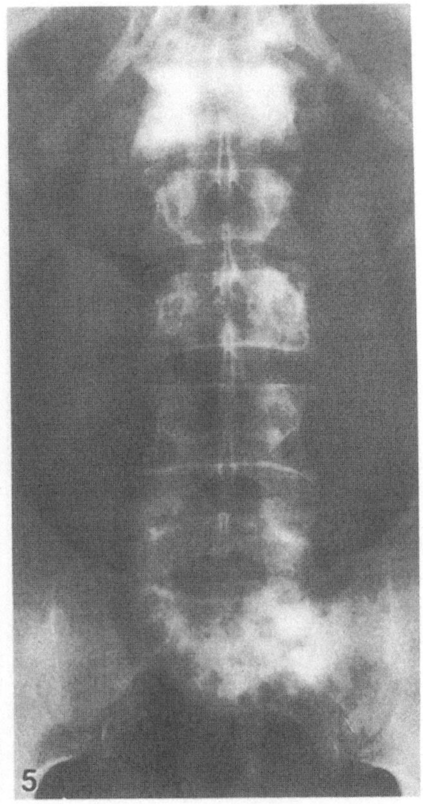

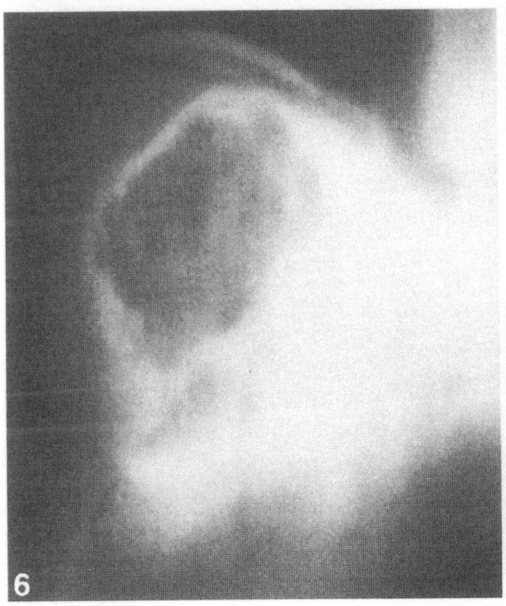

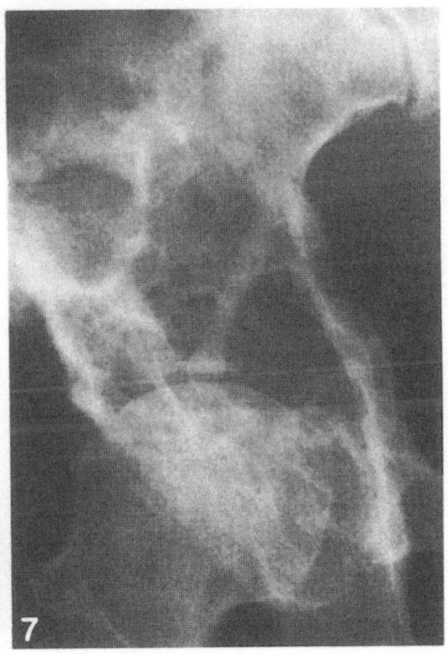

Fig. 4 a, b. The wedge-shaped L1 vertebra was the presenting feature but the underlying vertebrae are doubtless involved in the process

Fig. 5. Sclerosing form of plasmocytic myeloma. Osteosclerosis of L1 and part of sacrum. In such cases, as in the sclerosing form of metastases, diagnosis is often difficult; the technique requires intensive decalcification and the spaces occupied by the tumour cell proliferation are very much reduced

Fig. 6. This radiological image of the iliac wing suggests a cartilaginous tumour, but is really that of a large amyloid deposit

Fig. 7. Ballooned and alveolar appearance of plasmacytoma of iliac wing

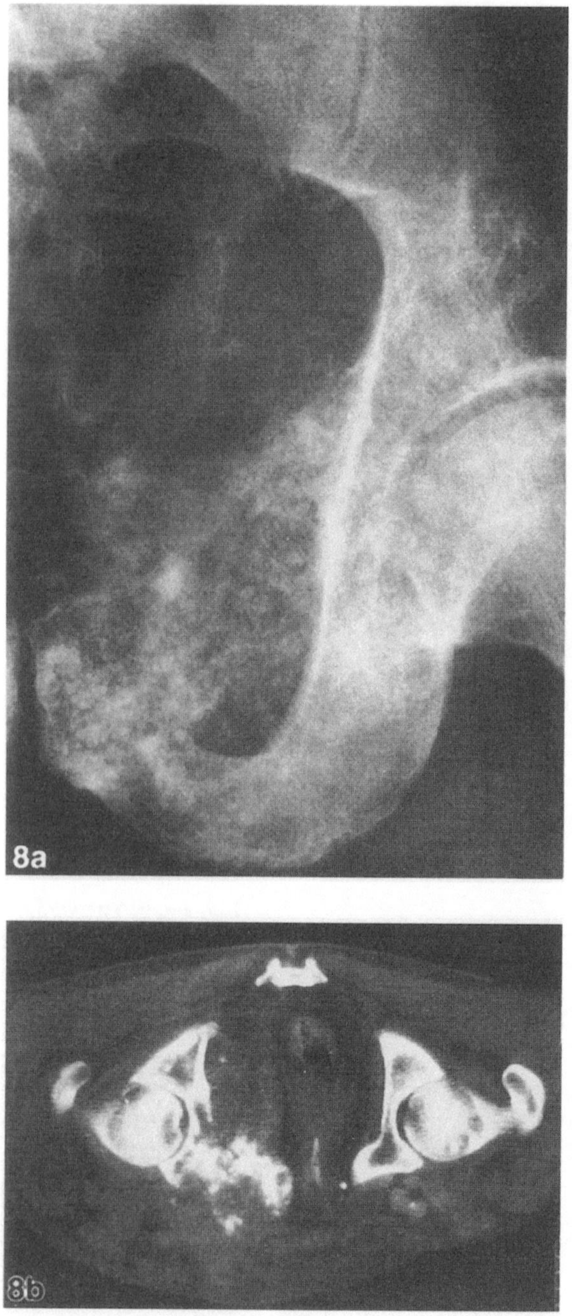

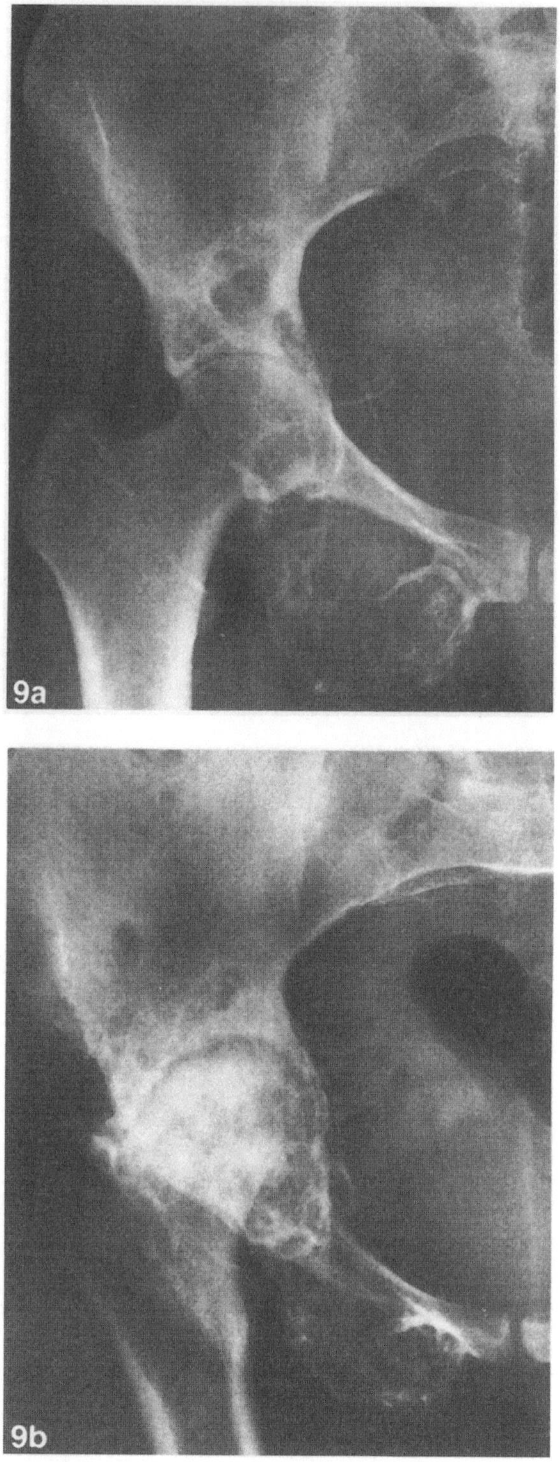

Fig. 8 a, b. Another appearance of amyloidosis (**a**) in a standard radiograph and (**b**) in CT

Fig. 9. a This solitary plasmacytoma was treated by radiotherapy. **b** 11 years later the lesion is stabilised with some bony sclerosis and acetabular protrusion

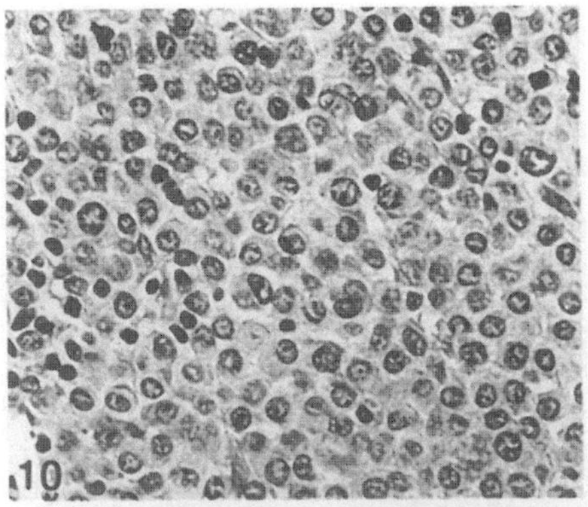

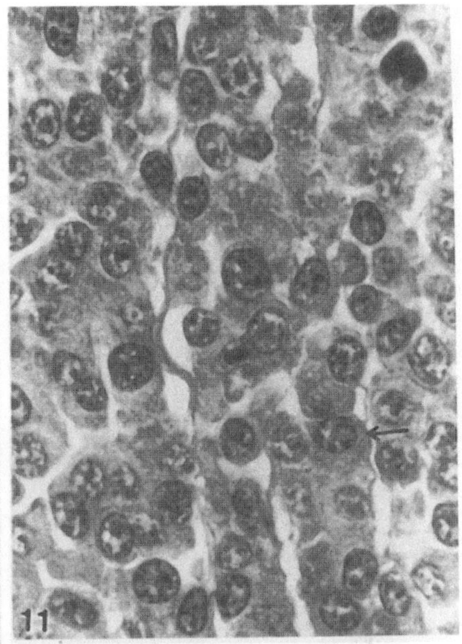

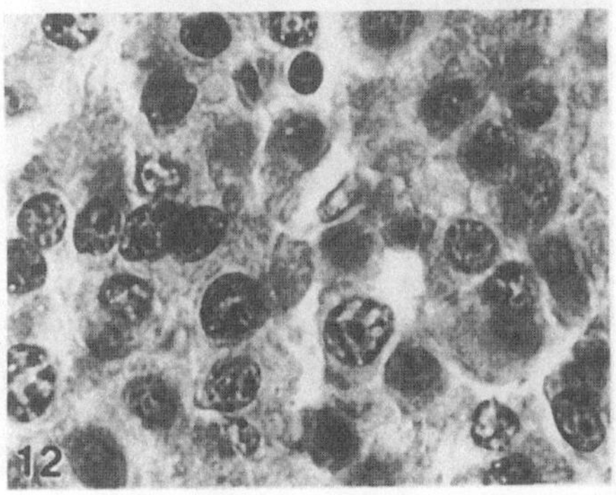

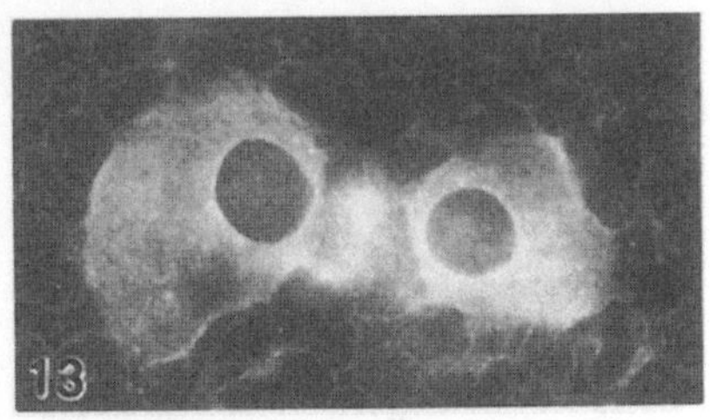

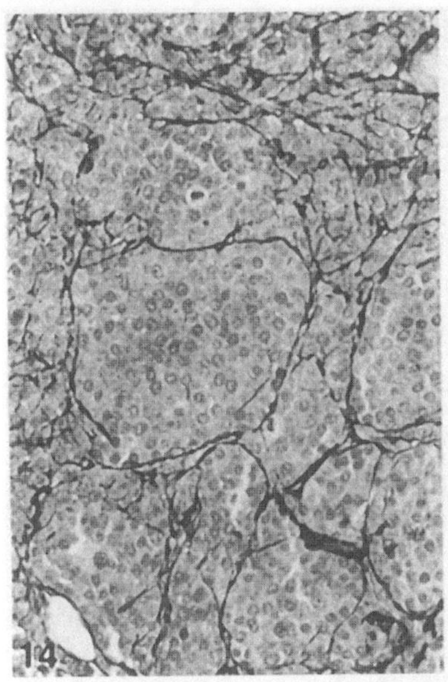

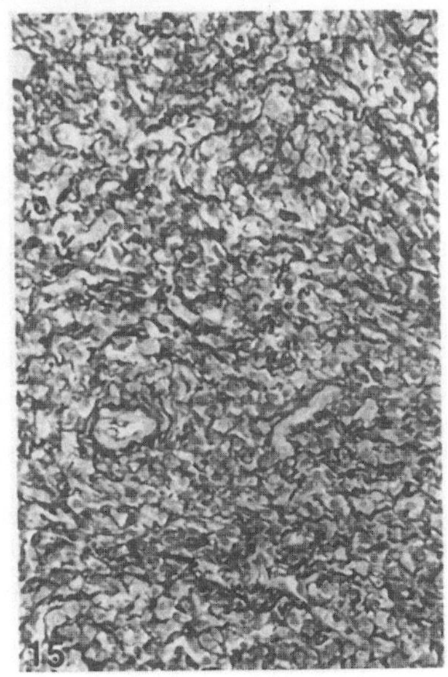

Fig. 10. Typical histological appearances: cells with rounded eccentric nuclei and clear cytoplasm. Moderate anisocytosis

Fig. 11. At higher magnification the cell characteristics appear more clearly. In the mature plasmocytes the chromatin is regularly distributed in small clumps at the periphery of the nucleus (*arrow*). The cytoplasm is sometimes separated from the nucleus by a clearer zone (archoplasm)

Fig. 12. This microphotograph shows coexistence of mature plasmocytes with regular chromatin and young plasmocytes in whose nuclei the nucleoli are plainly visible

Fig. 13. The cytoplasmic fluorescence indicates the presence in the ergastoplasm of a monoclonal IgA revealed by an antibody coupled with fluorescein (Courtesy Prof. Diebold)

Figs. 14, 15. Two varieties of reticulin networks in plasmacytoma: (14) lobular and (15) a denser network surrounding small cell groups

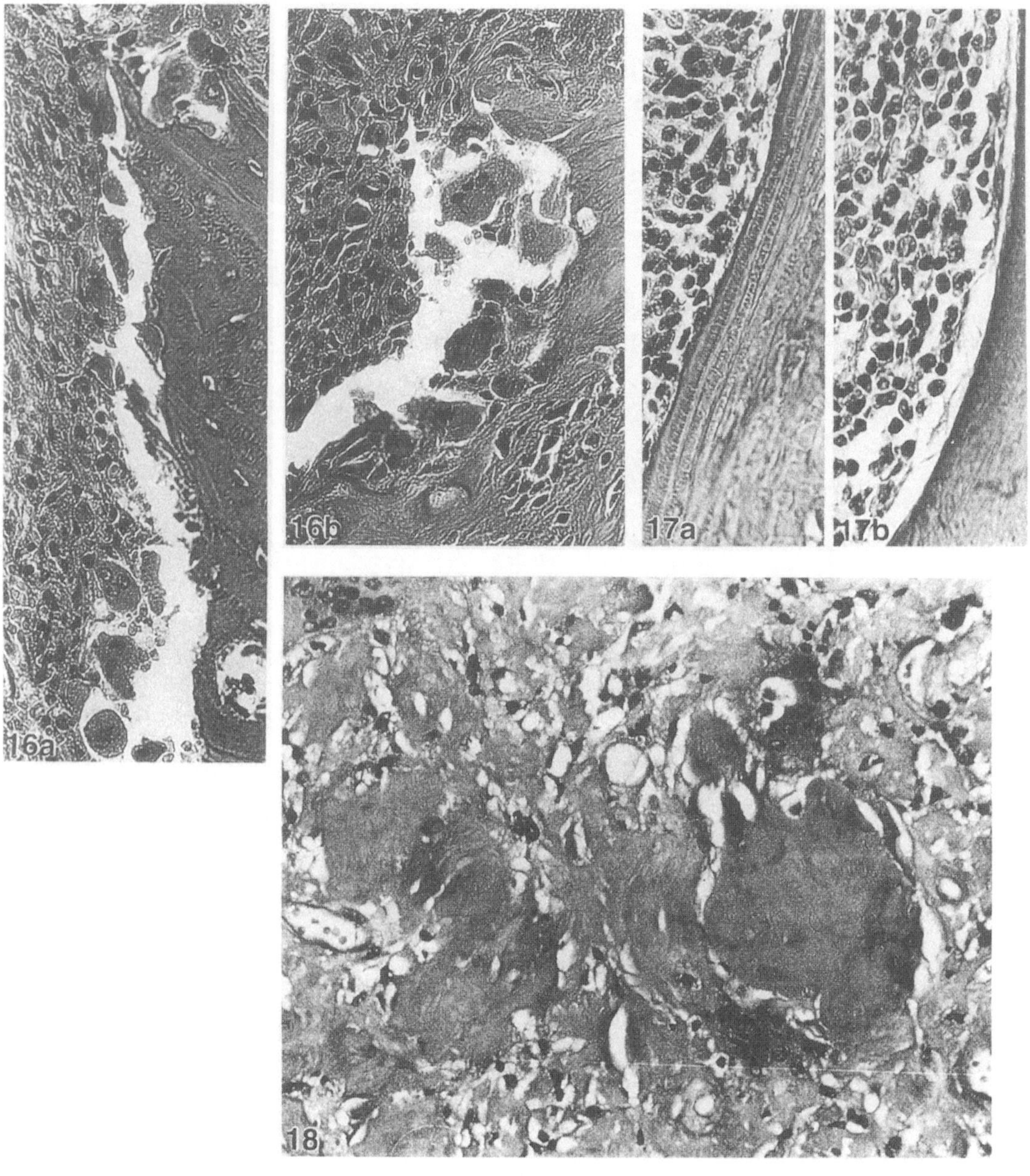

Fig. 16 a, b. This osteoclastic resorption develops at the periphery of a plasmocytic nodule

Fig. 17 a, b. On contrast to the preceding image, the smooth borders of these two bony trabeculae in contact with plasmocytic tumour nodules suggested another modality of bone resorption, resorption in which pressure from the proliferating plasmocytes plays an important part

Fig. 18. Large amyloid plaque in a biopsy of a tumour of the iliac bone

37. Leiomyosarcoma and rhabdomyosarcoma

Leiomyoarcoma

Primary leiomyosarcoma of bone is very rare and it is generally accepted that it arises from the vascular media. Even before the availability of immunohistological reactions, pathologists had noted quite distinctive appearances in what they classified under the term "primary fibroblastic sarcoma of bone". The malignant fibrous histiocytomas accounted for a large part of these sarcomas, but others were rare leiomyosarcomas as shown by immunohistological reactions and ultrastructure. The rather attractive hypothesis of a metaplasia of a fibroblastic sarcoma has also been advanced. Could it be the case that a tumour of unknown origin might express characteristics specific to the smooth muscle cell? The cell is totipotent and when neoplastic it is autonomous and is free to develop as it will.

General considerations

In the reported cases, now some 40 or so, there is a male predominance. Though the tumour is seen from the first to the ninth decade, the mean age is between 40 and 50. The preferential locations are the metaphyses of the long bones of the limbs; the femur, tibia, fibula, but the tumour also occurs in the jaws.

Clinical features and course

The presenting features are pain, intense in some cases, or swelling, sometimes known to have been present for several years. In the case of Shamsuddin (1980) the fibular swelling had been present for 10 years; such long intervals have suggested the malignant transformation of a preexisting leiomyoma, but given the rarity of diagnosed cases of leiomyoma this hypothesis seem unlikely. The tumour may be discovered at the time of a fracture produced by minimal trauma. In a curious case reported by Berlin et al (1987), the tumour developed in a zone adjacent to one from which a giant-cell tumour had been removed 31 years previously.

On examination, the swelling is often palpable, sometimes with increased local warmth and obvious dilatation of the venous network. The published cases are too few to allow any definition of the prognosis of this tumour. In the 19 cases collected from the literature by Young (1991) the outcome was known in 16 patients: 3 had died in 18 months and one patient was living with metastases 32 months after amputation and chemotherapy. Only one of the 5 patients of Angervall et al (1980) was followed up for 6 years without metastases. According to some reported figures, survival without metastasis (in the short term) is of the order of 30-40%.

Imaging

Imaging techniques demonstrate a lytic tumour with ill-defined boundaries (fig. 1). The osteolysis sometimes assumes the appearance of moth-eaten bone. Depending on its stage, the tumour may erode the inner aspect of the cortex, which becomes thickened, or even destroy the cortex completely and infiltrate the periosseous soft tissues. Angiography and scintigraphy provide valuable information with regard to the vascularisation and the extent of the tumour, information which is essential before operation.

Pathological anatomy and histopathology

On section the tumour is fleshy, reddish and relatively soft, though it may be whitish and firm. Study of the operative specimen makes it possible to decide whether the tumour has developed predominantly or entirely within the bone.

Examination of slides at low magnification shows interlacing bundles of fusiform cells surrounded by an abundant vascular plexus (figs. 3-6). Silver impregnation demonstrates a rich network of reticulin fibers. The fusiform cells have an eosinophil cytoplasm. Mitoses vary in number, but there is some polymorphism and atypical nuclei. It is not rare to observe palisaded appearances formed by these cigar-shaped nuclei with rounded ends. Some large cells have a large nucleus which is often notched. A small clear space around the nucleus has been described which has been variously interpreted.

Another appearance, usually passed over without mention, but easy to note in the majority of microphotographs of leiomyosarcomas, is the presence of clear zones where neither nuclei nor stainable cytoplasm persist. These irregularly distributed zones suggest the streaks of light of some watercolors, a sort of gum that obscures the design; it is probably an artefact but one which is curiously repeated in this tumour. There is usually no collagen which may be detected at the ultrastructural level as rare fibers in the acellular spaces. There is no osteogenesis or chondrogenesis.

The reaction to anti-desmin antibodies, which is positive in healthy muscle may be negative in tumour muscle. Reaction with the anti-actin of smooth muscle is more often positive. Cases of a positive anti-keratin reaction have also been reported but of very variable intensity.

Ultrastructural study demonstrates fusiform cells containing myofilaments, dense bodies, vesicles of pinocytosis and a basal layer surrounding the cells [Shamsuddin et al 1980].

Diagnosis

The histological appearances may initially suggest a diagnosis of leiomyosarcoma; once the muscular nature is demonstrated it is necessary to determine whether it is a primary tumour of intraosseous origin. The presence of local clinical features dating back for several months, the solitary lesion, the absence of pathological antecedents (such as hysterectomy for "suspect" fibroma), lead one to consider that the osteolysis is primary. In cases where the cortex is respected, but also when it is breached and associated with obvious ballooning, it is logical to acknowledge that the tumour is of intraosseous origin and that it is not a leiomyosarcoma of the soft tissues that has invaded the bone. Masson's trichrome stain, the Van Giesen stain and the immunological reactions will confirm the diagnosis suggested by standard staining.

It is not always thus; woven or overlapping appearances may suggest a malignant fibrous histiocytoma, other arrangements of the fusiform cells may logically suggest a fibroblastic sarcoma or a malignant neurinoma. Some authors have stressed the value of ultrastructural study [Sanerkin 1979, Shamsuddin et al 1980, Chomette et al 1984], but others consider that the immunohistological reactions allow diagnosis without recourse to ultrastructural study.

Rhabdomyosarcoma

Some very rare cases of rhabdomyosarcoma originate within bone; this fact is not always evident in the published photographs of macroscopic specimens, whether of very well developed tumours or of flat bones. Ghosez et al (1993) reports a case of rhabdomyosarcoma of the second dorsal vertebra; careful study excluded a metastasis, invasion by an adjacent tumour (the paravertebral muscles being macroscopically and microscopically normal) or invasion by a rhabdomyosarcoma developing in the central nervous system.

References

Angervall L, Berlin O, Kindblom LG, Steiner B (1980) Primary leiomyosarcoma of bone: a study of five cases. Cancer 46: 1270-1279

Berlin O, Angervall L, Kindblom LG, Berlin IC, Steiner B (1987) Primary leiomyosarcoma of bone. A clinical, radiographic, pathologic anatomic and prognostic study of 16 cases. Skeletal Radiol 16: 364-376

Chomette G, Auriol M, Princ G, Guilbert F (1984) Le léiomyosarcome osseux. Etude ultrastructurale et histoenzymologique. A propos d'un cas de siège mandibulaire. Arch Ana Cytol Pathol 32: 20-25

Evans DMD, Sanerkin NG (1965) Primary leiomyosarcoma of bone. J Pathol Bacteriol 90: 348-350

Fornassier VL, Paley D (1983) Leiomyosarcoma in bone: primary or secondary? Skeletal Radiol 10: 147-153

Ghosez JP, Himmer O, Lootvoet L, Beugnies A, Devyrer B (1993) Rhabdomyosarcome osseux primitif. A propos d'une localisation vertébrale. Rev Chir Orthop 79: 70-73

Hilpert Pl, Radecki PD, Edmonds P (1986) Primary leiomyosarcoma of the mandible. Skeletal Radiol 15: 570-574

Kawai T, Suzuki M, Mukai M, Hiroshima K, Shinmei M (1983) Primary leiomyosarcoma of bone. Arch Pathol Lab Med 107: 433-437

McLean RG, Murray IPC (1984) Alveolar rhabdomyosarcoma, metastatic to the right femur, primary site undetermined. Skeletal Radiol 12: 288-293

Myers JL, Arocho J, Bernreuter W, Dunham W, Mazur MT (1991) Leiomyosarcoma of bone. A clinicopathologic, immunohistochemical, and ultrastructural study of five cases. Cancer 67: 1051-1056

Overgaard J, Frederiksen P, Helmig O, Myhre Jensen O (1977) Primary leiomyosarcoma of bone. Cancer 39: 1664-1671

Pasquel PM, Levet SM, De Leon B (1976) Primary rhabdomyosarcoma of bone. A case report. J Bone Joint Surg 58A: 1176-1178

Pavlakis E, Augereau B, Lecomte D, Gintzburger S, Jagueux M (1982) Les leiomyosarcomes primitifs de l'os. Ann Pathol 4: 327-331

Sanerkin NG (1979) Primary leiomyosarcoma of the bone and its comparison with fibrosarcoma. A cytological, histological and ultrastructural study. Cancer 44: 1375-1387

Shamsuddin AK, Reyes F, Harvey JW, Toker C (1980) Primary leiomyosarcoma of bone. Hum Pathol 11: 581-583

Wang TY, Erlandon RA, Marcove RC, Huvos AG (1980) Primary leiomyosarcoma of bone. Arch Pathol Lab Med 104: 100-104

Young MPA, Freemont AJ (1991) Primary leiomyosarcoma of bone. Histopathol 19: 257-263

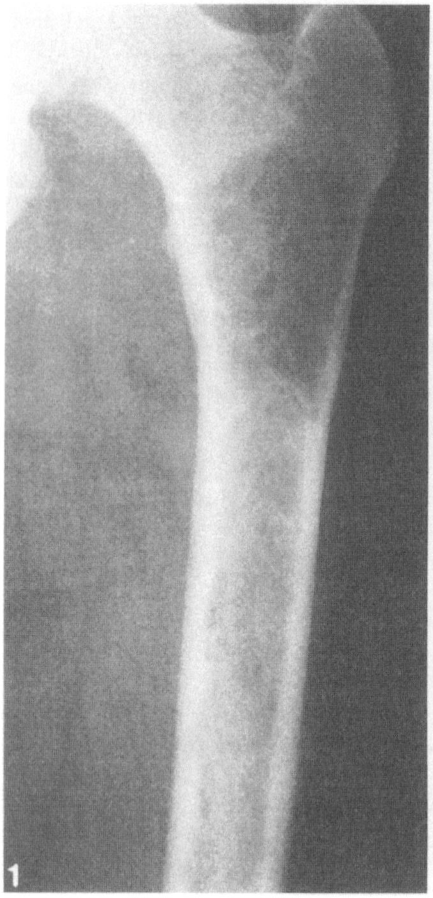

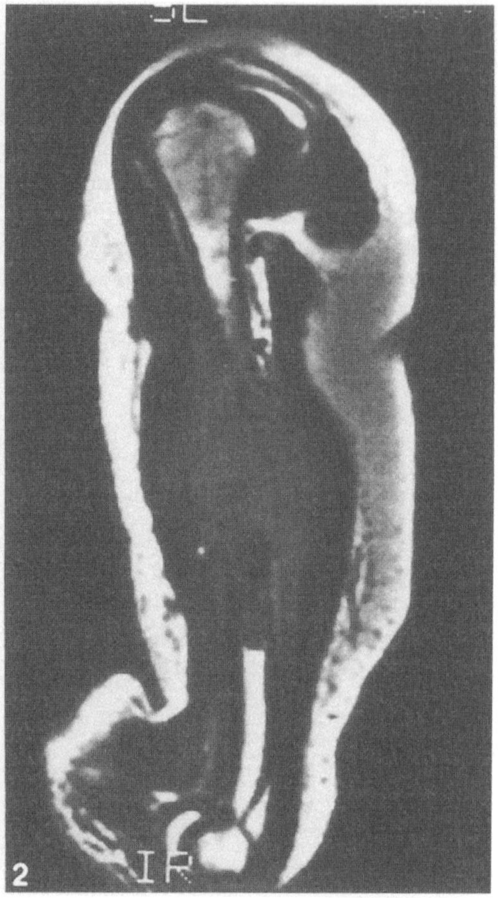

Fig. 1. Leiomyosarcoma of upper end of femur, revealed by pain of neuralgic type in a woman of 56. The metaphyseo-diaphyseal osteolysis is poorly defined. The deep aspect of the cortex, in part destroyed, gives a marbled veined appearance to the entire radiographical image. Examination of the resection specimen confirmed that the cortex was not breached. (Courtesy of Prof. Jagueux, Hôpital Saint-Antoine, who provided this radiograph [Pavlakis et al 1987])

Fig. 2. This extensive leiomyosarcoma of the humeral shaft has destroyed the cortex and invaded the soft tissues

Fig. 3. At low magnification bundles of fusiform cells are seen, between which large vessels are reduced to a simple endothelium

Fig. 4. The cell proliferation shows major anisocytosis and anisonucleosis

Fig. 5. An oedematous, less cellular zone

Fig. 6. This quasi-endocrinoid appearance is sometimes seen in areas where the bundles of myoblasts, cut at right angles to their axes, are surrounded by actual vascular sinuses (this is from a leiomyosarcoma of the ulna in an adolescent boy; histological sections by courtesy of our colleague, Dr Bouadhef, Hôpital Parnet, Alger)

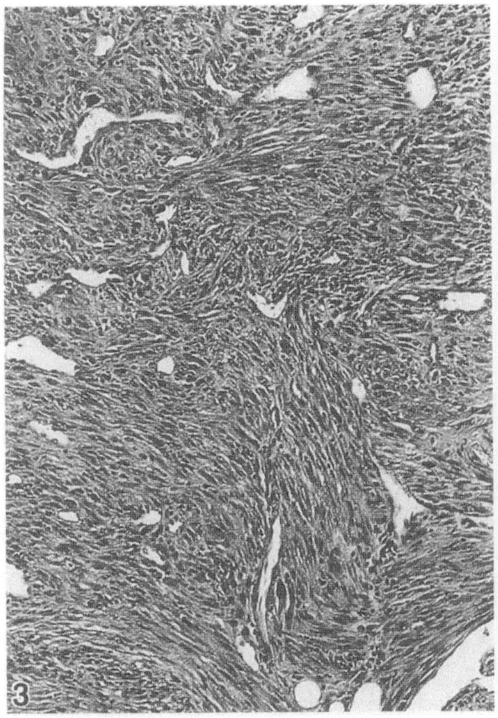
3

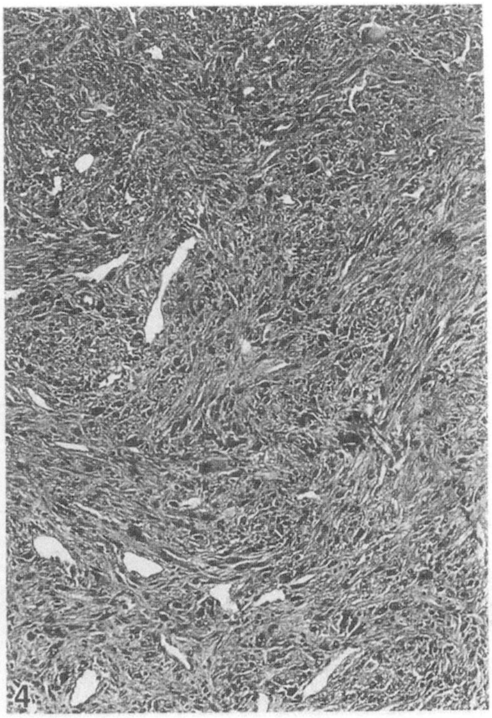
4

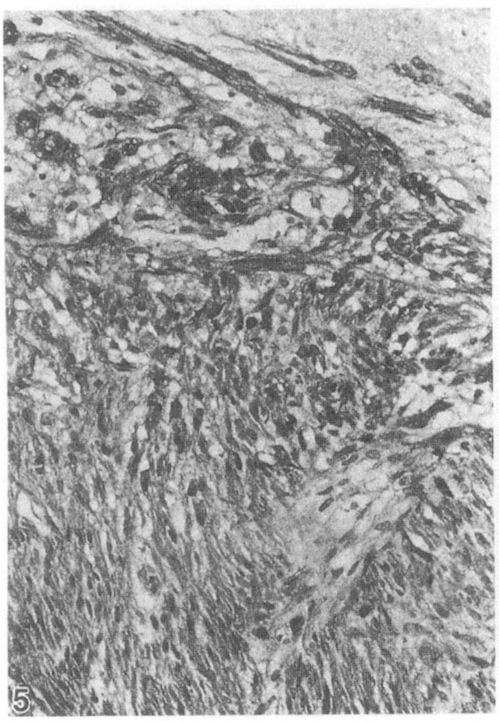
5

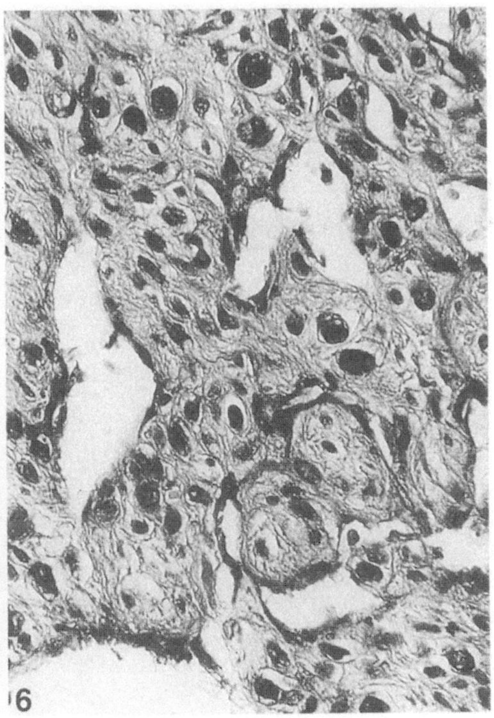
6

38. Craniofacial tumours and pseudotumours

μTwo special features of the bony tissue of the craniofacial skeleton impart a specific nature to tumours and pseudotumours at this site. There are the embryological origin of these bones, which for the most part are membrane bones derived from neuromesenchyme, and the presence in the jaws of dental rudiments as the source of specific lesions. The lesions whose special characteristics have been mentioned in the previous chapters will form the subject of only a short review of essential concepts in a craniofacial context.

Craniofacial tumours and pseudotumours of non-dental origin

Fibrous dysplasia

There is a craniofacial form without involvement of the long bones (fig. 1). The diagnosis is based entirely on study of the biopsy. This histological diagnosis from ossifying fibroma is often difficult (if one admits the existence of this entity, which seems virtually restricted to the craniofacial region). The hypertrophic variant has been accused of being a possible cause of leontiasis ossea. Dysplasia may be both hypertrophic and cystic, so that histological differential diagnosis may need to include an angioma or an aneurysmal cyst [Derome & Visot 1983].

Craniofacial fibrous dysplasia is a serious disorder because of its local complications manifest as compression of the nerves by narrowing of their exit foramina (optic fissure, facial canal).

Ossifying fibroma

The importance of diagnosing this tumour relates to the fact that its prognosis is favourable after complete excision, and thereby quite different from that of fibrous dysplasia, which is unpredictable and often serious (Chapter 32). The characteristics of this strange ossifying fibroma make it possible that it is a monostotic ossifying variant of fibrous dysplasia. A non-ossifying periosteal desmoid fibroma (fig. 2) in the mandible whose cellular component is quite different from that of ossifying fibroma is found [Crisi et al 1986, Mascrès & Vauclair 1989].

Paget's disease

The cranial onset of Paget's disease is suspected, if not diagnosed, from a radiograph showing considerable increase in the vascular network of the bone (fig. 3). This is succeeded by an osteolytic zone which may result in biopsy of the bone. This is not really lytic but is undergoing pagetic transformation: a general thickening involving the diploë and both inner and outer tables. Failure to calcify this new "bone" causes the lytic or porotic appearance, both terms being inaccurate - this is hypertransparency of a thickened bone.

Paget's disease does not exist in children; it is a purely adult disorder. At the apices of teeth lying in a zone of remodelling, there is a considerable and characteristic hypercementosis.

Histiocytosis X

Histicytosis X may occur as the commonplace lacunar cranial form. Quaraishi et al (1995), reviewing 73 cases of Langerhans'cell histiocytosis in children, found involvement of the head and neck in 67% of cases; the cranial bony lesion is more common. The biopsy sample is often sent to the pathologist with the label "abscess", given its macroscopic appearance. The more severe forms, the Letterer-Siwe and Hand-Schüller-Christian syndromes, are quite characteristic clinically (cf Chapter 31).

Idiopathic osteolysis

Idiopathic osteolysis, like other vascular lesions - angioma, angiosarcoma - may be localised to the bones of the craniofacial skeleton. It is discussed in Chapter 26, where I express my opinion, in agreement with many authors - that from all appearances it is a lymphangiomatosis.

As for the so-called idiopathic solitary bone cyst, like that of the long bones (Chapter 29) its origin is debatable. Its wall consists of layers of connective tissue not covered by an epithelium. The cavity is empty and devoid of any fleshy growth.

Epidermoid cyst

Epidermoid cysts of bone have two sites of election, the cranial vault and the phalanges, but they are also relatively common in the jaws. They may be located in any part of the cranial vault (figs. 6, 7). Sometimes the cyst is situated in the diploë, sometimes in the outer table, more rarely in the inner table. It may be found from childhood; it is a small firm swelling, attached to the bone and elevating the scalp. The radiographs of these cysts show a clear image bounded by a sclerosed border. Maroteau, who has studied their development, states that some disappear spontaneously and that continued growth is rare.

Cysts of the jaws are solitary and must be distinguished from ameloblastomas and cysts of dental origin, which may be multiple [Cernéa et al 1969] and form part of the syndrome of nevomatosis or basocellular carcinomatosis of Gorlin (skin carcinomas and bone anomalies, particularly cranial).

Histologically, the cyst consists of a malpighian epithelial wall with desquamated cells filling the cavity. Usually there are no inflammatory phenomena, but their appearance may become more complex when these develop and deposits of cholesterol are added.

In orbital sites, an epidermoid cyst or an aneurysmal cyst may be difficult to differentiate from a chronic blood cyst of the orbit. The latter is a late complication of an asymptomatic orbital haemorrhage which has become encapsulated, destroys the adjacent structures, including the bony tissues, and simulates an orbital neoplasm.

Fissural cyst

Fissural or inclusion cysts develop from the epithelial vestiges along the lines of suture; they include nasopalatine cyst, cysts of the nasal margin or nasolabial cyst, and median palatine cyst.

In the radiographs these cysts present as a clear space whose outlines are sometimes symmetrical (like that of a playing-card heart for nasopalatine cysts). They are true cysts, bordered by a malpighian lining, sometimes associated with mucin-secreting cells.

Osteoma

The bones of the skull and face may produce the same types of osteomas as do the other bones of the skeleton (Chapter 10).

Simple osteomas

Simple primary osteomas belong to two main types (figs. 8, 9) of dense and massive bone or of spongy bone, and angio-osteoma, a sort of bony telangiectatic growth.

Reactive osteomas

These are essentially the manifestations of a primary or secondary tumour (figs. 10, 11). But the craniofacial skeleton, which is the commonest site of osteomas, imparts particular anatomical and clinical features to the lesions. The sites of election are the cranial vault, the facial sinuses and the mandible. Osteoma is the commonest tumour of the orbit.

Deformation of the skull vault by an osteoma is easily recognised, even in the complete absence of pain. The visible and palpable swelling, bony in consistency and smooth of surface, is continuous with the underlying bone. These osteomas of the skull vault are sometimes manifestations of a meningioma or a metastasis.

Fronto-ethmoidal osteomas, if not detected early, become complicated by mucocele, sinusitis, even orbital invasion with exophthalmos [Earwaker 1993]. In children and adolescents the discovery of osteomas of the skull and jaw should suggest the possibility of Gardner's syndrome.

Histologically, some osteomas are formed by relatively regular apposition of bony lamellae in considerable number, the whole resembling bone of haversian type. Others are calcifications in osteoid or fibro-osteoid tissue (figs. 12, 13). Others still are represented by a construction of fine bony trabeculae arranged in a fan-shape in bundles of capillary arterioles which they separate from one another; these are true angio-osteomas (fig. 9).

It is clear that treatment is governed by the site and nature of the osteoma; whether it is simple or reactive to a primary or secondary tumour.

Torus

There are localised thickenings, a sort of sessile exostoses, which develop on the inner aspect of the mandible and in the median palatine zone and are known by the name of torus. "Exostoses" may develop on the mandible or at the zones of muscle attachments to the cranial bones, but they are really osteophytic structures rather than to true exostoses.

Primary osteogenic sarcoma

Primary osteogenic sarcoma of the bones of the skull and face is rare (figs. 14-18). Those of the maxillofacial massif represent less than 4% of osteosarcomas and are usually situated on the mandible. Their mean age of occurrence, around 35, is higher than that for sarcomas of the long bones.

Although different types of osteosarcoma have been described in the mandible [Brocheriou et al 1974, Clark et al 1983, Chan et al 1986], I have chiefly observed the fibroblastic type of a low grade of malignancy [Millar et al 1990]. In contrast, those cases I have diagnosed on the skull were of osteoblastic type, some very differentiated, and the diagnosis from osteoblastoma was difficult. Others, typified by cytological anomalies, were obvious sarcomas of a high grade of malignancy (cf Chapter 11).

Cartilaginous tumours

Cartilaginous tumours are rare in membrane bones [Brocheriou-Payen 1975] but exhibit certain special features.

Chondrosarcoma

Chondrosarcomas at these sites are 4 times as common in men as in women [Coltrera et al 1986, Garrington et al 1988, Hackney et al 1991]. They occur at an earlier age than those of the long bones; the mean age is around 30-35 years but they may affect patients from the first to the eighth decade of life. Most are sited at the maxilla and mandible, where they are commoner than benign cartilaginous tumours (fig. 19). Involvement of the base of the skull in the spheno-ethmoidal region is rare, but extremely serious.

The clinical picture is usually that of the painless development of a tumour mass. Some rare cases present after local trauma.

Development is dominated by the frequency of recurrence. Local spread is the main cause of death [Tran et al 1992]. In general these chondosarcomas have a worse prognosis than those in other parts of the skeleton; it is even worse than that of osteosarcomas of the bones of the skull and face.

The radiographical appearances do not differ notably from those of chondrosarcomas of other bones of the skeleton: poorly defined osteolysis spotted with opacities due to calcification is seen. In mandibular lesions the chondrosarcoma most often develops in the molar region.

Histological examination of a biopsy sample allows a diagnosis of chondrosarcoma in virtually all cases. In an apparently mature proliferation, Lichtenstein's criteria help to identify a chondrosarcoma of grade 1 malignancy: bulky nuclei - or increased nucleo-cytoplasmic ratio, numerous cells with double nuclei, some giant cells. The peripheral zones of chondrosarcomas of grades 2 and 3 are zones of tumour extension, rich in young and poorly differentiated cells and often containing cells in mitosis. Calcification and ossification are not rare, and in cases where there is a doubt between chondrosarcoma and osteosarcoma the nodular architecture of the tumour will point to the cartilaginous nature of the lesion.

Chondroma, chordoma

The problem of differential diagnosis between chondroma and chordoma of the base of the skull has been discussed in Chapter 20. We repeat only that some chordomas exhibit striking histological resemblances to cartilaginous tumours. These tumours, identified by the pathologists of the Mayo Clinic, have a more favourable prognosis. The immunological characteristics of these chondroid chordomas are more similar to those of chondrosarcomas; thus, they are better classed with chondrosarcomas of low-grade malignancy.

Chondroblastoma

According to statistics from the Mayo Clinic [Bertoni et al 1987], the localisation of 30 chondroblastomas to the bones of the skull and face represents 7% of all chondroblastomas. Two-thirds of the patients were male. The tumour was situated in the temporal bone in 21 cases and the mandible in 6. Histological examination of these chondroblastomas showed a frequent association of the tumour with appearances of giant-cell granuloma, aneurysmal cyst and giant-cell tumour. Even more notable was the virtually constant presence of mitoses and invasion of the zone of peri-neoplastic osteosclerosis.

Malignant histiocytofibroma

The prognosis of the few cases of malignant histiocytofibromas reported was most unfavourable.

Ewing's sarcoma

The prognosis of Ewing's sarcoma at this site is significantly worse than elsewhere.

Osteoid osteoma and osteoblastoma

Osteoid osteomas and osteoblastomas have been reported; the diagnosis of the latter from well-differentiated osteosarcoma may be extremely difficult.

Aneurysmal cyst

Aneurysmal cyst is rare at this site.

Angioma

Angiomas of the flat bones of the skull are quite common (cf Chapter 25).

Haemangioendothelioma

I have observed several malignant haemangioendotheliomas where the skull was the first site of the tumour.

Tumours and pseudotumour like giant-cell lesions

Though it is very artificial, it is possible to group under this heading different lesions with the common histological feature of the presence of numerous giant cells.

Giant-cell tumour (cf Chapter 21)

There have been possibly true reports of giant-cell tumours of the bones of the skull and face [Wolfe et al 1983]. Bertoni et al (1992) reported 11 cases in the sphenoid, 1 at the occiput and 1 in the temporal bone. While the histology was typical of a giant-cell tumour, the authors nevertheless mention the predominance of fusiform cells in 5 cases.

The stage of evolution can be assessed according to the classical schemas; but some give 4 grades of malignancy and others only 3. My own view is that the grade 3 is a sarcoma, perhaps a histiocytofibrosarcoma; but the important fact is the need for close liaison with our surgical colleagues. The relatively guarded prognosis depends on the surgical possibilities, sometimes supplemented by irradiation; hence the need to distinguish giant-cell tumour from a simple reparative granuloma. I have seen a giant-cell tumour in the ramus of the mandible, which recurred and proved fatal due to vascular ulceration.

Recklinghausen's brown tumour

This lesion has been discussed in connection with giant-cell tumours of the long bones. We recall that a giant-cell tumour of the jaws represents a "tumour" of parathyroid osteosis in about one case in twenty. Consequently, to make the diagnosis of giant-cell tumour at this site requires a study of calcium-phosphorus metabolism so as to avoid needless operation.

Giant-cell tumour of the alveolar margin (fig. 21 a, b)

This is regarded as an anatomo-clinical variety of epulis, from which it cannot be distinguished histologically.

Giant-cell granuloma (fig. 20 a, b)

Identified by Jaffe as "giant cell reparative granuloma", this obviously suggest a reactive process (cf Chapter 21). It is a benign lesion of young subjects which is cured by curettage.

The histological appearance resembles that of a fleshy granulation in its vascular richness, the presence of histiocytofibroblastic cells, also of giant cells and small deposits of haemosiderin. Mitoses are often numerous but without anomalies. Small bony or osteoid formations can be seen in places, but it is difficult to say whether they properly belong to the "tumour" [Rogers et al 1984, Flanagan et al 1988, Harman et al 1990].

Cherubism

This disorder was described by the Canadian Jons in 1933. It develops in children between 2 and 4 years of age and stabilises at puberty. Clinically, it is characterised in its typical form by the chubby appearance of the face. Radiographic examination demonstrates a multicavitary appearance of the enlarged rami and angle of the mandible. Its clinical appearance, characterised by its bilaterality and usual association with dental anomalies, allows diagnosis more easily than does examination of the histological sections. If there are no clinical aspects, the diagnosis becomes much more difficult and has to be based on the presence of an haemorrhagic fibrous tissue, variably rich in histiocytes and fibroblasts and with giant cells, often in clusters. From the genetic viewpoint, the disorder has dominant autosomal transmission.

Tumours developing from normal or heterotopic intraosseous elements

Melanic neuroectodermal tumour of infancy (fig. 22)

This tumour has been given various names, related to arguments about its origin which may be from *retinal anlage*, *melanotic progonoma* or retinal choristoma. It is a rare tumour, without gender predominance and is recognised in the first months of life, usually before the age of 1 year. Its elective site is in the maxilla (70% of cases), followed by the mandible, cranial bones and brain. It develops rapidly and may hinder suckling. Cure is obtained by surgical excision of the lesion. Some cases of local recurrence have been reported, as well as a case of a malignant type in the maxilla.

In the radiographs there is an ill-defined lytic image which displaces the dental rudiments.

Macroscopically, the tumour is bluish-gray. The larger part displaces the mucosa, often without ulcerating it, while the deep part is lodged in an irregular cavity hollowed out in the maxilla.

Histologically, there are two types of cells: small "lymphocytoid" cells of neuroblastic appearance grouped in clumps or thick strands; and larger polyhedral cells of epithelial nature laden with melanic pigment (Fontana +). These cells are dispersed in the collagenous stroma or arranged in pseudoglandular formations bordering narrow clefts. There are also some fusiform cells in the stroma. According to reports, there are various degrees of cell maturation; sometimes an abundant neurofibrillary material is mentioned.

Ultrastructural study [Cutler et al 1981] allows identification of two types of small dark cells and two types of large melanin-forming cells; biochemical studies [Johnson et al 1983] performed on tissue from maxillary tumours reveal a considerable level of dopamine in these tissues.

Diagnosis of the tumour is suspected from the time of its clinical discovery. This tumour, described by Krompecher in 1918, has given rise to diverse histogenetic interpretations, but the biochemical and ultrastructural studies suggest a neuroectodermal origin from cells migrating from the neural crest. The microphotographs illustrating this case (courtesy of one of our colleagues, Dr Epardeau of the Hôpital Foch) show positive immunohistological reactions for keratin and vimentin in the large cells and neuro-enolase in the small cells. Ultrastructural examination demonstrates melanosomes in the large cells and neurosecretory granules in the small cells.

Schwannoma and leiomyosarcoma

Schwannomas and leiomyosarcomas originate from the components of the neurovascular bundle of the inferior dental canal. The diagnostic problem of the cellular origin of a fusiform-cell tumour has been discussed in connection with tumours of the long bones belonging to the same category.

Neurofibromatosis

Neurofibromatosis very often has a maxillofacial expression and only poses any radiological or clinical problem when a bony tumour is solitary in a case with neural lesions.

Muco-epidermoid carcinoma

Primary intraosseous muco-epidermoid carcinoma develops preferentially in the premolar and molar regions of the maxilla after the age of 50. It is commoner in women than in men. Its origin is usually ascribed to an ectopic salivary gland.

Secondary tumours

It must be borne in mind that there is a possibility of secondary as well as primary tumours.

Sarcomas developing on a preexisting lesion

(cf Chapter 11)
(Paget's disease, osteoma)

Post-irradiation sarcoma

In the series of Sagerman et al (1969) dealing with 243 cases of retinoblastoma at 5-year follow-up, the frequency of radiation-induced cancers was 8.6%. In the statistics of the Institut Curie [Bataini et al 1979] dealing with 112 children irradiated for retinoblastoma, there were 10 malignant tumours, of which 7 were osteosarcomas and one a chondrosarcoma. The proportion of tumours is much the same. In adults, osteosarcomas induced by irradiation of soft tissue tumours can also be observed. In 1988, Lee et al listed 4 post-irradiation sarcomas in 46 osteosarcomas of the skull and face, of which 32 were primary: 8 cranial and 24 maxillary. Dickens et al (1990) studied maxillary osteosarcomas in 1000 patients in Hong-Kong treated by irradiation for nasopharyngeal cancer, and found 4 cases. The latent period was between 8 and 11 years. These authors considered that the small risk (0.4%) did not contraindicate this treatment.

It is clear that the enormous differences reported as to percentage incidence can be explained by the particular nature of clinical departments, the types of populations they serve and doubtless other factors (types of treatment, mean age of patients, perhaps certain genetic features).

Metastatic sarcoma

When osteolysis is the presenting feature, its nature and whether its origin is primary or secondary must be considered (cf Chapter 33). The histological appearance of the metastatic lesion may depart widely from that of the known primary tumour. Haematopoietic tumours (cf Chapters 34, 36) and disseminated angiomatoses (cf Chapter 25) are quite often the source of cranial osteolyses. Whether or not the lesion is attributable to a complex syndrome may be difficult to resolve; this is the case with the aggressive papillary temporal tumour [Thomas et al 1993] where some tumours have been reported in patients suffering from von Hippel-Lindau disease.

Odontogenic tumours and pseudotumours

Following the generally accepted classification, we may distinguish between cysts, purely epithelial tumours, epithelial-connective tumours and mesenchymal tumours.

Very generally, biopsies arrive at the laboratory with a label of "cyst" or "tumour" as suggested by the clinical and radiographic features, but such labels do not always correspond to the realities of the histological findings.

Cysts (figs. 23, 24)

Radiculo-dental or periapical cyst

This is common, and is an inflammatory lesion, the infection occurring via either the apex of a devitalised tooth or the alveolo-dental ligament. In the cyst wall, inflammatory cells may be associated with macrophages and giant cells and often crystals of fatty acids. The epithelialisation of the cyst is explained by hyperplasia of preexisting epithelial remnants (the epithelial remnants of Malassez) or possibly from the mucosa, into which they may open.

Corono-dental or follicular cyst

This develops from certain structures of the dental follicle, in contact with a partly or completely embedded tooth whose crown it surrounds. It is usually solitary. It may undergo major development (fig. 23), particularly in the region of the angle of the mandible, which accounts for the symptoms. This cyst is often remodelled by inflammatory changes. Its wall is bordered by an epithelium, either cubical or more often metaplastic malpighian, without keratinisation. The possible, but very rare, development of an ameloblastoma in this relatively common cyst has been reported.

Epidermoid cyst

At this site in the jaws, this cyst is usually attached to one of the epithelial invaginations of the dental buds. If multiple, the cysts form part of a basocellular nevomatosis.

Purely epithelial tumours (little or no induction of connective tissue response)

Ameloblastoma (adamantine epithelioma, adamantinoma)

This is the commonest of dental tumours. Adamantinoma occurs more often in men, chiefly between 20 and 50, but cases have been reported in young children and the elderly. Its elective site is the molar region and the angle of the mandible, extending to the ramus. More rarely, it is located in the premolar and incisor regions of the mandible as well as in the maxilla. Because its growth is slow and indolent, the tumour is often discovered late and its prognosis is impaired by frequent recurrences. Some surgeons prefer resection beyond the tumour bounds to simple curettage for this reason. Rare cases with pulmonary metastases have been reported [Dorner et al 1988, Seward et al 1975].

In the radiographs, the tumour presents as a clear image, usually multilocular, developing in the posterior part of the body of the mandible (figs. 25, 26) with varying encroachment on the ramus. The cortex remains intact for a long time, but as the lesion progresses and increases and if there are recurrences the cortex may be seen to be breached, usually at the level of the mylohoid and temporalis muscles.

The macroscopic appearance is of a tumour that is partly solid and grayish-white and partly a uni- or multilocular cyst whose extent needs to be carefully assessed. Ackermann et al (1988) reported 57 cases of unicystic ameloblastomas, representing 15% of all ameloblastomas observed over a period of 30 years; 52 had developed in the mandible in patients who were mostly Black and with a mean age of 23.8 years.

Several histological appearances have been described.

Typical (or follicular) form

The tumour is characterised by the formation of lobules and epithelial strands surrounded by a fibrous stroma (fig. 27). At the margins of the strands the cells assume a cubical or cylindrical appearance; they have a central nucleus and contain some glycogen droplets at their basal pole. This is the appearance of adamantoblasts. In the central part of the lobules and strands the cells are separated by a mucoid substance, but usually retain some points of union between themselves and assume a stellate shape. Immunological studies have shown that these stellate cells are strongly marked by the antikeratin antibody, whereas the columnar cylindrical cells are only weakly marked. Cystic modifications are seen In the midst of these epithelial strands (fig. 29), sometimes rudiments of keratinising maturation (fig. 27 c); when these appearances are predominant they justify the identification of histological subtypes.

Particular types classified by predominant cell type or by overall architecture

- Cystic type

An initial difficulty for the pathologist relates to these cystic types. The arrangement of the centro-follicular epithelial clumps leads to the formation of cavities, without cholesterol crystals, bordered by a thin multilayered epithelium, which must be distinguished from a epidermoid cyst. This epithelial membrane should be examined in numerous sections in the search for some more characteristic zones of cubical ameloblastic cells. Small epithelial outgrowths which infiltrate the connective tissue and adjacent bone outside the cyst(s) should be sought for.

- Plexiform type

The epithelial strands are inter-anastomosed, forming a sort of network of stellate cells bounded by prismatic cells. The type with malpighian metaplasia or differentiated epidermoid epithelium (acantho-ameloblastoma) is characterised by malpighian metaplasia of varying maturity. The abundance of malpighian foci is very variable; their presence does not influence the prognosis unfavourably.

- Granular cell type (fig. 28)

This is marked by the sometimes massive transformation of epithelial cells into granular cells whose cytoplasm is laden with eosinophil granules [Navarette et al 1971, Yamamoto et al 1989]. This form has a greater tendency to recur. A tumour has been described in the mandible with granular cells whose plexiform monophasic architecture should allow differentiation from granular cell ameloblastoma [Siar et al 1991].

- Basal cell carcinoma type (so-called)

The appearance is altogether comparable to that of basal cell carcinoma. In this poorly differentiated form the course is more unfavourable and recurrences are more frequent.

- Type with cylindrical remodelling

This may be confused with a tumour metastasis from a salivary gland or a tumour developing in a heterotopic gland embedded in the jaw.

- Clear-cell "desmoplastic" ameloblastoma

Clear-cell ameloblastoma [Odukoya et al 1992] and "desmoplastic" ameloblastoma [Eversole et al 1984] are characterised by a particularly dense fibrous stroma accompanying the typical appearances of ameloblastoma. Radiologically, there is a lytic image sited anteriorly, more often mandibular than maxillary. The two cases reported by Tamimoto et al (1991) and Ashman et al (1993) were also situated in the anterior part of the mandible. Waldrom and El-Mofty (1993) studied 116 cases of ameloblastoma and detected this "desmoplastic" variant in 214 cases (13%) always with a marked tendency to develop in the anterior part of the mandible.

Some rare cases of ameloblastoma have a malignant course with pulmonary metastases. Therefore it is wise to study the adamantoblasts very carefully, since they may exhibit cytological evidence of malignancy in these cases, resembling a more or less differentiated epidermoid carcinoma.

Intramandibular malpighian epithelioma

A ballooning and lytic tumour of the mandible is sometimes seen in which histological examination shows a usually mature malpighian epitheliomatous character. This type of epithelioma has developed either from epithelial remnants without clinical expression, or on an ameloblastoma or preexisting cyst. Some authors regard the keratinisation of the malpighian lining of a non-epidermoid mandibular cyst as suspicious.

The histological diagnosis poses no particular problems but the radiological image suggests a more specifically mandibular lesion in view of its strictly intraosseous development and its sometimes considerable size (fig. 34).

Three other rare epithelial tumours should be mentioned.

Cystic odontogenic tumour

Previously named adeno-ameloblastoma, this usually manifests in the second decade. It is commoner in women and occurs more often in the maxilla than the mandible, mainly in its anterior part. Its course is slow and excision is not followed by recurrence. Radiologically and clinically it can be interpreted as a cyst.

Histologically, there are strands and plaques of epithelial cells, sometimes grouped as tubular pseudocanalicular structures. The cylindrical cells have a basal nucleus and clear cytoplasm and a marked basement membrane separates them from a sometimes lax hyaline stroma which may contain some calcifications.

Calcified odontogenic epithelial tumour (Pindborg's tumour)

This is rare. In two-thirds of cases it is situated in the molar region of the mandible [Pindborg 1958, Page et al 1975, Chomette 1986, Brocheriou 1987]. It is seen mainly before the age of 40.

The radiographs show a clear image with scattered opacities of varying density. This structure is often related to an embedded tooth. The prognosis is excellent.

Histologically, it consists of plaques and strands of epithelial cells joined by cell bridges. Mitoses are rare but large nuclei with irregular outlines are frequent. In the cellular areas there are unstructured deposits in concentric layers (fluorescent to thioflavine T). These acidophil deposits may become calcified and the neighbouring cells in contact with them degenerate. The fibrous stroma may contain small irregular basophil formations, sometimes confluent. Depending on the predominance of certain aspects, diagnosis may have to be made from follicular or radicular cyst, certain cementomas, osteoma or ameloblastic fibroma.

Calcified cystic odontogenic tumour

This is bounded by a layer of cubical cells, overlaid towards the cyst cavity by proliferating epithelial cells recalling a stellate reticulum, but in which areas of mummified or even calcified cells are observed. The whole suggests the calcified epithelioma of Malherbe, with which it shares a favourable prognosis.

Epithelio-connective tumours

Ameloblastic fibroma (fig. 30)

This is a benign structure not containing calcified material. It is seen in the first two decades of life. It is located preferentially in the premolar region of the mandible and is seen in radiographs as a clear image easily confused with that of an ameloblastoma.

The epithelial component presents as narrow strands bordered by a layer of cylindrical cells. The surrounding mesenchymal tissue is more cellular than that of a pure ameloblastoma. Hyaline transformation of this mesenchymal tissue may be seen, particularly at the immediate periphery of the epithelial strands.

Ameloblastic fibrosarcoma

Very rare ameloblastic fibrosarcomas have been reported, either malignant from the outset or after recurrence of a fibro-ameloblastoma.

Dentinoma

Dentinoma (fig. 31), a very rare tumour, is seen in the same age-group as ameloblastic fibroma, from which it differs histologically only in the presence of dentine elaborated in irregularly dispersed zones. This dentine is poorly calcified. In some cases only dentine surrounded by mesenchyme persists, to the exclusion of epithelial cells.

Ameloblastic fibro-odontoma

This is histologically and clinically an ameloblastic fibroma in which reciprocal induction leads to the formation of dentine and enamel. This tumour is evidenced in the radiographs as a clear zone dotted with small opacities.

Odontoma

The odontomas reproduce the dental tissues in a relatively well-differentiated and interconnected form.

Complex odontoma

The different dental tissues contract close interrelations, as in the tooth, but do not reproduce the general architecture of that organ.

Organoid or composite odontoma

Elaboration of the different tissues leads to the formation of atypical teeth that crudely reproduce the architecture of those organs. This dental production may be considerable. These odontomas are really more like hamartomas than true tumours.

During the period of dental formation there is the possibility of observing an adamantine epithelioma which may be mistaken for an ameloblastoma, but the prognosis is excellent.

Mesenchymal tumours

Myxoma

This is a lesion of young subjects which affects the maxilla and mandible. It is a benign but poorly circumscribed invasive lesion, which may breach the cortex and infiltrate the soft tissues. If operative removal is incomplete these myxomas recur readily. The radiographic appearance is that of an ill-defined osteolysis, often with a bullous appearance.

Histologically the lesion consists of an abundant mucoid substance, which is weakly positive to PAS and alcian-blue. The fusiform or stellate cells are scattered in this matrix, which is poor in collagen fibers. Mitoses are rare, but some nuclear anomalies may be seen. The presence of epithelial remnants in some myxomas justifies considering these lesions as induced odontogenic tumours; Chomette and Auriol (1986) invoke the high phosphatase and ATPase activity of these connective tissue cells in support of this hypothesis.

Fibroma or fibromyxoma

This represents a form richer in collagen fibers than myxoma.

Cementomas

These are rare tumours, probably akin to dysplasias, and may be classified as follows:

True benign cementoblastoma or cementoma

This apically situated benign tumour, usually molar or premolar, is seen mainly between the ages of 10 and 30, but also in later decades. There is no gender predominance. The tumour is manifest by the appearance of a slowly progressive swelling or by pain. Radiographs show a rounded opaque tumour with a narrow clear border, attached to the apex of a tooth.

In histological sections the tumour is well-defined and uniform in appearance. It consists of wide trabeculae of osteoid and cement traversed by very irregular lines of arrested growth of pagetoid pattern. These trabeculae and partly calcified areas imprison small ovoid cells. Between the trabeculae there develops a very vascular fibrous tissue, quite rich in cells; cementoblasts and multinucleate cells which are either osteoclasts or cementoblasts. From the histological aspect this pattern may cause confusion with benign tumours such as osteoid osteoma and osteoblastoma but the latter tends to be extensive and is readily recurrent if the entire lesion has not been removed, a course different from that of the completely benign cementoma. The extent of the irregular lines of arrest, vascularisation and giant cells may also suggest a diagnosis of Paget's disease, the prognosis of which is quite difficult to predict.

The most serious error is to confuse this lesion with a well-differentiated osteoblastic osteosarcoma. In fact, the radiological and clinical features of cementoblastoma are quite specific; in multiple sections osteosarcoma does not have the same uniformity or the same definite boundaries and is evidenced by an occasional abnormal mitosis.

Fibrocementoma (fig. 32)

This develops in older persons that those affected by cementoblastoma. Radiologically, the lesion begins as a clear image which gradually opacifies. The fibrocementoma consists of small round or oval areas resembling cement, scattered in fibrous tissue. Such an appearance may raise the problem of histological diagnosis from fibrous dysplasia.

Multiple cementoma

Also termed giant cementoma, this may reach a considerable size and balloon the mandible. The histological appearance is similar to that of fibrocementoma but the development of zones of cement is considerable and the round or oval areas are almost acellular. This dysgenetic lesion, possibly bilateral, is sometimes hereditary.

Cementifying fibrous dysplasia

This occurs in menopausal women and is evidenced radiographically at the apices of the incisor region as clear images laden with denser nodules which tend to become confluent. Its structure is similar to that of cementifying fibroma, but the progressive development of cement masses which fuse together leaves only rare persistent zones of connective tissue.

References

Craniofacial tumours and pseudotumours unconnected with the dental organ

Idiopathic osteolysis (cf Chapter 26)

Bullough PG, Goodfellow JW (1976) Solitary lymphangioma of bone. J Bone Joint Surg (Am) 58: 418

Frederiksen NL, Wesley RK, Sciubba JJ, Helfrick J (1983) Massive osteolysis of the maxillotacial skeleton: a clinical, radiographic, histologic and ultrastructural study. Oral Surg Oral Med Oral Pathol 55: 470-480

Heffez L, Doku HC, Carter BL, Freeney JE (1983) Perspeectives on massive osteolysis: report of a case and review of the literature. Oral Surg Oral Med Oral Pathol 55: 331-343

Imbert JC, Picault C (1974) Ostéolyse massive idiopathique ou maladie de Jacksson-Gorham. A propos d'une nouvelle observation. Rev Chir Orthop 60: 73-80

Jumbelic M, Feverstein IM, Dorfman HD (1984) Solitary intraosseous lymphangioma. J Bone Joint Surg 66A: 1479-1481

Murphy JB, Doku HC, Carter BL (1978) Massive osteolysis: phantom bone disease. J Oral Surgery 36: 318-322

Quaraishi MS, Blayney AW, Walker D, Breatnach FB, Bradley PJ (1995) Langerhans'cell histiocytosis: Head and neck manifestations in children. Head & Neck 17: 226-231

Thomas CB, Kveton JF, Poe DS, Zamani AA, Tarlov EC (1993) Aggressive papillary tumor of temporal bone in von Hippel-Lindau disease. Surg Pathol 5: 63-71

Van Den Houten BR, Ten Kate LP, Gerding JC (1985) The Hajdu-Cheney syndrome. A review of the literature and report of 3 cases. Int J Oral Surg 14: 113-125

White AA (1971) Disappearing bone disease with arthropathy and severe scarring of the skin. A report of four cases seen in South Vietnam. J Bone Joint Surg 53B: 303-309

Osteosarcoma (cf Chapter 11)

Osteoma (cf Chapter 10)

Bataini JP, Chavanne G, Brugère J, Mazabraud A (1979) Radiocancers maxillo-faciaux. Rev Stomalol Chir Maxillofac 80: 178-182

Bertoni F, Dallera P, Bacchini P, Marchetti C, Campobassi A (1991) The Istituto Rizzoli-Beretta experience with osteosarcoma of the jaw. Cancer 68: 1555-1563

Blodi FC (1976) Pathologic changes of the orbital bones. Am Acad Ophthalmol Otolaryngol Jan-Feb, pp 26-57

Brocheriou C, Guilbert F, Rouchon C, Benoist M, Chikhani P (1974) Sarcomes d'Ewing à localisation mandibulaire, deux observations. Rev Stanotol 75: 877-884

Cernéa P, Payen J, Brochériou CL (1974) Sarcomes osseux des maxillaires. Etude statistique de 41 observations. Bull Cancer 61: 151-160

Chan CW, Kung TM, Ma AL (1986) Telangiectatic osteosarcoma of the mandible. Cancer 58: 2110-2115

Chomette G, Auriol M (1986) Histopathologie buccale et cervico-faciale. Ostéome, pp 262-263

Clark JL, Unni KK, Dahlin DC, Devine KD (1983) Osteosarcoma of the jaw. Cancer 51: 2311-2316

Dahlin DC, Unni KK (1986) Bone tumors general aspects and data on 8542 cases. 4th edn. Charles Thomas, Springfield, p 84

Dickens P, Wei WI, Sham JST (1990) Osteosarcoma of the maxilla in Hong-Kong Chinese postirradiation for nasopharyngeal carcinoma. A report of four cases. Cancer 66: 1924-1926

Earwaker J (1993) Paranasal sinus osteomas a review of 46 cases. Skeletal Radiol 22: 417-423

Goodman MA, McMaster JH (1976) Primary osteosarcoma of the skull. Clin Orthop 120: 110-114

Hendee RW (1976) Primary osteogenic sarcoma of the calvaria. J Neurosurg 45: 334-337

Hilpert PL, Radecki PD, Edmonds P, Friedman AC (1986) Primary leiomyosarcoma (LMS) of the mandible. Case report. Skeletal Radiol 15: 570-574

Huvos AG, Sundaresan N, Bretsky SS, Butler A (1985) Osteogenic sarcoma of the skull. A clinicopathologic study of 19 patients. Cancer 56: 1214-1221

Lee YY, Tassel PV, Nauert C, Raymond AK, Edeiken J (1988) Craniofacial osteosarcomas: plain film, CT, and MR findings in 46 cases. AJNR 9: 379-385

Marks MP, Marks SC, Segall HD, Schwinn CP, Forrester DM (1987) Parosteal osteosarcoma (case report). Skeletal Radiol 16: 246-251

Millar BG, Browne RM, Flood TR (1990) Juxtacortical osteosarcoma of the jaws. Br J Oral Surg 28: 73-79

Sagerman RH, Cassady JR, Tretter P, Ellswoth RH (1969) Radiation induced neoplasia following external form therapy for children with retinoblastoma. Am J Roentgenol 105: 529-535

Salvati M, Ciappeta P, Raco A (1992) Osteosarcoma of the skull. Cancer 71: 2210-2216

Sundaresan N, Galicich JH, Rosen H, Huvos AG (1985) Primary osteogenic sarcoma of the skull. Five-year disease-free survival following surgery and high dose methotrexate therapy. NY State J Med 85: 598-599

Tran LM, Mark R, Meier R, Calcaterra TC, Parker RG (1992) Sarcoma of the head and neck. Cancer 70: 169-177

Cartilaginous tumours and pseudotumours (cf Chapters 2 and 20)

Bertoni F, Unni KK, Beabout JW, Harner SG, Dahlin DC (1987) Chondroblastoma of the skull and facial bones. Am J Pathol 88: 1-9

Boorstein JM, Spizamy DL (1988) Chondrosarcoma of base of skull (CBS). Skeletal Radiol 17: 208-211

Brochériou C, Payen J (1975) Tumeurs cartilagineuses des maxillaires: à propos de 11 observations. Ann Anat Pathol 20: 23-34

Coltrera MD, Gonge PB, Harrist TJ, Hyams VJ, Schiller AL, Goodman ML (1986) Chondrosarcoma of the temporal bone. Diagnosis and treatment of 13 cases and review of the literature. Cancer 58: 2689-2696

Evans HL, Ayala AG, Romsdahl MM (1977) Prognostic factors in chondrosarcoma of bone. Cancer 40: 818-831

Fu YS, Perzin KH (1974) Non-epithelial tumors of the nasal cavity, paranasal sinuses, and nasopharynx: a clinicopathologic study. Cancer 34: 453-463

Garrington GE, Collett WK (1988) Chondrosarcoma. I. A selected literature review. II. Chondrosarcoma of the jaw: analysis of 37 cases. J Oral Pathol 17: 1-20

Gay I, Elidan J, Kopolovic J (1981) Chondrosarcoma at the skull base. Ann Otol Rhinol Laryngol 90: 53-55

Hackney FL, Aragon SB, Aufdemorte TB, Holt GR, Van Sickels JE (1991) Chondrosarcoma of the jaws: clinical findings, histopathology, and treatment. Oral Surg Oral Med Oral Pathol 71: 139-143

Heffelfinger MJ, Dahlin DC, McCarty CS, Beabout JW (1973) Chordomas and cartilaginous tumors at the skull base. Cancer 32: 410-419

Korbi S, Kochtali K, Mokni M, Ladeb F, Kraiem C, Hamza F, Bakir A, Bouzakoura C (1991) Le chondrosarcome de la mandibule. Etude anatomoclinique d'un cas. Ann Pathol 11: 113-116

Massarelli G, Gandolfo L, Tanda F, Ghiselli F, Manunta V (1988) Maxillary chondrosarcoma (report of two cases). J Laryngol Otol 102: 177-181

Sen CN, Sekhar LN, Schramm VL, Janecka IP (1989) Chordoma and chondrosarcoma of the cranial base: an 8-year experience. Neurosurg 25: 931-941

Wyatt RB, Schochet SS, McCormick WF (1971) Ecchordosis physaliphora an electron microscopy study. J Neurosurg 34

"Fibroblastic" tumours and pseudotumours
(cf Chapter 16)

Abdul-Karim FW, Ayala AG, Chawla SP, Jing BS, Goeffert H (1985) Malignant fibrous histiocytoma of jaws. A clinicopathologic study of 11 cases. Cancer 56: 1590-1596

Akai M, Ohno T, Sugano I, Matsuzaki O, Nagao K, Takigawa K (1990) Malignant fibrous histiocytoma of skull and face presenting with massive osteolysis. Skeletal Radiol 19: 154-157

Crisi G, Calo M, Mauri C (1986) Desmoid tumor of the greater wing of the right sphenoid bone. Skeletal Radiol 15: 247-250

Deroma PJ, Visot A (1983) La dysplasie fibreuse crânienne. Neurochirurgie 29 (suppl I): 1-117

Earwaker J (1993) Paranasal sinus osteomas: a review of 46 cases. Skeletal Radiol 22: 417-423

Ford KB, Palmer PES, Teslu KH (1985) Fibrous dysplasia of calvaria (multiple sclerotic lesions). Skeletal Radiol 13: 68-71

Mascrés C, Vauclair R (1989) Le fibrome desmoïde maxillo-mandibulaire. Synthèse des connaissances sur une entité rare. A propos de trois cas. Ann Pathol 9: 182-188

Remagen W, Nidecker A, Prein J (1986) Gigantic benign fibrous histiocytoma (nonossifying fibroma). Skeletal Radiol 15: 251-253

Schamaman A, Smith I, Ackerman LV (1970) Benign fibro-osseous lesions of the mandible and maxilla a review of 35 cases. Cancer 26: 303-312

Schultz E, Hermann G, Irwin GAL, Shih H (1986) Desmoplastic fibroma of the mandible. Skeletal Radiol 15: 560-564

Sherman NH, Rao VM, Brennam RE, Edeiken J (1982) Fibrous dysplasia of the facial bones and mandible. Skeletal Radiol 8: 141-143

Giant-cell tuour (cf Chapter 21)

Bertoni F, Unni KK, Beabout JW, Ebersold MJ (1992) Giant cell tumor of the skull. Cancer 70: 1124-1132

Chomette G, Auriol M, Tranbaloc P, Vaillant JM (1980) Contribution à l'histogenèse des tumeurs à cellules géantes des os. Etude comparative, ultrastructurale et histo-enzymologique de tumeurs ostéoformatrices et de tumeurs à cellules géantes et malignes. Ann Anat Pathol (Paris) 25: 231-243

Flanagan AM, Nui B, Tinkler SMB, Horton A, Williams DM, Chambers TJ (1988) The multinucleate cells in giant cell granulomas of the jaw are osteoclasts. Cancer 62: 1139-1145

Harman SA, Pribram H (1990) Giant cell tumor of sphenoid bone. Skeletal Radiol 19: 212-215

Maroteaux (1982) Maladies osseuses de l'enfant chérubisme. Flammarion Médecine-Sciences, Paris, pp 123-124

Rogers LF, Mikhael M, Christ M, Wolff A (1984) Giant-cell (reparative) granuloma of the sphenoid bone. Skeletal Radiol 12: 48-53

Wolfe JT, Schetthauer BW, Dahlin DC (1983) Giant-cell tumor of the sphenoid bone. Review of 10 cases. J Neurosurg 59: 322-327

Melanotic progonoma

Atkinson GJ, Davis PC, Patrick LE, Winn KJ, Ball TI, Wyly JB (1989) Melanotic neuroectodermal tumor of infancy. MR findings and a review of the literature. Pediatr Radiol 20: 20-22

Bignold LP, Nicks R (1980) Melanotic neuroectodermal tumour of infancy arising in anterior fontanelle. Pathology 12: 473-477

Carlier G, Donazzan M, Vandenbussche F, Gosselin B (1974) The neurocristopathies. A unifying concept of disease arising in neural creast maldevelopment. Hum Pathol 5: 409-429

Causeret M, Saint-André JP, Cerez-Pham H, Rousselet MC, Guy G, Simard CP (1987) Progonome mélanotique intra-crânien. Rapport d'un cas avec une étude immunohistochimique et ultrastructurale. Arch Anat Cytol Pathol 35: 45-48

Cutler LS, Chaudhry AP, Topazian R (1981) Melanotic neuroectodermal tumor of infancy: an ultrastructural study, literature review, and reevaluation. Cancer 48: 257-270

Dechaume M, Cauhepe J, Payen J, Peri G (1966) A propos d'un cas de mélanotic progonome. Rev Stomatol 67: 321-327

Johnson RE, Scheithauer BW, Dahlin DC (1983) Melanotic neuroectodermal tumor of infancy. A review of seven cases. Cancer 52: 661-666

Jones HH, Parker BR, Ballerio CG, Silverman FN, Kempson RL (1990) Melanotic neuroectodermal tumor of infancy (melanotic progonoma) involving the calvaria. Skeletal Radiol 19: 527-530

Kuhn R, Cabanne F, Garneau R (1954) Le rétinoblastome pigmentaire hétérotopique. Sem Hop Paris 30: 178-185

Lamping KA, Albert DM, Lack E, Dickersin GR, Chapman PH, Walton DS (1985) Melanotic neuroectodermal tumor of infancy (retinal anlage tumor). Ophthalmology 92: 143-149

Le Douarin N, Teillet MA (1973) Recherches sur le déterminisme de la migration des cellules issues de la crête neurale. CR Acad Sci Paris 277: 1929-1932

Melano-ameloblastoma, retinal anlage tumor, melanotic neuroectodermal tumor of infancy. A propos d'un cas. Revue de la littérature. Thèse de doctorat en médecine n° 9 février 1984, Patrick Chenet, Université de Clermont-Ferrand-I

Mugnier A, Bordais P, Croisier N (1974) Tumeur pigmentée du maxillaire supérieur chez l'enfant. Rev Stomatol Paris 75: 771-782

Navas Palacios JJ (1980) Malignant melanotic neuroectodermal tumor: light and electron microscopic study (Eng). Cancer 146: 529-536

Odontogenic tumours and pseudotumours

Ackerman GL, Altini M, Shear M (1988) The unicystic ameloblastoma: a clinicopathological study of 57 cases. J Oral Pathol 17: 541-546

Ashman SG, Goria RL, Eisele DW, Murphy MT (1993) Desmoplastic ameloblastoma. A case report and literature review. Oral Surg Oral Med Oral Pathol 75: 479-482

Aufdermaur M (1981) Pindborg tumor. J Cancer Res Clin Oncol 101: 227-230

Brochériou C, Roquancourt (de) A (1987) Anatomie pathologique dentaire et stomatologique. Editions CdP, Paris, p 58

Browne RM, Cough NG (1972) Malignant change in the epithelium lining odontogenic cysts. Cancer 29: 1199-1207

Cernéa P, Kuffer R, Baumont M, Brochériou C Guilbert F (1969) Naevomatose baso-cellulaire. Association de nævi baso-cellulaire de la peau, de kystes épidermoïdes des maxillaires, de malformations osseuses et d'autres anomalies; 7 observations. Rev Stomatol Chir Maxillofac 70: 181-226

Chomette G, Auriol M (1986) Histopathologie buccale et cervico-faciale. Masson, Paris, pp 58-62

Crawley WA, Levin LS (1978) Treatment of the ameloblastoma. A controversy. Cancer 42: 357-363

Dorner L, Sear AJ, Smith GT (1988) A case of ameloblastic carcinoma with pulmonary metastases. Br J Oral Maxillofac Surg 26: 503-510

Eversole LR, Leider AS, Hansen LS (1984) Ameloblastomas with pronounced desmoplasia. J Oral Maxillofac Surg 42: 735-740

Gardner DG (1977) Peripheral ameloblastoma. A study of 21 cases, including 5 reported as basal cell carcinoma of the gingiva. Cancer 39: 1625-1633

Goldstein G, Parker FP, Slaughter Fitz Hugh G (1976) Ameloblastic sarcoma. pathogenesis and treatment with chemotherapy. Cancer 37: 1673-1678

Gordeeff M (1987) Etude des kystes odontogènes des maxillaires. Thèse diplome d'état de docteur en chirurgie dentaire. Université de Nantes

Gordeeff M, Clergeau-Guerithault S, Gordeeff A (1989) L'histopathologie des kystes odontogènes. J Biol Buccale 17: 131-145

Hammer JE, Scofield H, Cornyn J (1968) Benign fibro-osseous jaw lesions of periodontal membrane origin. An analysis of 249 cases. Cancer 22: 861-878

Hodgkinson DG, Woods JE, Dahlin DC, Tolman DE (1978) Keratocysts of the jaw. Clinicopathology study of 79 patients. Cancer 41: 803-813

Maroteaux P (1982) Maladies osseuses de l'enfant. Flammarion Médecine-Sciences, Paris, pp 433-434

Navarette VR, Smith M (1971) Ultrastructure of granular cell ameloblastoma. Cancer 27: 948-955

Odukoya O, Arole O (1992) Clear-cell ameloblastoma of the mandible (a case report). Int J Oral Maxillofac Surg 21: 358-359

Page DL, Weiss SW, Eggleston JC (1975) Ultrastructural study of amyloid material in the calcifying epithelial odontogenic tumor. Cancer 36: 1426-1435

Pindborg JJ (1958) A calcifying epithelial odontogenic tumor. Cancer 11: 838-843

Sehdev MK, Huvos AG, Strong EW, Gerold FP, Willis GW (1974) Ameloblastoma of maxilla and mandible. Cancer 33: 324-333

Seward GR, Beales SJ, Johnson NW, Lumsden S (1975) A metastasising ameloblastoma associated with renal calculi and hyperealeaemia. Cancer 36: 2277-2285

Siar C, Ng N, Jalil N (1991) Plexiform granular cell odontogenic tumors: unicystic variant. Oral Surg Oral Med Oral Pathol 72: 82-85

Tamimoto K, Takata T, Suei Y, Wada T, (1991) A case of desmoplastic variant of a mandibular ameloblastoma. J Oral Maxillofac Surg 49: 94-97

Vap DR, Dahlin DC, Turlington EG (1970) Pindborg tumor: the so-called calcifying epithelial odontogenic tumor. Cancer 25: 629-636

Waldrom CA, El-Mofty SK (1987) A histopathologic study of 116 ameloblastomas with special reference to the desmoplastic variant. Oral Surg Oral Med Oral Pathol 63: 441-451

Yamamoto G, Yoshitake K, Tada K, Yoshida K, Yokota H, Fukuda Y, Ishida T (1989) Granular cell ameloblastoma. A rare variant. Int J Oral Maxillofac Surg 18: 140-141

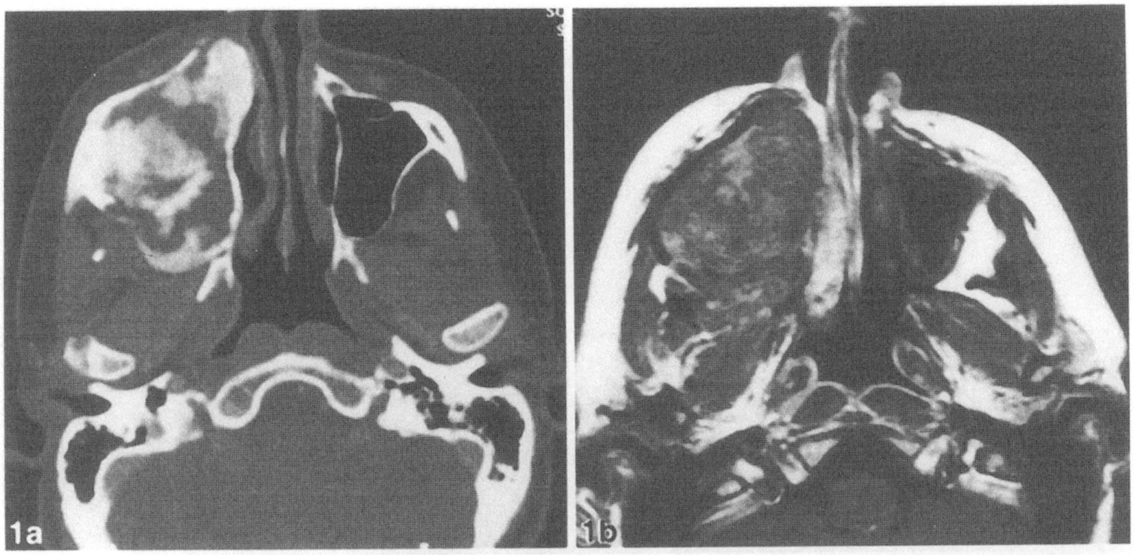

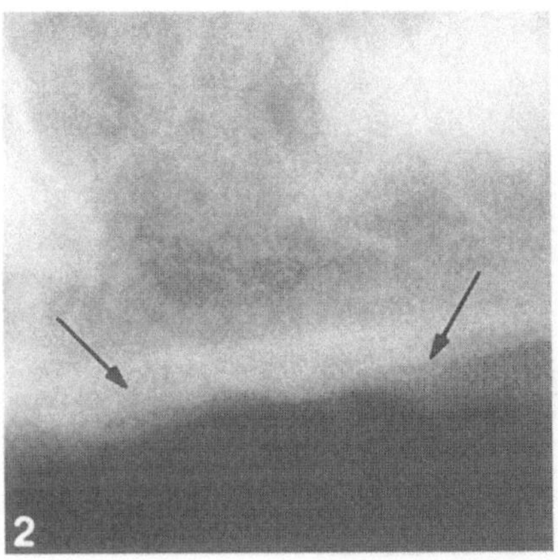

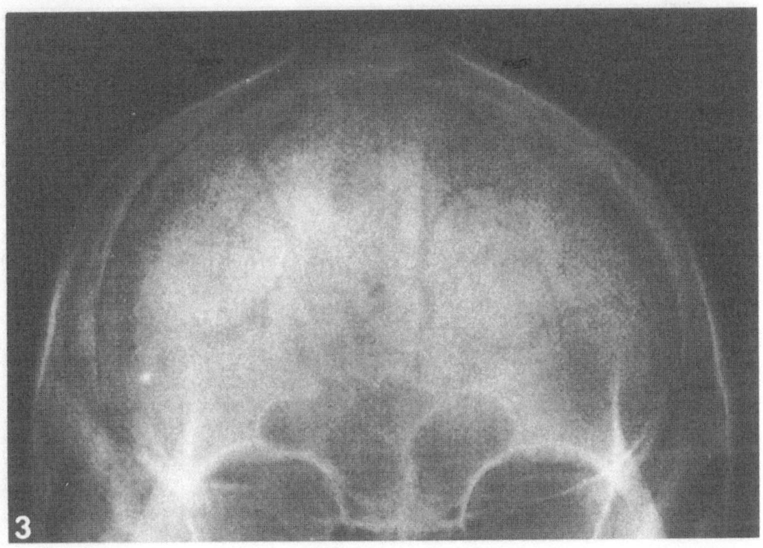

Fig. 1 a, b. Fibrous dysplasia of the maxilla had been developing in this woman of 43 for over 15 years. **a** In the CT images the right maxillary sinus is enlarged; it contained partly ossified fibrous tissue. Its wall is partly destroyed. **b** In MRI (axial section), T1 weighted (TR500, TE12) after contrast injection the mass of the sinus is heterogeneous. The wall (black line) is partly interrupted. The calcifications are less well analysed than in CT (Case of Dr Vanel)

Fig. 2. Periosteal fibroma developing in contact with inferior border of mandible in a child of 4. Local resection removing the bony attachment was followed by cure at 20-year follow-up

Fig. 3. Cranial hypervascularity, evidence of commencing Paget's disease

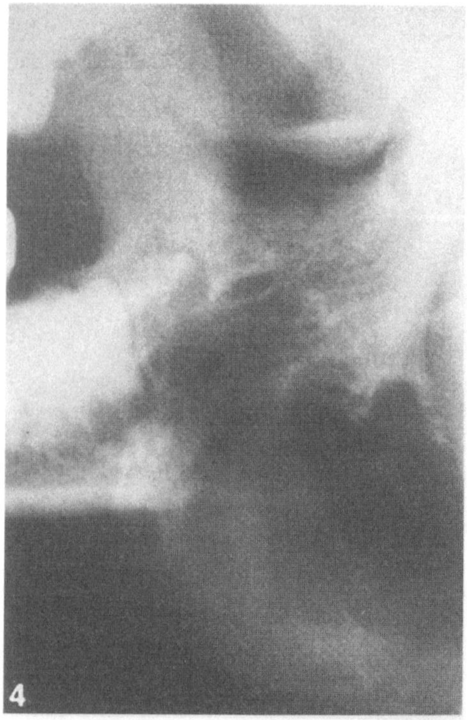

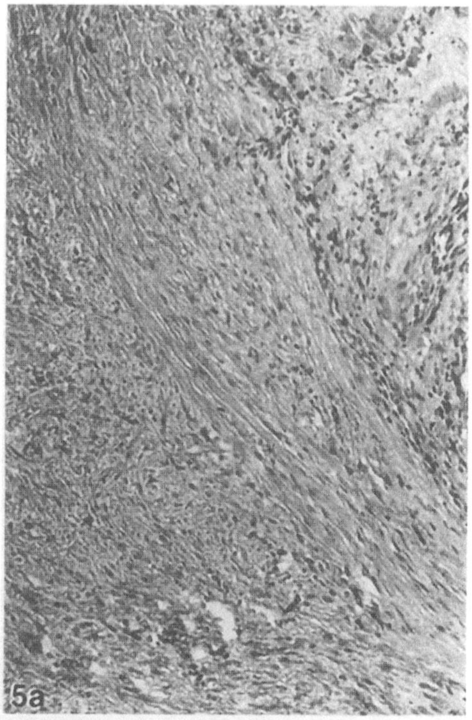

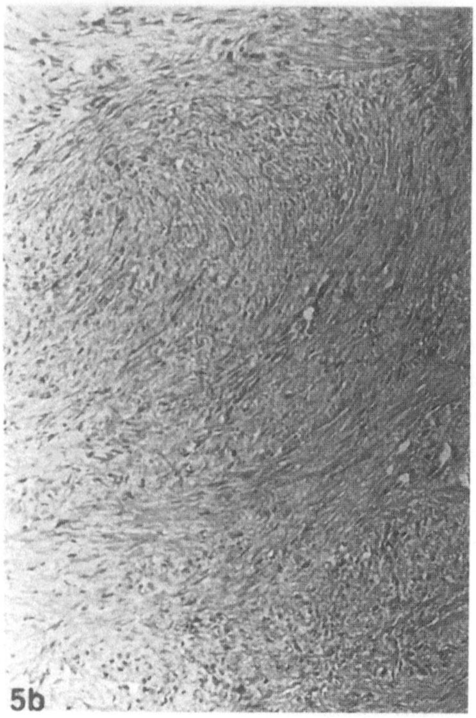

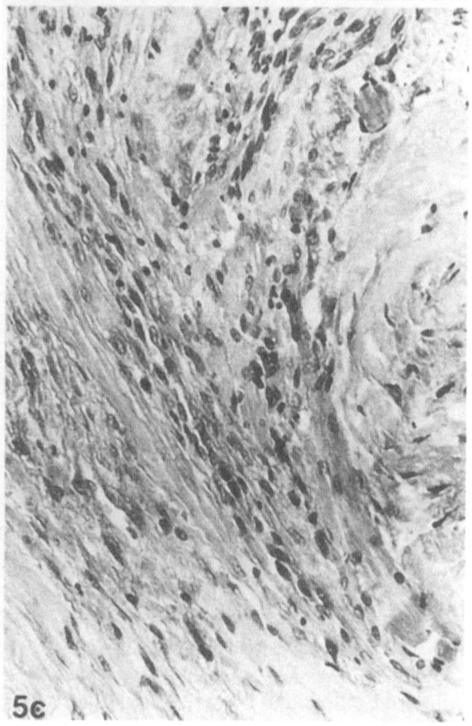

Fig. 4. Non-ossifying fibroma of angle of mandible, boy of 11. The angle is partly absorbed while the tumour is spreading towards the soft tissues, which it displaces: a very characteristic image

Fig. 5. a, b The microphotographs of the histological sections of this fibroma (fig. 4) demonstrate proliferation of fusiform cells and their grouping in bundles. **c** At higher magnification, note absence of nuclear anomalies and formation of moderately abundant collagen without osteogenesis

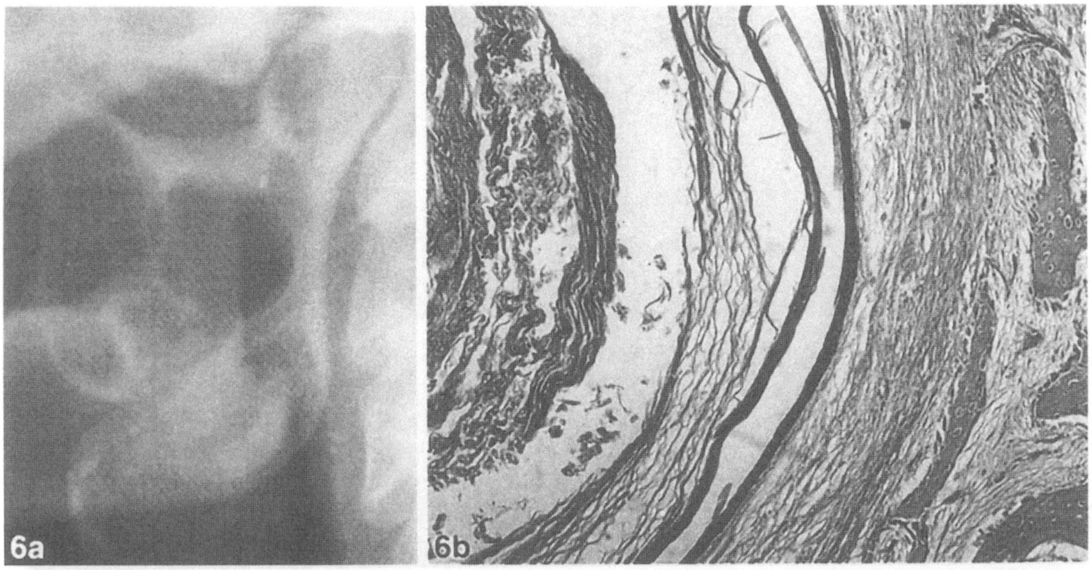

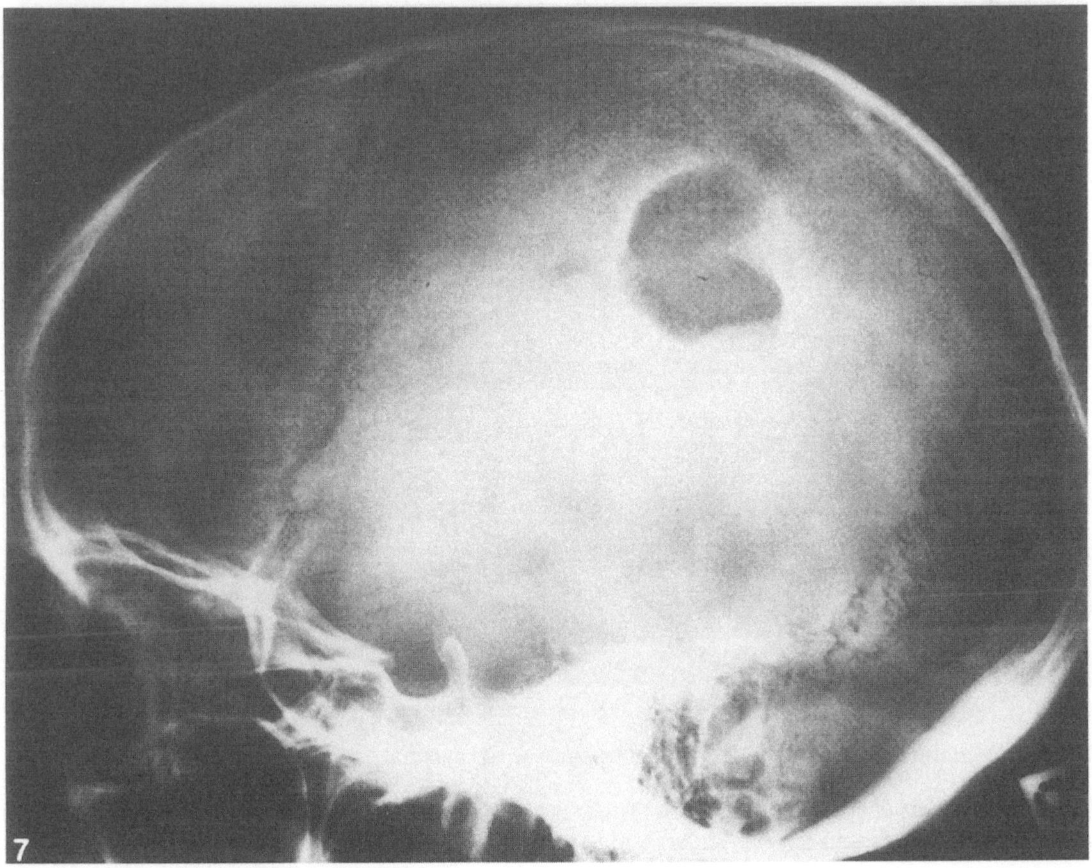

Fig. 6 a, b. Multilocular epidermoid cyst of ramus of mandible. **a** Some cavities are bordered by a sclerotic margin. **b** At low magnification this cavity appears filled with layers of desquamated epithelial cells. Peripherally, the cyst is bordered by newly-formed bony trabeculae in a fibrous marrow

Fig. 7. Epidermoid cyst of cranial vault, with sharp borders and surrounded by marked bony sclerosis (courtesy of Dr Derome, Hôpital Foch)

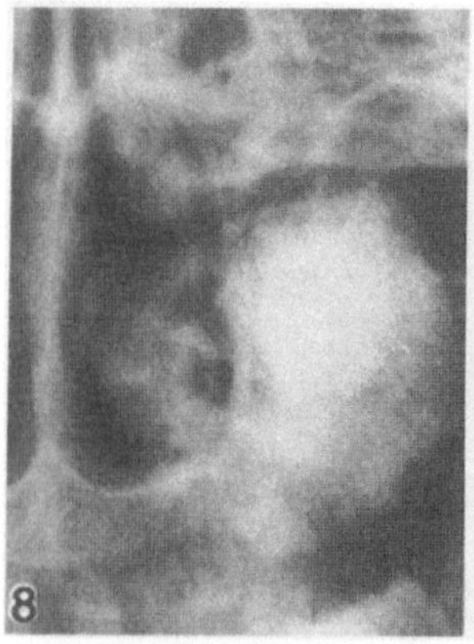

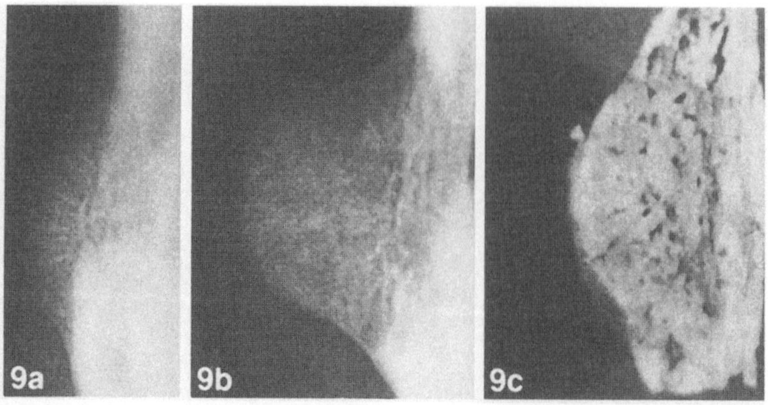

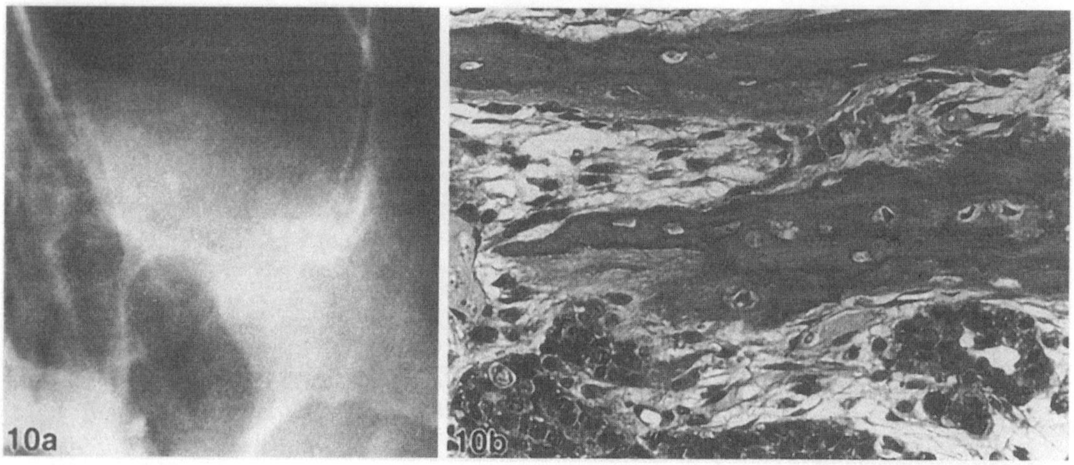

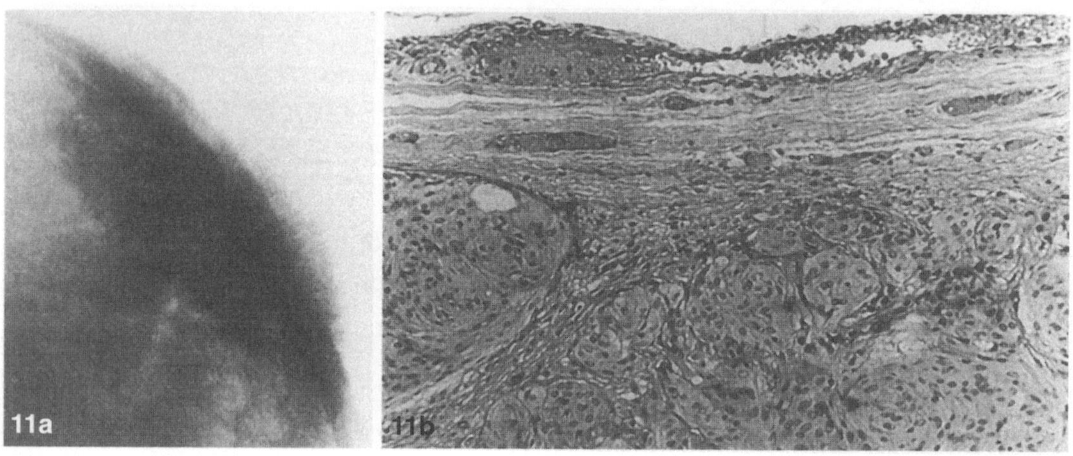

Fig. 8. No definite aetiology was found for this osteoma of the maxilla

Fig. 9 a-c. Osteoma of zygomatic bone. **a** In 1958, the osteoma was notable for the "cart-wheel" or "sunburst" arrangement of its newly-formed bony trabeculae. **b** 10 years later. **c** The resection specimen in frontal section demonstrates this patterned appearance. The sections show the close connection between vascular outgrowth and the formation of bone trabeculae. This fan-shaped vascular pattern, identical to what is seen in a fleshy granulation, suggests that this is an angio-osteoma

Fig. 10. a This bulky densification of the maxilla is not a true osteoma but a hypertrophy with bony sclerosis "induced" by (**b**) an epitheliomatous metastasis

Fig. 11. a Major occipital bony reaction, manifestation of a meningioma (**b**)

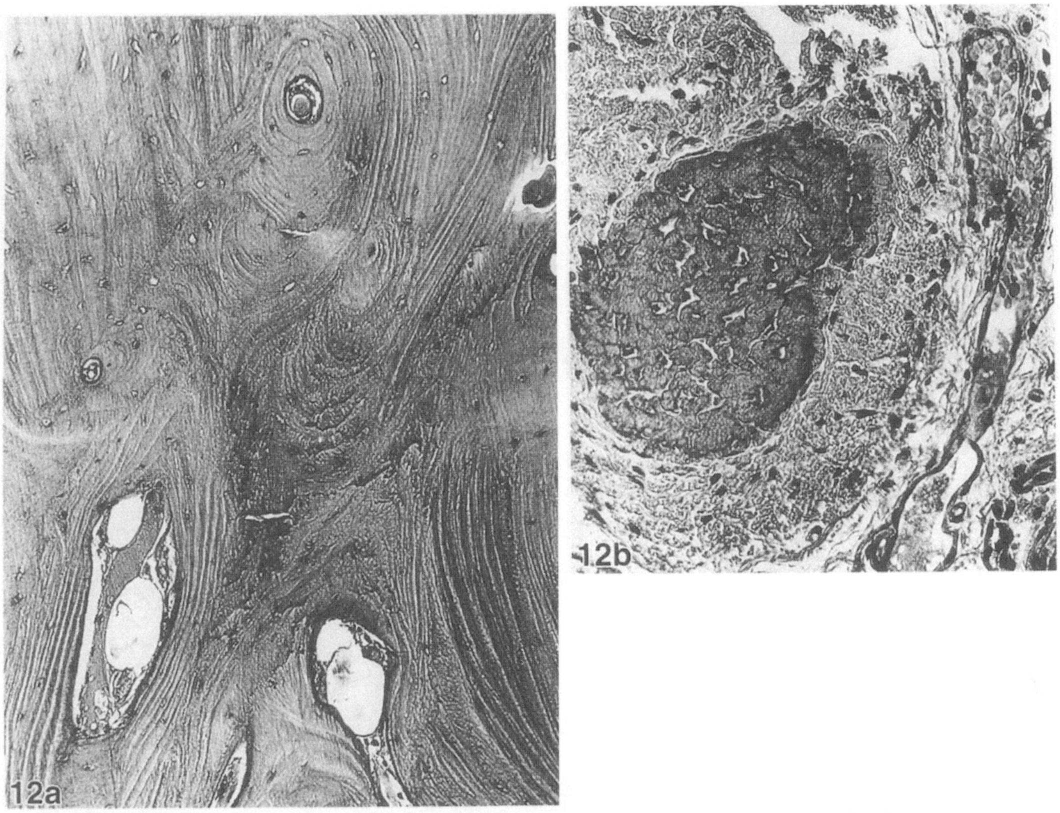

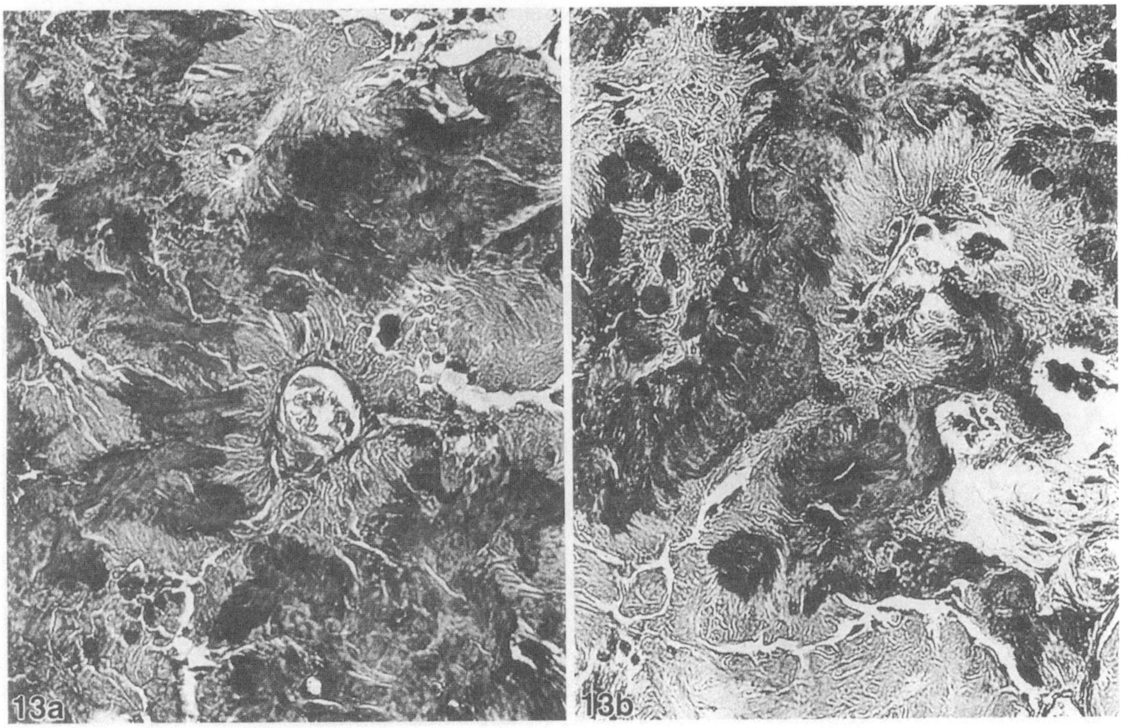

Fig. 12. a Histological appearance of osteoma of maxilla of unknown aetiology in a woman of 67. The osteoma is formed by juxtaposition of irregular haversian systems with abnormally numerous lamellae, arranged around some vascular channels of very reduced size. **b** In the vicinity of the lamellar osteosclerosis, in the connective tissue, there are zones of bony metaplasia

Fig. 13 a, b. Very dense "radiological" osteoma of the ethmoidal region of unknown aetiology. Histologically, there is production of markedly and irregularly calcified collagen. It seems unlikely that the course of such a lesion inevitably leads to the building of lamellar bone

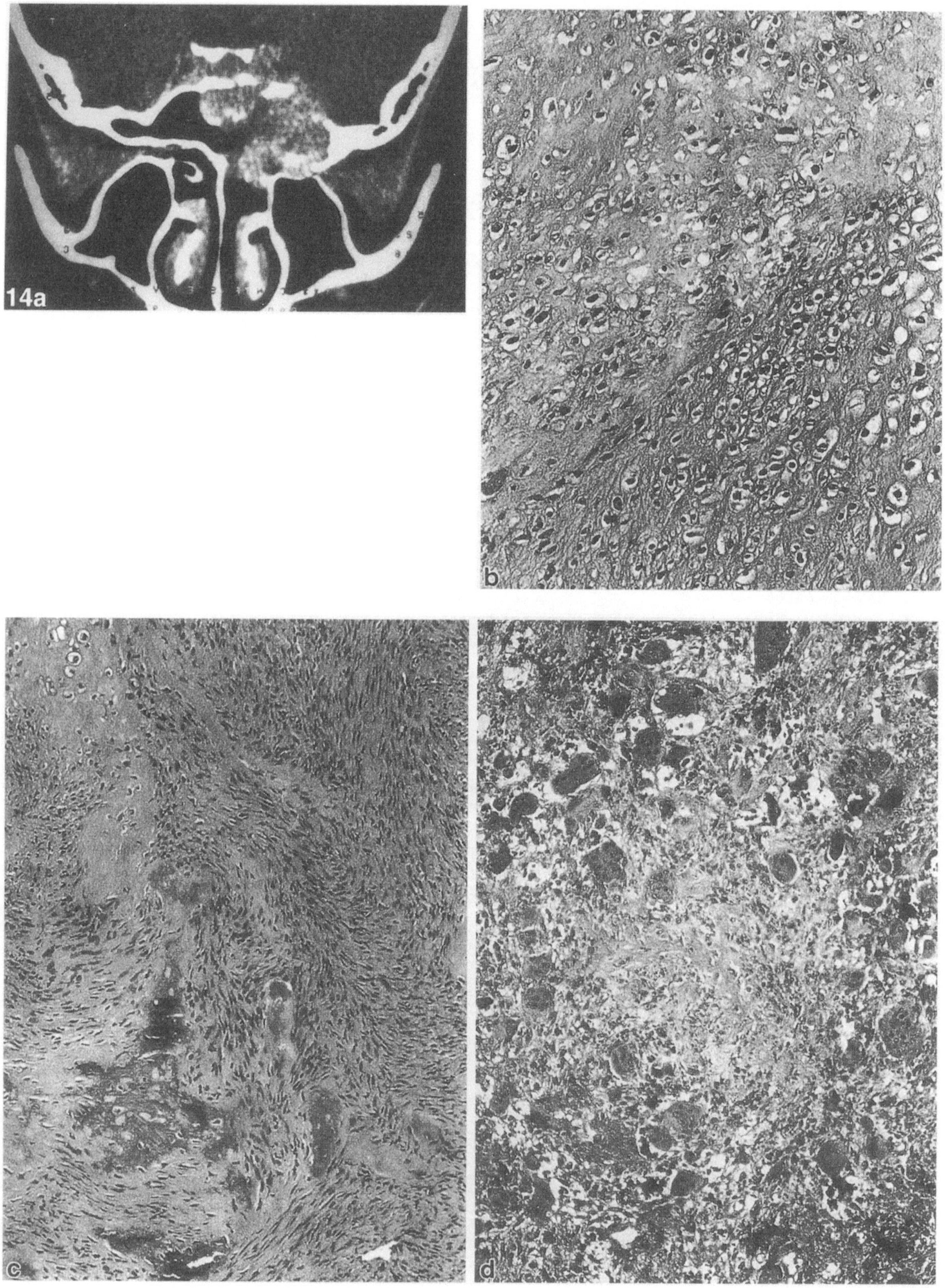

Fig. 14 a-d. This osteosarcoma of the sphenoid developed in a woman of 52. The tumour consists predominantly of fusiform cells; with chondroid zones and areas with abundant giant cells. The diagnosis of osteogenic sarcoma is based on the fact that in some sections osteoid or osseous development is seen, either from the collagenous substance or the cartilaginous tissue (Courtesy of Dr Vignaud, Nancy)

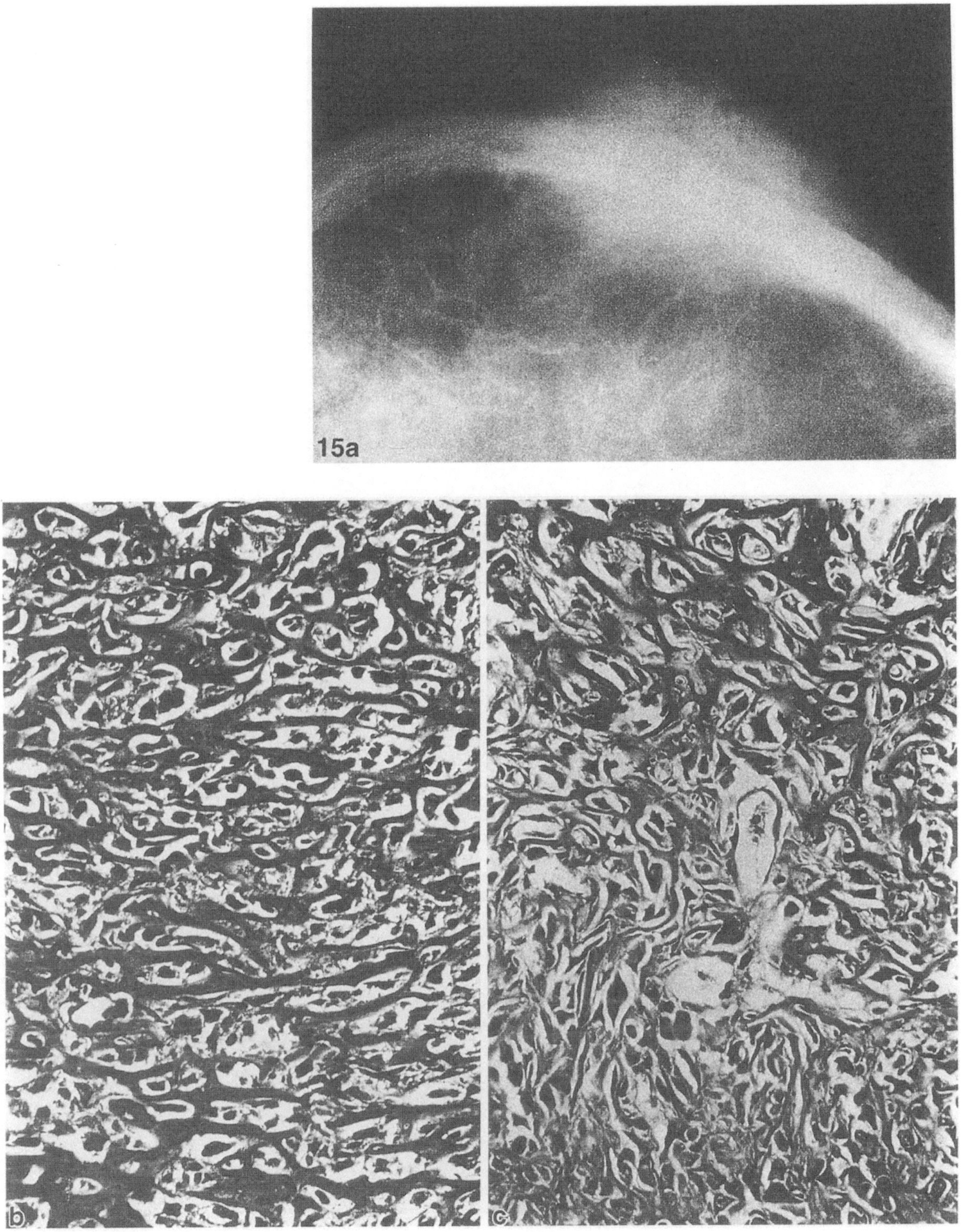

Fig. 15. a A palpable hard swelling in the parietal region associated with rather moderate pain was the presenting feature of this osteosarcoma in a young girl of 15. The very dense tumour osteogenesis traverses the outer and inner tables. Biopsy confirmed the diagnosis of osteogenic sarcoma. A second cranial lesion appeared very soon. Radio-cobalt and chemotherapy produced a "cure" which has lasted for over 14 years. **b, c** The tumour osteogenesis consists of fine bony or osteoid trabeculae between which are osteoblasts of very varied shape and size

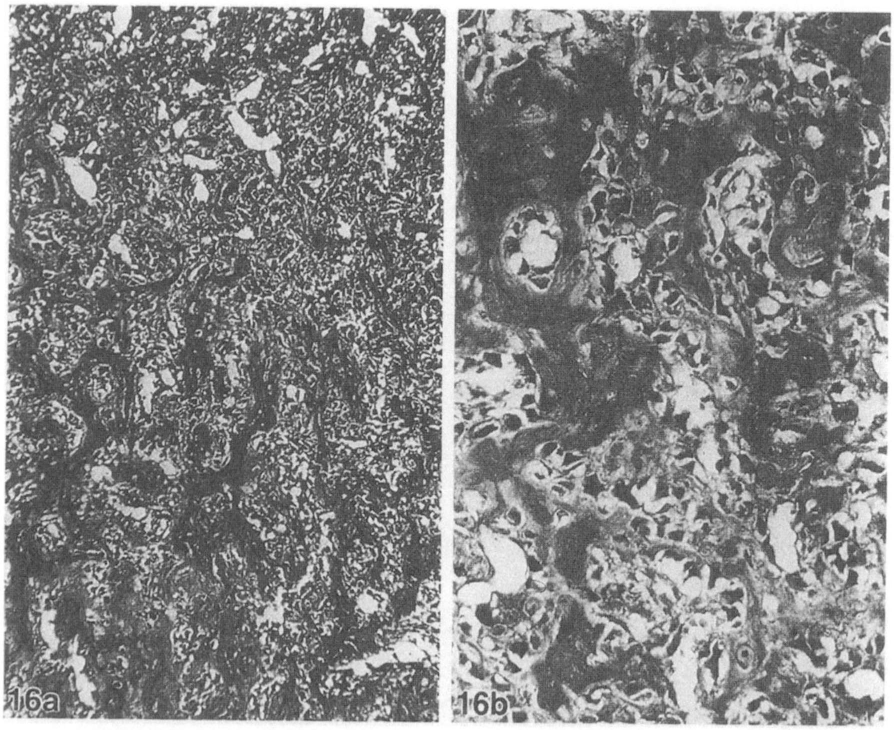

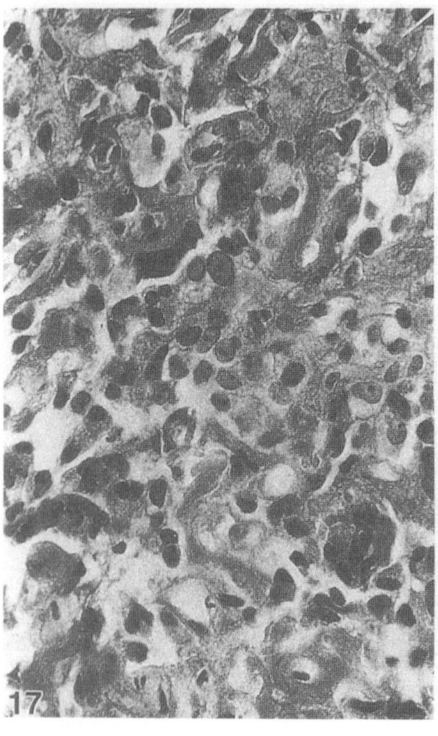

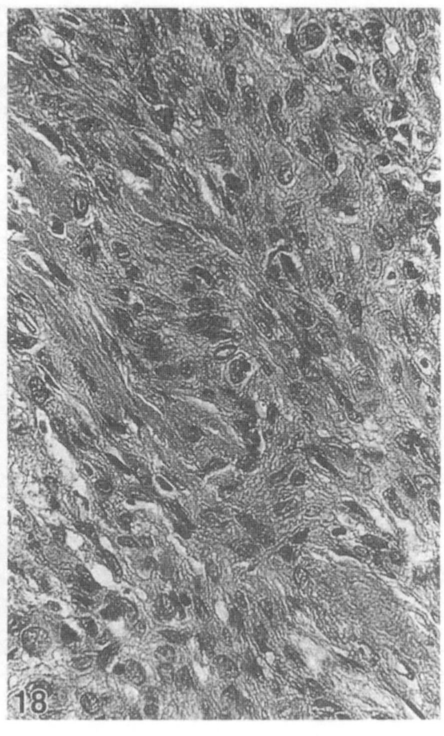

Fig. 16 a, b. Cranial osteosarcoma of typical histological appearance: partly calcified osteoid trabeculae (**a**) in a dense cell proliferation. **b** At higher magnification: newly-formed trabeculae of tumour bone surrounded by osteoblastic cells

Fig. 17. Osteosarcoma of parietal region in a man of 30. The differential diagnosis with an osteoblastoma was difficult to make from a small sample

Fig. 18. This fusiform-cell appearance of a low grade of malignancy in another osteosarcoma is more likely to be found in the facial bones, particularly the mandible

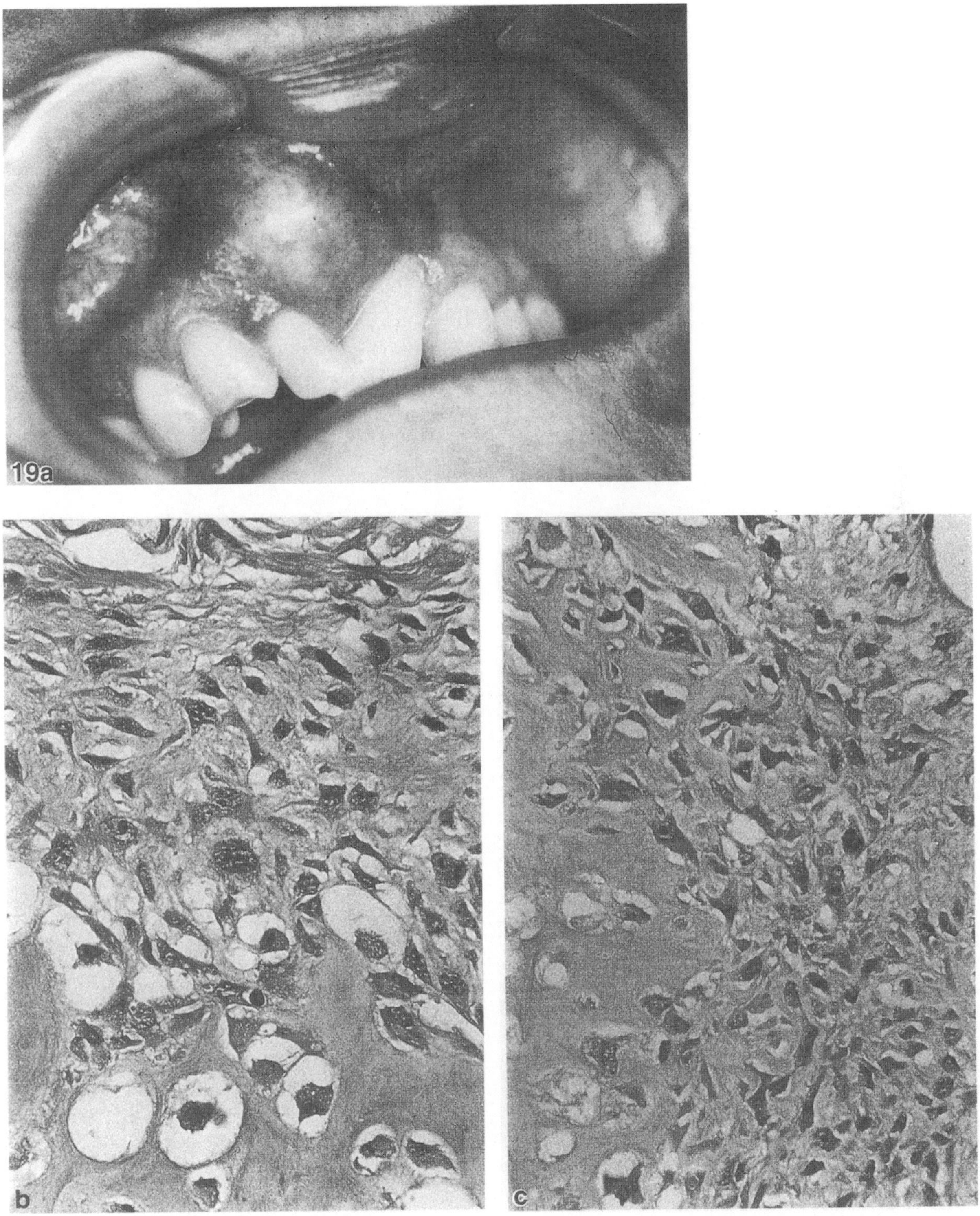

Fig. 19. a Swelling of anterior part of maxilla. **b, c** Biopsy shows its chondrosarcomatous nature

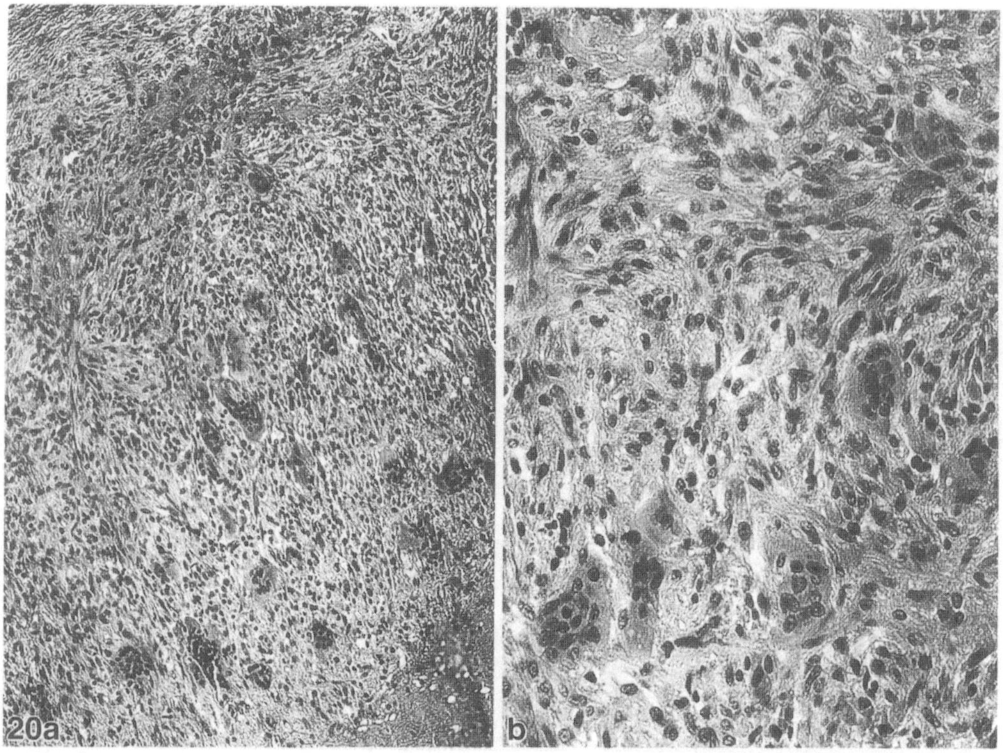

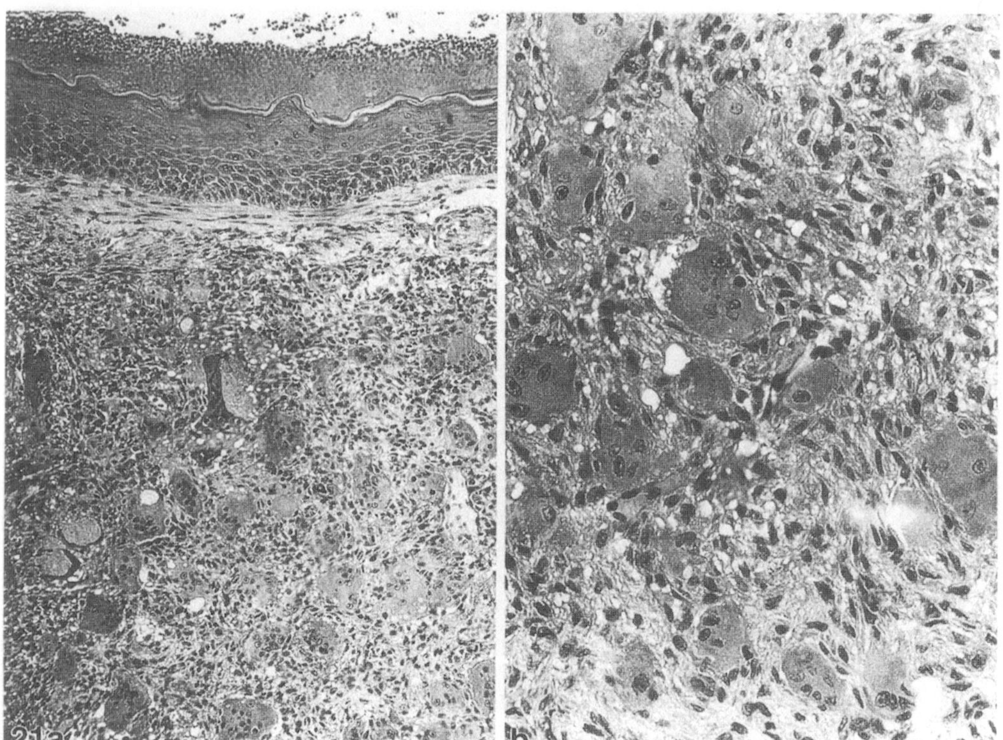

Fig. 20 a, b. Reparative granuloma with giant cells. It consists of fusiform cells, rare inflammatory cells and giant cells. In this case there were also minute trabecular osteoid formations

Fig. 21 a, b. Gingival epulis. Beneath a thickened gingival epithelium this lesion is predominantly fibroblastic with scattered giant cells and is usually very vascular and sometimes very inflammatory. The bone in contact with it is often remodelled (osteolysis); hence the interpretations of gingival lesion or exteriorised reparative granuloma

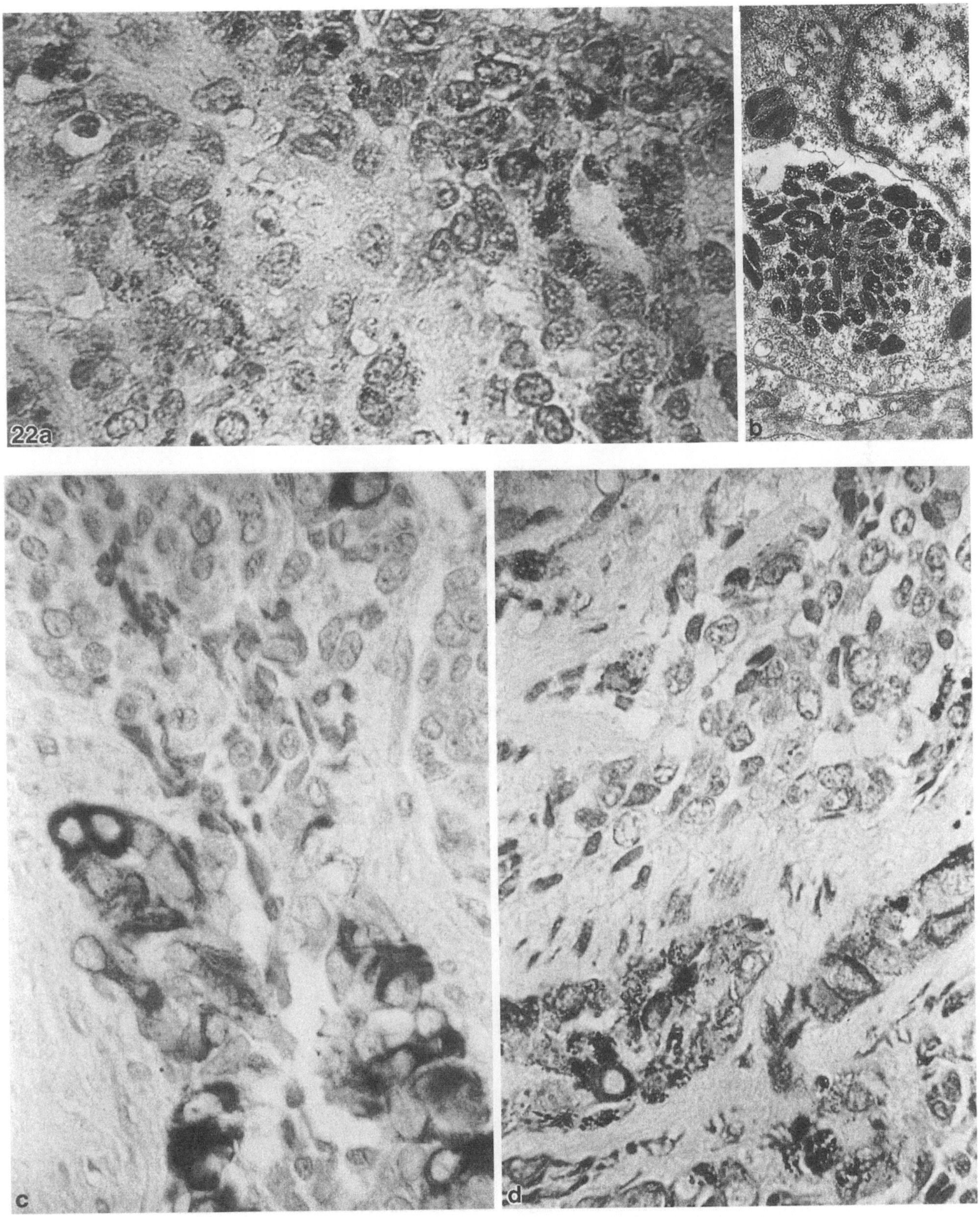

Fig. 22. **a** Presence of melanin pigment in the large cells of this neuroectodermal tumour of an infant. **b** Cell with melanosomes. **c** In the large cells the reaction with anti-keratin antibody is positive, as is (**d**) the reaction to the anti-vimentin antibody (Microphotographs by courtesy of Dr Epardeau, Hôpital Foch)

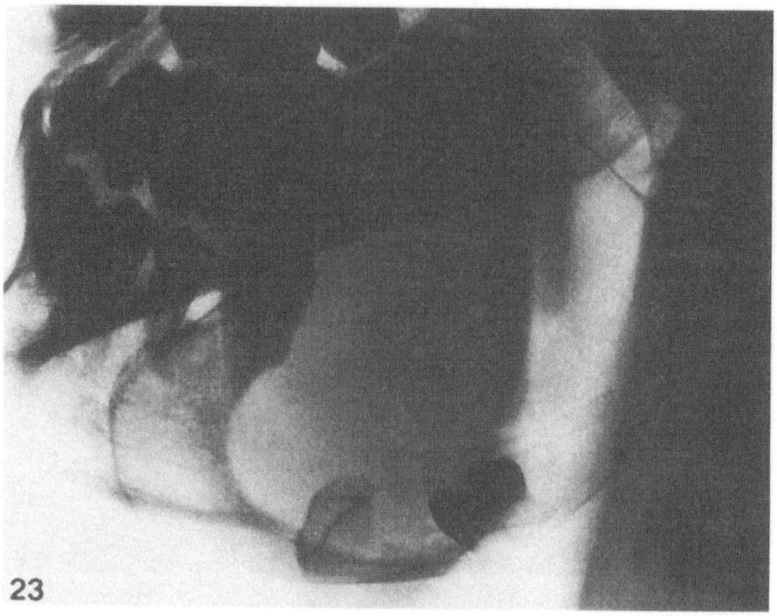

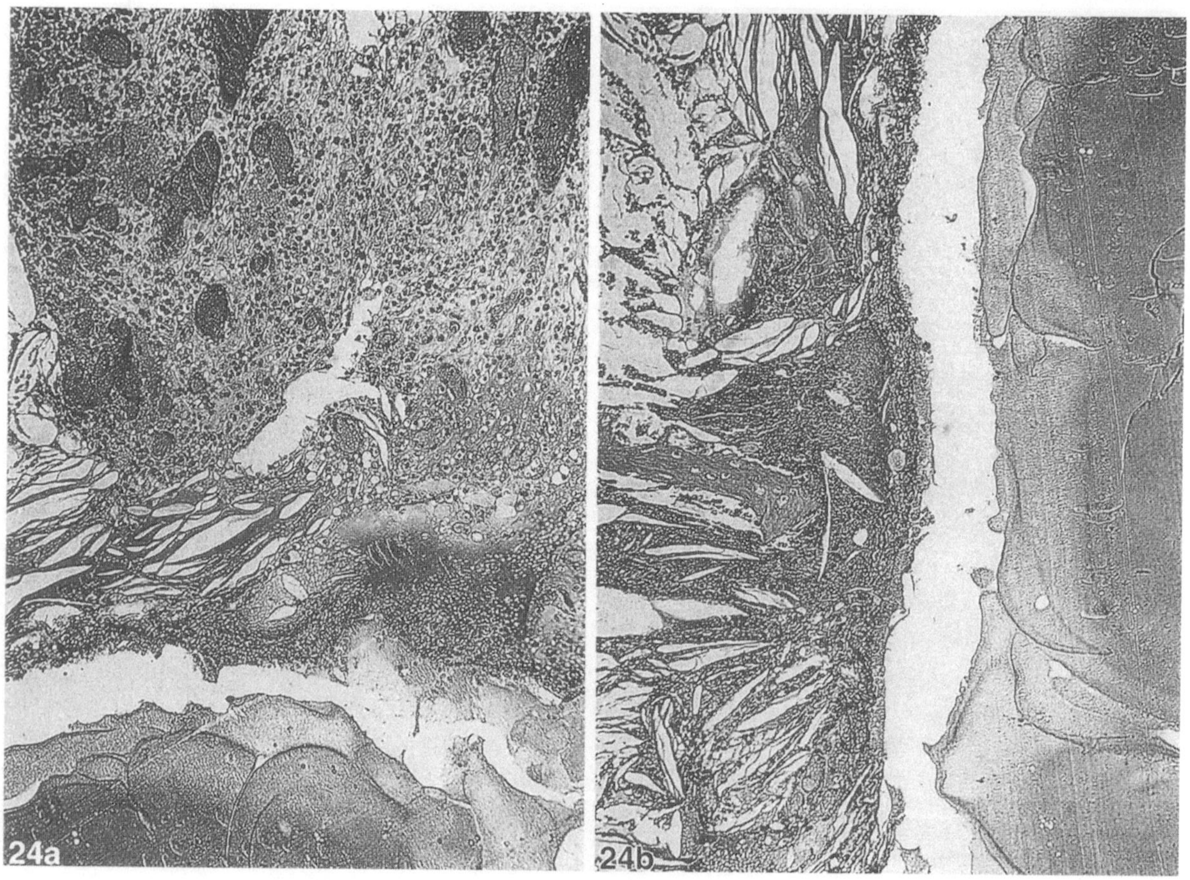

Fig. 23. Corono-dental cyst originating from germ of wisdom tooth: boy of 15

Fig. 24 a, b. Mandibular cyst remodelled by major inflammatory changes. No epithelial layer is seen in this section

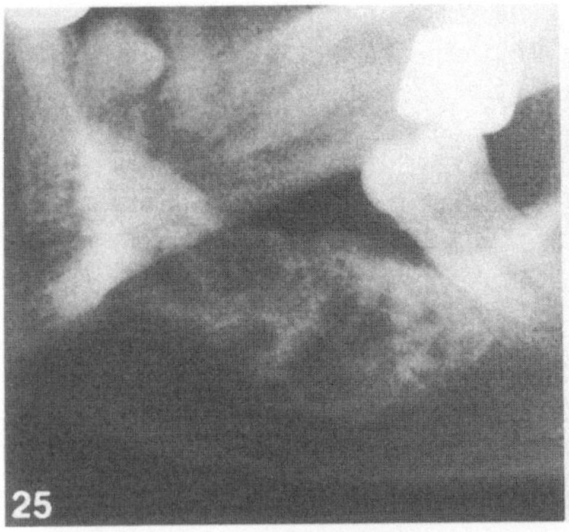

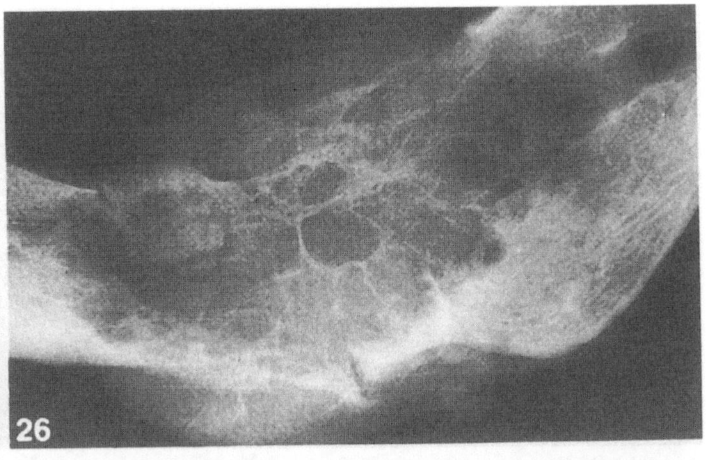

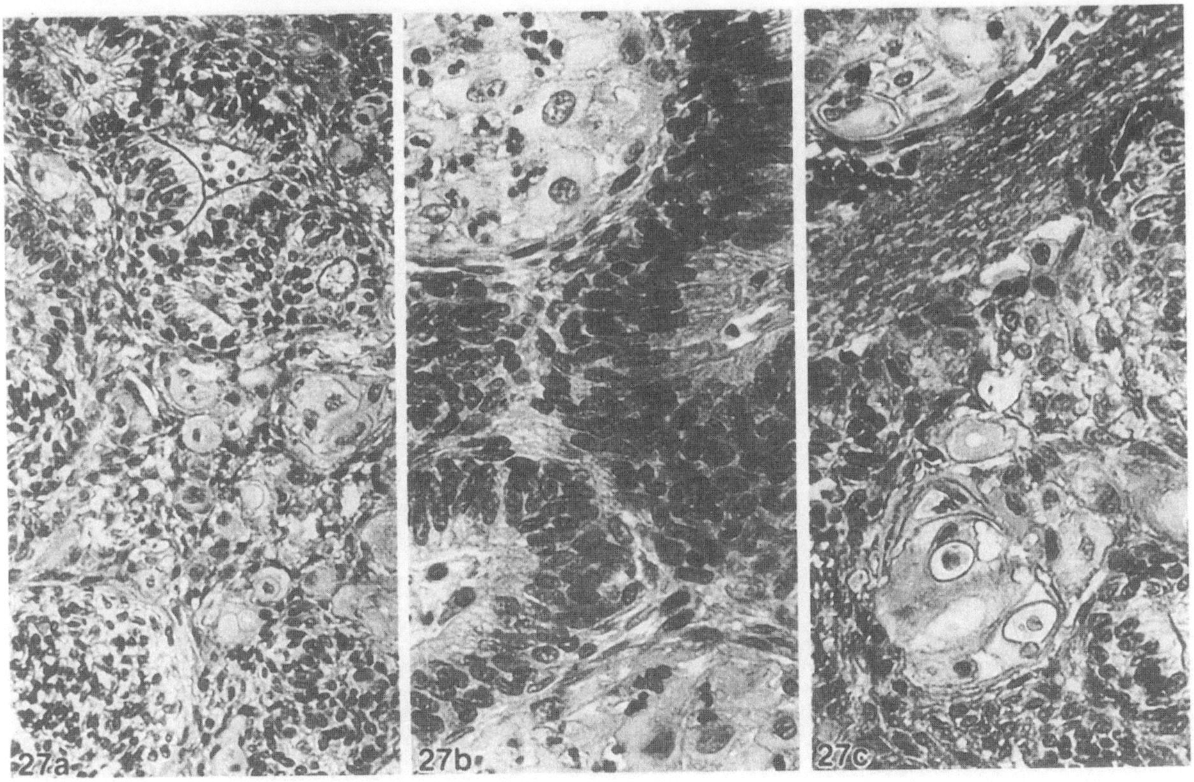

Fig. 25. Ameloblastoma of mandible: microcavitary appearance with bony sclerosis around the cavities

Fig. 26. Radiograph of resection specimen of recurrence of ameloblastoma. Large zone of multicavitary osteolysis reaching posterior part of body of mandible and lower half of ramus. The hemi-mandible has fractured obliquely below and to the right (radiograph by courtesy of Prof. Payen)

Fig. 27 a-c. Ameloblastoma of mandible. **a** Cellular and architectural polymorphism. **b** Palisaded arrangement of ameloblasts: nuclei surmounted by clear cytoplasm. **c** Rudiment of malpighian maturation at center of a tumour trabeculum

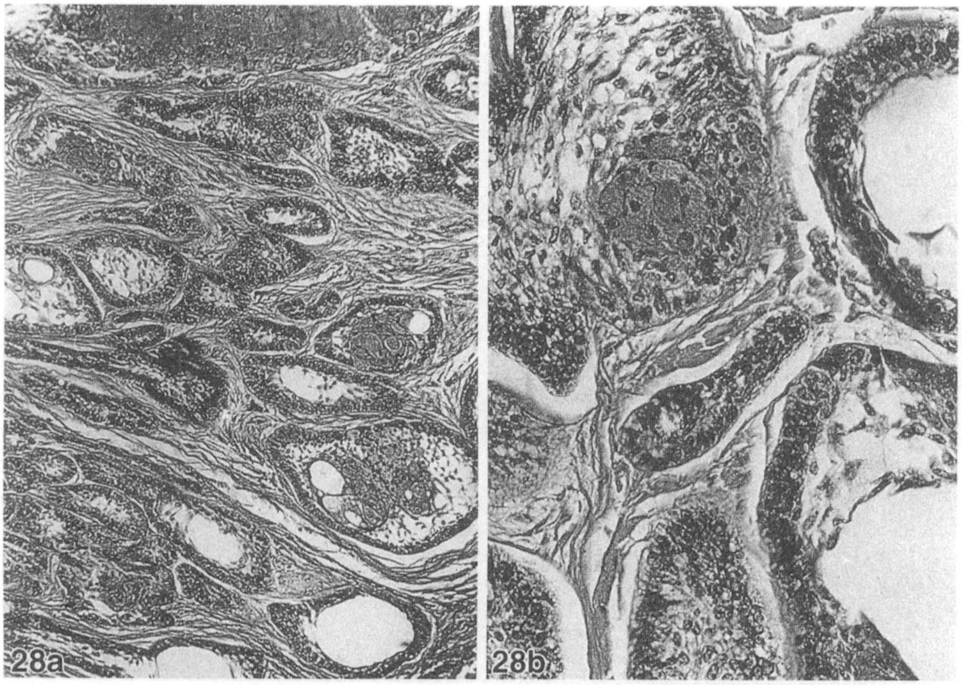

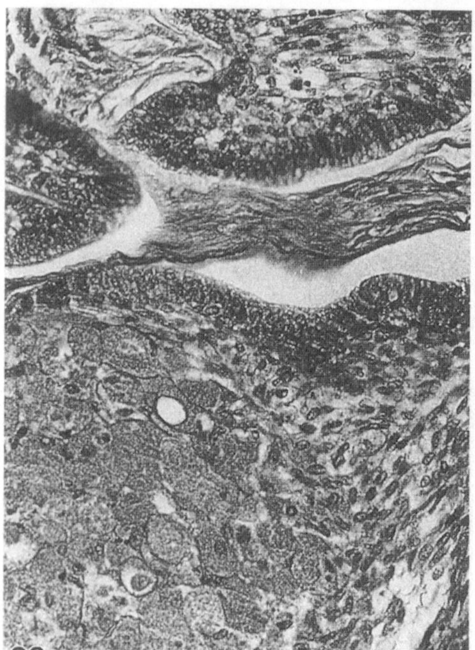

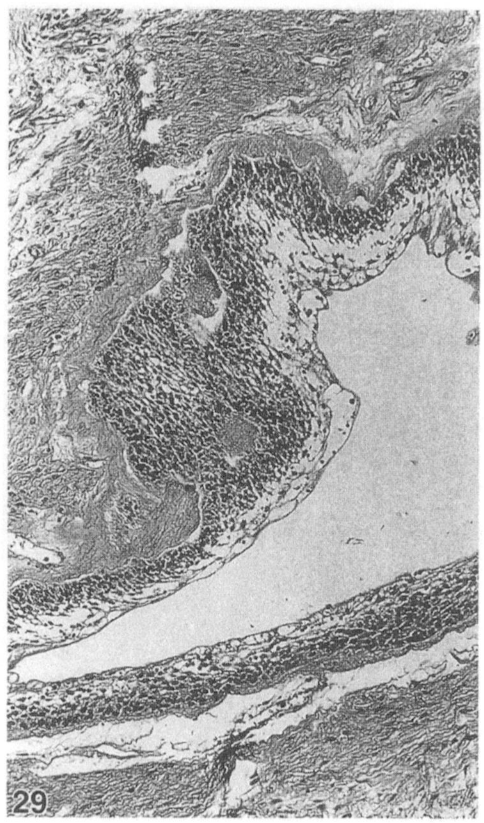

Fig. 28 a-c. Ameloblastoma with granular cells. **a** At low magnification the unequally sized strands are bounded by a layer of dark cells. The central part of the strands has either become cystic or occupied by clearer cells. **b, c** In the midst of these cellular areas are grayish islands of large cells with granular cytoplasm. Between the tumour strands the stroma is reduced to a few dense collagen fibers

Fig. 29. Cystic remodelling in an ameloblastoma

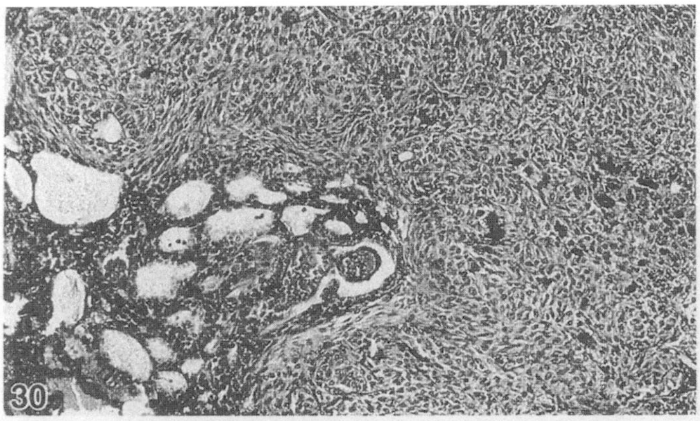

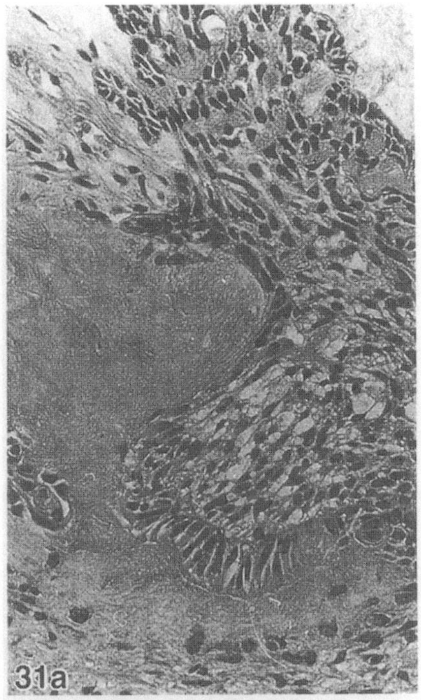

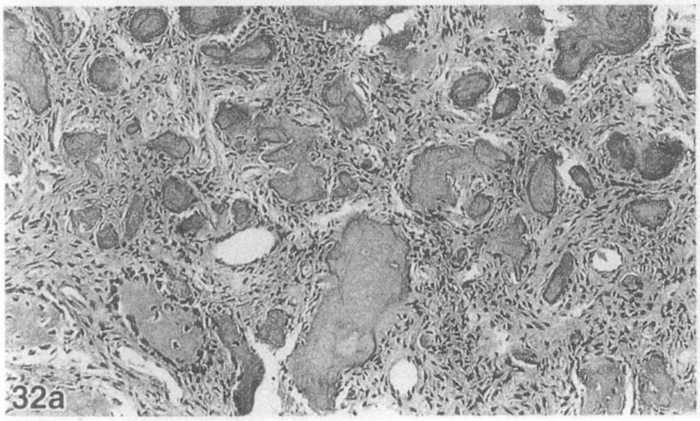

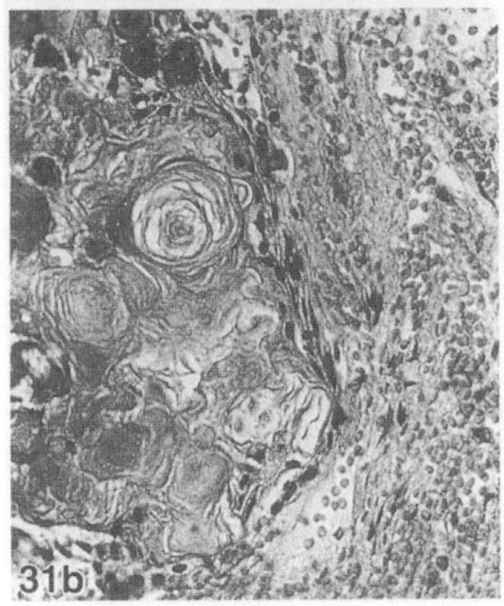

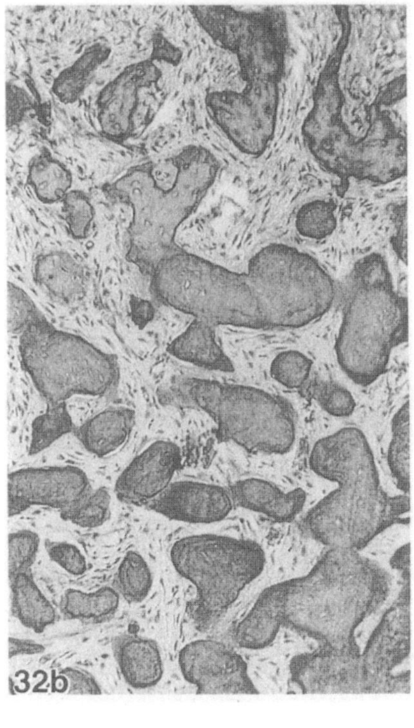

Fig. 30. Ameloblastic fibroma. Richly cellular aspect of mesenchymal portion in direct contact with an epithelial proliferation, which here forms a sort of network, the probable outcome of the phenomenon of cyst-formation

Fig. 31 a, b. Dentinoma. **a** Plaque of connective tissue which resembles that of the dental papilla. At the margin of the dentine the cells assume an appearance resembling that of odontoblasts. Some cells are immured in this poorly calcified dentine. There is no enamel secretion. **b** Dysplastic dentine formed of small nodules of stratified appearance

Fig. 32 a, b. Two cases of fibrocementoma. The tumour is characterised by the differentiation of numerous cementoid islands in a lax fibrous tissue

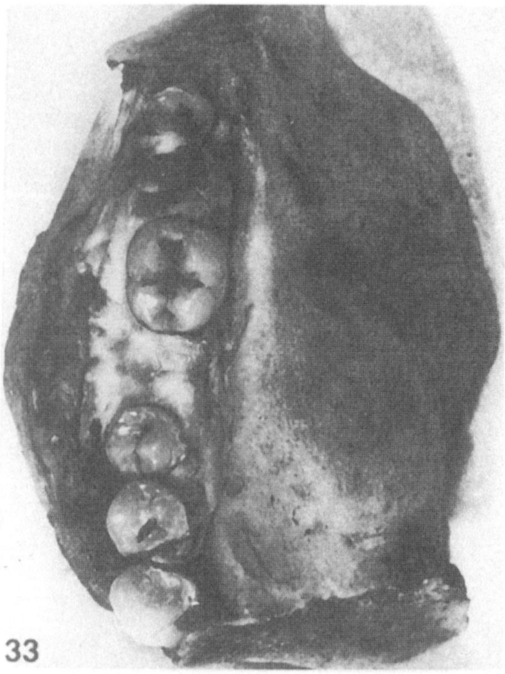

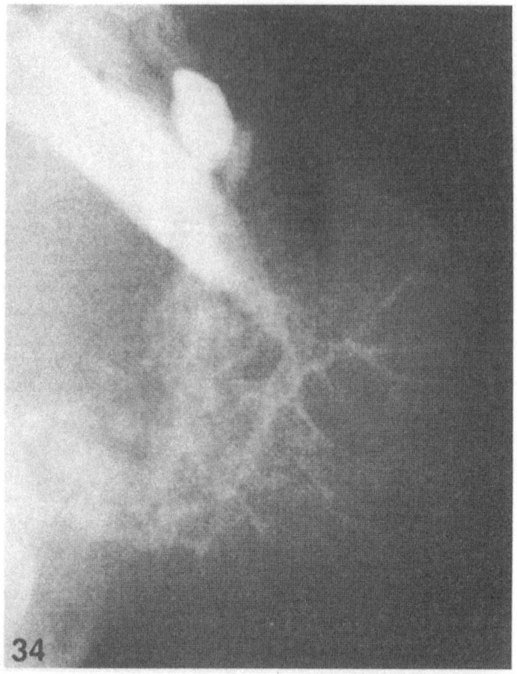

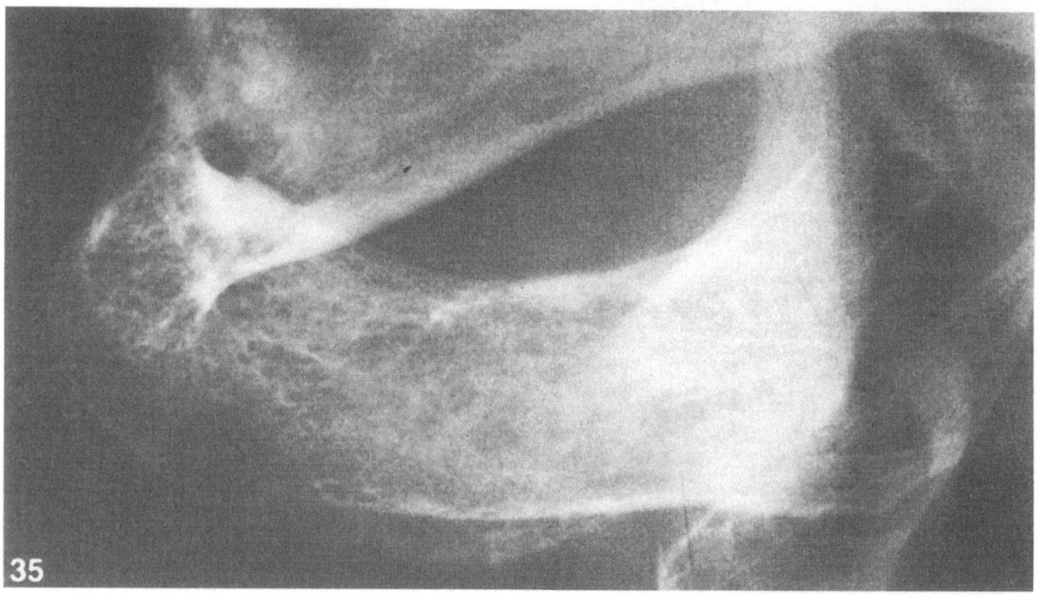

Fig. 33. Hypertrophy of body of mandible, the expression of a fibrous dysplasia

Fig. 34. Biopsy of this large mandibular tumour in an octogenarian demonstrated a malpighian epithelioma (possibly arising in an adamantinoma)

Fig. 35. The "moth-eaten" appearance of this mandible, with a clearly visible periosteal reaction at the lower border, is quite different from that of the sharply-bounded lacunae of plasmacytoma of the cranial vault; nevertheless, this is a plasmacytoma. Examination of the radiographs is an integral part of the pathological investigation, but the membrane bones have their own way of responding to neoplastic aggression

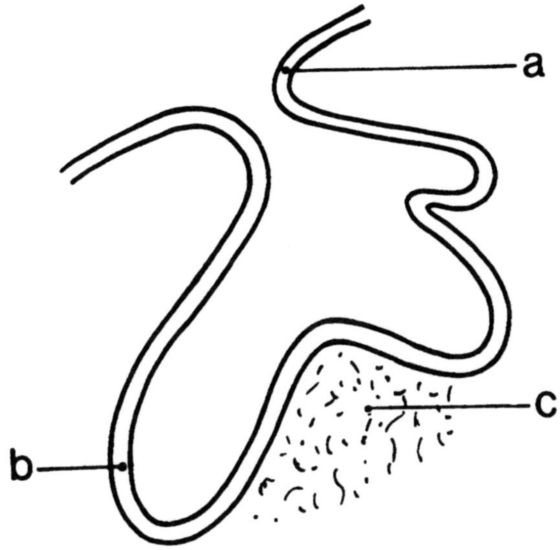

1

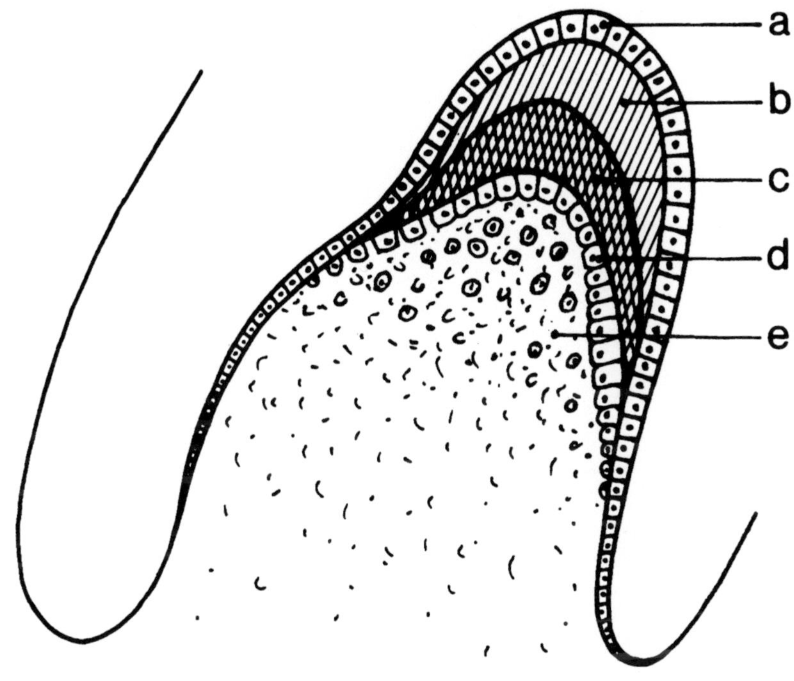

2

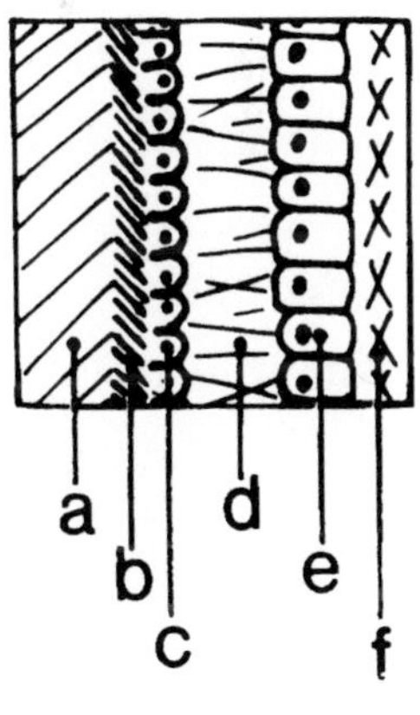

3

Diagrammatic review of the embryology of a tooth

Diagram 1. *a* Buccal epithelium, *b* invagination of buccal epithelium, *c* mesenchyme

Diagram 2. *a* Ameloblasts, *b* enamel, *c* dentine, *d* odontoblasts, *e* Mesenchyme (dental pulp)

Diagram 3. Relations of dental root and bony tissue. *a* Dentine, *b* cement, *c* cementoblasts, *d* Sharpey's fibers, *e* osteoblasts, *f* alveolar bony tissue

39. Extraskeletal skeletogenic tumours

Chondroma, osteochondroma

(figs. 1, 2)

The interpretation of small biopsies made from tumours developing in pre-existing cartilage (hamartochondroma) is difficult and has serious implications. Whatever the interpretation of the biopsy, the magnitude of the tumour at some sites (larynx, bronchi) may call for a major surgical intervention.

General considerations

Chondromas of the soft tissues are commoner in men. More than 90% of cases are sited peripherally, in the hands and feet, and therefore develop in periarticular regions, often related to tendino-aponeurotic and capsular tissues.

Clinical features and course

The tumour is slowly-growing and causes little or no pain. Often, the patient seeks advice several years after its discovery. Complete excision is followed by permanent cure of this benign tumour; too sparing an excision carries a risk of recurrence. Bansal et al (1993) report three cases (two in the feet and one of the hand) in patients aged 55, 57 and 78 years.

Imaging

Insofar as the chondroma is partly calcified, the radiographs may show the tumour at a distance from the underlying bone. In some cases there is a periosteal reaction of sclerosing type or, in contrast, an impression hollowed out in the bony cortex at the level of the tumour.

Pathological anatomy and histopathology

Macroscopically, the cartilaginous nodule is knobbly; its surface is smooth and shiny.

Histologically, the cartilage is normally hyaline; but some large nuclei and cellular polymorphism are not formal evidence of malignancy, as the microphotographs illustrating the reports of various authors prove. Some chondromas are associated with a chondroblastic proliferation with giant cells, suggesting an extraskeletal chondroblastoma. The presence of these zones of chondroblastic proliferation may also be seen in some intraskeletal cartilaginous tumours. Other chondromas exhibit large zones of bulky cells whose cytoplasm is filled with lipid vacuoles [Chan et al 1986]. Together with relatively large zones of calcification, there may be zones of necrotic adipose tissue [Bansal et al 1993], this is possibly commoner in chondromas of the feet, which are inevitably subject to trauma.

Differential diagnosis

Differential diagnosis is from benign lesions, including haemopigmented villonodular synovitis, when this contains large areas of chondrohyaline tissue, heterotopic calcification of unknown cause if the cartilage nodule is markedly calcified and an aponeurotic fibroma. Keasby's juvenile aponeurotic fibroma poses no real diagnostic difficulties; it is seen almost exclusively in children and adolescents and affects the palms of the hands and fingers, the soles of the feet, ankles, more rarely the toes.

In radiographs the fibrous mass (1-3 cm in diameter) is dotted with calcification.

In sections the fibrous nodule contains cartilaginous foci and calcifications surrounded by large fibroblasts. Excision leads to cure, often after a recurrence. It is much more serious to confuse this cartilaginous nodule with a chondrosarcoma. At least two appearances may encourage this diagnosis: proliferation of chondroblasts and myxoid zones. The specific arrangement of cells in small chains or alveolar formations which are usual in myxoid chondrosarcomas are not seen in chondromas. There may be cell anomalies in benign chondromas, but the well-circumscribed tumour and the hyaline appearance of the ground substance argue in favor of a benign lesion. But it is difficult, as stressed by Reiman and Dahlin (1986), to recognise the benign nature of these extraskeletal tumours of hyaline cartilage "if the histological criteria of intraosseous lesions are strictly applied". As with all histological diagnoses, a knowledge of the clinical aspects is of the greatest importance.

Para-articular chondroma and osteochondroma

Some authors have described para-articular chondromas and osteochondromas. The essential features applied to this identification are usually that it is a solitary lesion, either ovoid or lobular, with a long axis reaching 5-8 cm, that the structure is free in the joint or in a serous bursa adjacent to the joint, that there is no chondroid metaplasia in the joint synovium and that calcification and ossification are irregularly distributed [Milosevic et al 1972, Milgram et al 1980]. In one of our cases ossification was not central but peripheral.

If this lesion is considered to be an entity, it must be distinguished from synovial chondromatosis, with numerous often pedicled nodules, or synovial osteochondromatosis, with nodules whose centers are ossified and which usually coexist with purely cartilaginous nodules. A nodule of osteochondritis (cf Chapter 40) must also be excluded as a broken-off osteogenic exostosis which has become secondarily embedded in a serous bursa; the distinction is easier, at least as far as language is concerned, in French rather than in English, where the confusing term "osteochondroma" designates both an osteogenic exostosis and an osteocartilaginous nodule.

Osteochondroma of the soft tissues

Li et al (1989) described three cases of osteochondromas, partly ossified cartilaginous tumours of the soft tissues which they regarded as an entity. The authors stressed that these tumours had developed in sheaths and tendons, and at a distance from the joints. Nevertheless, though the first two developed in the subcalcaneal soft tissues, the third was connected with the capsule of the ankle joint.

In this context, one must identify these osteochondromas of the soft tissues, represented by a cartilaginous mass some centimeters in diameter, non tender, mobile, lobulated and well-circumscribed, in which there are some areas of calcification. This lesion must be distinguished from a synovial chondromatosis, myositis ossificans, a bizarre parosteal osteochondromatous proliferation which essentially affects the long bones of the hands and feet, and even more from a malignant tumour. These osteochondromatous structures develop like the first two cases, by metaplasia of the soft tissues. In the two cases reported by Li et al there was no history of trauma but it should be noted that both tumours were subcalcaneal.

Synovial chondromatosis: nodular type

(figs. 3-10)

The synovium of joints, tendons and serous bursae may be the origin of cartilaginous metaplasia. It is very probable that no articulation is exempt; Milchgrub et al (1992) report a case of relatively exuberant chondromatosis developing in the synovium of the first costovertebral joint.

Diagnostic problems

Identification of a chondromatosis at an unusual site

This is usually an easy problem to resolve. The presence of rounded or ovoid cartilaginous structures formed of concentric layers, free in the joint and coexisting with small cartilaginous nodules embedded in the synovium leaves no doubt. In the majority of cases it is obvious that the nodules are numerous (sometimes over 100); neither the radiologist nor the surgeon can fail to make the diagnosis.

Distinguishing a solitary intra-articular nodule of cartilaginous appearance from a nodule of osteochondritis

An osteochondritic nodule is identifiable by macroscopic and histological features. Importantly, one of its surfaces is covered by articular cartilage, a simple point which is clearly critical. Importantly, one of its surfaces is covered by articular cartilage, a simple point which is clearly critical.

Histologically, the chondrocytes are quite regularly distributed and even the deep zone of calcified cartilage can be recognised. This cartilage covers a small zone of spongy bone, whose remodelled marrow is fibrous. The deep aspect of this bony area is covered in turn with newly-formed fibrocartilage. This appearance is markedly different from that of a nodule of chondromatosis; even if its central zone is ossified there is no structural orientation in this small cartilaginous sphere.

It may be difficult to distinguish between a nodule of superficial osteochondritis or an old nodule. When the osteochondritis is very superficial only a fine bony layer remains united with the fragment of articular cartilage. If several years have passed between the time when this fragment became detached from the joint surface and the time when it was removed from the joint, its remodelling may be such that the articular cartilage is no longer identifiable. The whole has become "coated" with a newly-formed fibrocartilage. Further, the niche which contained this small focus of osteocartilaginous necrosis has also been filled in by fibrocartilage and may be invisible or barely visible in a standard radiograph. In some cases a remnant of articular cartilage may be identified in the midst of a nodule consisting of newly-formed cartilage. This is striking by virtue of its more marked staining affinity and the oriented arrangement of the chondrocytes.

It may be more difficult to distinguish between a fragment derived from articular surface and secondarily embedded in synovial tissue. Although there is no difficulty if the fragment has retained its typical morphology as a sequestrum from osteochondritis, there is a problem if only the cartilaginous tissue remains. Here the chondrocytes may retain their viable appearance, perhaps indefinitely. The presumptive features in favor of a secondarily embedded fragment are images of macrophage absorption of its outlines, absence of concentric appositions of cartilage layers and absence of chondrogenesis in the other synovial fragments examined.

If the clinical diagnosis is that of malignant chondromatosis, there will be considerable osteoporosis, probably related to the functional impairment created by a luxuriant, even aggressive, chondromatosis, but which the pathologist does not usually recognise as malignant. The presence of cellular anomalies of a dystrophic nature does not permit diagnosis of a sarcoma developing from chondromatosis.

The commonest lesion associated with synovial chondromatosis of a large limb joint is arthrosis. Even in cases of exuberant chondromatosis, developing over many years and sometimes associated with periosteal ossification, as in the case reported by Lagier (1987), histological study shows no evidence of malignancy.

Cases of true sarcomatous transformation are exceptional [Hamilton et al 1987]; they usually develop only after a long course. However, it is not impossible for a chondrosarcoma to coexist with a chondromatosis, requiring open biopsy of the suspect zones [Benoit et al 1990] which is usually more reliable than arthroscopic biopsy. The mean age of 21 reported cases was 40 [Hamilton et al 1987, Bertoni et al 1991, Kenan et al 1993, Auract et al 1996, Bascoulergue et al 1996]. Auract et al (1996) stress the rarity of sarcomatous change, which can be considered only after having excluded a synovial chondrosarcoma and the coexistence of a chondrosarcoma and of a synovial chondromatosis, either pre-existing or secondary to the chondrosarcoma.

Diffuse oncocytic chondromatosis of synovium and tendon sheaths is a special type of synovial chondromatosis (figs. 3-6) manifest by a proliferation of large chondroblastic cells enclosed in a thick, usually safranophil, border. These cells are sometimes joined in small groups of 5 or 6 components and sometimes isolated, scattered in a lax connective tissue which in no way resembles the intercellular chondroid ground substance of chondromas. This particular tissue may be the only one included in the biopsy (fig. 9 a, b); in other cases associated clearly identifiable chondrocytic areas are seen (fig. 10 a). Such lesions pose a difficult surgical problem in view of their diffuseness, enclosing not only a tendon but possibly also a neurovascular bundle. Operation is tricky and does not always succeed in avoiding functional complications or recurrences. This oncocytic type may coexist with or give origin to genuine extraskeletal chondrosarcomas of the synovium and tendon sheaths.

Bizarre parosteal osteochondromatous proliferation (figs. 11-17)

These rare parosteal lesions were described in 1983 by Nora, Dahlin and Beabout.

General considerations

They are sited juxtacortically and develop mainly on the long bones of the hands and feet, but excluding the terminal phalanges. The authors report 35 cases of this entity, localised to the hands and feet, but also mention two other cases situated at the lower ends of the humerus and the lower end of the radius. There was no sex predominance: 16 male and 19 female cases were reported. The extremes of age were 14 and 74 years but the maximum incidence was between 20 and 40, with a median age of 34 years.

Clinical features

The lesion is occult, but slight sensitivity may be associated with a rapidly growing swelling.

Imaging

There is an opaque formation situated either a few millimeters away from the phalanx or in contact with it, but without periosteal reaction.

Pathological anatomy and histopathology

Macroscopically, the tumour is clothed with cartilage of irregular thickness. On section the appearance is partly cartilaginous and osseous, partly fibrous. There are also some zones of fatty marrow.

Quite characteristic histologically are irregular cartilage boundaries and the coexistence of cartilaginous islands and zones of osteoid and bony differentiation, without any identifiable architectural pattern. The marrow is frankly fibrous and fusiform cells proliferate in places in the peripheral zones. The cartilage cells are bizarrely shaped and of unequal size; sometimes they are isolated in a chondroplast, sometimes stellate or fusiform and immature in appearance. Some binuclear chondrocytes can be seen.

Differential diagnosis

Differential diagnosis is from an osteogenic exostosis but this has a very characteristic architecture, whether pedicled or sessile; the spongy bone of an exostosis is continuous with that of the parent bone, as are the cortices of that bone and the exostosis. Even in exostoses whose morphology is somewhat deranged the distribution of bone and cartilage does not lead to this heterogeneous anarchic appearance. This tumour must also be distinguished from osteochondroma of the soft tissues, as described by Li et al.

It is more difficult, and more important, to exclude a juxtacortical sarcoma, chondrosarcoma or osteosarcoma but neither necrosis nor atypical mitoses have been reported. Moreover, while the chondrocytes are "bizarre", the osteoblasts and osteocytes are more or less normal. No case of malignant transformation has been reported but recurrence is common, of the order of 50%, and 20% of cases have recurred twice.

Extraskeletal chondrosarcoma (figs. 18-23)

Extraskeletal chondrosarcomas

These may develop in the soft tissues, either de novo (often in the thighs and arms) or in a preexisting cartilaginous tissue (larynx and bronchi mainly), or in newly-formed cartilaginous tissue (chondroma, hamartoma, synovial chondromatosis).

Chondrosarcomas have also been reported in several organs (synovium, meninges, breasts), either in isolation or associated with a carcinoma or a sarcoma. Insofar as chondrosarcomas reproduce the usual histological appearances of intraosseous sarcomas they pose the same diagnostic difficulties (cf Chapter 2). A separate place is accorded to mesenchymal chondrosarcoma, since about two-thirds of cases of this lesions develop outside bone, usually in the vicinity of a joint (cf Chapter 4).

Myxoid chondrosarcoma of the soft tissues

General considerations

This is a rare tumour, without doubt the rarest of myxoid tumours of soft tissues. Most authors accord it a male predominance. The mean age of the patients is between 45 and 50 years, but some cases have been reported in children and also in nonagenarians. The sites of election are the pelvic girdle, the proximal part of the lower limbs, then the shoulder-girdle and popliteal fossa. The deep forms are often related to tendons and aponeuroses.

Clinical features and course

Pain is responsible for consultation in a third of the cases and the discovery of a mass, either superficial or muscular, in two-thirds. In 25% of patients there is a history of previous trauma. Slowly growing and causing little or no pain, many months or even years elapse between the onset of the tumour and its detection. In a third of the cases the course is complicated by pulmonary, bony or nodal metastases; these last have been reported in 25% of metastasising cases.

Imaging

Imaging techniques show a quite well circumscribed non-calcified ovoid mass in the muscles, or more often near a joint in the groin, popliteal fossa or axilla.

Pathological anatomy and histopathology

At macroscopic examination the tumour consists either of a solitary nodule or a multinodular mass, adherent to ligaments or to tendino-aponeurotic tissue. Its longest axis varies from a few centimeters to more than 20. The pseudo-capsule gives it a firm consistency, but on section it is mucoid, grayish-white or grayish-pink, sometimes haemorrhagic or cystic. In the sections the small round or ovoid cells have scanty cytoplasm which is markedly eosinophil, sometimes hollowed out by one or two small vacuoles. The nucleus is very chromophil, mitoses are usually rare and some binuclear forms may be seen. These cells are surrounded by a mucoid material rich in sulfated mucopolysaccharides (PAS+, alcian blue+ at a concentration of 0.6 M $MgCl_2$, without appreciable variations after treatment with hyaluronidase). The entire structure is surrounded by dense collagen fibers, which form a pseudo-capsule; on its deep aspect this gives off some fibrous septa which partition the tumour. The vascularisation is reduced and very different from that of a myxoid liposarcoma.

One important feature is architectural polymorphism, which is doubtless partly responsible for its relatively late identification by Stout and Verner in 1953. This polymorphism is related to both remodelling of the mucoid material and to varied patterns of cell distribution. Fibrous remodelling, haemorrhage, hyalinisation, cyst formation and the development of clefts impart great architectural diversity on this tumour. In addition to these modifications of the mucoid material there are modalities of cell distribution, with several appearances usually coexisting in the same lesion. In one place the cell pattern assumes a typically myxoid character, in another the small eosinophil cells form long chains or relatively very cellular areas, or else they border clefts in the mucoid substance and simulate glandular formations. They are also capable of anastomosing in a network or forming dense zones of undifferentiated or fusiform elements which confuse the diagnosis, especially since in about half the cases characteristic cartilaginous differentiation cannot be demonstrated.

Ultrastructural study confirms the chondroblastic nature of the tumour cells. The ovoid nucleus is slightly indented, the chromatin marginalised, and the Golgi apparatus well developed; some glycogen granules are present here and there in the cytoplasm. Lastly, rare and rudimentary junctions connect some of the cells.

Differential diagnosis

Differential diagnosis is from an intramuscular myxoma, which is virtually avascular and whose fusiform or stellate cells are quite different from chondroblastic cells, a myxoid liposarcoma, which has characteristic vascularity and cells whose nucleus is displaced as a peripheral crescent by a fatty vacuole and a malignant fibrous histiocytoma in which the cell polymorphism, the presence of more cellular zones with a storifom arrangement and the rich vascularity are relatively characteristic differential features.

In these three tumours - myxoma, myxoid liposarcoma, malignant myxoid fibrous histiocytoma - staining with alcian blue is abolished by treatment with hyaluronidase. Ueda et al (1992) demonstrated collagen of type II in the stroma of extra- and intraskeletal myxoid chondrosarcomas whereas there was none in myxoid liposarcoma, malignant myxoid schwannoma and myxoma (1 case). It would be useful to confirm these results in a greater number of cases. In the same study the reaction with anti-protein S100 was frankly negative only in the myxoma.

Other differentials include a myxoid chondroma; initially this is a chondroma without histological evidence of malignancy and with adequately differentiated zones in most cases. A mesenchymal chondrosarcoma, a highly malignant tumour, is characterised by its very cellular areas of small undifferentiated elements, whose arrangement is often compared to the architecture of angiopericytoma. The cartilaginous zones may be very much reduced in extent (cf Chapter 4). A histiocytoid (or epithelioid) haemangioma may cause confusion in cases where the biopsy comes from a lax myxoid zone; but the endothelium formed of large atypical cells projecting into the vessel lumina should suggest the diagnosis. A chordoma will only be relevant where the tumour presents in the vertebral axis (cf Chapter 20).

For cartilaginous tumours in general, the current treatment is surgical as far as this is practicable.

Comments: Martin et al (1973) reported, under the name of chordoid sarcoma, a tumour identical to that which Enzinger et al had described in 1972 by the name of myxoid chondrosarcoma. Immunohistological and ultrastructural studies have demonstrated the identity of the two tumours [Weiss 1976, Dardick et al 1983]. Meis and Enzinger identified a chondroid lipoma in 1993 which is often confused with myxoid chondrosarcoma or myxoid liposarcoma. The rare cases of this tumour that some colleagues and I have observed led us to question the term lipoma used in association with chondroid metaplasia or mesenchymoma. Meis and Enzinger's report dealt with 20 cases (16 female) in which the tumour consisted of eosinophilic cells and clear cells whose vacuoles contain glycogen and lipids. The cells resembled those of brown fat, but lipoblasts and chondroblasts like cells where also seen. The stroma of the tumour is myxoid, hyaline and fibrous in places; it contains acid mucopolysaccharides generally resistant to digestion by hyaluronidase. The immunohistological reactions are positive for S100 protein, vimentin and the CD68 antigen. Ultrastructural study of two cases of chondroid lipoma led Nielsen at al (1995) to conclude that the tumour consists of adipocytes without cartilaginous differentiation, as optical microscopy might suggest. In the same year Kindblom et al in a study of 13 cases by electron microscopy found adipocytic and chondrocytic differentiation of the tumour cells.

Surgical excision of this well-circumscribed tumour is followed by definitive cure, usually without recurrence; hence the importance of not confusing this chondroid lipoma with myxoid liposarcoma. Meis and Enzinger (1993) interpret the tumour as a lipo-hibernoma with myxoid zones and chondroid differentiation.

Primary extraskeletal skeletogenic sarcoma (figs. 24-29)

Sarcomas of the soft tissues

General considerations

The incidence of skeletogenic sarcomas of the soft tissues is about 20-25 times less than that of skeletogenic sarcomas of skeletal origin. Although heterotopic bony metaplasia is commonplace, osteogenic sarcomas of soft tissues do not seem to develop in a preexisting ossification. The malignant transformation of an osteoma, osteochondromatosis or myositis ossificans is very rare [Jarvi et al 1958]. There does not seem to be marked predominance of either sex. In the series of Sordillo et al (1983) there were 23 men and 25 women; in that of Chang et al (1987), relating to 88 tumours, 58% were in men. The age of development is later than that of bone sarcomas, the mean age being between 45 and 55 years. In the study of Huvos (1986), of 117 osteogenic sarcomas in patients aged over 60, there were 16 extraosseous cases (cf Chapter 11). In most cases no aetiology can be found, but in 10-12% of cases an injury may be alleged. In Sordillo's series, 5.7% of cases were osteosarcomas secondary to irradiation. The commonest sites are the thighs: 11 out of 26 cases in the report of Bane et al (1990). The pelvic and shoulder girdles are the next common sites where the tumour is usually paraarticular. Then follow thoracic and lumbar lesions. The tumour sometimes develops in the deep connective tissue and sometimes subcutaneously.

Clinical features and course

The usual presenting features are an insidiously growing tumour and progressive and increasing pain. The latent period may extend over several years, as in the case of a cervical osteosarcoma developing 30 years after an injection of thorotrast for arteriography (with probable local extravasation) reported by Hasson et al (1975).

The course of currently reported cases is generally grave. The metastatic locations are identical with those of bone sarcoma, the lungs, lymph nodes, bones and viscera.

Imaging

The radiographs reveal an opaque mass of some centimeters in its main axis, the irregular opacity having no point of contact with adjacent organs, particularly muscles and neurovascular bundles.

Pathological anatomy and histopathology

There may be a typical macroscopic and microscopic appearance very similar to that of skeletogenic sarcomas of skeletal origin. The fusiform or osteoblastic sarcoma cells, in which anisocytosis and atypical mitoses are seen, form a disordered osteoid and chondroid tissue. The tumour displaces the adjacent issue and may seem to be surrounded by a pseudo-capsule, but actually it is infiltrating and invasive. In a sarcoma of the inner aspect of the thigh it may completely ensheath the femoral artery.

In another possible form there is osteoid or bone which is apparently regular and organoid. Some authors even regard this as mature osteogenesis, but the published illustrations do not seem to me to justify this qualification. What is certain is the organoid architecture, at least in my observations; a very "calm" bony tissue of benign appearance. Nevertheless, the marrow is not that of an osteoma since it too may become mature. The intertrabecular spaces are filled with a lax connective tissue with little fibrosis, in which the fusiform or rounded cells assume an osteoblastic appearance at the margins of strands of primary bone to which they have given rise.

Examination of the whole circumference of the tumour mass reveals marked cellular density, relatively intense mitotic activity and here and there cells whose nuclear-cytoplasmic ratio is manifestly increased, and some atypical mitoses.

Differential diagnosis

It is generally considered that myositis ossificans (cf Chapter 31) poses a difficult problem, at least in some cases. But we need only recall the importance of zonation if an adequate and suitably oriented sample is available, the fact that metaplastic osteogenesis develops in a non-sarcomatous tissue, and the rapidity of development of the lesion which usually occur in young subjects.

I find it much more difficult to recognise an osteosarcoma of low-grade malignancy, which calls for formal exclusion of a somewhat atypical osteoma, possibly traumatised or developing in tissue damaged by previous infective or surgical insults.

Another possibility is to confuse this tumour with a juxtacortical sarcoma (cf Chapter 11), which is connected to the underlying bone by a base of varying size. Lastly, in many soft tissue tumours, if the biopsy is made in a zone of bony metaplasia, it may pose some problems and be confused with liposarcoma, synovial sarcoma, malignant fibrous histiocytoma (particularly its giant cell form) or metastases. We should bear in mind that in general the zones of ossification are localised and relatively small; one must ensure that it is a non-tumour, metaplastic osteogenesis and retain the term appropriate to a tumour of the soft tissues. In these cases the osteogenesis may be associated with a better prognosis than that normally considered for such tumours (perhaps because it allows earlier diagnosis).

Osteogenic sarcoma of the viscera

These are very rare. They may develop either solitarily or in association with a sarcoma or carcinoma which is the usual cause for consultation and supplementary investigations; the discovery of an osteogenic sarcoma in a viscus is often a pathological surprise, either in the biopsy or even at autopsy. Nojima et al (1986) report the curious case of an intestinal haemorrhage revealing a jejunal lesion in a man of 23 who had several lesions in the soft tissues. However, some cases have been reported in most of organs including breast, thyroid, lungs, large vessels, kidneys, bladder, uterus, ovary and uterine tubes.

General considerations

The descriptions and illustrations sometimes show osteogenic sarcomas which are very similar to those of bony origin, sometimes in very fibroblastic forms. As for osteogenic sarcomas developing in association with another tumour, this may be a sarcoma or carcinoma, but also a benign tumour such as an adenoma or phylloides tumour.

Usually, the tumour is discovered after the age of 40 but some cases have, exceptionally, been reported in much younger patients. In the thesis of Pinston (1958) on skeletogenic sarcomas of the thyroid, the youngest patient was 21. Lowry et al (1972) reported a case of cardiac osteosarcoma in a man of 25, but in most cases of osteogenic sarcoma of the kidney, thyroid or mammary gland the patients are over 45.

Aetiology

The aetiology of these extraskeletal osteogenic sarcomas is a mystery; however, it is possible to incriminate previous irradiation for some sorts of tumour, often a carcinoma, in some cases. A study by Wiklund et al, in 1991, deals with the findings of an enquiry based on the Cancer Registry in Finland. Of 33 sarcomas attributed to irradiation, they found 10 osteosarcomas of which 6 were skeletal and 4 extraskeletal. These 4 extraskeletal osteosarcomas had developed after a latent period varying from 4 to 13.2 years after the irradiation. Hures et al (1985) reported 66 cases of radiation-induced osteosarcoma (cf Chapter 11).

References

Chondroma, osteochondroma

Bansal M, Goldman AB, Di Carlo EF, McCormack R (1993) Soft tissue chondromas: diagnostic and differential diagnosis. Skeletal Radiol 22: 309-315

Catalano F, Fanfani F, Taccardo G (1988) Lésions tumorales et pseudo-tumorales cartilagineuses des parties molles de la main. Ann Chir Main 7: 314-321

Chan JKC, Lee KC, Saw D (1986) Extraskeletal chondroma with lipoblast-like cells. Hum Pathol 17: 1285-1287

Chung EB, Enzinger FM (1978) Chondroma of soft parts. Cancer 41: 1414-1424

Dahlin DC, Salvador AH (1974) Cartilaginous tumors of the soft tissues of the hand and feet. Mayo Clinic Proc 49: 721-726

Heiple KG, Elmer RM (1972) Chondromatous hamartomas arising from the volar digital plates. A case report. J Bone Joint Surg 54A: 393-398

Keasby LE, Fanselau HA (1961) The aponeurotic fibroma. Clin Orthop 19: 115

Kermarec J, Ayrau N (1968) Fibrome aponévrotique juvénile: forme anatomoclinique spéciale de fibromatose pseudo-sarcomateuse. Arch Anat Pathol 16: 43

Kindblom LG, Meis-Kindblom JM (1995) Condroid lipoma: an ultrastructural and immunohistochemical analysis with further observations regarding its differentiation. Hum Pathol 26: 706-715

Li C, Arger PH, Dalinka MK (1989) Soft tissue osteochondroma. Skeletal Radiol 18: 435-437

Lichtenstein L, Goldman RL (1964) The cartilage analogue of fibromatosis: a reinterpretation of the condition called "juvenile aponeurotic fibroma". Cancer 17: 810

Milgram JW, Dunn EJ (1980) Para-anicular chondromas and osteochondromas. A report of three cases. Clin Orthop 148: 147-151

Milosevic D, Ukropina D (1972) Les chondromes para-articulaires. Rev Chir Orthop Suppl I T58: 241-244

Nielsen GP, O'Connel JX, Dickersin GR, Rosenberg AE (1995) Chondroid lipoma, a tumor of white fat cells. A brief report of two cases with ultrastructural analysis. Am J Surg Pathol 19: 1272-1276

Reiman HM, Dahlin DC (1986) Cartilage-and bone-forming tumors of the soft tissues. Semin Diagn Pathol 3: 288-205

Synovial chondromatosis

Auract Ph, Katabi M, Forest M, Benoit J, Witvoët J, Tomeno B (1996) Chondromatose synoviale et chondrosarcome, étude des rapports entre les deux affections. Rev Chir Orthop 82: 216-224

Bascoulergue G, Gougeon F, Lecomte-Houcke M, Baviera E, Mazabraud A (1996) "Chondromatose" synoviale maligne d'emblée ou évolution chondrosarcomateuse d'une chondromatose synoviale du genou. Bull Cancer 83: 951-956

Benoit J, Arnaud E, Moulucou A, Hardy PH, Got CL, Judet O (1990) Ostéochondromatose synoviale du genou et chondrosarcome synovial. A propos de 2 cas. Rev Chir Orthop 76: 198-203

Christensen JH, Poulsen JO (1975) Synovial chondromatosis. Acta Orthop Scand 46: 919-925

Hamilton A, Davis RI, Nixon JR (1987) Synovial chondrosarcoma complicating synovial chondromatosis. Report of a case and review of the literature. J Bone Joint Surg 69A: 1084-1088

Kenan S, Abdelwahab IF, Klein MJ, Lewis MM (1993) Synovial chondrosarcoma secondary to synovial chondromatosis (case report). Skeletal Radiol 22: 623-626

Lagier R (1987) Primary synovial osteochondromatosis of the knee with extensive bone formation observed over a period of 13 years. Skeletal Radiol 16: 660-665

McCarthy EF, Dorfman HD (1982) Primary synovial chondromatosis an ultrastructural study. Clin Orthop 168: 178-186

Milchgrub S, Mulhollan T, Vuiteh MF, Wheatherall PT (1992) Synovial chondrometaplasia of the 1st costovertebral joint. Case report. Skeletal Radiol 21: 45-48

Milgram JW (1977) The classification of loose bodies in human joints. Clin Orthop 124: 282-291

Pope TL, Keats TE, Lange (de) EE, Fechner RE, Harvey JW (1987) Idiopathic synovial chondromatosis in two unusual sites: inferior radioulnar joint and ischial bursa. Skeletal Radiol 16: 205-208

Bizarre parosteal osteochondromatous proliferation

Nora FE, Dahlin DC, Beabout JW (1983) Bizarre parosteal ostecchondromatous proliferation of the hands and feet. Am J Surg Pathol 7: 245-250

Extraskeletal chondrosarcoma

Angervall L, Enerback L, Knutson H (1973) Chondrosarcoma of soft tissue origin. Cancer 32: 507-513

Benoit J, Arnaud E, Moulucou A, Hardy PH, Got CL, Judet O (1990) Ostéochondromatose synoviale du genou et chondrosarcome synovial. A propos de 2 cas. Rev Chir Onhop 76: 198-203

Bertoni F, Unni KK, Beabout JW, Sim FH (1991) Chondrosarcomas of the synovium. Cancer 67: 155-162

Bleiweiss Ll, Kaneko M (1988) Chondrosarcoma of the larynx with additional malignant mesenchymal component (dedifferentiated chondrosarcoma). Am J Pathol 12: 314-320

Chetty R (1990) Extraskeletal mesenchymal chondrosarcoma of the mediastinum. Histopathol 17: 261-278

Dardick I, Lagace R, Carlier MT, Jung RC (1983) Chordoid sarcoma (extraskeletal myxoid chondrosarcoma). A light and electron microscopic study. Virchows Arch (A) 399: 61-78

Dabska M (1977) Parachordoma. A new clinicopathologic entity. Cancer 40: 1586-1592

Enzinger FM, Shiraki M (1972) Extraskeletal myxoid chondrosarcoma. An analysis of 34 cases. Hum Pathol 3: 421-435

Enzinger FM, Weiss SW (1988) Soft tissue tumors. 2nd edn. Mosby, St Louis, pp 861-881

Kahn LB, Uys CJ, Dale J, Rutherford S (1978) Carcinoma of the breast with metaplasia to chondrosarcoma: a light and electron microscopic study. Histopathology 2: 93-106

Lichtenstein L, Goldman RL (1964) Cartilage tumors of soft tissues, particularly in the hand and foot. Cancer 17: 1203-1208

Mackenzie DH (1983) The unsuspected soft tissue chondrosarcoma. Histopathol 7: 759-766

Manivel JC, Dehner LP, Thompson R (1988) Synovial chondrosarcoma of the left knee. Case report. Skeletal Radiol 17: 66-71

Meis JM, Enzinger FM (1993) Chondroid lipoma. A unique tumor simulating liposarcoma and myxoid chondrosarcoma. Am J Surg Pathol 17: 1103-1112

Mullins F, Berard CW, Eisenberg SH (1965) Chondrosarcoma following synovial chondromatosis. A case study. Cancer 18: 1180-1188

Smith MT, Farinacci CJ, Carpenter HA, Bannayan GA (1976) Extraskeletal myxoid chondrosarcoma. Cancer 37: 821-827

Stout AP, Verner EW (1953) Chondrosarcoma of the skeletal soft tissues. Cancer 6: 581-590

Sun CCJ, Kroll M, Miller JE (1982) Primary chondrosarcoma of the lung. Cancer 50: 1864-1866

Sundaram M, Percelay S, McDonald DJ, Janney C (1993) Extraskeletal chondrosarroma. Case report. Skeletal Radiol 22: 449-451

Trono D, Stalder J, Cox JN (1983) Extraskeletal myxoid chondrosarcoma. A case report with histochemical and ultrastructural features. Appl Pathol 1: 139-148

Ueda Y, Okada Y (1992) Cellular variant of extraskeletal myxoid chondrosarcoma of abdominal wall: a case report with comparative immuno-histochemical study on cartilaginous collagenous proteins in various myxoid mesenchymal tumors. J Cancer Res Clin Oncol 118: 147-151

Weiss SW (1976) Ultrastructure of the so-called "chordoid sarcoma". Evidence supporting cartilaginous differentiation. Cancer 37: 300-306

Wu KK, Guise ER (1981) Synovial chondrosarcoma: a case report. Orthopedics 4: 291-294

Primary extraskeletal skeletogenic sarcoma

Sarcoma of the soft tissues

Allan CJ, Soule EH (1971) Osteogenic sarcoma of the somatic soft tissues. Clinicopathologic study of 26 cases and review of literature. Cancer 27: 1121-1133

Amendola BE, Amendola MA, McClatchey KD, Miller CH (1989) Radiation-associated sarcoma: a review of 23 patients with postradiation sarcoma over a 50 year period. Am J Clin Oncol (CCT) 12:411-415

Bane BL, Evanss HL, Ro YJ, Carrasco CH, Grignon DJ, Benjamin RS, Ayala AG (1990) Extraskeletal osteosarcoma - a clinicopathologic review of 26 cases. Cancer 66: 2762-2770

Belasco JB, Meadows AT, Chatten J, Borden S, Schinaufer L (1982) Extraskeletal osteogenic sarcoma after treatment for Wilms' tumor. Cancer 50: 1894-1898

Chung EB, Enzinger FM (1987) Extraskeletal osteosarcoma. Cancer 60: 1132-1142

Eckardt JJ, Ivins JC, Perry HO, Unni KK (19781) Osteosarcoma arising in heterotopic ossification of dermatomyositis: case report and review of the literature. Cancer 48 : 1256-1261

Fine G, Stout AP (1956) Osteogenic sarcoma of extra-skeletal soft tissues. Cancer 9: 1027-1043

Greenspan A, Steiner G, Norman A, Lewis MM, Matlen J (1987) Osteosarcoma of the soft tissues of the distal end of the thigh. Skeletal Radiol 16: 489-492

Grignon DJ, Ayala AG, Carrasco CH, Ames FC, Meis JM (1989) Extraosseous intra-abdominal osteosarcoma. Case report. Skeletal Radiol 18: 147-151

Hasson J, Hartman KS, Milikow E, Mittelman A (1975) Thorotrast-indused extraskeletal osteosarcoma of the cervical region. Report of a case. Cancer 36: 1827-1833

Jarvi OH, Kvist HTA, Vainio PV (1958) Extraskeletal retroperitoneal osteosarcoma probably arising from myositis ossifiacans. Acta Pathol Microbiol Scand 74: 11-25

Kauffman SL, Stout AP (1963) Extraskeletal osteogenic sarcomas and chondrosarcomas in children. Cancer 16: 432-439

Present D, Bertoni F, Laus M, Bacchini P, Bocanera M (1989) Low-grade osteosarcoma of soft tissues (popliteal fossa). Skeletal Radiol 18: 471-474

Rao U, Cheng A, Didolkar MS (1978) Extraosseous osteogenic sarcoma. Clinicopathological study of eight cases and review of literature. Cancer 41: 1488-1496

Salm R (1959) A case of osteogenic sarcoma of the extraskeletal soft tissues. Br J Cancer 13: 614-617

Smith BH, Taylor HB (1969) The occurence of bone and cartilage in mammary tumors. Am J Clin Pathol 51: 610-618

Sordillo PP, Hajdu Sl, Magill GB, Golbey RB (1983) Extraosseous osteogenic sarcoma. A review of 48 patients. Cancer 51: 727-734

Osteogenic sarcoma of the viscera

Adler CP (1979) Extraosseous osteoblastic osteosarcoma of the right breast. Skeletal Radiol 4: 107-110

Allan CJ, Soule EH (1971) Osteogenic sarcoma of the somatic soft tissues: clinicopathologic study of 26 cases and review of the literature. Cancer 27: 1121-1133

Axelrod R, Naidech HJ, Myers J, Steinberg A (1978) Primary osteosarcoma of the kidney. Cancer 41: 724-727

Cabanne F (1960) Les sarcomes ostéogeniques des parties molles et des viscères. Arch Anat Pathol 8: 131-148

Cabanne F, Dargent M, Leclere F, Pinston M (1959) Le sarcome squelettogène du corps thyroïde. Revue Générale. Ann Anat Pathol 4: 136-153

Colby TV, Bilbao JE, Battifora H, Unni KK (1989) Primary osteosarcoma of the lung: a reappraisal following immunohistologic study. Arch Pathol Lab Med 113: 1147-1150

Fruhling L, Batzenschlager A, Blum E (1959) Epithéliosarcomes vrais (tumeurs mixtes malignes) et cancers doubles didermiques de la vessie. Ann Anat Pathol 4: 5-42

Fruhling L, Le Gal Y (1951) Les sarcomes vrais primitifs de la mamelle. Bull Cancer 38: 477-496

Greenwood SM, Meschter SC (1989) Extraskeletal osteogenic sarcoma of the mediastinum. Arch Pathol Lab Med 113: 430-433

Hirakawa T, Tsuneyosh M, Enjoji M, Shigyo R (1988) Ovarian sarcoma with histologic features of telangiectasic osteosarcoma of the bone. Am J Surg Pathol 12: 567-572

Llombart-Bosch A, Peydro A (1975) Malignant mixed osteogenic tumours of the breast an ultrastructural study of two cases. Virchows Arch A 366: 1-14

Lowry WB, McKee EE (1972) Primary osteosarcoma of the heart. Cancer 30: 1068-1073

Martin JF, Guichard A (1945) Les tumeurs squelettogènes du sein. Lyon Chir 40: 325-341

Mathew T, Prabhakaran K (1981) Osteosarcoma of the testis. Arch Pathol Lab Med 105: 38-39

McConnell TH (1970) Bony and cartilaginous tumors of the heart and great vessels. Report of an osteosarcoma of the pulmonary artery. Cancer 25: 611-617

Nojima T, Gelhan MC, Mankin HJ, Schiller AL (1986) Extraosseous osteosarcoma presenting with intestinal hemorrhage: case report and literature review. Hum Pathol 1 7: 85-87

Pinston M (1958) Le sarcome squelettogène du corps thyroïde. Thèse n° 29, Lyon

Reingold IM, Amromin GD (1971) Extraosscous osteosarcoma of the lung. Cancer 28: 491-498

Reznik M, Lenelle J (1991) Primary intracerebral osteosarcoma. Cancer 68: 793-797

Sumyoschi A, Niho Y (1971) Primary osteogenic sarcoma of the liver: report of an autopsy case. Acta Pathol Jpn 21: 305-312

Syrjanen KJ (1979) An osteogenic sarcoma of the thyroid gland (report of a case and survey of the literature). Neoplasma 26: 623-628

Von Hochstetter AR, Hättenschwiller J, Vogt M (1987) Primary osteosarcoma of the liver. Cancer 60: 2312-2317

Young RH, Rosenberg AE (1987) Osteosarcoma of the urinary bladder. Report of a case and review of the literature. Cancer 59: 174-178

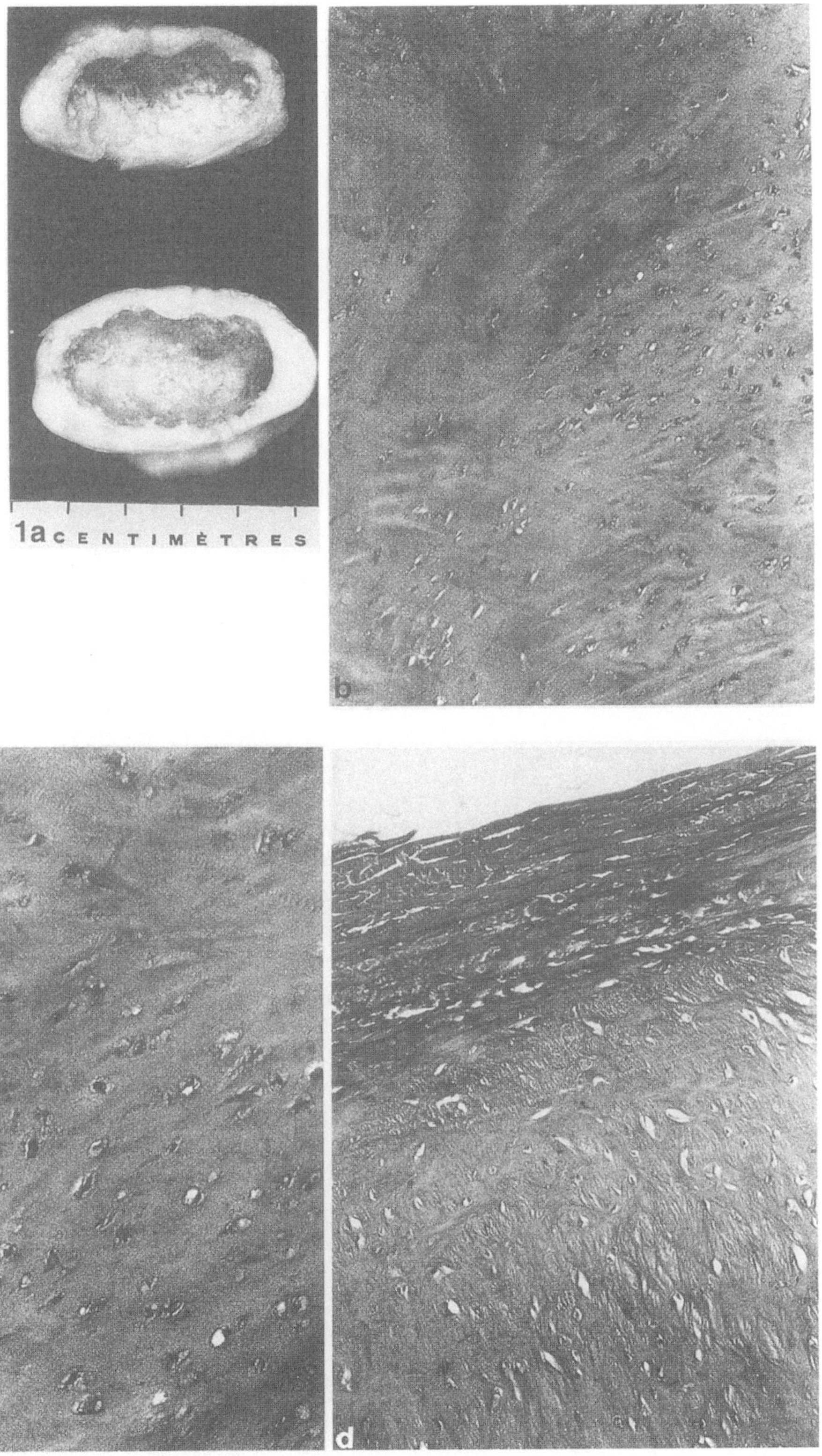

Fig. 1 a-d. Chondroma excavated from the sole of the foot, unconnected with the bony arch. The three microphotographs show the irregularly distributed chondrocytic proliferation of small chondrocytes and at the surface the orientation of fibers of aponeurotic appearance

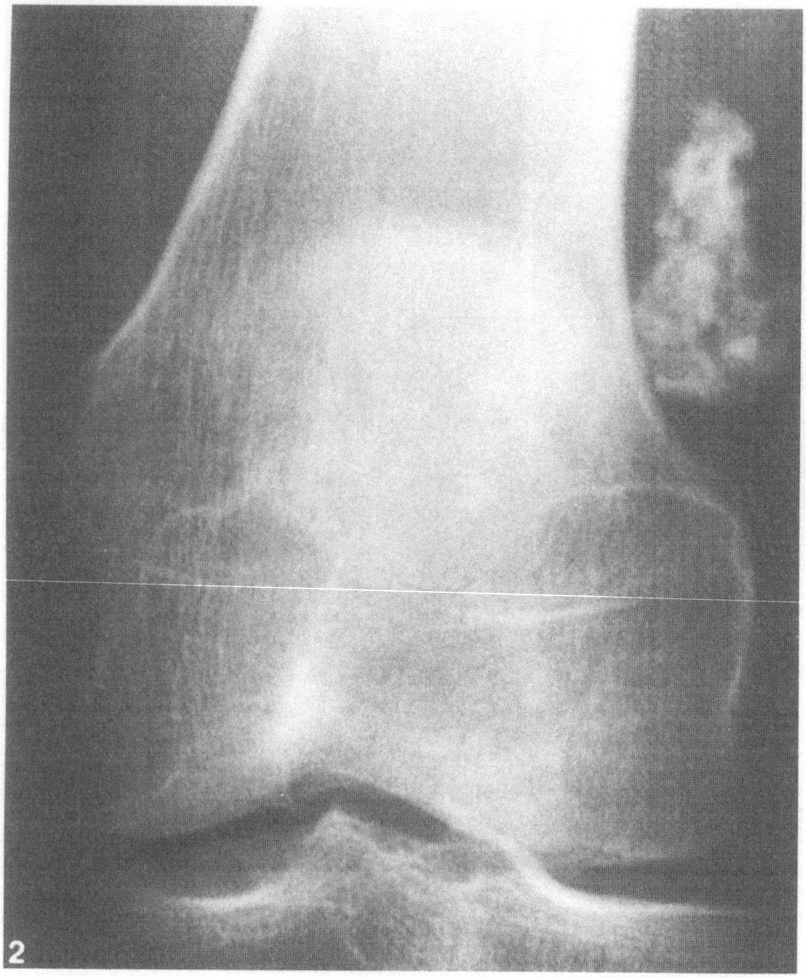

Fig. 2. Radiographic appearance of osteochondroma developing adjacent to the knee joint, possibly from a synovial recess. The tumour consists of agglomerated rounded nodules

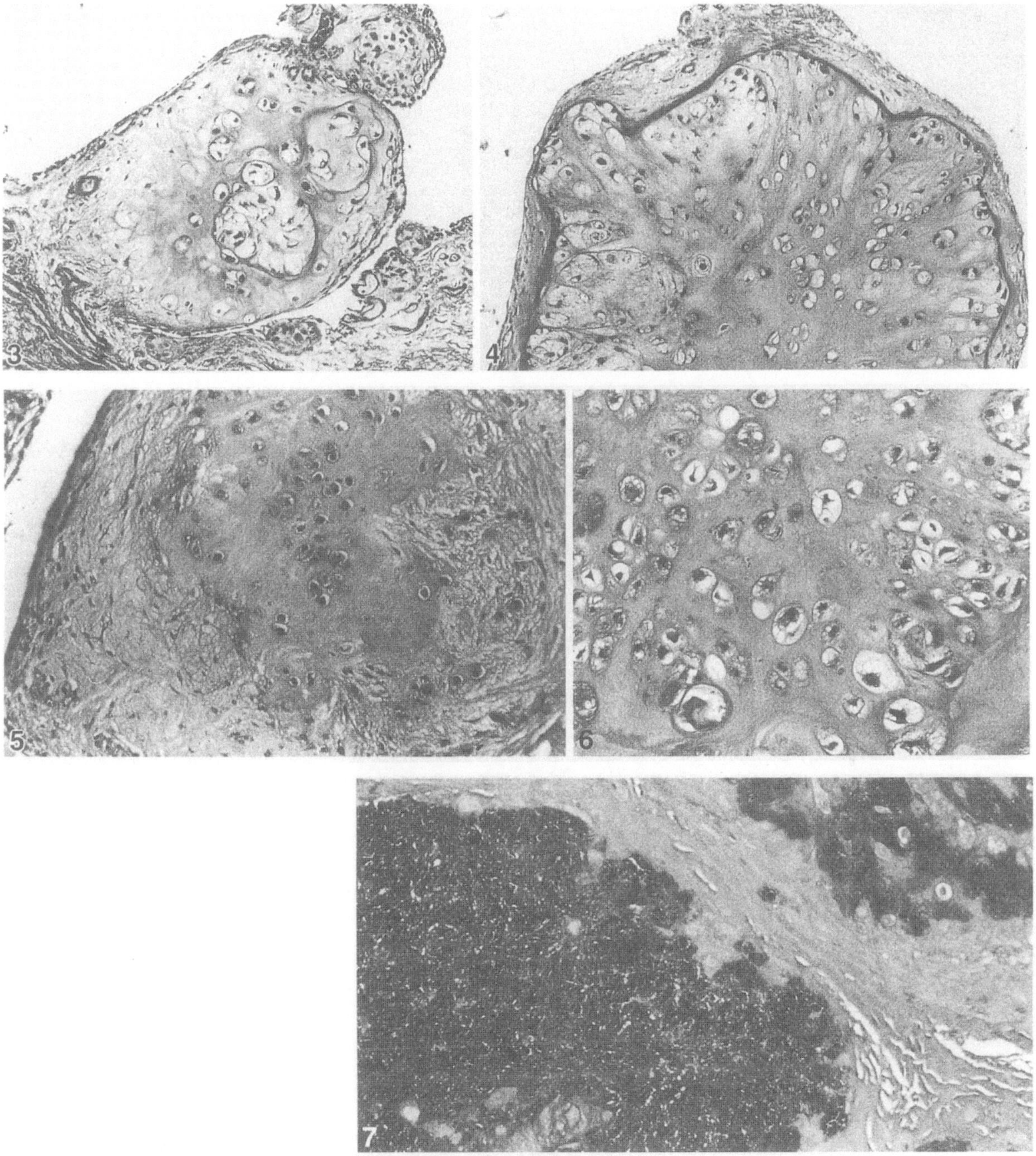

Figs. 3, 4. Well-individualised chondromatous nodules in synovial villi

Fig. 5. Metaplastic phenomena in a synovial villus

Fig. 6. Nuclear and cellular irregularities and inequalities in a chondromatous nodule. These appearances should be interpreted as "degenerative" and not as tumour proliferation

Fig. 7. Patches of calcinosis in a chondromatosis

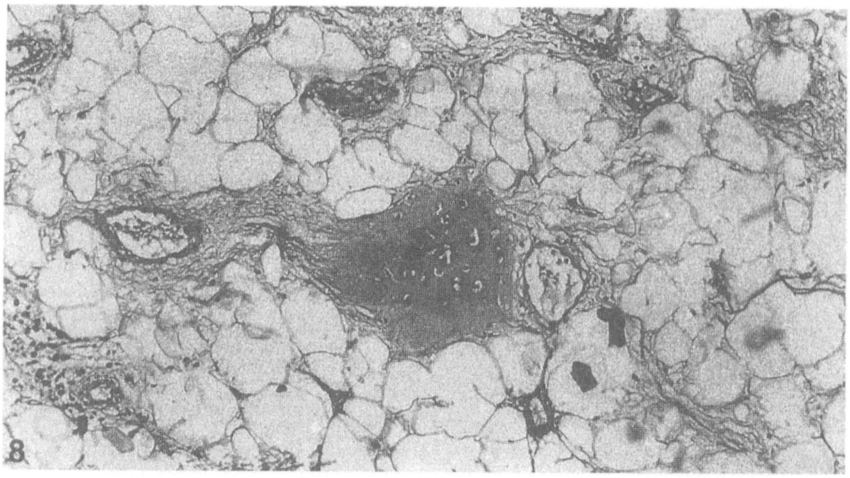

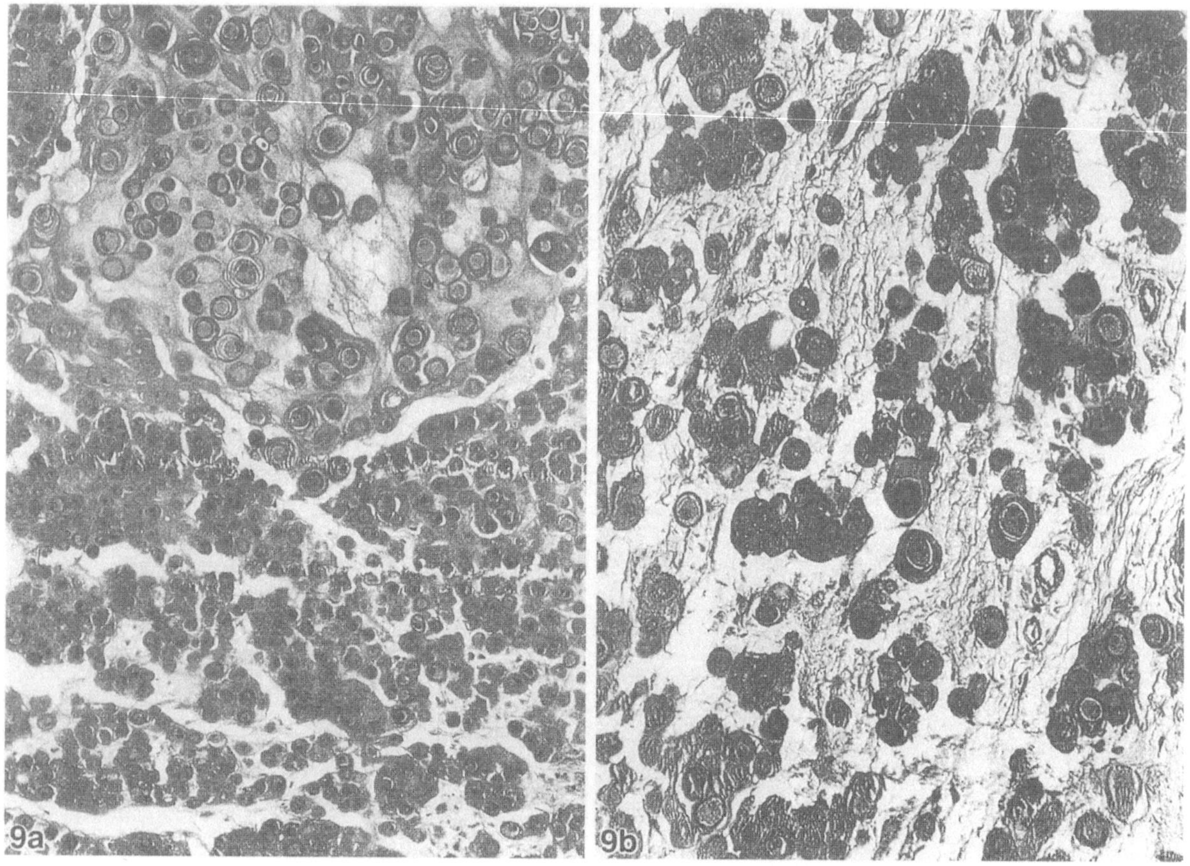

Fig. 8. A solitary metaplastic cartilaginous nodule in an intra-articular "arborescent lipoma"

Fig. 9 a, b. Recurrent synovial chondromatosis of oncocytic type of the sheath of the interossei. The large, bounded chondrocytic cells, independent from one another, often without intercellular hyaline substance, suggest certain chondrocytes of clear-cell chondrosarcomas. This appearance is found quite often in these cartilaginous formations of the synovium and tendon sheaths of the hands. It differs notably from the rounded or ovoid metaplastic formations developing in the synovial villi and formed by the successive apposition of cartilaginous layers

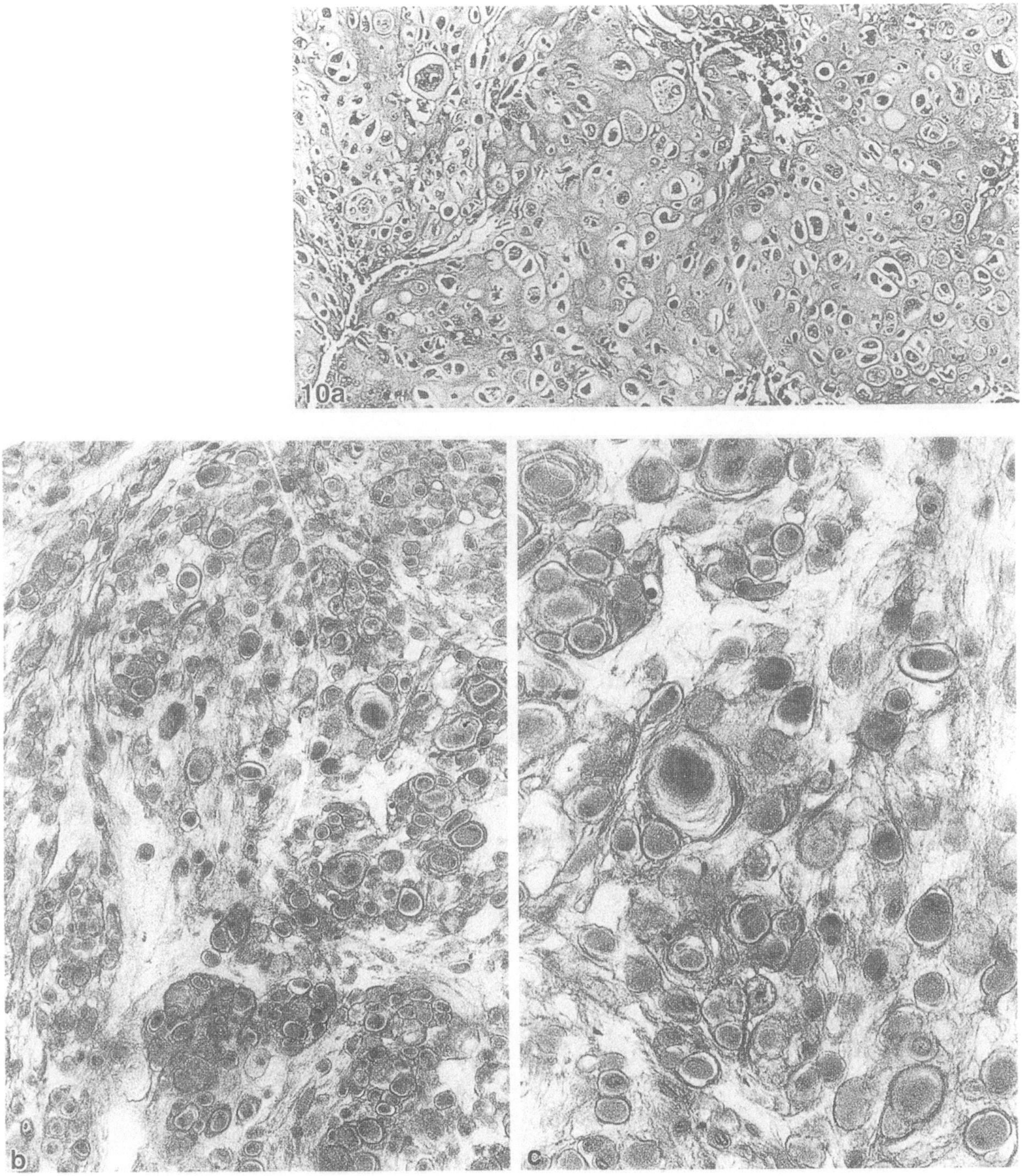

Fig. 10. a Cartilaginous zone of a synovial tumour of the wrist (low magnification). Considerable nuclear variation and anisocytosis. **b, c** Apart from this appearance there are large areas of oncocytosis. The cells are scattered in a lax connective tissue, bounded by a thick safranophil layer, a structure which in our experience is quite characteristic of a particular type of tenosynovial oncocytic chondromatosis

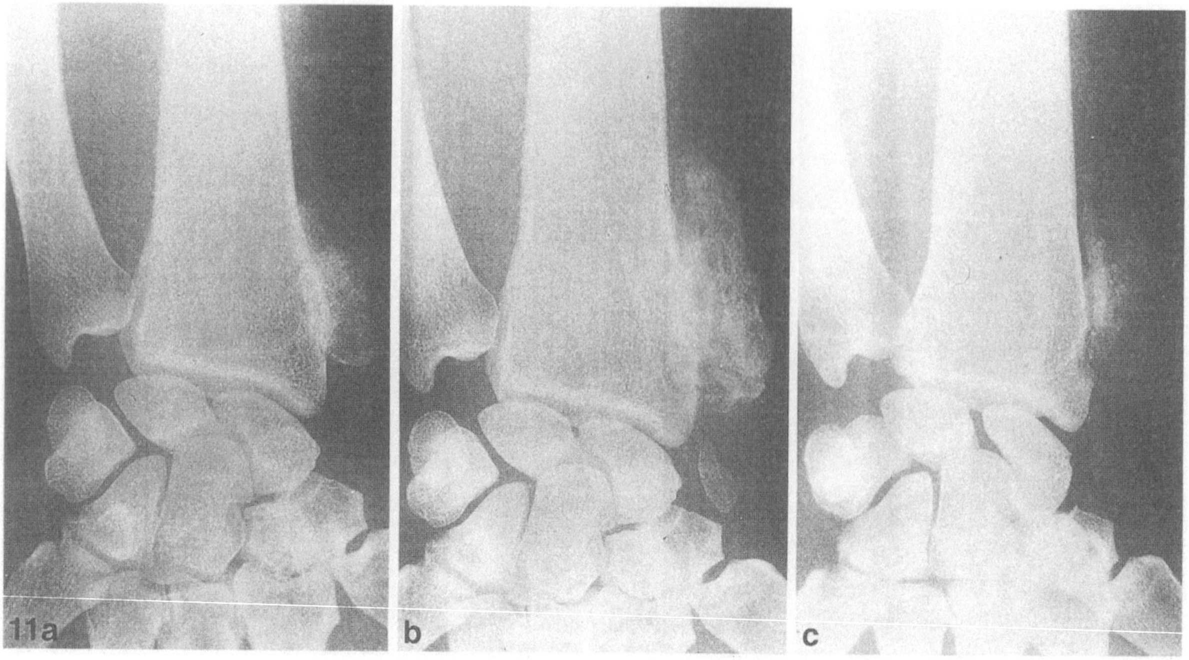

Fig. 11. a This woman of 35 has developed a juxtaosseous tumour of the lower end of the radius. At operation a tumour that was both bony and cartilaginous was removed. **b** 18 months after the first excision the tumour has recurred. **c** A second operation was followed by a small recurrence detected 6 months later. (This case, which we owe to Drs. Pouget and Rethers of Orléans, was shown at the meeting of the Société Orthopédique de l'Ouest on 8 June 1990 at Limoges. To my knowledge, this was the first published French case of this entity). The microphotographs 12-17 belong to this "bizarre parosteal osteochondromatosis"

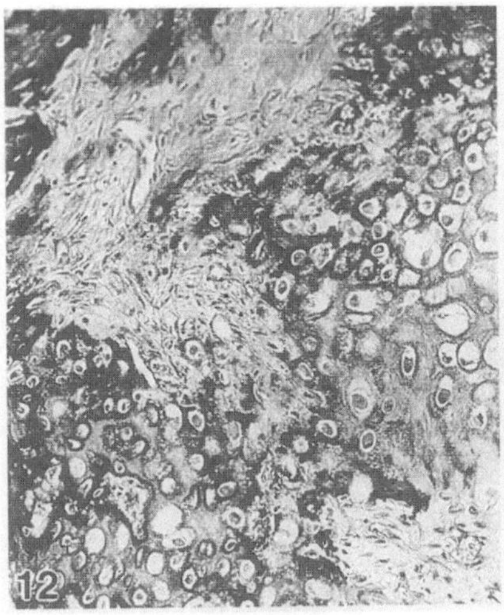
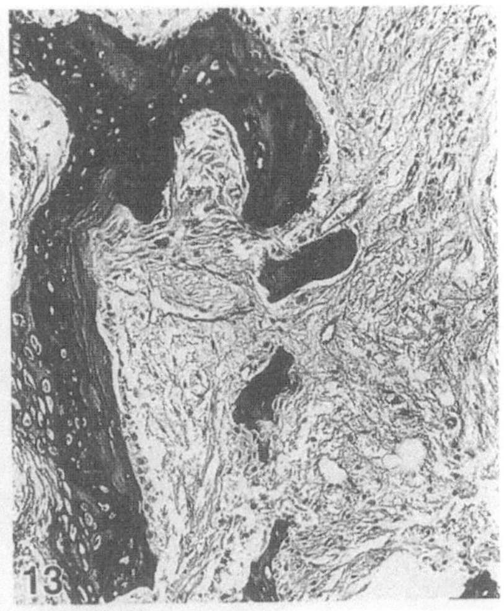
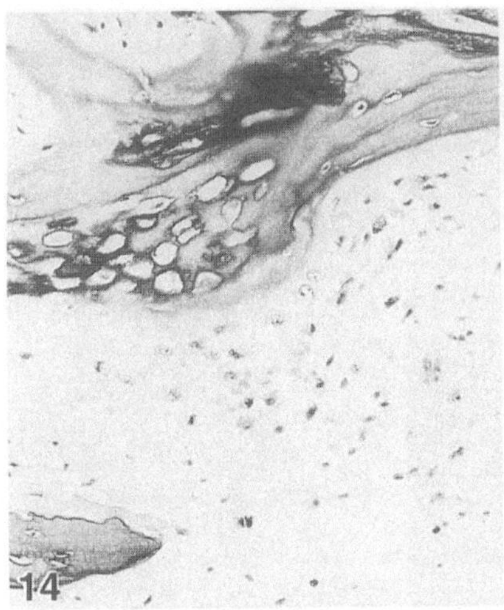
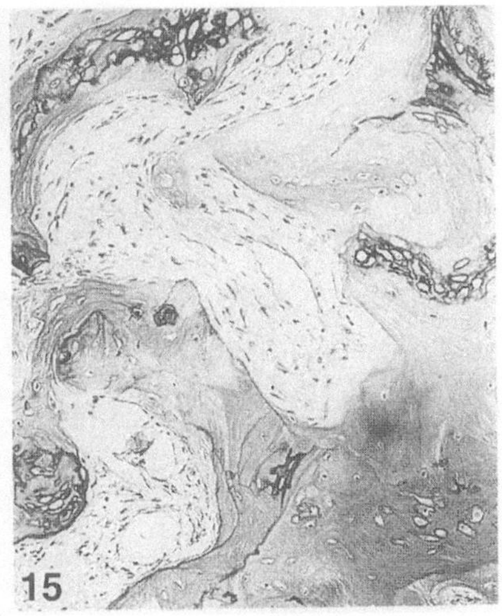
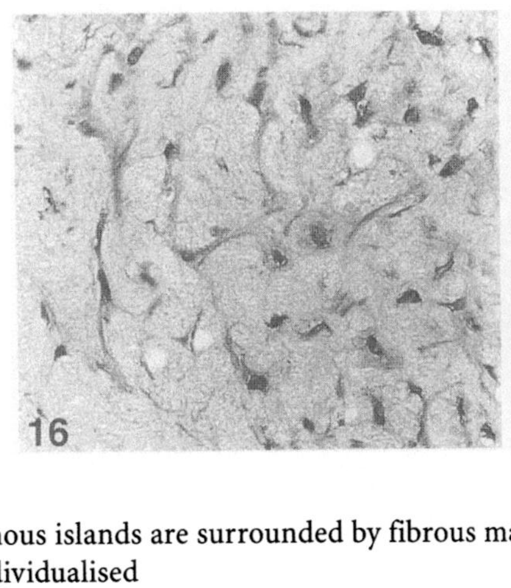
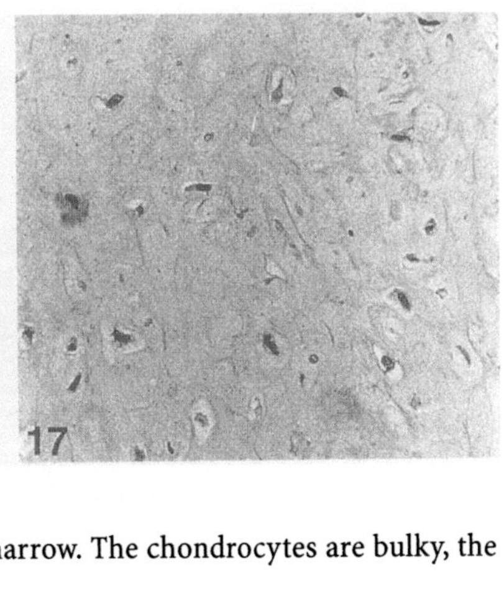

Fig. 12. Well-differentiated cartilaginous islands are surrounded by fibrous marrow. The chondrocytes are bulky, the chondrocytic compartments well individualised

Fig. 13. Elaboration of markedly calcified bony strands, partly bordered by osteoblasts

Figs. 14, 15. The osteogenesis is preceded by a cartilaginous stage

Figs. 16, 17. In places the cartilage is less well differentiated; the chondrocytes are of variable shape and irregular size

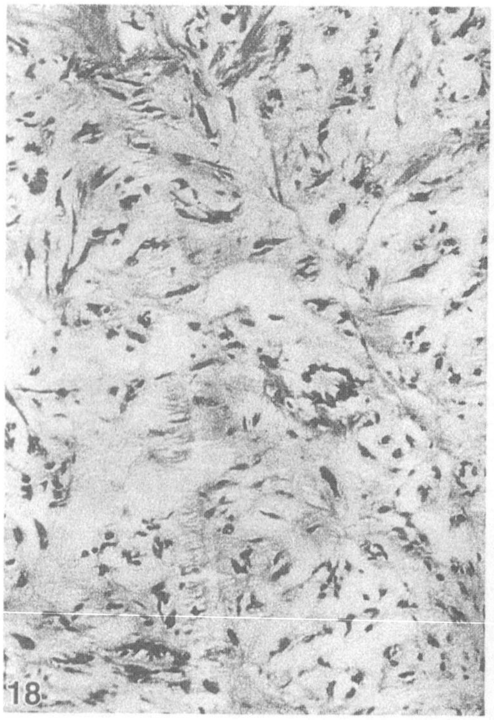
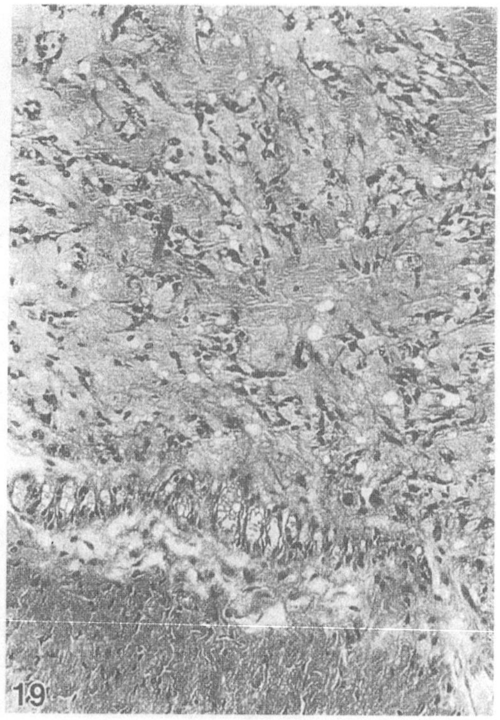
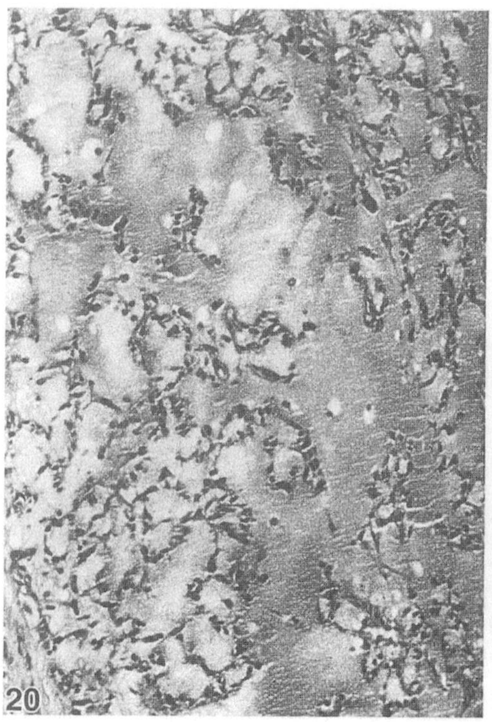
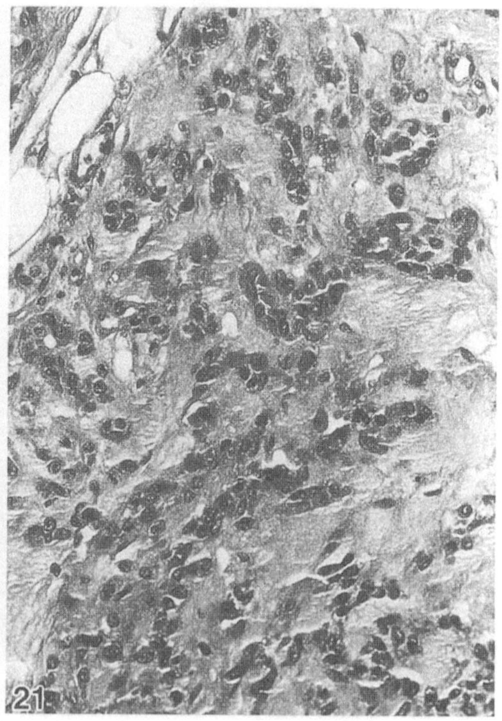

The next four microphotographs belong to a myxoid chondrosarcoma developing in the proximal part of a lower limb

Fig. 18. The cells of very unequal size are solitary or joined in small groups of 3-4

Fig. 19. Arrangement in chains and alignments at the edge of a nodule

Fig. 20. The cell pattern forms a network in the mucoid substance

Fig. 21. Numerous, only slightly differentiated cells. They are arranged in islands in the upper half and in chains in the lower half of this microphotograph

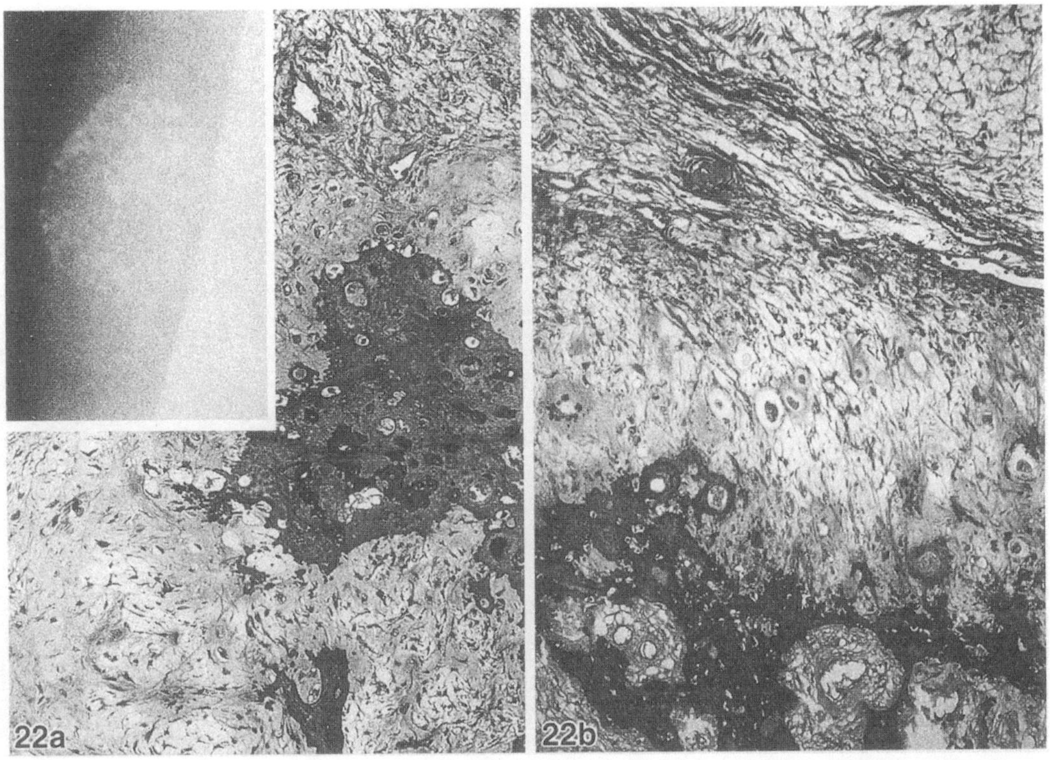

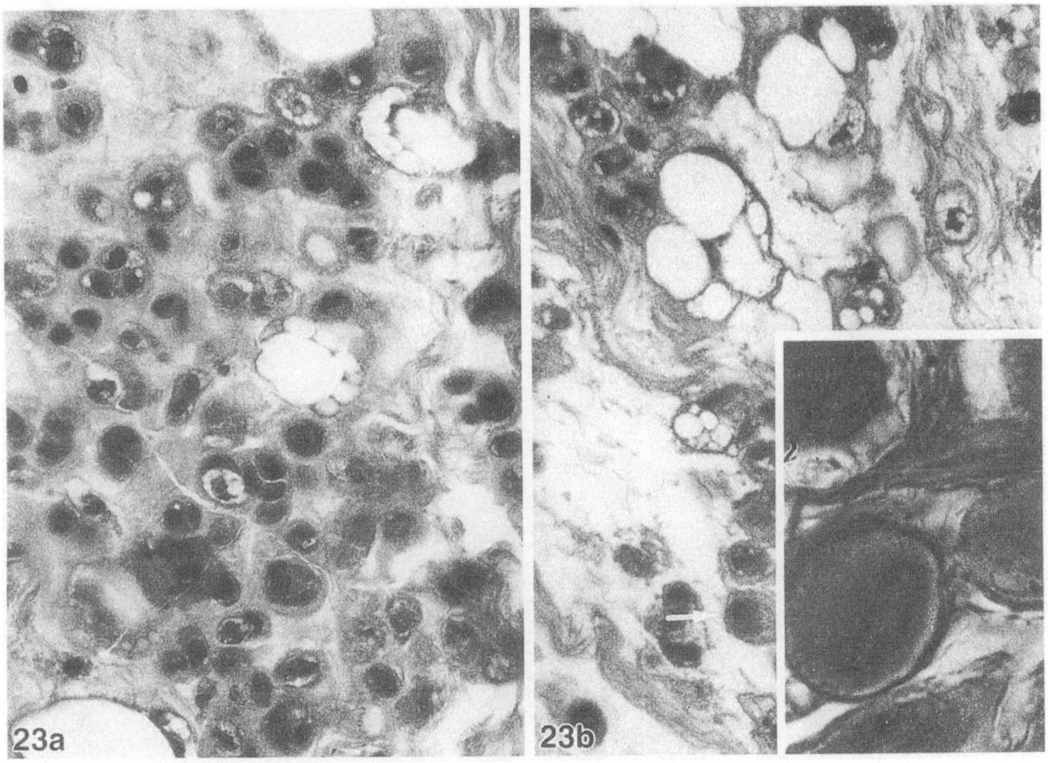

Fig. 22 a, b. Chondrosarcoma developing in the soft tissues of the arm, outer border of humerus (inset). **a** Myxoid appearance with calcification. **b** Above the calcified zone, cells of irregular size, binuclear and with large nuclei. Excision of this tumour was followed by local recurrence with the same histological appearance

Fig. 23 a, b. (**a**) Chondrosarcoma of popliteal fossa: anisocytosis, binuclear cells and cells with large nuclei are common, beside (**b**) small cell groups, isolated chondrocytes in a lax fibrillary ground substance. Below and left: cell with double nucleus (*arrow*), many cells are vacuolated. Inset: some large cells surrounded by a thick border; this appearance in this very localised case is seen in clear-cell sarcomas but more often still in a particular form of chondromatosis

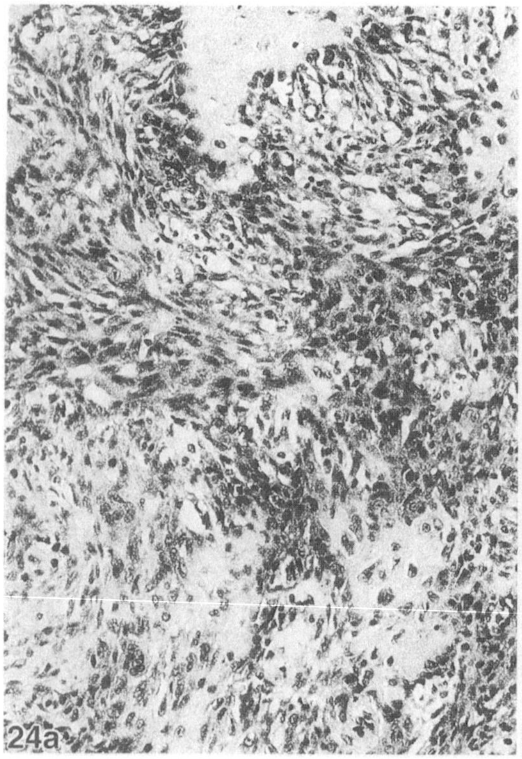

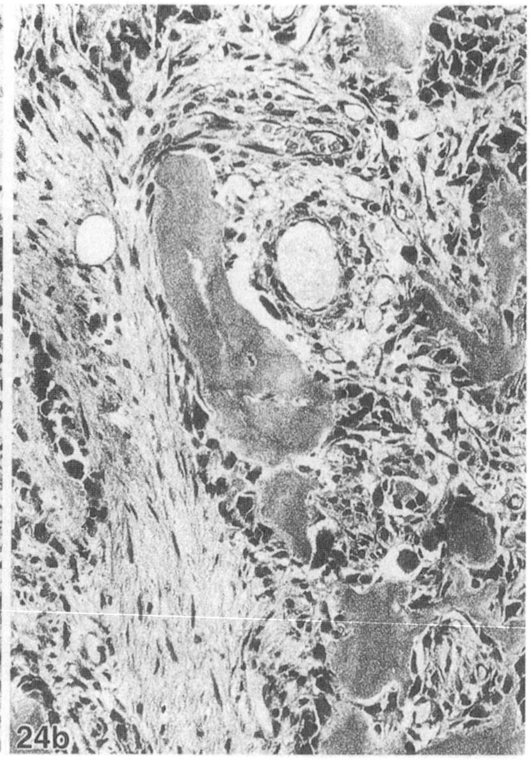

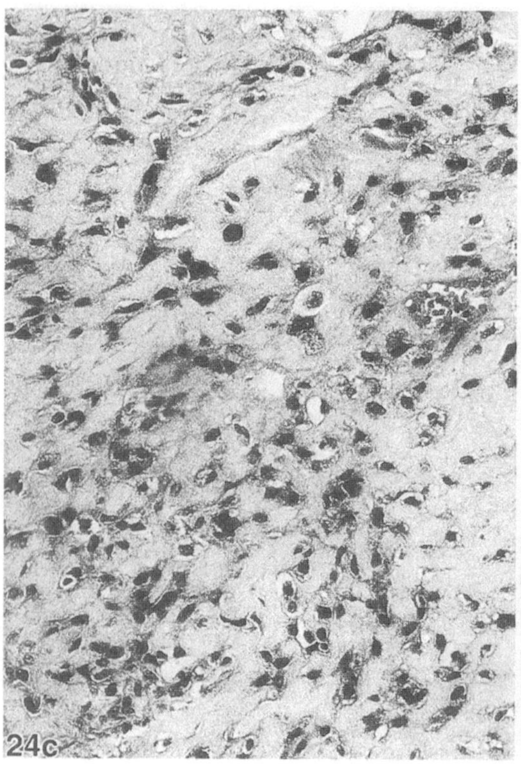

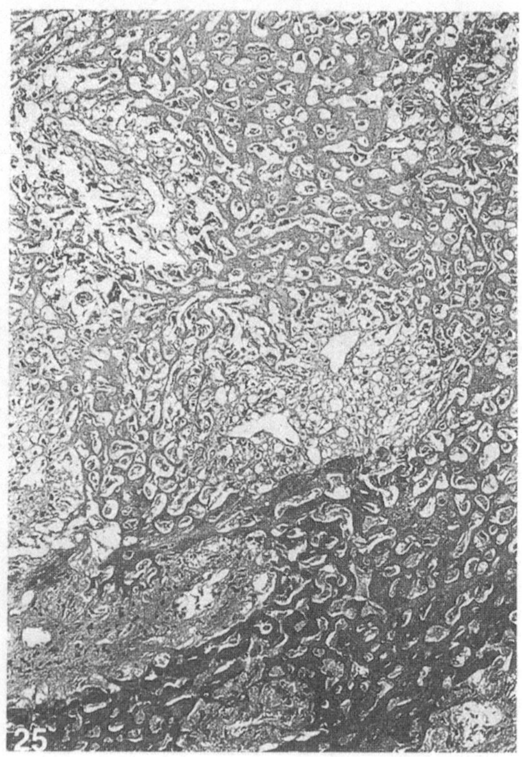

Fig. 24 a-c. Osteosarcoma of breast; the tumour is heterogeneous. **a** The predominantly fusiform cell proliferation is arranged in bundles. **b** Partly calcified osteoid strands bordered by tumour cells lie adjacent to chondroid areas (**c**). The cell polymorphism is evident in these osteochondroid areas

Fig. 25. Osteosarcoma of the bladder formed of osteoid strands composing a partly calcified network

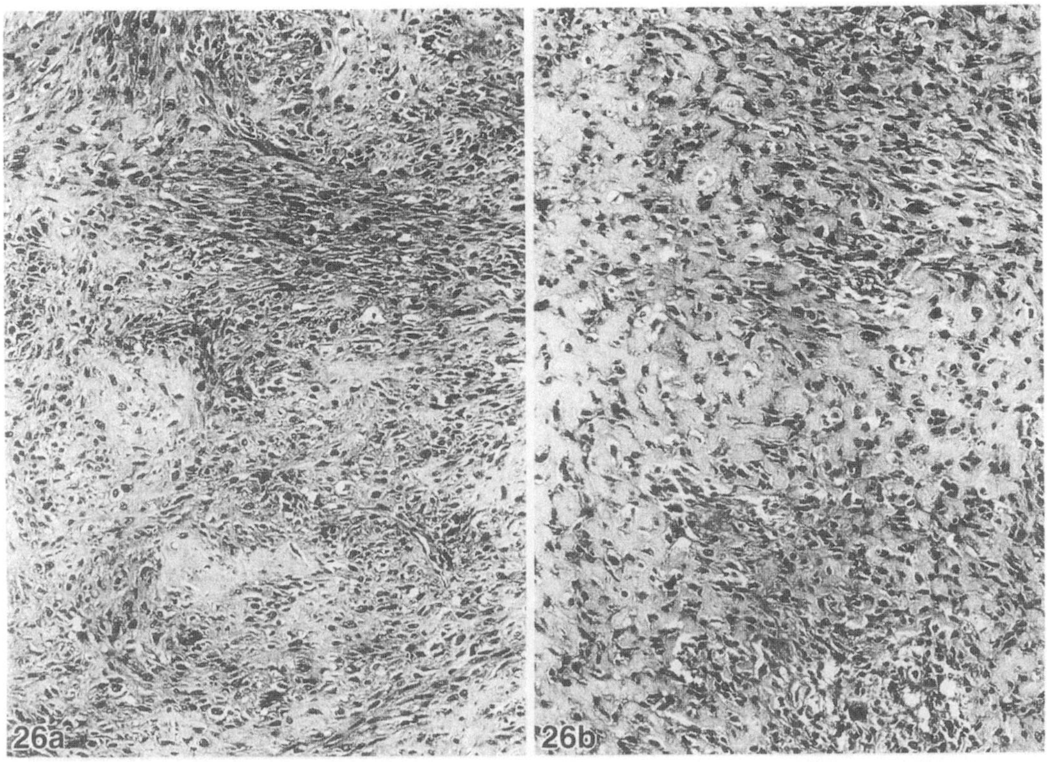

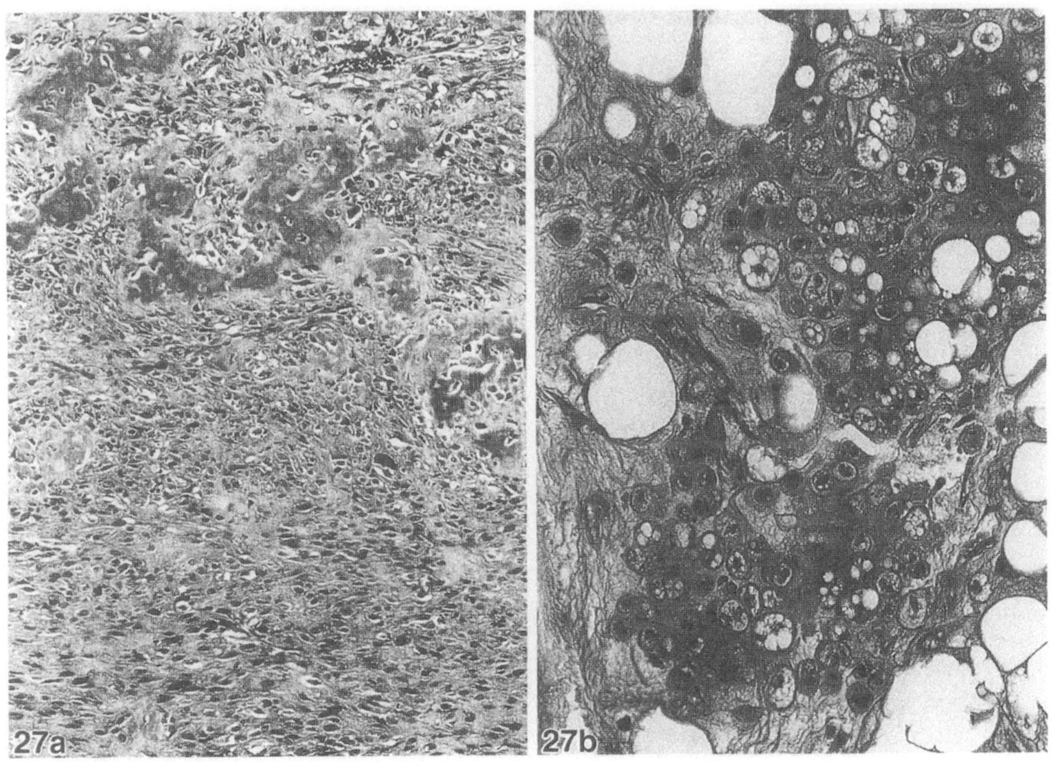

Fig. 26 a, b. Cell polymorphism, large nuclei and osteochondroid formation characterise this osteogenic sarcoma of the soft tissues of the foot

Fig. 27 a, b. Osteosarcoma of popliteal fossa. **a** Osteogenesis and cytonuclear anomalies are clearly visible. This chondroid zone suggests a particular form of diffuse oncocytic chondromatosis, from which this osteosarcoma has probably developed (**b**)

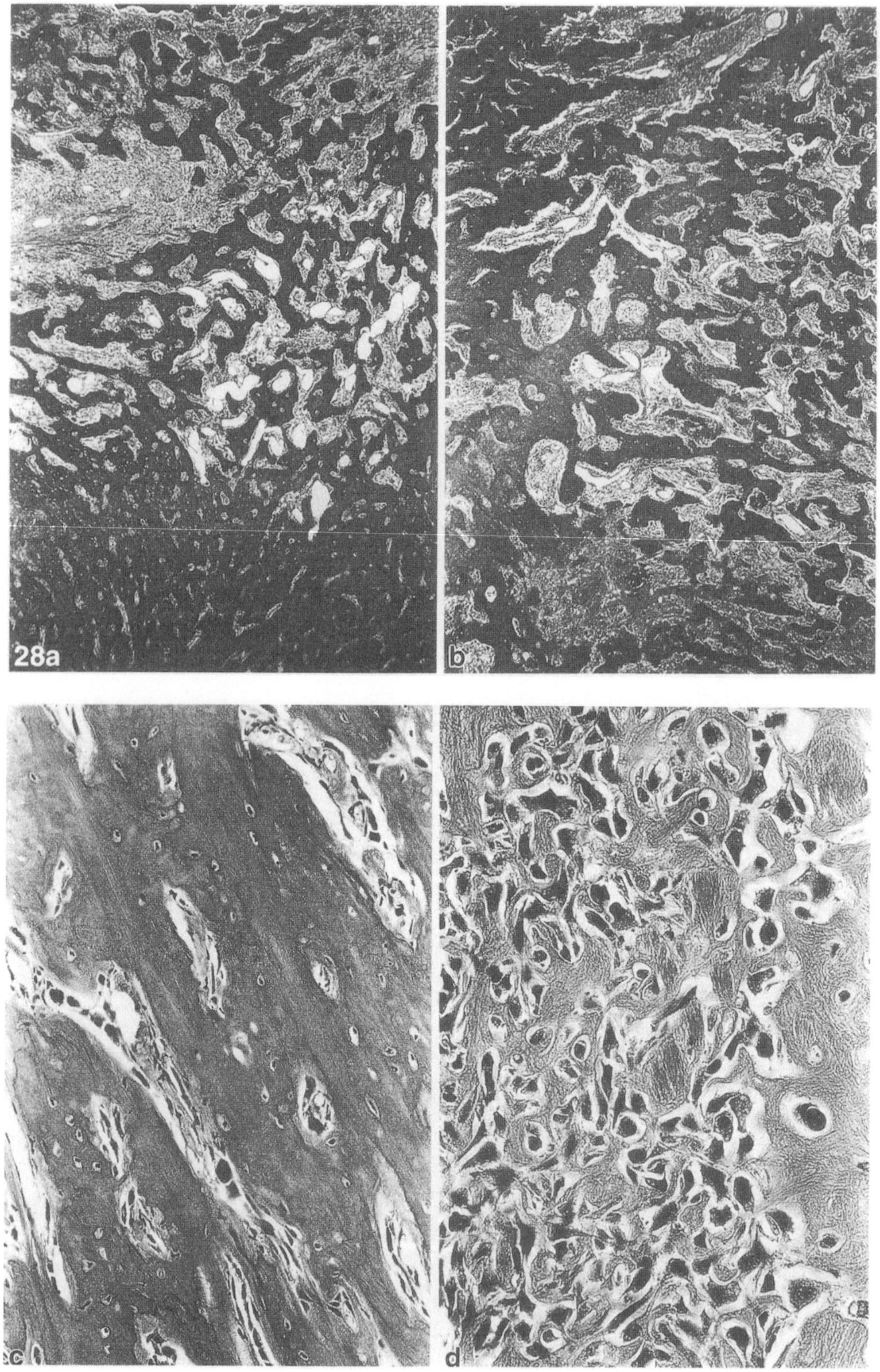

Fig. 28 a-d. The sections in figs. 28 and 29 concern an osteosarcoma of the nape of the neck. **a, b** At low magnification osteogenesis is quite regular, formed of apparently mature bony trabeculae; this osteogenesis represents the greater surface of the sections and may suggest an osteoma. **c** In other zones the osteogenesis is atypical and immature but the small osteocytes do not have a tumour like appearance, though between the strands the osteoblasts and their precursors are clearly pathological. **d** At a further stage the osteoid tissue is elaborated by a sarcomatous cellular component

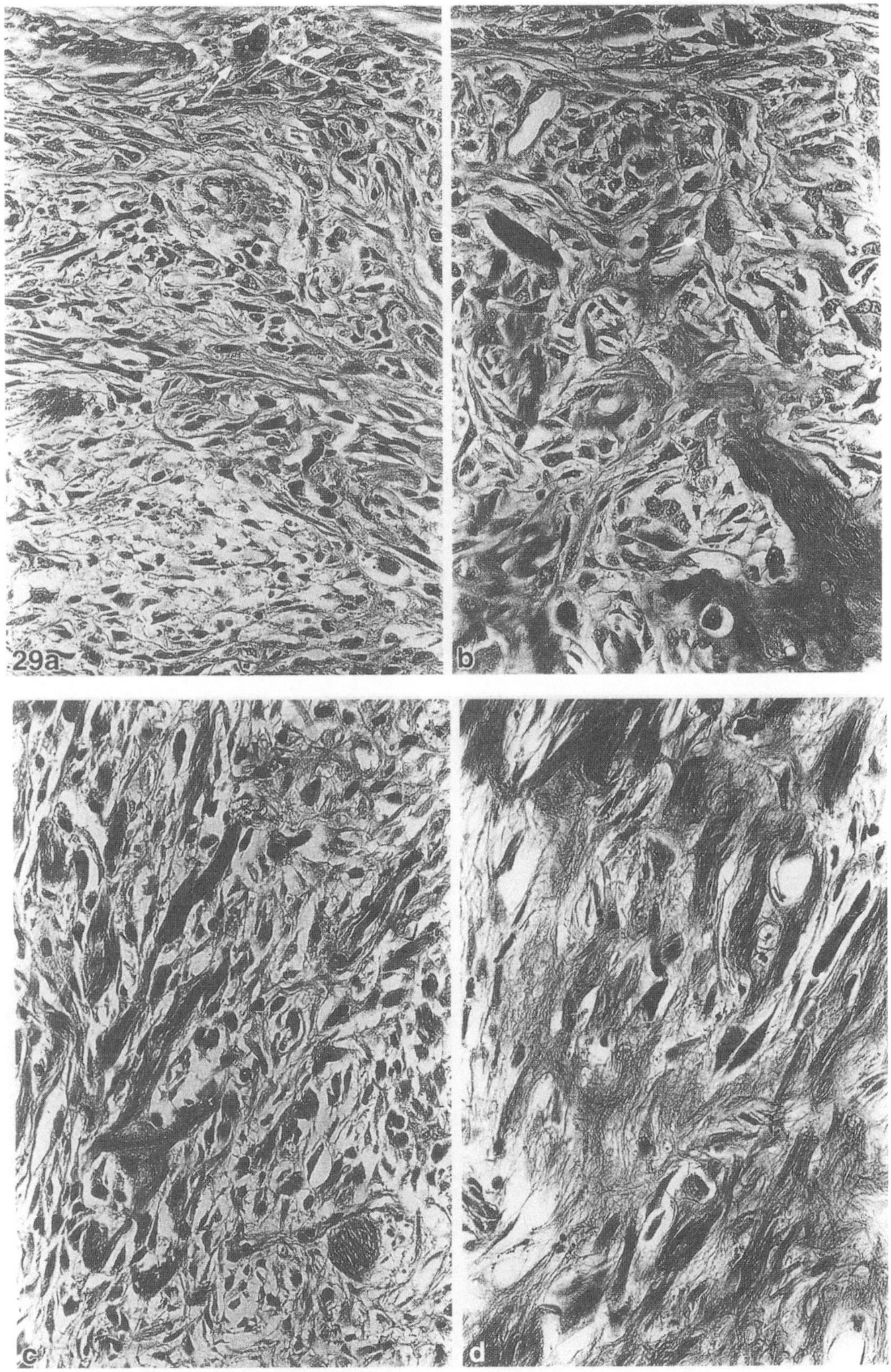

Fig. 29. a, b At the periphery of the tumour the cells have a very irregular size and shape and are generally more fusiform, with abnormal mitoses (*arrows*). **c, d** Moreover, the tumour shows no boundaries from the adjacent tissues, whether ordinary connective or fibrotendinous. This is therefore an osteogenic tumour unrelated to the underlying occipital bone, developing in a sarcomatous tissue (Courtesy of Mme Professeur Lecomte-Houcke)

40. Bony and osteoperiosteal pseudotumours

Periosteal fasciitis (figs. 1-3)

The nodular fasciitis described by Konvaler et al in 1955 in the subcutaneous soft tissues, often in connection with a superficial or muscular aponeurosis, sometimes develops in contact with the periosteum or even arises from it [Hutter et al 1962].

General considerations

Though common in the soft tissues, this lesion is rare in its periosteal site. The rapidly growing nodular structure measures 2-3 cm in diameter, rarely more, and is not encapsulated. It may create an impression on the adjacent cortex. A cranial lesion in children aged from a few weeks to six years [Lauer & Enzinger 1980] may be disconcerting for the pathologist. The growth of the fasciitis is rapid, about two months, and in the radiographs the lesion involves the subjacent bone, the outer table, and in some cases the inner table and adheres to the dura mater.

Pathological anatomy and histopathology

The macroscopic and microscopic appearances are identical with those described for the tumour of the soft tissues. Its consistency is firm when it is rich in collagen, soft or gelatinous when it is oedematous. There is no reason why this lesion should not reproduce the various characteristics of the soft tissue tumour in its periosteal location, but to our knowledge there has been no major series of cases of nodular periosteal fasciitis to confirm this assumption.

Histological study reveals a structure of fibroblastic nature, with the fibroblasts arranged in short intermingled bundles. Collagen formation is more or less abundant and separates the fibroblastic bundles. However, in some forms the cell bundles are spread apart by a substance rich in mucopolysaccharides which is alcian-blue positive, a reaction abolished by hyaluronidase treatment. The fibroblasts have a relatively large nucleus and a plainly visible nucleolus. Some mitoses are seen but these are not atypical. There is also a discrete lymphocytic infiltration.

Differential diagnosis

Depending on the macroscopic and microscopic findings, the pathologist must exclude a juxtacortical sarcoma, fibromatosis, myxoma or a myxoid schwannoma. There is no feature that argues seriously in favor of a juxtacortical sarcoma (cf Chapter 11).

A myxoma is avascular (or nearly so) and its slender cells are dispersed in a mucopolysaccharide substance. We may add that any confusion would not be serious for the patient since excision, as with fasciitis, is normally followed by cure.

A fibromatosis may be difficult to exclude, but in fasciitis the fibroblastic bundles are short, the collagen is usually less dense than in fibromatosis, and lastly there are nearly always myxoid zones in fasciitis. In the cases of musculo-aponeurotic fibromatosis we have examined, the lesion was usually more extensive, without definite boundaries and markedly richer in collagen.

As for schwannoma, this may be suggested, but apart from the positive immunohistological reaction (PS 100) a search must be made for vessels with a thick hyaline wall and palisades and cell whorls, features which are not present in fasciitis.

Table 1. Periostosis, associated periostitis

Differential diagnosis
Primary or secondary bone tumours and non-tumour bone lesions (infective, infarcts, stress fractures)
Risk: superficial biopsy which misses the underlying lesion
Juxtaosseous tumours or pseudotumours (angioma, fasciitis, myositis)
Risk: confusing these lesions with an osteoperiosteal lesion (juxtacortical sarcoma)
Affections characterised by contingent periosteal reaction (rheumatic, neurological, bronchial tumour)
In these cases the only problem posed by the periostosis is lack of specificity

Periostosis, periostitis (figs. 4-15)

In the preceding chapters we have mentioned the main tumours, which may develop at a juxtacortical site whether of bony origin or not, and their differential diagnosis has been discussed.

General considerations

It must be accepted that, apart from certain well-defined tumours, some biopsies of periosteal osteogenesis cannot be specifically identified. The terms "periostosis" or "periostitis" of unknown aetiology then amount to a pathological description which adds little information to that provided by imaging.

Numerous causes may give rise to periosteal osteogenesis (see Tables 1 and 2 and Chapter 41 on heterotopic ossification). The periosteum is quick to react to the least provocation. Experiment readily shows that the necrosis of some superficial osteocytes in a diaphyseal cortex provokes the onset of periosteal osteogenesis in a few hours. Subperiosteal haemorrhage, whatever the cause (avitaminosis, neurofibromatosis), may give rise to extensive periostosis. The patient usually attends because of pain.

The search for an aetiology

When there is periosteal elaboration of bone or osteoid which is not neoplastic, one must ensure that this is a local lesion and not a variably diffuse periosteal reaction. The causes of this are numerous (haemodialysis, vascular lesions, secondary hyperparathyroidism, avitaminosis, lung tumours and falciform-cell anaemia [Guerra et al 1984]. Once it is certain that the lesion is purely local, it is essential to ascertain by imaging that there is no deeply situated tumour which may be inaccessible to superficial biopsy.

The clinical and radiographic study may demonstrate a fatigue fracture [Arrivé et al 1988], circulatory disturbance (varices, angiomas) or a local infection. Though unproved, an unnoticed local injury is often regarded as responsible for the periostosis. Despite the lack of a demonstrable cause, cure is often definitive after surgery; but in many cases caution demands careful and prolonged local surveillance. In the case reported by Yoshida et al (1988) an amyloid periosteal tumour in a woman of 66 remained solitary for 7 years without any general disorder of protein metabolism.

Insertional disorders; strain osteotendinitis

(figs. 16-29)

General considerations, case history

The problem facing the pathologist usually arises in a stereotyped fashion. A young patient between 12 and 16 complains of vague pain of some weeks' duration in one knee, then more localised to the posterior aspect. A radiograph reveals a lytic lesion behind and above the medial condyle of the femur with "invasion of the soft tissues". Two or three days later the pathologist receives a biopsy marked "urgent" accompanied by the above information.

The time required for the histological examination can be used to obtain some complementary details. It will be found that the osteolytic zone is slightly tender to pressure, that the young patient is a keen sportsman (or woman), the pride of his club and the third piece of information, if available, provides the diagnosis; a radiograph of the opposite knee, requested by the pathologist, shows an identical lesion. A simple radiograph of both knees often reveals a completely asymptomatic symmetrical lesion, without having recourse to more sophisticated techniques (fig. 19).

Pathological anatomy and histopathology

Histological examination demonstrates a major, but very localised, bony remodelling. There are osteoclastic phenomena, with minute sequestra in a richly cellular and sometimes very vascular connective tissue. The cortex on this small surface is destroyed and the invasion of the soft tissues described in the radiologist's report corresponds to the ossification of some tendinous and aponeurotic fibers. This osteogenesis is bordered by small rows of osteoblasts but there are no cell anomalies, nuclear monstrosities or atypical mitoses.

At the onset this is a cellular and vascular reaction which becomes fibrous, with the eventual elaboration of chondroid and finally bony tissue. This last condition may be interpreted as an attempt at the repair of fragmentary avulsion of the tendon insertion.

Other sites

The problem posed is less formal in other sites such as the ankle, elbow or pubis, and at particular sites subjected to overstrain associated with occupational activities.

Course

Prolonged monitoring of the patient will dispel any anxiety but it must be realised that restoration to normal as followed on the radiographs usually takes many months.

Various terms have been used to designate these lesions, but what matters in the pathological report is to describe the benign reactive nature of this lesion developing in a zone of osteotendinous attachment, probably as a result of excessive traction.

Justification for biopsy and diagnosis

Apart from cases with bilateral lesions, surgical biopsy is justified because of the anxiety aroused by the radiological report, and also because of the fact that very similar images may pertain to a cortical fibrous defect, a juxtacortical sarcoma or a so-called stress fracture, as in the case of Pistolesi et al (1991). This was a young girl of 13 with pain in the lower end of the femur after several falls from a bicycle; only MRI revealed the presence of a transverse fracture. Overall, two manifestations of overstrain are relatively common in the lower limb; ligamentous avulsion and fatigue fracture. The first is perhaps commoner in adolescence, the second in young adults (the so-called conscripts' fracture).

Bone infarction, osteonecrosis and osteochondritis (figs. 30-50)

General considerations

The causes of osteomedullary necrosis are many and the pathogenic mechanisms diverse. The maximum incidence for detection of infarcts is around the 40th year. Necrosis of the femoral head, necrosis due to barotrauma, necrosis in irradiated territory or after fracture are all usually diagnosed before pathological study or are strongly suspected in renal dialysis, uraemia and patients submitted to prolonged corticosteroid treatment [Paologgi 1980-1983]. Those given antimitotic agents or affected by metabolic disorders (storage illnesses), haemoglobinopathies (drepanocytosis)and vasculitis may also develop infarctions.

Clinical features

In 15% of cases the infarct is clinically asymptomatic [Zizic et al 1986]. In the same series, dealing with 169 cases, 59% of the patients had several lesions, so that 310 bones were affected. In 20 patients suffering from metaphyseal and diaphyseal idiopathic aseptic necrosis studied by Lafforgue et al (1990), the lesion was painful in 6. The infarcts were situated mainly in the lower limbs and were multiple and symmetrical in 12 patients; of the 65 lesions listed, 77% were situated around the knee.

In cases where the necrosis is asymptomatic, the lesion is a radiological discovery. Conversely, it may develop suddenly with intense localised pain which is the motive for biopsy; whereas standard radiography supplies little or no information, CT and MRI usually provide important data. Studies of the intraosseous arterial and especially venous pressures may provide proof of a circulatory anomaly but these examinations are not routinely practicable.

Lastly, the pathologist is faced with a complex problem; to identify the infarct and recognise the associated lesions with the aim of arriving at an appropriate aetiology and treatment.

Pathological anatomy and histopathology

In a recent necrosis, the pathological examination reveals an unchanged bony framework and stainable osteocytes, but early medullary remodelling related to the necrosis of the adipose tissue is seen. This necrosis of fatty cells is associated with a marked macro-

Table 2. Periostoses and periostitis as first manifestation

The periostitis or periostosis is pathologically non-specific (common). Clinical examination discloses aetiology
The periostitis is inflammatory with necrotic foci. Bacterial or mycotic cause. More precise diagnosis rests on culture and the histochemical and immunohistological reactions
The periostosis is the outcome of an underlying bony lesion. The cortical bone is usually modified (enlarged Haversian canals, cellular activity). A deposit of fibrin, a cartilaginous island, point to a missed fracture (osteomalacia, stress fracture)
The periostosis (or periostitis) is connected with a soft tissue juxtaosseous lesion (vascular anomalies, angioma, neurovascular hamartoma, neuroma)

phage histiocytic cellular reaction but also, in our experience, with an attempted lipoblastic regeneration doomed to virtually total failure, fibrosis finally suppressing any restoration to normal.

Early biopsies made using a trocar do not permit proper examination of the surrounding tissues [Arlet et al 1968].

At a more advanced stage of necrosis, the standard radiographs may show heterogeneous opacities of different types; investigation with MRI, which is much more sensitive than CT examination [Lafforgue et al 1990] may provide near-characteristic images, sometimes associated with periostitis. In cases where the necrotic zone is examined after a period such that ostemedullary remodelling has occurred, not only is the marrow replaced by fibrous tissue (strongly calcified in places) but the remaining fragments of the partly absorbed bony trabeculae are also hypercalcified. Local physico-chemical phenomena provoke a marked calcium deposition which is shown by very dense radiological opacity.

It is important to make the pathological diagnosis of infarction since in over 50% of cases the lesions are multiple; further, various malignant tumours (malignant fibrous histiocytoma, osteosarcoma) have developed on an old infarction. Torres and Kyriakos (1992) found 50 cases of osteosarcoma developing in an infarct. In 38 well-documented cases, there were 26 men and 12 women. Several years had elapsed between the infarction and the development of osteosarcoma. The mortality of these osteosarcomas was of the order of 60-70% at 5 years. Malignant fibrous histiocytoma develops on a bony infarct relatively more often than does osteosarcoma.

Another problem is to recognise the resumption of activity of a previously treated tumour in contact with an infarct. In standard films an infarct may suggest an osteoma, osteoid osteoma or calcified cartilaginous tumour, mistakes easily corrected by histological examination.

Osteochondritis

It is necessary to consider metaphyseo-diaphyseal ostemedullary infarctions, with osteochondritides of various joints. Osteochondritis of the knee often results in material submitted to the pathologist to resolve the following problem; "is this solitary intra-articular nodule of the knee, a nodule of osteochondritis or osteochondromatosis?". There is a difficulty in relation to old osteochondritis, when the niche in which the sequestrum was lodged is almost filled by newly-formed bony and fibrocartilaginous tissue and the nodule of osteochondritis has been remodelled over the years and its deep aspect is entirely covered by fibrocartilage. Although it is possible to recognise the articular cartilage with its calcified basal line for a long time and to distinguish it from newly-formed fibrocartilage, this becomes impossible in a really old nodule. The difficulty is compounded when the nodule of osteochondritis is very superficial, since the few bony trabeculae which supported the articular cartilage may be totally eliminated by repeated friction in the joint.

If the surgeon has removed some synovial fringe at the same time as the solitary nodule, the presence of intrasynovial metaplastic cartilaginous zones will suggest the diagnosis of osteochondromatosis (cf Chapter 39).

Mastocytosis with bony presentation

(figs. 51, 52)

General considerations and case history

The bony lesions of mastocytosis may form part of a complex clinical picture of systemic mastocytosis, usually developing in an adult [de Sèze et al 1968, Deshayes et al 1969, Duriez 1975, Brunning et al 1983]. However, some rare cases of mastocytosis with bony presentation have been reported; I have observed only two cases of this type.

Case history

A colleague aged 60 complained of spinal pain and an increase in kyphosis. There were no relevant previous illnesses. The radiographs revealed diffuse vertebral decalcification and a wedge-shaped collapse of the first lumbar vertebra. Suspicion of a malignant metastasis or plasmocytic lesion called for vertebral biopsy by trocar, which allowed the diagnosis of mastocytosis.

Clinical features

Those patients without cutaneous features have a higher average age than those who do, and splenomegaly is more common [Brunning et al 1983]. The preferentially affected bones are the skull, ribs, vertebrae, pelvis and more rarely the long bones of the limbs. These are mainly bones with a marked haematopoietic activity, which are the site of osteosclerotic and osteolytic remodelling [Meister & Rablers 1987]. Mastocytosis in the absence of pigmented urticaria and any other cutaneous manifestation often presents with bone pain, in 3 cases out of 6 in the thesis of Prier (1972).

Imaging

The radiological features are sometimes those of bony lysis, rarely sclerosis, more often a mixture of sclerosing and lytic changes. The patient of Schweitzer et al (1989), a man of 55 who had no skin lesions, presented with multiple areas of vertebral osteosclerosis; that of Rodenberg et al (1986), who did have skin changes, also exhibited multiple lytic and sclerotic bony lesions. The lesions may be diffuse or localised, particularly in children.

Pathological anatomy and histopathology

Examination of sections allows identification of the presence of mastocytes, sometimes in a very fibrous marrow. The mastocytes, abnormally numerous, are grouped around the vessels or arranged at the margins along the bony trabeculae. They may assume very varied forms but their cytoplasm contains fine granules metachromatic to toluidin blue. Even in specimens fixed in formol or Zinker's agent and then decalcified, the toluidin blue test is positive. However, it is simpler to make smears on slides in the operating room, which allows testing with toluidin blue (pH between 4 and 7) and the demonstration of chloroacetate esterase. The mastocytes are also well shown by the reactive antibody CD68 (KP1) and even though this reaction is non-specific, strong positivity of the suspect cells plus the demonstration of chloroacetate esterase virtually establishes the diagnosis. Some reports mention a considerably increased number of osteoclasts associated with the osteolysis. Rare cases of osteomalacia have been reported associated with mastocytosis [Coindre et al 1983) and it is well known that the number of mastocytes is increased in osteomalacia, whether experimental [Urist & McDean 1957] or human [Rebel et al 1974]. The cause of the osteomalacia is to be sought in terms of intestinal malabsorption and not in the hyper-mastocytosis, which is reactive. The pathogenesis of the osteosclerosis is still not clear.

Pagetic and pagetoid remodelling

(figs. 53-60)

Undiagnosed Paget's disease

Imaging does not always allow the diagnosis of an isolated bony remodelling, whether vertebral, iliac or in a long bone of the limbs. This diagnostic uncertainty logically calls for biopsy.

Pathological anatomy and histopathology

Examination of the sections may reveal a number of changes.

There may be an appearance definitely characteristic of progressive Paget's disease which combines medullary fibrosis and hypervascularity, osteoclastic activity which gives rise to poorly calcified bone, and osteoblastic activity which forms lines of arrested growth in basophil arabesques (fig. 53 a). If the decalcification has been excessive these lines of arrest are replaced by dehiscences which mark out a real jigsaw puzzle (fig. 59). Superficially, the periosteum, sensitive to the underlying turmoil, rapidly lays down an envelope of normal bone (fig. 54 a, b).

In some cases, when there are radiological and/or clinical changes in an established case the pathologist has to distinguish an active advancing phase from sarcomatous transformation.

Alternatively, an appearance of stabilised, arrested Paget's disease may be seen (fig. 49). The storm has subsided but the landscape has changed; the cellular activity is extinct. The pattern of the lines of arrest persists, the osteoid is calcified, sometimes heavily, leading to radiological images of densification (black ver-

Table 3. Paget's disease and pagetoid remodelling

The Paget's disease is clearly characterised by:
- poorly calcified bone
- appositions, irregular destruction (jigsaw appearance)
- hypercellularity, hypervascularity, fibrosis

The Paget's disease is stabilised:
- persistent anarchic architecture of the bone
- subsidence of excessive cellularity and vascularity

The Paget's disease is hyperactive:
- little bony tissue
- cellularity ++, vascularisation ++

A rapid bony remodelling localised to a Pagetic bone raises problems of:
- sarcomatous transformation
- giant-cell tumour
- localised focus of hyperactivity (exclude osteoclastoma, osteoblastoma)
- metastatic lesion
- chance association with other tumours

tebra, ivory vertebra). The fibrous marrow is "normally" vascularised.

An appearance of hyperactive Paget's disease is less common and here the osteoblastic and osteoclastic activity are such that they leave no hope of calcification of the newly-formed trabeculae, which are incessantly remodelled and devoid of lines of arrest (fig. 56). The histological image of hyperactive Paget's disease may suggest an osteoblastoma or a giant-cell tumour (fig. 57).

The rare cases of Paget's disease of porotic type are extensive in my experience, but their diagnosis was difficult radiologically and histologically. From the histological aspect the dominant feature was osteoporosis. The marrow was more fatty than fibrous. The fine, rarefied bone trabeculae were traversed by a packed network of lines of arrest. Osteoblastic and osteoclastic activity were very reduced.

"Spontaneous" fracture in Paget's disease is commonplace and progress to consolidation is the rule. The osteoclastic and osteoblastic activity characteristic of the Paget's disease persists in the vicinity of the fracture. A zone of necrosis and haemorrhage is usual in the fracture region. Medullary fibrosis, common in Paget's disease, does not signify a fibroblastic sarcoma. It is quite possible that hyperactivity of the lesion, localised in time and space, has given rise to the fracture.

Pseudo-pagetic (pagetoid) appearances

The characteristic radiographic features are enlargement of a vertebra or thickening of a long bone. But if the clinical information is inadequate and the imaging is not available to the pathologist, his report must be particularly cautious. Pagetic and pagetoid remodelling are very difficult to distinguish and remodelling may conceal a metastasis (from the prostate or breast in particular). These metastatic lesions are probably commoner than the rare published cases would suggest [Taillandier et al 1984, Larbre et al 1991].

Pseudo-pagetic appearances may be seen adjacent to an inflammatory focus, or in a bony infarct, an osteogenic sarcoma, or the nidus of an osteoid osteoma.

Skeletogenic sarcoma

Every type of skeletogenic sarcoma has been described, including a form rich in giant cells, fibroblastic sarcomas and malignant fibrous histiocytomas. Given the inevitable architectural anarchy of a fracture in hyperactive Paget's disease, the diagnosis of sarcoma cannot be confirmed unless the findings of cytological and mitotic anomalies are beyond doubt. In 82 tumours developing in a pagetic bone, Haibach et al (1985) listed 77 osteosarcomas, 3 fibrosarcomas, 1 chondrosarcoma and one giant-cell tumour. In 43 cases where radiological study was possible, the authors identified 69% mixed forms, 21% "osteoblastic forms" and 10% osteolytic forms. The series of Hadjipavlou et al (1992), dealing with 1078 patients affected by Paget's disease, revealed a rate of malignant transformation of 0.7%. In half the patients such transformation was heralded by a pathological fracture with osteolysis. The extent of the periosteal reaction is very variously assessed, and non-existent for Moore et al (1991); on the contrary, Khraishi et al (1991) find it suggests a diagnosis of sarcoma.

The problem posed by a giant-cell "tumour" in a pagetic bone is not particularly difficult. Whatever its degree of mimicry, the particular accompanying circumstance do not allow it to be considered as a true giant-cell tumour (cf Chapter 2). We repeat that osteoclastic hyperactivity does not signify progressive malignancy.

Chance associations

The appearance of a zone of osteolysis in Paget's disease may be due to other causes: a drug effect [Roudier et al 1984], hyperparathyroidism [Bhate et al 1979], the chance association of a lymphoma [Molle et al 1983] or a desmoid fibroma [Hillmann et al 1988].

References

Fasciitis

Callahan DJ, Walter NE, Okoye MJ (1985) Florid reactive periostitis of the proximal phalanx. J Bone Joint Surg 67A: 968-970

Hutter RVP, Foote FW, Francis KC, Higinbotham NL (1962) Parosteal fasciitis. A self-limited benign process that simulates a malignant neoplasm. Am J Surg 104: 800-807

Konvaler BE, Keasby L, Kaplan L (1955) Subcutancous pseudosarcomatous fibromatosis (fasciitis). Am J Clin Pathol 25: 241-252

Kwitthen J, Branche M (1969) Fasciitis ossificans. Am J Clin Pathol 51: 251-255

Laver DH, Enzinger FM (1980) Cranial fasciitis of childhood. Cancer 45: 401-406

Price EB, Silliphant WM, Shuman R (1961) Nodular fasciitis: a clinicopathologic analysis of 65 cases. Am J Clin Pathol 35: 122-136

Spjut HJ, Dorfman HD (1981) Florid reactive periostitis of the tubular bones of the hands and feet. A benign lesion which may simulate osteosarcoma. Am J Surg Pathol 5: 422-433

Periostosis

Arrivé L, Sellier N, Kalifa G, Seringe R (1988) Difficultés diagnostiques des appositions périostées unilamellaires symptomatiques isolées. Forme inhabituelle des fractures de fatigue de l'enfant. J Radiol 69: 351-356

Fauré C (1969) Diagnostic radiologique des hyperostoses cortico-périostées du tout jeune nourrisson. Concours Med 5: 3799-3810

Guerra J, Resnick D, Cone R, Saltzstein S (1984) Periosteal (parosteal, juxta cortical) vascular malformation. Skeletal Radiol 11: 303-306

Jougeward RH, Martel W, Louis DS, Okoye MI, Walter N (1985) Florid reactive periostitis proximal phalanx of the left 5th finger. Case report. Skeletal Radiol 13: 169-173

Lequesne M, Barreau J, Mazabraud A, Lemoine A, Djian A, Lapresle CL (1981) Images trompeuses au cours des pasteurelloses digitales. Du liseré périosté à l'image pseudotumorale. Rev Rhum 48: 163-168

Meem HE, Orcopoulos DG, Rabinovich S, Hesdan H, Rapoport A (1974) Periosteal new bone fornation (periosteal neostosis) in renal osteodystrophy. Radiology 110: 513-522

Tamarozzi R, Bedani PL, Scutellari PN, Orzincolo C, Pinna L, Farinelli (1984) Periosteal new bone in uraemic osteodystrophy. Skeletal Radiol 11: 50-53

Wiggins T, Bohrer SP (1986) "Ulcer osteoma" associated with sickle cell disease. Skeletal Radiol 11: 303-306

Yoshida SD, Karjoo R, Jonhnstone MR (1988) Periosteal amyloid tumor. Skeletal Radiol 17: 226-230

Insertional disorders

Catonne Y (1990) Table ronde SOFCOT. Nov 89: Lésions traumatiques des tendons des membres inférieurs chez le sportif. Rev Chir Orthop 76 (suppl 1): 131-149

Dunoyer J (1991) Les enthésites. Ann Orthop Ouest 23: 62-63

Pistolesi GF, Caudana R, d'Attoma N, Residori E, Pregarz M (1991) Stress fracture at distal end of femur simulating "periosteal desmoid". Skeletal Radiol 20: 454-457

Bone infarction, osteonecrosis, osteochondritis

Arlet J, Ficat P, Lartigue G (1968) Mode de début de l'ostéonocrose fémoro-capitale primitive. Etude de 20 observations histologiquement prouvées par le forage-biopsie. Rev Rhum 35: 239-256

Cruess RL (1986) Osteonecrosis of bone. Current concepts as to etiology and pathogenesis. Clin Orthop 208: 30-39

Dang Vu V, You B, Bresson A, Claudon M, Grilliat JP (1990) Infarctus osseux et maladie de Behçet. Rhumathol 42: 173-177

de Sèze S, Jaffres R, Merer P, Mitrovic D, Mazabraud A (1963) Aspects histologiques de l'ostéonécrose aseptique barotraumatique. Sem Hop Paris 39: 869-878

Delaunay C, Le Balc'h, Mazas F (1986) Ostéonécrose aseptique non traumatique de la tête fémorale. Considérations étiopathogéniques, évolutives et thérapeutiques. Revue de la littérature. Rev Chir Orthop 72: 127-138

Gregg PJ, Walder DN (1986) Caisson disease of bone. Clin Orthop 210: 43-54

Hall MC, Elmore SM, Bright RW, Pierce JC, Hume DM (1969) Skeletal complications in a series of human renal allografts. JAMA 208: 1825-1829

Hardy PH, Hinojosa JF, Coudane H, Sommelet J, Benoit J (1992) L'ostéochondrite disséquante du cotyle. A propos d'un cas. Rev Chir Orthop 78: 134-137

Heater K, Collins PA (1987) Osteosarcoma in association with infarctus of bone. Report of two cases. J Bone Joint Surg 69A: 300-302

Jaffres R, Merer P (1964) Les localisations extra-épiphysaires de l'ostéonécrose barotraumatique. Rev Rhum 31: 272-276

Kahlstrom SC, Burton CC, Phemister DB (1939) Aseptic necrosis of bone. II. Infarction of bones of undetermined etiology resulting in encapsulated and calcified areas in diaphyses and in arthritis deformans. Surg Gynecol Obstet 68: 631-664

Lafforgue P, Schiano A, Acquaviva PC (1990) Les infarctus osseux, ou ostéonécroses aseptiques métaphysaires et diaphysaires "idiopathiques" des os longs. Mise au point et apport des nouvelles imageries. Rev Rhum 57: 359-366

Lecestre P, Dabos N, Benoit J, Ramadier JO (1977) L'ostéonécrose aseptique chez le transplanté rénal. A propos de 27 cas opérés. Rev Chir Orthop 63: 373-391

Marymont JV, Kaufman EE (1986) Osteonecrosis of bone associated with combination chemotherapy without corticosteroids. Clin Orthop 204: 150-153

Merle d'Aubigné R, Postel M, Mazabraud A, Massias P, Gueguen J (1965) Idiopathic necrosis of the femoral head in adults. J Bone Joint Surg 47A :612-633

Mirra JM, Bullough PG, Marcove RC, Jacobs B, Huvos AG (1974) Malignant fibrous histiocytoma and osteosarcoma in association with bone infarctus. Report of four cases, two in caisson workers. J Bone Joint Surg 56A :932-940

Paologgi JB (1983) Ostéonécroses cortisoniques. Rhumatologie 35: 183-188

Paologgi JB, Le Parc JM, Durigon M, Barrés D, Paolaggi F, Arfi S, Auquier L (1980) Ostéonécroses cortisoniques: acquisitions tirées de l'observation chez l'homme et confrontation avec les résultats de l'expérimentation animale. Rev Rhum 47: 719-729

Péré P, Adolphe J, Delgoffe C, Gaucher A (1984) Ostéonécroses épiphysaires, infarctus osseux multiples et histiocytome fibreux malin. Rev Rhum 51: 427-430

Rossleigh MA, Smith J, Strauss DJ, Engel IA (1986) Osteonecrosis in patients with malignant lymphoma: a review of 31 cases. Cancer 58: 1112-1116

Torres FX, Kyriakos M (1992) Bone infarct-associated osteosarcoma. Cancer 70: 2418-2430

Wuisman P, Erleman R, Roessner A, Bosse A, Kusniez-Glaz C (1991) Osteonecrosis of bone associated with intraarterial therapy using cisplatin. Skeletal Radiol 20: 294-298

Zizic TM, Marcoux C, Hungerford DS, Steven MB (1986) The early diagnosis of ischemic necrosis of bone. Arthritis Rhum 29: 1177-1186

Mastocytosis

Brunning RD, McKenna RW, Rosai J, Parkin JL, Risdall R (1983) Systemic mastocytosis. Extracutaneous manifestations. Am J Surg Pathol 7: 425-438

Coindre JM, Goudet-Lunel G, David-Chausse J, Mascarel (de) A, Meuge-Moraw C (1983) Mastocytose osseuse et ostéomalacie. A propos d'un cas avec étude histodynamique sur un os non décalcifié. Ann Pathol 3: 69-71

Deshayes P, Arinal C, Dreyfus P, Dryll A, Hubault A, Matrajt H, Sèze (de) S (1969) Les localisations osseuses de la mastocytose. Sem Hop Paris 45: 524-530

Duriez J (1975) L'atteinte osseuse au cours de la mastocytose cutanée. A propos de deux observations. Rev Rhum 42: 71-74

Hills E, Dunstan CR, Evans RA (1981) Bone metabolism in systemic mastocytosis. A case report. J Bone Joint Surg 63A: 665-669

Homy HP, Parwaresch MR, Lennert K (1985) Bone marrow in systemic mastocytosis. Hum Pathol 16: 808-814

Lortholary O, Audouin J, Le Toumeau A, Diebold J (1991) Le mastocyte et sa pathologie. 2ème partie: histopathologie des mastocytoses. Ann Pathol 11: 92-100

Meister HP, Rabben V (1987) Systemic mastocytosis. Skeletal Radiol 16: 158-162

Prier A (1972) Mastocytose osseuse. Revue de la littérature à propos de 6 cas. Thèse, Paris

Prost A, Malkani K, Cottin S, Rebel A (1974) Etude au microscope électronique des mastocytoses de l'os dans un cas d'ostéoporose associé à une mastocytose cutanée. Pathol Biol 22: 483-490

Rafii M, Firooznia H, Golimbu C, Balthazar E (1983) Pathologic fracture in systernic mastocytosis. Radiographic spectrum and review of the literature. Clin Orthop 180: 260-267

Rebel A, Riberi P, Bregean P, Malkani K (1974) Mastocytoses et remaniements du tissu osseux. Pathol Biol 22: 213-220

Rodenberg JC, Macgaard KK, Sranholm H (1986) Systemic mastocytosis. Case report. Skeletal Radiol 15: 334-337

Schweitzer ME, Irwin GAL (1989) Systemic mastocytosis. Case report. Skeletal Radiol 18: 411-413

Sèze S (de), Hioco D, Matrajt H, Tunchot S, Hubault A, Dreyfus P (1968) Ostéoporose et mastocytose. Sem Hop Paris 44: 1609-1615

Urist M, McLean F (1957) Accumulation of most cells in endosteum of bones calcium-deficient rats. Arch Pathol 63: 239-251

Pagetic and pagetoid remodeling

Basle M, Rebel A, Pouplard A, Kouyoumdjian E, Filmon R, Lepatezour A (1979) Mise en évidence d'antigènes viraux de rougeole dans les ostéoclastes de la maladie de Paget. CR Acad Sci Paris Série D 289: 225-228

Basle MF, Audran M, Rebel A (1991) Aspects actuels de la maladie de Paget. Rev Med Interne 12: 424-428

Bhate DV, Supan WAP, Sparagana M, Jablokow VR, Gonzales A (1979) Paget's disease and primary hyperparathyroidism. Skeletal Radiol 4: 115-118

Dubost JJ, Galtier B, Ristori JM, Sauvezié B, Bussière JL, Rampon S (1987) Maladie de Paget et cancer prostatique. Un difficile problème diagnostique illustré par 30 observations. Rev Rhum 54: 771-774

Hadjipavlou A, Lander P, Srolovitz H, Enker P (1992) Malignant transformation in Paget's disease of bone. Cancer 70: 2802-2808

Haibach H, Farrel C, Dittrich FJ (1985) Neoplasm arising in Paget's discase of bone. A study of 82 cases. Am J Clin Pathol 83: 594-600

Hillmann JS, Mesgarzadeh M, Tang CK, Bonakdarpour A, Reyes TG (1988) Benign intraosseous fibroma (desmoplastic fibroma) associated with Paget's disease of the iliac bone. Case report. Skeletal Radiol 17: 356-360

Khraishi M, Howard B, Fam AG (1991) Paget's pseudosarcoma (letter). Arthritis Rhum 34: 241

Labre JP, Collet P, Fournier S, Biron P, Llorca G (1991) Métastase osseuse d'un adénocarcinome mammaire du sein dans un os pagétique. Sem Hop Paris 67: 467-469

Lander P, Hadjipavlou A (1986) A dynamic classification of Paget's disease. J Bone Joint Surg 68B: 431-438

Molle D, Bard H, Kuntz D, Voisin C, Farcet JP, Delepine D, Ryckewaert A (1983) Ostéolyse révélatrice d'un lymphome développé sur un os pagétique. Rev Rhum 50: 217-221

Moore TE, King AR, Kathol MH, El-Khoury GY, Palmer R,

Downey PR (1991) Sarcoma in Paget's disease of bone. Clinical, radiologic, and pathologic features in 22 cases. Am J Roentgenol 156: 1199-1203

Potter HG, Schneider R, Ghelman B, Healey JH, Lane JM (1991) Multiple giant cell tumors and Paget's diseasse of bone. Radiographic and clinical correlations. Radiology 180: 261-264

Rebel A, Basle M (1981) Maladie osseuse de Paget et virus. Ann Pathol 1: 21-26

Rebel A, Malkani K, Basle M, Bregeou CH (1974) Particularités ultrastructurales des ostéoclastes de la maladie de Paget. Rev Rhum 41: 767-771

Roudier J, Huchet B, Cayla J (1984) Ostéolyse pseudo-sarcomateuse chez un pagétique traité par l'étidronate disodique (EHDP). Rev Rhum Mal Osteoartic 51: 49-54

Schajowicz F, Araujo ES, Berenstein M (1983) Sarcoma complicating Paget's disease of bone a clinicopathological study of 62 cases. J Bone Joint Surg 65B: 299-307

Schajowicz F, Velan O, Aranjo ES, Plantalech L, Fongi E, Ottolenghi E, Fromm GA (1988) Metastases of carcinoma in the pagetic bone. A report of two cases. Clin Orthop 228: 290-296

Taillandier J, Cohen de Lara A, Manigand G (1984) Métastase osseuse d'un adénocarcinome simulant, au cours d'une maladie de Paget, une dégénérescence sarcomateuse. Sem Hop Paris 60: 2019-2021

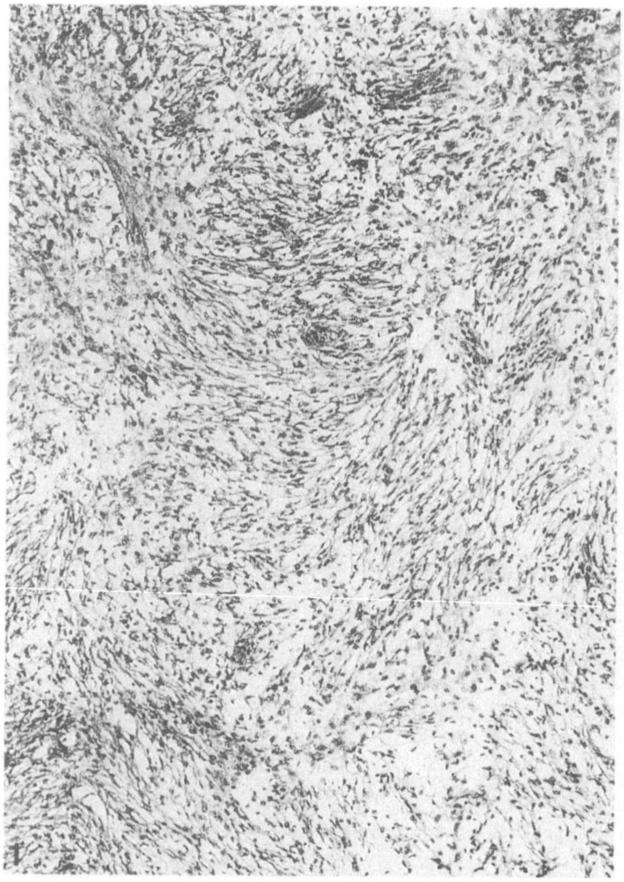

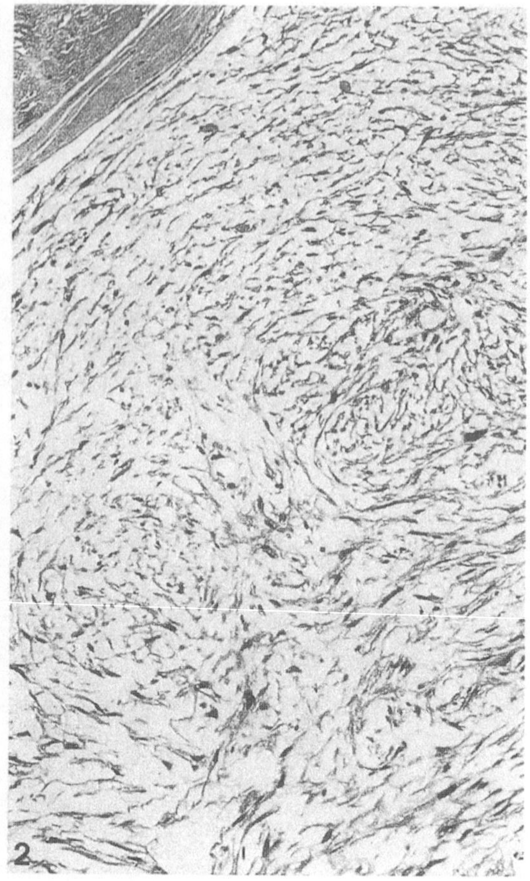

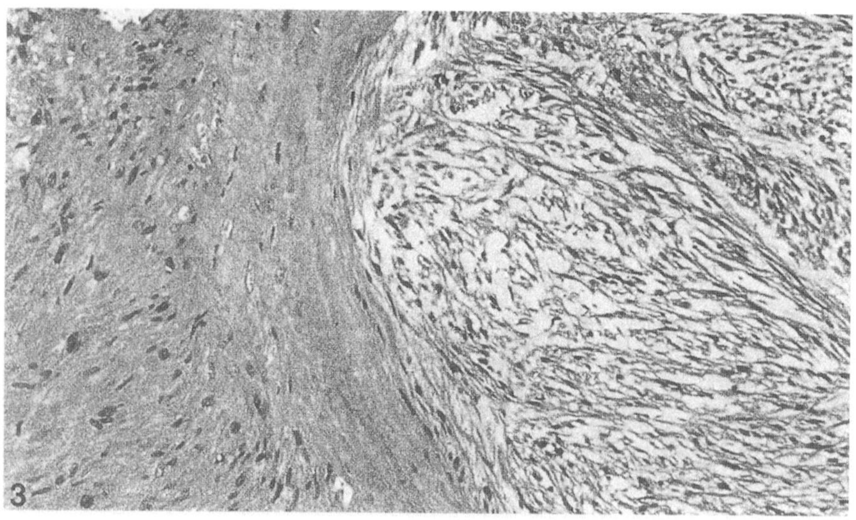

These three microphotographs, figs. 1-3, are of periosteal fasciitis

Fig. 1. Relatively cellular zone of oriented fusiform cells, mostly in bundles. Here and there macrophages with large or multiple nuclei are seen

Fig. 2. In this more lax zone with some nodular whorls the cell bundles are separated by a mucoid substance

Fig. 3. Sharp limits of this fasciitis in contact with dense fibrous bundles

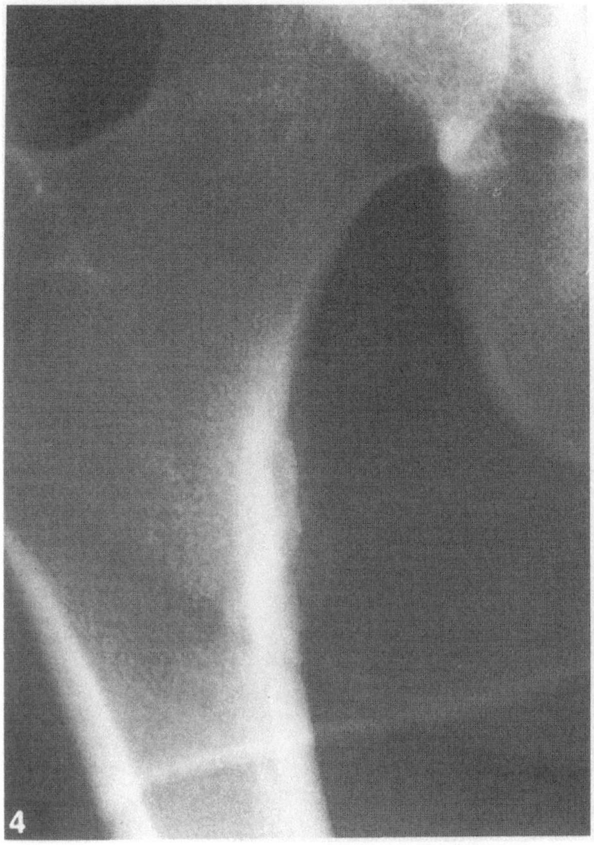

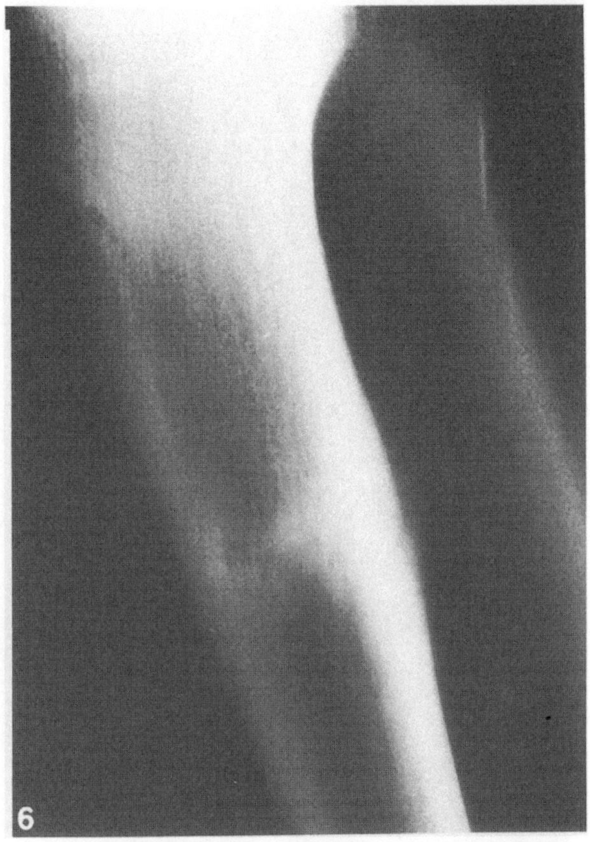

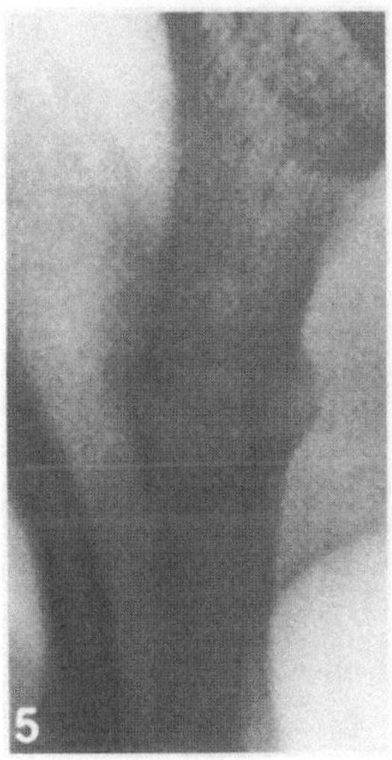

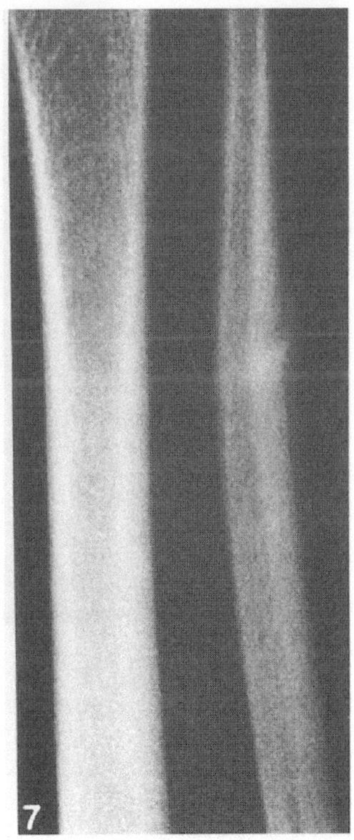

Fig. 4. Periosteal osteoma in contact with lesser trochanter. No known aetiology. Excision was followed by definitive cure

Fig. 5. Undisplaced fracture of body of scapula with major cartilaginous and osteoid reaction in a women with osteomalacia

Fig. 6. Fatigue fracture of tibia, man of 21

Fig. 7. Fracture of fibula in boy of 4, aetiology unknown

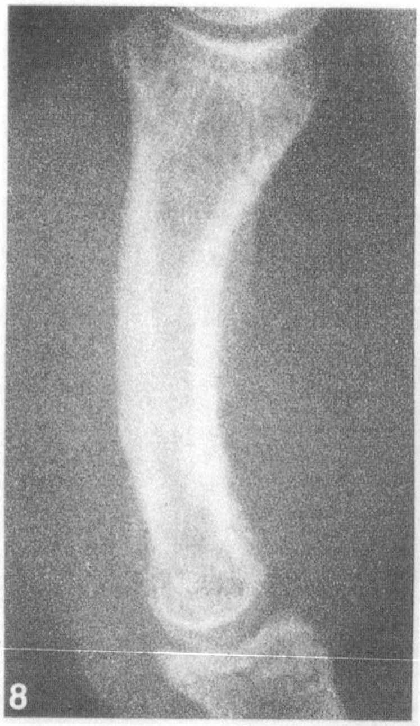

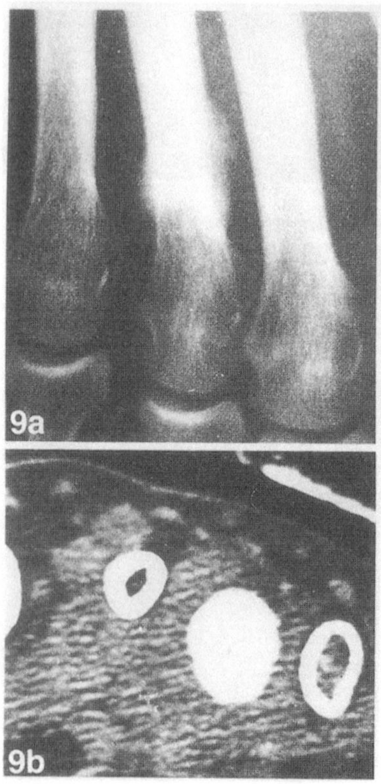

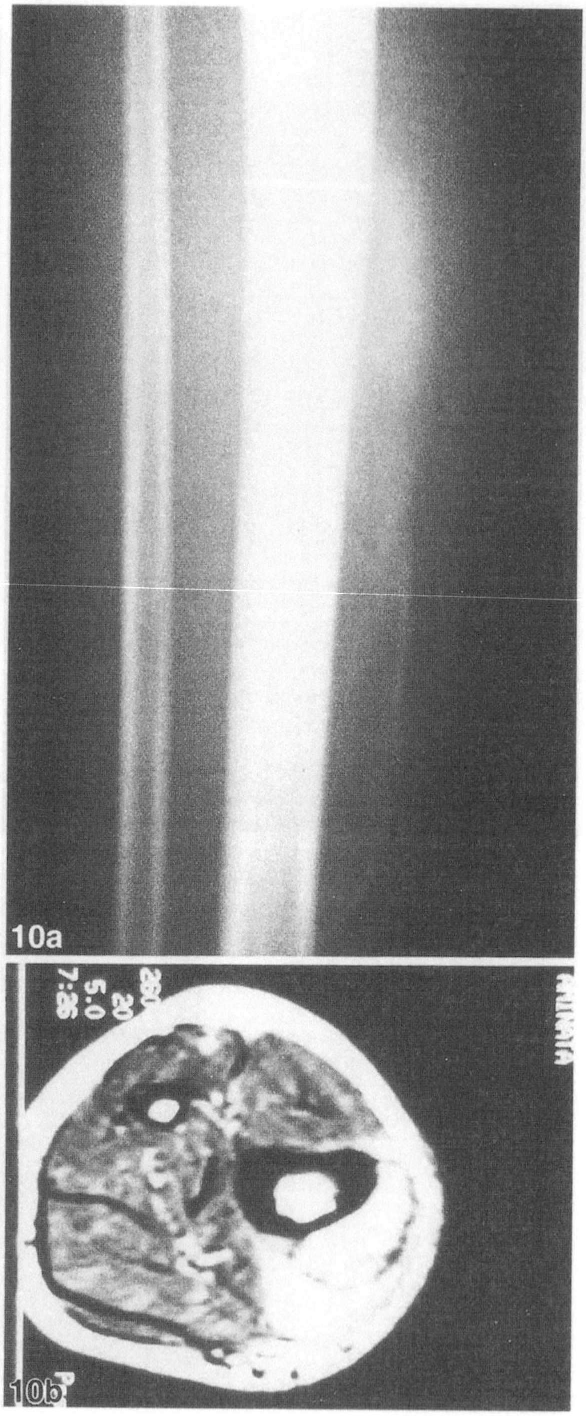

Fig. 8. Synovial chondromatosis of sheath of ring finger with periosteal reaction

Fig. 9 a, b. Missed fracture of metatarsal. The delayed discovery of (**a**) periosteal and (**b**) endosteal osteogenesis often leads to biopsy

Fig. 10 a, b. This tibial periosteal reaction revealed a neurofibromatosis. Examination of the biopsy specimen (Chapter 41) showed only neurofibromatous proliferation without haematoma or visible sequel of haematoma

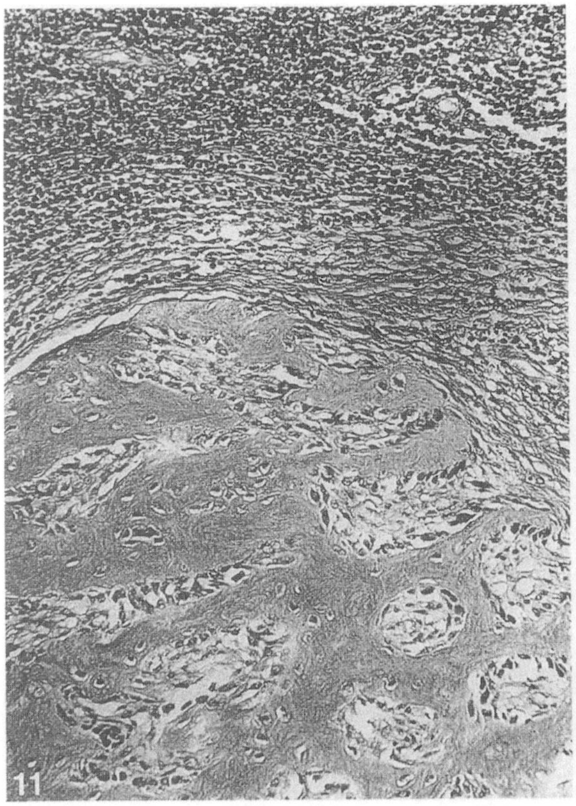

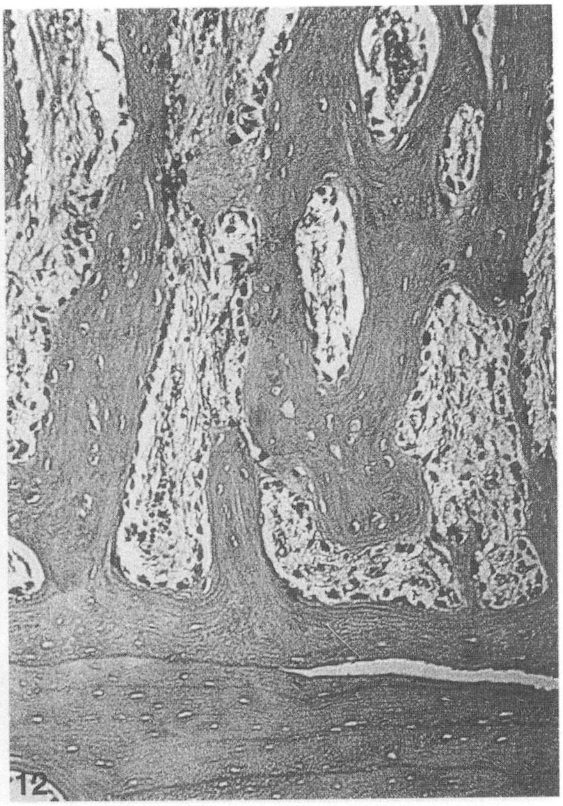

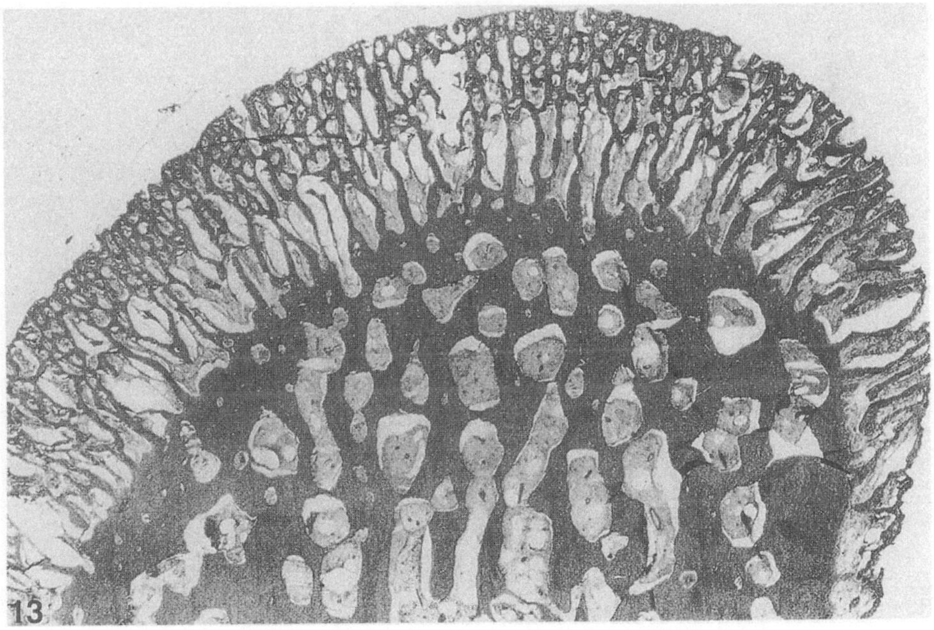

Fig. 11. Apposition of immature bone. The trabeculae are generally parallel to the cortex

Fig. 12. Here the newly-formed periosteal trabeculae are, unlike the previous case, at right angles to the cortex

Fig. 13. Section perpendicular to axis of bone, a little away from the site of fracture, which was missed. Such appearances are often seen in the metatarsals and ribs

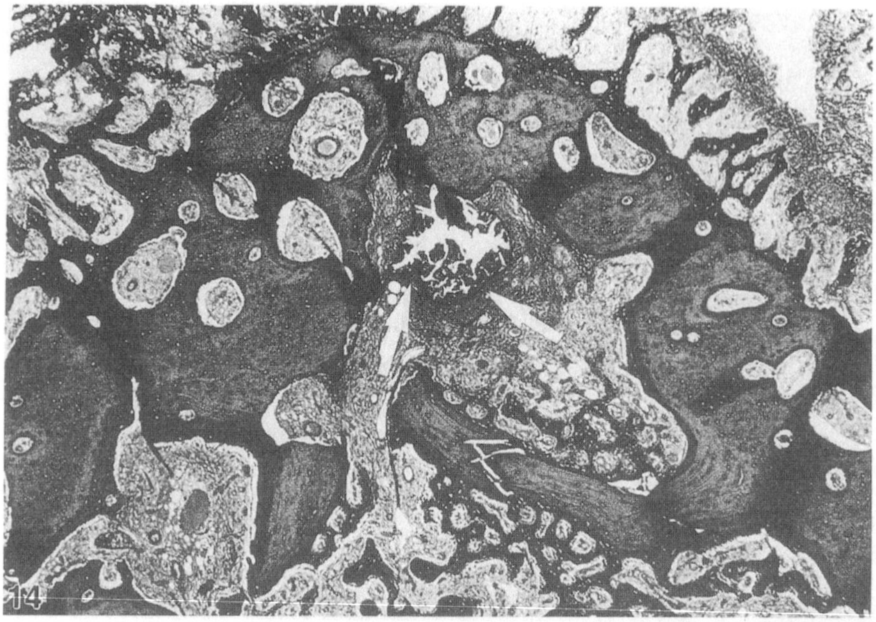

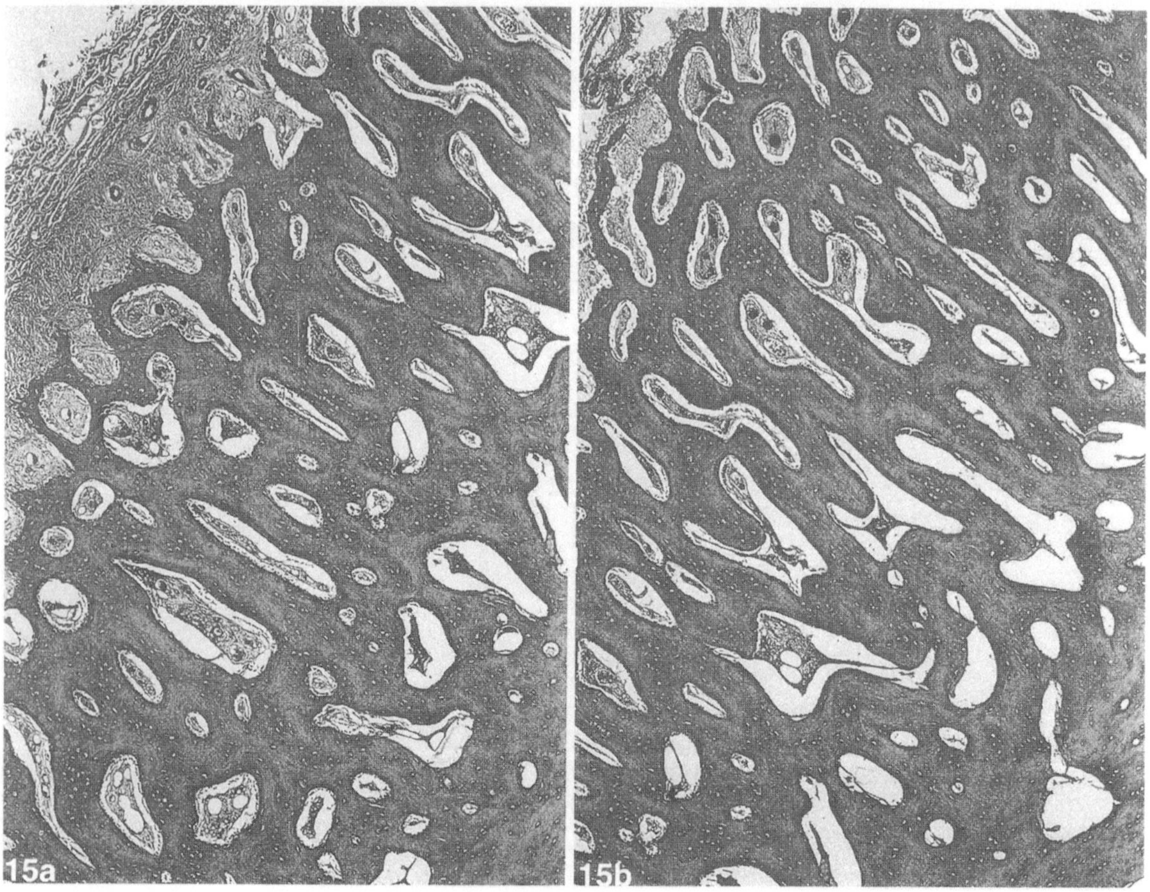

Fig. 14. Fatigue fracture. In this section of the fibula a focus of haemorrhagic necrosis is seen (*white arrows*). There is endosteal bony reaction and a sheath of periosteal bone

Fig. 15 a, b. Periosteal reaction, regular and harmonious, in vicinity of nidus of an osteoid osteoma. The original cortex is seen in the lower right part of these two microphotographs. Superficially, the osteogenesis continues to grow in a thickened and very vascular periosteum, visible in upper left part of (**a**) (low magnification)

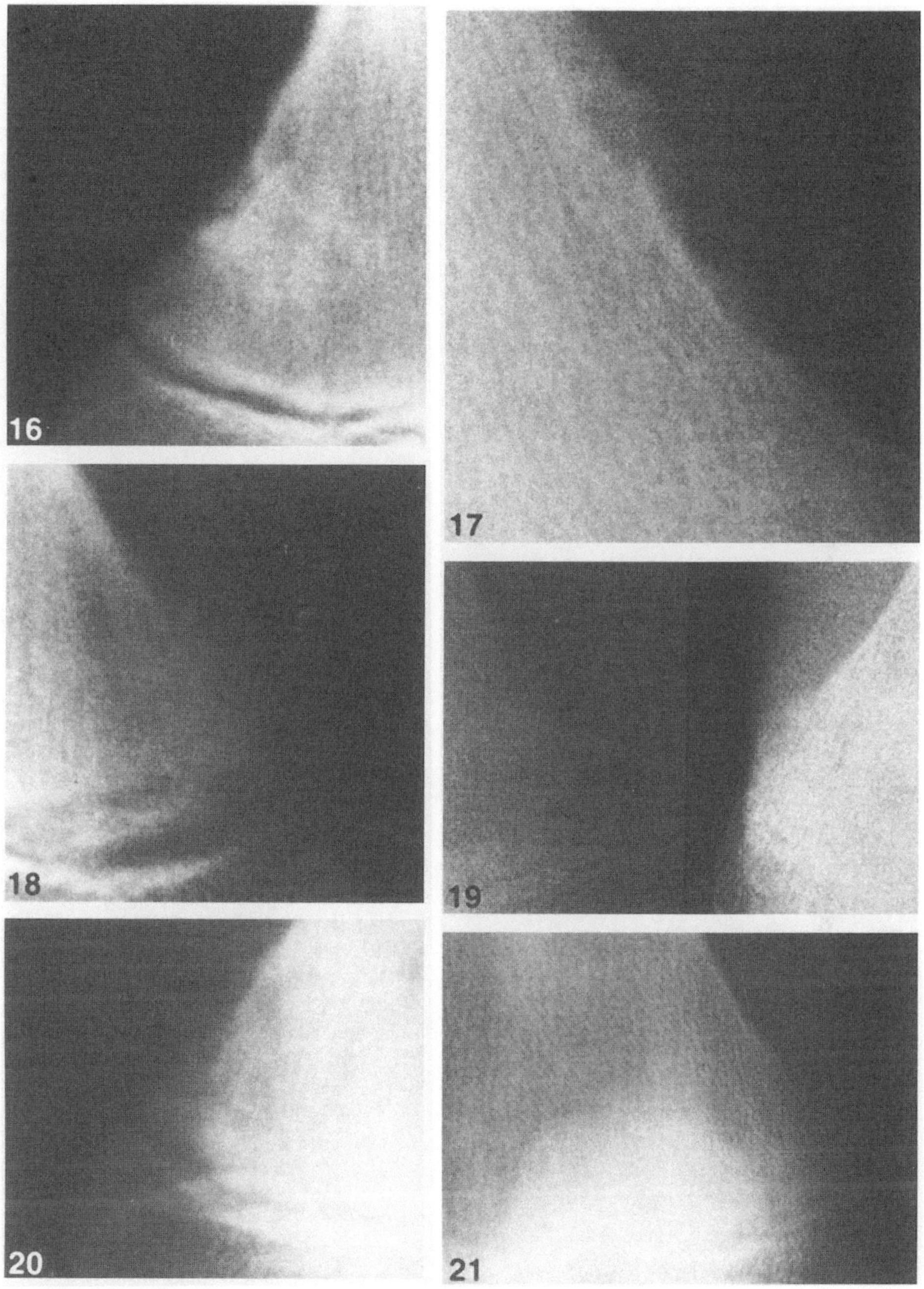

Figs. 16, 17, 18. The lesions shown in these 3 radiographs are quite suggestive - in the light of the clinical findings - of an insertional disorder. Such images sometimes give rise to reports in which the terms "osteolysis" and "ossification of the soft parts" are used, which may suggest a malignant tumour

Fig. 19. In this adolescent male the bilaterality of the lesions is a further argument supporting the diagnosis

Figs. 20, 21. These two radiographs are not very characteristic. If fig. 20 is carefully examined, there is a remodelling of the cortex of a lytic type but also, at the upper part of this lysis, there is a discrete periosteal reaction which is not reassuring. In fig. 21 there is only a discrete osteolysis. These are standard films; well-chosen views may provide sharper images and if need be recourse to more effective imaging may provide a better analysis of these entities

22

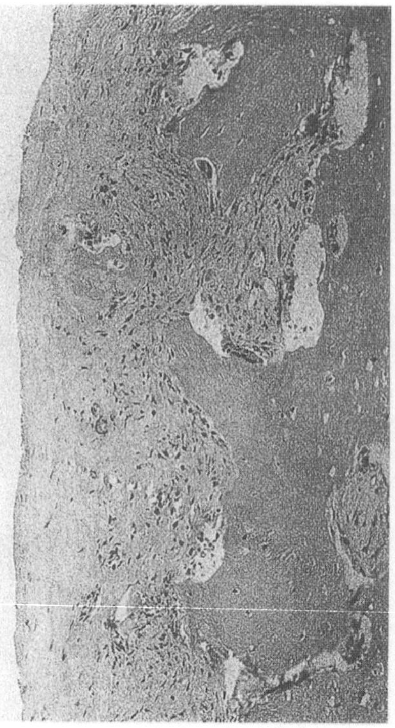

23

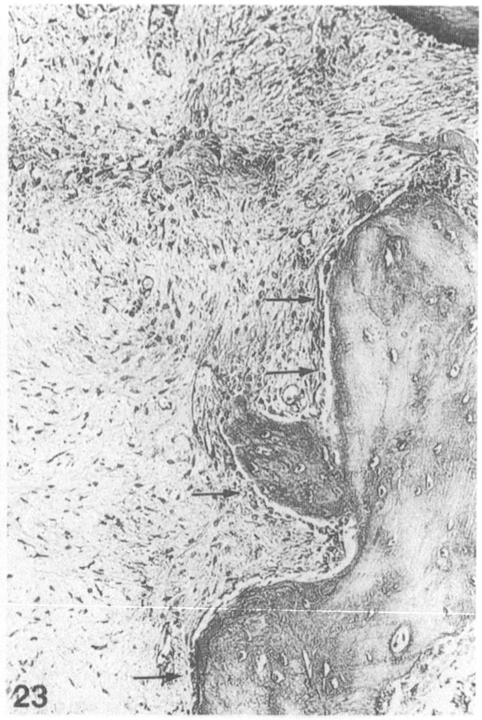

24

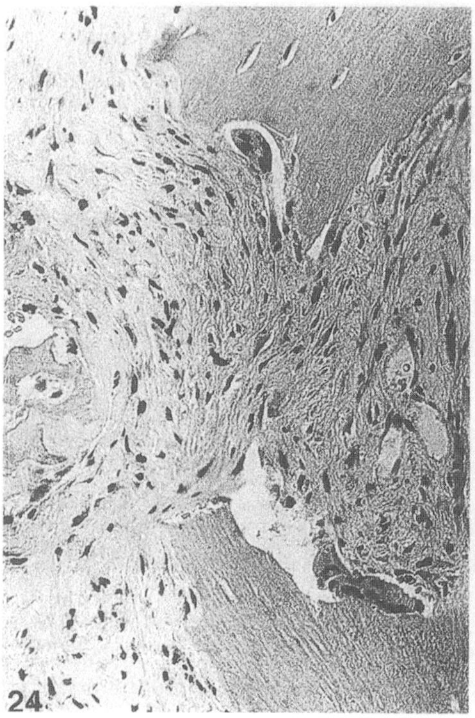

25

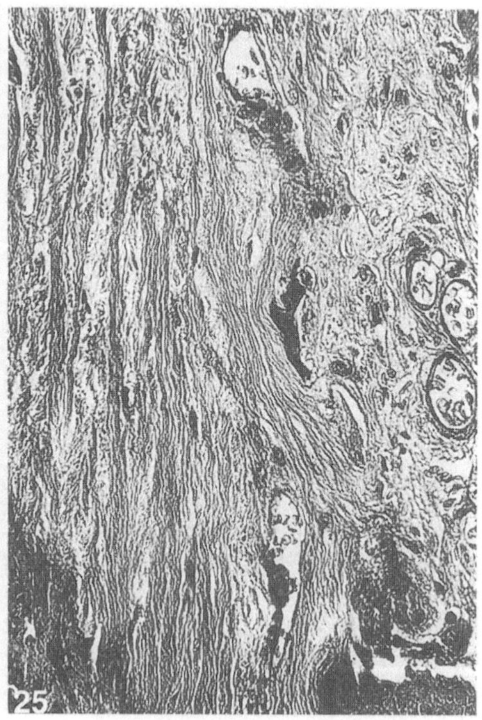

Fig. 22. The cortex is slashed and crenellated by osteoclastic absorption. The deep aspect of the periosteum is transformed into dense fibrous tissue

Fig. 23. Another zone of cortical destruction; an endosteum is being differentiated on the remaining trabecula (*arrows*)

Fig. 24. At this enlargement the lamellar bony trabecula situated at the base of the figure is necrotic; the osteoplasts are uninhabited and enlarged. In the bony trabecula of the upper part of the figure, some osteocytes persist whose nuclei still stain, but are greatly retracted and pyknotic. Near the left margin of the figure, at the middle, a small sequestrum is partly enclosed in newly deposited osteoid tissue

Fig. 25. Remodelling of the osteotendinous junction. The tendon fibers are spread apart but their pattern is still clearly recognisable in the left half of the figure. In the right half, vascular penetration has destroyed the pattern of the architecture. Below, the tendon fibers are calcified

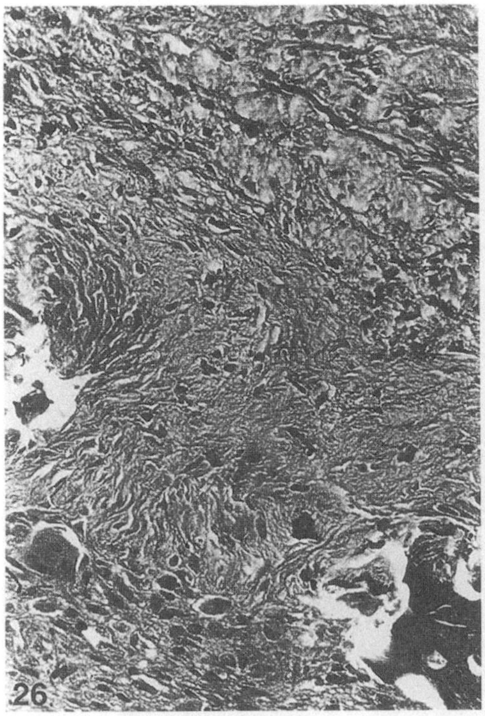

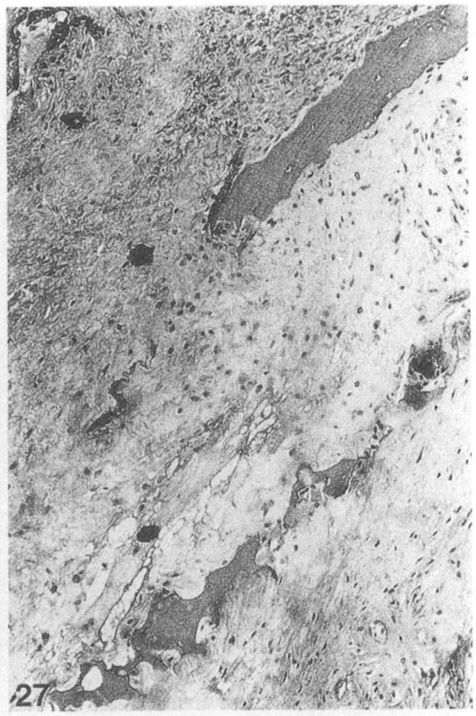

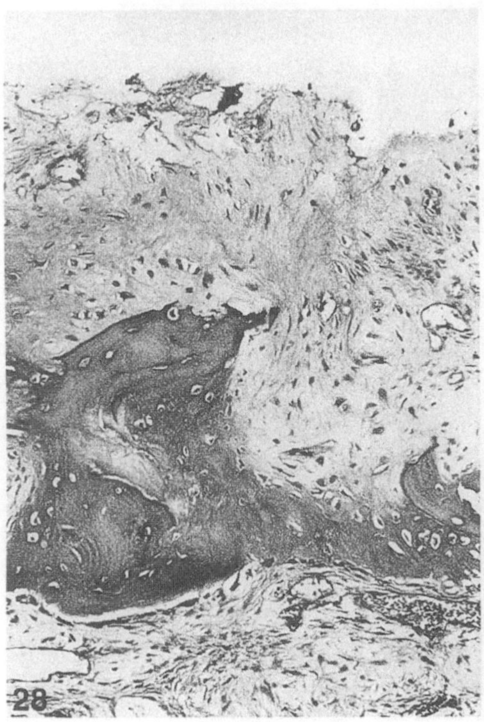

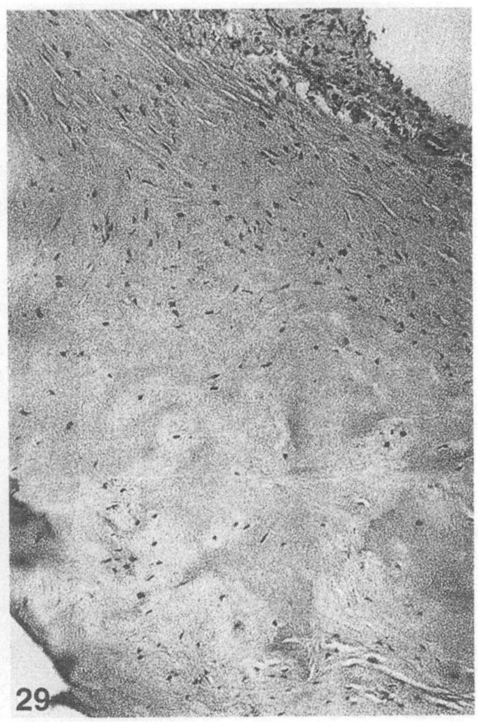

Fig. 26. In the lower part of this microphotograph a fragment of cortical bone is "cut out" by osteoclastic absorption

Fig. 27. Fragments of lamellar bone detached from the subjacent cortex and immersed in a fibrochondroid matrix

Fig. 28. Bony fragments avulsed from the cortex and partly calcified osteoid tissue formed in contact with them are responsible for this radiological "invasion" of the soft tissues

Fig. 29. Remodelling of a tendino-periosteal insertion zone into a fibrochondroid material shadowed with cloudy calcifications. However non-specific these different appearances, and despite a somewhat alarming radiological report, there is no histological evidence to support a diagnosis of osteogenic sarcoma

The microphotographs 22-29 correspond to the insertional disorders of figs. 16-21

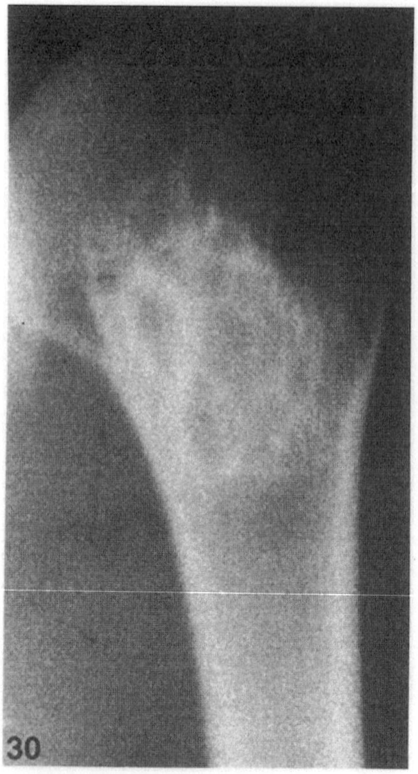
30

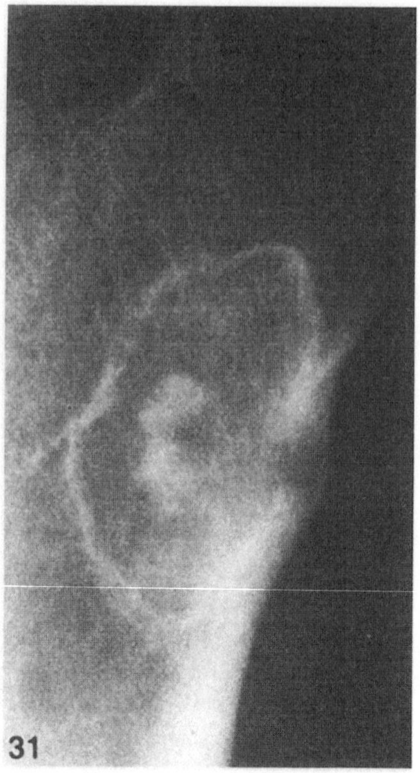
31

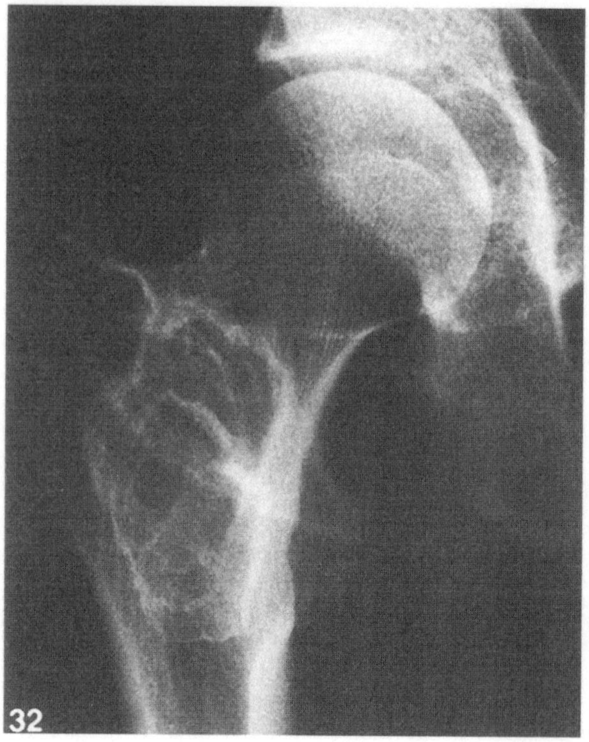
32

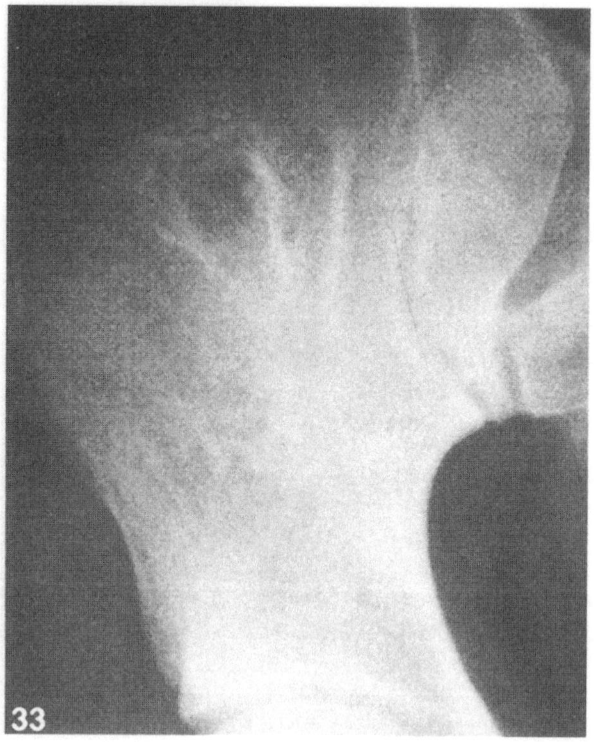
33

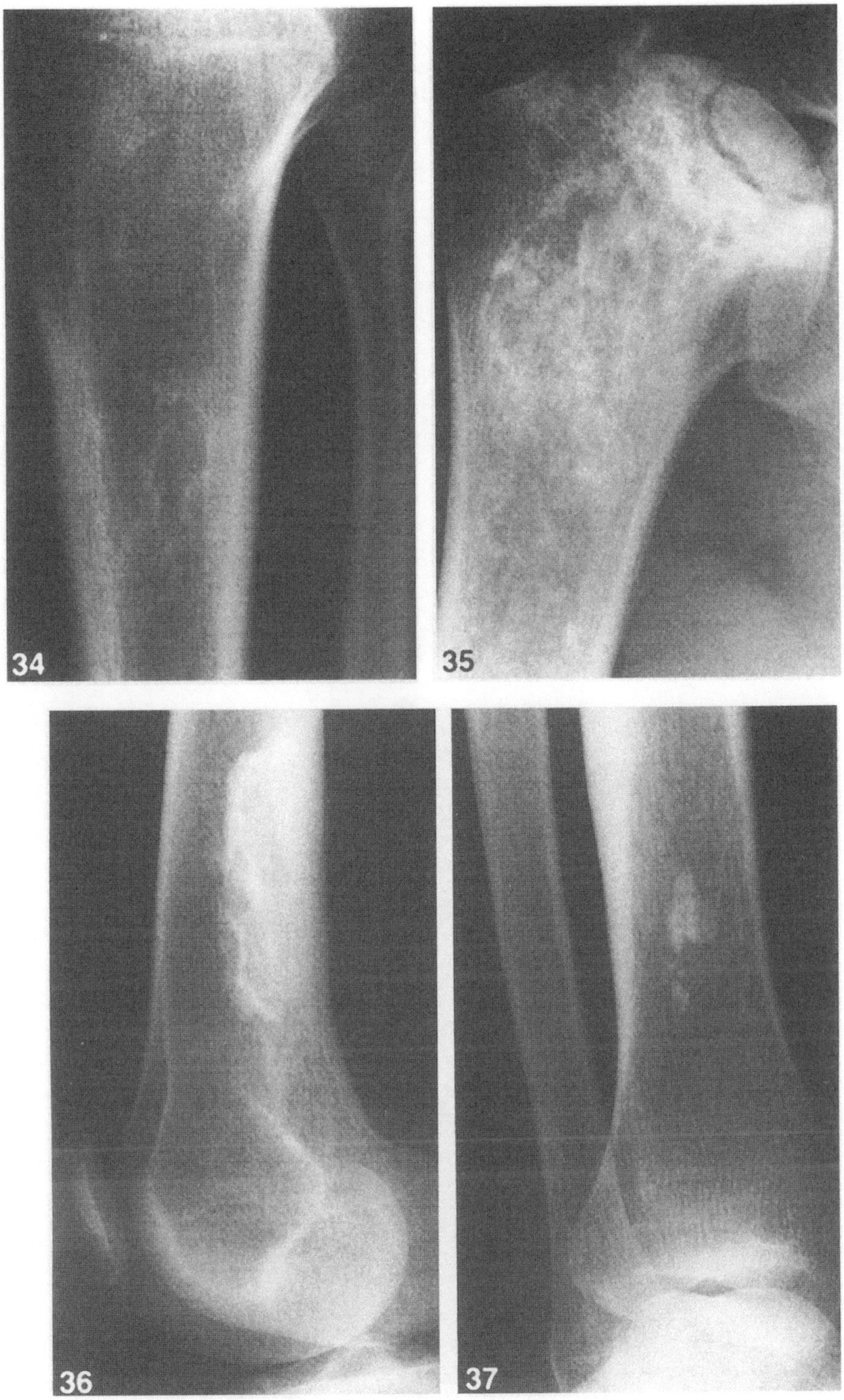

Figs. 30-37. These bone infarcts of the humerus (30, 35), femur (31, 32, 36) and tibia (34, 37) developed in young men working in caissons to repair bridge piles (films by courtesy of Dr Jaffrès, Brest). The infarct of the ilium (33) was revealed by pain in a young man who had dived some years previously, almost every day for a year, when installing telephone cables. The radiographic image of these infarcts is rounded, with irregular outlines, with calcified areas and small opaque patches. At an epiphyseal site the infarct produces marked articular damage, here of the osteochondritic type (35)

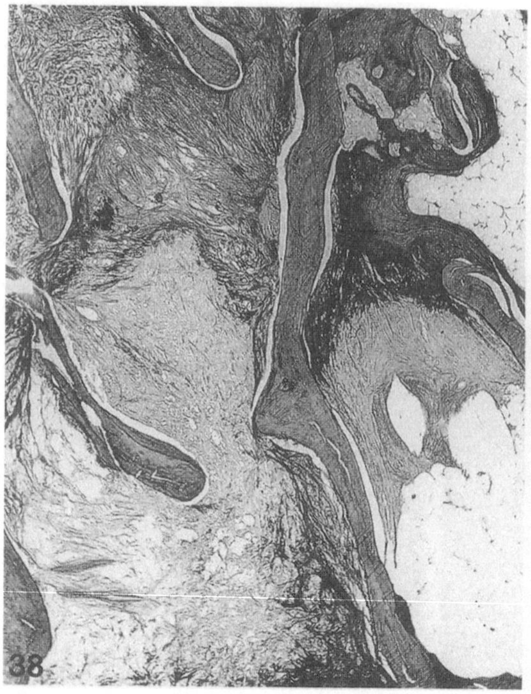

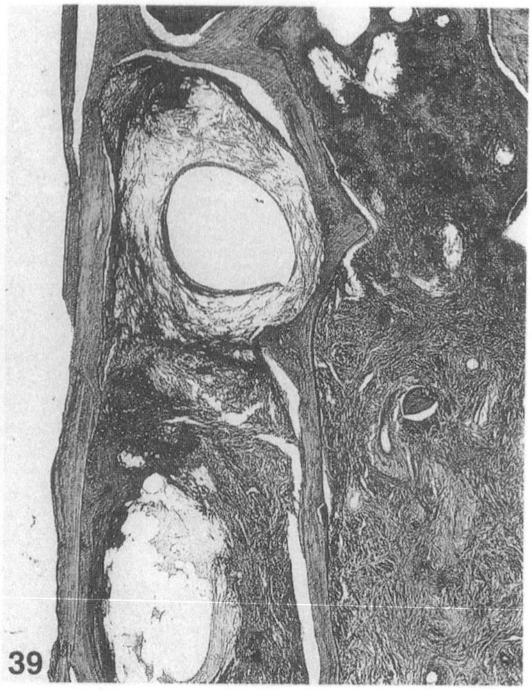

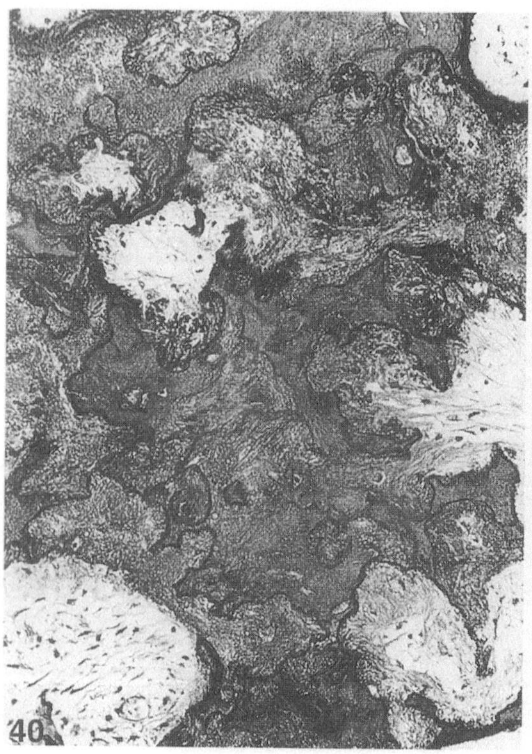

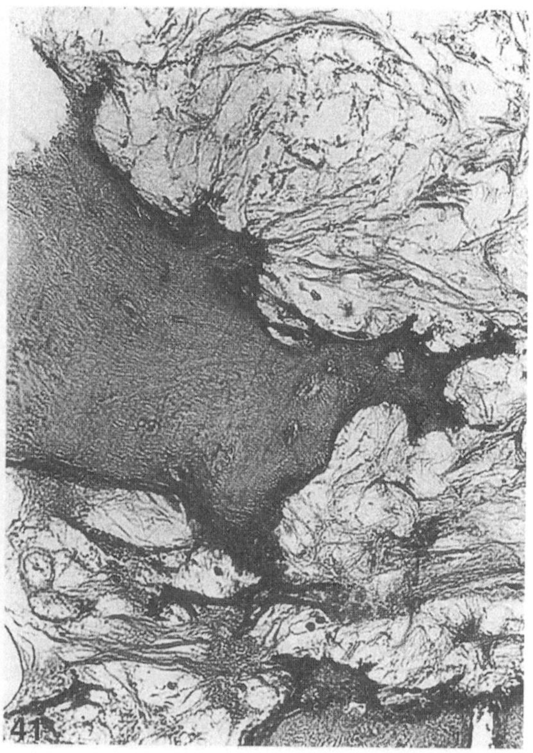

Figs. 38-40. Microphotographs of bone infarction at low and high magnification. Medullary fibrosis replaces the fatty marrow; its calcification, in places very dense, is reinforced at the lines of osteoclastic arrest (**40**)

Fig. 41. Post-irradiation bone necrosis. The marrow is fibrillar and paucicellular. The osteoclastic absorption has been followed by calcium deposits which enclose the relics of the bony trabeculae. These calcifications explain the hyperdense radiological images which accompany bone necrosis

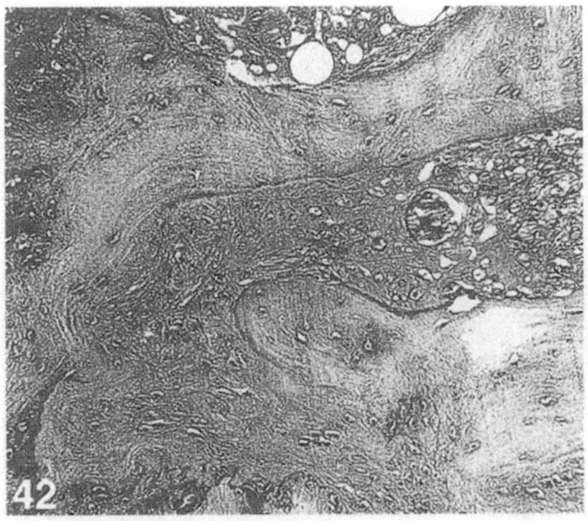

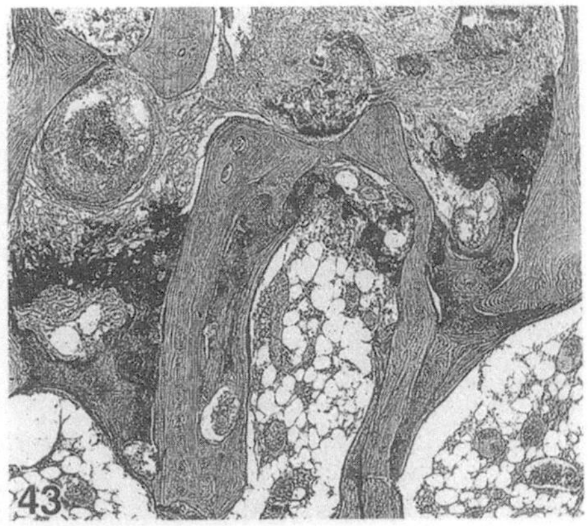

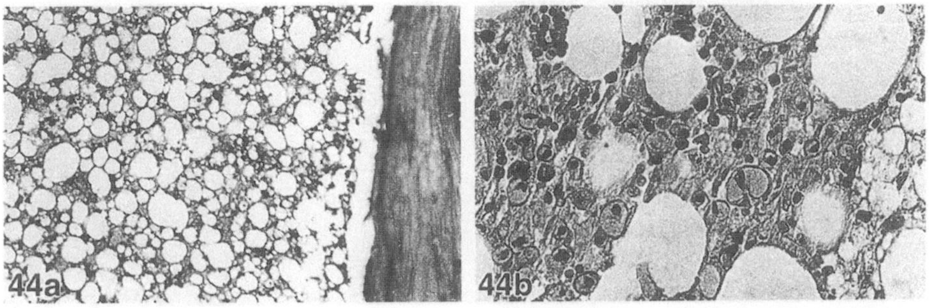

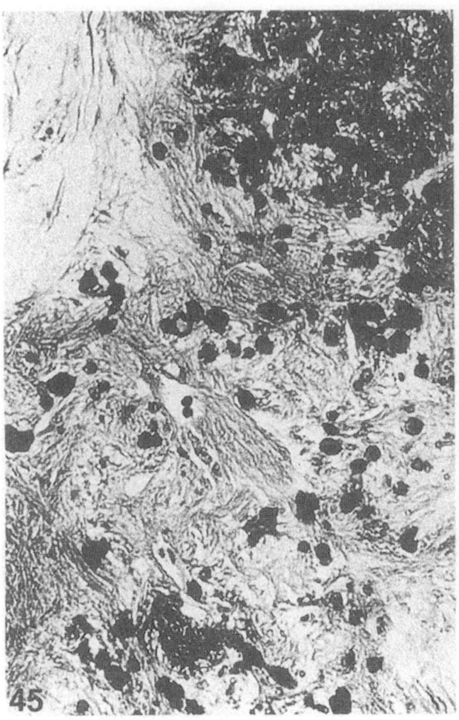

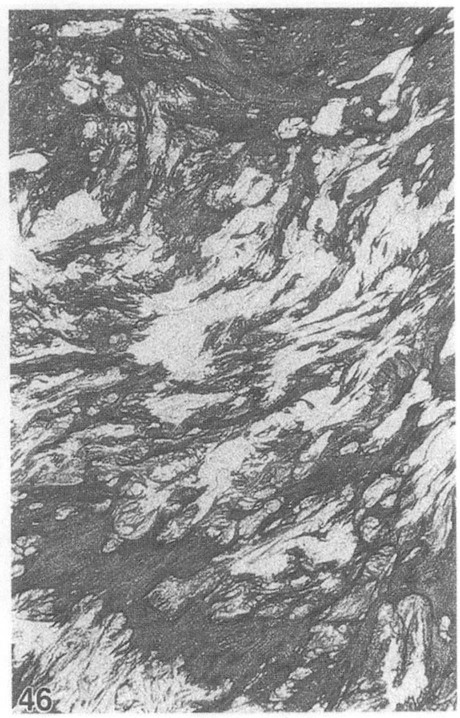

Fig. 42. Between two necrotic bony trabeculae the medullary spaces are occupied by a partly calcified fibrocartilaginous tissue

Fig. 43. Junctional zone between dead bone (above) and living bone (below) in a necrosis of the upper pole of the femoral head. The osteomedullary reaction of this "boundary line of the bone" is represented by a partly calcified fibrous band and by thickening of the living trabeculae by apposition of bony lamellae

Fig. 44 a, b. Marrow biopsy in recent infarct. Between the clear "lacunae" of liponecrosis the cell proliferation includes histiocytes, lymphocytes and some lipoblasts

Figs. 45, 46. Two quite different appearances of a necrotic area. **45** Infarct in a young man (caisson disease). Multiple rounded calcium deposits, confluent in places, in an only slightly fibrous marrow. **46** Infarct of upper end of femur in an octogenarian. Within the medullary fibrosis the calcification is arranged as if laid on by a brush along the collagen fibers

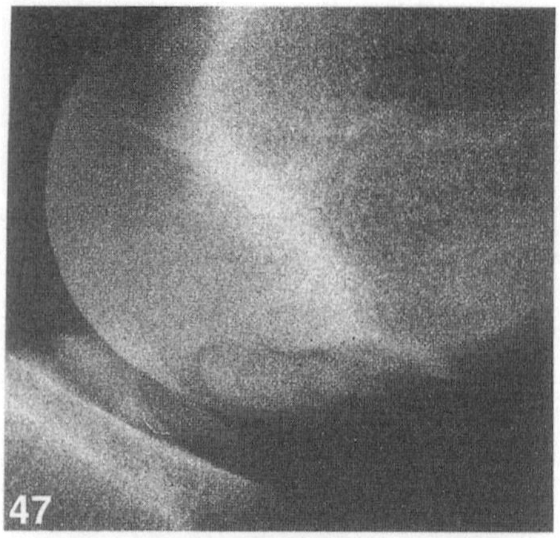

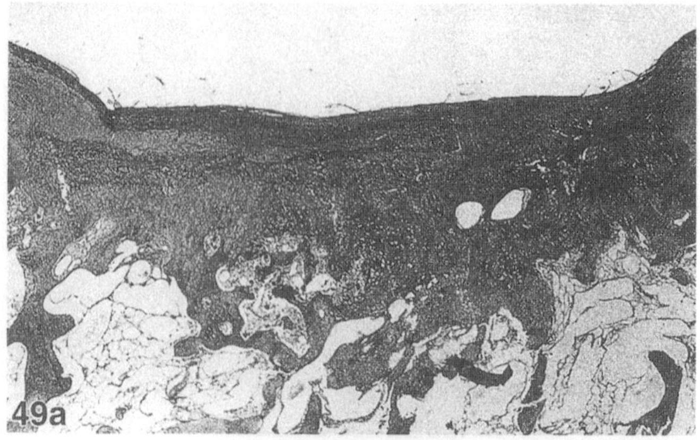

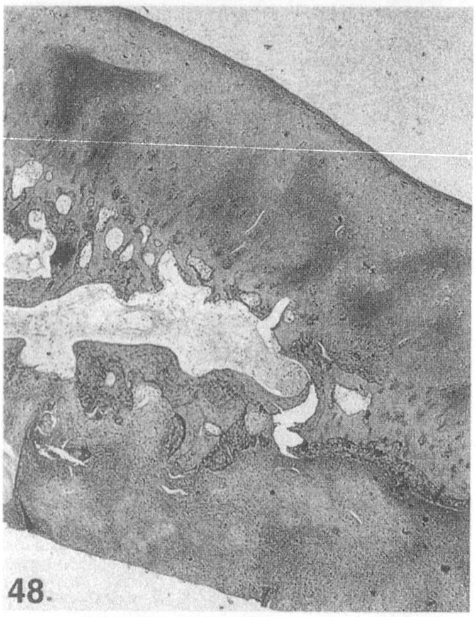

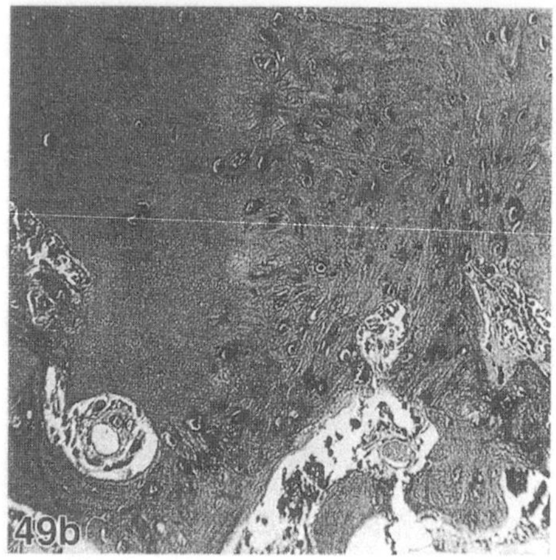

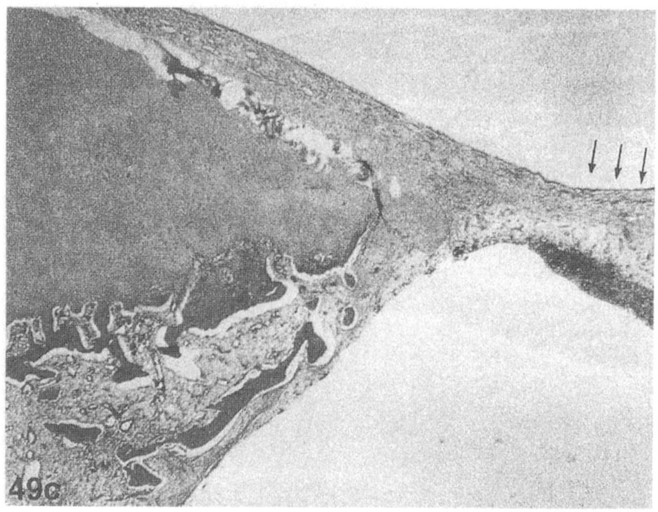

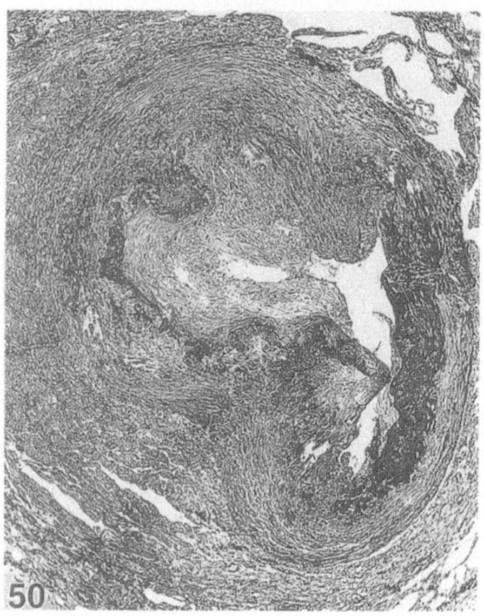

Fig. 47. An osteochondritic nodule in its compartment, circumscribed by a radiolucent fibrocartilaginous layer. The nodule may stay connected to the living bone by one of its poles for a long time (fig. 49c)

Fig. 48. Fibrocartilaginous nodule free in the joint. It is probable that before it was detached from its base there was a fibrous remodelling of some medullary areas of what was to become an osteocartilaginous sequestrum. The newly-formed fibrocartilage covering the inferior (deep) face of this nodule is quite different from the articular cartilage which covers the opposite face, particularly as regards the arrangement of the chondrocytes

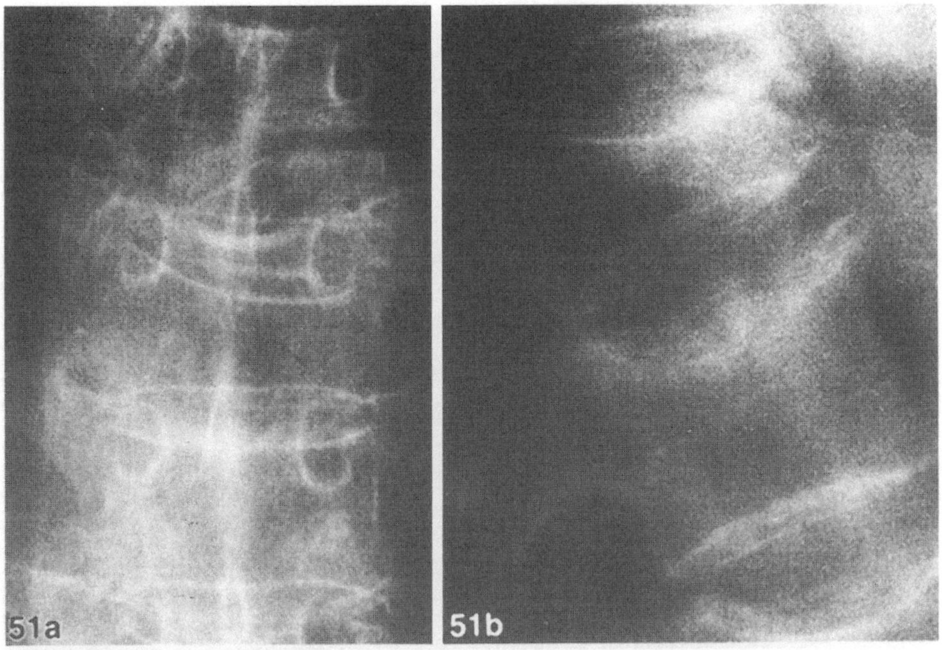

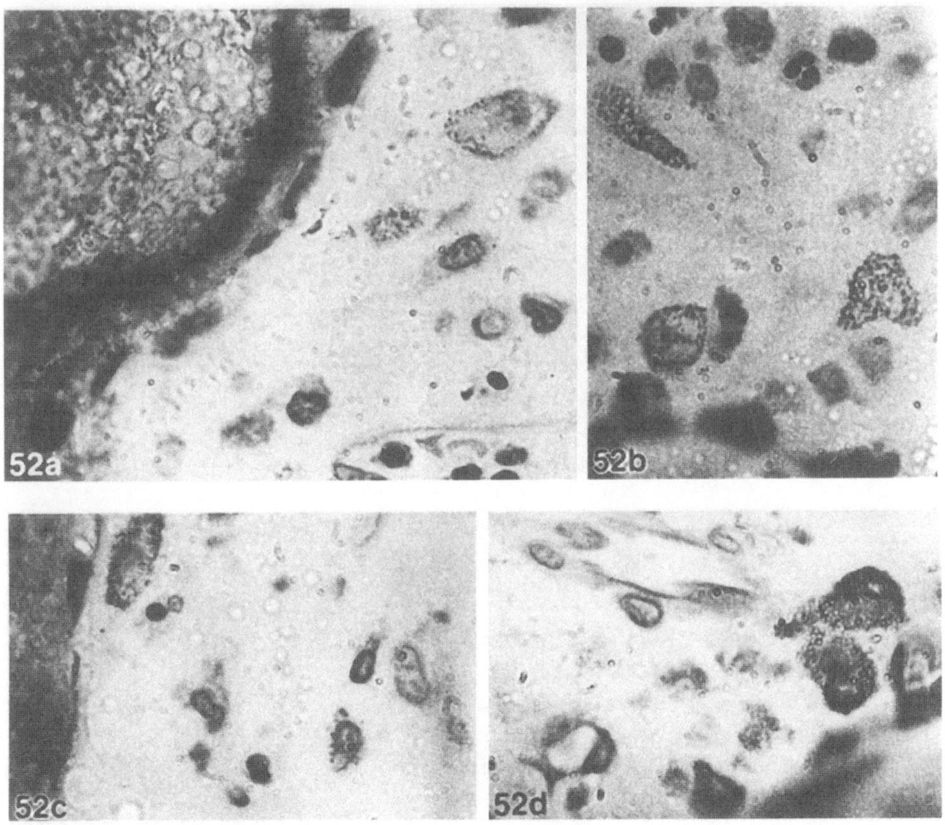

Fig. 51 a, b. Vertebral osteoporosis, wedge-shaped L1 vertebra, evidence of bony mastocytosis without skin lesions

Fig. 52. Mastocytes in bone marrow of varied shape and size, either dispersed (**a, b**) or in contact with or very close to a bony trabecula. **c, d** Undecalcified sections stained with toluidin blue

←

Fig. 49. a Bony and fibrocartilaginous regeneration in a pocket of osteochondritis. **b** At higher magnification the zone of junction between articular cartilage and newly-formed fibrocartilage. **c** Pedicle (*arrows*) connecting the detached osteocartilaginous fragment to the peripheral zone of the articular surface

Fig. 50. Partly calcified endothelial thickening in a capsular vessel of a necrotic femoral head

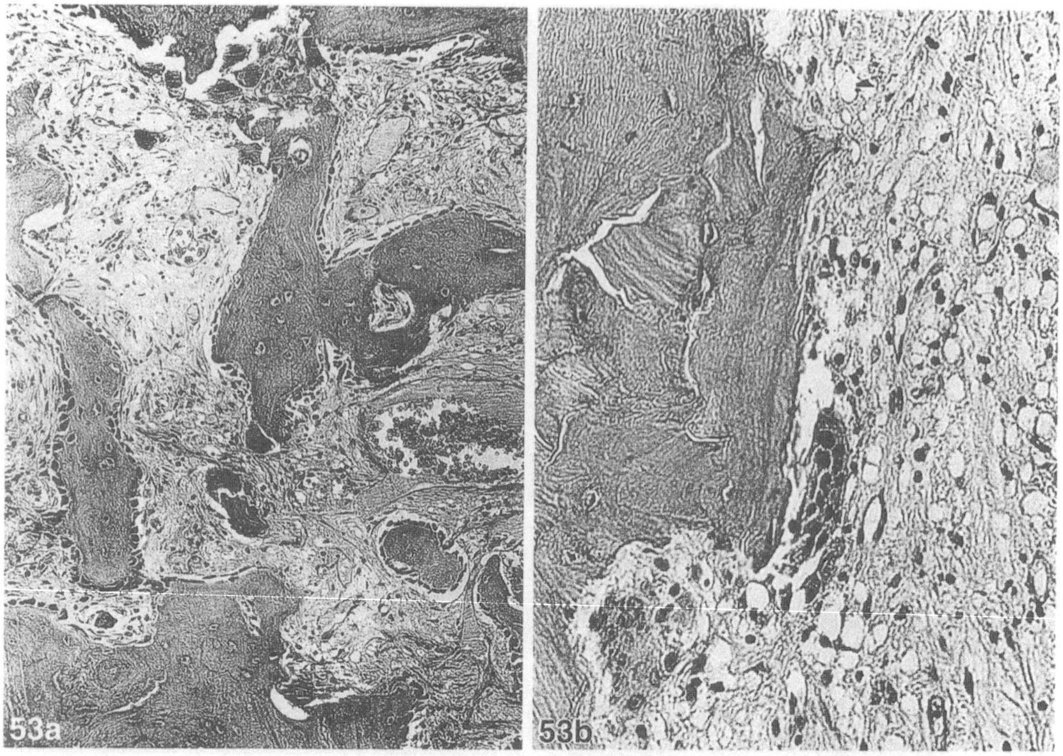

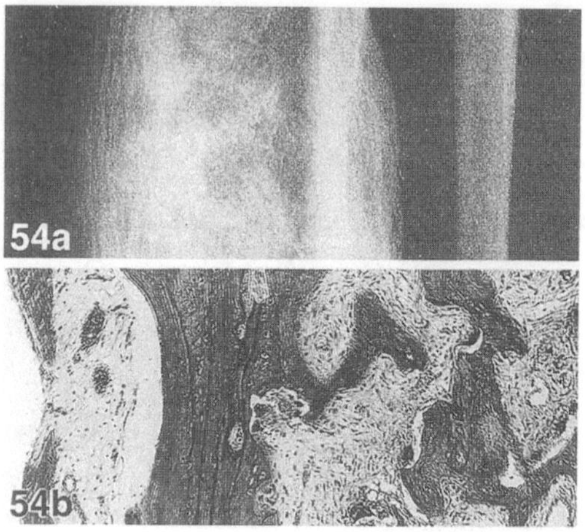

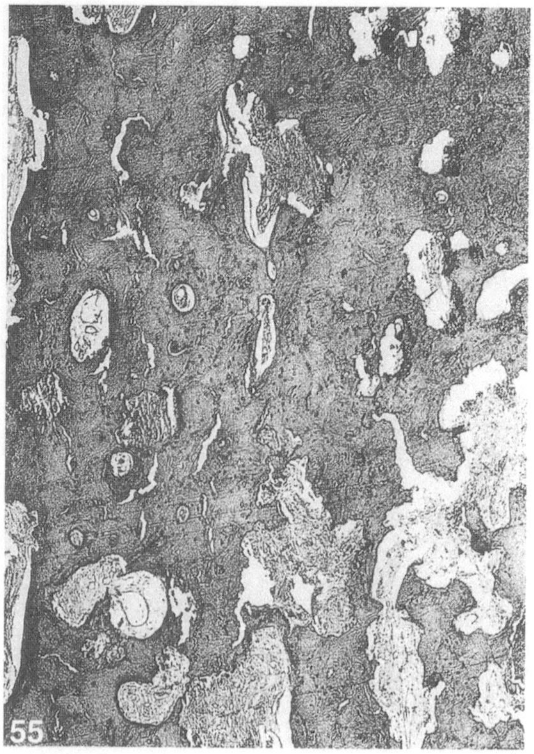

Fig. 53. a Moderately active Paget's disease: formation of bone trabeculae of unequal thickness, bordered by a row of osteoblasts and some osteoclasts. The fibrous marrow is very vascular. **b** "Cutting-out" of a bony trabecula by lines of arrest which form arabesques, jigsaw images (de Sèze) and with two large osteoclasts in contact with the bone. The marrow is fibro-fatty

Fig. 54. a Pagetic thickening of tibia. **b** Note the lamellar flaky non-Pagetic appearance of the periosteal apposition by a well-vascularised periosteum

Fig. 55. Stabilised or not very progressive Paget's disease. The bony trabeculae are calcified; very reduced osteoblastic and osteoclastic activity in this fibrous marrow

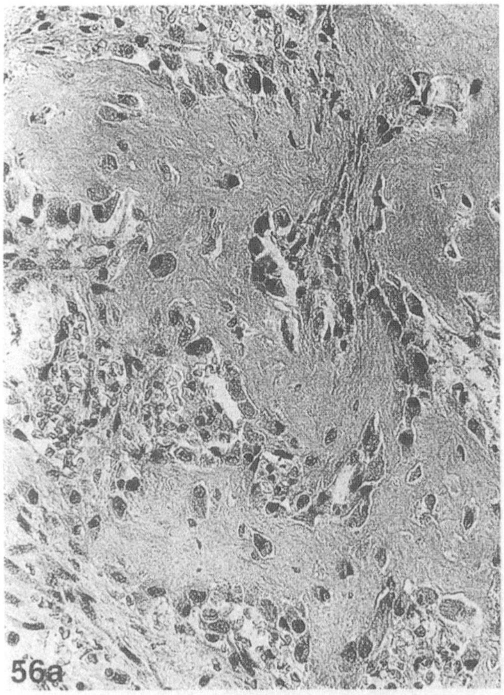

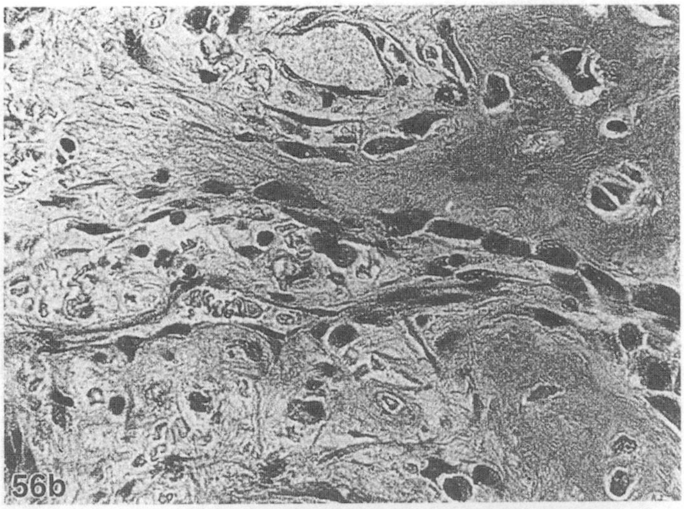

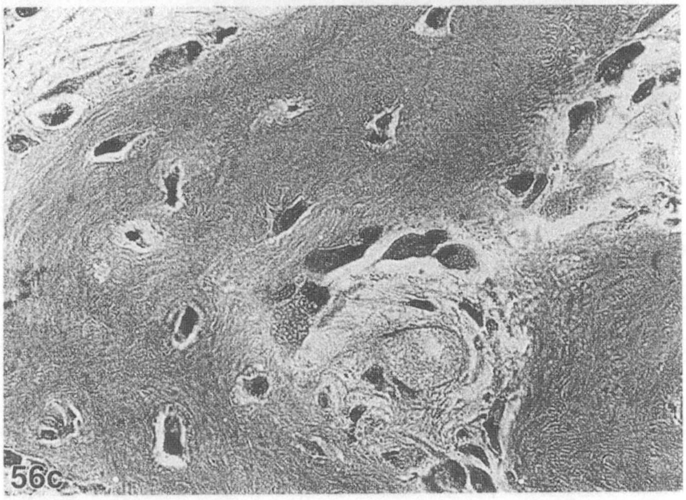

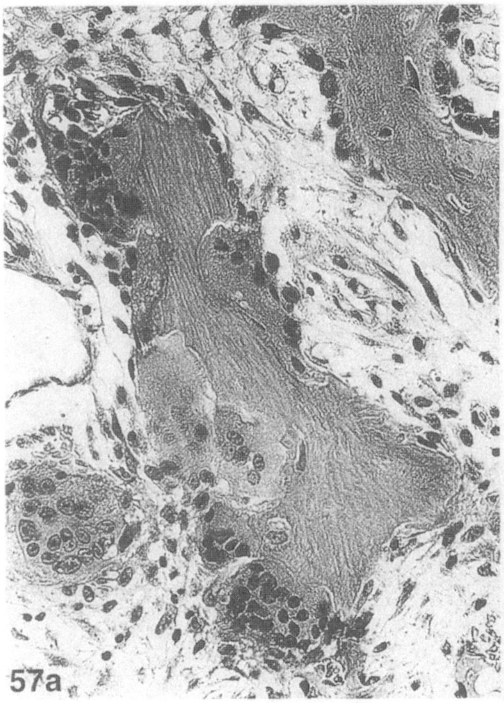

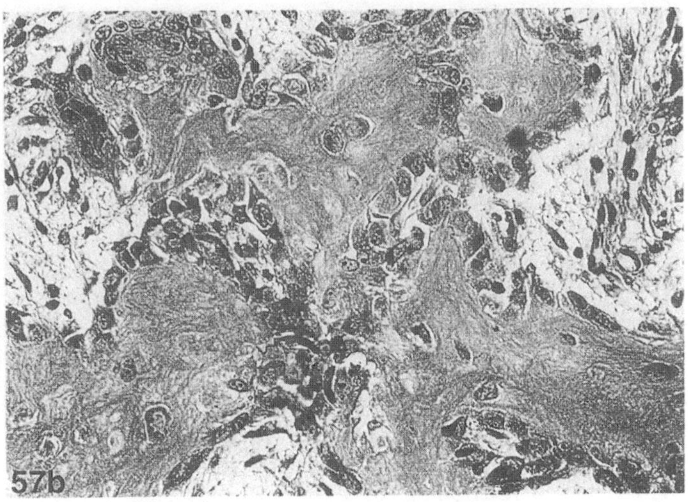

Fig. 56 a-c. Hyperactive Paget's disease: the bony or more precisely the osteoid trabeculae are devoid of lines of arrest. The osteoblasts are bulky but without atypical nuclei. Pagetic bone is normally only slightly calcified but in this case there is a sort of pagetic osteomalacia

Fig. 57 a, b. Hyperactive Paget's disease. **a** Sometimes the predominance of osteoclasts is considerable, almost amounting to an osteoclastoma. **b** Sometimes osteoblastic predominance suggests a diagnosis of osteoblastoma

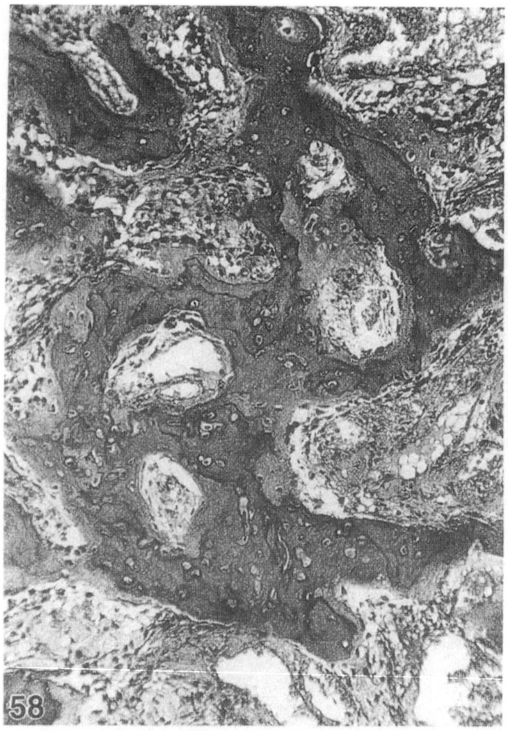

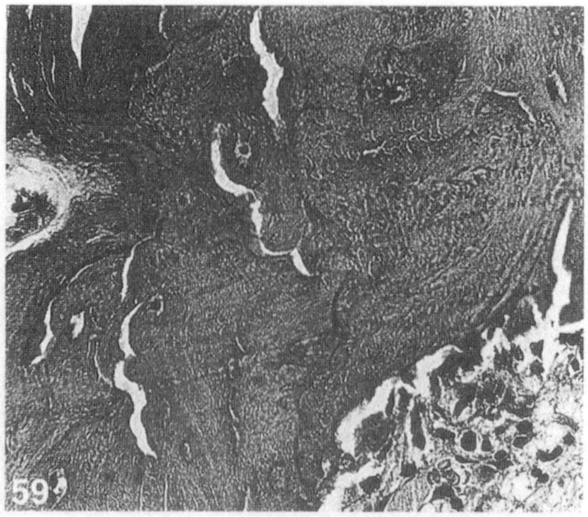

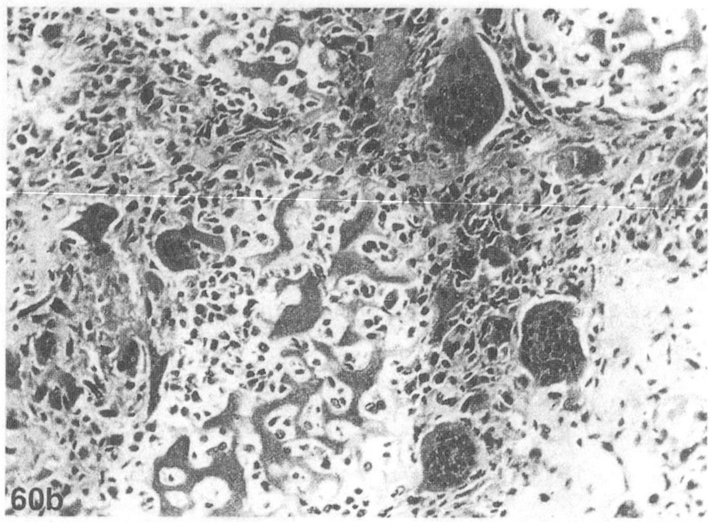

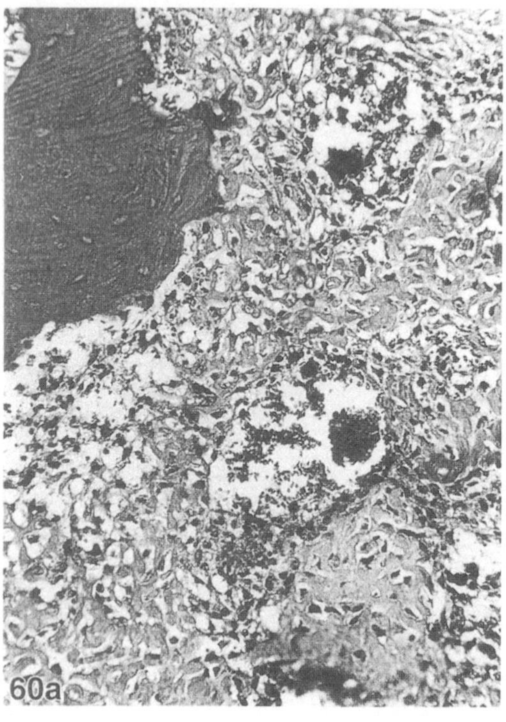

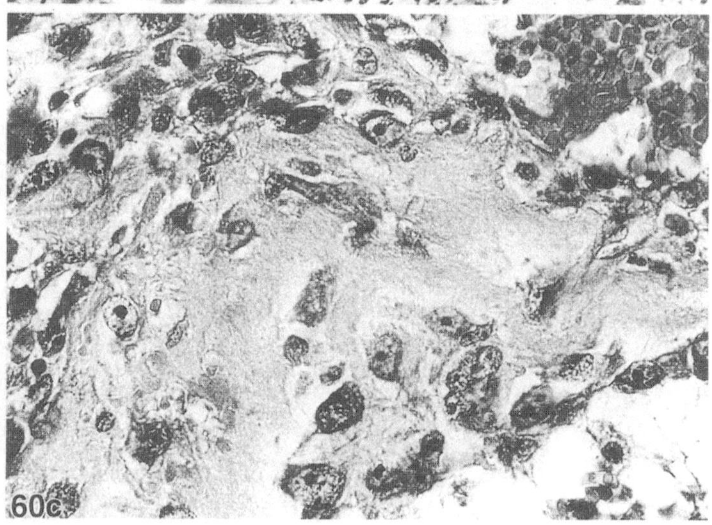

Fig. 58. Pagetoid osteogenesis in an osteogenic sarcoma

Fig. 59. The pagetic bone is only slightly calcified and too often the decalcification overshoots its mark. In this case the lines of arrest have lost their basophilia and are replaced by fine dehiscences

Fig. 60 a-c. Sarcomatous transformation in Paget's disease of bone. **a** A pagetic island persists. The sketchy trabecular osteogenesis (**b**) and the deposition of osteoid tissue (**c**) differ from pagetic formations. The osteoclasts remain numerous and may suggest hyperactive Paget's disease, but at higher magnification (**c**) they are seen to be cellular anomalies and in themselves exclude simple hyperactive Paget's disease

41. Calcified and/or ossified lesions of the soft tissues and various disorders affecting bone

Circumscribed myositis ossificans and related lesions (pseudo-malignant bony tumour of the soft tissues, ossifying haematoma, osteoma, circumscribed benign ossification of the soft tissues)

(figs. 1-17)

Nomenclature

The term "circumscribed myositis ossificans" designates a benign limited heterotopic ossification developing in muscle tissue usually secondary to trauma. In practice this label is less restrictive, as it may be argued that the lesion is not always situated in a muscle, and that in some cases development of the lesion is preceded by a quite characteristic infective process. In other cases there is neither a traumatic nor an infective history. These qualifications explain the numerous terms under which the lesion has been reported. Even if the term myositis ossificans is arrived at arbitrarily, it properly describes the majority of cases and recognition of its essentially benign nature avoids long arguments.

General considerations

This is a rare lesion, commoner in boys than in girls. It particularly affects older children and young adults; the mean age at diagnosis is around 18-20 years. The commonest sites are the brachialis, quadriceps and hip adductors, but it also affects the glutei, deltoid, pectoralis major and muscles of the hand.

Clinical features

Moderate pain or a palpable intramuscular mass brings the patient to consultation. In most cases the history reveals the nature of the original injury, which may be no more than violent physical exertion. The most remarkable fact is the rapidity of development of this ossification, which may reach 5-7 cm along the muscle axis and 4-5 cm in thickness within 6-8 weeks. This rapid development is very suggestive of circumscribed myositis ossificans. The firm and slightly tender palpable mass forms part of the muscle. The sedimentation rate may be raised but the blood count is usually normal.

The progress of this lesion is benign; without surgical intervention it may persist or be spontaneously reabsorbed and disappear.

Myositis ossificans at around the 8th week

- Imaging

In the typical case, seen around the 8th week of development, imaging shows an ovoid mass, lumpy and dense peripherally, with quite marked boundaries. Its central part shows little or no ossification. Current imaging techniques clearly demonstrate this zone phenomenon, confirmed histologically, and the increased vascular network if angiography is performed. It is important to note the independence of the tumour from the underlying bone although in some cases the presence of minor periosteal osteogenesis opposite this intramuscular ossification may be noted.

- Pathological anatomy and histopathology

Macroscopically, the tumour is firm and smooth with muscle and aponeurotic fibers adherent to its surface, despite the ease with which it can be separated from the surrounding tissue often mentioned in the operation findings. On section the peripheral zone is ossified, the central part is soft and reddish.

Histological examination of an adequate and suitably sited biopsy shows, from center to periphery the

Table 1. Myositis ossificans

Young patients, generally between 15 and 25 year Rapid on set 6 to 8 weeks Zonation with ossified periphery
Main differential diagnosis: extraskeletic osteosarcoma - Rare - Older patients - Slower evolution - Active peripheral extension zone - Myositis ossificans at its onset, a few weeks
Differential diagnoses: sarcomas: synovial, periosted, muscular; malignant fibrous histiocytoma - Very young children
Differential diagnosis: progressive myositis ossificans - Localisation mainly cervical, associated malformations of thumb and first toe

following appearances. There is a cellular fibrohistiocytic zone in which traces of fibrin may be observed and cases with abundant fibrin have suggested the diagnosis of ossifying haematoma. Between the central and peripheral zones there is an intermediate zone in which there form bundles of fibroblasts and collagen fibers which anastomose. These safranophil collagen bundles stand out boldly against the histiocyto-fibroblastic background; they represent the beginnings of osteoid metamorphosis. In the peripheral zone the bony trabeculae evolve towards maturity and are implanted on a fine cortical shell which bounds the lesion and separates it from the muscular and musculo-aponeurotic tissue. Some striated muscle fibers are usually included in this structure and adjacent to this ossification the muscle fibers exhibit degenerative changes. Though the fibroblasts which border the bundles of collagen fibers are large and herald osteoblastic metamorphosis, mitoses are not very numerous and there is no atypical mitosis.

At this stage and with good material there is no question of a differential diagnosis, especially since the clinical history of rapid development only confirms the histological diagnosis. More advanced lesions resemble a true mature osteoma, bounded over its entire periphery by a fine bony cortex, unless all is spontaneously reabsorbed as I have had the opportunity of observing.

As a summary it may be said that the myositis ossificans behaves like a callus built around a non-existent fracture, which closes in on itself.

Myositis ossificans: initial stage

- Imaging

When the patient attends early because of severe pain, osteogenesis is not detectable either clinically or radiologically. The radiographs show only a vague opacity corresponding to a swollen zone, an ill-defined thickening without bony consistency. If the films show some irregular cloudy opacities, this will probably suggest the diagnosis of osteosarcoma or synovial sarcoma.

- Pathological anatomy and histopathology

Biopsy of this early lesion involves a very vascular reddish tissue, mainly represented by a histiocytic and fibroblastic cell proliferation, rich in mitoses. In places giant cells and fine fibrin layers complete the histological picture. In addition to numerous mitoses there are often cellular anomalies, so that the general picture is disturbing; it is best to delay for a few weeks rather than to make a rash diagnosis of sarcoma.

Differential diagnosis

The main differential diagnosis is from osteosarcoma. This diagnosis may be particularly difficult in a biopsy made at an early stage, for example, around the 2nd or 3rd week.

In osteogenic sarcoma, apart from the cellular and particularly the mitotic atypias, the cell proliferation is usually more undifferentiated peripherally, in the zone of extension, than at the center, which is sometimes spontaneously necrotic. Osteogenesis in myositis ossificans resembles the osteogenesis in a fracture callus, an osteogenesis which begins at the periphery and gradually reaches the central fibrinous zone which has in part undergone a chondroid metaplasia; cartilaginous tissue is readily seen in myositis ossificans. The speed of development is a fundamental aid to diagnosis. Osteosarcoma does not develop as rapidly as myositis ossificans. The myositis grows like a mushroom and it is the immature mushrooms which lead to fatal mistakes. Three weeks later the radiology and the histological appearances of a second biopsy will allow the diagnosis of myositis ossificans without much difficulty. But at the onset stage other types of sarcoma may possibly be suggested including synovial sarcoma, rhabdomyosarcoma, malignant histiocytofibroma, periosteal sarcoma. Immunohistology, particularly for synovial sarcoma and muscle sarcoma, are of the greatest importance.

In the very young child, circumscribed myositis ossificans is extremely rare, but the diagnosis may then have to be made from a commencing progressive myositis ossificans (Muenchmeyer's disease). This is seen in children before the age of 12 and is localised mainly in the regions of the neck, shoulders and back. It is usually associated with malformations of the thumbs and great toes; it is a dominant autosomal disease with a grim prognosis.

We mentioned at the start of this chapter that the term circumscribed myositis ossificans included in practice ossification not connected with the muscles, for which various causes have been suggested, particularly infection. In 1969, Angervall et al reported 5 cases of pseudomalignant ossifying tumour of the soft tissues. Four of these five tumours were situated at the base of the limbs, the fifth in the paravertebral muscles. The radiological and histological appearances were identical to those of myositis ossificans and consequently posed the same diagnostic problems. But Angervall et al pointed out that no injury could be related to their origin and that all the patients exhibited an infective syndrome at the start of the disorder (raised sedimentation rate, fever, local pain and in some a raised titer of antistreptolysin O). Further, the lesion developing in the fat (case 2) under the gluteal muscles was quite unconnected with those muscles. The authors concluded that such lesions are not necessarily of traumatic origin and may be unrelated to the muscles. They consider that the term "pseudo-malignant bony tumour of the soft tissues" is preferable to that of circumscribed myositis ossificans [Kuttner 1910, Liebig 1929]. Ackman et al (1995), in connection with some cases of periarticular ossification in patients with respiratory distress given muscular relaxants, suggest the possible role of these agents in patients on assisted respiration.

Ossifying haematoma

The term ossifying haematoma should normally be applied to a well defined lesion: a haemorrhagic focus, usually traumatic, in process of organisation with peripheral osteogenesis. The osteoma of horse-riders might correspond to this definition, but the term has sometimes been extended to intramuscular ossifications where the pathologist would find it quite impossible to prove their origin.

Certain pathologists extend the scope of ossifying myositis not only to ossifications that develop in the fatty tissue but also to para-articular ossifications that may complicate post-traumatic coma, tetanus, extensive burns, paraplegia, and operations to insert prostheses. Traumatic dislocations of the hip, with or without fracture of the acetabulum, studied in 106 cases by Hougaard et al in 1994, were followed in 28% of cases by heterotopic bone formation. Goutallier et al (1986, 1993) stressed the prevention of these ossifications by anti-inflammatory agents.

The context in which such ossification develops points to the diagnosis at the outset. The periarticular ossification fairly common in paraplegics may end in total ankylosis of the joint. Probably arising at the musculo-tendinous junctions, it invades the fibrous capsulo-ligamentous system. Such ossification evolves towards maturity, forming very dense osteomas which, say some authors, it is unwise to remove prematurely if the risk of recurrence is to be avoided.

Some cases of malignant transformation of a myositis ossificans have been reported. Reading these reports, it is to be noted that sometimes the diagnosis of myositis was made clinically, without histological evidence. The so-called myositis had sometimes been irradiated, and often the diagnosis of skeletogenic sarcoma of the soft tissues followed that of myositis so rapidly as to leave a doubt about the original diagnosis of a benign lesion. It emerges from reading different publications that, though malignant transformation of a genuine myositis ossificans is possible, it is quite exceptional.

Osteofibrous pseudotumour of the digits

[Duprée & Enzinger 1986]

Grouped with myositis ossificans, this lesion like the osteoma of paraplegics, raises the issue of development in a site where striated muscle fibers are rare or absent.

General considerations

This is a rare benign lesion of the hands and feet. Given the rarity of the cases it is difficult to assess the sex ratio with any degree of certainty, but there is probably a slight female predominance. This parosteal formation is seen mainly in young adults, the mean age being around 20; but some cases have been reported throughout the first five decades. It is chiefly localised to the proximal and middle phalanges of the digits, the great toes and sometimes a metacarpal.

Clinical features

A localised painless swelling, sometimes slight tenderness, more rarely cutaneous erythema may attract attention; but it is often 2-3 months after the first signs that the patient seeks help. In 40% of cases an injury is invoked as the cause of the lesion. Excision of the lesion is usually followed by definitive cure.

Imaging

Imaging techniques demonstrate an ovoid shadow, a sort of half-spindle, quite well-defined, sometimes resembling that of an exostosis.

Pathological anatomy and histopathology

Macroscopically, the whitish-gray tumour is of fibrous or predominantly bony consistency.

Histologically, it is a loose fibroblastic proliferation, sometimes both cellular and fibrous, in which osteoid or bony trabeculae are differentiated, surrounded by osteoblasts. A key feature is the absence of atypical cells, despite mitoses which may be numerous. There are also some osteoclasts and giant cells and, in a third of the cases, inflammatory lymphocytes and plasmocytes. In some cases fibrosis preponderates. In very few cases are included muscle fibers seen.

The various histological reports are inconsistent as to the presence or not of a zonation phenomenon, as described for myositis ossificans. Actually, this phenomenon can be recognised only by examination of a sample of sufficient size (if from a biopsy) and one which is perfectly located. There is no correlation between the duration of symptoms and osteoid maturation.

Diagnosis

The differential diagnosis includes a periosteal sarcoma (rare in this phalangeal site), a chondrosarcoma (this has atypical cells), an osteoblastoma (where the architecture is different and a mistake is not serious), and a fracture callus or a bony fissure after injury. Here too there is a zonation, but this is more clearly defined.

Heterotopic ossification

As we have mentioned, some pathologists assign periarticular ossification of various origins to the category of myositis ossificans. These ossifications should perhaps be linked to calcification or ossification (one may precede the other) to be observed in the intervertebral disks, menisci and cartilage.

Various reports refer to more or less extensive zones of ossification in most viscera, the meninges, liver, kidney, lung, lymph nodes, retina, vessel walls, bladder and so on, but also in benign or malignant sarcomatous or epithelial tumours. Though myositis ossificans may pose the pathologist a difficult problem of diagnosis, this does not apply to these heterotopic ossifications, usually of mature bone, and whose bony trabeculae often retain some elements of fatty marrow. Nor does it apply to benign osteogenesis, an epiphenomenon during the development of a benign or malignant tumour or other specific disorder such as melorheostosis [Yu et al 1995].

Tumour calcinosis (pseudotumour calcinosis, lipocalcino-granulomatosis, Teutschlaender's disease)

(figs. 18-23)

This rare disorder was identified by Durer in 1899, who considered it a lesion of the serous bursae; Teutschlaender (1935) named it "lipocalcino-granulomatosis" and Inclan described it by the name of "tumour calcinosis" in 1943. It is characterised by the development of calcified masses in the vicinity of one or more large joints.

The familial cases studied have shown a dominant autosomal transmission [Lyles et al 1985]. Further, biochemical studies have revealed hyperphosphataemia, particularly evident in cases with multiple lesions. This hyperphosphataemia is associated with a normal or raised level of 1-25-dihydroxycholecalciferol [Prince et al 1982, Bard et al 1984].

There has also been noted, in several patients, the presence of angioid retinal striae, an anomaly often found in pseudoxanthoma elastica, and in 1980 Kaplan et al published a case which combined tumour calcinosis with such a pseudoxanthoma.

General considerations

This is a rare disorder, commoner in Blacks. Both sexes are equally affected, possibly with a slight male predominance. The disease is manifest in the first decades of life. Haddad et al (1989) reported a case in a white child aged 6; that of Serre et al (1969) was aged 7, and the second case of Rodriguez-Peralto et al (1987) was a child of 10 days. However, adults are also affected and familial forms represent 30% of the reported cases. The "tumours" are situated in the vicinity of the large limb joints, on their extensor aspect; the hips, elbows, shoulders, more rarely the knees and ankles are affected.

Clinical features and course

The tumour grows slowly and is usually painless, often reaching several centimeters in diameter by the time of the first examination. Thus the first attendance may be brought about by limitation of movement, as was the case reported by Bishop et al (1982) of a man of 50 who had been aware of the existence of the lesion of his right shoulder for some years.

On examination there is a firm lobular mass, not tender to palpation; it is adherent to the deep planes and is covered by normal skin; the range of movement of the adjacent joint may be limited.

The spontaneous course is towards sinus formation and infection; surgical excision must be complete to prevent recurrence.

Imaging and paraclinical investigations

Calcium deposits form opaque islands, most often at the surface of the extensor aspect of the joint. The initial image is heterogeneous, and Bard and Perez (1990) specify that diagnosis is possible when the radiographs show "nodular calcifications and cystic images containing an opaque fluid which sediments". CT and MRI provide supplementary information about the relations hips of the calcified deposits to the underlying bones, which may be the site of diverse reactions. It is important to look for other sites of calcification and here scintigraphy is particularly effective.

Supplementary studies may demonstrate a hyperphosphataemia, probably due to a primary renal tubular anomaly, a normal plasma calcium, and an increased sedimentation rate in forms with multiple lesions [Feldman et al 1981, Bard et al 1984].

Pathological anatomy and histopathology

The mineral deposits vary greatly in size in the same patient. In the case of Traca et al (1965) the greatest diameters of the gluteal tumour were 12 and 15 cm. Firm in consistency and multilobular, it is surrounded by a fibrous pseudo-capsule continuous with the septa which lobulate the entire mass. On section, multiple cavitary necrotic foci contain a clear sterile or milky fluid.

In histological sections the calcific concretions are obvious. Particular techniques (Von Kossa) allow the detection of the presence of calcium in the giant cells of the granuloma which surrounds the necrotic calcific foci. This polymorphous inflammatory granuloma consists of giant cells, polynuclears, plasmocytes and histiocytes. In the adjacent collagen there persist numerous elastic fibers, with hyaline degeneration in places. The incineration technique for sections reveals numerous necrotic zones with multiple small rounded or oval formations of calcific deposits.

Dryll et al (1984) studied a case of chondrocalcinosis by electron microscopy, electronic diffraction and X-ray micro-analysis and noted the existence of two types of macrophages, mono- or multinucleate, and cells of fibroblastic type. The calcific deposits were identified as consisting of hydroxyapatite. They noted no changes in the vessels or the collagen which could be incriminated in the physiopathological process of hydroxyapatite deposition. Slavin et al (1993) presented a histopathological and ultrastructural study of familial tumour calcinosis and made a pathogenic hypothesis.

Differential diagnosis

The concordance of the histological lesions around the hydroxyapatite deposits with the radio-clinical and biochemical data is what allows the pathologist to confirm the diagnosis. However, the question of differential diagnosis may arise in certain other conditions with para-articular calcification and ossification belonging to specific disorders.

In hyperparathyroidism, calcification may not only be visceral but also periarticular, around the large joints. These clinical and biochemical syndromes (such as the hypercalcaemia and chronic renal failure in secondary hyperparathyroidism, which is probably the only condition that may pose a real diagnostic problem) differ markedly from that of idiopathic pseudotumour calcinosis. Tezelman et al (1993) reported 17 cases of "tumour calcinosis" of which 11 were connected with primary hyperparathyroidism and 2 with secondary hyperparathyroidism. Three other patients mentioned an injury as the origin of the calcified deposits. The authors could find no cause in only two patients. It is clear that different disorders with more or less identical clinical and radiological appearances are reported under the names of tumour or pseudotumour calcinosis, whereas the biochemical mechanisms are different. This is also the opinion of Frere et al (1983). Sissons et al (1989) reported two quite exceptional cases of large pseudotumour like deposits of calcium pyrophosphate, one digital, the other near the hip, which were at first considered to be genuine tumours. The calcifying fibrous pseudotumour described by Fetsch et al (1993), which affects the extremities in particular, poses no real diagnostic problem.

We may mention here the diffuse calcinoses of children which are associated with muscle and joint phenomena and, in 40% of cases, with scleroderma, and the circumscribed lesions of adults in superficial sites, often associated with Raynaud's syndrome.

Ossifying fibromyxoid tumour of the soft tissues

In 1989, Enzinger et al identified this pseudotumour on the basis of 59 cases.

General considerations

It is commoner in males. Though mainly situated in the subcutaneous tissues, in a third of the cases it is placed more deeply, related to muscles and aponeuroses.

Pathological anatomy and histopathology

Its size varies in the reported cases between 1.5 and 17 cm. It is firm and whitish or whitish-gray in color.

On section it is lobulated, of mucoid appearance, and partly encapsulated by a peripheral osteogenesis which may resemble that of myositis ossificans. The nodules are composed of small round or ovoid cells with frankly eosinophil cytoplasm and an eccentric nucleus. These cells are arranged in columns or a network, or scattered in the mucoid ground substance. In about a fourth of the cases there are changes to fusiform or clear cells. Vascularisation is usually abundant. In places the metamorphism of the ground substance leads to the formation of hyaline areas, fibrosis and osteoid trabeculae. In some cases there are also cartilaginous areas and calcifications.

In two-thirds of 59 cases of this entity [Enzinger et al 1989], the reaction to the anti-S100 antibody was positive but varied in intensity from one patient to another; 9 cases were positive to anti-keratin.

Complete removal, sometimes amounting to a wide excision after one or two recurrences, leads to cure. The origin of this lesion is debatable; therefore Enzinger et al (1989) prefer not to be dogmatic and propose the term of ossifying fibromyxoid tumour, suggesting, only as hypotheses either a cartilaginous origin or one from the cells of the nerve sheaths. This schwannian origin is supported by Miettinen (1991) and Donner (1992). In the case reported by Lax et al (1995), in a prethyroid location 20 years after thyroidectomy, the authors suggest schwannian proliferation as a possible cause of the tumour. Positive immunoreactions with antibodies PS100 and GFAP seem to argue in favor of what remains an hypothesis.

Pigmented villonodular synovitis

(figs. 25-38)

This lesion of the synovial membranes and tendon sheaths was distinguished from sarcomas by Heurtaux in 1891. Bonhomme recognised its inflammatory origin in 1897. In 1924, Lecène and Moulonguet confirmed its inflammatory aetiology in these terms: "... these are all the elements that are habitually encountered in chronic inflammation of long standing". The disorder has been described under numerous designations: giant-cell tumour, myeloplaxoma and benign synovioma among others. In 1941, Jaffe et al first described it by the name of pigmented villonodular synovitis, clearly indicating the inflammatory origin of the lesion. Schematically, several anatomo-clinical forms may be distinguished.

Synovitis, a cryptogenic disease

General considerations

From lack of knowledge of the real cause of the disorder, numerous aetiological hypotheses have been advanced; haemorrhage in an angioma, repeated microtrauma, a chronic haemorrhagic disorder, and so on. It is quite a common affection and may involve any joint, but predominates in the finger joints (80-90% of cases) and in the large joints (knees, hips, elbows). Though usually monoarticular, there are multiple lesions in 4-5% of cases, sometimes symmetrical. This synovitis also occurs in children [Bruns et al 1993, Curtin et al 1993], in whom there seems to be a female predominance.

Clinical features

The presenting features are pain, swelling and joint effusion.

In most cases the diagnosis is made at operation; the villous appearance, nodular or villonodular, of a rust-colored proliferation leaves hardly any doubt, as for the origin of the cavitary lesion which may be associated with it.

This bony lesion may be the presenting feature and the synovial proliferation only slightly pigmented or not at all. It is then for the pathologist to make the diagnosis of the synovial lesion which is the origin of the bony cavities formed in this non-arthrotic joint. The forms with predominantly bony involvement are discussed later.

The course of the disorder depends on the surgical possibilities; complete resection prevents recurrence but is not always possible.

Imaging

Gaubert et al (1974) gave a minute description of the radiological appearances; sometimes marginal "fingernail" erosions situated at the osteo-articular junction, sometimes cavities with sharp outlines surrounded by a fine layer of osteosclerosis. These cavities are often multiple and peripheral. By eroding the articular cartilage they may communicate with the joint-space. Together with these positive signs the absence of calcification in the soft parts argues against an angioma, a very rare juxta-articular myxoma [Daluiski et al 1995], a synovial sarcoma or a cartilaginous tumour; the negative quality of this characteristic however, makes its value relative. In advanced forms the severity of bone destruction strongly suggests a tumour process or a cyst.

Hernigou et al (1990) have shown the value of magnetic resonance imaging. Compared with other investigations (CT scan, arthrography, arteriography) it has proved markedly superior in demonstrating the bony lesions and the infiltration of the soft tissues.

Pathological anatomy and histopathology

The operative and arthroscopic findings and macroscopic examination of resection specimens allows the distinction of localised, diffuse and pseudotumour-like forms.

The localised forms are villous, nodular or mixed. They may be reduced to a few nodules or even only one, which may reach several centimeters in size. The diffuse forms may extend to the entire synovium in some joints, rendering complete excision virtually impossible.

The exuberant pseudotumour-like forms, of firm fibrous consistency or soft and haemorrhagic, may reach a considerable size, as we had the opportunity to see in a boy of 10 whose synovium of the knee weighed over 300 g. It is only natural that, faced with such lesions which penetrate the bony tissue and invade the soft tissues, the operative report should end with a question-mark as to the benign or malignant nature of the lesion.

The histological appearance is characteristic in most cases, presents some difficulties in 15-20% of cases and is frankly difficult in 2-3%. In most cases the compact histiocytic proliferation is dotted with giant cells and traversed by thick-walled vessels. The whole lesion is lobulated by connective tissue septa. There are also fine deposits of haemosiderin, irregularly distributed inflammatory lymphocytic infiltrations and above all foamy histiocytes, either grouped in small clumps or scattered in the cellular proliferation. Sometimes the picture of massive pseudotumour synovitis is completed by deposits of cholesterol and a macrophage reaction. Mitoses are usually rare but occasionally more common but without atypia. There may also be some large nuclei which should not give rise to anxiety if the other appearances correspond to those described above.

Table 2. Pigmented villonodular synovitis

Villous, nodular, mixed cellularity
Easy diagnosis, often by arthroscopy
- Massive forms
Hyalino-osteoid zones, some big nuclei, giant cells, together with: well differentiated vessels, zones of foamy histiocyts and absence of mitotic anomalies
Differential diagnosis
- Synovitis and bony lesions
Easy anatomopathological diagnosis
- Multifocal synovitis
Aetiology can be established only by the context
- Reactive synovitis
Often on arthrosis, minimal cellular proliferation
- Synovitis in contact with prostheses
Necrosis (either extensive of limited) is not by itself a sign of malignancy: nevertheless, it is necessary to exclude a synovialosarcoma and a malignant fibrous histiocytoma

The vascularisation of the synovial villi is often striking. The winding arteries are sectioned many times in the villi and their walls are thickened and hyaline. In some cases the appearance is markedly angiomatous and there is an implied relationship between this vascularity and the haemosiderin deposits. However, Devaney et al (1993) who studied 20 cases of synovial haemangiomas, concluded that their material did not suggest any relationship between the two lesions. However, these massive forms may pose some diagnostic problems. Sometimes the cellular proliferation is monomorphous and pseudo-epithelial, reduced to histiocytic layers with well-marked cell membranes, or pseudo-sarcomatous with giant cells evocative of malignant fibrohistiocytoma. The mitoses may be numerous and their somewhat irregular appearance may stimulate a vain search for a frankly pathological mitosis.

Some rare deposits of haemosiderin (Perls or Turnbull positive) are not formal evidence of a benign lesion but study of the section should reveal the existence of those areas of foamy cells important for the diagnosis. Moreover, the well-individualised thick-walled vessels, the absence of definite cytological signs of malignancy and the general absence of necrosis permit no other diagnosis than that of aggressive but histologically benign haemopigmented synovitis.

Diagnosis

In its villous form the synovitis poses no diagnostic problems, but villous or massive recurrence is always possible. In the diffuse extensive forms (knee, hip, spine) complete excision is rarely practicable and postoperative surveillance is indicated. Recurrences in themselves are no proof of malignancy.

Association of haemopigmented synovitis and bony lesions

Motivated by joint pain in the knee, hip or elbow the radiological examination shows one or more cavities situated in one of the bones of the joint or in both articular bone-ends (acetabulum and femoral head, femoral and tibial condyles). Classically, these relatively rare bony lesions are commoner in nodular synovitis than in diffuse synovitis; however a number of major bony lesions have been reported in diffuse synovitis [Scott 1966, Schajowicz & Blumenfeld 1968]. CT and MRI allow not only a detailed analysis of the synovial lesions but also reveal bony involvement much more often than might have been assessed from conventional radiographs [Spritzen et al 1987, Butt et al 1980].

In the six cases reported by Lequesne et al (1980) in patients aged 19 to 43, the synovitis had several times hollowed out acetabular and femoral cavities. The development of these cavities is very insidious; whereas 62% of the 58 patients studied by Cottent et al (1995) exhibited multiple bony lesions, pain provoked by movement was the presenting feature in only 47%. This bony involvement may simulate a sarcomatous tumour radiologically [Jergesen et al 1978, Kang et al 1992] or raise the diagnosis of a malignant giant-cell tumour [Nielsen & Kiaer 1989].

In my own experience, in practice limited to the hip and knee joints, and that of some fellow pathologists, it seems that at least for some cavities bony penetration takes place to the bone-cartilage boundary and perhaps more probably (and more inevitably) into the zones of capsulo-synovial attachment to the subjacent bones. The location of these cavities in the femoral neck and in non-weightbearing zones of the femoral head and acetabulum is relatively characteristic of the disorder.

Multifocal forms

The rare multifocal forms raise other problems of aetiology. The clinical findings and supplementary investigations may exclude lesions such as haemangiomatosis [Lindenbaum & Hunt 1977] but I have seen in a child confusion with the manifestation of acute articular rheumatism. Dryll et al (1983) made a comparative ultrastructural study of two cases of haemopigmented villonodular synovitis of the knee and two cases of haemophilic synovitis of the elbow and suggested that chronic haemarthrosis may be a mechanism common to both disorders.

Haemopigmented reactive synovitis

Synovitis as a disease must be distinguished from the reactive synovitis which often accompanies an arthrosis. It consists of short markedly pigmented villi which are oedematous or fibrous. In places, the vessels are surrounded by inflammatory cells. In such cases the histiocytic proliferation is usually minimal. Much more rarely, a very cellular form is observed which resembles the synovial disease and poses the same diagnostic problems and in which the part played by various drug injections of the underlying arthrotic joint may play a part.

Synovial proliferation in contact with prostheses

During the operative "revision" of a prosthesis, as at the hip, the pathologist sometimes receives a large specimen which some authors [Griffiths et al 1987] qualify as a pseudotumour. In this compact histiocytic proliferation no villous appearance is seen; if there are any villi they are completely adherent to one another and not identifiable. This is more probably a massive histiocytic reaction which separated the periarticular soft tissues; however this may be, it is necessary to exclude the diagnoses of malignant synovioma and malignant fibrous histiocytoma which may be suspected clinically.

More rarely, we are asked to examine synovial reactions in which the histiocytes assume an epithelioid appearance and form follicular groupings. It is very likely that these appearances are connected with a particular prosthetic material when one considers the extensive range of foreign substances employed. In most cases, the follicles are centered around a fragment of foreign body; but sometimes one may suspect the provocation of a reaction of the Besnier-Boeck-Schaumann type and more rarely tuberculosis; a knowledge of the case history is essential. Some macrophagic synovitides are qualified as giant-cell synovitis; the presence of foreign bodies makes the diagnosis obvious. They are often haemopigmented [Abdul-Karim et al 1992]. Voluminous synovial proliferation may also be seen during the course of subacute lympho-plasmocytic infections.

Synovial sarcoma (figs. 39-46)

General considerations

The tumour is usually localised to the vicinity of a joint, where it may - if only rarely - infiltrate the bone-ends. Intratumour calcification, ossification and chondrogenesis were reported in 17% of the 35 tumours studied by Schmidt et al (1991) in children under the age of 18 years. Ladensteins et al (1993) remind us that synovial sarcoma is the third commonest of the soft tissue tumours in children and adolescents.

The essential prognostic factor is the size of the tumour. The 5-year survival is of the order of 85% if the tumour does not exceed 5 cm in diameter, but is only 21% if its diameter exceeds 10 cm [Brodsky et al 1992]. Sex, age, tumour site and histological type (mono- or biphasic) are without prognostic value.

According to Hashimoto et al, a raised level of nuclear antigen of the cellular proliferation is a bad prognostic factor. In contrast, extensive calcification is a favourable element [Varela-Duran & Enzinger 1982].

Differential diagnosis

In the majority of cases the biphasic tumour poses no real histological problem. The question that may arise at certain sites, for example at the inguinal region, is to know if this is a primary tumour or a lymph node destroyed by invasion, a problem not confined to bone pathology. More specific problems are raised by calcified and osseous tumours, however Milchgrub et al (1993) reported 4 cases of synovial sarcoma with major calcification and formation of osteoid and bone. Radiologically, the tumour being well-circumscribed, three of these cases suggested a benign tumour, but the fourth case, by reason of a subjacent bony erosion, looked very much like a juxtacortical sarcoma. Of the four sarcomas, three were biphasic and only one monophasic, with fusiform predominance. Even more rarely, the tumour is intra-articular [McKinney et al 1992]. The only (unreported) case which I have examined with my colleagues at the pathology department at Bièvres was initially identified as chondromatosis since the intra-articular calcification naturally pointed to that diagnosis. Arthroscopic biopsy allowed histological study and immunohistology of this intra-articular synovial sarcoma (figs. 45, 46). However, if the tumour is monophasic with fusiform cells, the diagnosis must necessarily be based on the immunohistological reactions. In about 50% of cases of monophasic fusiform-cell synovial sarcoma the immunohistological reactions demonstrate keratin and epithelial membrane antigen in a very variable number of cells, at least 10-50% [Corson et al 1984]. But positivity to the antikeratin antibody does not allow the formal exclusion of a leiomyosarcoma. Again, positivity for S100 may be found in synovial sarcoma, even if only rarely, but such positivity does not formally imply a diagnosis of schwannoma.

Monophasic epithelioid synovial sarcoma raises difficult problems. An epithelioid sarcoma must be excluded (but the nodular architecture with central necrosis is quite characteristic) as must a clear-cell sarcoma, in whose cells melanin may be demonstrable in 50% of cases. Some malignant epithelioid schwannomas may also cause difficulty. In these cases comparison of the tests carried out with several antibodies will point to the diagnosis.

The cytogenetic analysis of several clear-cell sarcomas shows the presence of a characteristic remodelling between chromosomes 12 and 22. In synovial sarcoma itself, several authors have reported a reciprocal translocation between the short arm of the X chromosome and the long arm of chromosome 18 [Turc-Carel et al 1986, Miozzo et al 1992]. Lee et al (1993) have used FISH (fluorescence in-situ hybridisation) to identify the translocation t(X;18) in three of five cases.

It is important to note these partly calcified or ossified synovial sarcomas which on the whole have a better prognosis. But it should also be remembered that some trabeculae resulting from benign osteogenesis and some calcification are without diagnostic value; the presence of these bony formations, as we have seen, in no way excludes the diagnoses of chondrosarcoma, giant-cell tumour, malignant fibrous histiocytoma or synovial sarcoma.

Tumour-like bony lesions related to central or peripheral neurological disorders

(figs. 47-54)

Cranial osteoma in meningioma

An osteogenic reaction in the vicinity of a meningioma of the skull vault is commonplace. The biopsy specimen usually consists of thick bony trabeculae between which there is a proliferation of tumour tissue surrounded by fibrous tissue. The sample may not include the meningioma; the remodelling or disappearance of the inner table in the radiographs, the medullary fibrosis, the overall architecture of this bone with its thick trabeculae, separated by wide fibrous spaces all argue against the diagnosis of a simple osteoma. It is prudent in such circumstances to mention the possibility of an underlying lesion not included in the biopsy in the report (cf p. 422).

Bone lesions in neurofibromatosis

Numerous appearances of lesions related to peripheral neurofibromas have been described, but some are related to complex tumours of the nervous system. There may be simple cortical notching of a long bone, a cavity, a congenital pseudarthrosis, repeated fractures, bowing, unequal limb length or scoliosis.

In the serious complex forms the diagnosis is obvious and it is precisely in these cases that a bone biopsy gives the opportunity of identifying the presence of intraosseous neurofibroma. In contrast, in formes frustes such as congenital pseudarthrosis of the tibia, the biopsy has little chance (in my experience) of confirming a neurofibroma as the origin of the lesion. More often, the sample demonstrates nothing more than fibrous tissue.

Subperiosteal haemorrhages are the cause of pseudocystic lesions and probably of most periostoses. They may be massive, as in the case of Gaghwai and Tafazoli (1977) or more discrete (Chapter 40, fig. 10 a).

Vertebral osteolysis in tumours of the spinal canal

The problem here is to identify the nature of the tumour and whether or not it is of bony origin. In principle, if there is a nonosteogenic and nonchondrogenic tumour (an undifferentiated tumour) or a small round-cell sarcoma, the histological examination will not be decisive. The distinction is more easily made from the clinical examination and from good imaging, which may show great extension in length of the lesion which would be improbable if its origin were bony.

Schwannoma: intra- and juxtaosseous

This rare tumour develops from nerves following an intraosseous course, as in the mandibular canal or from the nerves supplying the periosteum. The tumour is observed mainly between the ages of 20 and 45 and in both sexes. Cases are distributed more or less equally among the long, short and flat bones (sacrum, face).

The clinical features are related to the site; an intratibial schwannoma may be revealed only by slight pain or even local swelling. The clinical picture is more definite if the origin is a dental or sacral nerve. The history of a benign schwannoma may precede operation by several years; excision is followed by definitive cure. This is very different from the course of a malignant schwannoma, where the chances of cure are limited.

Imaging of benign intraosseous schwannomas reveals a clear round or oval luscency with regular outlines often bordered by a layer of sclerotic bone. In the long bones this clear image is often eccentric and the persistence of bony ridges may give a multilocular appearance; there is usually a bony bulge at the level of the lesion. The radiological image of juxtacortical schwannoma is both lytic, due to the notch it hollows out in the cortex, and osteogenic, due to the periosteal reaction which develops some bony spicules. Imaging reveals an ovoid tumour attached to a bone, elevating the soft musculo-aponeurotic tissues (fig. 49).

On gross section, a schwannoma is yellowish-brown, red in places, and the entire lesion is spherical or ovoid. Its consistency is elastic, or soft if it contains haemorrhagic areas. Its relation to the nerve from which it arises is not always obvious.

In histological sections, the tumour consists of bundles of fusiform cells, classically separated from each other by a fine reticulin network. The palisaded nuclear arrangement, the whorled bundles (nodules of Verocay) and the vessels with their thick hyaline walls are characteristic. There may also be some areas of oedema. Periosteal osteogenesis, where present, consists of newly-formed bony trabeculae of regular architecture.

The diagnosis of schwannoma is uncommon. It is only at certain sites (facial nerve, sacral nerve roots) that this diagnosis will be suggested by the appearances on imaging. Though, the diagnosis of benign schwannoma is relatively easy from the histological viewpoint, despite possible secondary remodelling, that of malignant schwannoma poses some problems with standard stains. Paradoxically, diagnosis is the more difficult when its malignancy is more obvious; possible alternative diagnoses include fibroblastic sarcoma, malignant fibrous histiocytoma and leiomyosarcoma, hence the importance of immunological testing.

Osteolysis of the sacral segments

While the pathologist faced with a tumour of the sacrum is often led to make a diagnosis of chordoma, chondroma or chondrosarcoma, giant-cell tumour, plasmocytoma, metastasis, invasion by a bowel carcinoma (some problems related to such tumours have been discussed in previous chapters), he is sometimes surprised to discover a tumour of the filum terminale or a meningocele. These lesions have histological appearances which raise no problems of differential diagnosis from a true bone tumour or from the tumours normally identified by the radiological or clinical evidence or during an operative procedure [Ozoux et al 1986, Duthel et al 1988].

Parathyroid osteosis (figs. 55-65)

The pathologist finds this a very protean disorder, and the diagnosis of solitary presentation of a bony lesion sometimes leads to a conclusion that is not clinically evident.

Case histories

Case 1. A woman of 50 was hospitalised for a fracture of the femoral shaft following minimal trauma. The radiographs showed a loss of substance at the fracture site and a biopsy was made during operation. Histologically, this was a giant-cell "tumour"; an osteoclastic reaction at a fracture site never reaches this degree of cellular proliferation although the only possible diagnosis was that of giant-cell tumour, true giant-cell tumour has a metaphyseo-diaphyseal location rather than diaphyseal. Another lesion was a possibility, the brown tumour of von Recklinghausen.

Case 2. Twenty-four hours after a relatively minor injury of the right knee, a man of 20 attended for pain and loss of function. A radiograph revealed a well-circumscribed tumour above the medial femoral condyle, ballooning the cortex. There were also small lytic lesions of the upper end of the tibia and fibula. A skeletal survey demonstrated other lesions. These radiological and clinical findings pointed initially to a diagnosis of hyperparathyroidism. The histological picture was that of osteolysis in an angiomatous and haemorrhagic setting. While this appearance is in no way specific, given the context it must suggest the diagnosis of hyperparathyroidism and exclude that of angiomatosis.

Case 3. A woman of 45 complained of rather ill-defined pain which she localised in the left iliac fossa. In the pelvic radiograph there was an irregular lacuna of the left ilium. This patient had no pathological history. Biopsy removed a haemorrhagic bone fragment which was diagnosed as angioma. Actually it was more representative of a state of hypervascularity than a true angioma. The well-formed vessels were associated with quite diffuse and irregular fibrosis, dense in places. The radiographs of the whole skeleton showed no other tumour-like lesions, but the skeleton had the washed-out appearance seen in osteomalacia, and despite the nonspecificity of the lesions the diagnosis of hyperparathyroidism was considered and then confirmed.

Case 4. A well limited lacuna of the outer part of the upper metaphysis of the tibia in a girl of 11 was subjected to biopsy (fig. 57). Histologically, the lesion presented fibrous tissue which suggested osteitis fibrosa or a fibrous cortical defect, but this small girl suffered from chronic renal failure complicated by secondary hyperparathyroidism.

Neither the extensive lesions of fibrocystic osteitis nor the biochemical features of primary or secondary hyperparathyroidism are involved here. While subperiosteal bony absorption is considered to be very suggestive, it is in no way specific for parathyroid osteosis. Much more suggestive are multiple lytic lesions. For the pathologist, the osteoclasis, osteolysis, medullary fibrosis, osteoid borders, often osteoblastic appositions and the radiological and clinical data are sufficient to direct him to a study of calcium/phosphorus metabolism and to seek the cause of any abnormality identified.

Problems

The problems posed by this disorder evoke two further remarks. The first concerns a particular aspect of the bone absorption, probably non-specific but which I have often found in parathyroid osteosis and rarely seen in osteolysis due to other causes (tumour, metastasis). This is an incomplete absorption, without interruption of the continuity of the bony trabeculae. The collagen framework of the decalcified portion persists in the form of fine fibrils which ensure continuity of the bone trabeculae (fig. 59 a, b). To some extent, this represents on the microscopic scale what is represented by fibrous callus between two fractured bone fragments. The essential difference is that the callus is newly formed, whereas in this type of osteolysis it is the decalcified collagen support which persists, at least partially. Everything happens as if the rapid decalcification markedly preceded the destruction of the collagen which supported the mineral substance. In fact, collagen fibers of the pre-existing bony matrix really do persist, and also a loose fibrosis develops which covers the still intact trabeculae very rapidly and thickens progressively;

The second point, commonplace for those with experience of these problems, concerns parathyroid adenoma. The presence of cells whose nuclei, though not monstrous, are much bulkier than usual, often suggests a diagnosis of carcinoma. But we must recall that parathyroid carcinoma is very rare, functional parathyroid carcinoma even rarer, and that the presence of some large nuclei in a parathyroid adenoma should not make too great an impression on the pathologist.

Sinus histiocytosis: Destombes-Rosai-Dorfman disease (figs. 66-71)

In 1965, Destombes defined this disorder, giving it an anatomical and clinical description based on 4 cases seen in the Antilles and Mali. In 1966, Marie et al described two other cases in young Antillese. In 1969, Rosaï and Dorfman described four new cases and termed it sinus histiocytosis with massive adenopathy, a new entity; in 1972 they added 34 new cases.

General considerations

Currently, the disorder is better known and more often diagnosed, and the existence of bony lesions seem relatively common according to Allegranza et al (1991). In the HML registry (Sinus histiocytosis with massive lymphadenopathy) 33 cases of skeletal involvement are listed; in 9 cases the first lesion was bony and in three there was a solitary lesion without adenopathy. The authors reported a fourth case in a girl of 14, where a lytic lesion of the temporal bone was the first and only manifestation. In the case reported by Unni (1988), the first biopsy was made on a lytic lesion of the sacrum - only two months large cervical lymphadenopathies developed, followed by a lesion of the sternum.

The bony involvement may be manifested by an articular syndrome associated with metaphyseal-epiphyseal involvement, as in the case reported by Delauche et al (1984) in a woman of 26 (figs. 66, 67). In a girl of 11, the clinical onset was with ankle pain [Heidelberger et al 1980]. The pain was rapidly followed by the appearance of lymphadenopathy, but after admission to hospital a skeletal study showed disseminated lesions. Ramos (1976) described the bony lesions, without specific features, in a boy aged only 3 years.

This anatomical and clinical entity, with its benign course, is rare. It affects children and young adults. As we have said, the first reported cases were of African origin (Mali, Transvaal, Senegal) but the sources have become more diverse as the number of cases increases.

What we are particularly concerned with here are forms with osseous or osteoarticular onset but it is important to note that the complete clinical picture comprises, in addition to bilateral cervical lymphadenopathy, an increased sedimentation rate, polyclonal hypergammaglobulinaemia and anaemia of unknown origin.

Diagnostic problems

The problems raised by sinus histiocytosis for the pathologist, as we see it, are as follows. When the bony lesion or lesions precede the adenomegaly by some months, a biopsy is needed as it will be when the bone involvement remains solitary, which is certainly exceptional. If the diagnosis has been made from a nodal biopsy, the development of bony lesions leads to the performance of a biopsy. In favourable circumstances, the diagnosis of sinus histiocytosis may be made from the biopsy if there are specific lesions.

The osteolytic zone is occupied by a polymorphous infiltration of lymphocytes, plasmocytes, neutrophils, few or no eosinophils, and large histiocytes with eosinophil cytoplasm, finely vacuolated. The nucleus of these histiocytes is solitary and the nucleolus small, but some reports mention larger nuclei with a large nucleolus. The cytoplasm of some histiocytes contains phagocyted lymphocytes, neutrophils and sometimes some plasmocytes.

Lymphophagocytosis is one of the characteristic features of this disease. There is no necrosis, but deposits of haemosiderin and some degree of fibrosis may be seen. Along with the osteolysis, moderate bony regeneration is evidenced by the thickening of some trabeculae bordered by osteoblasts.

Immunohistological reactions with antibodies anti-PS100 and CD68 are positive in some histiocytes. Some authors even report a strong positivity of some histiocytes for the anti-PS100 antibody, which is in no way specific to this disorder. The histological lesions in bone do not always allow diagnosis of sinus histiocytosis, but may suggest it when there is a lymphohistiocytic predominance. It is still necessary to exclude histiocytosis X, by the rarity or total absence of eosinophils, the absence of Langerhans cells and especially the absence of necrosis, and osteomyelitis in which the metaphyseal location in a child may be suggestive clinically. In osteomyelitis, the cellular infiltration is more abundant; there is cellular necrosis, and the search for organisms in sinus histiocytosis is negative.

In other cases, the predominantly fibrous histological appearance of the bony lesion does not permit a valid diagnosis [Ramos 1976]. It must be admitted that if the clinical picture is not characteristic or at least suggestive, solitary or primary extranodal lesions rarely permit the diagnosis. In the 17 cases located in the soft tissues reported by Montgomery et al (1992), only one had been diagnosed.

Currently, no cause has been formally demonstrated for this disorder but despite this ignorance the relatively favourable prognosis of Destombes-Rosai-Dorfman disease is clear including cases with bone lesions. Whenever a complete study has been made, it has shown that deaths were usually secondary to intercurrent disease [Ramos 1976, Rosai 1984].

Erdheim-Chester disease (figs. 72-75)

In 1930, William Chester published a study he had made in the department of Professor Erdheim in Vienna, under the title *Über Lipoidgranulomatose*, in which he defined the disorder that was to be named after him. The two cases he studied in great detail were a woman aged 44, dying from cardiopulmonary failure, who exhibited no bony symptoms but an extensive bilateral periorbital xanthelasma, and a man of 69. In both patients Chester described autopsy findings of bilateral bony lesions, with lipogranulomatous infiltration of the tibial and femoral medullary cavities and of various viscera.

General considerations

This is a rare disorder which seems slightly commoner in men than in women. It is discovered around the 5th or 6th decade, but there is nothing to exclude a much earlier and asymptomatic true onset.

The clinical appearances are very polymorphous and related to the extent of the bony lesions, but even more to the visceral involvement, hence the diversity of presenting features. The bony lesions are relatively characteristic: a bilateral and virtually symmetric osteosclerosis, usually sparing the epiphyses and axial skeleton.

Diagnosis is based on the imaging and histologic examination of a biopsy specimen.

The disease raises problems of aetiology, clinical presentation and, in severe forms, of treatment.

Clinical features and course

The purely bony forms, about 50% of cases, may present with pain, usually moderate but sometimes severe [Boulanger et al 1992]; this is sometimes associated with swelling of the soft parts, eg pretibial or periarticular.

In many cases the clinical manifestations are related to the lipogranulomatous infiltration: bilateral exophthalmos due to intraorbital infiltration [Rozenberg et al 1986, Sellami 1991], diverse skin lesions, xanthelasma [Miller et al 1986, Boulanger et al 1992, Brower et al 1984], visceral or perivisceral infiltration evidenced by pulmonary, hepatic or cardiac features; splenomegaly is rare and there is no lymph node involvement, but there may be a retroperitoneal lipogranulomatous tumor and, in some cases, diabetes insipidus, with or without changes in the sella turcica, which precedes diagnosis of the bony lesions by 5-10 years.

Involvement of the nervous system has rarely been reported : signs of pyramidal irritation [Boulanger et al 1992], cerebral images on CT examination [Farre et al 1995]. Modification of the platelet count has also been reported [Bellin et al 1993]. These systemic multivisceral forms are usually associated with a raised sedimentation rate and fever of 38 -38.5°, without any detectable infection.

The course of the purely bony forms is quite unpredictable; some appear to become stabilised, while others progress to virtual generalisation. In the multivisceral forms, the prognosis is worsened by pericardial, vascular or pleuropulmonary involvement and the disease may be fatal.

Imaging

This demonstrates bilateral symmetric metaphyseal or metaphyseo-diaphyseal osteosclerosis sparing the epiphyses. This osteosclerosis may, rather rarely, be associated with a periosteal reaction. In most cases, the long bones of the lower limbs are affected, more rarely those of the forearm.

Exceptionally, osteosclerosis is reported in the axial skeleton, face, cranium or iliac ala [Fink et al 1991]; despite the diabetes insipidus, the sella turcica is described as normal.

Although osteosclerosis is markedly predominant, in places this is obliterated by zones of osteolysis.

In all cases the extent of the bony and visceral lesions must be determined by a complete study (CT, MRI, as indicated). All the affected areas are positive to technetium scintigraphy.

Histology

Histologic examination of bony and visceral biopsies led Chester to designate this condition as lipidogranulomatosis. The lesion is marked by a histiocytic proliferation, in which the cytoplasm shows finely scattered lipid vacuoles giving a foamy appearance; it invades the zones of osteolysis, and at least partially the medullary canal and the perivisceral or visceral tissues of the affected organs. The nuclei are of reduced size in an abundant cytoplasm. There are no cell anomalies and mitoses are very rare. There are also some multinucleate giant cells, lymphocytes, and rare polynuclear cells without any predominance of eosinophil granulocytes.

To date, immunohistologic studies have not demonstrated any cell specificity. In the case reported by Ono et al (1996), the foamy histiocytes exhibited a positive reaction to antibodies anti-Kp1, anti-S100 alpha and beta, anti-neuron specific enolase, anti-alpha1 antitrypsin and anti-alpha1 antichymotrypsin. However, Boulanger et al (1992), Molnar et al (1988) and Fink et al (1991) found a negative reaction to anti-S100.

Ultrastructural study shows numerous lipid droplets in the cytoplasm of the foamy histiocytes, but Birbeck granules have not been demonstrated.

Laboratory findings

In the absence of a specific test, it should be noted that in the majority of cases the plasma phosphorus and calcium are normal and that there are no specific anomalies of plasma lipids. Repeated estimations of cholesterol and triglycerides [Fink et al 1991] gave normal figures but in the patient of Bohne et al (1979), affected by a diffuse form, the neutral fats in the plasma were markedly elevated.

The sedimentation rate is often raised, particularly in forms with visceral involvement. Changes in the platelet count have also been reported.

Diagnosis

This should be suspected when virtually symmetric osteosclerosis sparing the epiphyses and axial skeleton is discovered in the long bones, mainly in the lower limbs, in patients aged 50-60. According to Pertuiset et al (1995), this osteosclerosis is discovered in 40% of cases during an examination performed for some other reason. It is of course the case that the florid symptomatology of this lipogranulomatosis - diabetes insipidus, exophthalmos, xanthelasma, visceromegaly - without lymph node involvement may also lead to the diagnosis. In the absence of a formal test, it is essentially the imaging (figs. 72-75) and the histologic findings which provide the most valuable information.

Apart from purely bony, or bony and multivisceral forms, atypical forms present problems difficult to resolve. This is the case with forms affecting very few bones, osteolytic forms and those affecting only the ribs [Palinka et al 1982] or with involvement of the epiphyses or axial skeleton; the histologic findings cannot be regarded as specific.

Only the circumstances suffice to exclude Gaucher's disease, Niemann-Pick disease, mastocytosis, Engelmann's disease or fluoride poisoning, each requiring the appropriate investigations. The diagnosis from Langerhansian histiocytosis is often difficult, but the absence of Birbeck granules and the negative immunoreaction to antibody CD1a are indicative [Amouroux et al 1993, Farre et al 1995].

Study of the previous history in the search for a cause is disappointing despite the frequency of hypertension, cardiac failure or diabetes insipidus, often detected several decades before the diagnosis of Erdheim-Chester disease is considered.

The disease is often classified with the histiocytoses, which is only a very restricted approach to a genuine nosologic classification.

As for the treatment, various methods have been tried (irradiation, antimitotic agents), not without some encouraging results.

References

Myositis ossificans

Ackerman LV (1958) Extra-osseous localized non-neoplastic bone and cartilage formation (so-called myositis ossificans). J Bone Joint Surg (Am) 40: 279-298

Ackerman LV, Ramamurthy S, Jablokow V, Van Drunen M, Kaplan E (1988) Post-traumatic myositis ossificans mimicking a soft tissue ncoplasm. Case report. Skeletal Radiol 17: 310-314

Ackman JB, Rosenthal DI (1995) Generalized periarticular myositis ossificans as a complication of pharmacologically induced paralysis. Skeletal Radiol 24: 395-397

Amir G, Mogle P, Sucher E (1992) Myositis ossificans and aneurysmal bone cyst. Skeletal Radiol 21: 257-259

Angervall L, Stener I, Ahren C (1969) Pseudomalignant osseous tumour of soft tissue. A clinical, radiological and pathological study of five cases. J Bone Joint Surg (B) 51: 654-663

Bronfen C, Touzet PH, Peuchmaur M, Prieur AM, Rigault P (1993) Myosite ossifiante non traumatique chez l'enfant. Revue de la littérature: à propos d'un cas simulant une tumeur maligne. Rev Chir Orthop 79: 229-234

Brooker AF, Bowerman JW, Robinson RA, Riley LH (1973) Ectopic ossification following total hip replacement. Incidence and a method of classification. J Bone Joint Surg 55A: 1629-1632

Chaplin DM, Harrison MHM (1972) Pseudomalignant osseous tumour of soft tissue. Report of two cases. J Bone Joint Surg 54B: 334-340

Chomette G, Crouzet J, Beraneck L, Akil N (1982) Myosite ossifiante circonscrite non traumatique. A propos d'une observation anatomoclinique. Arch Anat Cytol Pathol 30: 313-316

Clapton WK, James CL, Morris LL, Davey RB, Peacock MJ, Byard RW (1992) Myositis ossificans in childhood. Pathol 24: 311-314

Crouzet J, Chomette G, Nguyen VH, Auriol M, Pere G (1983) Myosite ossifiante circonscrite non traumatique. Difficultés diagnostiques à propos d'une observation. Rev Rhum Mal Osteoartic 50: 213-216

Ducloyer PH, Tomeno B, Forest M, Belloir C, Wybier M (1988) La myosite ossifiante circonscrite non traumatique. A propos de 14 observations et revue générale. Rev Chir Orthop 74: 659-668

Dupree WB, Enzinger FM (1986) Fibro-osseous pseudotumor of the digits. Cancer 58: 2103-2109

Fauré C, Vialas M (1975) Myosite ossifiante circonscrite. A propos d'un cas. Rev Chir Orthop 61: 663-671

Goldman AB (1976) Myositis ossificans circumscripta: a benign lesion with a malignant differential diagnosis. AJR 126: 32-40

Gougeon J, Dousset H, Labram C, Caulet T, Adnet JJ, Boulle J, Rosemberg A (1970) La myosite ossifiante circonscrite non traumatique. Observation anatomaclinique d'un cas et revue générale. Rev Rhum Mal Osteoartic 37: 367-373

Jarvi OH, Kvist HTA, Vaino PV (1968) Extraskeletal retropritoneal osteosarcoma probably arising from myositis ossificans. Acta Pathol Micobiol Scand 74: 11-25

Jeffreys TE, Stiles PJ (1966) Pseudomalignant osseous tumour of soft tissue. J Bone Joint Surg 48B: 488-492

Lagier R, Cox JN (1975) Pseudomalignant myositis ossificans. A pathological study of eight cases. Hum Pathol 6: 653-665

Nuovo MA, Norman A, Chumas J, Ackerman LV (1992) Myositis ossificans with atypical clinical, radiographic, or pathologic findings: a review of 23 cases. Skeletal Radiol 21: 87-101

Ogilvie-Harris DJ, Fornassier VL (1980) Pseudomalignant myositis ossificans: heterotopic newbone formation without a history of trauma. J Bone Joint Surg 62A: 1274-1283

Pack GT, Braund RR (1942) The development of sarcoma in myositis ossificans. Report of three cases. JAMA 119: 776-779

Paterson DC (1970) Myositis ossificans circumscripta. Report of four cases without history of injury. J Bone Joint Surg 52B: 296-301

Pazzaglia UE, Beluffi G, Colombo A, Marchi A, Coci A, Ceciliani L (1986) Myositis ossificans in the newborn. Case report. J Bone Joint Surg 68A: 456-458

Valette C (1985) A propos d'un cas de myosite ossifiante du creux axillaire avec réaction périostée. Ann Orthop Ouest 17: 83-84

Yaghmai I (1977) Myositis ossificans: diagnostic value of arteriography. Am J Roentgenol 128: 811-816

Yu JS, Resnick D, Vaughan LM, Haghighi P, Hughes T (1995) Melorheostosis with an ossified soft tissue mass: MR features. Skeletal Radiol 24: 367-370

Osteoma

Abdelwahab IF, Lewis MM, Klein MJ (1987) Malignant schwannoma of soft tissue of the thigh. Skeletal Radiol 16: 573-576

Benassy J, Boissier JR, Patte D, Divems JC (1960) Ostéomes des paraplégiques (contribution à l'étude de l'ossification neurogène). Presse Med 68: 811-814

Bidard Y, Maury M (1970) Les para-ostéo-arthropathies. Etat actuel du problème. Presse Med 78: 2245-2248

Bitter MA, Komaiko W, Franklin WA (1985) Giant lymph node hyperplasia with osteoblastic bone lesions and POEMS (Takatsukits) syndrome. Cancer 56: 188-194

Brooker AF, Bowerman JW, Robinson RA, Riley LH (1973) Ectopic ossification following total hip replacement. J Bone Joint Surg 55A: 1629-1632

Chatten J, Cromie WJ, Duckett JW (1980) Ossifying tumor of infantile kidney. Report of two cases. Cancer 45: 609-612

Collina G, Annessi G, Di Gregorio C (1991) Cellular blue naevas associated with osteoma cutis. Histopathol 19: 473-475

Engelstad BL, Gilula LA, Kyriakos M (1980) Ossified skeletal muscle hemangioma radiologic and pathologic features. Skeletal Radiol 5: 3540

Fabre J, Bouissou H, Sendrail-Presqué M (1959) Ossifications disséminées du poumon. Ann Anat Pathol 4: 343-360

Fauré C, Vital C, Guériot JC (1972) Calcifications et ossifications des parties molles para-articulaires chez les enfants brûlés. Ann Radiol 15: 733-738

Goutallier D, Lèche PH (1986) Les ossifications périprothétiques après prothèse totale de hanche. Facteurs de risques prévention par l'indométacine. Rev Chir Orthop 73 (suppl II): 211-215

Goutallier D, Colmar M, Penot P (1993) Les ossifications périprothétiques de hanche: influence de la durée du traitement post-opératoire par l'indométacine sur la prévention des ossifications et influence du cotyle vissé sur l'apparition des ossifications. Rev Chir Orthop 79: 22-28

Hougaard K, Kuur E, Kjaersgaard-Andersen P (1994) Heterotopic bone formation after traumatic dislocation of the hip with or without fractures of the acetabulum. Orthop Int 2: 507-511

Le Minor JM, Kempf JF (1989) Ossicule intraméniscal du genou (Lunula) à propos d'un cas. Revue de la littérature. Rev Chir Orthop 75: 501-505

Louis DS, Dick HM (1973) Ossifying lipofibroma of the median nerve. J Bone Joint Surg 55A: 1082-1084

Lubbers PR, Chandra R, Markle BM, Downey EF, Malawer M (1987) Calcified leiomyoma of the soft tissues of the right buttock. Case report. Skeletal Radiol 16: 252-256

Randall JC, Morris DC, Tomita T, Anderson HC (1989) Heterotopic ossification: a case report and immunohistochemical observations. Hum Pathol 20: 86-88

Rhone DP, Horowitz RN (1976) Heterotopic ossification in the pulmonary metastases of gastric adenocarcinoma. Report of a case and review of the literature. Cancer 38: 1773-1780

Royer J, Oppermann, Rollin JP, Pageaut G, Carbillet JP (1969) Ossification choroïdienne. Ann Anat Pathol 14: 239-242

Silverman JF, Fu YS, Williams NB, Kays S (1975) An ultrastructural study of mixed hepatoblastoma with osteoid elements. Cancer 36: 1436-1443

Sodemann B, Persson PE, Nilsson O (1988) Etiology and treatment of periarticular heterotopic ossification after total hip replacement. Rev Chir Orthop 74 (suppl II): 329-332

Warter J, Mantz JM, Otteni JC, Kempf F (1965) L'ossification para-ostéo-articulaire complication fréquente du tétanos (à propos de 9 observations personnelles). Presse Med 73: 1203-1208

Tumoural calcinosis

Baldurson H, Evans EB, Dodge WF, Jackson WT (1969) Tumoral calcinosis with hyperphosphatemia. A report of family with incidence in four siblings. J Bone Joint Surg 51A: 913-925

Bard H, Kuntz D, Molle D, Witvoet J, Ryckewaert A (1984) Etude du métabolisme du phosphore dans un cas de calcinose tumorale. Rev Rhum Mal Osteoartic 51: 63-68

Bard H, Perez CL (1990) La calcinose tumorale. Actualités Rhumatol 7: 183-192

Basex A, Salvador R, Dupre A, Parant M, Christol B (1962) Lipocalcino-granulomatose de Teutschlander. Bull Soc Franc Dermatol Syph 69: 113-116

Bishop AF, Destouet JM, Murphy WA, Gilula LA (1982) Tumoral calcinosis: case report and review. Skeletal Radiol 8: 269-274

Croock AD, Silver RM (1987) Tumoral calcinosis presenting as adhesive capsulitis: case report and literature review. Arthritis Rheum 30: 455-458

Duret MH (1899) Tumeurs multiples et singulières des bourses séreuses. Bull Soc Anat Paris 74: 725-731

Dryll A, Bardin T, Lansaman J, Tran Van P, Hard H, Ryckewaert A (1984) Tumoral calcinosis: light and electron diffraction and X-ray microanalysis of the mineral deposit. J Submicrosc Cytol 16: 577-583

Feldman S, Dalinka MK, Schumacher HR (1981) Diffuse soft tissue calcification in tumoral calcinosis. Skeletal Radiol 7: 33-35

Fetsch JF, Montgomery EA, Mels JM (1993) Calcifying fibrous pseudotumor. Am J Pathol 17: 502-508

Frere D, Kinnaert P, Van Geel P, Van Geertruyden J (1983) Calcinose tumorale et calcifications métastatiques. Pathogénie et essai de classification. Rev Rhum 50: 545-551

Geirnaerdt MJA, Kroon HM, Van der Heul RO, Herfkens HF (1995) Tumoral calcinosis. Skeletal Radiol 24: 148-151

Hacihanefiuglu U (1978) Tumoral calcinosis. A clinical and pathological study of eleven unreported cases in Turkey. J Bone Joint Surg 60A: 1131-1135

Haddafd SN, Ghossain MA, Jebara VA, Roucos S, Kharrat K, Boustany FN (1989) Calcinose tumorale revue de la littérature. A propos d'un cas. Rev Chir Orthop 75: 340-344

Harkess J, Peters HJ (1967) Tumoral calcinosis. J Bone Joint Surg 49A :721-731

Inclan A, Leon P, Camejo MG (1943) Tumoral calcinosis. JAMA 121: 490-495

Kaplan G, Vinceneux PH, Grossin M, Kahn MF (1980) Calcinose tumorale associée à un pseudoxanthome élastique. Rev Rhum 47: 657-660

Kwittken J Branche M (1969) Fasciitis ossificans. Am J Clin Pathol 51: 251-255

Lambrozo J, Boughon JP, Vignalou J, Michaud G (1979) Calcinose tumorale chez un homme de race blanche. Nouv Presse Med 8: 765-767

Lyles KW, Burkes EJ, Ellis, Lucas KJ, Dolan EA, Drezner MK (1985) Genetic transmission of tumoral calcinosis: autosomal dominant with variable expressivity. J Clin Endocrinol Metab 60: 1093-1096

Manaster BJ, McDowell Anderson T (1982) Tumoral calcinosis: serial images to monitor successful dietary therapy. Skeletal Radiol 8: 123-125

Martinez S, Volger JB, Harrelson JM, Lyles KW (1990) Imaging of tumoral calcinosis: new observations. Radiology 174: 215-222

Martini-Benkeddache Y, Martini M, Chlap Z (1974) Calcinose tumorale multiple: un nouveau cas. Rev Chir Orthop 80: 81-87

Masse L, Rousseau M, Masse CL, Chassaigne JP, Mesnier F (1961) La calcinose interstitielle diffuse à propos d'un cas. Presse Med 69: 1384-1387

Peller PJ, Ho VB, Kransdorf MJ (1993) Extraosseous Tc99mMDP uptake: a pathophysiologic approach. Radiographics 13: 715-734

Prince MJ, Schaeffer PC, Goldsmith RS, Chausmer AB (1982) Hyperphosphatemic tumoral calcinosis. Association with elevation of serum 1-25 dihydroxycholecalciferol concentrations. Ann Intern Med 96: 586-591

Rodriguez-Peralto JL, Lopez-Barea F, Torres A, Rodriguez-Gonzalez JI, Diaz-Faes J (1989) Tumoral calcinosis in two infants. Clin Orthop 242: 272-276

Serre H, Izarn P, Simon L, Sany, Baldet P, Pnvat JM (1969) Calcinose circonscrite idiopathique. Presse Med 8: 765-767

Sissons HA, Steiner GC, Bonar F, May M, Rosenberg ZS, Samuel SH, Present D (1989) Tumoral calcium pyrophosphate deposition disease. Skeletal Radiol 18: 79-87

Slavin RE, Wen J, Kumar D, Burke Evans E (1993) Familial tumoral calcinosis: a clinical, histopathologic and ultrastructural study with an analysis of its calcifying process and pathogenesis. Am J Surg Pathol 17: 788-802

Teutschlaender O (1951) Zur Kenntnis der Lipoido-caecinosis progrediens. Zentralb F Allg Path 87: 1-15

Teutschlaender O (1935) Über progressive Lipogranulomatose der Muskulatur zugleich ein Beitrag zur Pathogenese der Myopathia osteoplastica progressiva. Klin Wochenschr 14: 451-453

Tezelman S, Siperstein AE, Duhry Clark OH (1993) Tumoral calcinosis controversies in the etiology and alternatives in the treatment. Arch Surg 128: 737-744

Traca G, Hennebert PN, Mazabraud A (1965) Considérations sur un cas de lipocalcinogranulomatose. Presse Med 73: 543-546

Yaghmai I Mirbod P (1971) Tumoral calcinosis. J Bone Joint Surg 111: 573-578

Zawin M, Katz LD, Lawson JP (1988) Tumoral calcinosis in area of the left hip. Skeletal Radiol 17: 450-453

Ossifying fibromyxoid tumour

Akai M, Azuma H, Ohno T, Kimura H, Sugano I, Nagao K (1991) Ossifying fibromyxoid tumor of the soft parts of the upper arm. Skeletal Radiol 20: 608-612

Donner LR (1992) Ossifying fibromyxoid tumor of soft parts: evidence supporting schwann cell origin. Hum Pathol 23: 200-202

Enzinger FM, Weiss SW, Liang CY (1989) Ossifying fibromyxoid tumor of soft parts a clinicopathological analysis of 59 cases. Am J Surg Pathol 13, 10: 817-827

Kyriakos M (1991) Ossifying fibromyxoid tumor. Something new to mull over (editorial). Am J Clin Pathol 95: 107-111

Lax SF, Ratschek M, Steindorfer P, Langsteger W, Harms D, Beham A (1995) Ossifying fibromyxoid tumour of the neck clinically mimicking a primary neoplasm of the tyroid gland. Pathol Res Pract 1991: 57-60

Miettinen M (1991) Ossifying fibromyxoid tumor of soft parts additional observations of a distinctive soft tissue tumor. Am J Clin Pathol 95: 142-149

Oda N, Yasui W, Ito H, Tahara E (1993) Ossifying fibromyxoid tumor of soft parts: a case report. Jpn J Clin Oncol 23: 64-68

Hemopigmented villonodular synovitis

Abdul-Karim FW, El-Naggar AK, Joyce MJ, Makley JT, Cartier JR (1993) Diffuse and localized tenosynovial giant-cell tumor and pigmented villonodular synovitis. Hum Pathol 23: 729-735

Abrahams TG, Pavlov H, Bansal M, Bullogh P (1988) Concentric joint space narrowing of the hip associated with hemosiderotic synovitis (HS) including pigmented villonodular synovitis (PVNS). Skeletal Radiol 17: 37-45

Amouroux J (1971) La synavite villonodulaire hémopigmentée. Rhumathologie 23: 287-294

Babin-Chevaye J, Mazabraud A (1969) Synovite villonodulaire pigmentée de la hanche. Rev Chir Orthop 55: 359-364

Bellamy HF (1901) The tumor of tendon sheaths. J Pathol Bacteriol 7: 465-480

Bergstrand H (1936) Notes on the genesis of giant-cell tumors. Am J Cancer 27: 701-706

Bonhomme (1897) Contribution à l'étude des tumeurs myéloïdes des gaines tendineuses. Thèse, Lyon

Bruns J, Schubert T, Egger-Stroeder G (1993) Pigmented villonodular synovitis in children. Arch Orthop Trauma Surg 112: 148-151

Butt WP, Hardy G, Ostlere SJ (1990) Pigmented villonodular synovitis of the knee: computed tomographic appearances. Skeletal Radiol 19: 191-196

Byers PD, Cotton RE, Deacon OW, Lowy M, Newman PH, Sissons HA, Thomson AD (1968) The diagnostic and treatment of pigmented villonodular synovitis. J Bone Joint Surg 50B: 290-305

Cotten A, Flipo RM, Chastanet P, Desvigne-Noulet M-C, Duquesnoy B, Delcambre B (1995) Pigmented villonodular synovitis of the hip: review of radiographic features in 58 patients. Skeletal Radiol 24: 1-6

Curtin WA, Lahoti OP, Fogarty EE, Dowling FE, Regan BF (1993) Pigmented villonodular synovitis arising from the sheath of the extensor hallucis longus in an eight-month-old infant. Clin Orthop 292: 282-284

Daluiski A, Seeger LL, Doberneck SA, Finerman GAM, Eckardt JJ (1995) A case of juxta-articular myxoma of the knee. Skeletal Radiol 24: 389-391

Devaney K, Vinh TN, Sweet DE (1993) Synovial hemangioma: a report of 20 cases with differential diagnostic considerations. Hum Pathol 24: 737-745

Dryll A, Lansaman J, Bardin T, Ryckewaert A (1983) Synovite villonodularre hémopigmentée: étude ultrastructurale et comparaison avec la synovite hémophilique. Rev Rhum 50: 87-93

Forest M, Courpied JP, Le Floch P, Carlioz A, Abelanet R, Postel M (1985) La hanche opérée: réactions tissulaires locales. Ann Pathol 5: 3-18

Gaubert J, Mazabraud A, Verdie JC, Cheneau J (1974) Les synovites villo-nadulaires hémopigmentées des grosses articulations. Rev Chir Orthop 60: 265-298

Grailly de R, Léger H, Loubet R (1953) Considérations biopathologiques concernant les articulations, les bourses séreuses, le milieu synovial et leurs affections inflammatoires et tumorales. Rev Path Gen Comp 53: 457-511

Greenfield MM, Wallace KM (1950) Pigmented villonodular synovitis. Radiology 54: 350-356

Griffiths HJ, Burke J, Bonfiglio TA (1987) Granulomatous pseudotumors in total joint replacement. Skeletal Radiol 16: 146-152

Hernigou PH, Marichez M, Voisin MC, Delepine H, Goutallier D (1990) Apport de l'imagerie par résonance magnétique dans le bilan de la synovite villonodulaire du genou à forme pseudo-tumorale. A propos d'un cas. Rev Chir Orthop 76: 218-221

Heurtaux A (1891) Myélome des gaines tendineuses. Arch Gen Med 27: 40-54 & 160-169

Jaffe, Lichtenstein, Surro (1941) Pigmented villonodular synovitis, bursitis and tenosynovitis. Arch Pathol 31: 730-765

Jergesen HE, Mankin HJ, Schiller Al (1978) Diffuse pigmented villonodular synovitis of the knee mimicking primary bone neoplasm. Report of two cases. J Bone Joint Surg 60A: 825-839

Kang GH, Chi JG, Choi IH (1992) Pigmented villonodular synovitis of the sacral joint with extensive bone destruction in a child. Pediatr Pathol 12: 725-730

Kindblom LG, Gunterberg B (1978) Pigmentod villonodular synovitis involving bone. J Bone Joint Surg 60A :830-832

Lequesne M, Nicolas JL, Kerboull M, Postel M (1980) La synovite villonodulaire de la hanche. Etude de six cas. Int Orthop 4: 133-144

Lindenbaum BL, Hunt T (1977) An unusual presentation of pigmented villonodular synovitis. Clin Orthop 122: 263-267

Locker B, Beguin J, Vielpeau C (1987) Synavite villonodulaire du genou. Ann Orthop Ouest 19: 51-54

Mac Master PE (1960) Pigmented villonodular synovitis with invasion of bone. Report of 6 cases. J Bone Joint Surg 42A: 1170-1183

Malherbe A (1896) Du myélome des gaines tendineuses et du tissu fibreux. Congrès Français de Chirurgie, 10e Session, Paris: 807-828

Mazabraud A (1954) Les vaisseaux dans la synovite et la tenosynovite hémopigmentée villonodulaire. Sem Hop Paris (Arch Ana Path) 2: 1-14

Monghal JP, Dorfman H, Caroit M, Ryckewaert A (1981) Contribution à l'étude de la synovite villonodulaire du genou. Rev Rhum 48: 397-402

Nielsen AL, Kiaer T (1989) Malignant giant-cell tumor of synovium and locally destructive pigmentod villonodular synovitis: ultrastructural and immunohistochemical study and review of the literature. Hum Pathol 20: 765-771

Pantazopoulos TH, Stavrou Z, Stamos C, Kehayas G, Hartofilakidis-Garofalidis G (1975) Bone lesions in pigmented villonodular synovitis. Acta Orthop Scand 46: 579-592

Present DA, Bertoni F, Enneking WF (1986) Pigmented villonodular synovitis arising from bursa of the pes anserinus muscle, with secondary involvement of the tibia. Skeletal Radiol 15: 236-240

Schajowicz F, Blumenfeld I (1968) Pigmented villonodular synovitis of wrist penetration into bone. J Bone Joint Surg 50B: 312-317

Scott PM (1968) Bone lesions in pigmented villonodular synovitis. J Bone Joint Surg 50B: 306-311

Spritzer CE, Dalinka MK, Kressel HY (1987) Magnetic resonance imaging of pigmented villonodular synovitis: a report of two cases. Skeletal Radiol 16: 316-319

Weidner N, Challa VR, Bonsib SM. Davis CH, Carroll TJ (1986) Giant-cell tumors of synovium (pigmented villonodular synovitis) involving the vertebral column. Cancer 57: 2030-2036

Synovial sarcoma

Brodsky DT, Burt ME, Hajdu SI, Casper ES, Brennan MF (1992) Tendosynovial sarcoma clinicopathologic features, treatment and prognosis. Cancer 70: 484-489

Buck P, MicKelson R, Bonfiglio M (1981) Synovial sarcoma. A review of 33 cases. Clin Orthop 156: 211-215

Corson JM, Weiss LM, Banks-Schlogel SP, Pinkus GS (1984) Keratin proteins and carcinoembryonic antigen in synovial sarcomas. An immunohistochemical study of 24 cases. Hum Pathol 15: 615-621

Dardick J, O'Brien PK, Diane Jeans MT, Massiah KA (1982) Synovial sarcoma arising in an anatomical bursa. Virchows Arch (Pathol Anat) 397: 93-101

El-Naggar AK, Ayala AG, Abdul-Karim FW, MacLemore D, Ballance WW, Garncey L, Ro JY, Batsakis JG (1990) Synovial sarcoma. A DNA flow cytometric study. Cancer 65: 2295-2300

Fievez M, Haas F (1965) Les sarcomes de la synoviale. Ann Anat Pathol 10: 351-362

Fischer C (1986) Synovial sarcoma. Ultrastructural and immunohistochemical features of epithelial differentiation in monophasic and biphasic tumors. Hum Pathol 17: 996-1008

Fisher C, Schofield JB (1991) S-100 protein positive synovial sarcoma. Histopathology 19: 375-377

Gabbiani G, Yao-Shi fu, Kaye GI, Lattes R, Majno G (1972) Epithelioid sarcoma. A light and electron microscopic study suggesting a synovial origin. Cancer 30: 486-499

Ghardially FN (1987) Is synavialosarcoma a carcinosarcoma of connective tissue? Ultrastructural Pathol 11: 147-151

Hajdu SI, Shiu MH, Fortner JG (1977) Tendosynovial sarcoma. A clinicopathological study of 136 cases. Cancer 39: 1201-1217

Ivanov-Dutescu R, Tomeno B, Mallet F, Laugier A, Forest M (1992) Synovialosarcome. Etude d'une série de 46 cas. Rev Chir Orthop 78: 1-7

Ladenstein R, Treuner J, Koscielniak E, d'Oleire F, Keim M, Gadner H, Jurgens H, Niethammer D, Ritter J, Schmidt D (1993) Synovial sarcoma of childhood and adolescence. Report of the German Cws-81 study. Cancer 71: 3647-3655

Leader M, Patel J, Collins M, Kristin H (1987) Synovial sarcomas true carcinosarcomas? Cancer 59: 2096-2098

Lee W, Han K, Harris CP, Shim S, Kim S, Meisner LF (1993) Use of FISH to detect chromosomal translocations and deletions. Analysis of chromosome rearrangement in synovial sarcoma cells from paraffin- embedded specimens. Am J Pathol 143: 15-19

Lejars, Rubens-Duval (1910) Les sarcomes primitifs des synoviales articulaires. Rev Chir 41: 751-783

McKinney CD, Mills SE, Fechner RE (1992) Intraarticular synovial sarcoma. Am J Surg Pathol 16, 10: 1017-1020

Miettinen M, Virtane I (1984) Synovial sarcoma. A misnomer. Am J Pathol 117: 18-25

Milchgrub S, Ghandur-Maymneh L, Albores-Saavedra J (1993) Synovial sarcoma with extensive osteoid and bone formation. Am J Surg Pathol 17: 357-363

Miozzo M, Sozzi G, Cariani CT, Di Palma S, Luksch R, Azzarelli A, Pierotti MA, Della Porta G (1992) A synavial sarcoma with t(X;-18)(pll;-qll) in a patient with Turner's syndrome. Genes Chrom Cancer 4: 192-193

Oda Y, Hashimoto H, Takeshita S, Tsuneyoshi M (1993) The prognostic value of immunohistochemical staining for proliferating cell nuclear antigen in synovial sarcoma. Cancer 72: 478-485

Oda Y, Hashimoto H, Tsuneyoshi M, Takeshita S (1993) Survival in synovial sarcoma a multivariate study of prognostic factors with special emphasis on the comparison between early death and long-term survival. Am J Surg Pathol 17: 35-44

Ordonez NG, Mahfouz SM, Mackay B (1990) Synovial sarcoma an immunohistochemical and ultrastructural study. Hum Pathol 21: 733-749

Panh MH, Aftimos G, Pasquier B, Couderc P, Mazabraud A (1976) Les synovialosarcomes cervicaux extra-articulaires. Revue de la littérature à propos de deux observations. Bull Cancer 63: 309-326

Parache R (1963) Contribution à l'étude histologique de la synoviale et de ses tumeurs. Thèse, Nancy

Raynal L, Fievez M, Collard, Cornil Y, El Banna S (1976) Sarcome synovial primitif intra-articulaire. Acta Orthop Belg 42 : 318-328

Sastre-Garau X, Bosq J, Carlu C (1989) Etude immunohistochimique de 20 sarcomes synoviaux de l'enfant. Ann Pathol 9: 109-114

Schmidt D, Thum P, Harms D, Treuner J (1991) Synovial sarcoma in children and adolescents. A report from the Kiel pediatric tumor registry. Cancer 67: 1667-1672

Steinberg BD, Gelberman RH, Mankin HJ, Rosenberg AE (1992) Epithelioid sarcoma in the upper extremity. J Bone Joint Surg 74A: 28-35

Stenman G, Kindblom LG, Angervall L (1992) Reciprocal translocation t(l2;-22) (q13;-q13) in clear-cell sarcoma of tendons and aponeuroses. Genes Chrom Cancer 4: 122-127

Turc-Carel C, Dal Cin P, Li F, Sandberg AA (1986) Translocation X;18 in a synovial sarcoma. Cancer Genet Cytogenet 23: 93

Van de Stadt J, Thoua Y, Spiegl G, Rasquin C, Bumy F (1984) Synoviosarcome, présentation d'un cas et revue de la littérature. Rev Chir Orthop 70: 643-648

Varela-Duran J, Enzinger FM (1982) Calcifying synovial sarcoma. Cancer 50: 345-352

Wright CSE (1952) Malignant synovioma. J Pathol Bacteriol 64: 585-603

Bone changes in neurologic lesions

Abdelwahab IF, Hemmann G, Stollman A, Wolfe D, Lewis M, Zawin J (1989) Giant intraosseous schwannoma. Skeletal Radiol 18: 466-469

Andersen KS (1976) Congenital pseudarthrosis of the leg late results. J Bone Joint Surg 58A: 657-666

Bitan F, Rigault, Padovani JP, Finidori G, Touzet PH (1987) Pseudarthroses congénitales du tibia et du péroné chez l'enfant. Résultats du traitement de 18 cas par enclouage et greffe. Rev Chir Orthop 73: 552-560

Crawford AH (1992) In: The child's foot and ankle. James Drennan (ed). Raven Press, pp 445-447

Crawford AH, Bagamery N (1986) Osseous manifestations of neurofibromatosis in childhood. J Pediatr Orthop 6: 72-88

De la Monte SM, Dorfman HD, Chandra R, Malawer M (1984) Intraosseous schwannoma: histologic features, ultrastructure, and review of the literature. Hum Pathol 15: 551-558

Debeyre J, Godlewski S, Mazabraud A, Ben Hamida M (1966) Ependymome du sacrum. Revue Neurologique 116: 265-268

Disimone RE, Berman T, Schwentker EP (1987) The orthopedic manifestation of neurofibromatosis a clinical experience and review of the literature. Clin Orthop 230: 277-283

Duthel R, Charret MC, Huppert J, Deluzarches Ph, Motuo Fotso MF, Barral F (1988) Méningocèle sacrée antérieure. A propos de onze cas. Neurochir 34: 90-96

Gordon EJ (1976) Solitary intraosseous neurilemmoma of the tibia. Review of intraosscous neurilemmoma and neurofibroma. Clin Orthop 117: 271-282

Gregg PJ, Price BA, Ellis HA, Stevens J (1982) Pseudarthrosis of the radius associated with neurofibromatosis. Clin Orthop 171: 175-179

Hensley CD (1953) The rapid development of a "subperiosteal bone cyst" in multiple neurofibromatosis. J Bone Joint Surg 35A: 197-203

Hooper G, McMaster MJ (1979) Neurofibromatosis with tibial cyst caused by recurrent hemorrhage. J Bone Joint Surg 61A: 274-275

Janecki CJ, Nelson CL, Dohn DF (1972) Intrasacral cyst. J Bone Joint Surg 54A: 423-428

Klenerman L, Merrick MV (1973) Anterior sacral meninogocele occuring in a family. J Bone Joint Surg 55B: 331-334

Kullmann L, Wouters HW (1972) Neurofibromatose, gigantisme et hématome sous-périostal. Deux cas accompagnés de formation osseuse extensive sous périostal sur les os longs. Rev Chir Orthop 58 (suppl 1): 237-240

Locht RC, Huebert HT, McFarland F (1981) Subperiosteal hemorrhage and cyst formation in neurofibromatosis: a case report. Clin Orthop 155: 141-146

Lorson EL, Delong PE, Obson B, Dolan KB (1977) Neurofibromatosis with central neurofibromas of the mandible. Review of literature and case report. J Oral Surg 35: 733-738

Mazingarbe A, Mazabraud A (1970) A propos d'un cas de neurinome du tibia. Rev Chir Orthop 56: 83-88

Morrissy RT, Riseborough EJ, Hall JE (1981) Congenital pseudarthrosis of the tibia. J Bone Joint Surg 63B: 367-375

Myers JL, Bernreuter W, Dunham W (1990) Melanotic schwannoma of bone. Clinicopathologic, immunohistochemical and ultrastructural features of a rare primary bone tumor. Clin Pathol 93: 424-429

Ozoux JP, de Calan L, Portier G, Burgot D, Brizon J, Lapierre F, Gouaze A (1986) Méningocèle sacrée antérieure. Présentation de ces 2 cas traités par voie abdominale. J Chir (Paris) 123: 424-427

Pitt JM, Mosher JF, Edeiken J (1972) Abnormal periosteum and bone in neurofibromatosis. Radiology 103: 143-146

Schenkein I, Bucker ED, Helson L, Alselrod F, Dancis J (1974) Increased nerve-growth-stimulating activity in disseminated neurofibromatosis. N Engl J Med 290: 613-614

Thierry A, Archimbaud JP, Fischer G, Freidel M, Mansuy L (1968) La meningocèle antérieure. Revue de la littérature et présentation d'un cas. Neurochirurgie 15: 389-412

Yaghmai I, Tafazoli M (1977) Massive subperiosteal hemorrhage in neurofibromatosis. Radiology 122: 439-441

Parathyroid osteosis

Barbier J, Kraimps JL, Denizot A, Henry JF (1992) Hyperparathyroïdisme primaire: résultats d'une étude multicentrique française. Bull Acad Natl Med 176: 1033-1048

Bardin T, Kuntz D (1988) Chondrocalcinose articulaire et hyperparathyroïdie primitive. Rev Rhum 55: 511-513

Buchanan WW (1990) L'hyperparathyroïdie primitive. Le premier cas décrit d'ostéite fibrokystique. Rev Rhum 57: 167-169

Carretier M, Barbier J (1992) L'hyperparathyroïdie primitive: étiologie, physiopathologie, histoire naturelle. Ann Chir 46: 646-652

Chigot JP, Lizana C, Chiche B, Dura C, Menegaux F (1990) Hyperparathyroïdie primaire analyse rétrospective de 645 observations. Sem Hop Paris 14: 726-730

Hayes CW, Conway WF (1991) Hyperparathyroidism. Radiol Clin North Am (Metabolic Bone Disease) 29: 85-96

Lièvre JA (1932) L'ostéose parathyroïdienne. Masson, Paris

Lièvre JA, Camus JP, May V (1971) Etude sur 30 cas récents d'hyperparathyroïdisme. Rev Rhum 28: 401-407

Meunier P, Vignon G, Bernard J, Edouard C, Coupron P, Porte J (1972) Lecture quantitative de la biopsie osseuse, moyen de diagnostic et d'étude de 106 hyperparathyroïdies primitives, secondaires et parancoplasiques. Rev Rhum 39 : 635-644

Oberlin F, Camus JP (1992) Petite histoire de l'hyperparathyroïdie primaire. Synoviale 8: 34-43

Parisien M, Silverberg SJ, Shane E, Dempster DW, Bilezikian JP (1990) Bone disease in primary hyperparathyroidism. Endocrinol Metab Clin North Am 19 :19-34

Robin C (1849) Sur l'existence de deux nouvelles espèces d'éléments anatomiques qui se trouvent dans le canal des os. CR Soc Biol 1: 149-150

Wémeau JL, Gilliot-Valtille E, Bizard JP, Leroy R, Marchandise X, Decoulx M, Proye C (1989) Current concepts in primary hyperparathyroidism. Horm Res 32: 93-96

Sinus histiocytosis

Allegranza A, Barbareschi M, Solero CL, Fornari M, Lasio G (1991) Primary lymphohistiocytic tumour of bone: a primary osseous localization of Rosaï-Dorfman disease. Histopathology 18: 83-86

Delauche MC, Clauvel JP, Tricot G, Laval-Jeantet M, Mazabraud A, Seligmann M (1984) Sinus histiocytosis with massive lymphadenopathy: one further case with osteoarticular presentation. J Rheumatol 11: 83-86

Destombes P (1965) Adenites avec surcharge lipidique de l'enfant ou de l'adulte jeune, observées aux Antilles et au Mali: quatre observations. Bull Soc Pathol Exot Filiales 58: 1169-1175

Do PL, Estes ML (1989) Immunohistochemical characterization of the histiocytes in sinus histiocytosis with massive lymphadenopathy: analysis of an extranodal case. Hum Pathol 20: 711-715

Heidelberger KP, Schnitzer B, Tilford D, Poznanski AK, Heyn R (1980) Sinus histiocytosis with massive lymphadenopathy and gross skeletal involvement. Skeletal Radiol 5: 42-46

Larkin DFP, Dervan PA, Munnelly J, Finucane J (1986) Sinus histiocytosis with massive lymphadenopathy simulating subacute thyroiditis. Hum Pathol 17: 321-324

Le Tinier M (1972) Histiocytose lipidique ganglionnaire et pseudo-tumorale. Une nouvelle observation antillaise. Thèse, Paris

Leroy JP, Reguer M, Parent P, Volant A, Castel Y (1985) Histiocytose sinusale hémocytophagocytaire avec lymphadénopathie ou maladie de Destombes-Rosaï. Rev Inter Pediatr 149: 29-35

Lewin JR, Das SK, Blumenlhal BI, D'Cruz C, Patel RB, Howell GE (1985) Osseous pseudotumor, the sole manifestation of sinus histiocytosis with massive lymphadenopathy. Am J Clin Pathol 408: 183-189

Marie J, Bernard J, Nezelof C, Leveque B, Scharson G, Desbois JC, Watchi JM, Lemaigre-Voreaux J (1966) Adénopathies chroniques avec prolifération réticulohistiocytaire et surcharge lipidique. Ann Pediatr 46: 2689-2697

Montgomery EA, Meis JM, Frizzera G (1992) Rosai-Dorfman disease of soft tissue. Am J Surg Pathol 16: 122-129

Nawroz IM, Wilson-Storey D (1989) Sinus histiocytosis with massive lymphadenopathy (Rosal-Dorfman disease). Histopathology 14: 91-99

Penneys NS, Ahn YS, McKinney EC, McCleod T, Byrne G. Byrnes J, Nadji M (1982) Sinus histiocytosis with massive lymphadenopathy. A case with unusual skin involvement and a therapeutic response to vinblastine-loaded platelets. Cancer 49: 1994-1998

Ramos CV (1976) Widespread bone involvement in sinus histiocytosis. Arch Pathol Lab Med 100: 606-608

Rosaï J, Dorfman RF (1972) Sinus histiocytosis with massive lymphadenopathy: a pseudolymphomatous benign disorder. Cancer 20: 1174-1188

Rosaï J, Dorfman RG (1969) Sinus histiocytosis with massive lymphadenopathy: a clinocopathologic entity. Arch Pathol 87: 63-70

Unni KK (1988) Sinus histiocytosis with massive lymphadenophathy (Rosai-Dorfman disease) presenting as lesion in the sacrum. Skeletal Radiol 17: 129-132

Walker PR, Rosai J, Dorfman RF (1981) The osseous manifestation of sinus histiocytosis with massive lymphadenopathy. Am J Clin Pathol 75: 131-139

Erdheim-Chester disease

Amouroux J, Guérin CL, Cywiner-Golenzer Ch (1993) Réticulohistiocytose multicentrique. L'actualité rhumatologique. Expansion Scientifique Française, Paris

Bellin MF, Cacoub P, Grellet J (1993) Erdheim-Chester disease associated with renal involvement and thrombocythemia. Eur Radiol 3: 266-269

Bohne ZHO, Goldman AB, Bullough P (1979) Erdheim-Chester disease. Case report. Skeletal Radiol 4: 164-167

Boulanger E, Talaska A, Le Monies de Sagazan (1992) Maladie de Chester-Erdheim. Une observation. Presse Med 21: 1714-1716

Brower AC, Worsham GF, Dudley AH (1984) Erdheim-Chester disease: A distinct Lipoidosis or part of the spectrum of histiocytosis. Radiology 151: 35-38

Chester W (1930) Über Lipoidgranulomaose. Virchow's Arch (Pathol Anat) 279: 561-602

Farre I, Copin M-Ch, Boulanger E, Remy J, Wallaert B, Gosselin B (1995) Maladie d'Erdheim-Chester. Etude anatomo-clinique à propos de deux cas. Ann Pathol 15: 59-62

Fink MG, Levinson DJ, Brown ND, Sreekanth S, Sobel GW (1991) Erdheim-Chester disease case report with autopsy findings. Arch Pathol Lab Med 115: 619-623

Guinebretière JM, Hatcherian G, Lesort A, Mechin J-F, Vandroux J-C (in press) Un cas de maladie d'Erdheim-Chester

Miller RL, Sheeler LR, Bauer TW, Bukowski RM (1986) Erdheim-Chester disease case report and review of the literature. Am J Med 80: 1230-1236

Molnar CP, Gottschalk R, Gallagher B (1988) Lipid granulomatosis: Erdheim-Chester disease. Clin Nucl Med 13: 736-741

Nezelof C, Barbet S (1985) Histiocytosis. Nosology and pathobiology. Pediatr Pathol 3: 1-41

Ono K, Oshiro M, Vemura K, Ota H, Matsushita Y, Ijima S, Iwase T, Uchida M, Katsuyama T (1996) Erdheim-Chester disease: a case report with immunohistochemical and biochemical examination. Hum Pathol 27: 91-95

Palinka MK, Turner ML, Thompson JJ, Lee RE (1982) Lipid granulomatosis of the ribs: Focal Erdheim-Chester disease. Radiology 142: 297-299

Pertuiset E, Guérin CL, Amouroux J, Cywinner-Golenzer (1995) Manifestations osseuses des histiocytoses. L'actualité rhumatologique. Expansion Scientifique Française, Paris, pp 141-155

Rozenberg I, Wechsler J, Koenig F, Brun B, Larde D, Ravlo Y, Hazard J, Pinaudeau Y, Coscas G (1986) Maladie d'Erdheim-Chester. Forme multiviscérale révélée par une exophtalmie. Rev Med Interne 7: 311-317

Sellami M, Sellami F (1991) Une cause rare d'exophtalmie, la maladie d'Erdheim-Chester. Presse Med 20: 607

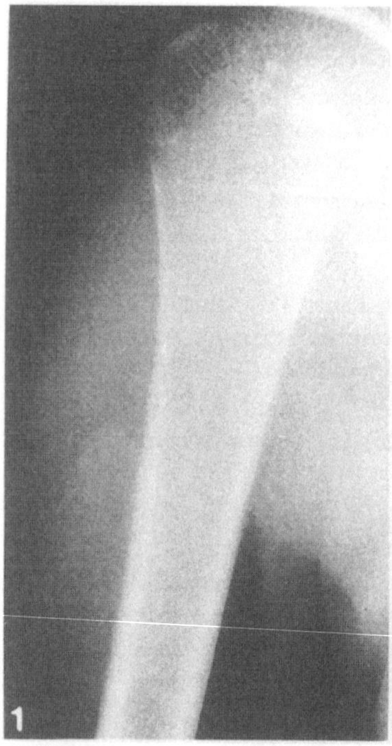

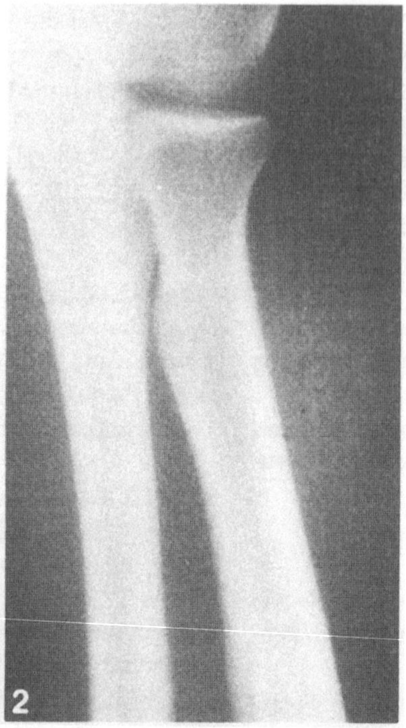

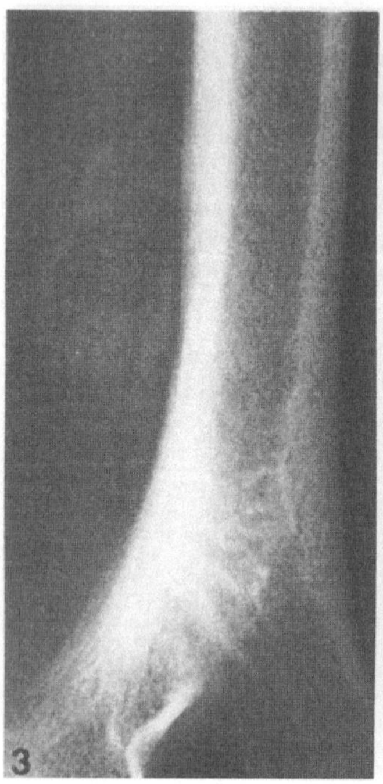

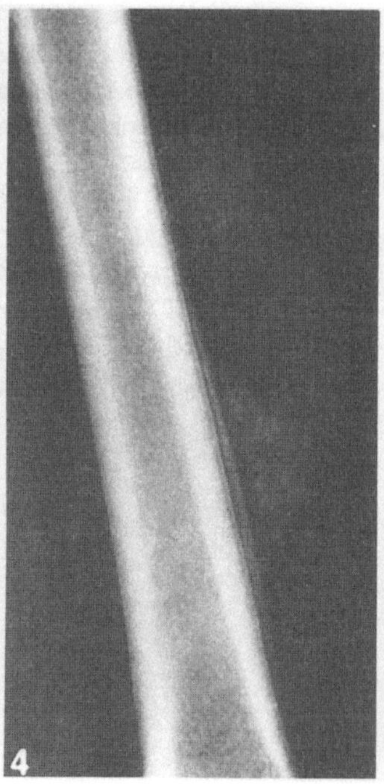

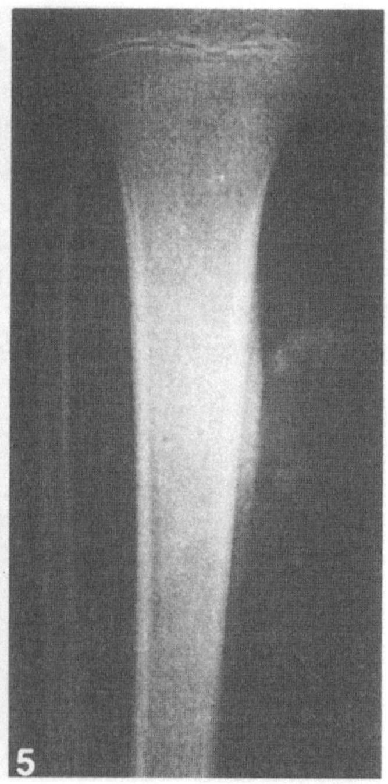

Fig. 1. Young girl aged 13: osteogenesis appearing as an ovoid shadow at the outer aspect of the arm is barely visible at this onset stage

Fig. 2. Adjacent to the radius a cloudy shadow evidences the first stages of ossification in this woman of 20

Figs. 3-5. Three cases of myositis ossificans adjacent to the humerus, femur and tibia in patients aged 15, 14 and 8 years, accompanied by major periosteal reaction. The opacity of the lesion is irregular and cloudy, but more marked peripherally, especially in (3)

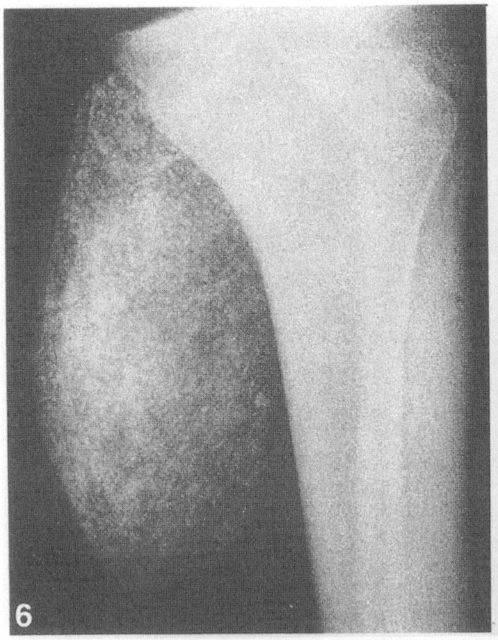

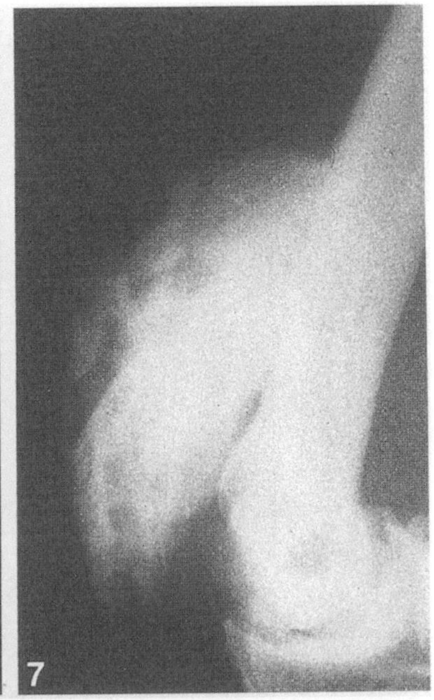

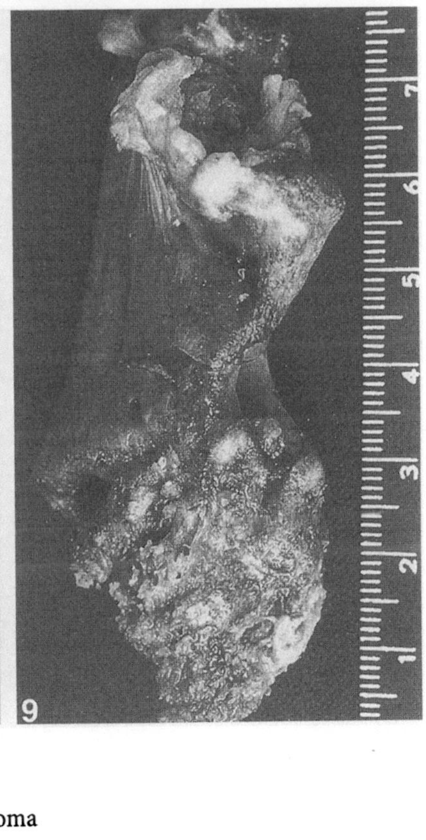

Fig. 6. Transformation of the soleus muscle into a sort of calcified angiofibroma

Fig. 7. This dense ossification at the postero-inferior part of the humerus may be regarded as a late mature stage of "myositis ossificans" in a man of 56

Fig. 8. Unusual appearance of myositis ossificans at outer aspect of thigh

Fig. 9. After an injury followed by coma, this patient developed several periarticular osteomas

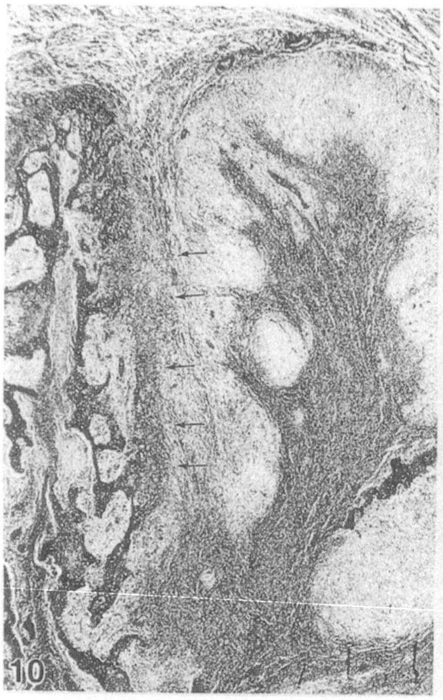
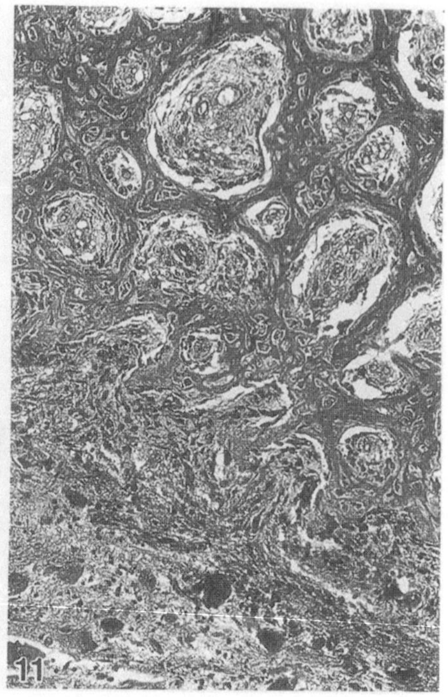
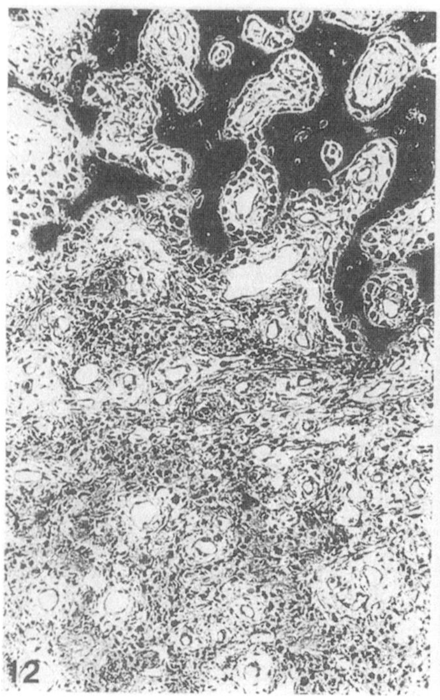
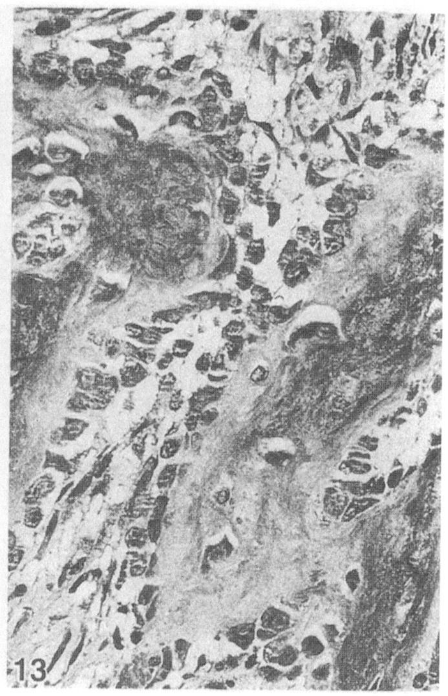

Fig. 10. Nodule of myositis ossificans: zonation. Central portion: loose non-ossified connective tissue. Periphery: newly-formed immature bony tissue, partly calcified. Between the central and peripheral zones: osteoid noncalcified tissue (*arrows*). No haemorrhagic or necrotic focus

Fig. 11. Inter-anastomosed trabeculae of metaplastic bone at periphery of nodule. More laterally (below and left) relics of muscle fibers in a dense connective tissue

Fig. 12. Noncalcified osteoid rudiments, intermediate between the calcified bony tissue and the central fibrous zone

Fig. 13. Osteoid trabeculae, under process of calcification, bounded by a row of osteoblasts. Loose connective tissue between trabeculae

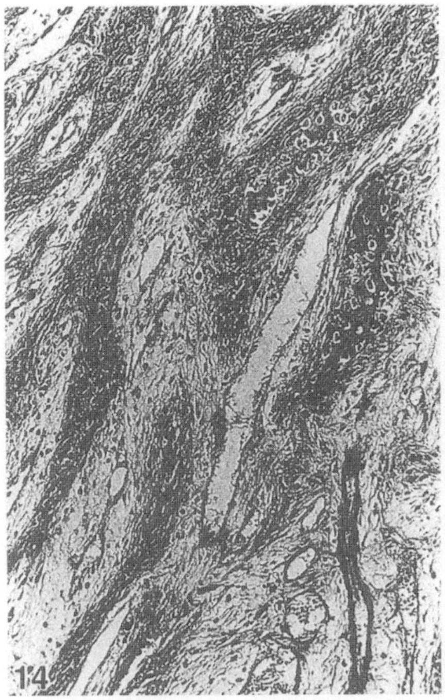

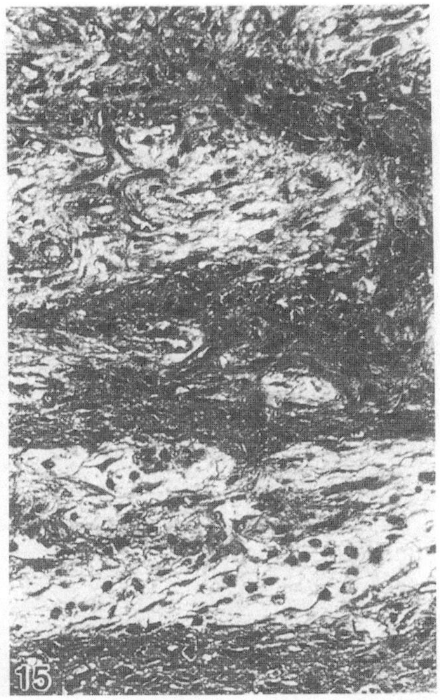

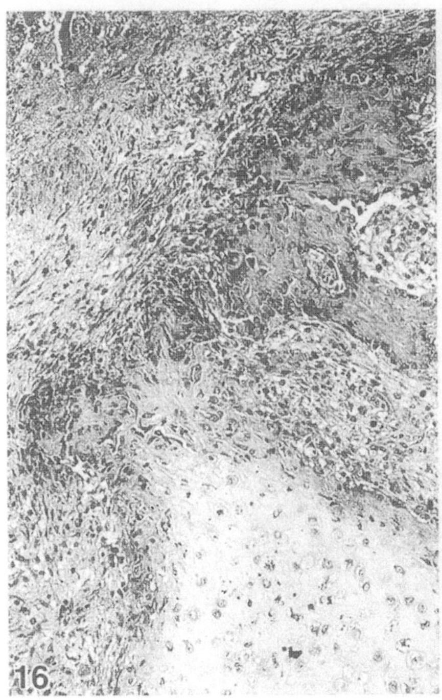

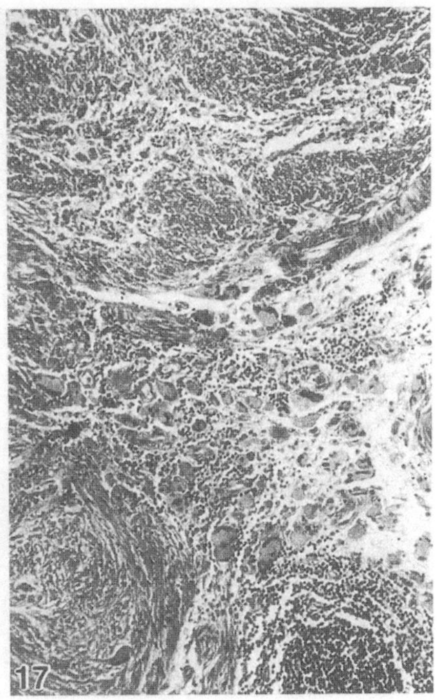

Figs. 14, 15. Relatively characteristic appearance of myositis ossificans. In the loose connective tissue, denser collageno-fibroblastic bands inter-anastomose, hyalinise and pack the cells in osteocytic metamorphosis, then calcify to form a network of primary bone. These zones are abundantly vascularised

Fig. 16. The ossification may pass through a chondroid stage. At the periphery of the nodule is a loose connective tissue infiltrated by inflammatory cells and numerous persistent relics of muscle fibers

Fig. 17. Peripherally, muscle tissue in process of necrosis and inflammatory infiltration

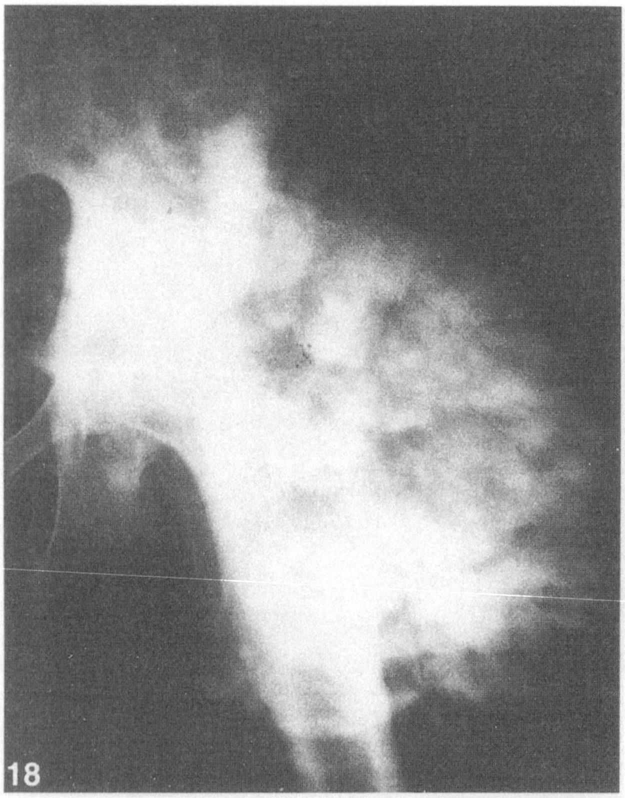

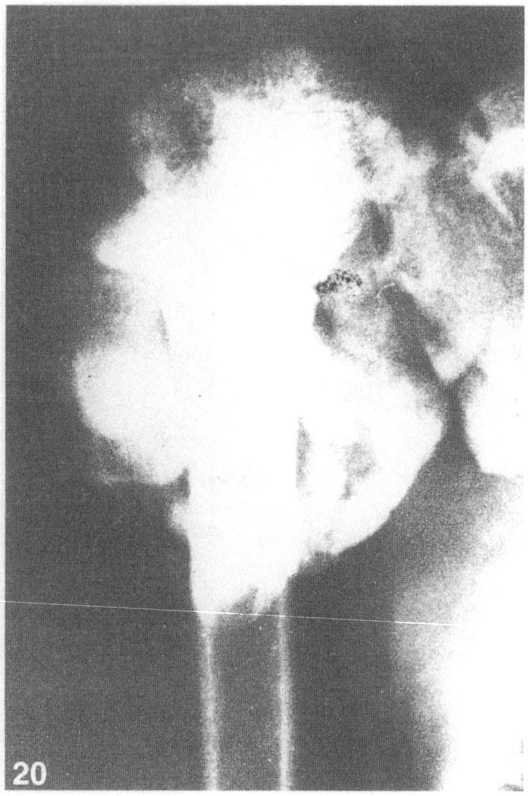

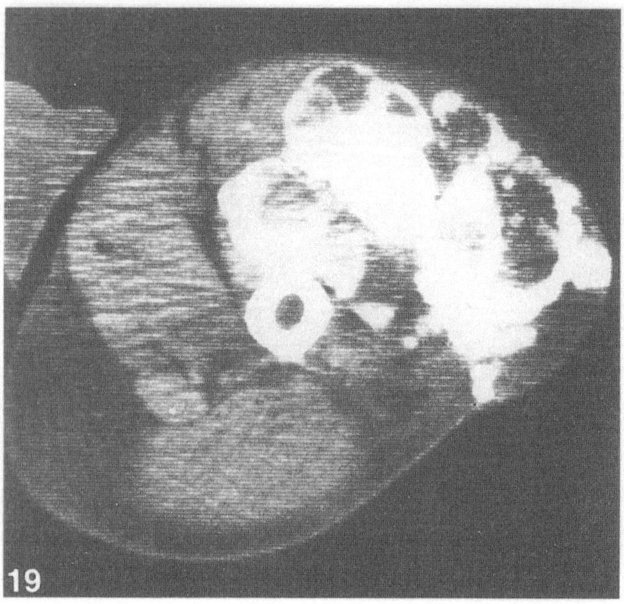

Fig. 18. Frontal view of hip showing voluminous calcification of soft parts. The tumour mass is multilobular and heterogeneous, and there is a hint of some fluid levels in its lower part

Fig. 19. CT of this tumour-like calcinosis confirms the presence in the perifemoral soft tissues of multiple calcified masses with well-defined walls and a mixed fluid and calcified content with fluid levels (films by courtesy of Prof. Laredo)

Fig. 20. This tumour calcinosis of the proximal end of the upper limb is formed by heterogenous nodules, separated by a few noncalcified fibrous septa (by courtesy of Dr Traca et al)

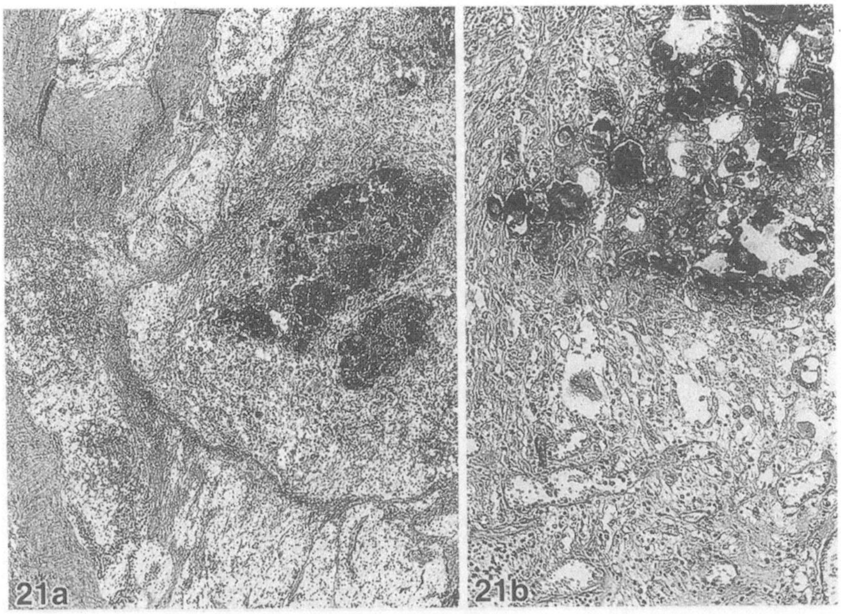

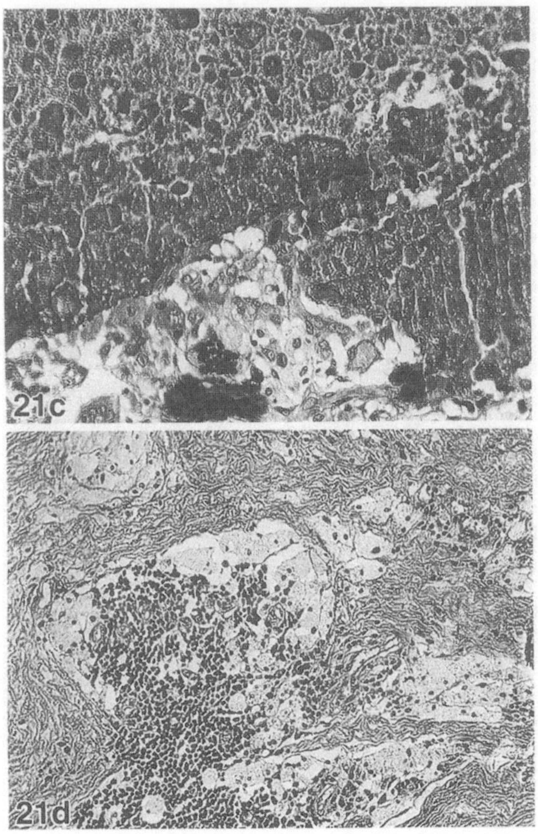

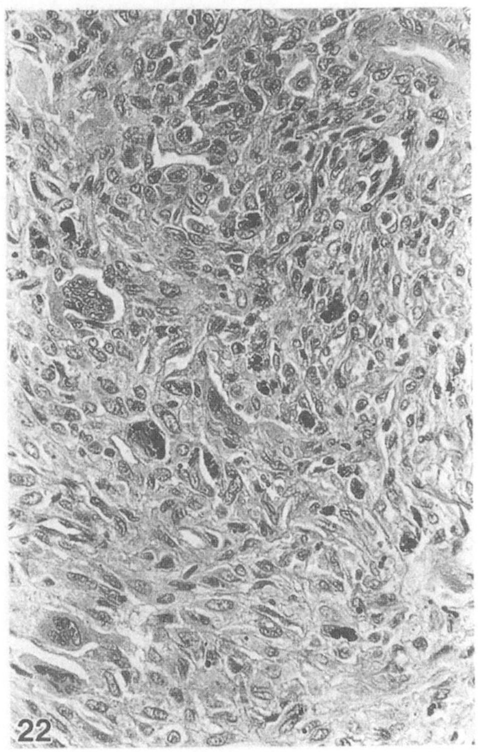

Fig. 21 a-d. These three microphotographs demonstrate (**a, b**) foci of calcified deposits surrounded by (**c**) foamy histiocytes, (**d**) inflammatory cells and collagen fibers (case published with Drs. Traca and Hennebert, Presse médicale, 1965)

Fig. 22. Another case of pseudotumour calcinosis: granuloma around the zone of calcified necrosis

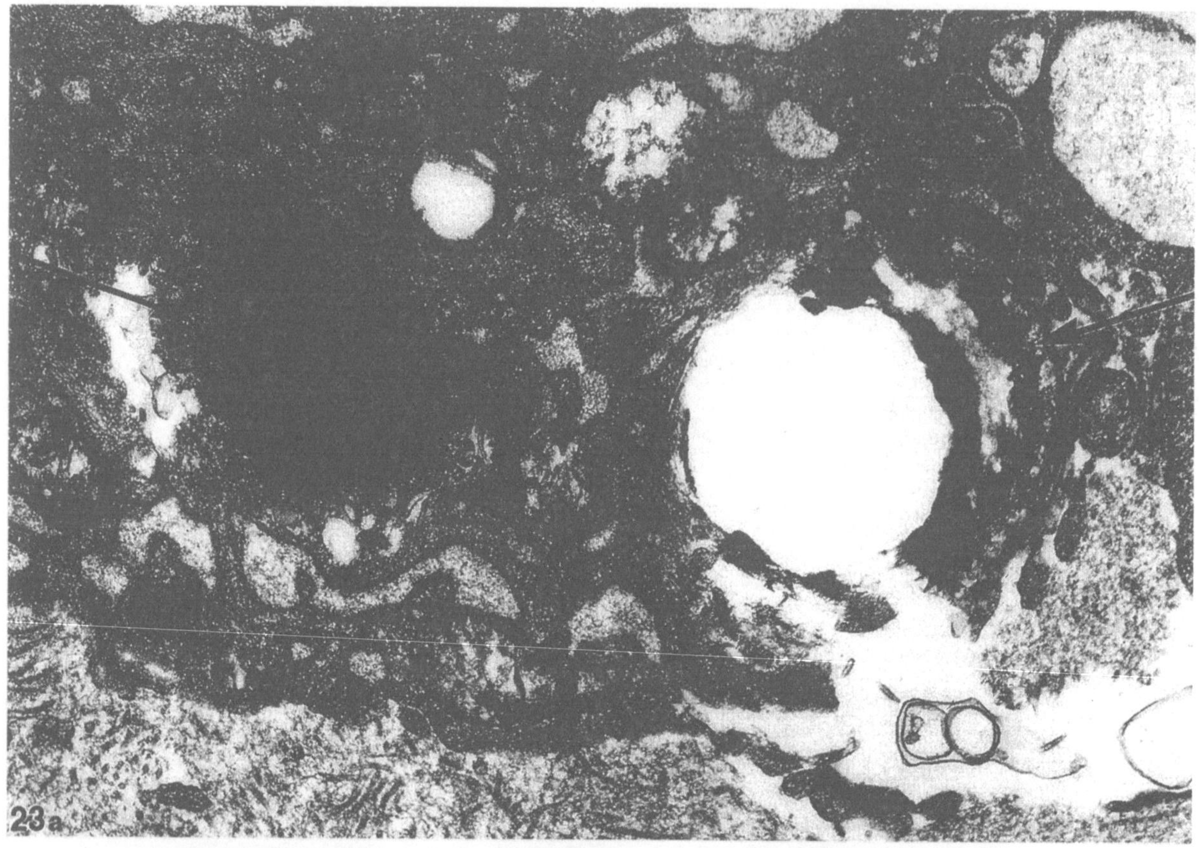

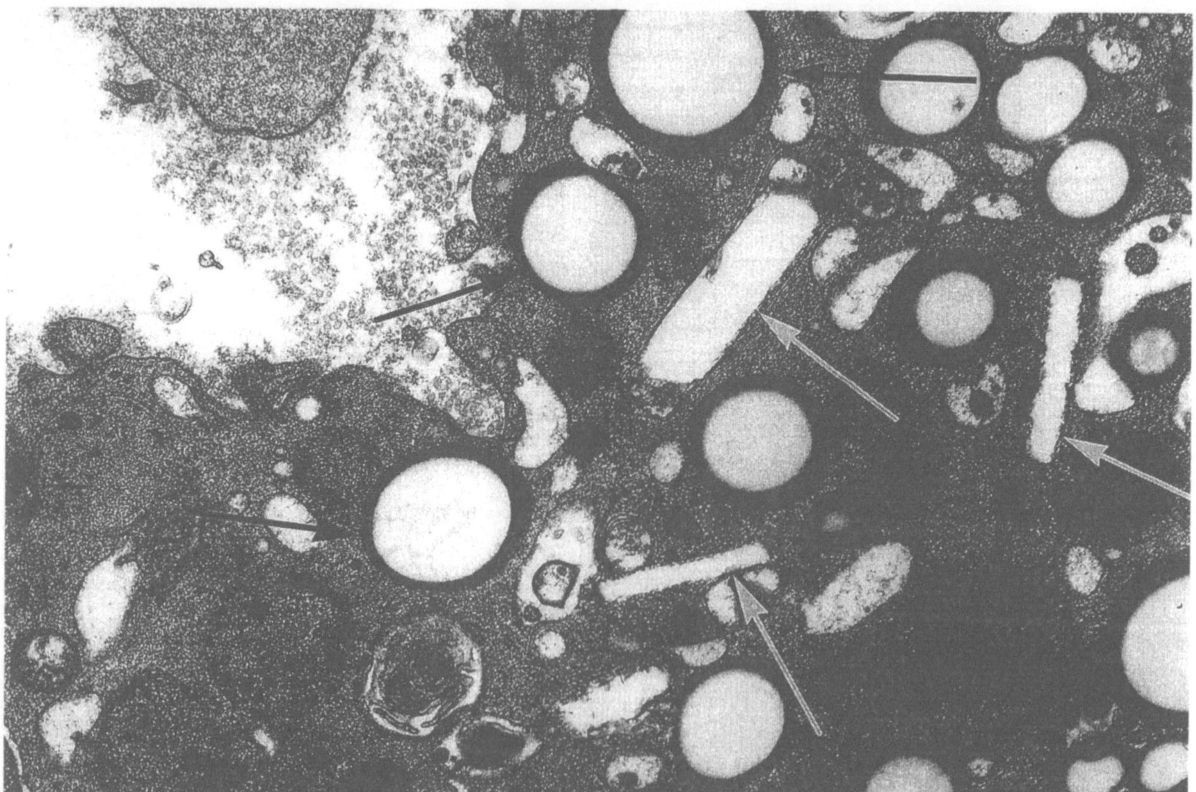

Fig. 23. a Intracellular hydroxyapatite (*arrows*) in a cell whose cytoplasm is enlarged and mitochondria ballooned (Magnif. 8,200 x 3). **b** Macrophages containing numerous lipid vacuoles (*black arrows*) some of which probably contain cholesterol crystals (*white arrows*) (Magnif. 6800 x 3) (by courtesy of Dr Dryll)

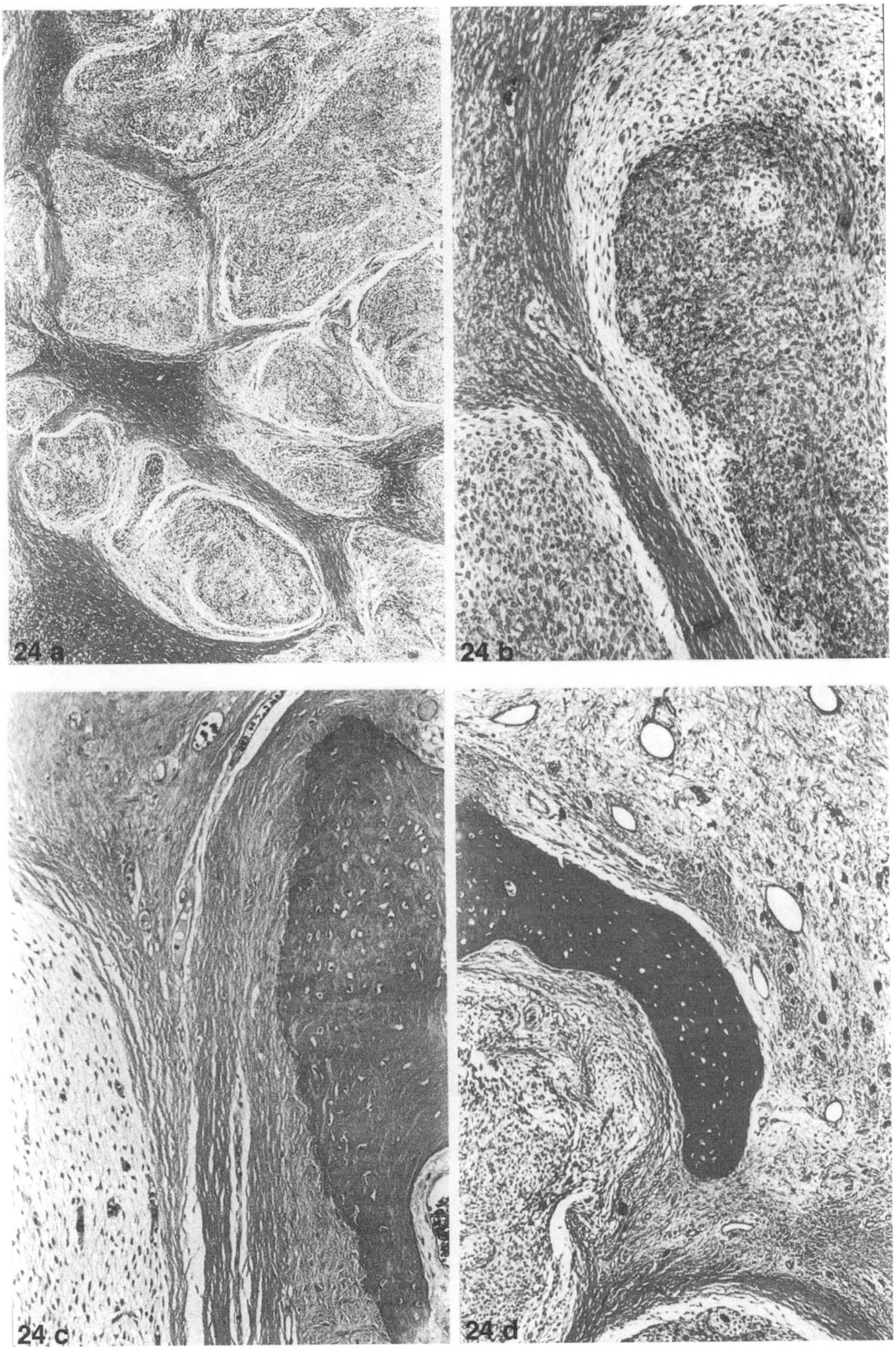

Fig. 24. a In this ossifying fibromyxoid tumour, the lobules are separated from each other by connective tissue trabeculae. **b** Ovoid cells are small and abound in the central part of the lobule; around some lobules a clear space develops which is less cellular. **c** Osseous metaplasia in collagen fibers. **d** A bony trabeculum is clearly calcified

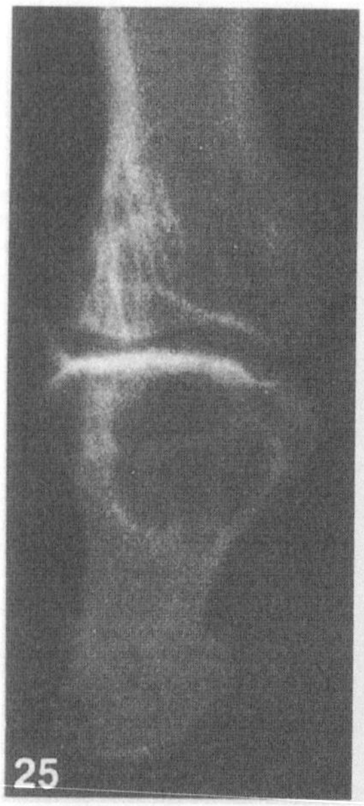

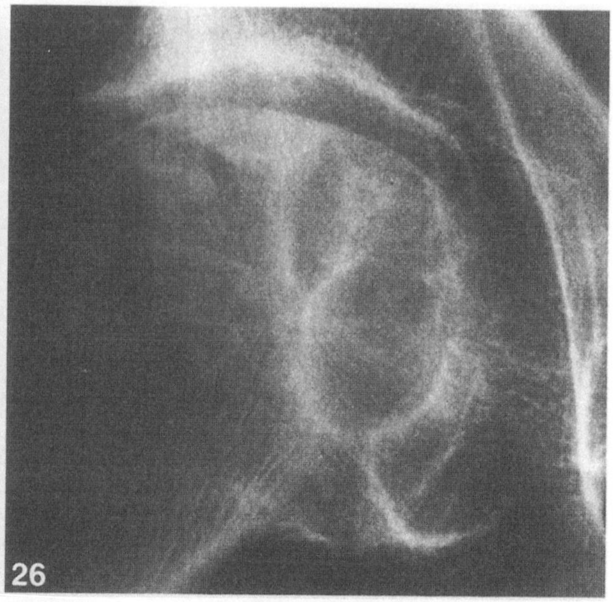

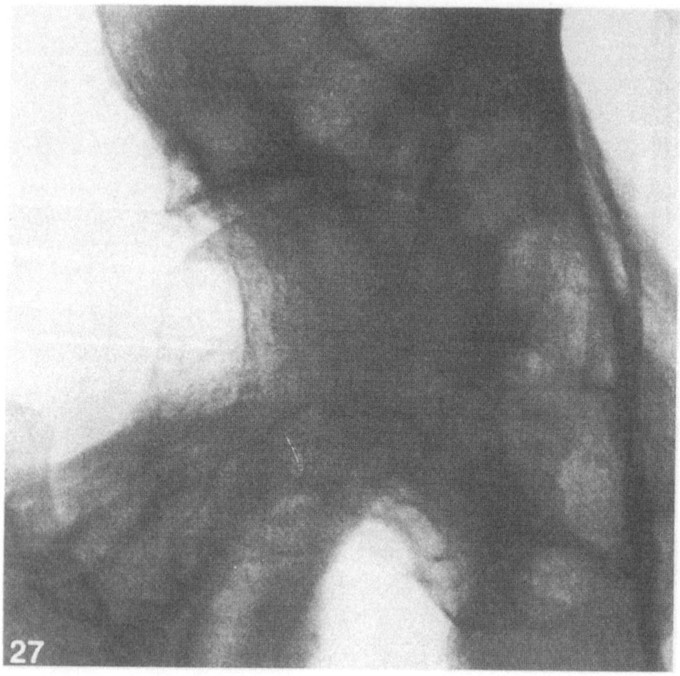

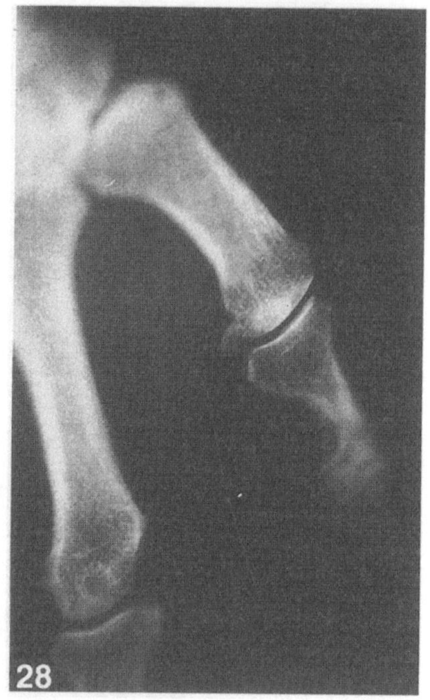

Fig. 25. Synovitis has hollowed out a cavity with sharp outlines in the distal phalanx of the thumb

Fig. 26. Large cavities with sharp outlines and dense borders in femoral head: the result of bony invasion by pigmented synovitis

Fig. 27. In this case the synovitis simultaneously infiltrates the femoral neck and head and the acetabulum

Fig. 28. A nodule of synovitis leaves its impression on the palmar aspect of the distal phalanx of the thumb

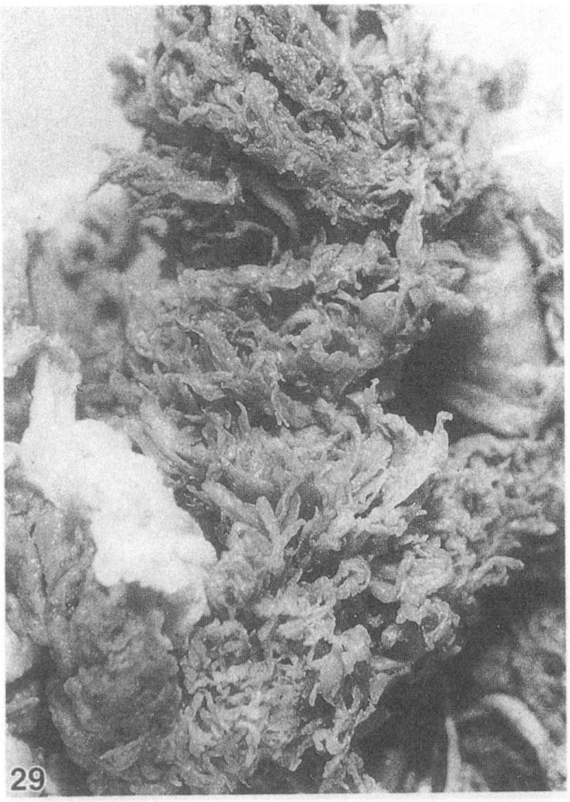

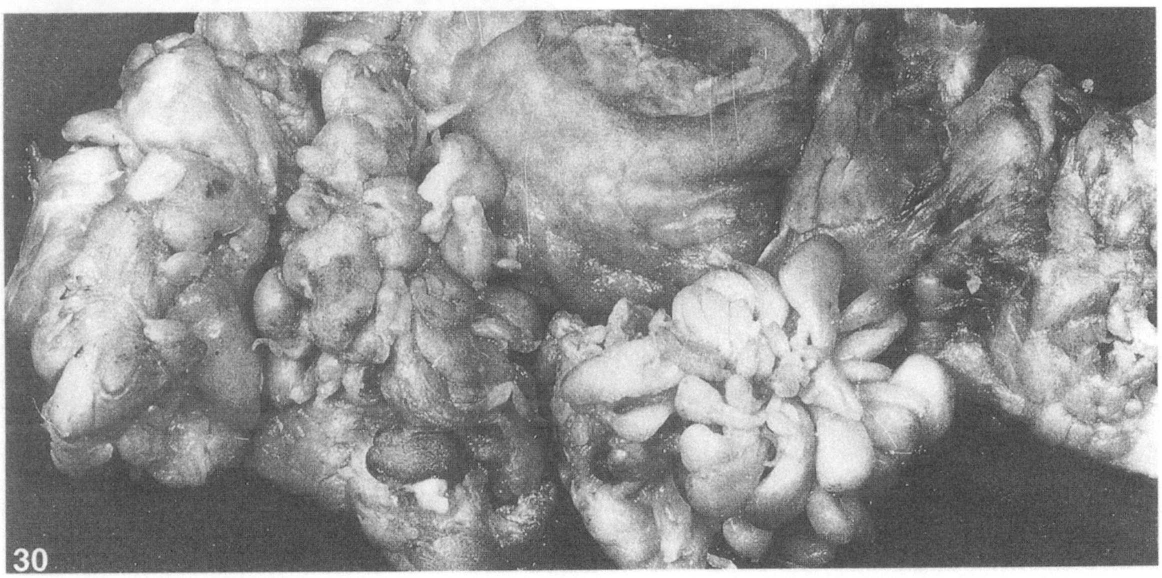

Fig. 29. Characteristic appearance of villous synovitis

Fig. 30. Adherent villi form small ovoid nodules in this synovitis. The darker aspect of some nodules is due to their marked rusty coloration

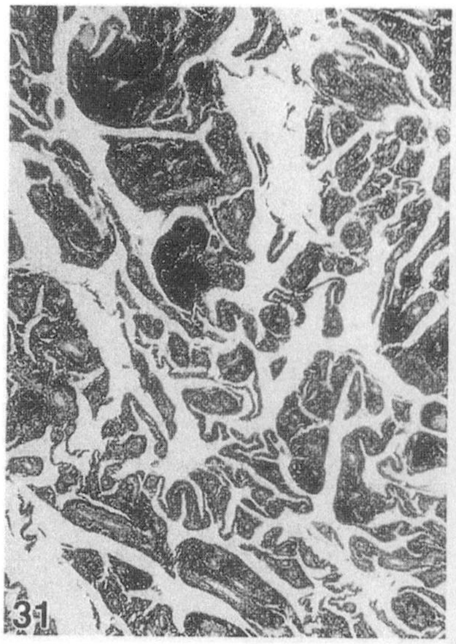

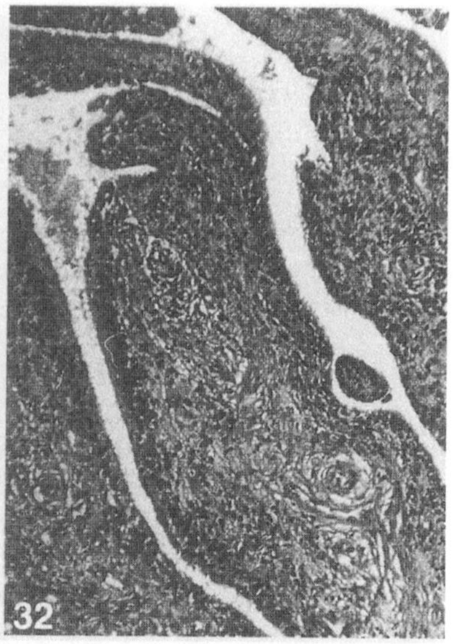

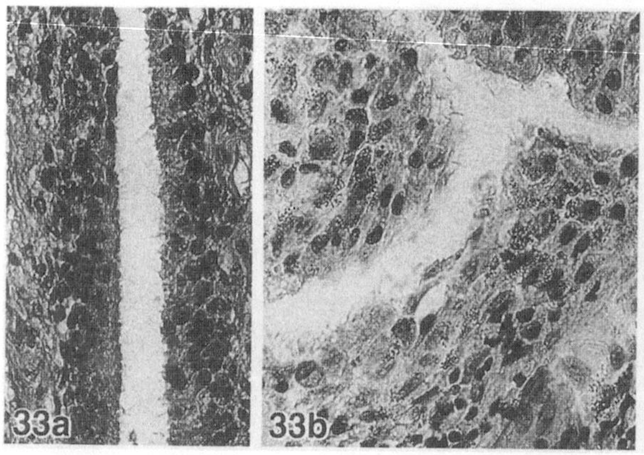

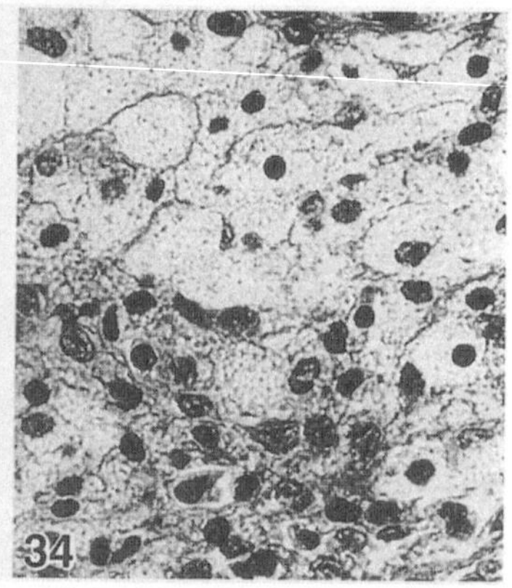

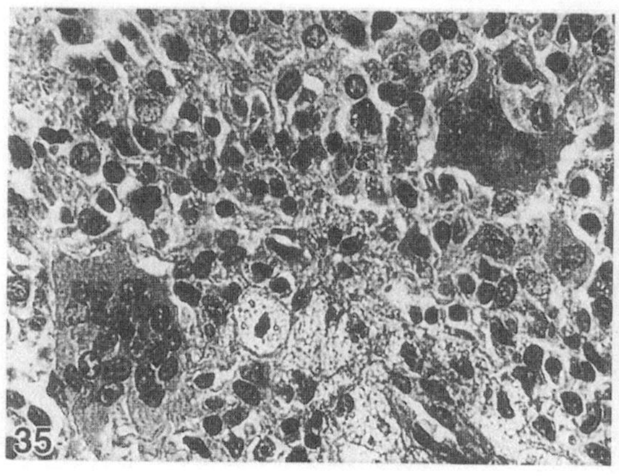

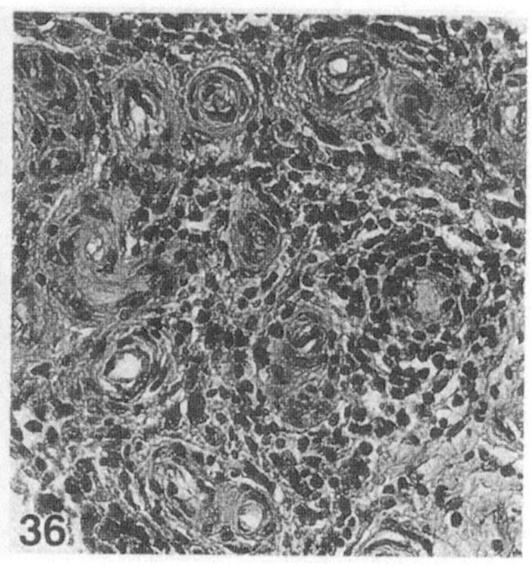

Fig. 31. Villi, some fine, some thick, laden with haemosiderin pigment (blackish in the photograph)

Fig. 32. Moderately fibrous villi traversed by some thick-walled vessels and with scattered inflammatory cells

Fig. 33. a The cells bordering the villi are arranged irregularly in several layers and (**b**) are often laden with pigment

Fig. 34. The presence of areas of foamy histiocytes is not a proof of a benign lesion, but their absence calls for a minute cytological study to exclude any sign of malignancy in a compact synovial proliferation

Fig. 35. Polymorphous appearance of histiocytic proliferation: giant cells, foamy cells, mononuclear histiocytes

Fig. 36. The numerous vascular sections shown in this section are surrounded by a discrete inflammatory infiltration. Further, the vessel walls in this villus are thick and hyalinised

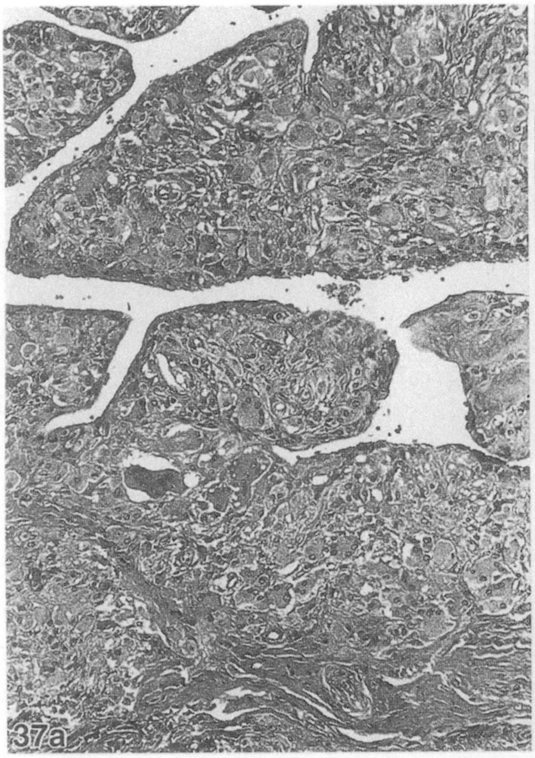

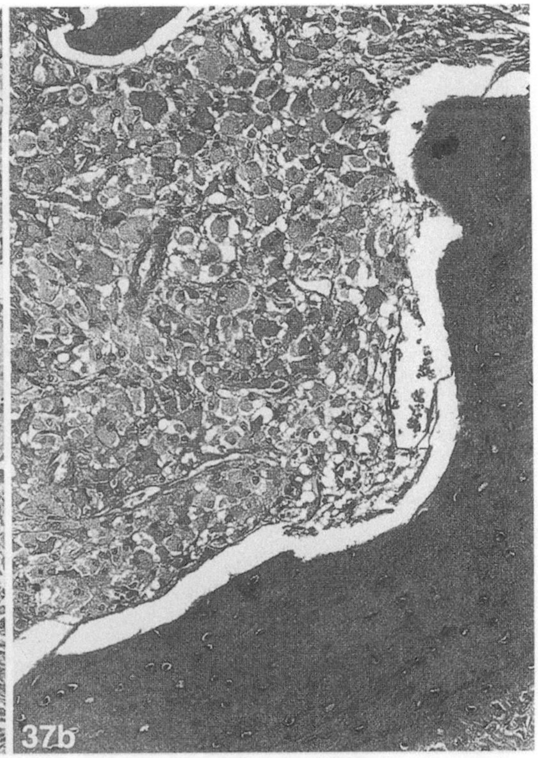

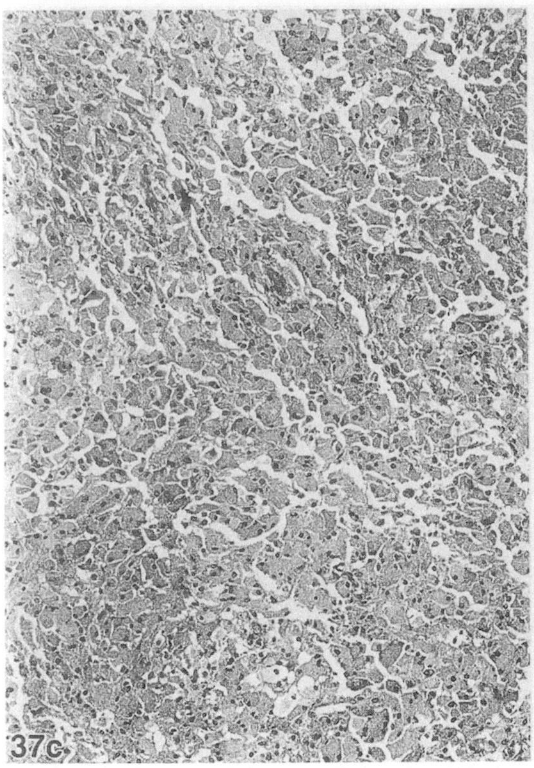

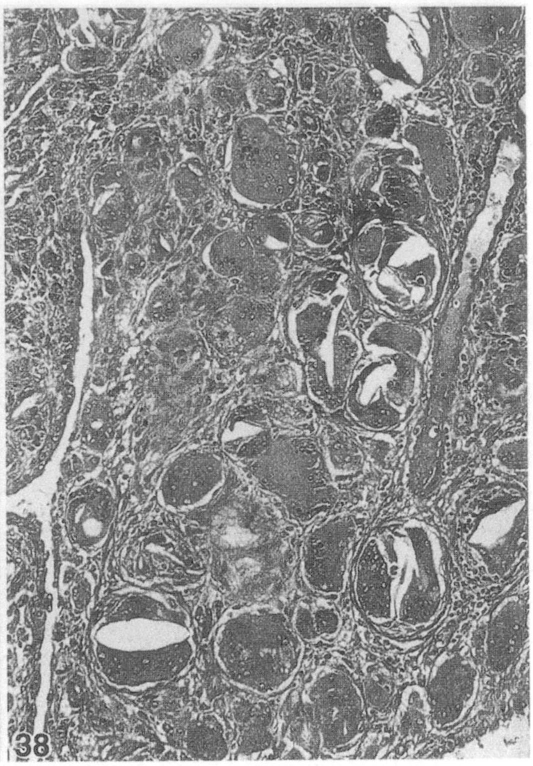

Fig. 37 a-c. Pseudotumour histiocytic synovites, prosthesis removal. **a** Numerous and large villi, mainly histiocytic. **b** The synovitis has invaded the medullary spaces and resorbed the bony tissue. **c** Massive and diffuse form of histiocytic reaction producing a pseudotumour around a hip prosthesis, where one can occasionally see some bands of villi placed side by side. Usually, mitoses are rare, but this varies widely with the zones examined. In these pseudotumour forms, histoimmunological reactions prove the histiocytic nature of almost all the cells

Fig. 38. Giant-celled and macrophagic type of synovitis

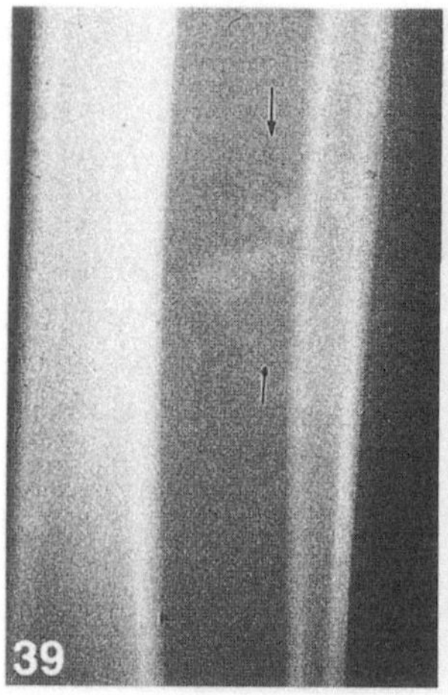

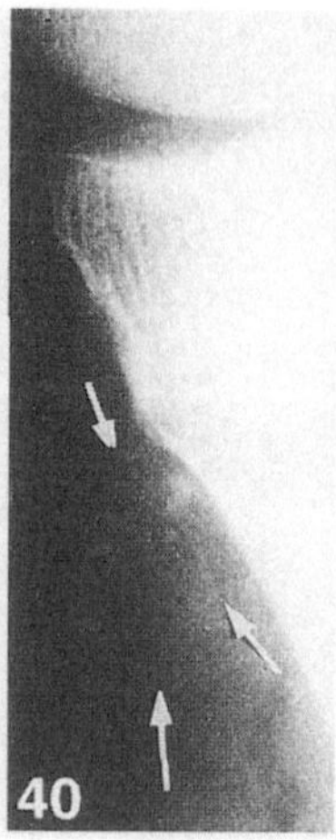

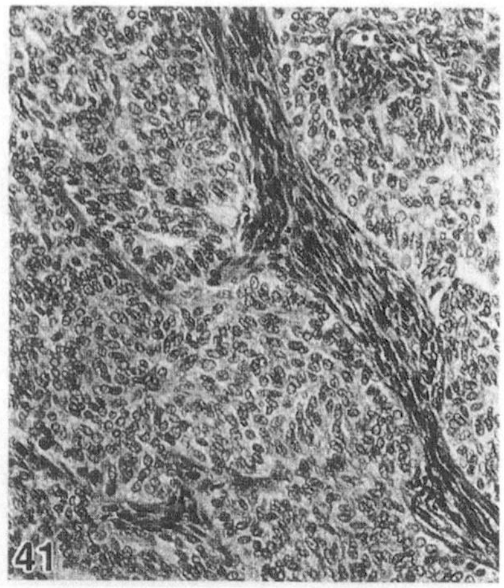

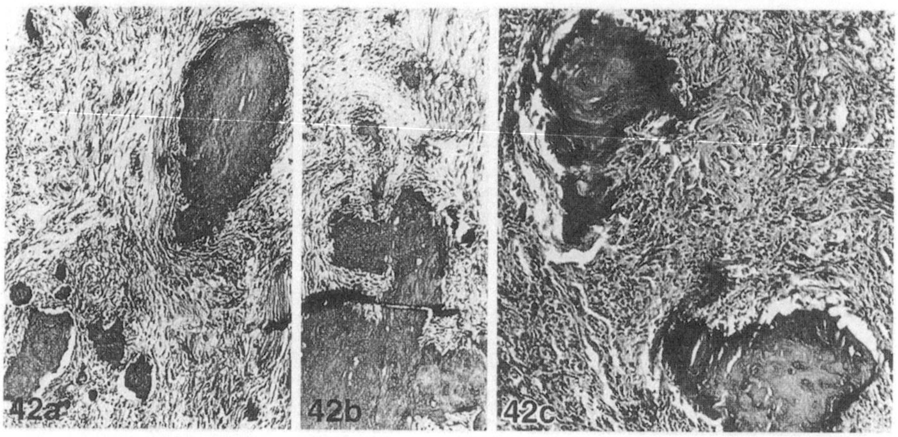

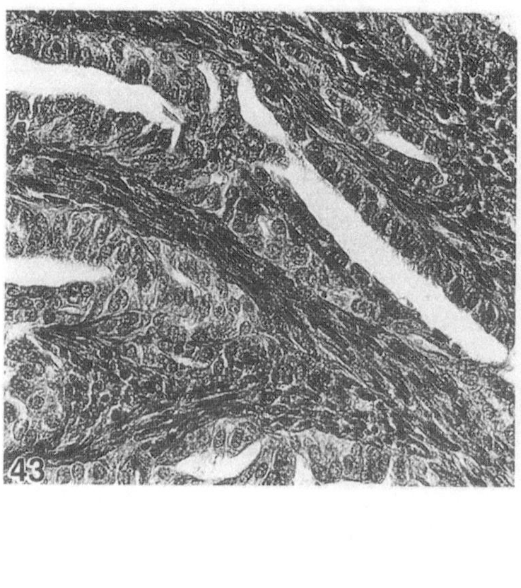

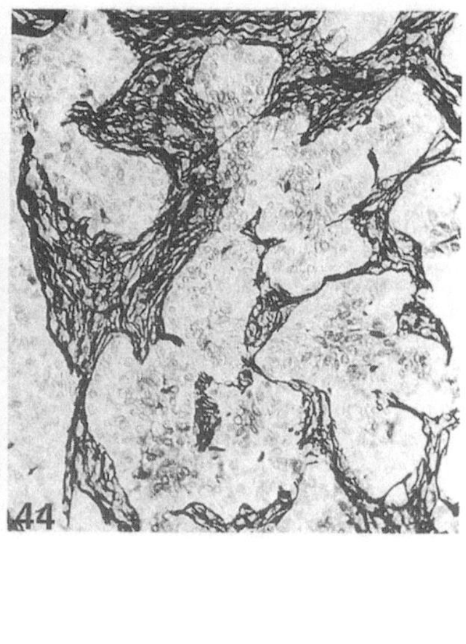

Figs. 39, 40. Presence of calcification (*arrows*) in these two synovial sarcomas, one developing in the tibio-fibular interspace, the other at the inner aspect of the upper end of the tibia

Fig. 41. At this low magnification, the biphasic appearance of this synovial sarcoma is obvious

Fig. 42 a-c. Calcification in neoplastic synovial tissue. These calcifications are usually situated at the periphery of the tumour

Fig. 43. In this synovial sarcoma of the forearm, the clefts are bordered by cubo-cylindrical cells of epithelioid appearance

Fig. 44. In the compact forms, silver impregnation of the reticulin fibers clearly outlines the epithelioid areas

→

Fig. 45. Standard lateral radiograph of left knee of a man of 52, complaining of moderate pain at the knee. The intra-articular calcifications suggest synovial chondromatosis

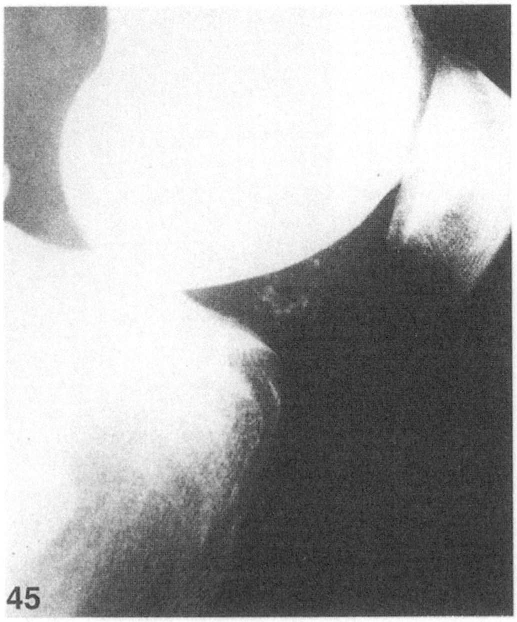

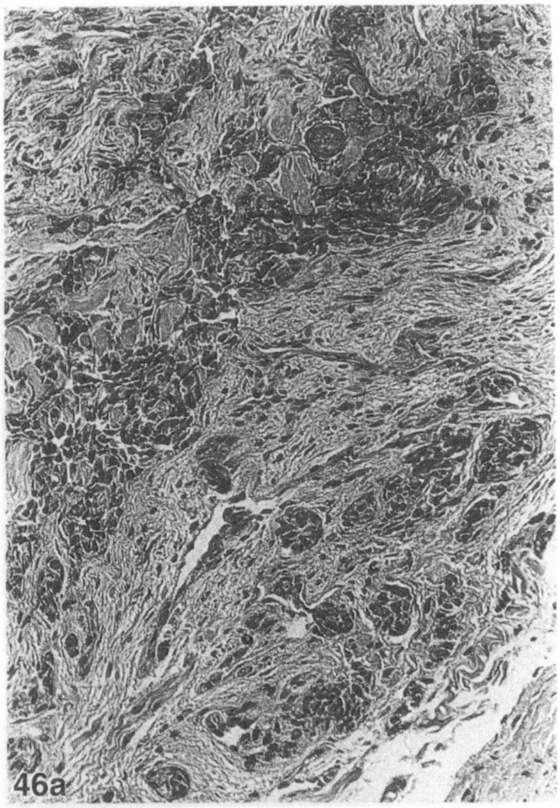

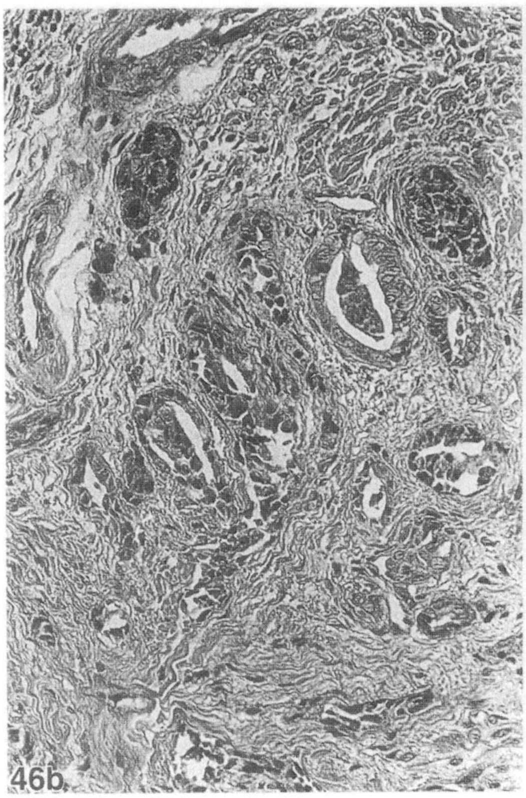

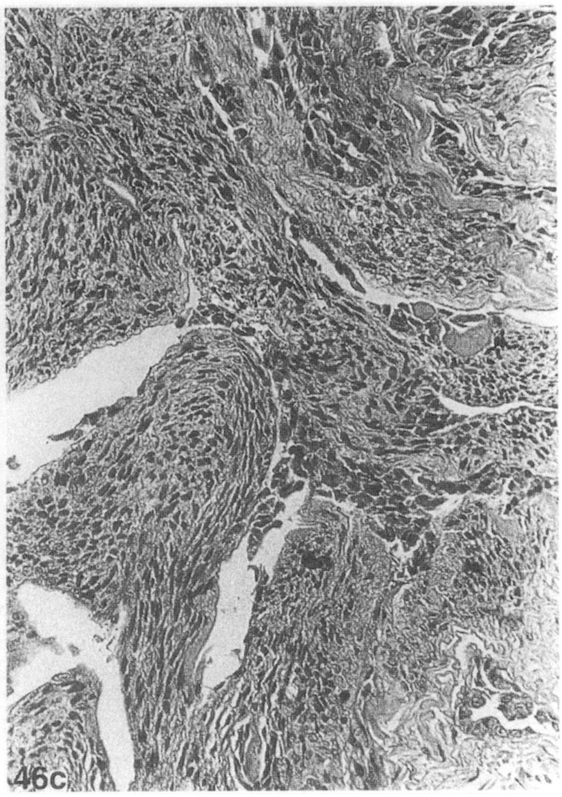

Fig. 46. a, b Histological examination of a synovial biopsy shows a cellular proliferation of epithelial glandular appearance in most fragments, strongly positive with antikeratin antibody and (**c**) zones of fusiform cells, the second cellular component of this intra-articular biphasic synovial sarcoma

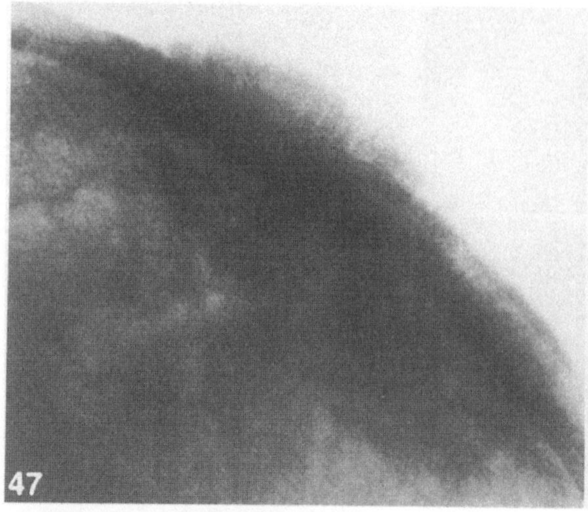

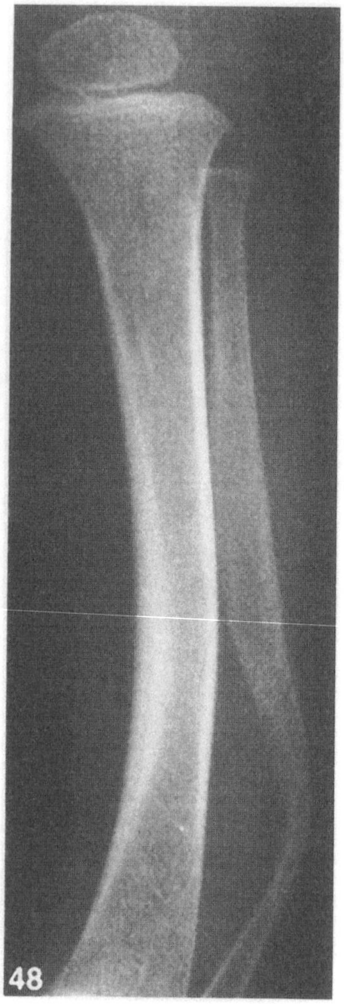

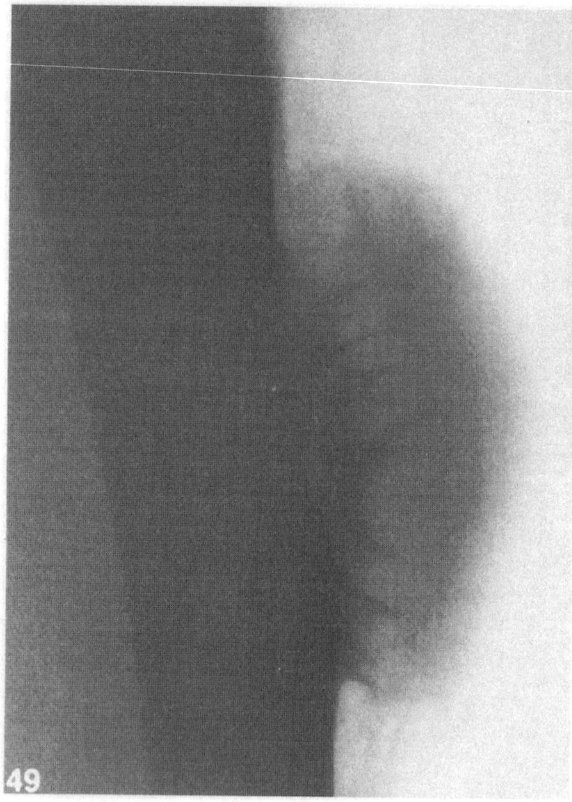

Fig. 47. Bony reaction of cranial vault to invasion by a meningioma

Fig. 48. In this neurofibromatosis there is bowing of the tibia with cortical thickening in the concavity and major deformity of the fibula

Fig. 49. Bony reaction to a periosteal schwannoma. The orientation of the bony trabeculae at right angles to the cortex is spectacular

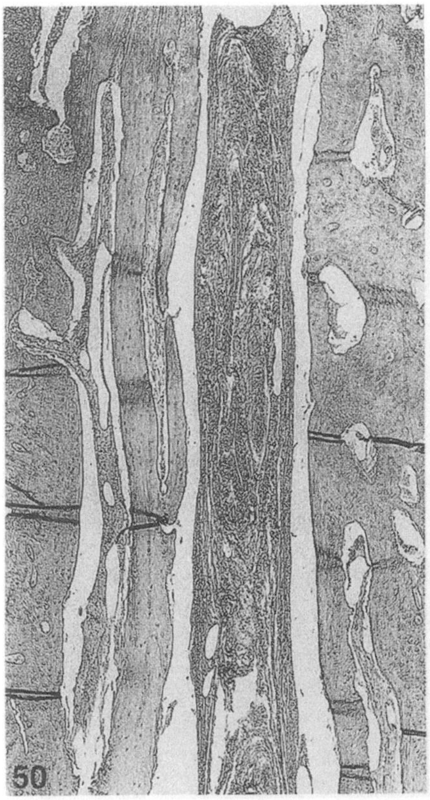

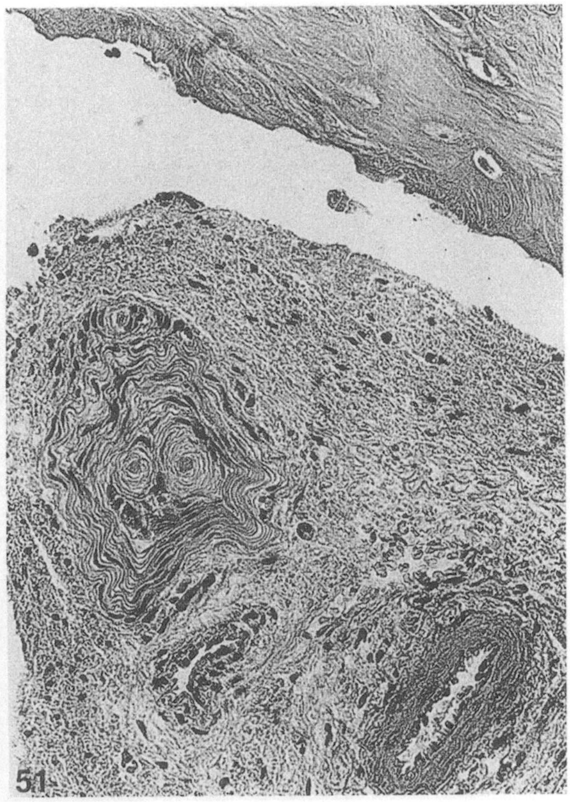

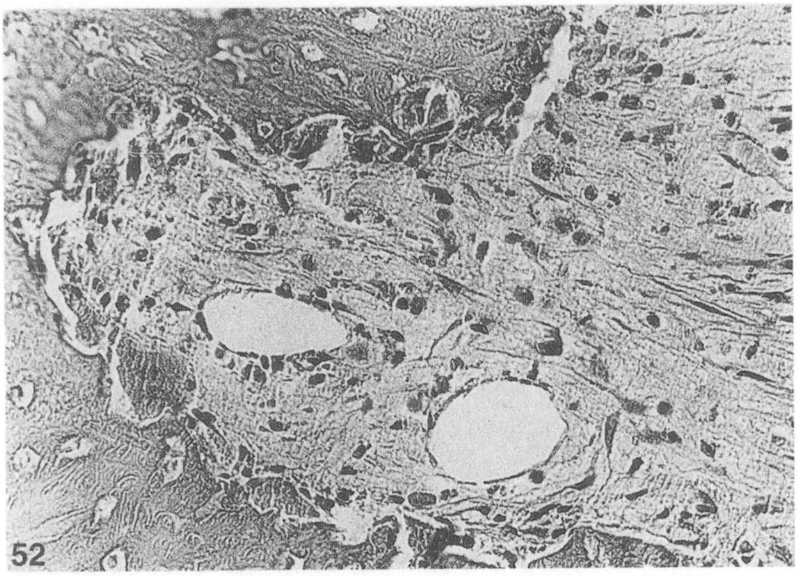

Fig. 50. Longitudinal section in pathological zone of fibula in severe neurofibromatosis. A fibrous connective tissue containing large vessels and neural structures is surrounded by haversian bone

Fig. 51. Layered lamellar appearance of a structure in the context of neurofibroma and thick-walled vessels

Fig. 52. In this neurofibromatosis the osteolysis is the outcome of intense osteoclastic activity

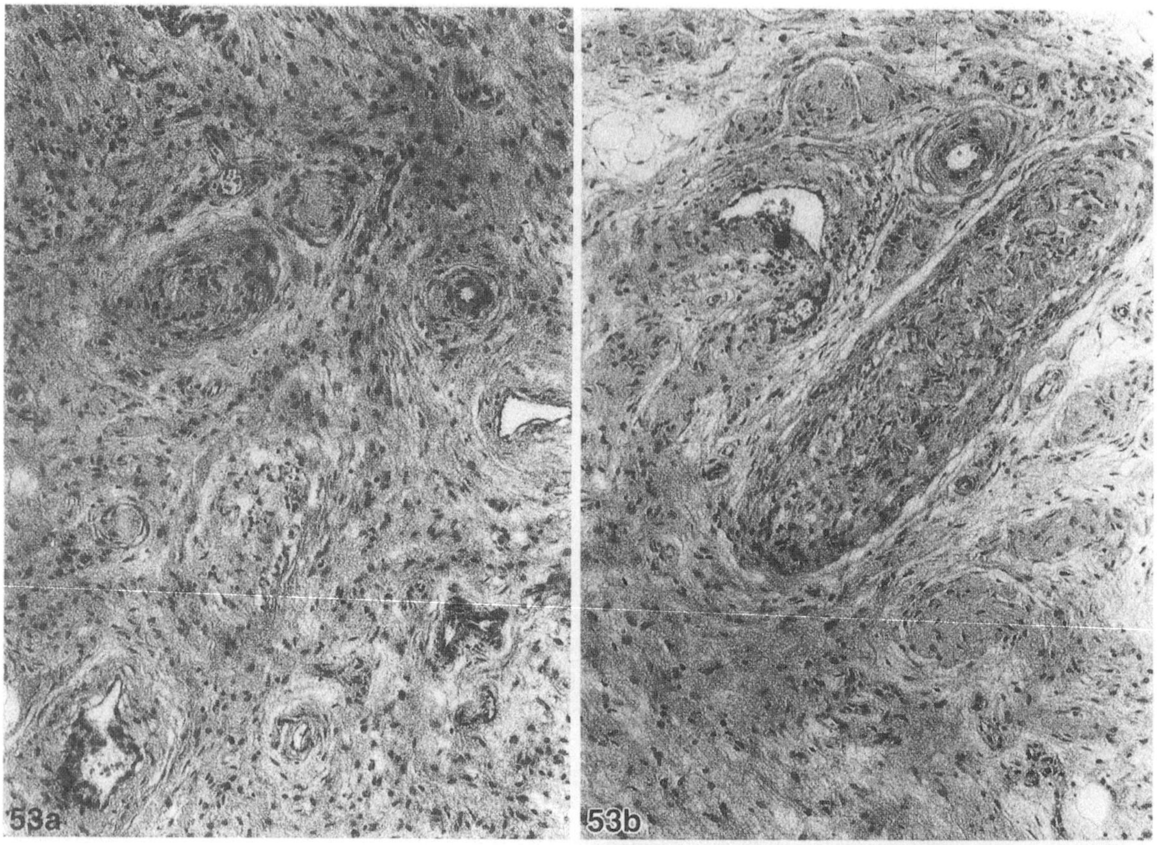

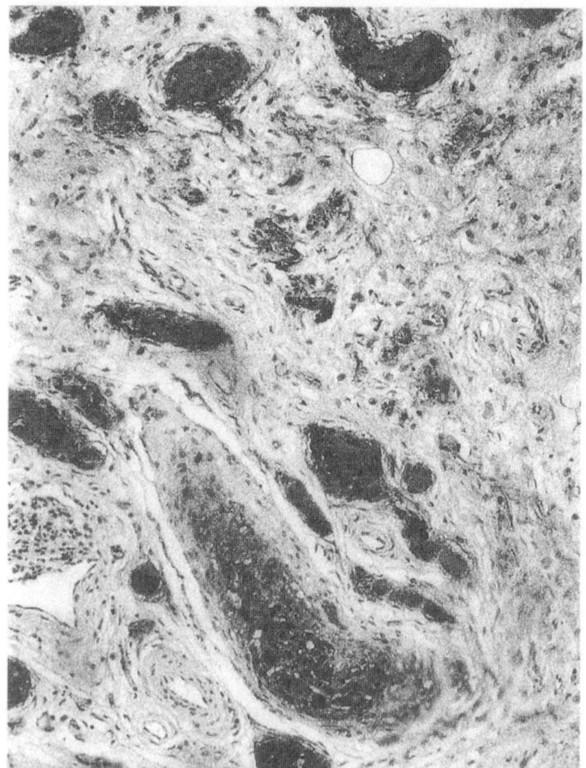

Fig. 53. a, b This neurofibromatosis was revealed by a major tibial periosteal reaction. The biopsy showed abundant neurofibromatous proliferation associated with thick-walled vessels. **c** Positive marking for protein S100

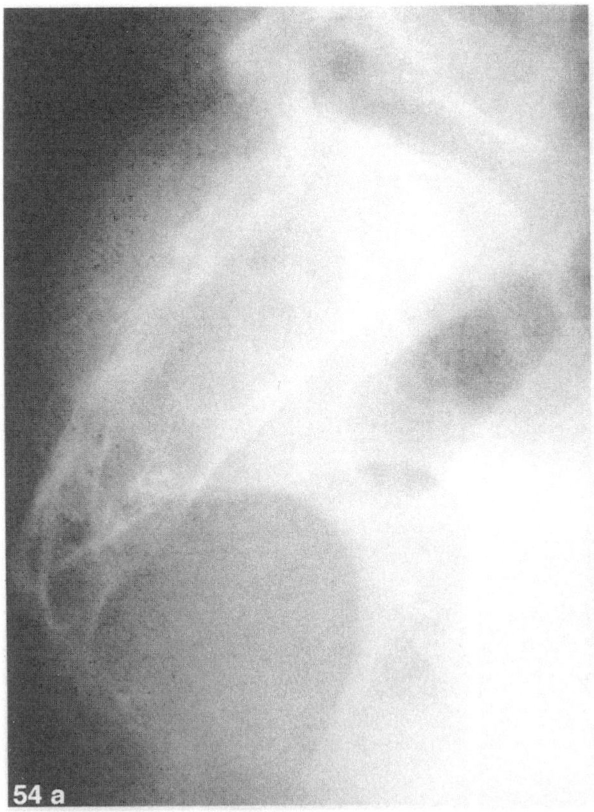

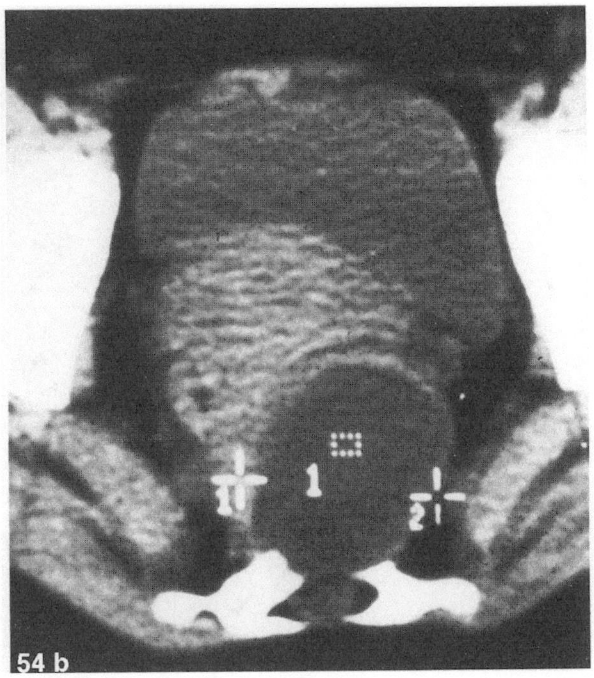

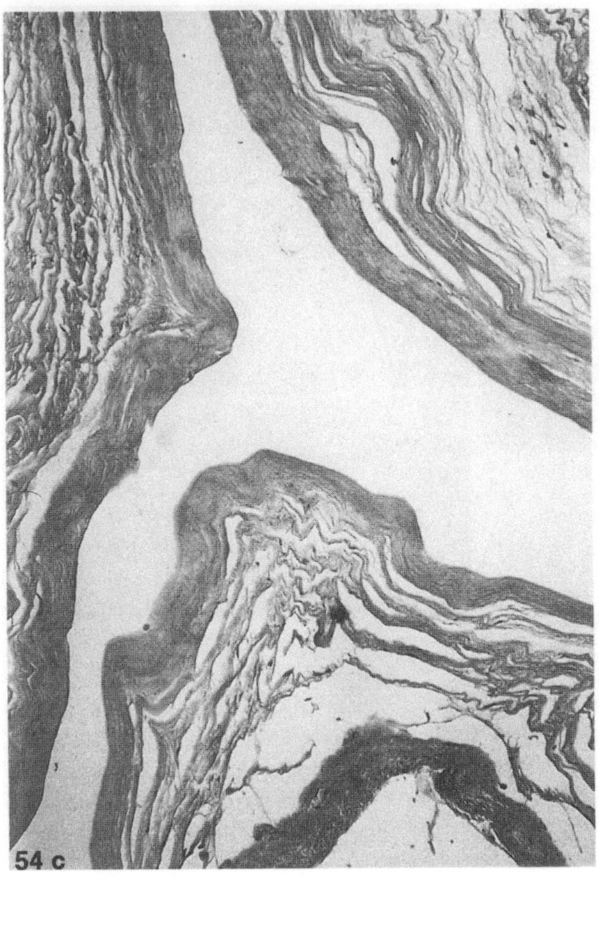

Fig. 54 a-c. This meningocele was diagnosed in a woman aged 39 by abdomino-pelvic ultrasound. The radiograph and the CT demonstrated a presacral fluid structure. Operation (Prof. Ravon) led to removal of this pelvic "cyst", which communicated with the subarachnoid spaces of the sacral dural sac. The sections made of this meningocele (Prof. Catanzano) show a wall of variable thickness, whose deep aspect is perfectly smooth

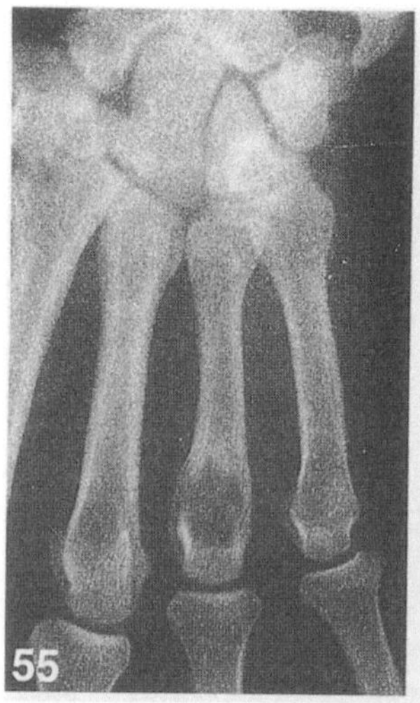

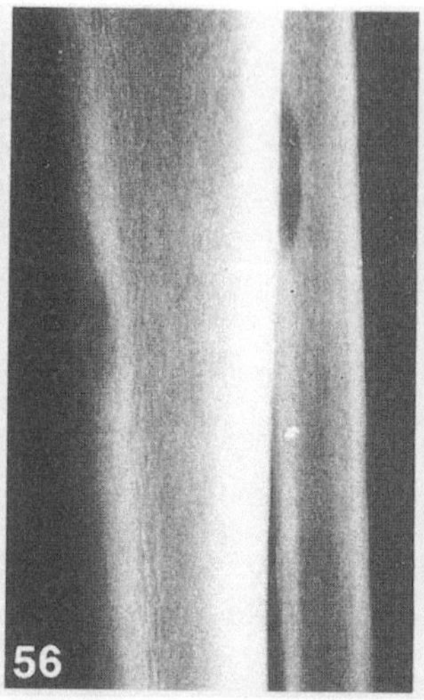

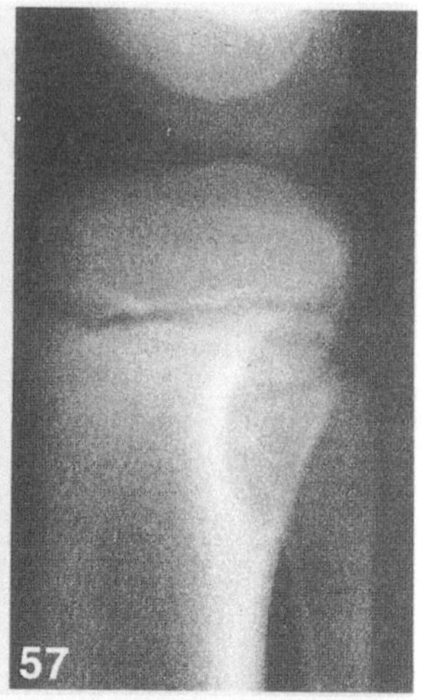

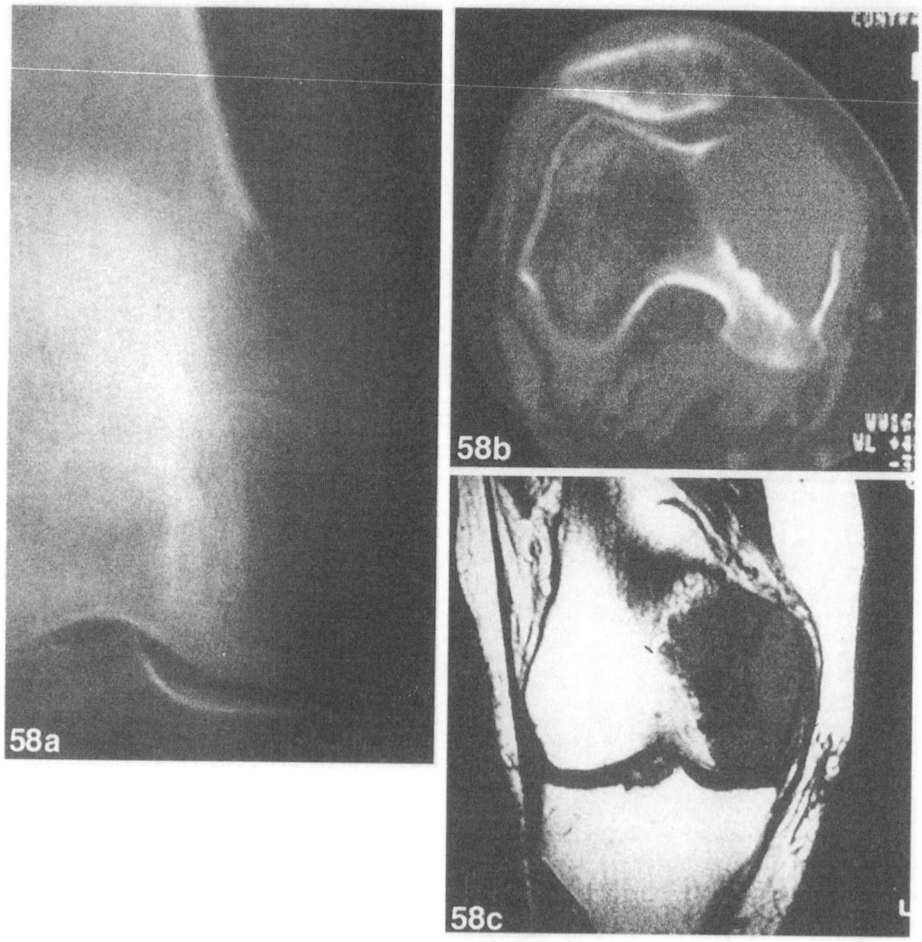

Figs. 55-64 relate to the lesions of parathyroid osteosis

Fig. 55. Limited osteolysis of distal end of 4th metacarpal

Fig. 56. Two sharply defined foci of osteolysis in the tibia and fibula. The bony texture of the tibial cortex is slightly remodelled

Fig. 57. Well-circumscribed lacunar image of upper end of tibial metaphysis in a young girl suffering from chronic renal failure (illustrations of this secondary hyperparathyroidism by courtesy of Prof. de Laguillaumie, Clermont-Ferrand)

Fig. 58 a-c. This giant-cell tumour is as typified by its location as by its histology. The relatively high number of mitoses is consistent with the purely lytic image of the tumour. **a** Standard view, **b** CT, **c** MRI. Despite the excellent preservation of the joint-space in a 74-year-old woman, the age of this patient was more than enough to justify a review of calcium/phosphorus metabolism, the results of which led to removal of a parathyroid adenoma. Consequently, every giant-cell tumour, even if histologically typical but which differs in some features (age, site) from the normal scheme of things, and even if it is the sole bony lesion, requires study of the calcium/phosphorus metabolism

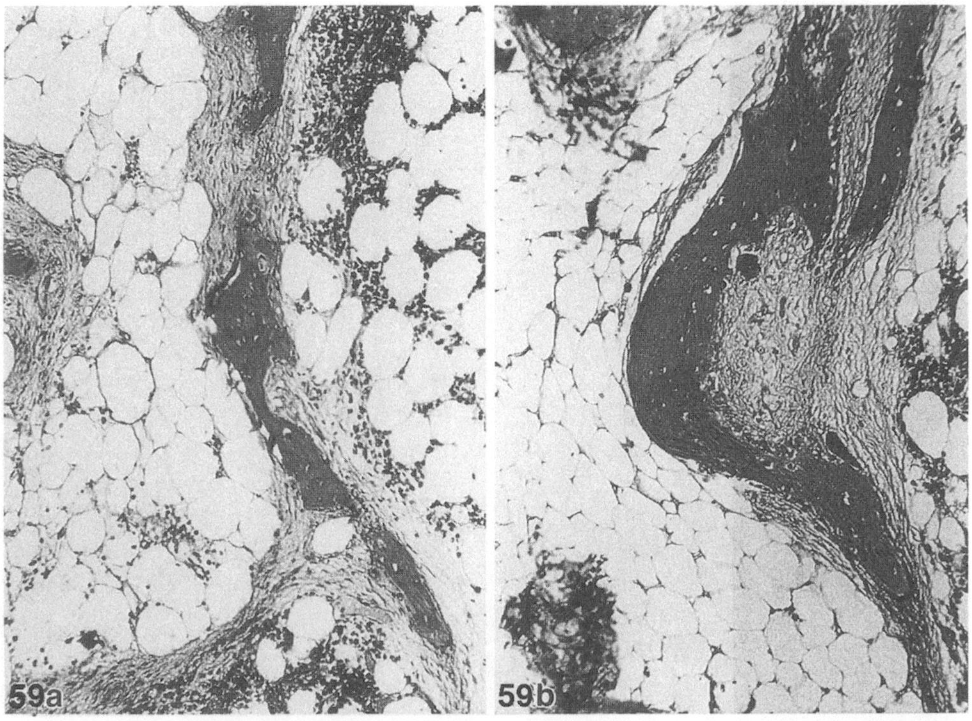

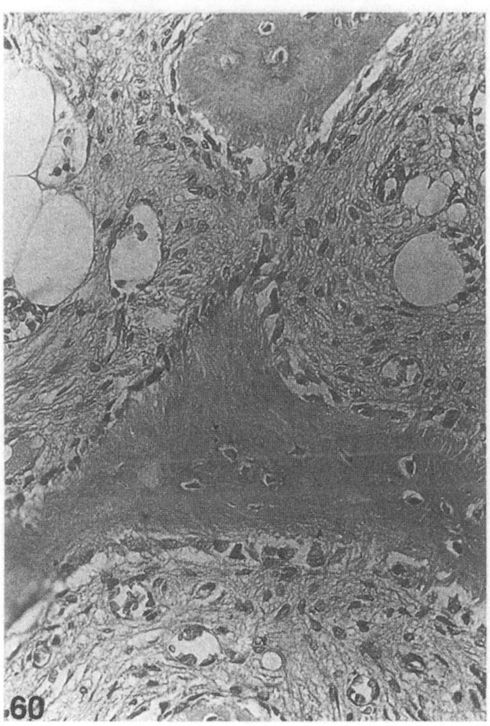

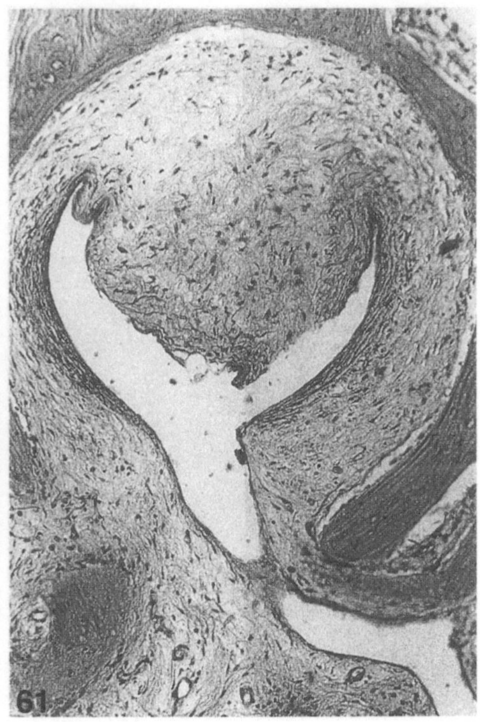

Fig. 59 a, b. Fibrosis occupies the absorbed zones of a partly destroyed bony trabecula. This fibrosis is partly of new formation but is probably also due to partial persistence of the collagenous bony framework

Fig. 60. Denser fibrosis in contact with bony trabeculae. The role of the cells bordering the bony tissue is difficult to define. These are sometimes mononuclear osteoclasts, sometimes osteoblasts

Fig. 61. In some lesions the dense fibrosis, traversed by numerous large vessels, readily suggests an angioma

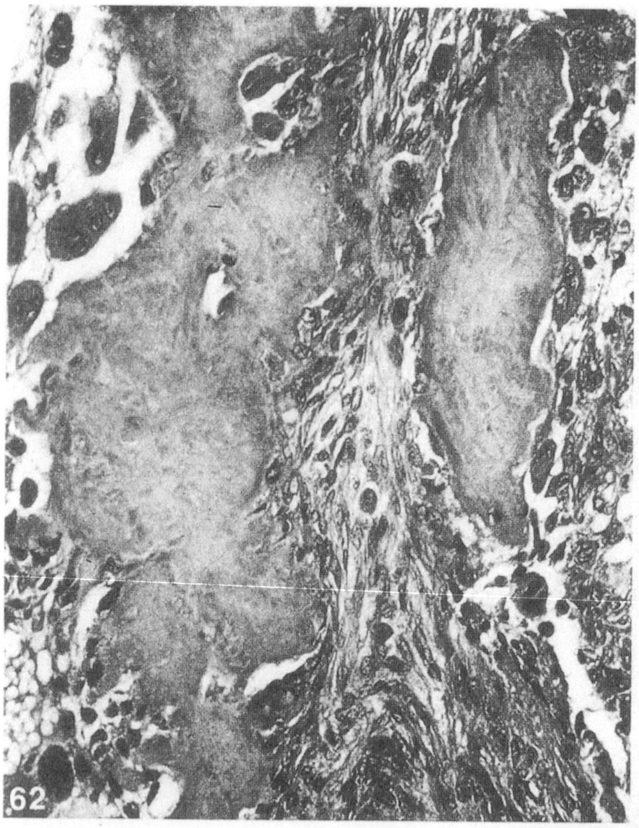

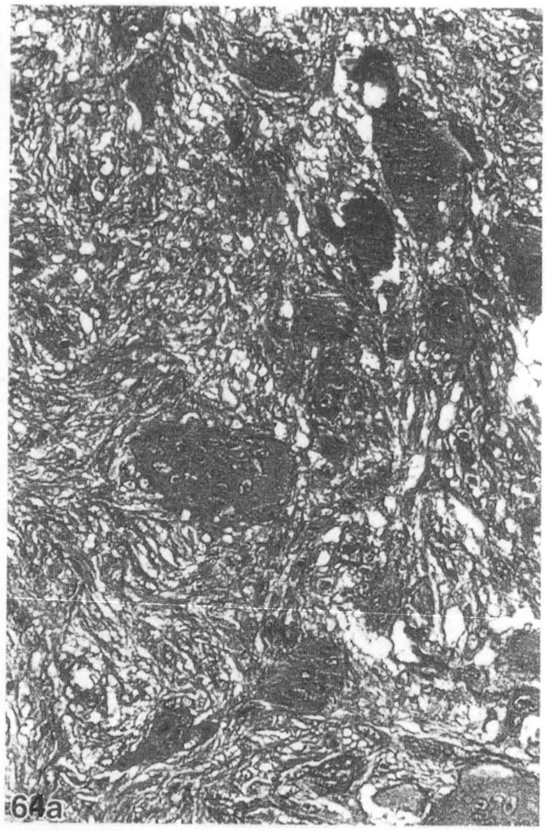

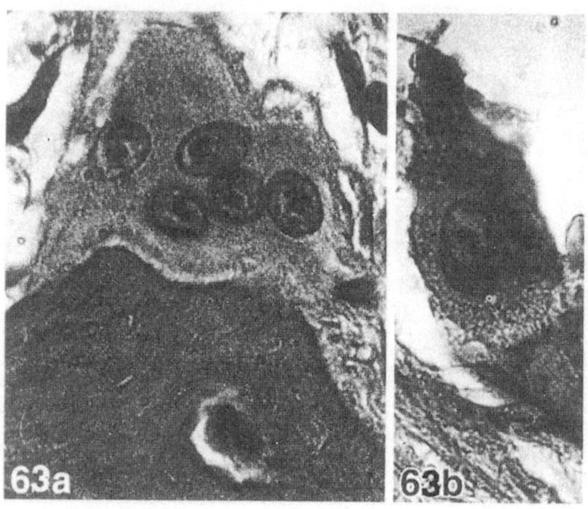

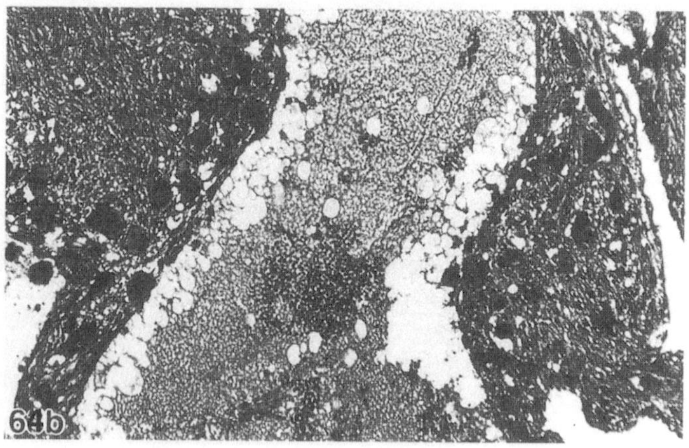

Fig. 62. When fibrosis and osteoclastic proliferation are so obvious they are more suggestive of parathyroid osteosis

Fig. 63. a Osteoclasts with few nuclei in contact with bony tissue. **b** The osteoclast has just liberated an osteoblast nucleus. Note the brush border of the osteoclasts in the zone of absorption

Fig. 64 a, b. Major fibrosis and giant cells of unequal size. **a** Another zone of the same case (**b**) hypervascular cystic appearance which may suggest an angioma or aneurysmal cyst

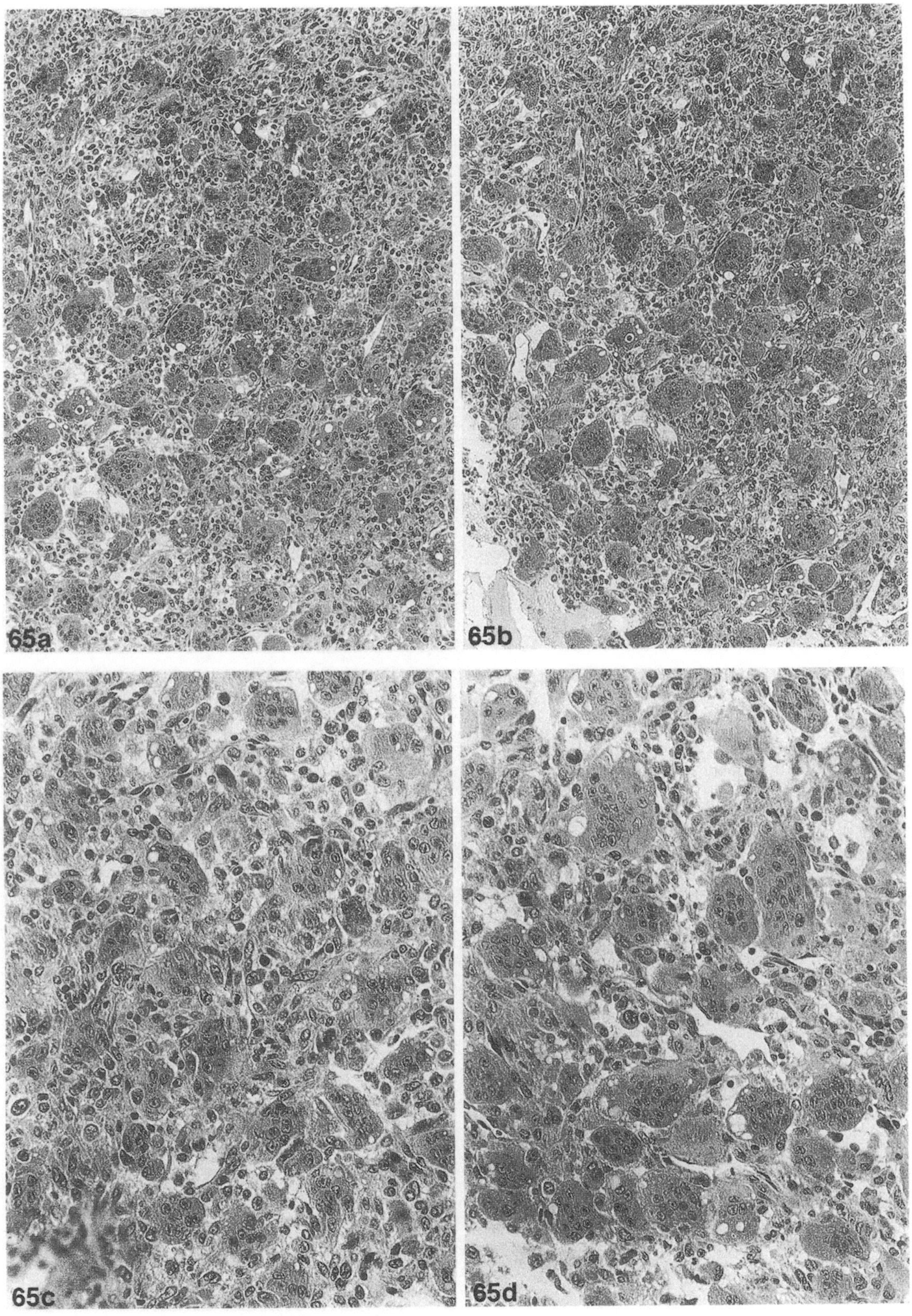

Fig. 65 a-d. Metaphyseo-epiphyseal tumour (fig. 57). In this homogeneous tumour the histological distinction between a giant-cell tumour and the brown tumour of von Recklinghausen is difficult or impossible, but the age of this woman (74) required a search for hyperparathyroidism (Case by courtesy of Drs Leroy and Terrade, Limoges)

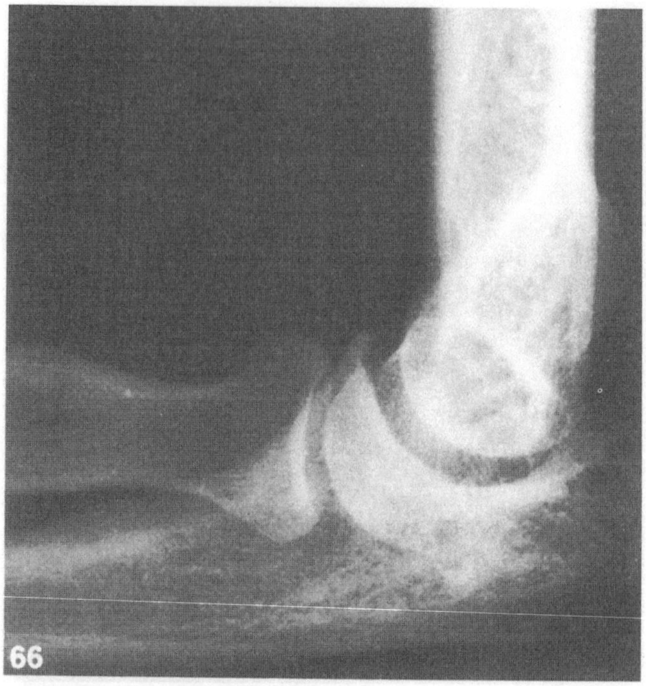

66

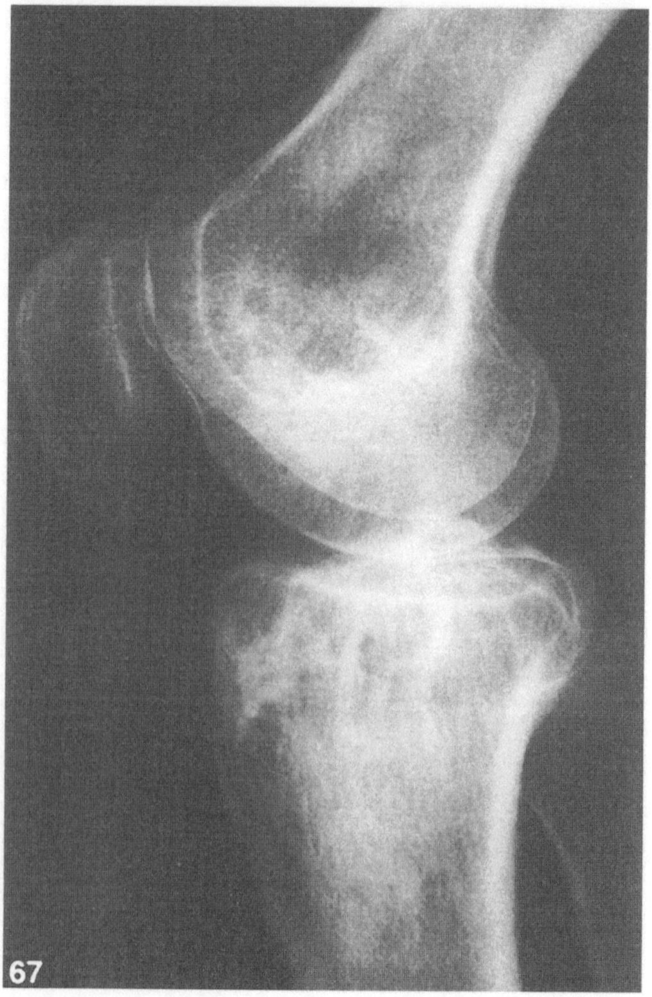

67

Figs. 66-71 relate to the lesions of Destombes-Rosai-Dorfman disease

Figs. 66, 67. In this woman of 26, the presenting features are essentially articular. In the radiographs of the elbow and knee the bony remodelling is marked, with simultaneous osteolysis and osteosclerosis

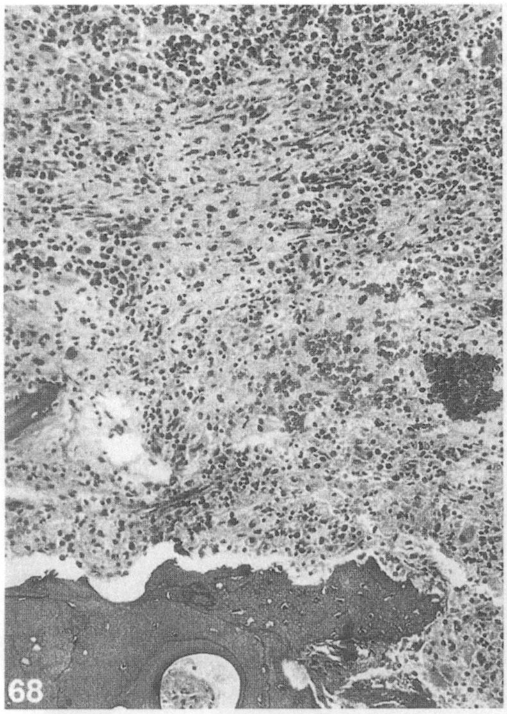

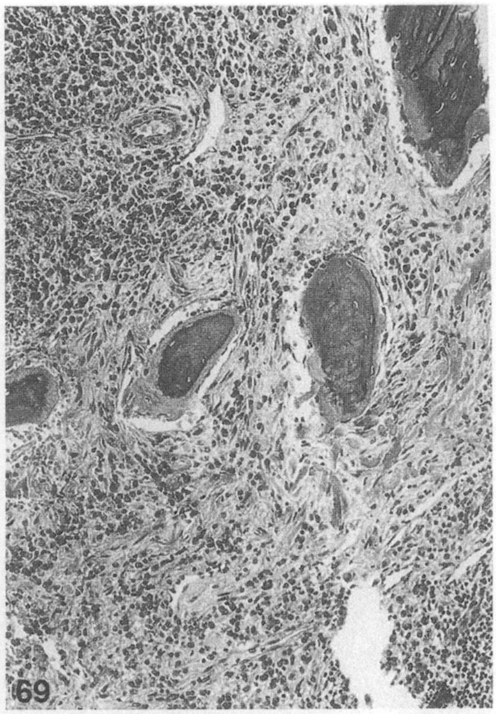

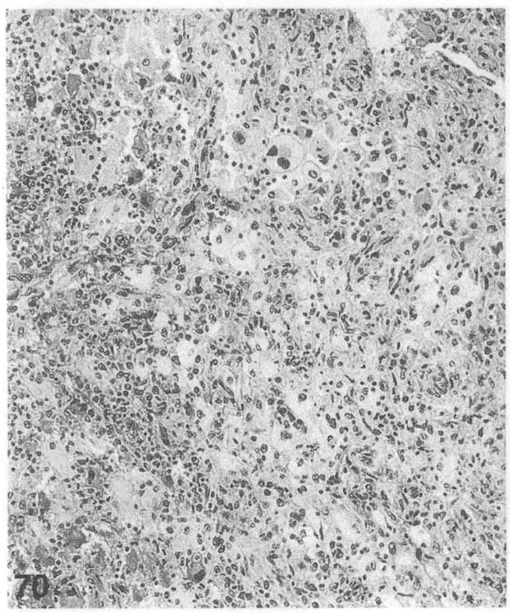

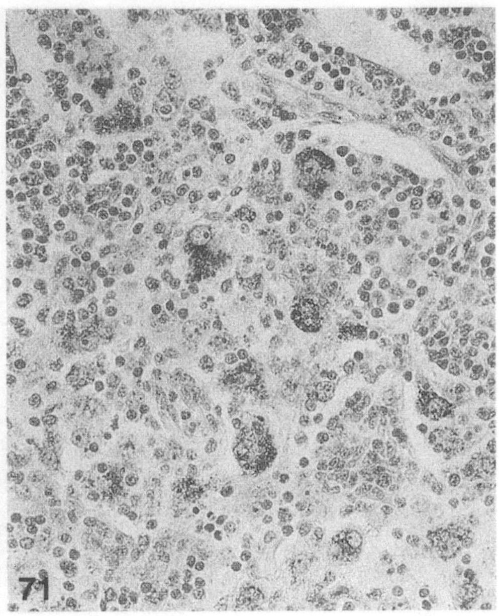

Fig. 68. Biopsy from a patellar lesion. On the partly destroyed old lamellar bone there is newly-formed bone whose margins are excavated by osteoclastic absorption. The marrow is traversed by numerous vessels and there are scattered inflammatory cells unidentifiable at this magnification

Fig. 69. In another section the calcified persistent bony fragments are surrounded by osteoid apposition bordered by osteoblasts. The cellular infiltration in this fibrous stroma primarily suggests a lesion of an osteomyelitic nature (sections by courtesy of Dr Baviera, Hôpital Saint-Joseph)

Fig. 70. Biopsy from an enlarged lymph node. The cellular polymorphism is seen to contain numerous unequally sized histiocytes, whose cytoplasm is sometimes eosinophil, sometimes foamy

Fig. 71. In this section, immunohistological reaction demonstrates the CD68 antigen in some large histiocytes (case kindly supplied by Prof. Leroy, CHU Brest)

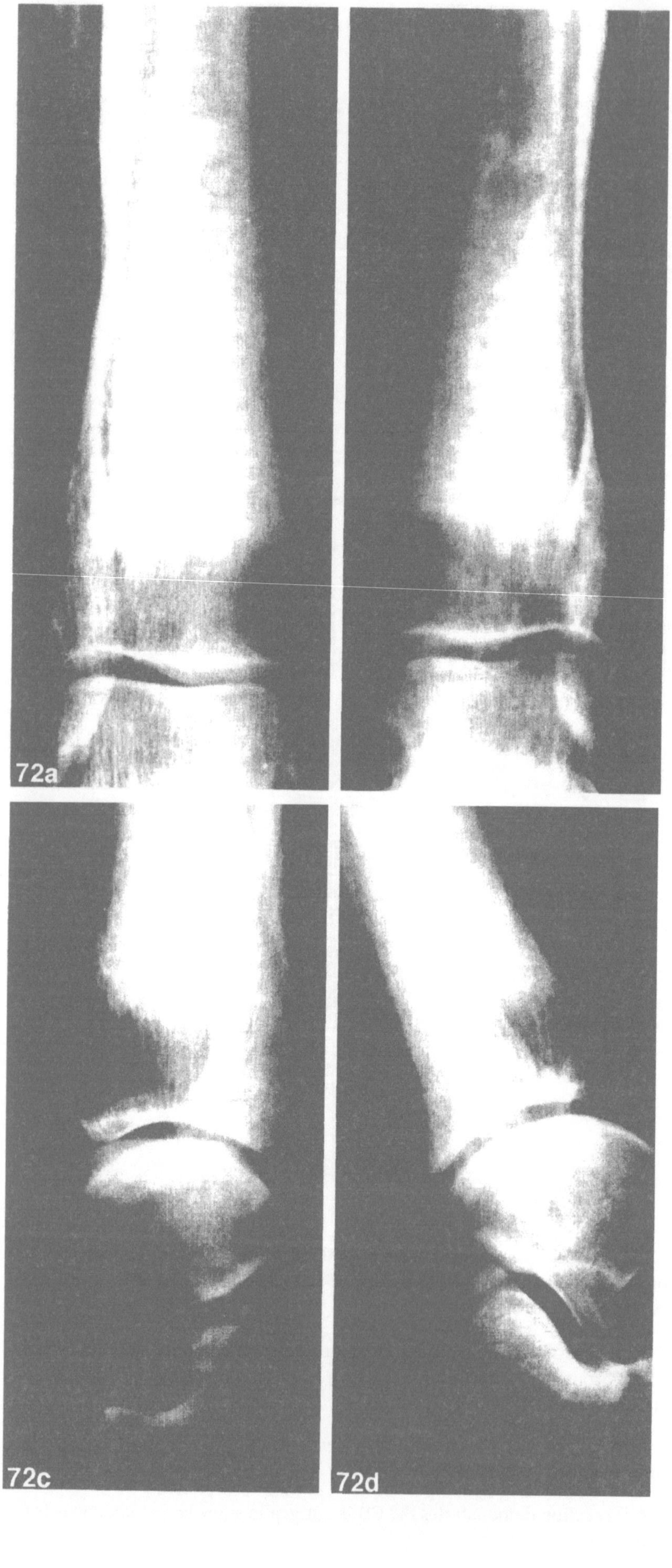

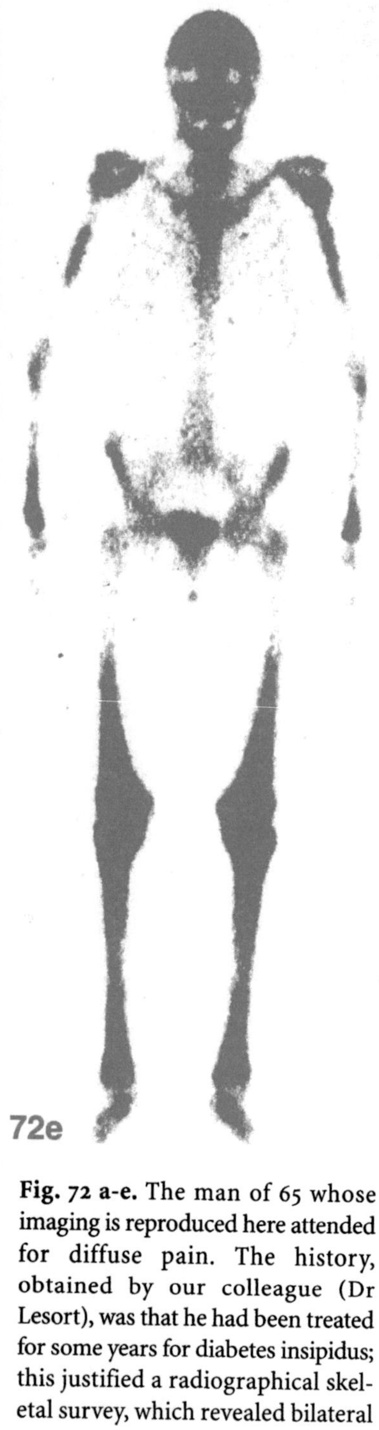

Fig. 72 a-e. The man of 65 whose imaging is reproduced here attended for diffuse pain. The history, obtained by our colleague (Dr Lesort), was that he had been treated for some years for diabetes insipidus; this justified a radiographical skeletal survey, which revealed bilateral symmetric osteosclerotic lesions of the metaphyses of the tibiae and the lower metaphyses of the femora extending toward the diaphysis (**a, b, c, e**), as well as the inferior metaphyses of the radii. There were also patchy condensations of the calcanea and an erosion of the inner table of the frontal bone. Scintigraphy used to supplement the radiographical findings (Prof. Vendroux) showed all the lesions to be hyperfixative (**e**)

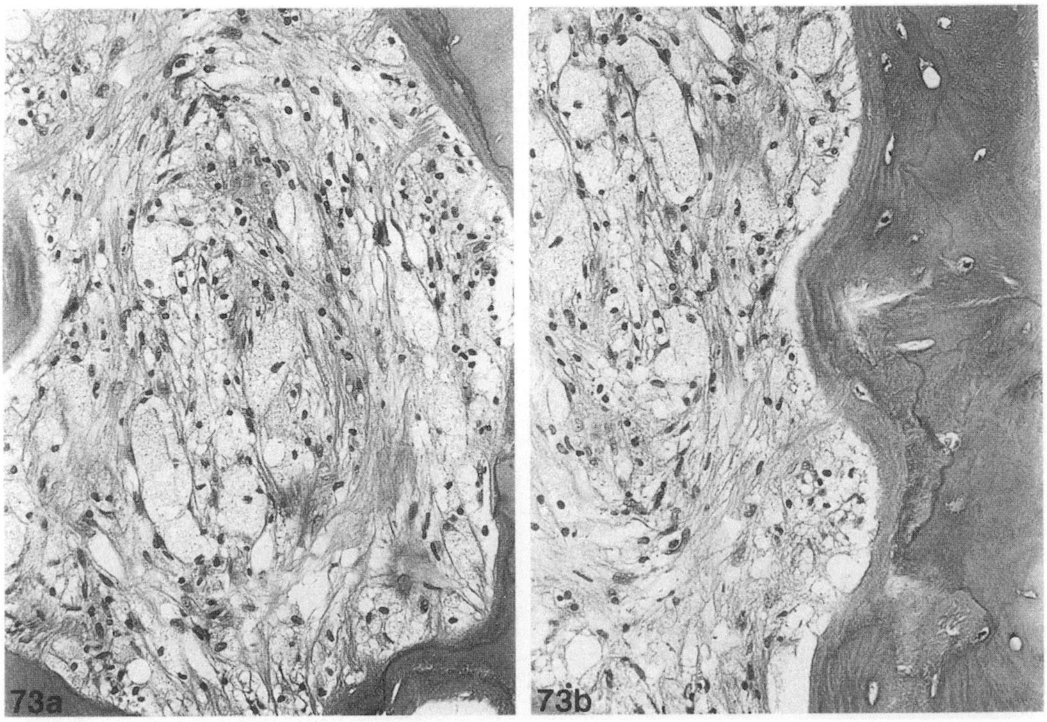

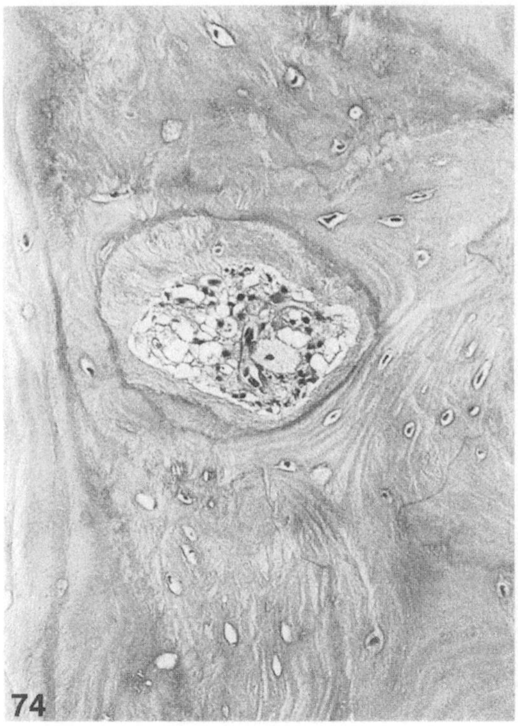

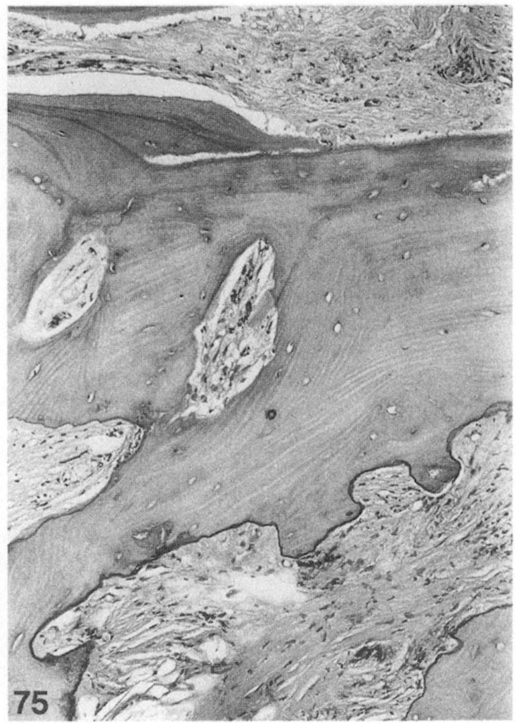

Fig. 73 a, b. At biopsy made on the lower end of the left tibia "the cortex is not smooth but striated, and the bone is very hard without differentiation between the cortex and the underlying bone" (Dr Méchin). In the sections, the lipogranulomatosis is represented by proliferation of histiocytes, some of which are large and have the appearance of foamy histiocytes, together with some inflammatory cells. In this predominantly cellular zone, the marrow shows some rudimentary fibrillary formations. The bony outlines show the traces of osteoclastic absorption

Fig. 74. Here the osteosclerosis is due to an inordinate lamellar apposition and to large-fiber osteo-genesis

Fig. 75. Zone of osteosclerosis and medullary fibrosis. Chester interpreted this type of lesion as an appearance of healing of the process. The bone consists of regular lamellae; there is no cellular activity along their margins and their hyperstaining indicates the presence of an abundant calcium deposit. In what remains of the medullary spaces the marrow is fibrous

Technical notes

Provided certain fundamental principles are observed, the technique of bone biopsy presents no major difficulty. It is evident that all the microscopic techniques applicable to tumours of the soft tissues are also applicable to tumours of bone. Thus measurement, weighing, identification of the borders with Indian ink are indispensable in assessing the quality of the resection, to define the distance of the line of section from the tumour and to evaluate the efficacy of the treatment program; this last point is specified in Chapter 11, which deals with osteogenic sarcoma.

In many cases it is important to study the relationships of the lesions to adjacent tissues, and consequently one must be careful not to "peel" the bone to examine it in a way which would make any assessment of these relationships impossible. This stripping of the bone is unfortunately very much to the liking of technicians, who realise only too well that it is more difficult to cut tendino-aponeurotic tissue correctly than suitably prepared bony tissue.

The need for decalcification calls for perfect and relatively rapid fixation, which can only be obtained by sectioning the bone into slices 3-4 mm thick. If a motor-saw is used, it is essential that the friction of the blade does not heat the tissues which would cause major cell changes. There are many types of saw: circular, diamonded or toothed, oscillating and ribbon, but the pathologist can find satisfactory instruments in the range of hand-saws, which extend from jewellers' instruments to classical metal saws. However, a small biopsy fragment can be cut with a fine slicing blade after decalcification without having recourse to a saw.

It is often possible to separate a fragment of "soft" tissue, in which a technique not requiring decalcification rapidly yields satisfactory sections. The bony fragments are immersed in a sufficient amount of fixing agent for a minimum of 24 hours.

Decalcification must not be too sudden or too slow; in either case the result obtained is poor. The fixed specimen is washed and is then immersed in the decalcifying agent. If there are small specimens obtained by trocar or fragments of spongy bone, a few hours will suffice. If it is a relatively large piece of bone incompletely decalcified after 24 hours in an adequate amount of the agent, it must be removed, washed, fixed and washed again before a second bath in the decalcifying agent. If the procedure is concluded by washing and fixation this greatly facilitates staining.

For many years I have been satisfied with decalcification by a 10-15% dilution of nitric acid. I have also obtained excellent results with the following classical formulation:

water	830 ml
formic acid	170 ml
caustic soda as pastille (pure)	20 g

Some precautions should be taken in preparing this decalcifying agent: to use the components in the order given and to introduce the soda cautiously.

Some suppliers suggest two types of decalcifiants: one "weak" for small samples, the other "strong" for larger bony specimens.

Some colleagues obtain satisfactory results by electrolytic decalcification; in this procedure the tank containing the electrolytic fluid must be constantly chilled.

Whatever the method used, the decalcification time depends on the size and nature of the specimen.

To sum up, the two most common current faults are:
• inadequate fixation, in which case no decalcification procedure is valid and there is a great risk of obtaining sections impossible to interpret;
• excessive decalcification, whose harmful effects may be less if fixation has been perfectly correct, but where cell and tissue damage introduce a supplementary factor tending to hinder interpretation of the sections.

Only attentive surveillance by our colleagues responsible for technical procedures can remedy these problems, which may have serious consequences.

Glossary

I hope that our colleagues who are not pathologists, and for whom this glossary is intended, will forgive the use of "private" terminology that I have not been able to completely discard; terms that pathologists use in a specific sense. Some of these, tricked out in a sense entirely open to criticism, are discussed in this glossary only from the viewpoint of osteoarticular pathology.

Anaplastic, dedifferentiated

These are used improperly, but I have yielded to usage and custom, as does WHO while making its excuses. Logically, the meaning of these words implies that a relatively differentiated tumour cell (for example a chondrosarcoma of grade 2 malignancy) will dedifferentiate and revert (ana) to its origin as an undifferentiated stem-cell. It is more likely that there are undifferentiated clones, together with the relatively differentiated cell majority, and that these clones are the origin of metastases or local recurrences in the form of a totally undifferentiated tumour.

Histologic examination of an entirely undifferentiated proliferation does not permit identification of the cell line to which it belongs. To justify the use of these terms we say that everything happens as if the differentiated tumour cells were capable of reverting to the stem cell. Therefore, the terms "anaplastic" and undifferentiated" are to be understood in a morphological and not a biological sense.

In his book General pathologic anatomy, among the excellent definitions given by Professor de Saint-Maur, a perhaps more justified sense of the term "dedifferentiated" is envisaged in the context of epithelial regeneration.

Aneurysmal cyst

In the field of bone pathology this term characterises a cavitary lytic and expansive lesion filled with fluid blood. This aneurysmal cyst is often partitioned by connective tissue membranes of varying thickness. Some of these aneurysmal septa are lined with osteoid and osseous trabeculae. (The term "aneurysm" may also be used.)

Chondro-osteoid

I have ventured to use several word combinations of this type. The simple reason is as follows: I confess myself incapable (and I am probably not alone in this) of formally distinguishing in every case, from the routine staining of tumours, the boundaries between chondroid, osteoid and sometimes hyalinised collagen.

Cyst

This term is normally applied to cavities bounded by an epithelial membrane, but in practice it is extended to all sorts of cavities. The "degenerative" cysts of the wrist or of an arthrotic femoral head are zones of necrosis where the tissue, tendino-aponeurotic or osteomedullary, is replaced by a mucoid material. The evident inappropriateness of the word "cyst" in these cases is partly masked by the term "pseudo-cyst".

Degenerative

The term is mainly employed in osteoarticular pathology to designate the degradation or catabolism of a tissue zone. This lesion deprives a tissue of its functional capabilities. It is shown by modification of staining affinity and very often by multiple vascular penetrations, small vessels around which fibrous tissue usually develops, incapable of functionally replacing the specialised degenerated tissue. Often, the expressions "disk degeneration" or "meniscal degeneration" are used inadvertently, by force of habit, when it would be preferable to speak of a degenerative state.

Differentiation

"A well-differentiated cancer is one which has an image close to that of a normal tissue" (General pathologic anatomy, Prof. de Saint-Maur). This differentiation allows the pathologist to identify the tissue origin of the tumour. Usually, well-differentiated tumours have a relatively slow spontaneous course. At the other extreme, completely undifferentiated tumours (so-called anaplastic) have a much more rapid spontaneous course. But the arrival of the antimitotic agents (once again I am only dealing with bone tumours) has upset these ideas and an "anaplastic" or even telangiectatic sarcoma currently has a transformed prognosis.

Eosinophil

This is the pinkish-red stain most used for cell cytoplasm. But this trichrome stain also includes haematoxylin, which stains nuclei blue or blue-violet. There is a sort of resulting conflict, essentially a competition between yellow and red on the one hand and red and blue on the other. Thus, collagen readily assumes an orange-yellow color and some so-called amphophil cytoplasm a mauve tint. Despite the rather disdainful description as "identification stains", it is clear that the different hues obtained are evidence of particular characteristics of the cytoplasm or the membranes or both. The often very marked variations of staining affinity are characteristic (non-specific) of degenerative aspects of cartilaginous and tendino-aponeurotic tissues.

Hamartoma

Structure of tumour-like appearance resulting from hyperproduction and atypical organisation of normal tissues in a region where they normally exist.

Hyperplasia

This is merely a quantitative increase in a tissue and the term in no way implies a neoplastic nature of the relevant tissue.

Hypertrophy, cellular

An increase in volume of a cell which does not imply a neoplastic nature but which may precede cell death in some conditions. However, in the description of malignant tumours, our reports often mention "the presence of large cells"; it would be better to speak of atypical tumour cell hypertrophy.

Juxtacortical

Juxtacortical sarcoma designates an anatomical and clinical entity. It is a sarcoma developing from the surface of a bone and of low-grade malignancy; this in no way excludes that a highly malignant sarcoma may develop in this situation. In the WHO international classification these sarcomas are described as superficial osteosarcomas of a high grade of histological malignancy.

Metamorphism

A modification of the ground substance: osteoid or chondroid metamorphism. These modifications of the ground substance are more specific and more easily assessed when they go hand in hand with cellular metamorphosis.

Metamorphosis, cellular

Modification, at least structural, of cells. Usually this refers to slightly differentiated connective tissue cells which evolve towards more specific types: chondroblasts, osteoblasts and so on.

Myxoid

With a myxomatous appearance, a soft tumour formed of ordinary poorly-differentiated connective tissue. The rare cells and few elastic fibers are embedded in a mucoid substance (which resembles mucus in its gelatinous appearance).

Oncosis, oncocytic

(Greek onkos: mass, volume) indicates swelling of a cell, a term used to designate tumours formed of large cells with granular cytoplasm. Oncosis, simple swelling of a cell, may precede normal cell death, particularly of osteocytes and chondrocytes.

Organelles

Generic term applied to various intracytoplasmic structures.

Organoid

When a tissue proliferation (usually benign) exhibits a recognisable architecture, the lesion is described as organoid. Thus the organoid appearance of osteoid osteoma contrasts with the disorderly architecture of osteoblastoma.

Osteogenic

Giving rise to bone; forms part of the very definition of osteosarcoma, osteogenic sarcoma. One can also quite properly use the term "skeletogenic' if it produces cartilaginous and bony tissue.

Osteoid

A pre-osseous tissue, still uncalcified, normally produced by osteoblasts. The osteoblasts in the hyperactive forms of Paget's disease or osteomalacia produce variably abundant amount of preosseous tissue - osteoid - which mostly remains uncalcified. In contrast, in a fracture callus in process of union the osteoid tissue evolves normally towards calcification.

Osteolysis

Destruction of bony tissue; normally, bone destruction is the work of the osteoclasts, large multinucleate cells which secrete acid phosphatase. Other mechanisms of destruction have been suggested for some tumours.

Osteosclerosis

Densification, either of spongy bone by thickening of the trabeculae at the expense of the medullary spaces, or of the haversian bone by apposition of concentric lamellae at the expense of the haversian canal and the medullary canal, with possible participation of the periosteum. This osteosclerosis can lead to a marble bone, an osteopetrosis; such bone is particularly fragile.

Periosteal sarcoma

Periosteal sarcoma refers to an entity, a sarcoma supposed to originate in the periosteum, with a major cartilaginous component.

Periostosis, periostitis

Terms applied to superficial, periosteal, bony apposition. Periostosis and periostitis are intended to represent a periosteal reaction to various insults (bone tumours, inflammations, superficial juxtaosseous lesions).

Skip metastasis

Indicates a metastatic lesion close to the parent tumour.

Stains and staining

We consider here only the so-called routine classic trichrome staining. To describe a tissue as being safranophil merely signifies that it is yellow. The hidden sense of the term is quite different. Collagen is a particularly safranophil structure; consequently, the translation of "safranophil tissue" might be: tissue rich in collagen, which suggests the intervention of collagen-producing fibroblasts.

Stroma

Connective-vascular tissue which supports the different tissues of the organism and of tumours. Tumour cells and stroma often produce reactions in each other. The relative proportions of tumour tissue and stroma are very variable. In the same type of tumour, the stroma may be virtually nonexistent or abundant, the latter characterising the fibrous forms (chordoma, adamantinoma of long bones, ameloblastoma, synovial sarcoma).

Index

D

E

F

G

H

K

L

M

N

O

P

R

S

MIX
Papier aus verantwortungsvollen Quellen
Paper from responsible sources
FSC® C105338

FSC
www.fsc.org

If you have any concerns about our products,
you can contact us on
ProductSafety@springernature.com

In case Publisher is established outside the EU,
the EU authorized representative is:
Springer Nature Customer Service Center GmbH
Europaplatz 3, 69115 Heidelberg, Germany

Printed by Libri Plureos GmbH
in Hamburg, Germany